Primer on the Rheumatic Diseases

Tenth Edition

Library of Congress Cataloging-in-Publication Data

Primer on the rheumatic diseases / editor, H. Ralph Schumacher, Jr.;
   associate editors, John H. Klippel, William J. Koopman.—10th ed.
        p.   cm.
   Includes bibliographical references and index.
   ISBN 0-912423-07-2: 25.00
   1. Rheumatism.   2. Arthritis.   I. Schumacher, H. Ralph, 1933–
II. Klippel, John H.   III. Koopman, William J.
   [DNLM: 1. Arthritis.   2. Rheumatic Diseases.   WE 344 P953 1993]
RC927.P67   1993
616.7'23—dc20
DNLM/DLC
for Library of Congress   93-31510
                                                               CIP

Copyright 1993 by the Arthritis Foundation, Atlanta, Georgia **ARTHRITIS FOUNDATION**

Managing Editor: Cynthia M. Kahn, Director, Professional Publications
Consulting Editor: Barbara Stapleton
Editorial Assistant: Elizabeth E. Axtell

Arthritis Foundation catalog number 3250. ISBN 0-912423-07-2

Primer on the Rheumatic Diseases

Tenth Edition

H. Ralph Schumacher, Jr., MD, Editor

John H. Klippel, MD, Associate Editor

William J. Koopman, MD, Associate Editor

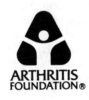

ARTHRITIS
FOUNDATION®

Published by the Arthritis Foundation
1314 Spring Street NW
Atlanta, Georgia 30309

CONTRIBUTORS

The following people contributed to this edition of the *Primer on the Rheumatic Diseases* by writing or revising chapters and sections for the publication of the tenth edition. Credits for illustrations are given in figure legends.

Steven B. Abramson, MD
Ronald S. Adler, PhD, MD
Graciela S. Alarcón, MD, MPH
Ronald J. Anderson, MD
William P. Arend, MD
Gene V. Ball, MD
Thomas Bardin, MD
C. Lowry Barnes, MD
Thomas G. Benedek, MD
Joseph J. Biundo, Jr, MD
Warren D. Blackburn, Jr, MD
Laurence A. Bradley, PhD
Kenneth D. Brandt, MD
Peter Brooks, MD
Robert B. Buckingham, MD
Ken J. Bulpitt, MD
Joel Buxbaum, MD
Philip L. Cohen, MD
Marta Lucia Cuéllar, MD
Thomas R. Cupps, MD
Paul A. Dieppe, MD
Bonnie B. Dorwart, MD
Robert A. Eisenberg, MD
Luis R. Espinoza, MD
Adel G. Fam, MD
Peng Thim Fan, MD
José Luis Ferreiro-Seoane, MD
Bruce Freundlich, MD
Eric P. Gall, MD
Lynn Gerber, MD
Dafna D. Gladman, MD
Victor M. Goldberg, MD
Duncan A. Gordon, MD
Leonardo Guzman, MD
Nortin M. Hadler, MD
E. Nigel Harris, MD
Peter Hasselbacher, MD
L. A. Healey, MD
David B. Hellmann, MD

Gary S. Hoffman, MD
Gene G. Hunder, MD
A. Huttenlocher, MD
Robert D. Inman, MD
Sergio Jimenez, MD
Herbert Kaplan, MD
Tomisaku Kawasaki, MD
Muhammad Asim Khan, MD
John H. Klippel, MD
William J. Koopman, MD
Franklin Kozin, MD
Steven M. Krane, MD
Phoebe R. Krey, MD
Richard L. Leff, MD
E. Carwile LeRoy, MD
Lawrence Leventhal, MD
Matthew H. Liang, MD, MPH
Worawit Louthrenoo, MD
Harvinder S. Luthra, MD
Maren L. Mahowald, MD
Henry J. Mankin, MD
William Martel, MD
Manuel Martínez-Lavín, MD
Daniel J. McCarty, MD
Thomas A. Medsger, Jr, MD
Robert F. Meenan, MD, MPH, MBA
H. Mielants, MD
Frederick W. Miller, MD
Pekka Mooar, MD
Larry W. Moreland, MD
Roland W. Moskowitz, MD
Haralampos M. Moutsopoulos, MD
Gregory R. Mundy, MD
Stanley J. Naides, MD
J. Desmond O'Duffy, MD
Susan M. Ott, MD
Richard M. Panush, MD
Harold E. Paulus, MD

Jean-Pierre Pelletier, MD
Johanne Martel-Pelletier, PhD
Robert S. Pinals, MD
David S. Pisetsky, MD, PhD
Paul H. Plotz, MD
A. Robin Poole, PhD, DSc
Parks W. Pratt, MD
Sally Pullman, MD
Reed E. Pyeritz, MD, PhD
Antonio Reginato, MD
Morris Reichlin, MD
Dwight R. Robinson, MD
Peter J. Roughley, PhD
Shaun Ruddy, MD
H. Ralph Schumacher, Jr, MD
Robert H. Shmerling, MD
Richard M. Silver, MD
Peter A. Simkin, MD
Bernhard H. Singsen, MD, MPH
Clement B. Sledge, MD
Charles W. Slemenda, DrPH
Virginia Steen, MD
Allen C. Steere, MD
Guillermo A. Tate, MD
Joel D. Taurog, MD
Robert Terkeltaub, MD
Murray B. Urowitz, MD
Frank B. Vasey, MD
E. M. Veys, MD
Zena Werb, PhD
Victoria Werth, MD
Patience White, MD
Ronald L. Wilder, MD, PhD
H. James Williams, MD
Robert J. Winchester, MD
Robert L. Wortmann, MD
Edward Yelin, PhD
David T. Y. Yu, MD

CONTENTS

FOREWORD

The Arthritis Foundation, publisher of this *Primer*, was founded in 1948 by a group of rheumatologists to raise money from patients to support research in the rheumatic diseases. Since then, the Arthritis Foundation has expanded its purpose so that its current mission is to "support research to find the cure for and prevention of arthritis and to improve the quality of life for those affected by arthritis."

Research remains a preeminent concern. In 1993 the Foundation will spend approximately $12 million to fund postdoctoral fellows, beginning investigators, biomedical and clinical research grants and health sciences research. The amount will increase significantly in succeeding years to reach $16 million by 1996.

The effort to improve the quality of life for people with arthritis involves many activities. Surveys of people with arthritis conducted for the Foundation both nationally and intensively in San Mateo, California, demonstrate the need to educate professionals, the public at large, and patients in the recognition and treatment of rheumatic diseases.

The treatment of arthritis involves a team approach. Many of the conditions described in this *Primer* require the knowledge and skill of a specialist, the rheumatologist, who still relies on the time-honored practice of a detailed physical examination to supplement a careful history and sophisticated immunologic and other tests. Rheumatology is a field that relies on cognitive skills, a long-term relationship with a patient who has a chronic disease, a commitment to educate patients about their disease, and the ability to coordinate a team of professionals that may include nurses, physical and occupational therapists, social workers, and orthopedic surgeons among others. Some conditions, such as osteoarthritis and low back pain, are so common that virtually all physicians will see patients with these problems. To educate physicians and medical students, the Arthritis Foundation produces not only this *Primer* but the *Bulletin on the Rheumatic Diseases* (free upon request), videotapes, interactive computer programs, and sponsors lectures, symposia and conferences. The Foundation also produces educational materials and programs for non-physician professionals.

The Arthritis Foundation, through its more than 60 chapters and by means of cooperative agreements with other agencies, provides programs and services for people with arthritis. These range from exercise programs to disease management courses for individuals and groups to advocacy programs. Other materials and programs are designed with special attention to the needs of children with arthritis and their parents and for individuals with the less common to rare diseases described in this book.

Very importantly, the Arthritis Foundation seeks to increase the awareness of arthritis as a serious health problem and to dispel the belief that little can be done to help people with arthritis. Disability as an outcome of disease can have profound economic and social costs, and disability from arthritis can be prevented. The Arthritis Foundation is working to convey that message to the public, to healthcare professionals, and to all levels of government. The Foundation seeks to increase funding for research in arthritis through the National Institute of Arthritis and Musculoskeletal and Skin Diseases, which it was instrumental in founding. The Arthritis Foundation has also worked to improve access to all necessary medical care including specialized care, long-term care, rehabilitation, and other needs for people with arthritis.

The Arthritis Foundation is especially proud of its role in publishing the *Primer on the Rheumatic Diseases*, now celebrating its tenth edition. The *Primer* has set the standard for similar publications in other diseases. It is recognized as a concise, authoritative, and timely summary of what physicians and students need to know about arthritis. The Foundation hopes that the *Primer* will inspire students to enter careers such as rheumatology and undertake the care of people with arthritis and that the *Primer* will enable physicians in all fields and in all countries to better understand and manage patients with rheumatic diseases, thus fulfilling the mission of the Arthritis Foundation to better the life of people with arthritis.

Arthur I. Grayzel, MD
Senior Vice President, Medical Affairs
Arthritis Foundation

INTRODUCTION

This tenth edition of the *Primer on the Rheumatic Diseases* is the result of an exciting collaborative effort of the editor; my two invaluable associate editors, John Klippel, MD, and William Koopman, MD, who kept to all deadlines despite their many other duties; Cynthia Kahn and her staff at the Arthritis Foundation; my own staff at the Veterans Affairs Medical Center in Philadelphia, and at the University of Pennsylvania; and the authors, chosen from the world's leading experts in each area. This edition continues our policy of revisions every five years. The rapid advances in basic sciences and increased understanding of many rheumatic diseases require such a pace to keep current. Every chapter has been extensively revised since the ninth edition or totally rewritten. You will notice some minor organizational changes but the general structure is as before with the basic science background followed by chapters on diagnostic methods, then discussion of the individual diseases, and finally frequently used therapeutic measures. Concise space limits have been required and referencing has been successfully limited by the authors of most chapters to keep this manageable and truly a "Primer", not a competitor for the textbooks. The index was compiled with attention to access of subjects that are addressed in several places throughout the text. Cross-references between chapters are also included where appropriate.

For the second time, the authors responsible for each chapter are individually identified. This acknowledges the major effort in initially preparing these concise chapters and in responding to our 1993 inquiries to keep the material as current as possible. We acknowledge and thank our current authors, but we also especially thank the many contributors to previous editions. The tremendous resource of superb contributors has allowed rotation of authors so that some new workers can share both the opportunities and duties. We hope many of our past contributors will allow us to call on them again in the future.

The international distribution of the *Primer* is paralleled by the expanding number of contributions from outside the United States. Foreign contributors to this edition are from Canada, Mexico, France, Belgium, Thailand, Greece, Spain, Japan, Argentina, Chile, the United Kingdom, and Australia. Such international collaboration seems appropriate as advances in laboratory and clinical research in rheumatic diseases increasingly come from the centers of excellence in rheumatology throughout the world.

To put this current *Primer* in perspective readers may be interested to know that it has evolved from two publications of the American Committee for the Control of Rheumatism, an early predecessor of the American Rheumatism Association (ARA) (1,2). The first of these, *What is Rheumatism?*, was issued in 1928; the second, *Rheumatism Primer: Chronic Arthritis*, was privately distributed in 1932. In 1934 the American Committee for the Control of Rheumatism published the next publication in this line, *Primer on Rheumatism, Chronic Arthritis*. This work, generally considered the first of the *Primers*, consisted of a brochure that had been prepared for distribution in connection with a scientific exhibit on arthritis at the Annual Convention of the American Medical Association. A revision, identified by its authors as the "Second Primer on Arthritis", appeared in the *Journal of the American Medical Association* in 1942 under the title *Primer on Arthritis* (3). The third through the seventh editions of the *Primer*, also published in the *Journal of the American Medical Association*, appeared in 1949 (third), 1953 (fourth), 1959 (fifth), 1964 (sixth), and 1973 (seventh) (4–8). The eighth edition (1983) and ninth (1988) were published by the Arthritis Foundation (9,10), as is this new edition.

The *Primer* is widely used in teaching programs throughout this country and in a number of countries abroad. More than 100,000 copies of the ninth edition were provided to medical schools and hospitals by the Arthritis Foundation for distribution to students and house officers. Previous editions of the *Primer* have been translated into Spanish, Japanese, Chinese, and Greek.

The chief purpose of the present edition of the *Primer* remains the same as that of previous versions: to provide a reasonably thorough yet concise description of the rheumatic diseases, with particular emphasis on clinical manifestations, pathogenesis, diagnosis, and management. We hope it will serve this purpose. Many of the changes in this and previous editions have come at the suggestion of our readers. We look forward to continued feedback from the users of this text.

H. Ralph Schumacher, Jr, MD
Editor

1. Stecher RM: The American Rheumatism Association-its origins, development and maturity. Arthritis Rheum 14–19, 1958
2. Rodnan GP: Growth and development of rheumatology in the United States: a bicentennial report. Arthritis Rheum 20:1149–1168, 1977
3. Jordan EP, et al: Primer on Arthritis. JAMA 119:1089–1076, 1942
4. McEwen C, et al: Primer on the Rheumatic Diseases. JAMA 139:1068–1076, 1139–1146, 1268–1273, 1949
5. Ragan C, Feldman HA, Clark WS, et al: Primer on the Rheumatic Diseases, JAMA 152:323–331, 405–414, 522–531, 1953
6. Crain DC, et al: Primer on the Rheumatic Diseases. JAMA 171:1205–1220, 1345–1356, 1680–1691, 1959
7. Decker JL, Bollet AJ, Duff IF, et al: Primer on the Rheumatic Disease. JAMA 190:127–140, 425–444, 509–530, 741–751, 1964
8. Rodnan GP, Schumacher HR, Zvaifler NJ: Primer on the Rheumatic Diseases. JAMA 224:661–812, 1973
9. Rodnan GP, Schumacher HR, Zvaifler NJ: Primer on the Rheumatic Diseases. Atlanta, Arthritis Foundation, 1983
10. Schumacher HR, Klippel JH, Robinson DR: Primer on the Rheumatic Diseases. Atlanta, Arthritis Foundation, 1988

1. HISTORY OF THE RHEUMATIC DISEASES

Recognition of rheumatic diseases as early as the 4th century BC is suggested by the fact that 18 of the aphorisms of Hippocrates refer at least partially to joint diseases. The term *rheuma* was introduced in about the first century AD. Its meaning resembled the Hippocratic *catarrhos*. Both terms indicated a substance that flows. They were conceived to be derived from *phlegm*, the primary humor believed to originate in the brain and cause various ailments, depending on the site to which they flowed. An early example of the association of rheuma with arthritis was advanced by Andrew Boorde. To paraphrase: The rheumatic humor, produced in the head, is viscous. Descending from the head to the inferior parts, it causes many infirmities. If it, in contrast to the coleric humor, causes joint disease, the affected parts become swollen and red, with engorged vessels (1547, London).

The concept of rheumatism as a systemic musculoskeletal syndrome was introduced by the Parisian physician Guillaume Baillou (Ballonius) (1558–1616) in a posthumously published work (1642). He claimed that "what arthritis is in a joint that is exactly what rheumatism is in the whole body." He wrote picturesquely that ". . . one may designate the condition we are considering inexactly as rheumatism, better as a sort of precipitation like a seasickness of the vessels (which vomit), until better terms offer themselves" (1). The term *rheumatologist* is recent, coined in 1940 by Bernard Comroe. Curiously, it preceded *rheumatology*, which was introduced in the textbook he edited by Joseph L. Hollander in 1949.

Ancient descriptions of diseases rarely permit a specific modern diagnosis. For centuries *gout* and *gouty diathesis* were used as nonspecifically as *arthritis* is used today. Thomas Sydenham began the process of identifying discrete diseases from the mix of rheumatism. Himself beset by gout, Sydenham distinguished an acute febrile polyarthritis ". . . chiefly attacking the young and vigorous" from gout. Most of the description is compatible with acute rheumatic fever, but it also alludes to a chronic phase in which the patient may become ". . . a cripple to the day of his death and wholly lose the use of his limbs whilst the knuckles of his fingers shall become knotty and protruberant . . ."—possibly rheumatoid arthritis. In addition to his portrayals of gout (1683) and acute rheumatism (1685), Sydenham described St. Vitus' dance (Sydenham's chorea, 1686), and in his discussion of *Hysteric Diseases* (1681) may have described fibrositis.

Some authors at the beginning of the 19th century realized how little progress had been made in distinguishing discrete diseases. For example, William Heberden (1802, London) wrote: "The rheumatism is a common name for many aches and pains, which have yet no peculiar appellation, though owing to very different causes. It is besides often hard to be distinguished from some, which have a certain name and class assigned them. . . ."

GOUT

Gutta in medieval medicine was a synonym for the Greek *podagra*. It meant a drop resulting from "a defluxion of the humors." *Podagra* was employed if the foot was affected, *chiragra* if the wrist, *gonagra* if the knee, and so forth. Little of significance was learned about gout between the 4th century BC and the end of the 18th century. Two concepts prevailed throughout the two millenia: that the disease occurred predominantly in sexually mature men, as pointed out by Hippocrates, and that gustatory and sexual excesses predisposed to its acute attacks. A huge folklore derived from these beliefs.

Antonj van Leeuwenhoek described the microscopic appearance of urate crystals from a tophus (1684, Delft). Nearly a century later, the Swedish pharmacist, Carl W. Scheele, demonstrated a hitherto unknown organic acid, originally called lithic acid, in urinary stones (1776). In 1797 at Cambridge, William H. Wollaston reported that the principal constituent of tophi is "a neutral compound consisting of lithic acid and mineral alkali."

The substance was renamed *acide ourique* by the French chemist, Antoine de Fourcroy, who also found it to be a constituent of normal urine (1798, Paris).

Half a century passed before uric acid was more convincingly related to gout. Alfred B. Garrod devised a quantitative gravimetric assay that could detect uric acid in hyperuricemic states such as gout and renal failure (1847, London). Because of its difficulty, the procedure was not adopted. He devised a qualitative test in 1854, in which uric acid precipitated on a thread. It received some use and along with his experiments led him to suggest: "Might it not, in doubtful cases, be possible to determine the nature of the affection from an examination of the blood?"

Garrod also demonstrated urate in subcutaneous tissue and articular cartilage in cases of gout. He hypothesized that gout might result either from a loss of renal excretory capacity or from increased formation of uric acid. These concepts were proved correct a century after the publication of Garrod's monograph on gout (1859). In 1876 he postulated that acute gout results from the precipitation of sodium urate in a joint or adjacent tissue. This was directly demonstrated in 1962 following intraarticular injection of monosodium urate by Joseph L. Hollander, Daniel J. McCarty, J. Edwin Seegmiller, and their collaborators (2).

Beginning in 1870 with the first of the methods devised by Ernst L. Salkowski, a German biochemist, numerous gravimetric assays of urinary uric acid were developed. However, the first technique that was sufficiently sensitive and practical to be applied to blood was colorimetric, one of several eventually developed by Otto Folin (1912, Boston). Folin's first method yielded results that were only about one-half of the actual values, but by 1938 sensitivity had been improved to the extent that the sex-related difference in the mean serum content of uric acid was established (Bernard M. Jacobson, Boston). Further analytic specificity and sensitivity were obtained with the enzymatic spectrophotometric technique developed by Praetorius and Poulsen (1949–1953, Copenhagen).

RHEUMATIC FEVER

Although Hippocrates mentioned an acute, migratory arthritis of young people, no definite descriptions of rheumatic fever were made until the contributions of Sydenham (1665, see above), and nothing further was added for more than a century. David Dundas published a good description of heart failure in patients with "acute rheumatism" and therein appears to have been the first to use the term *rheumatic fever* (1808, London). He concluded that "the knowledge that this [heart] disease is always the consequence of, or is connected with, rheumatic affection, points out the necessity of attending to the translation of rheumatism to the chest . . ."

Both Matthew Baillie and William C. Wells credited David Pitcairn, another London physician, for first having noted ". . . that persons subject to rheumatism were attacked more frequently than others with symptoms of an organic disease of the heart" (1788, unpublished). In his pathology text of 1797 Baillie noted "an ossification or thickening of some heart valves" of patients who had suffered from acute rheumatism. Wells then confirmed the clinical findings of Dundas and added the description of subcutaneous nodules (1810). James Hope explained the origin of valvular murmurs (1831, London). Jean-Baptiste Bouillaud concluded that "in the great majority of cases of acute articular rheumatism with fever, there exists in a variable degree a rheumatism of the serofibrinous tissue of the heart . . ." (1840, Paris), an observation that became known as the *law of coincidence*. Angel Money (1883, London) noted the myocardial granuloma, which was later described in greater detail by Ludwig Aschoff (1904, Marburg). The *Aschoff nodule* came to be considered diagnostic of rheumatic carditis (3).

Chorea was introduced as a medical term by Paracelsus (1493–1541, Switzerland), derived from the Greek for dance. In 1686

Sydenham, using the designation St. Vitus' dance, described the type of chorea that is now associated with his name. Richard Bright appears to have been the first to associate this behavior with rheumatic fever (1831, London), a suggestion which George Sée substantiated with an epidemiologic study (1850, Paris) (4).

James K. Fowler reported that tonsillitis is a common precursor of rheumatic fever (1880, London). Although Frederick J. Poynton and Alexander Paine of London had isolated a streptococcus from the tonsils of a patient with rheumatic fever in 1900, this was only one of several bacteria implicated as pathogens. Homer F. Swift advanced the hypothesis that rheumatic fever results from the development of hypersensitivity to streptococci (1928, New York), but he considered non-hemolytic strains to be the most probable pathogens. The epidemiologic studies of Alvin F. Coburn in New York and of William R. Collis in London, both published in 1931, led to the final identification of the beta-hemolytic streptococcus as the causative organism. The first evidence to support the hypothesis of an immune pathogenesis of rheumatic fever was the discovery of antistreptolysins by Edgar W. Todd (1932, London) (5).

RHEUMATOID ARTHRITIS

The appearance and distribution of lesions in ancient skeletons suggests that rheumatoid arthritis (RA) may have existed in North America at least 3000 years ago (6). However, the first clinical description of RA usually is credited to Augustin-Jacob Landré-Beauvais who, in his Paris thesis of 1800, described nine women who had a disease he considered to be a variant of gout and therefore called *goutte asthenique primitive*. He believed that a "primary weakness" predisposed the disease to develop and that it was associated with poverty, while true gout occurred generally in affluent persons who were robust. While RA may have been less common previously, it undoubtedly existed and was misdiagnosed as a variety of rheumatism.

Rheumatoid arthritis was clearly described by Benjamin C. Brodie (1819, London). He stressed its typically slow progression and pointed out that not only joints, but bursae and tendon sheaths might be affected. His most important contribution was to recognize that the disease begins as a synovitis that may lead to destruction of articular cartilage.

Jean-Martin Charcot made excellent clinical differentiations among gout, rheumatic fever, RA, and osteoarthritis. He felt, however, that "it is quite impossible to make an actual distinction between the various forms of rheumatism, but on the contrary, it is frequently possible to show that they all procede from one and the same cause." He perpetuated Landré-Beauvais' sociologic error, but may have been the first to recognize that RA is not rare: "While gout is almost unknown in the Salpetriere, chronic rheumatism is, on the contrary, one of the commonest infirmities in this institution; and indeed, this disease prevails among women and among the least favored classes of society" (1867, Paris).

AB Garrod coined the term *rheumatoid arthritis* in 1858. He explained his reasoning in 1892: "The study of articular affections some thirty years ago led me to the conclusion that the majority of cases then called "rheumatic gout" were related neither to true gout nor true rheumatism, and that they had an independent pathology of their own; and if such is the case, the term "rheumatic gout" was doubly wrong. . . . I propose the name of "rheumatoid arthritis"—a name which does not imply any error, but assumes the disease to be an arthritic or joint disease having some of the external characters of rheumatism. . . . Arthritis deformans [Rudolf Virchow (1869, Berlin)] has been applied to the malady, and this again is not an erroneous name, though in the earlier stages of the disease it is by no means a characteristic one. The term *rheumatic arthritis* is nearly, or at least half, as bad as that of *rheumatic gout*, as it implies the existence of one error instead of two . . ." Nosologic conflicts continued even after the British Ministry of Health in 1922 adopted rheumatoid arthritis as the official designation, a step the American Rheumatism Association (now American College of Rheumatology) did not take until 1941.

The first roentgenogram of joints affected by RA was published

by Gilbert A. Bannatyne (1896, Bath). Joel E. Goldthwait devised the first American classification of arthritides and included the roentgenographic appearance among the criteria in order to differentiate atrophic (rheumatoid) arthritis from hypertrophic (osteo) arthritis (1904, Boston). Edward Nichols and Frank Richardson (1909, Boston) differentiated proliferative arthritis, which begins with synovitis and affects articular cartilage secondarily, from degenerative arthritis in which the primary lesion is in articular cartilage. However, they did not correlate these pathologic observations with rheumatoid and osteoarthritis, respectively (1,7).

The discovery of *rheumatoid factor* ultimately began with the hypothesis popularized by Frank Billings that RA is a response to various chronic focal infections (1912, Chicago). Bacteriologic research stimulated by this hypothesis led Russell L. Cecil et al to conclude that RA "is a streptococcal infection, caused in a large proportion of cases by a biologically specific strain of this organism." They reported culturing this streptococcus from the blood or joints of two-thirds of RA patients and observed that serum from one-half of all cases agglutinated suspensions of these bacteria (1929, New York). The nonspecificity of this finding was demonstrated by Martin H. Dawson, who was unable to confirm the bacteriologic findings, but showed that rheumatoid serum agglutinated suspensions of various bacteria (1932, New York).

Erik Waaler (1940, Oslo), while studying complement fixation, observed that sheep erythrocytes incubated with rabbit anti-sheep cell serum were agglutinated by some rheumatoid sera. In 1947 this observation was unknown in the laboratory of Harry M. Rose in New York where serologic studies of Q fever were being conducted. A technician with RA used her own serum in a control test and found that it agglutinated sheep erythrocytes in high titer. This serendipitous observation led Rose and Charles A. Ragan to develop the sensitized sheep erythrocyte agglutination reaction as a diagnostic procedure (1948). Numerous modifications were subsequently devised to improve the specificity and sensitivity of the procedure. The most widely used variation, in which a suspension of polystyrene latex particles coated with human gamma globulin is used, was described by Jacques M. Singer and Charles M. Plotz (1956, New York) (8).

JUVENILE CHRONIC POLYARTHRITIS

The report by George F. Still concerning "a form of chronic joint disease in children" was antedated by several brief descriptions, but his was the first detailed investigation of this ailment (1897, London). Still described 12 children with a polyarthritis, which he argued should be distinguished from RA, and six other children with a disease that was clinically indistinguishable from the disease in adults. The distinctive findings in the former group included lymphadenopathy and splenomegaly, the frequent occurrence of pericarditis, and an unusual predilection for involvement of the cervical spine. Still also pointed out the febrile component of the disease and the tendency toward growth retardation. The characteristic rash was not described until 1933 by the London pediatrician Harold E. Boldero. Eric L. Bywaters (1971, London) first reported the occurrence of this form of polyarthritis in adulthood (9).

ANKYLOSING SPONDYLITIS

In retrospect it is clear that several clinical and osteologic descriptions of ankylosing spondylitis were published prior to the 1890s. However, interest in this disease was stimulated by a series of publications (1893–1899) by Vladimir von Bechterew in St. Petersburg, Russia. The first cases he described were a woman and two of her daughters, and he hypothesized that the principal etiologic factors were a hereditary predisposition and post-traumatic myelopathy. Adolf Strümpell (1897, Erlangen) and Pierre Marie (1898, Paris) disagreed. They considered spondylitis to be a rheumatic disease, probably distinct from RA, in which neither trauma nor heredity were of pathogenetic importance. The male predominance of the disease was recognized in 1901 and proposed as a differentiating criterion from *spondylitis deformans* (degenerative spondylosis) by F. Glaser (Berlin).

A case of iritis with an arthropathy that probably was ankylosing spondylitis was described in 1861 by James Jackson in Boston. The association was mentioned by Bechterew (1893), but iritis as a manifestation of ankylosing spondylitis was first suggested by E. Kunz and E. Kraupa, German ophthalmologists, in 1933. The first study of heart disease in ankylosing spondylitis included six cases of aortic insufficiency, but this was attributed to rheumatic fever (L. Bernstein and OJ Bloch, 1949, Oslo). Attention was called serendipitously to the association between this arthropathy and aortic insufficiency when the first 100 patients with aortic insufficiency into whom Charles A. Hufnagel (1956, Washington, DC) had inserted a prosthetic aortic valve were reviewed. Five were found to have ankylosing spondylitis, a frequency that far exceeded chance. Peter Kulka et al differentiated this form of aortic insufficiency pathologically from that of rheumatic fever (1957, Boston). Despite numerous publications dealing with roentgenographic findings in ankylosing spondylitis, the characteristic obliteration of the sacroiliac joints was not reported until 1934 (Walter Krebs, Aachen).

Epidemiologic evidence of a heritable predisposition to the development of ankylosing spondylitis led Lee Schlosstein et al (Los Angeles) and Derek Brewerton et al (London) to study the HLA antigen distribution in patients with this disease. Both reported in 1973 that 88% and 96%, respectively, of their subjects carried the antigen now designated HLA–B27, which normally occurs in 4% to 8% of the white population. The finding of such a strong association stimulated numerous studies of the relationship between histocompatibility antigens and the various rheumatic diseases. The decision of the American Rheumatism Association in 1963 to adopt the term *ankylosing spondylitis* in preference to rheumatoid spondylitis has been supported by the lack of an association between the HLA phenotypes of patients with RA and spondylitis (10).

OSTEOARTHRITIS

The term *osteoarthritis* (OA) was introduced by John K. Spender (1886, Bath) in preference to rheumatoid arthritis and not to designate the conditions to which it is now applied. The modern usage and the clinical differentiation from RA were introduced by Archibald E. Garrod (1907, London). Aside from the older age of onset of OA, Garrod was impressed by an even stronger female predominance than he found with RA, as well as a heritable tendency. However, he was unable to make consistent distinctions. The first differentiation was made by William Heberden (1802, London), who distinguished nodules on the fingers from tophi. His description clearly identified "Heberden's nodes." Charles J. Bouchard (1884, Paris) described nodes adjacent to the proximal interphalangeal joints that are identical to those Heberden had described distally. Garrod related Heberden's nodes to OA. Robert M. Stecher (1944, Cleveland) demonstrated the strong genetic predisposition and female preponderance of the digital nodes, but questioned their relationship with other characteristics of OA. Osteoarthritis is now recognized as an imprecise diagnosis; variants such as "generalized osteoarthritis" (Jonas H. Kellgren, 1952, Manchester, UK) and "inflammatory" or "erosive" osteoarthritis (Darrell C. Crain, 1961, Washington, DC) have been described.

LUPUS ERYTHEMATOSUS

Ferdinand von Hebra described an eruption that occurs ". . . mainly on the face, on the cheeks and nose in a distribution not dissimilar to a butterfly" (1845, Vienna). *Lupus erythemateux* was introduced by Pierre A. Cazenave to identify a skin disease that probably was discoid lupus erythematosus (1851, Paris). Although Moritz Kaposi described cases with fever and pneumonia, he also used *lupus erythematosus* to designate the cutaneous findings and not to differentiate a multisystem disease (1872, Vienna). Many of the visceral features were described by William Osler under the name *exudative erythema* (1895–1904, Baltimore). Emanuel Libman and Benjamin Sacks added nonrheumatic verrucous endocarditis to the syndrome (1923, New York). In 1935 George Baehr et al (New York) published a study of 23 autopsied cases, the largest series to that time, and described the exacerbating effect of sunlight and the "wire loop" glomerular lesions (11).

In 1948 Malcolm M. Hargraves (Rochester, MN) described the *LE cell*, which he found in marrow aspirates from several cases of acute systemic lupus erythematosus. Soon thereafter, John H. Haserick (Cleveland) demonstrated that the LE cell may be induced by a serum factor, and in 1950 Hargraves demonstrated LE cell formation in peripheral blood. Efforts to elucidate the mechanism of LE cell formation led to the observation by Peter A. Miescher and M. Fauconnet (1956, Lausanne) that the LE cell-inducing factor can be absorbed from serum by exposure to isolated cell nuclei. Therefore, they suggested that this factor was an anti-nuclear antibody. A method to detect anti-nuclear antibodies by labeling with fluorescent antihuman globulin subsequently was described by George J. Friou et al (1958, West Haven, CN) (12).

The term *diffuse collagen disease* was introduced by Paul Klemperer (1942, New York). Based on pathologic studies of systemic lupus erythematosus and scleroderma, he concluded that there are some "acute and chronic maladies that are characterized anatomically by generalized alterations of the connective tissue, particularly by abnormalities of its extracellular components." Klemperer built on the work of Fritz Klinge (1927–1934, Leipzig), who concluded from his pathologic studies that some of the manifestations of rheumatic fever and RA may reflect a disturbance in the connective tissues. The concept of *collagen diseases* gained rapid acceptance, even though the number of diseases it encompassed remained in dispute. Following the suggestion of William E. Ehrich (1952, Philadelphia), the term *connective tissue diseases* gradually replaced collagen diseases in usage (13).

SYSTEMIC SCLEROSIS

Hippocrates commented, "In those persons in whom the skin is stretched, parched and hard, the disease terminates without sweats;" (aphorism V:71). However, the earliest definite descriptions of scleroderma were published by WD Chowne (1842, London), pertaining to a child, and in an adult by James Startin (1846, London). Several cases were described by French clinicians in 1847, and Elie Gintrac (1791–1877, Bordeaux) suggested the designation *sclerodermie*.

Maurice Raynaud described the vasospastic phenomenon that bears his name (1862, Paris), and commented on its occurrence in a patient with scleroderma in 1863. Jonathan Hutchinson pointed out the consistent association between Raynaud's phenomenon and scleroderma (1899, London). Heinrich Auspitz described death due to renal failure in scleroderma (1863, Vienna), but this was considered a chance association until 1952 (HC Moore and HL Sheehan, Liverpool). Albrecht von Notthafft (1899, Munich) described parenchymatous and vascular pulmonary fibrosis, and Salomon Ehrmann suggested that dysphagia was due to the occurrence of the same process in the esophagus as in the skin (1903, Vienna). Georges Thibierge and Raymond J. Weissenbach associated the development of calcinosis with scleroderma (1910, Paris). To these were added Raynaud's phenomenon, esophageal dysfunction and telangiectasias in a case reported by Prosser Thomas (1942, London), and the acronym CRST (later CREST) was coined for this syndrome by Richard H. Winterbauer (1964, Baltimore). Despite several descriptions of myocardial fibrosis, beginning with that of Carl F. Westphal (1876, Berlin), this form of cardiac involvement only became recognized as a manifestation of scleroderma by the work of Soma Weiss et al (1943, Boston). Due to the extensive visceral involvement in this disease, RH Goetz (1945, Capetown) proposed *progressive systemic sclerosis* as more descriptive than scleroderma. Since the disease may stabilize, the modifier "progressive" has recently been discarded (14,15).

POLYMYOSITIS

Introduction of the term *polymyositis* is credited to Ernst L. Wagner (1886, Leipzig), although a definite case had been described by Potain (1875, Paris). Heinrich Unverricht coined the term *dermatomyositis* in describing a case (1891, Dorpat, Estonia). An association between dermatomyositis and cancer was first reported by Rudolf Bezecny (1935, Prague). A patient who underwent resection of an ovarian carcinoma experienced regression of her skin lesions within a few days, despite peritoneal metastases, and the myopathy improved during subsequent roentgen therapy. The feasibility of evaluating disease activity biochemically was first demonstrated by RG Siekert and GA Fleisher (1956, Rochester, MN), who measured serum glutamic oxalacetic transaminase (16).

POLYARTERITIDES

From the earliest descriptions of polyarteritis to the present, both the etiologies and classifications that may be valid on clinical or pathologic grounds have remained in dispute. The first certain case was described by Karl Rokitansky in a general pathologic study of arterial aneurysms (1852, Vienna). This case was in part reexamined microscopically by Hans Eppinger (1887, Graz). Adolf Kussmaul and Rudolf Maier published one case with autopsy findings (1866, Freiburg). They called the disease *periarteritis nodosa* because of the presence of aneurysmal dilatations in most of the medium size and smaller arteries. Enrico Ferrari (1903, Trieste) preferred *polyarteritis nodosa* in describing a patient with severe arteritis without aneurysms.

Giant cell arteritis was described by Jonathan Hutchinson in 1890 and rediscovered by Bayard T. Horton et al (1934, Rochester, MN) as *arteritis of the temporal vessels*. The association between this arteritis and *polymyalgia rheumatica* was suggested by J.W. Paulley (Ipswich, UK) in 1956. The latter ailment had been described by William Bruce, a Scottish physician, in 1888 and rediscovered by L. Bagratuni (1953, Oxford). The term was introduced by Stuart Barber (1957, Manchester, UK).

Heinz Klinger (1931, Berlin) reported another distinctive form of arteritis, which was described in greater detail by Friedrich Wegener (1936, 1939, Breslau) and now is called *Wegener's granulomatosis*. Jacob Churg and Lotte Strauss described *allergic granulomatosis*, a variant characterized by bronchospasm and eosinophilia (1951, New York) (17).

GONOCOCCAL ARTHRITIS AND REITER'S DISEASE

The early history of gonococcal arthritis and of Reiter's disease must be considered together because, before the discovery of the gonococcus by Albert Neisser (1879, Breslau), it would have been impossible to differentiate the two diseases. An association between arthritis and urethritis (blennorrhagia) was first described by Francois X. Swediaur (1784, Paris). When Luigi Petrone (1883, Bologna) demonstrated gonococci in the urethral exudates and synovial fluid of two men, the disease was well known. The culture of gonococci from synovial fluid was first accomplished in an infant by Heinrich Höck (1893, Vienna) and in an adult by Neisser a year later. The unity of gonococcal urethritis and arthritis was proved by Ernst Finger (1896, Vienna). A culture made from joint fluid obtained from a patient with gonococcal arthritis was innoculated into the urethra of a man who, thereupon, developed typical gonorrhea.

The recurrence of arthritis and/or ocular inflammation with urethritis following totally asymptomatic intervals provided a clue that some of the early descriptions of arthritis with urethritis did not represent gonococcal disease. The first such case report probably was that of Thomas Whateley (1801, London). Benjamin Brodie, beginning in 1818, described several men with recurrent episodes of urethritis, conjunctivitis, and arthritis. One had nine attacks in 20 years. Adolf Vossius (1855–1925), a German ophthalmologist, reported the first case that began with bacillary dysentery. In 1916 Noel Fiessinger and Edgar Leroy published a report concerning dysentery among French troops, incidentally providing a brief description of a "conjunctivo-urethro-synovial syndrome," of which they had seen four cases. One week later Hans Reiter published his first report about the disease with which his name has become associated. His patient, a German officer on the Balkan front, developed urethritis, conjunctivitis, and a febrile polyarthritis after a bout of dysentery (18).

Emil Vidal described a man who had suffered two bouts of a heretofore unknown hyperkeratotic eruption in association with presumed recurrent gonorrheal arthritis (1893, Paris). The term *keratodermia blennorrhagica* was introduced by Anatole M. Chauffard and Georges Froin (1894, Paris) in describing such a case. Despite little evidence in support of a gonococcal etiology, Wiedmann (1934, Vienna) was the first to suggest that keratodermia blennorhagica was a manifestation of Reiter's disease.

U.S. RHEUMATOLOGY ORGANIZATIONS

Organization of the specialty of rheumatology in the United States began in 1928 with the American Committee for the Control of Rheumatism. This was enlarged into the American Association for the Study and Control of Rheumatic Diseases in 1934. It was renamed the American Rheumatism Association in 1937, and the American College of Rheumatology in 1988. The first certification examination in rheumatology was administered in 1972. The evolution of rheumatology in America has recently been reviewed (19).

Thomas G. Benedek, MD

1. Parish LC: An historical approach to the nomenclature of rheumatoid arthritis. Arthritis Rheum 6:138–158, 1963
2. Rodnan GP: Early theories concerning etiology and pathogenesis of the gout. Arthritis Rheum 8:599–609, 1965
3. Benedek TG: Subcutaneous nodules and the differentiation of rheumatoid arthritis from rheumatic fever. Sem Arthritis Rheum 13:305–321, 1984
4. Schechter DC: St. Vitus dance and rheumatic disease. NT St J Med 75:1091–1102, 1975
5. Murphy GE: The evolution of our knowledge of rheumatic fever. Bull Hist Med 14:123–147, 1943
6. Rothschild BM, Woods RJ: Symmetrical erosive disease in Archaic Indians: The origin of rheumatoid arthritis in the New World? Sem Arthritis Rheum 19:278–284, 1990
7. Short CL: Rheumatoid arthritis: historical aspects. J Chron Dis 10:367–387, 1959
8. Fraser KJ: The Waaler–Rose test: Anatomy of the eponym. Sem Arthritis Rheum 18:61–71, 1988
9. Baum J, Baum ER: George Frederic Still and his account of childhood arthritis–a reappraisal. Amer J Dis Child 132:192–194, 1978
10. Spencer DG, Sturrock RD, Buchanan WW: Ankylosing spondylitis: Yesterday and today. Med Hist 24:60–69, 1980
11. Smith CD, Cyr M: The history of lupus erythematosus from Hippocrates to Osler. Rheum Dis Clin N Amer 14:1–14, 1988
12. Hargraves MM: Discovery of the LE cell and its morphology. Mayo Clin Proc 44:579–599, 1969
13. Bywaters EG: The historical evolution of the concept of connective tissue diseases. Scand J Rheumatol 5(suppl 12):11–29, 1976
14. Rodnan GP, Benedek TG: An historical account of the study of progressive systemic sclerosis (diffuse scleroderma). Ann Intern Med 57:305–319, 1962
15. Benedek TG, Rodnan GP: The early history and nomenclature of scleroderma and of its differentiation from sclerema neonatorum and scleroedema. Sem Arthritis Rheum 12:52–67, 1982
16. Pearson CM: Polymyositis. Ann Rev Med 17:63–82, 1966
17. Lie JT: Vasculitis, 1815 to 1991: Classification and diagnostic specificity. J Rheumatol 19:83–89, 1992
18. Benedek TG: The first reports of Dr. Hans Reiter on Reiter's disease. J Alb Einstein Med Cent 17:100–105, 1969
19. Benedek TG: A century of American rheumatology. Ann Intern Med 106:304–312, 1987

2. THE MUSCULOSKELETAL SYSTEM
A. Joints

Human bones join with each other in a variety of ways to serve the functional requirements of the musculoskeletal system. Foremost among these needs is that of purposeful motion. The activities of the human body depend on effective interaction between normal joints and the neuromuscular units that drive them. The same elements also interact reflexively to distribute mechanical stresses among the tissues of the joint. Muscles, tendons, ligaments, cartilage, and bone all do their share to ensure smooth function. In this role, the supporting elements both unite the abutting bones and position the cartilages in the optimal relationship for low-friction load-bearing.

CLASSIFICATION

Differing designs of human joints usually are classified according to a scheme based on the histologic features of the union and the range of motion it permits. *Synarthrosis* describes the suture lines of the skull where adjoining cranial plates are separated only by thin fibrous tissue as they interlock to prevent detectable motion but to still provide for orderly growth. When cranial growth ceases, synarthrodial joints have no further role and they regularly close.

In *amphiarthroses*, adjacent bones are bound by flexible fibrocartilage that permits modest motion to occur. In the pubic symphysis and in a portion of the sacroiliac joint, amphiarthroses permit minor rotary motion of the pelvic bones. Between the vertebral bodies, the intervertebral disc has developed into a more mobile, highly specialized amphiarthrodial articulation, which is discussed in Chapter 47, Disorders of the Back.

The third class, the *diarthroses*, includes the most mobile joints and is, by far, the most common of the articular design patterns. Because these joints all possess a synovial membrane and contain synovial fluid, diarthrodial joints are more commonly referred to as *synovial joints*. These joints are the focus of this section.

Synovial joints are further subclassified according to shape as in *ball and socket* (hip), *hinge* (interphalangeal), *saddle* (first carpometacarpal), and *plane* (patellofemoral) joints. These widely varying configurations reflect the fact that form parallels function in the design of diarthrodial joints. In every case, a well-lubricated bearing develops from essentially congruent cartilaginous surfaces that slide freely against each other. The direction and the extent of the permitted motion are defined by the shape and the size of the opposing surfaces (Fig. 2A–1). Within these limitations, a wide variety of designs permit motion in flexion (bending), extension (straightening), abduction (away from the midline), adduction (toward the midline), and rotation. Individual joints thus can act in one (humero-ulnar joint), two (wrist), or even three (shoulder) axes of motion.

ARTICULAR TISSUES

Articular cartilage comprises the low-friction facing that surfaces the opposing members of synovial joints. It is described in Chapter 2B. Synovial joints are surrounded by a capsule that defines the boundary between articular and periarticular tissues. The capsule varies in thickness from a thin membrane in some areas to a strong ligamentous band in others. A reinforced capsular plate, for instance, serves as an effective check to prevent hyperextension of most hinge joints. Over extensor aspects of the same joints, the capsule is a much less consequential structure. Reinforcing the capsule are additional ligaments that are sometimes extracapsular. Further, the tendons of those muscles acting across the joint provide periarticular support. Capsule, ligaments, and tendons all are formed primarily from bundles of type I collagen fibers aligned with the axis of tensile stress (1).

The synovium, containing lining cells that are one to three cells deep, surfaces all intracapsular structures other than the contact areas of cartilage (2). This highly flexible, well-lubricated lining is normally collapsed on itself and on articular cartilage to minimize the volume of the joint space it encloses. In fact, most normal human joints, when opened, reveal moist, tacky synovial and

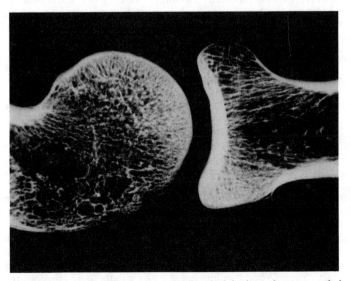

Fig. 2A–1. Radiograph of a 3-mm sagittal slab through an extended elbow joint. The convex distal humerus has a thin subchondral plate and honeycombed underlying trabeculation, whereas the concave, proximal radius has a thick subchondral plate over coarse, vertical trabecular bone. Comparable convex-concave differences are regularly seen in other large human joints (from reference 7).

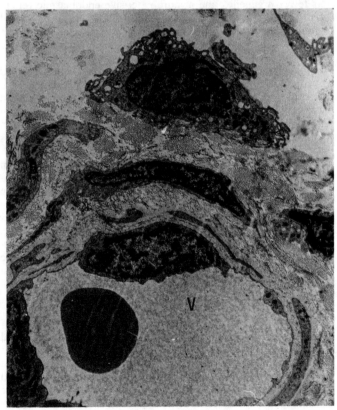

Fig. 2A–2. Electron micrograph showing a type A synovial lining cell at the top. The type B cell is deeper and contains rough endoplasmic reticulum. V indicates a superficial synovial vessel (courtesy of Dr HR Schumacher).

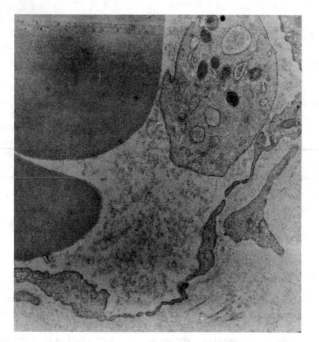

Fig. 2A–3. Higher magnification electron micrograph of a synovial vessel shows red cells and a platelet in the lumen. The endothelium has fenestrations closed by diaphragms (courtesy of Dr HR Schumacher).

cartilaginous surfaces but contain no obvious pool of synovial fluid.

The synovial lining cells reside in a matrix rich in collagen fibrils and proteoglycans. In most areas, the cells do not abut directly on each other but are separated by interstitium. The principal cells of the normal synovium come in two forms, type A and type B (Fig. 2A–2). The monocyte-derived type A cell resembles a macrophage in its high content of cytoplasmic organelles, which include lysosomes, smooth-walled vacuoles, and micropinocytotic vesicles. In contrast, the fibroblastic type B cell has fewer organelles and a more extensive endoplasmic reticulum. A number of other cells are sometimes seen in normal synovial tissue. These include apparent antigen-processing cells with a dendritic configuration, mast cells, and occasional white blood cells.

The synovial lining is supported by a rich bed of fenestrated microvessels (Fig. 2A–3), which, for the most part, lie close to the surface of the joint space (3). The tissue is also supplied with lymphatic vessels and nerve fibers. The blood supply comes from an arterial plexus that also supports the capsule and the juxtaarticular bone. The innervation derives from all of the nerve roots supplying the muscles that cross the joint.

Synovial tissue overlies a spectrum of matrices ranging from fibrous capsule through loose areolar connective tissue to organized structures composed mainly of fat. The tissue may take the form of fat pads, which serve as highly flexible, space-occupying structures to accommodate the changes in geometry during articular motion. In other locations, a somewhat similar role is played by much more solid fibrocartilaginous structures. Examples of the latter are found in the temporomandibular joints, the wrists, and in the knees, where the medial and lateral menisci help to preserve alignment and distribute loads (4).

STRESS DISTRIBUTION

In active motion, substantial loading forces cross each normal joint. If these forces exceed the inherent limits of a tissue, that structure will fracture or fail. Normal joints distribute these forces and minimize the likelihood that any one component will fail. The greatest share of loading energy is taken up within the muscles and tendons crossing each joint. Effective reflexes normally ensure that impact forces are delivered to flexed joints, which bend further under the acute load. Most persons have experienced the surprise of finding one more step than expected when descending a flight of stairs. The sudden jolt of that moment

results from landing on a hip and knee that have not flexed in anticipation of the impact. Appropriate flexion of these joints distributes the stress in time by prolonging the deceleration of landing and in space by loading a larger surface area of each convex joint member as it slides within the embrace of its concave mate.

Loading stress that is not absorbed by surrounding muscles, tendons, and ligaments impacts directly on the opposing articular cartilages and their underlying trabecular bone. The firm, resilient articular cartilage has viscoelastic properties that allow it to serve as a hydraulic shock absorber analogous to those found in automobiles (5). Despite these desirable characteristics, the cartilage is so thin that most loading energy is transmitted directly into bone (6).

Immediately beneath the cartilage is a continuous plate of subchondral bone supported by a complex meshwork of underlying trabeculae. In convex members such as the femoral and humeral heads, this plate is a thin shell supported by a honeycombed structure of interconnecting bony chambers. In contrast, the opposing concave acetabulum and the glenoid fossa have much thicker subchondral plates supported by a coarser and more open framework of trabecular struts (7). This structural difference in bone is matched by a corresponding difference in the thickness of overlying cartilage. In cartilage, however, the thicker layer is on the convex side, while the thinner layer is concave. It tends to have more of a fibrous than a hyaline composition. These concave-convex differences in structure provide for stiff concave joint members in opposition to more flexible convex mates. Clinically significant patterns of injury occur where overwhelming stresses regularly explode the stiff, concave side but do not crush its more flexible convex opponent. Similarly, raised subchondral pressures in loaded convex bones may play a role in their special vulnerability to ischemic necrosis of bone (osteonecrosis) (8).

STABILITY

A number of factors interact to confer stability, while permitting motion in active human joints. First among these is the shape of the component parts. In the hips, for example, weight bearing drives the femoral head into a relatively deep socket, the acetabulum. The articular members are configured and positioned so that normal loading enhances the closeness of their fit.

Ligaments provide a second major stabilizing influence as they guide and align normal joints through their range of motion. An excellent example is the pair of collateral ligaments along each side of interphalangeal joints. These strong, relatively inelastic structures limit articular motion to flexion and extension. In addition, the broad, ligamentous posterior capsule serves as a check that prevents hyperextension.

Within the axes of motion, however, more flexible constraints are required. This need is met by muscles and tendons. Muscular stabilization is perhaps most obvious in the shoulder, which is the quintessential polyaxial joint. The rotator cuff muscles approximate and stabilize the articular surfaces of the shoulder as larger muscles with better leverage provide the power for effective shoulder motion (9).

The synovial fluid contributes significant stabilizing effects as an adhesive seal that freely permits sliding motion between cartilaginous surfaces while effectively resisting distracting forces. This property is most easily demonstrated in small articulations such as the metacarpophalangeal joints. The common phenomenon of "knuckle cracking" reflects the fracture of this adhesive bond. Secondary cavitation within the joint space causes a radiologically obvious bubble of gas that requires up to 30 minutes to dissolve before the bond can be reestablished and the joint can be "cracked" again (10). This adhesive property depends on the normally thin film of synovial fluid between all intraarticular structures. When this film enlarges as a pathologic effusion, the stabilizing properties are lost.

The intraarticular pressure is about −4 mmHg in the resting, normal knee, and this pressure falls farther when the quadriceps muscle contracts. The difference between atmospheric pressure on overlying tissues and subatmospheric values within the joint helps to hold the joint members together and thus provides a stabilizing force. In a pathologic effusion, however, the resting pressure is above that of the atmosphere and it rises farther when surrounding muscles contract. Thus, reversal of the normal pressure gradient is an additional destabilizing factor in joints with effusions (11).

LUBRICATION

Synovial joints act as mechanical bearings that facilitate the work of the musculoskeletal machine. As such, normal joints are remarkably effective with coefficients of friction lower than those obtainable with manufactured journal bearings. Furthermore, the constant process of renewal and restoration ensures that living articular tissues have a durability far superior to that of any artificial bearing. No arthroplastic implant can equal the performance of a normal human joint.

The mechanics of joint lubrication have provided a focus of investigation beginning with the unique structure of the bearing surface. Articular cartilage is elastic, fluid-filled, and backed by a relatively impervious layer of calcified cartilage and bone. This means that load-induced compression of cartilage will force interstitial fluid to flow laterally within the tissue and to surface through adjacent cartilage. As that area, in turn, becomes load-bearing, it is partially protected by the newly expressed fluid above it. This is a special form of *hydrodynamic lubrication*, so-called because the dynamic motion of the bearing areas produces an aqueous layer that separates and protects the contact points (5).

Boundary layer lubrication is the second major low-friction characteristic of normal joints. Here, the critical factor is proposed to be a small glycoprotein called *lubricin*. The lubricating properties of this synovium-derived molecule are highly specific and depend on its ability to bind to articular cartilage where it retains a protective layer of water molecules. Lubricin is not effective in artificial systems and thus does not lubricate artificial joints (12).

Other lubricating mechanisms have been proposed; some remain under investigation. Interestingly, hyaluronic acid, the molecule that makes synovial fluid viscous (*synovia* means "like egg white"), has largely been excluded as a lubricant of the cartilage-on-cartilage bearing. Instead, hyaluronate lubricates a quite different site of surface contact—that of synovium on cartilage. The well-vascularized, well-innervated synovium must alternately contract and then expand to cover non-loaded cartilage surfaces as each joint moves through its normal range of motion. This process must proceed freely. Were synovial tissue to be pinched, there would be immediate pain, intraarticular bleeding, and inevitable functional compromise. The rarity of these problems testifies to the effectiveness of hyaluronate-mediated synovial lubrication.

SYNOVIAL FLUID

In normal human joints, a thin film of synovial fluid covers the surfaces of synovium and cartilage within the joint space. The volume of this fluid increases when disease is present to provide an effusion that is clinically apparent and may be easily aspirated for study. For this reason, most knowledge of human synovial fluid comes from patients with joint disease. Because of the clinical frequency, volume, and accessibility of knee effusions, our knowledge is largely limited to findings in that joint.

In the synovium, as in all tissues, essential nutrients are delivered and metabolic by-products are cleared by the bloodstream perfusing the local vasculature. Synovial microvessels contain fenestrations that facilitate diffusion-based exchange between plasma and the surrounding interstitium. Free diffusion provides full equilibration of small solutes between plasma and the immediate interstitial space. Further diffusion extends this equilibration process to include all other intracapsular spaces including the synovial fluid and the interstitial fluid of cartilage. Synovial plasma flow and the narrow diffusion path between synovial lining cells provide the principal limitations on exchange rates between plasma and synovial fluid (13).

This process is clinically relevant to the transport of therapeutic agents in inflamed synovial joints. Many investigators have made serial observations of drug concentrations in plasma and synovial fluid after oral or intravenous administration. Predictably, plasma levels exceed those in synovial fluid during the early phases of absorption and distribution. This gradient reverses during the subsequent period of elimination when intrasynovial levels exceed those of plasma. These patterns reflect passive diffusion alone, and no therapeutic agent is known to be transported into or selectively retained within the joint space (14).

Metabolic evidence of ischemia provides a second instance when the delivery and removal of small solutes becomes clinically relevant. In normal joints and in most pathologic effusions, essentially full equilibration exists between plasma and synovial fluid. The gradients that drive net delivery of nutrients (glucose and oxygen) or removal of wastes (lactate and carbon dioxide) are too small to be detected. In some cases, however, the synovial microvascular supply is unable to meet local metabolic demand, and significant gradients develop. In these joints, the synovial fluid reveals a low oxygen pressure (PO_2), low glucose, low pH, high lactate, and high carbon dioxide pressure (PCO_2). Such fluids are found regularly in septic arthritis, often in rheumatoid disease, and infrequently in other kinds of synovitis. Such findings presumably reflect both the increased metabolic demand of hyperplastic tissue and impaired microvascular supply.

Consistent with this interpretation is the finding that ischemic rheumatoid joints are colder than joints containing synovial fluid in full equilibration with plasma (15). Like other peripheral tissues, joints normally have temperatures lower than that of the body's core. The knee, for instance, has a normal intraarticular temperature of 32°C. With acute local inflammation, articular blood flow increases and the temperature approaches 37°C. As rheumatoid synovitis persists, however, microcirculatory compromise may cause the temperature to fall as the tissues become ischemic.

The clinical implications of local ischemia remain under investigation. Decreased synovial fluid pH, for instance, was found to correlate strongly with radiographic evidence of joint damage in rheumatoid knees (16). Other work has shown that either joint flexion or quadriceps contraction may increase intrasynovial pressure and thereby exert a tamponade effect on the synovial vasculature. This finding suggests that normal use of swollen joints may create a cycle of ischemia and reperfusion that leads to tissue damage by toxic oxygen radicals (17).

Normal articular cartilage has no microvascular supply of its own and, therefore, is at risk in ischemic joints. In this tissue, the normal process of diffusion is supplemented by the convection induced by cyclic compression and release during joint usage. In immature joints, the same pumping process promotes exchange of small molecules with the interstitial fluid of underlying trabecular bone. In adults, however, this potential route of supply is considered unlikely, and all exchange of solutes may occur through synovial fluid. This means that normal chondrocytes are farther from their supporting microvasculature than are any other cells in the body. The vulnerability of this extended supply line is clearly shown in synovial ischemia.

The normal proteins of plasma also enter synovial fluid by passive diffusion. In contrast to small molecules, however, protein concentrations remain substantially less in synovial fluid than in plasma. In aspirates from normal knees, the total protein was only 1.3 g/dL, a value roughly 20% of that in normal plasma (18). Moreover, the distribution of intrasynovial proteins differs from that found in plasma. Large proteins such as IgM and α_2-macroglobulin are underrepresented, whereas smaller proteins are present in relatively higher concentrations. The mechanism determining this pattern is reasonably well understood. The microvascular endothelium provides the major barrier limiting the escape of plasma proteins into the surrounding synovial interstitium. The protein path across the endothelium is not yet clear; conflicting experimental evidence supports the fenestrae, intercellular junctions, and cytoplasmic vesicles as the predominant sites of plasma protein escape. What does seem clear is that the process follows diffusion kinetics. This means that smaller proteins, which have fast diffusion coefficients, will enter the joint space at rates proportionately faster than those of large proteins with relatively slow diffusion coefficients.

In contrast, proteins leave synovial fluid through lymphatic vessels, a process that is not size-selective. Protein clearance may vary with joint disease. In particular, joints affected by rheumatoid arthritis (RA) experience significantly more rapid removal of proteins than do those of patients with osteoarthritis (19). Thus, in all joints, there is a continuing, passive transport of plasma proteins involving synovial delivery in the microvasculature, diffusion across the endothelium, and ultimate lymphatic return to plasma.

The intrasynovial concentration of any protein represents the net contributions of plasma concentration, synovial blood flow, microvascular permeability, and lymphatic removal. Specific proteins may be produced or consumed within the joint space. Thus, lubricin is normally synthesized within synovial cells and released into synovial fluid where it facilitates boundary layer lubrication of the cartilage-on-cartilage bearing. In disease, additional proteins may be synthesized, such as IgG rheumatoid factor in RA, or released by inflammatory cells, such as lysosomal enzymes. In contrast, intraarticular proteins may be depleted by local consumption, as are complement components in rheumatoid disease.

Synovial fluid protein concentrations vary little between highly inflamed rheumatoid joints and modestly involved osteoarthritic articulations. Microvascular permeability to protein, however, is more than twice as great in RA as in osteoarthritis. This marked difference in permeability leads to only a minimal increase in protein concentration, because the enhanced ingress of proteins is largely offset by a comparable rise in lymphatic egress. These findings illustrate that synovial microvascular permeability cannot be evaluated from protein concentrations unless the kinetics of delivery or removal are concurrently assessed.

Peter A. Simkin, MD

1. Amiel D, Frank C, Harwood F, et al: Tendons and ligaments: A morphological and biochemical comparison. J Orthop Res 1:257–265, 1984

2. Henderson B, Edwards JCW: The Synovial Lining in Health and Disease. London, Chapman and Hall, 1987

3. Knight AD, Levick JR: Morphometry of the ultrastructure of the blood-joint barrier in the rabbit knee. Q J Exper Physiol 69:271–288, 1984

4. Thompson WO, Thaete FL, Fu FH, et al: Tibial meniscal dynamics using three-dimensional reconstruction of magnetic resonance images. Am J Sports Med 19:210–215, 1991

5. Mow VC, Roth V, Armstrong CG: Biomechanics of joint cartilage, Basic Biomechanics of the Skeletal System. Edited by VH Frankel, M Nordin. Philadelphia, Lea & Febiger, 1980, pp 61–86

6. Radin EL: Mechanics of joint degeneration, Practical Biomechanics for the Orthopedic Surgeon. Edited by EL Radin, SR Simon, RM Rose, et al. New York, John Wiley & Sons; 1979

7. Simkin PA, Graney DO, Feichtner JJ: Roman arches, human joints, and disease: Differences between convex and concave sides of joints. Arthritis Rheum 23:1308–1311, 1980

8. Downey DJ, Simkin PA, Taggart R: The effect of compressive loading on intraosseous pressure in the femoral head in vitro. J Bone Joint Surg 70A:871–877, 1988

9. Jobe CM: Gross Anatomy of the Shoulder, The Shoulder. Edited by Rockwood CA, Matsen FA. Philadelphia, WB Saunders, 1990, pp 34–97

10. Unsworth A, Dowson D, Wright V: "Cracking joints": A bioengineering study of cavitation in the metrcarpophalangeal joint. Ann Rheum Dis 30:348–358, 1971

11. Levick JR. Joint pressure-volume studies: Their importance, design and interpretation. J Rheumatol 10:353–357, 1983

12. Swann DA, Silver FH, Slayter HS, et al: The molecular structure and lubricating activity of lubricin isolated from bovine and human synovial fluids. Biochem J 225:195–201, 1985

13. Levick JR: Blood flow and mass transport in synovial joints, Handbook of Physiology Vol. IV, Microcirculation, Part 2. Edited by EM Renkin, CC Michel. Bethesda, MD, American Physiological Society, 1984, pp 917–947

14. Wallis WJ, Simkin PA: Antirheumatic drug levels in human synovial fluid and synovial tissue: Observations on extravascular pharmacokinetics. Clin Pharmacokinet 8:496–522, 1983

15. Wallis WJ, Simkin PA, Nelp WB: Low synovial clearance of iodide provides evidence of hypoperfusion in chronic rheumatoid synovitis. Arthritis Rheum 28:1096–1104, 1985

16. Geborek P, Saxne T, Pettersson H, et al: Synovial fluid acidosis correlates with radiological joint destruction in rheumatoid arthritis knee joints. J Rheumatol 16:468–472, 1989

17. Stevens CR, Williams RB, Farrell AJ, et al: Hypoxia and inflammatory synovitis: Observations and speculations. Ann Rheum Dis 50:124–132, 1991

18. Weinberger A, Simkin PA: Plasma proteins in synovial fluids of normal human joints. Semin Arthritis Rheum 19:66–76, 1989

19. Wallis WJ, Simkin PA, Nelp WB: Protein traffic in human synovial effusions. Arthritis Rheum 30:57–63, 1987

B. Articular Cartilage

Articular cartilage is a specialized avascular and neural connective tissue that provides covering for the osseous components of diarthrodial joints. It serves as a load-bearing material, absorbs impact, and is capable of sustaining shearing forces. The unique properties of this tissue are related to the composition and structure of its extracellular matrix, which is composed mainly of a high concentration of proteoglycans entangled in a dense network of collagen fibers and a large amount of water.

CARTILAGE STRUCTURE

The different molecular components of the articular cartilage form a highly ordered structure that changes with depth from the joint surfaces (1,2). From top to bottom, the cartilage has been classified into four zones (Fig. 2B–1): superficial zone, middle or transitional zone, the deep or radial zone, and the calcified cartilage zone located immediately below the tidemark and above the subchondral bone. By electron microscopy, the surface of the articular cartilage demonstrates small mounds that cover the superficial cells (3). The superficial zone is the thinnest of the four zones and consists primarily of fine collagen fibrils with a tangential orientation, a low content in proteoglycans, and elongated chondrocytes. In the middle zone, comprising 40% to 60% of the total cartilage height, the collagen fibrils are thicker and organized into radial bundles or layers, and the chondrocytes have a spheroidal shape. Deep zone chondrocytes have a similar shape to those in the middle zone and are perpendicular to the articular surface. The latter zone contains the largest collagen fibrils; these have a radial disposition. The calcified cartilage zone separates

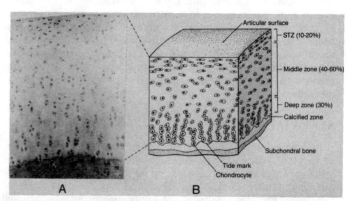

Fig. 2B–1. Photomicrograph (left) and schematic representation (right) of the arrangement of the different zones of articular cartilage (reproduced with permission, Mow et al In: Basic Biomechanics of the Musculoskeletal System, 2nd edition, 1989). STZ = superficial zone.

the hyaline cartilage from subchondral bone. It appears to serve as an anchor of the cartilage to the bone as collagen fibrils from the radial zone penetrate into the calcified cartilage. In this zone, the cell population is very scarce and chondrocytes are usually smaller.

The pericellular area surrounding the chondrocytes is made of a thin layer of nonfibrillar material that most likely represents the synthetic products of the chondrocytes such as proteoglycans and glycoproteins (1,2,4; Fig. 2B–2). Immediately adjacent to the pericellular area is the territorial cartilage matrix that has been

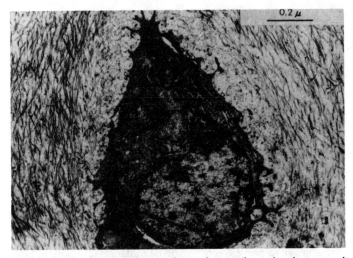

Fig. 2B–2. Electron micrograph of articular cartilage chondrocyte and the surrounding matrix from dog femoral condyle (original magnification ×6396). Illustrated is the extracellular matrix surrounding a chondrocyte, the pericellular compartment consisting of a narrow halo of nonfibrillar molecules, and the territorial matrix consisting of a dense network of collagen fibers (reproduced with permission, Pelletier et al, Arthritis Rheum 26:866–874, 1983).

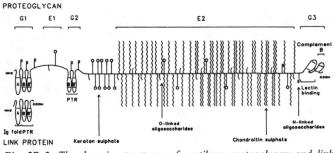

Fig. 2B–3. The domain structures of cartilage proteoglycan and link protein. The globular (G_1, G_2, and G_3) and extended (E1, E2) domains are shown (from reference 10, reproduced with permission).

shown by ultrastructural study to contain a dense meshwork of thin collagen fibers forming a capsule-like structure around the cells, and providing mechanical protection to the chondrocytes (1,3,5). The interterritorial matrix, which immediately follows the territorial matrix, is composed of larger collagen fibrils with a more parallel orientation. It is the largest matrix compartment and is responsible for the mechanical properties of cartilage.

COMPOSITION

Normal cartilage is composed of a sparse population of specialized cells, named *chondrocytes*, that are responsible for the synthesis and maintenance of the intercellular matrix. The matrix consists mainly of collagen and proteoglycans (1,2,6). Most of the collagen is type II collagen, which forms a fiber network that provides the shape and form of the tissue. The high content of proteoglycans, principally of the large aggregating type, is responsible for the compressive properties associated with load bearing. Collagen, proteoglycans, other proteins, and glycoproteins represent only about 20% of the tissue wet weight. Water and inorganic salts represent most of the remaining tissue. The water content of cartilage plays an important role in maintaining the resiliency of the tissue and contributing to the nutrition and lubrication system.

Chemistry of Cartilage

Collagen. Collagen makes up about 50% to 60% of the dry weight of articular cartilage (see Chapter 3A). Type II collagen is specific for cartilage and is the primary collagen of articular cartilage (about 90% to 98% of the total tissue collagen) (1,6). The extracellular collagen unit is the tropocollagen made of three polypeptide chains organized into a triple helix. The triple helix consists of three identical polypeptide chains α 1 (II). These molecules assemble to form fibrils and larger fibers, stabilized by covalent interfibrillar cross-links. The most important mechanical properties of collagen fibers are tensile stiffness and strength.

A small portion of cartilage collagen is composed of other types of collagen fibers called minor collagens including types V, VI, IX, X, XI and perhaps some other types (1,6,7). The functions of minor collagens in articular cartilage are not well understood, but these could make an important contribution to the structure of the matrix. Analyses have demonstrated that the helical domain of type IX collagen forms cross-links with telopeptide domains of type II collagen (7). The function of this covalent bond at the surface of fibrils is not known, but is believed to link fibrils together or bind fibrils to other matrix mol-

ecules. Cross-links between collagen molecules and other extracellular matrix proteins seem to be common, and are probably important in maintaining cartilage architecture. Type XI collagen is possibly involved in controlling the diameter of type II fibrils.

Proteoglycans. The proteoglycans constitute the second largest portion of the solid phase in articular cartilage accounting for 5% to 10% of the wet weight (see Chapter 3B). The proteoglycans in articular cartilage are complex supramolecular aggregates (6,8,9). The proteoglycan aggregate consists of a central hyaluronic acid (HA) filament to which multiple monomers are noncovalently attached. Proteoglycan monomers of varying size arise laterally at regular intervals from the opposite side of the hyaluronic acid chain. A low molecular weight protein called link protein stabilizes the bond between the monomer and the hyaluronate. The chemical structure of the monomer can be compared to a "test tube brush". Proteoglycans of the cartilage matrix are mainly of the large aggregating type (50% to 85%) and the large nonaggregating type (10% to 40%). An aggregating proteoglycan is composed of a monomer that in turn consists of a protein backbone, the core protein. Numerous glycosaminoglycan chains radiating from the core at a right angle and stiffly extending in space are linked to this protein core (Fig. 2B–3). The glycosaminoglycan molecules are a long chain of repeating polydimeric saccharides: chondroitin 4-sulfate, chondroitin 6-sulfate, and keratan sulfate, in which chondroitin sulfates are the most abundant (60% to 90%). The average length of a chondroitin sulfate chain consists of 25 to 30 repeating disaccharide units. Keratan sulfate chains are shorter and consist of only 5 to 6 repeating dimeric units.

Six different structural domains of cartilage proteoglycans (8) were recently identified (Fig. 2B–3). There are three globular (G_1, G_2, G_3) domains and two extended regions on the core protein. The N-terminal globular domain (G_1) contains a site for interacting with HA and also with the link protein and function as the HA-binding region. The G_2 domain does not interact with HA, link protein, or other matrix protein. Its precise functional role remains unknown. The third globular domain (G_3) is located at the carboxy terminal of the proteoglycans and may be involved in interactions with other extracellular matrix glycoproteins. At present, the exact function of the G_3 domain remains unclear. Two extended regions occur in the core protein of proteoglycans; a short extended domain (E_1) between the G_1 and G_2 and a larger extended region (E_2) between G_2 and G_3 incorporates the keratan sulfate and chondroitin sulfate attachment regions.

The composition and size of proteoglycan aggregates in cartilage is not uniform. Differences in chain lengths of HA, glycosaminoglycans, and the core protein, as well as the amount of glycoaminoglycans and aggregates, are important factors contributing to the variation of proteoglycan composition and structure in cartilage (9). The content in proteoglycan also varies within the tissue. The highest concentration is found in the middle and deep zones, and the lowest is found in the superficial layer. The composition of cartilage proteoglycan monomers changes with aging (10). These include a decrease in the proportion of chondroitin sulfate, while the amount of keratan sulfate and hyaluronate increases. These changes are related to a decrease in the size and number of chondroitin sulfate chains with a decrease in the length of the chondroitin sulfate-rich region, and a concomitant increase in the size and number of keratan sulfate chains.

Low molecular mass non-aggregating proteoglycans have also been identified in articular cartilage (8). These proteoglycans are biglycan (DS–PG–I) and decorin (DS–PG–II). Their structure consists of a core protein of about 40 kDa to which is attached a single (DS–PG–II) or two (DS–PG–I) dermatan sulphate chains. Although they account for only a very small portion of the total cartilage glycosaminoglycans, they are present in similar molar proportions to the large aggregating proteoglycans.

Chondrocytes are responsible for the synthesis and assembly of the proteoglycan molecule. While individual monomers are synthesized within a single cell and secreted extracellularly, the aggregation with the HA backbone takes place extracellularly (8,9). The monomers are most likely synthesized in a low affinity form for HA and need to transform into a high affinity form before they can interact with HA (8). Current work suggests that the maturation process involves a conformational change in the HA-binding region of the proteoglycan monomer. The role of the link protein in this process remains unknown. A possible mechanism decreasing the rate of conversion in situ is the fall in the matrix pH during cartilage compression created by the increase in proteoglycan concentration. This could have a beneficial function in cartilage homeostasis allowing the monomer to diffuse from the chondrocyte well into the matrix before it can form aggregates.

The distribution, architecture, and organization of the aggregates serve to maintain a high concentration of nondiffusible negative charges within the cartilage. They condition the penetration of solutes through the matrix conferring rigidity and elasticity to the tissue (9). The repelling forces of the negatively charged groups make the proteoglycans spread out and expand until the elastic forces are balanced by the tensile forces of collagen fibers.

Other Materials. There are at least other two proteins (chondronectin and anchorin CII) that appear to be involved in the organization of the matrix structure and to have established links between the chondrocytes and the matrix (1). Chondronectin is a 150 kDa molecule found in articular cartilage. It is presumed to make the type II collagen fibrils adhere to the cartilage surface and possibly help stabilize the chondrocyte phenotype. Anchorin CII (11), a 34 kDa protein found in the pericellular space of cartilage matrix appears to be responsible for the binding of type II collagen to chondrocytes. However, its exact function is still poorly understood.

Lipids are present as less than 1% of the cartilage wet weight. These consist mainly of triglycerides, cholesterol, glycolipids, and phospholipids and are found both intra and extracellularly, particularly at the superficial zone in younger individuals (6). With aging, lipids are more diffusely distributed through the matrix.

Water. Water is the most abundant component of articular cartilage and accounts for about 70% to 80% of the tissue wet weight (6). The matrix water content of cartilage is unevenly distributed through the cartilage. Its highest concentration, 80%, is found near the articular surface. Concentration decreases gradually with increasing depth to reach about 65% in the deep zone (2). Water plays an important role in the material properties of cartilage and also in joint lubrication (12). Most of the water is contained in the extracellular compartment. Inorganic salts, such as sodium, calcium, and potassium chloride, are dissolved in the tissue water. The maintenance and flow of the water in the tissue relies on its interaction with the matrix macromolecules. The diffusion of water through the cartilage helps move the nutrients from the synovial fluid through the tissue, contributing to the nutrition of chondrocytes (2,6).

Chondrocytes and Cartilage Nutrition. The homeostasis of the extracellular matrix depends on the function of chondrocytes. These cells are responsible for the synthesis and maintenance of the matrix. The chondrocytes are surrounded by a dense extracellular matrix forming a functional unit called *chondron* (3). The intracytoplasmic organelles of these mesenchymal cells include an abundant rough endoplasmic reticulum and Golgi apparatus as part of the matrix synthesis pathway (4). In normal conditions, chondrocytes rarely divide, and the cell population tends to decrease with aging.

Adult cartilage is an avascular tissue and its function depends on the diffusion of nutrients through the matrix, in which interstitial water content plays a primordial role (2,6). The electrolytes and nutrients necessary for the chondrocytes to maintain their normal metabolic activity are derived from the synovial fluid. These are transported through the extracellular matrix by diffusion or by convection, which is caused by the interstitial fluid flow occurring during joint loading. The synthetic activity of chondrocytes respond to various factors such as growth factors and cytokines (13). These factors play an important role in the rate of matrix turnover (see below).

MATRIX TURNOVER

In normal articular cartilage, the extracellular matrix components slowly but continually turn over as the aged molecules are replaced by newly synthesized ones. Of the major components, proteoglycans have a faster turnover rate than collagen, as they are more susceptible to enzymatic degradation (2). Normal turnover involves the release of large proteoglycan fragments indicating that the major cleavage site of the protein core takes place close to the G_1 and G_2 domains, separating the HA binding region from the glycosaminoglycan-bearing regions (10).

The degradation of macromolecules appears to be under the control of proteolytic enzymes, which are synthesized by the chondrocytes. Metalloproteases, such as collagenase and stromelysin, are very likely to play an important role in this process (14). The degradation rate is determined by the level of enzyme synthesis and activation in the tissue (6,14–16). In normal cartilage, the synthesis and degradative process must be coordinately regulated in order to maintain the tissue macromolecule content. Several factors are capable of influencing both the synthesis and degradation of matrix macromolecules and may play an important role in keeping the metabolic balances of cartilage (13,14); however, the exact factors involved in the in vivo biologic control of these mechanisms remain largely unknown.

Certain anabolic and catabolic factors known to be capable of influencing the chondrocyte metabolism may be involved in matrix turnover. Cytokines, such as interleukin-1 (IL–1) and tumor necrosis factor-α (TNF–α) stimulate the synthesis of proteolytic enzymes, induce the degradation of collagen and proteoglycans, and simultaneously inhibit the synthesis of proteoglycans (14). These cytokines, which are mainly synthesized by macrophages, are more likely to be involved in conditions where joint inflammation is present. Growth factors, such as tumor growth factor-β (TGF–β) and insulin-like growth factor-1 (IGF–1) usually have an anabolic effect on chondrocyte metabolism. The effect of these factors is particularly interesting as they not only can stimulate proteoglycan synthesis but can also counteract the action of IL–1 on chondrocyte metabolism by inhibiting its catabolic effects on cartilage (13,17).

MARKERS OF CARTILAGE DEGRADATION

Over the last decade, efforts have been made to set up assays that could detect the breakdown of articular cartilage extracellular matrix. In most arthritic conditions, including osteoarthritis (OA), there are increases in the degradation of the extracellular matrix accompanied by increased release of collagen and proteoglycan fragments into synovial fluid. These eventually reach the blood. Several assays have been developed to measure their levels in body fluids and to use these methods as diagnostic assays or to monitor treatment. For example, monoclonal antibodies that can detect epitope present on the keratan sulfate (KS) chains of proteoglycan have been developed (18). Because articular cartilage is one of the main sources of KS in mammals, the measurement of KS levels in serum and synovial fluid can provide useful information about proteoglycan degradation in cartilage. Studies have shown that the rate of proteoglycan turnover does not change during the day or from day to day for one individual. However, the level of KS could vary markedly from one individual to another and may show a tendency to increase with age. The measurement of KS epitope level in serum has provided useful information in assessing tumor grade in patients with chondrosarcomas, as well as in assessing the rate of growth in children. Serum KS levels are higher in patients with polyarticular OA, supporting the suggestion that proteoglycans in OA cartilages are degraded at an accelerated rate.

In addition, recent work has shown that the detection of type II collagen using a monoclonal antibody in biologic fluid could also be used to evaluate cartilage erosion in patients with OA and rheumatoid arthritis (RA), as indicated by the demonstration of type II collagen in synovial phagocytes in these diseases (19). Similarly, an increased level of type II collagen as measured by ELISA assay was also demonstrated in the synovial fluid and serum of patients with OA and RA (20).

Jean-Pierre Pelletier, MD
Johanne Martel-Pelletier, PhD

1. Buckwalter J, Hunziker E, Rosenberg L, et al: Articular cartilage: composition and structure, Injury and Repair of the Musculoskeletal Soft Tissues. Edited by Woo SLY, Buckwater JA, (1987, Savannah, GA), Chicago, American Academy of Orthopaedic Surgeons, 1991, pp 405–425

2. Mow VC, Settan LA, Ratcliffe A, et al: Structure-function relationships of articular cartilage and the effect of joint instability and trauma on cartilage function, Cartilage Changes in Osteoarthritis. Edited by Brandt KD, Indianapolis, University Press, 1990, pp 22–42

3. Stockwell RA: Morphology of cartilage, Methods in Cartilage Research. Edited by Maroudas A, Kuettner K, San Diego, Academic Press, 1990, pp 61–63

4. Sheldon H: Transmission electron microscopy of cartilage, Cartilage Vol 1, Structure Function and Biochemistry. Edited by Hall BK, New York, Academic Press, 1983, pp 87–104

5. Schenk RK, Eggli PS, Hunziker EB: Articular cartilage morphology, Articular Cartilage Biochemistry. Edited by Kuettner KE, Schleyerbach R, Hascall VC, New York, Raven Press, 1986, pp 3–22

6. Mankin HS, Brandt KD: Biochemistry and metabolism of cartilage in osteoarthritis, Osteoarthritis Diagnosis and Management. Edited by Moskowtiz RW, Howell DS, Goldberg VM, et al. Philadelphia, WB Saunders, 1992, pp 109–154

7. Eyre DR, Wu JJ, Woods PE: The cartilage collagens: Structural and metabolic studies. J Rheumatol (suppl 27) 18:49–51, 1991

8. Hardingham T, Dudhia J, Fosang AJ: Domain structure and sequence homologies in cartilage proteoglycan, Methods in Cartilage Research. Edited by Maroudas A, Kuettner K, San Diego, Academic Press, 1990, pp 187–190

9. Rosenberg L: Structure and function of proteoglycans, Arthritis and Allied Conditions. Edited by McCarty DJ, Philadelphia, Lea & Febiger, 1989, pp 240–255

10. Hardingham T, Bayliss M: Proteoglycans of articular cartilage: Changes in aging and in joint disease. Semin Arthritis Rheum (suppl 1) 20:12–33, 1990

11. von der Mark K, Mollenhauer J, Pfäffle M, et al: Role of anchorin CII in the interaction of chondrocytes with extracellular collagen, Articular Cartilage Biochemistry. Edited by Kuettner KE, Schleyerbach R, Hascall VC, New York, Raven Press, 1986, pp 125–141

12. Mow V, Rosenwasser M: Articular cartilage: Biomechanics, Injury and Repair of the Musculoskeletal Soft Tissues. Edited by Woo SLY, Buckwater JA, (1987; Savannah, GA), Chicago, American Academy of Orthopaedic Surgeons, 1991, pp 427–463

13. Howell DS, Treadwell BV, Trippel SB: Etiopathogenesis of osteoarthritis, Osteoarthritis Diagnosis and Medical/Surgical Management, 2nd ed. Edited by Saunders WB, Howell DS, Goldberg VM, et al, Philadelphia, WB Saunders Company, 1992, pp 233–252

14. Pelletier JP, Roughley P, DiBattista JA, et al: Are cytokines involved in osteoarthritis pathophysiology? Semin Arthritis Rheum (suppl 2) 20:12–25, 1991

15. Dean DD: Proteinase-mediated cartilage degradation in osteoarthritis. Semin Arthritis Rheum 20 (suppl 2) 2–11, 1991

16. Zafarullah M, Martel-Pelletier J, Cloutier JM, Gedamu L, Pelletier JP: Expression of c-fos, c-jun, jun–B, metallothionein and metalloproteinase genes in human chondrocyte. FEBS Lett 306:169–172, 1992

17. Fosang AJ, Tyler TA, Hardingham TE: Effect of interleukin-1 and insulin-like growth factor-1 on the release of proteoglycan components and hyaluronan from pig articular cartilage in explant culture. Matrix 11:17–24, 1991

18. Thonar EJMA, Glant T: Serum keratan sulfate—A marker of predisposition to polyarticular osteoarthritis. Clin Biochem 25:175–180, 1992

19. Moreland LW, Stewart T, Gay RE, et al: Immunohistologic demonstration of type II collagen in synovial fluid, phagocytes of osteoarthritis and rheumatoid arthritis patients. Arthritis Rheum 32:1458–1464, 1989

20. Stewart TE, Mestecky J, Moreland LW, et al: Immunoassay for collagen type II (CII) in synovial fluid and serum of patients with erosive joint diseases. Arthritis Rheum (suppl) 32:R43, 1989 (Abstract)

C. Bone

Bone is a novel type of mineralized connective tissue. It is comprised of two distinct subtypes, *cortical* (or compact) bone and *cancellous* (or trabecular) bone. Cortical bone comprises about 80% of the skeleton and is enriched in the long bone shafts. Cancellous bone is the flat platelike bone in sheets that crisscross the bone marrow cavity. Cancellous bone is in intimate contact with the cells of the marrow cavity. It is relatively enriched in the vertebral bodies, the pelvis, and the proximal ends of the femora, all of which are subject to fracture following trivial injury in the elderly. Both cortical and cancellous bone are remodeled by specific types of cells. The mineral within bone comprises 99% of the body's calcium, 80% of the phosphate and large amounts of sodium, magnesium, and carbonate.

BONE REMODELING

Bone is continuously renewed by the process of bone remodeling. Remodeling is comprised of cycles of bone resorption and bone formation, which lead to renewal of replaced bone. Remodeling occurs in discrete packets throughout the skeleton known as bone remodeling units. In young adult life, there is balance between the processes of bone resorption and bone formation, so that total bone mass remains constant. With advancing age, there is a relative increase in bone resorption compared with bone formation, and bone is progressively lost. Thus, bone mass declines progressively with advancing age (Fig. 2C–1).

NATURAL HISTORY OF THE SKELETON

During growth and adolescence, bone formation is greater than bone resorption. Consequently, bone mass increases until the age of about 20. Bone mass remains constant between the ages of 20 and 35, because there is balance between the processes of resorption and formation. After the middle of the fourth decade, there is a relative increase in resorption compared with formation so that bone mass progressively decreases thereafter. In women

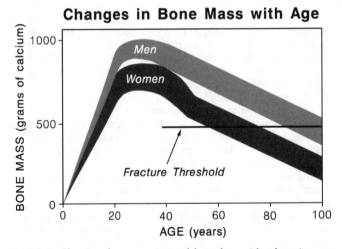

Changes in Bone Mass with Age

Fig. 2C–1. Changes that occur in total bone loss with advancing age. During growth, total bone mass progressively increases in both men and women and reaches a zenith in early adult life. After mid-adult life, there is a progressive decline in total bone mass in both men and women. In women there is a marked acceleration of bone loss occurring at the time of the menopause and lasting for about ten years. The fracture threshold is a theoretical concept. It occurs when total bone loss declines to a level where fractures can occur after trivial injury.

there is a rapid phase of bone loss in the postmenopausal period due to estrogen withdrawal. This is characterized by a marked increase in osteoclastic bone resorption. In both sexes, there is decreased bone formation in later life with an impairment of bone formation relative to bone resorption. In some patients, this decline in skeletal mass concurrent with advancing age means that the skeleton is no longer able to provide adequate structural support for the body, and fractures occur following trivial injury. This is the condition known as osteoporosis. Those bones most

Normal Bone Remodelling

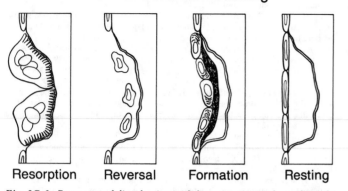

Resorption   Reversal   Formation   Resting

Fig. 2C–2. Bone remodeling begins with bone resorption by multinucleated osteoclasts. This is followed by a reversal phase, where resorption ceases and multinucleated osteoclasts are replaced by mononuclear cells. The mononuclear cells are replaced by bone forming osteoblasts, which lay down new bone at the sites of previous resorption. This bone is then mineralized. At the end of the remodeling sequence, the bone which has been removed by the action of osteoclasts is completely replaced by osteoblasts, and the resorption defect is replaced by new bone.

likely to fracture are enriched in cancellous bone and include the vertebral bodies and the proximal ends of the femora (1).

CELLULAR EVENTS INVOLVED IN BONE REMODELING

The cellular sequence of events involved in bone remodeling is always the same, whether cortical bone or cancellous bone is being considered (2). These cellular events are shown diagrammatically in Fig. 2C–2. The cellular remodeling sequence occurs in the Haversian canals of cortical bone, and on the endosteal surfaces of cancellous bone. The initial event is an increase in osteoclastic bone resorption. The signal responsible for this initial activation of osteoclasts is still unknown. Osteoclasts form from their mononuclear precursors on bone surfaces, become multinucleated by fusion, and are then polarized to form a special area of the cell membrane adjacent to the bone surface called the ruffled border. Next, they resorb bone by secreting hydrogen ions and lysosomal enzymes across this ruffled border. At cessation of resorption, osteoclasts break up into mononuclear cells and leave the resorption lacunae. Teams of osteoblast precursors are then attracted to the resorption site, proliferate, and differentiate into mature osteoblasts. Subsequently, these mature osteoblasts make new bone by synthesizing and secreting the structural proteins of bone including type I collagen, and are responsible for mineralizing this bone matrix.

On a normal human adult endosteal bone surface, the osteoclastic resorption phase takes 7 to 10 days, and the new bone formation phase takes approximately 3 months. Since the cellular events involved in resorption and formation are very complex, and lead to relative balance between these two processes, these must be under exquisite regulatory control. It appears most likely that factors produced locally are responsible for controlling the cellular events involved in bone remodeling. Cytokines generated by bone cells or mononuclear cells in the marrow cavity have powerful effects on osteoclast formation and activation. Growth factors within the bone matrix released as a consequence of the resorption process have powerful effects on osteoblast bone formation. The systemic hormones, parathyroid hormone and 1,25 dihydroxyvitamin D also influence both resorption and formation, but their major function is to control calcium homeostasis rather than bone remodeling (3). Bone remodeling is regulated by mechanical loading (4). Immobilization or loss of weight bearing leads to rapid bone loss, due to both increased resorption and decreased formation.

CELLS IN BONE

There are three distinct cell types in bone—osteoclasts, osteoblasts, and osteocytes. These will now be considered in turn.

Osteoclasts

The osteoclast is a unique multinucleated cell that contains 10–20 nuclei and may reach a size of 100 μm in diameter (2). It is the only cell in the body that can form bone resorption lacunae. Osteoclasts are found in Haversian systems and on the endosteal surfaces of cancellous bone. They are found only on bone surfaces. Osteoclasts are derived from hematopoietic precursors in the marrow, and osteoclast precursors have the capacity to circulate in the peripheral blood. The precursors of the osteoclast have the capacity to form other cells such as monocytes, but under the direction of specific growth regulatory factors, these pluripotent precursors differentiate along the osteoclast lineage to form the mature multinucleated osteoclast. The mature multinucleated cell is a polarized cell with a specialized area of the cell membrane adjacent to the bone surface known as the ruffled border.

Osteoclasts contain lysosomal enzymes and tartrate-resistant acid phosphatase, which is often used as a histochemical marker for this cell. They also contain a vacuolar ATPase that acts as a proton pump to acidify the area under the ruffled border, where bone is demineralized and degraded. The bone is probably demineralized by the highly acidic micro-environment under the ruffled border. Calcium released from the mineral may act to inhibit continued osteoclast activity and is available to enter the extracellular fluid. Osteoclasts attach firmly to bone surfaces by interactions between osteoclast proteins known as integrins, which traverse the cell membrane, and the proteins of the bone matrix. Tyrosine kinase enzymes have recently been found important both in osteoclast formation and osteoclastic resorption of bone. These tyrosine kinases include the receptor for the cytokine colony stimulating factor–1 (CSF–1), which is required for normal osteoclast formation, and the proto-oncogene src, which encodes a tyrosine kinase required for osteoclasts to form ruffled borders.

Osteoclasts require help from accessory cells to resorb bone (5–7). These accessory cells may be the bone lining cells (also called surface osteocytes) or mononuclear cells in the marrow cavity. The bone lining cells arise from the stromal cell system. Osteoclastic bone resorption is under the control of local cytokines such as interleukin–1 (IL–1), tumor necrosis factor (TNF), and interleukin–6 (IL–6), and systemic hormones such as parathyroid hormone and 1,25 dihydroxyvitamin D. The bone resorption that occurs in disease states such as osteoporosis, malignant diseases of bone, and Paget's disease is associated with an increase in osteoclast activity. Drugs used in the treatment of these disorders are inhibitors of osteoclast activity. These drugs include calcitonin, bisphosphonates, gallium nitrate, estrogen, and plicamycin.

Osteoblasts

Osteoblasts represent a heterogeneous family of cells that are derived from the stromal cell system (8). This family includes mature osteoblasts, which synthesize the proteins of the bone matrix, or osteocytes, which are buried within bone and communicate with each other via the canalicular system, and the bone lining cells (see above), which cover bone surfaces. Cells in the osteoblast lineage have a common precursor, which they share with adipocytes, reticular cells, fibroblasts, and chondroblasts. The factors involved in differentiation of cells along the osteoblast lineage have not yet been characterized.

Mature Osteoblasts. Mature osteoblasts are cuboidal cells that have a single eccentric nucleus and a well developed endoplasmic reticulum and Golgi apparatus. They have the capacity to synthesize the proteins of the bone matrix such as type I collagen and the bone Gla protein (osteocalcin). They also contain a membrane-bound ectoenzyme alkaline phosphatase, which probably plays an essential role in bone mineralization and which is used as a marker for the osteoblast phenotype.

Osteoblasts are responsible for the production of the proteins of the bone matrix including type I collagen and osteocalcin. They also are responsible for the production of growth factors that are stored in the bone matrix, such as transforming growth factor β (TGF-β), bone morphogenetic proteins, platelet-derived growth factor (PDGF), and the insulin-like growth factors (IGF) (9). Osteoblasts are capable of mineralizing newly formed bone matrix. This may be mediated by subcellular particles generated from osteoblast cytoplasm known as matrix vesicles. Matrix vesicles are enriched in alkaline phosphatase. Osteoblasts also produce other bone matrix constituents that may be important in the mineralization process such as phospholipids and proteoglycans. Osteoblasts may be required for normal bone resorption to occur. Experimental data suggest that osteoblasts or their progeny (bone lining cells) may act as accessory cells for osteoclastic resorption. These interactions may occur either by cell–cell contact with osteoclast precursors, by the production of soluble mediators, which are required for osteoclasts to resorb bone, or by preparing the bone surface for osteoclastic resorption by the production of proteolytic enzymes.

Osteocytes. Osteocytes are buried within the mineralized matrix of bone. They probably represent osteoblasts that have successfully synthesized bone matrix and then become buried within the matrix. Osteocytes communicate with each other and with cells on the bone surface via a canalicular system. Their normal function is unknown. One function that has long been ascribed to them is the capacity to resorb bone by enlarging osteocyte lacunae. More recent evidence suggests that this "osteocytic osteolysis" may represent fixation artefact (10). Osteocytes have been shown to produce TGF-β and possibly other growth factors. Whether this observation has physiologic significance requires further study. Bone lining cells, which are probably osteocytes present on the bone surface, have been implicated as accessory cells in the bone resorption process (see above).

There is a specific bone fluid that circulates through the canalicular system and bathes the bone surface. It is separated from the extracellular fluid by a bone "membrane" that is probably comprised of bone lining cells. These lining cells function to keep calcium in the extracellular fluid, where it is supersaturated with respect to bone (11). Their overall function may be to buffer changes in extracellular fluid calcium concentrations. It is unknown whether this process of exclusion of calcium from the bone fluid by the bone lining cells is regulated.

CONTROL OF BONE FORMATION

Bone formation is controlled by a series of systemic hormones and growth factors in the bone matrix. The major systemic hormone that controls bone formation is 1,25 dihydroxyvitamin D, which is responsible for mineralization of newly formed bone. In the absence of 1,25 dihydroxyvitamin D, bone mineralization is impaired and as a consequence there is accumulation of unmineralized matrix (also called osteoid tissue). This condition is known as rickets in children or osteomalacia in adults.

The formation of bone is also regulated by a series of growth factors, which have been recently identified in the bone matrix. These include TGF-β, the bone morphogenetic proteins, IGFs I and II, PDGF, and the heparin-binding fibroblast growth factors (9). TGF-β and IGF-1 are powerful stimulators of bone collagen synthesis and the formation of new bone. The bone morphogenetic proteins have major effects on repairing bone defects and causing ectopic bone formation in experimental systems. Their role in normal bone formation has still to be defined. All of these factors stored in bone are likely released during the process of osteoclastic resorption and thereby made available to influence subsequent events involved in bone remodeling (Fig. 2C–3).

CONTROL OF BONE RESORPTION

Bone is resorbed by the activity of osteoclasts. Osteoclasts produce protons that release the mineral from bone and lysosomal enzymes that degrade the bone matrix (12). Release of bone mineral occurs as a consequence of proton production by the osteoclasts. In turn, this is due to generation of intracellular hydrogen ions by osteoclastic carbonic anhydrase type II isoenzyme, and these hydrogen ions are then pumped across the ruffled border of the osteoclast by the action of a vacuolar ATPase. Once the bone is demineralized, it can be degraded by

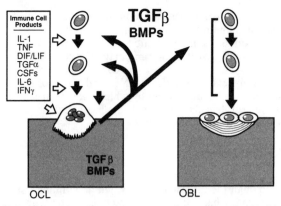

Fig. 2C–3. *Diagrammatic representation of the events involved in bone remodeling, with osteoclastic bone resorption shown at left and osteoblastic bone formation shown at right. Cytokines such as IL-1 modulate the process of osteoclastic bone resorption. (OCL = osteoclasts, OBL = osteoblasts, TGFβ = transforming growth factor β, BMPs = bone morphogenetic protein).*

the activity of proteolytic enzymes produced by the lysosomes of the osteoclasts, which are then transported to the ruffled border by the mannose-6 phosphate receptor pathway. These lysosomal enzymes include β-glucuronidase, β-galactosidase, and cathepsin D (12).

Bone resorption is controlled by a number of systemic hormones and local factors or cytokines (13). The systemic hormones that control bone resorption are parathyroid hormone, calcitonin, and 1,25 dihydroxyvitamin D. Parathyroid hormone stimulates osteoclastic bone resorption by increasing the formation of osteoclasts and then activating the mature multinucleated cell. It probably works directly on osteoclast precursors and indirectly on the mature cell via bone lining cells or osteoblasts (15). 1,25 dihydroxyvitamin D is a differentiation agent for osteoclasts. It causes fusion of committed precursors to form mature multinucleated cells and then activates the mature multinucleated cells indirectly through the accessory cells required for osteoclastic bone resorption. 1,25 dihydroxyvitamin D receptors have not been found as yet in mature osteoclasts (2,14).

Calcitonin is a peptide hormone that transiently inhibits osteoclastic bone resorption. It inhibits the formation of the osteoclast, causes contraction of the mature osteoclast cell membrane so that the resorbing cell withdraws from bone and discontinues resorption, and also causes fission of the multinucleated cell into mononuclear cells. These effects are mediated through the second messenger, cyclic AMP. However, the effects of calcitonin on the osteoclast are transient, and in its continued presence, there is down-regulation of calcitonin receptors and "escape" from the inhibitory effects of calcitonin on bone resorption.

CYTOKINES AND BONE RESORPTION

A number of local factors generated in the microenvironment of bone resorbing surfaces capable of stimulating osteoclast activity have recently been described (13). These include IL–1, TNF, and lymphotoxin, the thyroid hormones and systemic sex hormones. Interleukin–1 is a powerful multifunctional cytokine produced by monocytes as well as by bone cells in response to inflammatory stimuli. It stimulates bone resorption by increasing the formation of new osteoclasts and activating mature osteoclasts to resorb bone. When administered systemically, it rapidly causes hypercalcemia because of its effects on osteoclast activity. It may be involved in a number of disease states, such as rheumatoid arthritis and periodontal disease, in which localized bone loss occurs. It has also been linked to the bone destruction associated with some cancers.

Tumor necrosis factor and lymphotoxin are also multifunctional cytokines produced by monocytes, other types of immune cells, and bone lining cells. These cytokines have similar effects to IL–1 on osteoclastic bone resorption. They have been implicated in the bone destruction that occurs in disease states such as myeloma and in the localized bone destruction that occurs in chronic inflammatory diseases.

Interleukin–6 is a multifunctional cytokine that functions as a powerful B-cell growth factor and may be involved in the pathogenesis of myeloma. It increases osteoclastic bone resorption and acts synergistically with IL–1, TNF, and lymphotoxin. It may explain in part the mechanism by which bone destruction occurs in myeloma. It has also recently been implicated in the bone loss associated with estrogen withdrawal (16).

SEX HORMONES

Estrogens are important inhibitors of osteoclastic bone resorption, although the mechanism by which they inhibit osteoclastic bone resorption has not been characterized. Estrogen withdrawal at the time of the menopause is associated with a rapid phase of osteoclastic bone resorption, and this osteoclastic bone resorption can be inhibited by estrogen therapy. Researchers are working actively on the mechanisms by which estrogens regulate osteoclastic bone resorption (17,18). Whether they have direct effects on osteoclasts, or whether their effects are indirect and mediated through other factors such as the cytokines generated by osteoblastic cells or monocytes is still being debated.

Gregory R. Mundy, MD

1. Mundy GR: Osteopenia. Disease A Month 33:537–600, 1987
2. Mundy GR, Roodman GD: Osteoclast ontogeny and function, Bone and Mineral Research, Vol 5. Edited by Peck WA. New York, Elsevier Science Publishers, 1987, pp 209–280
3. Mundy GR: Calcium Homeostasis: Hypercalcemia and Hypocalcemia, 2nd Ed. London, Martin Dunitz, 1990
4. Rubin CT, Lanyon LE: Regulation of bone mass by mechanical strain magnitude. Calcif Tiss Int 37:411–417, 1985
5. Rodan GA, Martin TJ: Role of osteoblasts in hormonal control of bone resorption—a hypothesis. Calcif Tiss Int 33:349–351, 1981
6. Chambers TJ. The pathobiology of the osteoclast. J Clin Pathol 38:241–252, 1985
7. Jones SJ, Boyde A: Scanning electron microscopy of bone cells in culture, Endocrinology of Calcium Metabolism. Edited by Copp DH, Talmadge RV. Amsterdam, Excerpta Medica, 1978, pp 97–114
8. Owen M: Lineage of osteogenic cells and their relationship to the stromal system, Bone and Mineral Research, Vol 3. Edited by Peck WA. New York, Elsevier Science Publishers, 1985, pp 1–26
9. Hauschka PV, Mavrakos AE, Iafrati MD, et al: Growth factors in bone matrix, isolation of multiple types by affinity chromatography on heparin-sepharose. J Biol Chem 261:12665–12674, 1986
10. Boyde A: Electron microscopy of the mineralizing front, Bone Histomorphometry, Third International Workshop. Edited by Jee WS, Parfitt AM. Paris, Societe Nouvelle de Publications Medicales et Dentaires, 1980, pp 69–78
11. Parfitt AM: Bone plasma calcium homeostasis. Bone 8(Suppl):S1–S8, 1987
12. Vaes G: On the mechanism of bone resorption: The action of parathyroid hormone on the excretion and synthesis on the lysosomal enzymes and on the extracellular release of acid by bone cells. J Cell Biol 39:676–697, 1968
13. Mundy GR. Cytokines of bone, Physiology and Pharmacology of Bone. Handbook of Experimental Pharmacology. Edited by Mundy GR, Martin TJ. Berlin, Springer, In press
14. Bell NH: Vitamin D—Endocrine System. J Clin Invest 76:1–6, 1985
15. McSheehy PM, Chambers TJ: Osteoblastic cells mediate osteoclastic responsiveness to parathyroid hormone. Endocrinology 118:824–828, 1986
16. Jilka RL, Hangoc G, Girasole G, et al: Increased osteoclast development after estrogen loss: Mediation by interleukin–6. Science 257:88–91, 1992
17. Komm BS, Terpening CM, Benz DJ, et al: Estrogen binding, receptor mRNA, and biologic response in osteoblast-like osteosarcoma cells. Science 241:81–84, 1988
18. Oursler MJ, Osdoby P, Pyfferoen J, et al: Avian osteoclasts as estrogen target cells. Proc Natl Acad Sci 88:6613–6617, 1991

D. Skeletal Muscle

MORPHOLOGY

Skeletal muscles are organs that contract for the purpose of generating force and movement in specific directions. Most skeletal muscles are connected at each end to bone by tendons. Skeletal muscle is composed of cells termed *fibers* that are structured in a highly ordered fashion (1). Fibers are anatomically grouped in fascicles so that different fibers within a fascicle are innervated by different motor neurons. The parallel arrangements of fascicles between the tendinous ends of muscles allow for the force of contraction to be additive. Functionally, muscle fibers are grouped in motor units that consist of a lower motor neuron originating in a spinal cord anterior horn cell and the muscle fibers it innervates. All muscle fibers within a motor unit are of the same type. Individual human muscles are heterogeneous with regard to fiber type.

Muscle fibers vary with respect to their metabolism and response to stimuli and may be typed accordingly. A variety of fiber-type classifications have emerged based on different biochemical and physiologic properties (2,3). For most purposes, fibers are divided among three types. Type 1 fibers, also called slow twitch oxidative (SO) fibers, respond to electrical stimulation more slowly with a moderate contractile intensity and are fatigue-resistant with repeated stimulation. Type 1 cells have greater numbers of mitochondria and higher lipid content. In contrast, type 2b fibers, known as fast twitch glycolytic (FG) fibers, respond more rapidly with greater force of contraction but fatigue rapidly. These fibers have higher activities of myophosphorylase and myoadenylate deaminase and more glycogen. Type 2a fibers, termed fast twitch oxidative glycolytic (FOG), have properties that are intermediate between those of type 1 and 2b. A type 2c fiber is included in some classification schemes and is believed to represent an undifferentiated cell. The characteristics of each fiber type are originally determined during development and are maintained through interaction with the motor neuron through which it is innervated. Fiber type specificity and

distribution can be altered by reinnervation with a different type of motor neuron, physical training, or disease processes (4,5).

Each muscle fiber is an elongated multinucleated cell surrounded by a plasma membrane, termed the *sarcolemma*. Fibers contain contractile proteins (actin, troponin, tropomyosin and myosin) termed myofilaments (Fig. 2D–1). The myofilaments are bathed in cytosol, termed *sarcoplasm*, and organized within fibrils, which are enveloped by the sarcoplasmic reticulum. Communication between the sarcolemma and sarcoplasmic reticulum is provided through a network of pores and channels called the *T-tubule system*.

CONTRACTION AND RELAXATION

Muscle contraction requires shortening of myofilaments located within muscle fibers. Contraction can result from electrical, chemical, or physical stimulation that initiates the orderly transmission of an action potential along the sarcolemma, then through the T-tubule system to the sarcoplasmic reticulum. As a result, calcium is released into the sarcoplasm. As sarcoplasmic calcium concentrations increase, actin is released from an inhibited state allowing actin myosin cross-linkage and shortening of the myofilaments. Shortening continues until calcium is actively pumped back into the sarcoplasmic reticulum, breaking the cross-linkages and allowing relaxation.

Both contraction and relaxation are active processes and require normal levels of electrolytes and adenosine triphosphate (ATP). Sodium, potassium, calcium, and magnesium are critical to the function of three ATPase proteins that must work effectively for normal fiber contraction and relaxation. Sodium–potassium ATPase activity maintains normal polarity of the sarcolemma. The ATPase that controls actin myosin cross-linking is magnesium-dependent. A calcium-dependent ATPase pumps calcium from the sarcoplasm into the sarcoplasmic reticulum permitting relaxation. Phosphorus levels are also critical, because

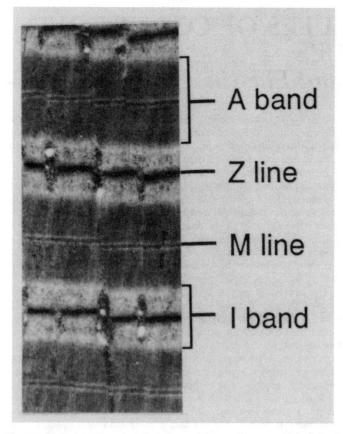

Fig. 2D–1. *The varying refractile indices of the myofilaments give skeletal muscle its characteristic ultrastructural cross-striated appearance. The functional contractile unit of the fiber is the sarcomere, defined as the area between two Z lines. Z lines transect the fibrils and connect the actin filaments. The A band is composed of the thick myofilaments (myosin) and the M line is due to the bulges in the middle of the myosin filaments. In cross-section, each myosin filament is surrounded by 6 actin filaments in a hexagonal pattern. At rest, the I band is the area occupied by the thin filaments (actin, troponin, and tropomyosin) not overlapped by myosin. With contraction, cross-bridges form between actin and myosin, Z lines move toward the M line, and I bands become smaller.*

phosphorus is the ion that forms the high energy bonds of ATP, the substrate for the three enzymes.

ENERGY METABOLISM

Energy required for the contraction and relaxation of muscle is derived from the hydrolysis of ATP. Skeletal muscle uses fatty acids and carbohydrates to produce ATP (6,7), with several pathways used to produce energy from each source. The importance of a particular pathway varies with the level of exertion and nutritional status of the individual. Working in concert, these pathways maintain intracellular ATP concentrations at constant levels under most conditions and restore them to normal levels if vigorous activity or hypoxia cause ATP concentrations to fall.

Free fatty acids provide the major source of ATP during fasting intervals, at rest, and for muscle activities of low intensity and long duration. They must enter mitochondria to be processed for energy (8). To enter mitochondria, long-chain fatty acids combine with the carrier molecule carnitine (9) and transfer across the mitochondrial membrane by a process that is catalyzed by two enzymes found on the inner membrane, carnitine palmitoyltransferase (CPT) I and CPT II (10). Once in the mitochondria, fatty acid and carnitine separate. Two carbon fragments of acetylCoA are split off the fatty acid by the process of β-oxidation. These are metabolized sequentially by the tricarboxylic acid cycle and the oxidative phosphorylation. By this metabolic route, one molecule of palmitate results in the net gain of 131 molecules of ATP.

Glycogen, the major storage form of carbohydrate, can be metabolized aerobically or anaerobically but provides the primary source of ATP when physical activity is intense or when anaerobic conditions exist. Under such conditions, glycogen is mobilized to form glucose–6–phosphate by the process of glycogenolysis, a process initiated by the activity of myophosphorylase (11). Glucose–6–phosphate is metabolized through the glycolytic pathway to lactate. Under aerobic conditions, this pathway produces pyruvate, which can enter the tricarboxylic acid cycle. The aerobic metabolism of one molecule of glucose nets 38 molecules of ATP, whereas the anaerobic processing results in the generation of only two molecules of ATP.

At rest, oxidative metabolism produces excess amounts of ATP, but intracellular levels of ATP remain constant. Creatine phosphokinase (CK) activity plays a pivotal role in maintaining constant intracellular ATP concentrations, functioning to buffer changes in cytosolic levels. Creatine phosphokinase catalyzes the reversible transphosphorylation of creatine and adenine nucleotides. At rest, the terminal phosphate of ATP is transferred to creatine forming creatine phosphate and ADP. The creatine phosphate acts as a reservoir of high energy phosphates. With muscle activity and ATP hydrolysis, CK catalyzes the transfer of those phosphates to adenosine disphosphate, rapidly restoring ATP levels to normal. The enzyme—along with its products, creatine and creatine phosphate—also serves as a shuttle mechanism for energy transport between mitochondria, where ATP is generated by oxidative metabolism, and the myofibrils, where ATP is consumed in the active processes of muscle contraction and relaxation (12).

The CK buffering system maintains ATP concentrations at usual levels during exercise until creatine phosphate concentrations are depleted by 50%. If activity continues, ATP concentrations fall and the purine nucleotide cycle begins to play a pivotal role. This tends to occur when glycolysis becomes the major route for ATP generation (13). The first step of the purine nucleotide cycle is conversion of adenosine monophosphate (AMP) to inosine monophosphate (IMP) by myoadenylate deaminase with the generation of ammonia. Both IMP and ammonia stimulate glycolytic activity. As ATP concentrations fall, IMP concentrations rise stoichiometrically. This process continues until muscle activity decreases and recovery can occur. During recovery, oxidative pathways resume a major functional role and AMP is regenerated from IMP by a two step process with the liberation of fumarate (14). Fumarate is converted to malate, which enters mitochondria and participates as an intermediate in the tricarboxylic acid cycle. The higher concentrations of malate thus act to "drive" the cycle causing efficient regeneration of ATP by oxidative phosphorylation.

Robert L. Wortmann, MD

1. Craig R: The structure of the contractile filaments, Myology, 1st ed. Edited by Engel AG, Banker BQ. New York, McGraw-Hill Book Company, 1986, pp 73–124
2. Tunell GL, Hart MN: Simultaneous determination of skeletal muscle fiber types I, IIA, and IIB by histochemistry. Arch Neurol 34:171–176, 1977
3. Pette D, Staron RS: Molecular basis of the phenotypic characteristics of mammalian muscle fibers. Ciba Found Symp 138:22–32, 1988
4. Haggmark T, Eriksson F, Jansson E: Muscle fiber type changes in human skeletal muscle after injuries and immobilization. Orthopedics 9:181–185, 1986
5. Edstrom L, Grimby L: Effect of exercise on the motor unit. Muscle & Nerve 9:104–126, 1986
6. Hochachka PW: Fuels and pathways as designed systems for support of muscle work. J Exp Biol 115:149–164, 1985
7. Layzer RB: How muscles use fuel. N Engl J Med 324:411–412, 1991
8. Lee CP, Schatz G, Dallner G (eds): Mitochondria and Microsomes. Reading, MA: Addison-Wesley, 1981
9. Robouche CJ, Paulson DJ: Carnitine metabolism and function in humans. Ann Rev Nutr 6:41–66, 1986
10. Zierz S, Engel AG: Regulatory properties of a carnitine palmitoyltransferase in human skeletal muscle. Eur J Biochem 149:207–214, 1986
11. Brown DH: Glycogen metabolism and glycolysis in muscle, Myology, 1st ed. Edited by Engel GA, Banker BQ. New York, McGraw-Hill Book Company, 1986, pp 673–698
12. Erikson-Viitanen S, Geiger P, Yang WCT, et al: The creatine-creatine phosphate shuttle for energy transport-compartmentation of creatine phosphokinase in muscle. Adv Exp Med Biol 151:115–125, 1982
13. Wy T-FL, Davis EJ: Regulation of glycolytic flux in an energetically controlled cell-free system: The effects of adenine nucleotide ratios, inorganic phosphate, pH, and citrate. Arch Biochem Biophys 209:85–99, 1981
14. Aragon JJ, Lowenstein JM: The purine nucleotide cycle: Comparison of the levels of citric acid intermediators with the operation of the purine nucleotide cycle in rat skeletal muscle during exercise and recovery from exercise. Eur J Biochem 110:371–377, 1980

3. STRUCTURAL MOLECULES OF CONNECTIVE TISSUES
A. Collagen and Elastin

COLLAGENS

The collagens comprise a family of specialized molecules with common structural features that provide an extracellular framework for all multicellular animals. The collagens are the most abundant body proteins, accounting for more than 20% of total body mass. At least 14 different collagens (types I to XIV) have been identified thus far, and it is likely that more will be discovered in the future (1–3). These different molecules represent homopolymers or heteropolymers of specific polypeptide products of at least 20 different collagen genes (4,5).

There is a high degree of specialization in the functions of the various collagens that requires maintenance of a delicate balance in the temporal and spatial expression of each collagen type synthesized in a given connective tissue. In addition, their precise supramolecular organization is essential for the adequate function of the tissues of which they are the principal structural components. By subtle control of the polypeptide structures synthesized and the numerous post-translational modifications that occur in the newly synthesized chains (see below), connective tissue cells can produce diverse support structures that arrange in structural arrays like ropes (tendons), woven sheets (skin), transparent lenses (the cornea), a scaffold for mineralization (bone), compressible shock absorbers (weight-bearing cartilage), and porous filtering structures (basement membranes).

In addition to structural functions, collagens have been implicated in morphogenesis and in the various complex regulatory processes that occur during growth, development, aging, and wound healing. Alterations in the structure and metabolism of collagen are widely believed to be involved, either directly or indirectly, in the pathogenesis of many disorders (6).

Common Structural Features

The definitive structural feature of all collagen molecules is the *triple helix* (7). This unique protein conformation is the result of the winding of three constituent polypeptide chains of the collagen molecule (known as α-chains) around each other at two levels of organization. Each chain is coiled into a left-handed helix with about three amino acid residues per turn. The three chains are then twisted around each other into a right-handed super helix to form a rigid structure similar to a thin segment of rope.

This unique three-dimensional conformation is made possible by a unique amino acid sequence in the polypeptide chains. With the exception of sequences of variable length at the ends of the chains and occasionally interspersed within the triple helix, every third amino acid residue in each collagen chain is glycine. Since the side-chain of this amino acid is a hydrogen atom, glycine is the only residue small enough to occupy the restricted space in which the helical α-chains cluster together in the center of the triple helix. Approximately 25% of the residues in the triple helical domains consist of proline and hydroxyproline, amino acids with ring structures that impose restrictions on the α-chain conformation and, thereby, strengthen the triple helix and stiffen the collagen molecule. In the most abundant interstitial collagens, the triple helical region is approximately 100 nm long and contains about 1,000 amino acid residues.

The helical region of the collagen α-chain of fibrous collagens can be represented by the molecular formula $(X-Y-Gly)_{333}$, where X and Y are residues other than glycine. In mammals, about 100 of the X positions are occupied by prolyl residues and about 100 of the Y positions by hydroxyprolyl residues. Hydroxyproline is produced during the collagen biosynthetic process by enzymatic hydroxylation of specific prolyl residues. This complex enzymatic reaction takes place because hydroxyproline can-

not be incorporated directly into the nascent collagen polypeptide chain due to the absence of hydroxyproline transfer RNA. The hydroxylation of peptide-bound prolyl residues involves a specific enzyme, prolyl hydroxylase, which requires O_2, Fe^{++}, α-ketoglutarate and ascorbic acid as cofactors. The presence of hydroxyproline residues in the collagen molecule is essential to the maintenance of the collagen conformation, because the hydroxyproline content determines the thermal stability of the collagen triple helix (8). A decrease in the hydroxyproline content of collagen, as occurs in scurvy, results in unstable molecules that loosen their triple helical conformation at normal body temperatures and, therefore, become susceptible to proteolytic degradation by nonspecific proteases.

The precise sequence of amino acid residues that fill the remaining X and Y positions differs among the various collagen types. This may partially account for the tissue-specific properties of the collagens of cartilage, skin and basement membranes. One characteristic residue that occupies these positions is hydroxylysine. Hydroxylysine is also produced by a post-translational enzymatic hydroxylation of some lysyl residues in the collagen molecules. The responsible enzyme is distinct from prolyl hydroxylase, although it exhibits the same cofactor requirements. Hydroxylysine is involved in many of the subsequent processes of fiber formation and stabilization as a precursor of cross-linking compounds and as a site for attachment of carbohydrate residues. In the latter instance, the hydroxyl group is involved in an O-glycoside linkage to a galactose or to glucosylgalactose.

In most collagens, both ends of the helical region are terminal sequences (telopeptides) that do not have glycine as every third residue and therefore lack the triple helical conformation. These regions represent the persistent peptide sequences remaining from the proteolytic cleavage of collagen precursors or procollagens after they have been processed by specific procollagen-peptidases. The regions have different lengths in the chains of the various collagen types and appear to be important in the formation of supramolecular aggregates as well as in their stabilization. In certain collagens, one or more non-triple helical segments are intercalated within the triple helix, imparting flexibility to the rigid domain. Variations of the common triple helical theme in terms of primary structure and post-translational modifications enable the collagens to participate in a vast array of structural complexes (3,9).

Collagen Polymorphism

Each collagen type has a unique amino acid sequence and has been firmly identified as a distinct gene product (1–3). The different collagen types can be classified according to their ability to aggregate into highly structured fibrils and to the presence of intercalated non-triple helical domains within their triple helical regions (Table 3A–1). The fibrillar interstitial collagens, forming the extracellular fabric of the major connective tissues, are the most abundant class. A second class comprises the fibril-associated collagens with interrupted triple helices (FACIT), and a third class comprises collagens forming specialized structures such as the basement membranes, anchoring fibrils of the dermo-epidermal junctions, beaded filaments of the dermis, or collagens performing specialized functions as, for example, in the cartilage of the growth plate.

In addition to these molecules that are classified as members of the collagen family, several unrelated proteins contain collagen-like sequences. These sequences presumably enable the molecules to maintain their steric conformation in order to perform their specialized biologic functions. For example, the collagenous sequences in the C1q subcomponent of the complement

Table 3A–I. *Genetic polymorphism of collagen*

Collagen Type	Chain Composition	Molecular Weight	Tissue Distribution
Interstitial collagens			
I	$\alpha_1(I)_2$, $\alpha_2(I)$	300,000	Skin, bone, tendon, synovium
I trimer	$\alpha_1(I)_3$	300,000	Tumors, fetal skin, liver
II	$\alpha_1(II)_3$	300,000	Hyaline cartilage, vitreous, nucleus pulposus
III	$\alpha_1(III)_3$	300,000	Fetal skin, blood vessels, intestine
V	$\alpha_1(V)_2$, $\alpha_2(V)$	300,000	Same as type I collagen
XI	1α, 2α, 3α	450,000	Hyaline cartilage
FACIT collagens			
IX	$\alpha_1(IX)$, $\alpha_2(IX)$, $\alpha_3(IX)$	500,000	Hyaline cartilage, vitreous, cornea
XII	$\alpha_1(XII)_3$	600,000	Same as type I collagen
XIV	$\alpha_1(XIV)_3$	?	Skin, tendon
Basement membrane collagen			
IV	$\alpha_1(IV)$, $\alpha_2(IV)$	450,000	Lamina densa of the basement membrane
Other non-fibrillar collagens			
VI	$\alpha_1(VI)$, $\alpha_2(VI)$, $\alpha_3(V)$	570,000	Aortic intima, placenta, skin, kidney, muscle
VII	$\alpha_1(VII)_3$	960,000	Amnion, dermo-epidermal anchoring fibrils
XIII	?	?	Endothelial Cells
Short-chain collagens			
VIII	$\alpha_1(VIII)_3$	500,000	Endothelial cells, Descemet's membrane
X	$\alpha_1(X)_3$	180,000	Growth plate cartilage

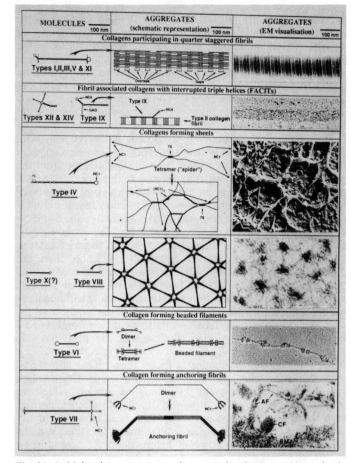

Fig. 3A–1. *Molecular structures and supramolecular assemblies of collagens. Schematic representations of collagen molecules are on the left panel with the molecules oriented with their NH_2 termini to the left. Triple helical (COL) domains are shown as thick black lines and nontriple helical (NC) domains are represented by double lines or empty circles. The larger circles at the ends of the molecules correspond to the globular domains visible on rotary shadowing electron micrographs of isolated intact collagens (or procollagens). Vertical arrows indicate the sites of action of the processing proteinases. A glycosaminoglycan chain attached to the α_2 chain of type IX collagen molecule is shown as GAG; 7S is the domain of antiparallel interaction of the type IV collagen triple helices to form a tetramer (spider). The middle panel contains diagrams of collagen aggregates and assemblies. The right panel illustrates actual collagen aggregates as observed by electron microscopy (courtesy of Dr M van der Rest).*

system are thought to provide the molecules with a rigid segment that enables them to self-aggregate, and those in acetylcholinesterase appear to anchor the enzyme to basement membranes. Two protein components of lung surfactant have also been found to contain collagenous sequences that appear to be responsible for the attachment of surface active phospholipids.

The structure and supramolecular organization of the various collagens are briefly described below and are illustrated in Figure 3A–1.

Fibrillar Collagens

The major fibrillar collagens are known as types I, II, III, V and XI. In electron micrographs these collagens exhibit a cross-striated pattern with a characteristic 64–67 nm periodicity. The periodicity of the collagen fibril is generated by the packing of the collagen molecules in a precise axial register that is usually described as a near-quarter-stagger with overlap. This axial stagger has been precisely defined at 234 ± 1 residues for type I collagen. No lateral substructure is obvious by electron microscopy, and it is not yet clear whether the side-to-side aggregation of molecules, ultimately responsible for the fiber diameter, is due to accretion of the molecules as microfibrillar subunits or whether the lateral organization is amorphous.

What is clear, however, is that the primary structure of the chains contains all the information needed to allow the folding of the native molecules and their packing into fibers. In addition, recent studies suggest that the ultimate diameter of the collagen fibers may be influenced by the presence of the amino-terminal noncollagenous extensions and by interactions with noncollagenous macromolecules such as the small proteoglycan decorin. The primary structure also appears to determine the type and number of intermolecular cross-links that will eventually be formed and the nature of the interaction of the collagen with the other connective tissue components, namely glycoproteins and proteoglycans.

Type I collagen, the most abundant and best characterized mammalian collagen, consists of two identical $\alpha_1(I)$ chains and a genetically distinct α_2 chain in the molecular form $\alpha_1(I)_2\alpha_2$. This species accounts for about 90% of the collagen in the body and is the major collagenous component of skin, tendon, bone, synovium, cornea, conjunctiva, and sclera. The type I collagen fibers observed by electron microscopy are usually wide cross-striated fibers.

A molecule apparently composed of three $\alpha_1(I)$ chains has been found in low concentrations in cornea, skin, embryonic bones and tendons, and rat dentin. This molecular species has also been identified as a product of various cell cultures and tumors. The α-chain of this molecular species appears to be identical, by peptide mapping, to the $\alpha_1(I)$ chain of type I collagen and has been designated α_1 type I trimer collagen. Although its functional role is not understood, this collagen appears in higher concentrations in healing wounds, inflammatory reactions, and embryonic tissues.

Type II collagen is a specific product of chondrocytes and vitreous cells. Its fibers appear much thinner than those of type I collagen in electron micrographs. Type II collagen consists of three identical α-chains and is designated $\alpha_1(II)_3$. These molecules contain a higher number of hydroxylysine residues and several-fold greater amounts of carbohydrate residues than type I collagen. Several properties of the $\alpha_1(II)$ chains of vitreous humor differ from those of the $\alpha_1(II)$ chains of cartilage. These differences strongly suggest that type II molecules are not a homogenous population, but they may represent a family of closely related molecules. Furthermore, recent studies of the gene encoding type II collagen have shown that this collagen exists in at least two separate molecular species that result from alternative splicing of certain portions of the gene. These isoforms appear to have special functional properties, because they are preferentially expressed at various stages of growth and development.

Type III collagen frequently associates with type I in skin, synovium, and vascular wall tissue. This collagen also contains three identical chains that are readily distinguishable from the previously described fibrillar types and is therefore designated $\alpha_1(III)_3$. Unlike the other interstitial collagens, type III collagen molecules contain intrahelical cysteine residues that form interchain disulfide bonds so that the native molecules are disulfide-bonded trimers. Because substantial quantities occur in fetal tissue, this molecular species was first thought to be a fetal type collagen. The fact that type III collagen forms fibrils of smaller diameter and of different fibrillar organization than type I collagen suggests that the relative levels of expression of separate collagen genes is an important step in establishing and maintaining the individual characteristics of a particular connective tissue. For example, the relative proportions of type I and type III change drastically in healing skin wounds and in keloid skin lesions.

Type V collagen is frequently found surrounding fibroblasts, smooth muscle cells, and other mesenchymal cells. This collagen type contains distinct chains known as αA and αB, which are minor components found in pepsin digests of placenta, cornea, skin, and blood vessels, and which have been identified in surface-associated materials of cells in culture. The type V molecules are comprised of homo or heteropolymers, depending on the tissue of origin. The most common molecular form of type V collagen consists of two αA-chains and one αB-chain. However, trimers of αA and αB-chains have also been described. What determines the relative proportion of these chains within the molecule and what is their exact role in tissue structure or function is not clear.

Type XI collagen is the designation recently assigned to collagen molecules composed of chains previously known as 1α, 2α, and 3α. Like type II collagen, type XI collagen is a specific constituent of cartilaginous tissues. Type XI collagen molecules are comprised of three chains that retain large globular domains at both ends. There is some controversy regarding the nature of the 3α chain, since it is not clear whether it represents a type II collagen chain with extensive post-translational modifications or a distinct gene product. In most cartilaginous tissues the proportion of the three chains is equimolar, suggesting that they are arranged in a heterotrimeric structure. Recent studies have shown that type XI collagen molecules are integral components of the cartilage collagen fibrils and appear to be located in their central axis. Despite their prominent presence in cartilaginous tissues, the exact function of type XI collagen molecules has not been determined.

Fibril-Associated Collagens with Interrupted Triple Helices

Three distinct collagens do not form the characteristic quarter-staggered fibrils of interstitial collagens. This subgroup is composed of types IX, XII, and XIV collagens. Structurally, these collagens contain alternating triple-helical (COL domains) and noncollagenous domains (NC domains) of various lengths and molecular masses. This structural arrangement provides greater flexibility to these molecules. Topographically, these collagens associate with the fibrils of types I and II collagens and may play important roles in the organization of the matrix in the immediate peri-fibrillar millieu.

The molecular structure of these collagens can be divided into three main functional regions. One region contains one or two triple helical domains and is responsible for the interaction and adhesion of these molecules to the surface of the interstitial collagen fibrils. A second region, consisting of another triple helical domain, serves as a rigid arm that projects out of the fibril. The third region, which does not include triple helices, may promote interaction with other matrix elements or with cells.

Type IX collagen, the prototype of the FACIT group of collagens is found almost exclusively in cartilaginous structures. Its function has not been determined. The type IX collagen molecule is composed of three chains containing four non-helical domains alternating with three helical regions. The individual chains are associated by disulfide bonds. The α_2 chain of type IX collagen contains a covalently bound glycosaminoglycan and, therefore, can be considered a proteoglycan core protein. The demonstration of a covalent interaction between a collagen and a glycosaminoglycan molecule in articular cartilage and other hyaline cartilages, suggests that type IX collagen may be involved in mediating the interaction of the collagenous matrix with the proteoglycans in these tissues. Rotary shadowing studies have shown that type IX collagen molecules are topographically localized to the surface of cartilage collagen fibrils, surrounding the type II collagen molecules with the COL3 and NC4 domains bent in an angle projecting out of the surface of the fibrils into the surrounding interfibrillar matrix. These studies led to the suggestion that the NC4 domain of the α_1 chain of type IX collagen may be involved in the formation of interfibrillar collagen interactions or in interactions with other components of the articular cartilage matrix. The highly positively charged composition of the NC4 domain may favor the establishment of non-ionic interactions with proteoglycans, glycoproteins, or other collagens, thus establishing the interfibrillar "glue" that maintains the structure of articular cartilage matrix (9). Although these suggestions are quite attractive, experimental evidence to prove their validity is still lacking. However, the nucleotide sequence of cDNAs corresponding to type IX collagen molecules in the cornea, hypertrophic cartilage of the growth plate and late developmental stages of the vitreous indicates that these molecules lack the NC4 domain (short form of type XI collagen). These observations suggest that this NC4 domain may play an important role in determining the structural organization of these tissues, particularly during development.

Type XII collagen. Because type IX collagen in tissues containing type II collagen provides possible means of attachment and new functionalities to the fibrils, the need for molecules with similar functions in tissues containing type I collagen was apparent. Studies conducted to search for homologs of type IX collagen in tissues containing type I collagen as their major fibrillar constituent were conducted, initially at the cDNA level and subsequently at the protein level. Molecules with striking similarities with type IX collagen (identically located cysteines and triple helix imperfections) were identified. However, further characterization of the intact protein molecule, designated type XII collagen, revealed major differences between the two molecules. Type XII collagen is a homotrimer with the molecular structure $\alpha_1(XII)_3$ and contains only two triple helical domains, COL1 and COL2, and three noncollagenous domains. The NH_2–terminal NC3 domain is very large (3 × 190 kDa). When visualized by rotary shadowing, the type XII collagen molecules have a characteristic morphology with three 60 nm arms projecting from a large central globule and a 70 nm rigid tail. The co-localization of type XII collagen with type I collagen suggests that type XII collagen interacts with fibrils containing type I collagen, although the precise nature of this interaction has not been determined. The homology between the COL1 domains of type IX and type XII collagens suggests that this domain may play a role in this interaction.

Type XIV collagen. The existence in skin and tendon of another homotrimeric molecule with the characteristic FACIT COL1 domain has recently been demonstrated. Characterization of the molecule at the cDNA and protein levels indicates that it is very similar but clearly distinct from type XII collagen. It has been suggested that it constitutes a distinct type of collagen termed type XIV collagen.

Basement Membrane Collagen

The collagens present in the basement membrane are probably responsible for the structural integrity of the membranes and act as anchors for other extracellular matrix components. Unlike the fibrillar collagens discussed above, the principal basement membrane collagen, termed type IV collagen, does not form fibrillar aggregates and appears to be incorporated directly into the membrane structure without prior excision of the pro-peptide extensions.

The structure of this molecular species has been a controversial matter; however, more recent work has identified two distinct α-chains as the molecular components of type IV collagen. These chains associate to form homo or heterotrimers with the compositions of $\alpha_1(IV)_3$, $\alpha_2(IV)_3$ or $\alpha_1(IV)_2\alpha_2(IV)$. Characterization of the structure of type IV collagen has been accomplished by rotary shadowing of intact molecules, demonstrating that these molecules contain several intrahelical noncollagenous domains that probably confer great flexibility to the main body of the molecule. The helical domains of type IV collagen chains display a distinct bend approximately 360 nm from the amino terminal end of the chains. In addition, a large globular domain is present at the carboxy–terminal end of the chains. A large number of cysteine residues are present at both the amino– and carboxy–terminal ends and are involved in intra- and inter-chain disulfide bonds.

The molecules of type IV collagen assemble into a very specific supramolecular network formed as a result of the association of similar ends of the molecules. Four molecules are associated through their amino terminal domains distal to the bend described above, forming a tetrameric pepsin-resistant domain known as the 7S aggregate. The C terminal globular domains connect two molecules with each other, resulting in a well-organized network arrangement.

Other Non-Fibril Forming Collagens

Several collagens that do not form the characteristic cross-striated pattern of the fibrillar collagens and that do not appear to have a FACIT molecular structure have been identified. Some of these collagens form highly specialized structures with specific functions such as the establishment of connections between cell surfaces and the extracellular matrix (type VI collagen) or the attachment of subepidermal structures to the dermo-epidermal basement membrane (type VII collagen).

Type VI collagen consists of chains containing a triple helical collagenous domain flanked by a large globular domain at each end of the chains. The globular domains account for approximately two-thirds of the total chain mass while the collagenous region represents only one-third. The type VI collagen chains have been found distributed in many connective tissues, but are predominantly localized in the skin and may represent the previously described "beaded filaments" found in embryonic tissues as well as in active lesions in scleroderma. The type VI collagen molecules form aggregates composed of two chains intertwined to form a dimer, and two dimers associate by criss-cross interactions between their ends to form a tetramer. Tetramers associate by head to tail attachment to form long fibrillar structures.

Type VII collagen also known as "long chain collagen", consists of chains containing a collagenous helical domain that is at least one and one-half times larger than that of the interstitial collagens. Type VII collagen molecules form the so-called anchoring fibrils responsible for the attachment of basement membranes to stromal tissues, particularly in the epidermal–dermal interphase. The type VII collagen molecules interact by anti-parallel dimeric arrangement, showing a 60 nm overlap between the interacting amino-terminal molecular ends. The carboxyl terminal ends are grouped in a tuft that appears to attach to the basement membrane and to form loops surrounding interstitial collagen fibrils. It has recently been shown that mutations in the genes encoding this collagen are responsible for certain forms of epidermolysis bullosa.

Short-Chain Collagens

Two distinct collagens characterized by the presence of short triple helical domains have been characterized in vascular tissues and in growth plate cartilage. The two members of this group are type VIII and type X collagens.

Type VIII collagen was originally described as a product of endothelial cells in culture and was termed EC collagen. This collagen is an important component of the corneal endothelium. Type VIII collagen has not been completely characterized, but the molecules may be composed of relatively short helical domains, interrupted by protease sensitive, non-helical domains with large globular domains at each end of the chains. These chains are stabilized by abundant disulfide bonds, and the intact molecule appears to have a molecular weight greater than 500 kDa under nonreducing conditions. The type VIII collagen molecules have a dumb-bell shape and appear to interact laterally and by their extremities to form regular hexagonal lattices.

Type X collagen is a specific biosynthetic product of growth plate hypertrophic chondrocytes and is exclusively found in the regions undergoing endochondral bone formation. Because of the close temporal and topographic relation of the initiation of type X collagen synthesis with the onset of tissue calcification, these chains may play a role in the process of endochondral ossification. The type X collagen chains are formed by short (45 kDa), triple helical regions containing a 15 kDa globular domain at the amino terminal end. The triple helical domain appears to be stabilized by disulfide bonds in certain mammalian species such as those present in calf cartilage. Recent interest has been focused on possible alterations in the metabolism of type X collagen in osteoarthritis. It has been found that in contrast to normal articular cartilage, osteoarthritic cartilage expresses this collagen.

Collagen Genes

Recent advances in recombinant DNA technology have permitted a greater understanding of the initial steps of collagen biosynthesis, and have allowed the isolation and characterization of the genes encoding for most of the collagenous molecules described above. At least 20 distinct genes encoding for the various collagen chains have been identified and studied (4,5). In particular, the genes for types I, II, and III collagens have been extensively analyzed and sequenced. The gene for the pro α_1-chain of type I collagen appears to be approximately 18,000 bases long, while the gene for the pro α_2-chain is much larger, containing approximately 38,000 bases. The collagen genes studied thus far contain coding sequences (exons) interrupted by large, non-coding sequences (introns). The genes encoding most of the collagens, like various other eukaryotic genes, contain regulatory sequences in the 5' region of the gene, including the so-called TATA and CAAT boxes (Table 3A–2). These two consensus sequences have been shown to be essential promoter components required for efficient transcription of several other eukaryotic genes. In addition, enhancer sequences, which act as long-range activators of gene transcription, have been identified within the first intron of several collagen genes.

The genes encoding the chains of the interstitial collagens appear to contain short exons of 54 or 108 bases in length, and it has been suggested that the 54 base exon represents the ancestral collagen gene that has evolved into the present collagen genes by duplication and expansion of the 54 base pair (bp) unit. This appears to be the case for most of the collagens; however, recent characterization of the genes for avian collagen types VIII, IX and X demonstrated substantial deviations from this structure, indicating that these genes may represent different families of genes developed by selective pressures exercised during evolution. For example, the gene for the α_2 chain of type IX collagen contains the 54 bp coding units only in the central portions of the sequence coding for the triple helix, whereas the genes for types VIII and X collagens contain only 4 and 3 exons, respectively, without the 54 bp repeat unit. For a more detailed description of the structure of the genes encoding the various members of the

Table 3A–2. *Sequence motifs present within the promoter elements and the first intron of several collagen genes*

	Promoters				
Motif	α1(I)	α2(I)	α1(II)	α1(III)	α1, α2(IV)
TATA	Yes	Yes	Yes	Yes	No
CCAAT	Yes	Yes	No	Yes	Yes
Ap1 (TGAC/GTCA)	No	No	Yes	No	Yes
Ap2 (CCCCAGGC)	Yes	No	No	No	No
Sp1 (GGGGCGG)	Yes	Yes	Yes	Yes	Yes
NF-1	Yes	Yes	No	No	No
Pyrimidine-rich	Yes	Yes	Yes	No	No

	First Introns			
Motif	α1(I)	α2(I)	α1(II)	α2(IV)
Functional enhancer	Yes	Yes	Yes	Yes
Enhancer sequence	Yes	Yes	Yes	Yes
Ap1 (TGAG/GTCA)	Yes	No	No	N/A
Ap2 (CCCCAGGC)	Yes	No	No	Yes
NF-1	Yes	No	Yes	Yes
Sp1 (GGGGCGG)	Yes	No	Yes	Yes
(GT)n	No	No	Yes	No
Pyrimidine-rich	Yes	No	Yes	No

Modified from Sandell and Boyd (5).

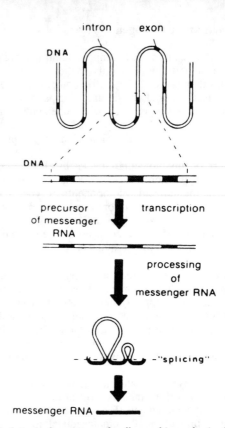

Fig. 3A–2. *Intranuclear steps of collagen biosynthesis. The DNA sequences in collagen genes, containing the coding sequences (exons) and the intervening noncoding sequences (introns), are transcribed into a precursor form of the messenger RNA (mRNA) molecule. The precursor molecule is then processed to functional mRNA by post-transcriptional modifications, including splicing which removes the intervening sequences (courtesy of Dr J Uitto and colleagues; reproduced with permission).*

collagen family of proteins, the reader is referred to recent reviews (4,5).

Collagen Biosynthesis

The biosynthesis of type I procollagen has been studied in most detail and can be used as an example of a general biosynthetic pathway for all collagens. A general scheme of type I collagen biosynthesis and processing is depicted in Figure 3A–2. The initial step involves the expression of a particular collagen gene that resides in the DNA of the cell producing these molecules (Fig. 3A–2). The collagen genes are transcribed into a complementary high molecular size messenger RNA (mRNA) precursor. These molecules are then processed to the mature mRNA by a complex series of post-transcriptional modifications including capping, splicing, methylation, and addition of a polyadenylated tail. Splicing is probably the most important of these reactions, because it is responsible for the precise excision of the noncoding, intervening sequences and the exact religation of the remaining sequences that encode the mature protein. Variations in the patterns of splicing (alternative splicing) can result in the production of polypeptide chains with subtle but important structural and functional differences. Thus, alternative splicing appears to be a versatile mechanism for the generation of a vast molecular diversity of the biosynthesized proteins and may play a crucial role in the temporal and topographic regulation of collagen gene expression. In addition, the genes for certain collagens appear to have more than one transcription initiation site. Selective use of these sites can result in the production of shorter chains with variable lengths and the inclusion or exclusion of specific molecular domains (see above). The mature mRNA molecules exit the nucleus and are transported to the rough endoplasmic reticulum where they associate with the polyribosomal apparatus and then undergo translation onto the growing polypeptide chains of the newly synthesized protein (Fig. 3A–3).

Studies of the translation of mRNA for procollagen type I in cell-free systems indicate that the molecule is synthesized on the ribosomes as pre-procollagen, and each chain contains a short (approximately 20 residue) leader sequence at the extreme amino terminus. This hydrophobic leader sequence is thought to channel the nascent polypeptide through the membrane into the cisternae of the rough endoplasmic reticulum. It is immediately cleaved off by a protease to yield procollagen.

Type I procollagen consists of two pro α_1 and one pro α_2 chains with estimated molecular weights of about 150,000 d compared with 95,000 d for the corresponding α-chains of the fully processed molecule. Each of the pro α-chains contains two polypeptide extensions, one at each end of the triple-helical region. The amino and carboxy-terminal extensions are estimated to be 20,000 d and 35,000 d, respectively. The carboxy terminal ends contain several cysteine residues involved in intra and interchain disulfide bonds. These extensions, or propeptides, appear to prevent the nonphysiologic formation of collagen fibrils before the molecules reach the extracellular space. They are also involved in directing the proper assembly of the collagen molecules from their constituent chains and in initiating triple-helix formation. Some evidence has suggested a role for the propeptides in feedback inhibition of collagen biosynthesis and in extracellular collagen fibrillogenesis. Shortly after synthesis of the individual procollagen polypeptide chains, specific association of three chains in a proper ratio (i.e. two proα_1-, and one proα_2-chains for type I collagen), formation of disulfide bonds and triple helix assembly occur. The crucial step of triple helix formation requires an adequate level of proline hydroxylation in order to take place at physiologic temperatures. As mentioned above, hydroxyproline-deficient collagen fails to form a stable triple helix at normal body temperatures and undergoes rapid intracellular degradation. Similarly, excess procollagen chains that are not assembled into a triple helical conformation are degraded intracellularly.

During the biosynthetic process, the polypeptide chains of procollagen are subject to at least six different enzyme-mediated modifications prior to secretion. Further post-translational modifications involving cross-link formation occur extracellularly. These enzyme-mediated modifications are not usually found in the biosynthetic pathways of other proteins. Intracellular post-translational modifications include hydroxylation of proline and lysine, addition of galactose to certain hydroxylysines and of glucose to certain galactose-hydroxylysines, and finally extrusion from the cell coupled with proteolytic cleavage of the extension peptides from the amino and carboxy termini of the molecule by specific proteases.

The post-translational microheterogeneity resulting from these

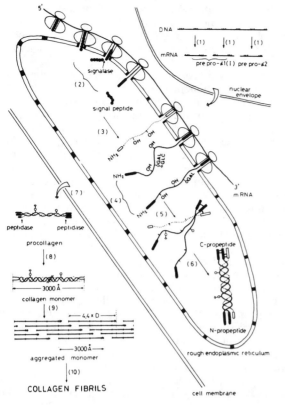

Fig. 3A–3. *Post-transcriptional steps of collagen biosynthesis. 1. Transcription of collagen genes resulting in synthesis of different mRNAs for each procollagen chain. 2. Translation of the mRNA for each procollagen chain. Procollagen mRNAs are transported from the nucleus to ribosomes lining the rough endoplastic reticulum. The procollagen is depicted as a polypeptide chain having a signal peptide which is cleaved by a signal peptidase. 3. Hydroxylation by peptidyl proline hydroxylase or peptidyl lysine hydroxylase. 4. Glycosylation of hydroxylysyl residues by galactosyl transferase and glucosyltransferase. 5. Formation of the interchain disulfide links in the C-terminal propeptides. 6. Triple-helix formation. 7. Secretion. 8. Procollagen-collagen conversion by limited proteolysis (pN-collagen aminopeptidase and pC-collagen carboxypeptidase). 9. Assembly into fibrils by a near quarter-stagger's shift. 10. Cross-linking of collagen fibrils (courtesy of Dr RI Bashey; reproduced with permission).*

enzyme-mediated modifications probably represents the fine-tuning that adapts the collagen molecule for its ultimate biologic function. The molecule is only secreted after hydroxylation, glycosylation, and triple helix formation are complete. Secretion appears to be a stepwise process, requiring packing into a Golgi vacuole before exocytosis.

Although almost all the procollagens of most tissues are converted to collagen molecules, some unprocessed procollagen molecules may be retained at the cell surface to interact specifically with various structural components of the interfibrillar matrix. Basement membrane procollagens appear to be incorporated into the membrane structure without prior processing.

Processed molecules destined to form extracellular matrix fibrils self-assemble into three-dimensional fibrillar complexes, which are then stabilized by a series of covalent inter and intrachain cross-links. Most of these bonds originate from lysine or hydroxylysine and from modified forms of amino acid residues derived by oxidative deamination. Control of the extent of polymerization and of cross-linking is poorly understood, but has multiple effects on the mechanical properties of collagen fibers.

Regulation of Collagen Biosynthesis

Under normal conditions, fibroblasts and other connective tissue-producing cells are capable of regulating extracellular matrix production according to the dynamic requirements of processes such as development, differentiation, and repair (10–13).

Remarkable methodologic advances in recent years have re-

sulted in an explosion of knowledge regarding the mechanisms that regulate gene expression in eukaryotic cells. It has become possible to clarify certain aspects of the intricate mechanisms responsible for the regulation of expression of the genes encoding multiple extracellular matrix proteins including several collagens, fibronectin, and proteoglycan core proteins. These advances will undoubtedly help to clarify the mechanisms responsible for the pathologic increase in tissue collagen in fibrotic diseases such as scleroderma.

There are three general mechanisms by which the production of collagen can be controlled: a) modulation of the steady state level of mRNA; b) control of mRNA translation; and c) variation in the fraction of the newly synthesized protein, which is degraded before it is secreted from the cell. In most normal and pathologic conditions, the levels of procollagen or collagen mRNA correlate with the rate of synthesis of the corresponding collagen polypeptides. The steady state mRNA levels are determined by a delicate balance between the transcription rates of the corresponding genes and the mRNA degradation rates. Transcription regulation is by far the most important mechanism determining the steady state mRNA levels; however, under certain conditions, particularly under the influence of growth factors and cytokines, alterations in mRNA stability or in the rates of mRNA degradation may play a substantial role.

Many mechanisms may be responsible for derangement of transcription regulation, including mutations in important promoter regulatory regions or in other specialized regulatory elements of the gene. These upstream elements are also principal targets for the action of promoter-specific transcription factors. These factors may regulate the initiation of transcription of their target genes by controlling the binding of RNA polymerases to preexisting transcription complexes or by the formation of the transcription complex itself. Several transcription factors that regulate the levels of expression of various collagen genes have been identified and characterized. They can exert either stimulatory or inhibitory effects on the rates of gene transcription. Some of these trans-acting factors recognize and bind to DNA sequences that are homologous to sequences in other genes, which are targets for transcription regulators such as Ap1, Ap2, NF–1, and Sp1 (Table 3A–2). The entire complement of DNA-binding proteins that specifically modulate the transcription of collagen genes has not been determined. The activity of many promoters is also modulated by enhancer elements located either upstream or downstream of the transcription start site. Transcription factors may also bind to enhancer elements to bring about transcription regulation. Recent studies of the effects of transcription/DNA-binding factors and of their interactions with collagen gene promoter regions or with other regulatory elements indicate that the transcription regulation of collagen gene expression is extremely complex and that these interactions will undoubtedly affect the tissue specificity and the levels of collagen production in response to intracellular or extracellular perturbations.

Post-translational events may also influence the levels of collagen production. An intriguing control mechanism has been suggested from the observations that the N-propeptides of type I or type III calf collagen can reduce the rate of collagen synthesis when added to cultures of calf dermal fibroblasts and can inhibit the translation of type I procollagen mRNA in a cell free system. This negative feedback process may be a means whereby the concentration of pro-peptides in the extracellular matrix can modulate the rate of collagen synthesis at a translation level. Other possible mechanisms of control may be exerted by regulation of the stability of mature messenger RNA molecules. Increased stability of these messages will result in increased production of a specific protein.

The observation that cultured fibroblasts can degrade a fraction of newly synthesized collagen before it is secreted represents another possible regulatory mechanism. The fraction of collagen that undergoes such degradation appears to be mediated by lysosomal enzymes and can be increased by a variety of agents that raise the level of intracellular cyclic AMP or cause disruption of triple helix formation. A decrease in the fraction of collagen that is degraded intracellularly could result in a net increase in production of this protein and lead to fibrosis.

In addition to these intrinsic mechanisms of control, it has recently been shown that extra-fibroblastic factors may influence the rates of collagen synthesized by these cells. The role of certain products of inflammatory cells in regulation of fibroblastic function has recently been emphasized (12). It has been shown that several well-characterized products of activated mononuclear cells can profoundly influence fibroblast function. Stimulation of fibroblast proliferation and collagen synthesis by cytokines and growth factors is well recognized (13). For example, interferons and tumor necrosis factor can produce a selective inhibition of fibroblast collagen production (14), whereas transforming growth factor β is a potent stimulator of fibronectin and collagen production by these cells (15).

Collagen Degradation

The native interstitial tissue contains collagen in the form of insoluble paracrystalline aggregates in close association with many other tissue components. Collagen degradation is thus extremely complex (16). The rate of degradation seems to depend, at any one moment, on the amount of active specific degradative enzymes present, on the degree of substrate susceptibility, and on the presence and activity of specific tissue or humoral inhibitors. Much current knowledge of collagenolytic enzymes that belong to the broad group of matrix metalloproteinases (MMP) relates to the enzyme responsible for the cleavage of the native type I collagen. This enzyme (MMP1) cleaves the collagen molecule at a single specific site within the triple-helical region producing two pieces: one, (the TC^A peptide) accounts for 75% of the molecule, the other (the TC^B peptide) for the remaining 25%. These peptides are unstable at physiologic temperatures and after denaturation become susceptible to the hydrolytic action of gelatinases or other nonspecific tissue proteases. All collagens are not susceptible to MMP1, however. Type-specific collagenases that are capable of specifically degrading types IV and V collagens have been identified. These type-specific collagenases may play important roles in vessel-wall basement membrane degradation, especially during inflammation or tumor cell invasion.

Several investigators have provided evidence that collagenases are secreted as inactive precursor molecules, while others suggest that these latent enzymes are in reality enzyme–inhibitor complexes. In fact, both mechanisms may be operating within a connective tissue, depending on the prevailing set of circumstances. Other proteins may regulate collagenase activity by either activation, such as the "collagenase activator protein" or inhibition such as α-2 macroglobulin and the tissue inhibitor of metalloproteases (TIMP) (17). Furthermore, regulation of collagenase production and activation may be influenced by hormones, cytokines such as interleukin–1, growth factors such as platelet-derived growth factor and transforming growth factor β, and other substances such as prostaglandins. These factors may play important but as yet not entirely defined operational roles in a variety of rheumatic diseases.

ELASTIN

Elastin fibers are easily identified by their characteristic tinctorial properties (with acid-orcein stain) and their ability to stretch when hydrated. These widely distributed fibers stretch and return to their original length after application and removal of a deforming force. Elastic fibers are the most prominent component of ligaments. They comprise 70% to 80% of the dry weight of ligamentum nuchae, and they contribute to the unique elastic properties of the lungs, skin, and walls of the larger blood vessels (aorta contains 30% to 60% elastin). Elastic fibers constitute 2% to 5% of the dry weight of dermis.

Main Structural Features

The structure, biosynthesis, and function of elastin have been reviewed (18). Electron microscopy reveals that elastic fibers consist of two distinct components. The major component has an amorphous appearance and demonstrates no distinct periodicity. This component, the protein elastin, forms 5 nm diameter ropes that are aligned in parallel to form a 5–6 μm diameter core in the elastic fiber. This core is surrounded by a sheath of microfibrillar structures that measure 10–12 μm in diameter.

The fibrous elastin core is a polymer of tropoelastin sub-units. Each tropoelastin monomer contains 850 amino acids and has a molecular weight of about 72,000 d. Four amino acids—glycine, alanine, proline, and valine—constitute 80% of all the amino acids of tropoelastin. Hydroxyproline is present in the molecule, but it is much less plentiful than in collagen. The protein lacks tryptophan, cystine, and methionine. This unusual composition leads to a unique primary structure containing repeating peptide sequences. For example, the pentapeptide (Val–Pro–Gly–Val–Gly) appears to be a dominant feature since it is repeated more than six times in a segment of the molecule and occurs elsewhere in the chain.

Biochemical characterization of the microfibrillar protein has shown that this component is totally distinct in composition from the elastin core. It contains smaller amounts of the amino acids glycine, alanine, and valine than elastin, and it does not contain hydroxyproline. It is relatively rich in those amino acids that are entirely lacking or only present in small amounts in elastin, such as cystine, methionine, and histidine. Indeed, the content of cystine in microfibrillar protein is particularly high (70–80 residues per 1,000 amino acid residues). The microfibrils also contain a large number of hexose and hexosamine sugar residues revealing the glycoprotein nature of this component.

When tropoelastin molecules associate to form a fiber, they do so in a way that favors juxtaposition of a limited number of the 38 lysine residues present in the polypeptide chain. This alignment process is probably brought about by pairing of like amino acid sequences and interlocking of particular chain segments. The lysine residues occur in alanine-rich sequences with two or three alanine residues between the two lysine residues that serve as cross-link precursors. Cross-linking involves two lysine residues from each of two chains. Thus the major cross-links, desmosine and isodesmosine, derive from the side chain of four lysine residues. These cross-links appear to be unique to elastin.

The resultant polymeric insoluble fibrous matrix is a twisted-rope structure held together by hydrophobic ridges stacked at 6 Å intervals that run at angles to the axis. Three well-defined regions can be recognized in the stabilized structure: a dynamic β-spiral region largely responsible for the elastometric properties, an interlocked β-spiral region, and the essentially α-helical cross-linking region that covalently binds the tropoelastin sub-units into the fibrous network.

Biosynthesis

The same essential principles apply to both collagen and elastin biosynthesis. The gene for elastin has been extensively studied. The hydrophobic and cross-linking domains are encoded in separate exons (19). These tend to be relatively small (27–114 base pairs) and are separated by large introns. Sequence analysis of the elastin gene has uncovered the presence of two cysteine residues not identified by protein analysis. They may be important in establishing disulfide interactions with other chains or with other matrix proteins. Translation of the mRNA for the monomer sub-units takes place in the rough endoplasmic reticulum resulting in the synthesis of the 72 kDa tropoelastin. After translation the newly synthesized tropoelastin polypeptides are passed through the cisternae, they are packaged and discharged into the extracellular space where they undergo chemical modifications in preparation for incorporation into polymeric elastin.

The first step in the formation of the cross-links, desmosine and isodesmosine, is the oxidative deamination of three lysine residues to form aldehydes. The fourth lysine is incorporated into the cross-link without modification.

Thus, the generation of activated cross-link precursors in elastin is similar to that which occurs with collagen. The oxidative deamination reaction is catalyzed by lysyl oxidase. In diseases with a genetic deficiency or a reduced level of activity of this enzyme, abnormal cross-linking of elastin appears to be partly responsible for the clinical manifestations. Deficient lysyl oxidase activities have been encountered, for example, in an inbred strain of mice demonstrating aortic aneurysms, reduced tensile strength of the skin, and bone abnormalities.

Degradation

Although the metabolic turnover of elastin in adult animals is relatively slow, a continuous degradation of small amounts of the protein normally takes place. A specific family of enzymes, the elastases, degrade elastin at neutral pH (20). They are serine proteases that appear to be inactivated by serum inhibitors such as α1-antitrypsin and α2-macroglobulin.

Although the first specific elastase was isolated from pancreatic tissue, elastolytic enzymes have been found in other tissues and in macrophages, leukocytes, and platelets. The leukocyte elastase is of particular interest because release of this enzyme, together with other lysosomal proteolytic enzymes, may contribute to the damage of blood vessels in diseases such as leukocytoclastic vasculitis. The elastases may play a role in other disease processes, such as arteriosclerosis, pulmonary emphysema, and the invasion of various tumors into adjacent connective tissues. Furthermore, a specific elastolytic activity in aortic tissue has been shown to increase with advancing age, suggesting that aging and degenerative changes of the cardiovascular system might be partly explained by an increased rate of degradation of elastic fibers.

OTHER PROTEINS OF CONNECTIVE TISSUE

The intracellular matrices and basement membranes contain several other important proteins in addition to collagens and elastin. Several of these have recently been characterized and can be considered part of a family of proteins with specific adhesive and other important properties. Among these, the best characterized are fibronectin, laminin, chondronectin, and osteonectin. In addition, there are many other proteins with unknown functions and poorly defined biochemical characteristics such as the matrix associated glycoprotein and the high molecular weight protein found in hyaline cartilage, and fibrillin, a protein found in soft connective tissues. These proteins represent important quantitative components of the extracellular matrix; however, their exact structures and their physiologic roles await further study.

Sergio A. Jimenez, MD

1. Miller EJ: The structure of fibril-forming collagens. Ann NY Acad Sci 460:1–13, 1985
2. Structure and Function of Collagen Types. Edited by Mayne R, Burgeson RE. New York, Academic Press, 1987
3. van der Rest M, Garrone R: Collagen family of proteins. FASEB J 5:2814–2823, 1991
4. Vuorio E, deCrombrugge B: The family of collagen genes. Ann Rev Biochem 59:837, 1990
5. Extracellular Matrix Genes. Edited by Sandell LJ, Boyd CD. New York, Academic Press, 1990
6. Krieg T, Hein R, Hatamochi A, et al: Molecular and clinical aspects of connective tissue. Eur J Clin Invest 18:105–123, 1988
7. Gay S, Miller EJ: What is collagen, what is not. Ultrastruct Pathol 4:365–377, 1983
8. Rosenbloom J, Harsch M, Jimenez SA: Hydroxyproline determines the denaturation temperature of chick tendon collagen. Arch Biochem Biophys 158:478–484, 1973
9. Gordon MK, Olsen BR: The contribution of collagenous proteins to tissue-specific matrix assemblies. Curr Opin Cell Biol 2:833–838, 1990
10. Bornstein P, Sage H: Regulation of collagen gene expression. Prog Nucleic Acids Res Mol Biol 37:66–106, 1988
11. Adams SL: Collagen gene expression. Am J Resp Cell Mol Biol 1:161–168, 1989
12. Bornstein P, Horlein D, McPherson J: Regulation of collagen synthesis, Myelofibrosis and the Biology of Connective Tissue. New York, Allan R. Liss, Inc., pp 61–80, 1984
13. Freundlich B, Bomalaski JS, Neilson E, et al: Regulation of fibroblast proliferation and collagen synthesis by cytokines. Immunol Today 7:303–307, 1986
14. Jimenez SA, Freundlich B, Rosenbloom J: Selective inhibition of human diploid fibroblast collagen synthesis by interferons. J Clin Invest 74:1112–1116, 1984
15. Varga J, Rosenbloom J, Jimenez SA: Transforming growth factor β (TGFβ) causes a persistent increase in steady state amounts of type I and type III collagens and fibronectin mRNAs in normal human dermal fibroblasts. Biochem J 247:597–604, 1987
16. Harris ED, Welgus HG, Krane SM: Regulation of the mammalian collagenases. Coll Relat Res 4:493–512, 1984
17. Woessner JF, Jr: Matrix metalloproteinases and their inhibitors in connective tissue remodeling. FASEB J 5:2146–2154, 1991
18. Rosenbloom J: Elastin: Relation of protein and gene structure to disease. Lab Invest 51:605–623, 1984
19. Yoon K, May M, Goldstein N, et al: Characterization of a sheep elastin cDNA containing translated sequences. Biochem Biophys Res Commun 11:261–264, 1984
20. Werb Z, Banda MJ, McKerrow JH, et al: Elastases and elastin degradation. J Invest Dermatol 79:1545, 1982

B. Proteoglycans

Proteoglycans are synthesized by all connective tissue cells, after which they either remain associated with the cells or are secreted into the extracellular matrix. These molecules are related to the family of glycoproteins, and like all members of this family, they usually possess N-linked and/or O-linked oligosaccharides. The additional presence of at least one sulfated glycosaminoglycan chain as part of their carbohydrate complement distinguishes proteoglycans from other glycoproteins. These glycosaminoglycans enable proteoglycans to be localized in tissue sections by the use of cationic dyes, such as safranin O and Alcian blue. A proteoglycan may thus be defined as a protein bearing one or more glycosaminoglycan chains. A vast array of different structures exist, with the largest proteoglycans possessing over 100 glycosaminoglycan chains. Proteoglycans are best classified according to their core proteins, which represent the products of distinct genes (Table 3B–1). To date, 12 such genes have been described, and it is likely that more exist. However, recognition of these gene products is not always easy, because the mRNA transcribed by different cells may vary due to alternative splicing and the use of different transcription start sites. Also, cells may process the same core protein in different ways post-translationally with respect to glycosaminoglycan structure, and the molecules may be further processed proteolytically once they leave the cells. Such processing variation may alter the functional properties of the proteoglycans, which can reside in both the protein and glycosaminoglycan moieties (1).

GLYCOSAMINOGLYCANS

Sulfated glycosaminoglycans are generally classified into five types, depending on their structural features: chondroitin sulfate, dermatan sulfate, heparan sulfate, heparin, and keratan sulfate (2). All are initially synthesized as polysaccharides based on a repeating disaccharide structure, which may then undergo several polymer modifications, including sulfation (Table 3B–2). As there is no template for either polymer elongation or modification, these parameters can vary with cell type, tissue site, age, and disease. Chondroitin sulfate consists of glucuronic acid and N-acetylgalactosamine, and the latter residue may be sulfated at either its 4- or 6-position. Dermatan sulfate differs from chondroitin sulfate by the presence of iduronic acid replacing some glucuronic acid residues. Since iduronate synthesis involves epimerization of glucuronic acid in the polymer, dermatan sulfate can be considered a derivative of chondroitin sulfate. Similarly,

Table 3B–1. *Structural features of proteoglycans*

Proteoglycan	Location	GAG[1] (Number)	Protein[2] (Species)
Syndecan	Cell surface	HS/CS (4)	293 (human)
Betaglycan	Cell surface	HS/CS (2)	829 (rat)
Serglycin	Intracellular	CS or Hep (8)	131 (human)
Perlecan	Basement membrane	HS (3)	3686 (mouse)
Aggrecan	Extracellular matrix	CS/KS (>100)	2297 (human)
Versican	Extracellular matrix	CS/DS (12)	2389 (human)
Decorin	Extracellular matrix	CS or DS (1)	343 (human)
Biglycan	Extracellular matrix	CS or DS (2)	349 (human)
Fibromodulin	Extracellular matrix	KS (4)	357 (bovine)

[1] Typical substitution of core protein by glycosaminoglycan (GAG) chains: HS, heparan sulfate; CS, chondroitin sulfate; Hep, heparin; KS, keratan sulfate; DS, dermatan sulfate.

[2] Number of amino acids in primary translation product, following signal peptide removal, but including any propeptide.

heparan sulfate and heparin are based on a repeating backbone of glucuronic acid and N–acetylglucosamine, which may be modified by epimerization of the glucuronic acid and sulfation of the hexosamine.

Unlike the other glycosaminoglycans, the hexosamines of heparan sulfate and heparin may have their N–acetyl moieties replaced by N–sulfation. In heparin, polymer modification occurs to a greater extent than in most heparan sulfate chains, resulting in heavily sulfated domains. Keratan sulfate differs from other glycosaminoglycans in not possessing any uronic acid. Its backbone consists of galactose and N–acetylglucosamine that may be modified by sulfation of both monosaccharides at their 6-positions. Furthermore, one of two linkage oligosaccharides joins keratan sulfate to its protein, and these are different from that utilized by the other sulfated glycosaminoglycans (Table 3B–2).

In addition to the five sulfated glycosaminoglycans, there is also one nonsulfated glycosaminoglycan, hyaluronic acid (Table 3B–2). This glycosaminoglycan is not covalently linked to a core protein and is therefore not present as a proteoglycan. Moreover, in contrast to the other glycosaminoglycans, it is not synthesized in the Golgi apparatus on a protein core, but rather at the plasma membrane of the cell with no lipid or protein primer being required. The molecule undergoes no polymer modification following synthesis, but consists solely of repeating disaccharides of glucuronic acid and N–acetylglucosamine. The molecule is also extremely long (M_r up to 6×10^6), approximately 300 times the length of a typical sulfated glycosaminoglycan (M_r 2×10^4). These unique structural features endow hyaluronic acid with distinct functional properties in the connective tissue matrix.

With the exception of the action of a heparanase in some tumors, glycosaminoglycan degradation ordinarily occurs within the lysosomes of cells by a series of glycosidases and sulfatases. For the sulfated glycosaminoglycans that reside outside the cell, this necessitates their initial release from a proteoglycan by the action of proteinases, thus allowing cellular uptake by endocytosis. Once within the cells, degradation commences by the action

Table 3B–2. *Structural features of glycosaminoglycans*

Glycosaminoglycan	Initial Disaccharide	Polymer Modification	Protein Linkage
Hyaluronic acid	GlcA–GlcNAc	None	None
Chondroitin sulfate	GlcA–GalNAc	GalNAc-SO$_4$	Yes[1]
Dermatan sulfate	GlcA–GalNAc	GlcA→IdA IdA-SO$_4$ GalNAc-SO$_4$	Yes[1]
Heparan sulfate/Heparin	GlcA–GlcNAc	GlcA→IdA IdA-SO$_4$ GlcNAc-SO$_4$ GlcNAc→GlcNSO$_3$ GlcNSO$_3$-SO$_4$	Yes[1]
Keratan sulfate	Gal–GlcNAc	Gal-SO$_4$ GlcNAc-SO$_4$	Yes[2]

[1] Linkage to serine by Xyl–Gal–Gal–GlcA.

[2] Linkage to serine or threonine in aggrecan and to asparagine in fibromodulin and lumican by distinct oligosaccharides.

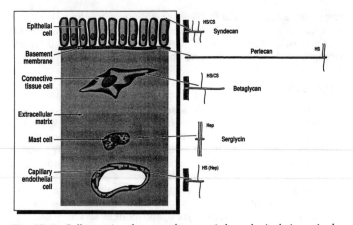

Fig. 3B–1. *Cell-associated proteoglycans. A hypothetical tissue is depicted with surface epithelial cells on an underlying basement membrane and connective tissue matrix. The matrix contains connective tissue cells, capillaries and mast cells. Proteoglycans typical of these various cell types are depicted, with their extended core proteins drawn to the same scale. The type of glycosaminoglycan chain present on each proteoglycan is indicated: HS/CS, heparan sulfate and chondroitin sulfate chains; Hep, heparin chains; HS(Hep), heparan sulfate chains with regions analogous to heparin. For the cell surface proteoglycans, the plasma membrane of the cell is also depicted.*

of endoglycosidases, such as hyaluronidase, followed by a series of exoglycosidases and sulfatases. These latter enzymes are only capable of acting at the terminus of the glycosaminoglycan fragments, and must do so in a sequential manner to permit complete degradation. If one of the enzymes is defective, glycosaminoglycan degradation cannot proceed, and storage of the partially degraded product occurs within the cells. This forms the basis of the mucopolysaccharidoses (3). The type of glycosaminoglycan affected will depend on the precise defective enzyme. This gives rise to the variety of clinical phenotypes observed. In all cases the disorders are characterized by hepatomegaly, as liver endothelial cells are the major site of glycosaminoglycan degradation.

CELL-ASSOCIATED PROTEOGLYCANS

Proteoglycans may be conveniently classified into those that remain associated with the cell following synthesis (Fig. 3B–1), and those that are secreted and reside within the extracellular matrix (Fig. 3B–2). The latter class is abundant in connective tissues. To some extent, the glycosaminoglycan type utilized by the two classes of proteoglycans differs. Cell-associated proteo-

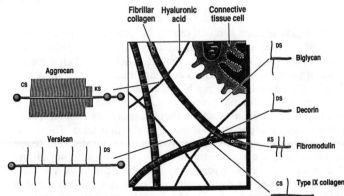

Fig. 3B–2. *Extracellular matrix proteoglycans. A hypothetical connective tissue matrix containing collagen fibrils and hyaluronic acid is depicted, together with part of a connective tissue cell in which a mitochondrion and rough endoplasmic reticulum are visible. Proteoglycans present in such a matrix are depicted, with their extended core proteins drawn to the same scale. In the case of aggrecan and versican, the sites of globular domains present along the core proteins are indicated. The type of glycosaminoglycan chain usually present on each proteoglycan is also indicated: DS, dermatan sulfate; KS, keratan sulfate; CS, chondroitin sulfate. In the case of type IX collagen only the $\alpha2(IX)$ chain is depicted.*

glycans commonly bear heparin/heparan sulfate or chondroitin sulfate, whereas the matrix proteoglycans bear chondroitin sulfate, dermatan sulfate, or keratan sulfate, although this distinction is not absolute. The cell-associated proteoglycans may be subdivided further into those that reside on the outer surface of the plasma membrane and those that are present in intracellular storage granules. The former category is present on all cells, but the latter is confined principally to cells of the myelocytic lineage, including mast cells. The cell surface proteoglycans may be subdivided according to the mechanism by which attachment to the plasma membrane occurs. This may be either via the core protein of the proteoglycan or the heparan sulfate chains. In the latter case association is via interaction with cell surface receptors.

A typical cell surface proteoglycan is represented by syndecan present on epithelial cells (4). It consists of a core protein bearing both heparan sulfate and chondroitin sulfate chains. There are commonly one or two chains of each type. The core protein of syndecan can be divided into three functional regions: a large N–terminal domain that resides outside the cells and bears the glycosaminoglycan chains, a short central hydrophobic domain that allows intercalation within the plasma membrane, and a short C–terminal cytoplasmic domain. The heparan sulfate chains on the extracellular domain allow interaction with matrix proteins such as collagen, fibronectin, and laminin, and may also permit cell–cell adhesion via self-association. In this manner the cell is localized in the tissue. The neoplastic phenotype has been associated with altered heparan sulfate structure and proteoglycan degradation, thus impairing cellular interaction. While syndecan is limited mainly to epithelial cells, proteoglycans having a similar structure have been characterized on other cell types, for example, fibroglycan (5), and it is likely that proteoglycans having similar features are also present on connective tissue cells. It should, however, be pointed out that cell surface proteoglycans do not necessarily require the structural features of syndecan for attachment to the plasma membrane. A heparan sulfate–proteoglycan from human lung fibroblasts, termed glypican, is anchored to the plasma membrane via a phosphatidylinositol linkage (5). This type of cell surface proteoglycan does not possess a transmembrane domain.

Betaglycan is a cell surface heparan sulfate–proteoglycan that contains functional domains equivalent to those of syndecan, with heparan sulfate and chondroitin sulfate chains being attached to the large extracellular domain. This proteoglycan corresponds to the type III TGF-β receptor (6). However, the glycosaminoglycan chains are not essential for the binding of TGF-β, since the latter binds to the core protein. Betaglycan is also able to bind bFGF via its heparan sulfate chains. There is considerable interest in the role of proteoglycans as potential mediators of growth factor action and their consequent roles in normal tissue physiology and pathology.

The intracellular proteoglycans are not structurally related to the cell surface proteoglycans, and appear to be the product of a single gene, which encodes the proteoglycan serglycin. This molecule derives its name from a central region of repeating serine/glycine residues to which either chondroitin sulfate or heparin may be bound. In the mature mast cell heparin is present, whereas less mature cells of the same lineage possess an oversulfated chondroitin sulfate. The region containing the glycosaminoglycan chains shows resistance to proteolysis, and varies in length between species (7). In man, the gene for serglycin consists of three exons, with the region encoding the serine/glycine repeat of 18 amino acids residing in exon 3. It was initially thought that the heparin proteoglycan of the mast cell provided for the natural anticoagulant needs of the body. However, it is now appreciated that heparan sulfate–proteoglycans present on the surface of vascular endothelial cells also possess heparin-like properties (8). Unlike most heparan sulfate chains, those of the vascular endothelial cells show regions of overmodification resembling the antithrombin III binding sequences of heparin.

Another proteoglycan that bears heparan sulfate chains is that present in basement membranes, designated perlecan because of its ultrastructural appearance. The core protein of this proteoglycan is very long and consists of a series of globular domains. The three probable attachment sites for heparan sulfate all reside

at the N–terminal end of the molecule (9). In man, perlecan is encoded by a gene on chromosome 1. The presence of heparan sulfate on this proteoglycan endows it with the capacity for interaction with other basement membrane components. In the glomerular basement membrane, perlecan is thought to limit protein permeability. A deficiency in this proteoglycan is observed in diabetes.

MATRIX PROTEOGLYCANS THAT INTERACT WITH HYALURONIC ACID

Proteoglycans that function in the extracellular matrix may be conveniently classified into those that interact with hyaluronic acid and those that interact with collagen. The former class have commonly been called aggregating proteoglycans, because the interaction of many proteoglycan molecules with a single hyaluronate molecule results in the formation of large proteoglycan aggregates. The best characterized member of this family is the large proteoglycan of articular cartilage, aggrecan (10) (Fig. 3B–2).

Aggrecan is characterized by its high abundance of glycosaminoglycan chains, which are commonly chondroitin sulfate but frequently include keratan sulfate. The core protein of aggrecan is long and may be divided into four regions based on its electron microscope appearance. Two globular domains (G1 and G2) are found at the amino terminus of the core protein and one (G3) at the carboxy terminus. The central portion of the molecule consists of a long extended domain to which over 100 glycosaminoglycan chains may be attached. There are differences in the sequence of the extended domain between species, which influence the relative degree of modification of the proteoglycans by chondroitin sulfate and keratan sulfate chains. The N–terminal globular domain is responsible for the interaction with hyaluronate and is commonly termed the hyaluronic acid binding region (HABR). The adjacent globular domain has homology with this region but does not participate in hyaluronate binding. The C–terminal globular domain has a variable structure due to alternative splicing and is commonly absent from the mature matrix proteoglycans due to proteolytic processing. The aggrecan gene contains 15 exons, with most of the glycosaminoglycan attachment region being encoded by the large exon 10.

Aggrecan is not unique to the matrix of hyaline cartilage, but is also present in other connective tissues subjected to compressive loads. It forms a major constituent of the intervertebral disc and those areas of tendons that pass over bone in a joint. However, the requirement for an aggregating proteoglycan need not necessarily be fulfilled by aggrecan in all connective tissues. A second aggregating proteoglycan, termed versican, has been described (11). Its core protein is similar in size to that of aggrecan, but it possesses only one globular domain at both its amino and carboxy termini. The N–terminal domain is homologous to the hyaluronate-binding domain of aggrecan. Versican also contains many less consensus sequences for glycosaminoglycan attachment than aggrecan, which presumably influences its functional role. The aggregating proteoglycan present in the aorta is likely versican, judging from its appearance on electron microscopy.

The interaction between aggrecan and hyaluronic acid is noncovalent and reversible. In the tissue, the interaction of each aggrecan molecule is stabilized by the additional interaction of a glycoprotein called link protein. A similar mechanism probably stabilizes versican aggregation also. Link protein is not a proteoglycan. It does not possess a glycosaminoglycan chain, but its core protein does show considerable homology with the hyaluronate-binding regions of aggrecan and versican (12). It consists of three disulfide-bonded loops. The central and C–terminal loops are homologous and are responsible for the interaction with hyaluronate, whereas the distinct N–terminal loop can interact with the proteoglycan. The structure of link protein changes throughout life due to proteolytic processing, although this does not appear to affect the function of the molecules. The link protein gene consists of four exons, with each functional region being encoded by a separate exon. In man, this gene is present on chromosome 5.

A molecule that exhibits structural homology with link protein is CD44, a cell surface glycoprotein that may exist in a proteoglycan form on some cells (13). It is present on fibroblasts as a chondroitin sulfate–proteoglycan. CD44 consists of multiple domains with multiple functions. One extracellular domain is homologous to the hyaluronate-binding loops of link protein, and gives CD44 the properties of a hyaluronate receptor. Such a function may have an important role in the binding of cells to hyaluronate in extracellular matrices or at the plasma membrane of other cells. In inflammation, CD44 may facilitate leukocyte homing to hyaluronate on the surface of vascular endothelial cells at the inflammatory site. CD44 may also play a role in regulating lymphocyte activation.

MATRIX PROTEOGLYCANS THAT INTERACT WITH COLLAGEN

This group of proteoglycans is distinct from the aggregating proteoglycans in both structure and function (Fig. 3B–2). They have much shorter core proteins and possess only a few glycosaminoglycan chains. Their widespread distribution among different connective tissues probably indicates a requirement for their presence wherever collagen fibrils are present. However, the abundance of the different members of the family varies among different tissues, suggesting unique functional roles.

Decorin, which is present in all connective tissues, possesses only one glycosaminoglycan chain, near the amino terminus of its core protein. In most connective tissues this is dermatan sulfate, although in bone, chondroitin sulfate is present because epimerization does not occur. In the tissues where dermatan sulfate is synthesized, the chain length and the degree of epimerization and sulfation can vary considerably. This may influence the functional role of the decorin molecules, for while interaction with the collagen fibrils is mediated via the core protein, the dermatan sulfate chain can promote self-association. These interactions have been postulated to aid in collagen fibril association to form fibers. A deficiency in decorin has been reported in a variant form of Ehlers–Danlos syndrome, whereas overproduction of decorin has been reported in some patients with scleroderma. In addition, a genetic defect that perturbs the synthesis of the dermatan sulfate chain of decorin has been reported in a patient with a progeroid syndrome (14).

Decorin shows considerable structural similarity to a second dermatan sulfate–proteoglycan, termed biglycan (15). In contrast to decorin, biglycan has two glycosaminoglycan chains near the amino terminus of its core protein. Both proteoglycans are the products of distinct genes that are present on different chromosomes in man. The decorin gene is on chromosome 12 and the biglycan gene is on the X chromosome. The biglycan gene consists of eight exons. The relative expression of the two proteoglycans varies between different connective tissues, as does their localization within the extracellular matrix. Biglycan is found mainly in the pericellular region. The difference in localization may relate to the low capacity of biglycan to interact with fibrillar collagens. This is surprising in view of the structural homology between the core protein of biglycan and decorin, and presumably indicates a unique functional role.

Structural homology with the core proteins of decorin and biglycan is also shown by fibromodulin (16). Unlike decorin and biglycan, however, fibromodulin does not bear dermatan sulfate chains near its amino terminus. Instead it possesses up to four keratan sulfate chains within its central region, attached to the core protein at asparagine residues. Additional collagen-binding N–linked keratan sulfate–proteoglycans also exist, particularly in the cornea where a proteoglycan termed lumican has been identified. At least in this tissue, it is apparent that the keratan sulfate–proteoglycans and dermatan sulfate–proteoglycans interact at different sites along the collagen fibrils, and probably fulfill different functional roles. Abnormalities in corneal organization are observed in macular corneal dystrophy, where defects in the structure of the glycosaminoglycans on either class of proteoglycan can occur. In contrast, lack of transparency in healing corneal scars is associated with an initial deficiency in the keratan sulfate–proteoglycans.

Another collagen-associated proteoglycan is a collagen itself.

Type IX collagen located along the periphery of type II collagen fibrils may bear a chondroitin sulfate chain on its $\alpha2(IX)$ chain (17). This molecule does not show any structural homology with other collagen-associated proteoglycans. It is of particular interest in hyaline cartilage because of its basic NC4 domain, which may serve as a link between the fibrillar collagen network and the surrounding anionic proteoglycans and hyaluronic acid. Type IX collagen also exists in the cornea and vitreous of the eye, although in both cases the NC4 domain is absent. The role of the chondroitin sulfate chain is unclear. In cartilage it may be present or absent from the type IX collagen, and in the vitreous it is exceedingly long in some species and may replace hyaluronic acid as the major carbohydrate constituent.

GROWTH FACTORS, CYTOKINES AND PROTEOGLYCAN METABOLISM

Proteoglycans and glycosaminoglycans can bind and modulate growth factor function. The reverse is also true, in that the interaction of a growth factor with its cell surface receptor can modulate both the quantity and structure of the proteoglycans produced by the cell. Both insulin-like growth factor (IGF–I) and transforming growth factor–β (TGF–β) increase the rate of aggrecan synthesis and decrease its rate of catabolism in articular cartilage. In osteoarthritis, there is increased synthesis of aggrecan and extensive replacement of degraded molecules (18). TGF–β is of particular interest as it can be synthesized by chondrocytes and sequestered in the cartilage matrix, presumably through interaction with resident proteoglycans. The expression of biglycan and versican by fibroblasts is also increased by the action of TGF–β. Not all proteoglycan synthesis is up-regulated by TGF–β. Levels of decorin are down-regulated and those of fibromodulin show little change in fibroblasts. However, the effect of a given growth factor on proteoglycan synthesis may vary with cell type and age. Finally, TGF–β may influence not only core protein expression, but in some cases may also affect the synthesis of the glycosaminoglycan chains, which in turn could potentially affect the function of the proteoglycan.

In contrast to IGF–I and TGF–β, the cytokine IL–1 downregulates the production of aggrecan by articular cartilage. Furthermore, this cytokine also increases the degradation of matrix proteoglycans by stimulating metalloproteinase synthesis. The metalloproteinase stromelysin has been considered a prime candidate for causing proteoglycan degradation, although this is not the only proteinase activity generated by IL–1. The effect of IL–1 on proteoglycan synthesis occurs at lower doses than its effect on degradation, and both processes occur by independent post-receptor mechanisms. In the case of inhibition of proteoglycan synthesis, it has been reported that induction of IL–6 is required in some systems. As a result of the adverse effects of IL–1 on proteoglycan metabolism, it has been suggested that IL–1 may have a role in the generation of arthritic lesions in cartilage. However, the effect of IL–1 appears more pronounced on young human cartilage than on old, which may provide some protection to the adult.

Because some growth factors have an opposite effect on proteoglycan synthesis from IL–1, the possibility exists that they can be used to counteract the detrimental influence of this cytokine. Both IGF–I and TGF–β can at least partially reverse the adverse effect of IL–1 on both proteoglycan synthesis and degradation (19). However, this does not necessarily mean that growth factors can be used to reverse the effects of IL–1 on arthritic cartilage. In an experimental arthritis model it has been shown that chondrocytes lose their responsiveness to IGF–I. Unfortunately, few of the antiinflammatory drugs used in the treatment of arthritis have a stimulatory effect on proteoglycan synthesis, and none can reverse the detrimental effects of cytokines (20). However, the possibility of future drug therapy is still feasible with new drug development, and the potential for inhibiting the detrimental effects of IL–1 on cartilage has already been demonstrated with the anti-tumor drugs, doxorubicin and methotrexate. In addition, it is likely that physiologic agents that directly interfere with cytokine/receptor interaction could be used in a therapeutic manner. Such agents include soluble forms of tumor necrosis factor–α and IL–1 receptors and the IL–1 receptor anatagonist.

PROTEOGLYCANS AS IMMUNOGENS

Immunity to proteoglycans involves both B and T lymphocyte recognition of these molecules. Only protein epitopes are recognized by T cells, including the G1 globular domain of aggrecan (21). Immunity to aggrecan, involving both B and T cells, leads to the development of an erosive polyarthritis and spondylitis in BALB/c mice. The disease can be passively transferred into irradiated recipients. Some of the most interesting antibodies to proteoglycans include those that recognize epitopes on chondroitin sulfate chains. Although several have been described, the chemical identities of the epitopes generally have not been studied. These epitopes are usually found in embryonic and fetal tissues, and are almost completely absent in the adult. However, in osteoarthritis, these epitopes can reappear both in experimental and human disease, and may serve as disease markers (22).

Peter J. Roughley, PhD
A. Robin Poole, PhD, DSc

1. Kjellén L, Lindahl U: Proteoglycans: Structures and interaction. Ann Rev Biochem 60:443–475, 1991
2. Jackson RL, Busch SJ, Cardin AD: Glycosaminoglycans: Molecular properties, protein interactions, and role in physiological processes. Physiol Rev 71:481–539, 1991
3. Hopwood JJ, Morris CP: The mucopolysaccharidoses: Diagnosis, molecular genetics and treatment. Mol Biol Med 7:381–404, 1990
4. Bernfeld M, Sanderson RD: Syndecan, a developmentally regulated cell surface proteoglycan that binds extracellular matrix and growth factors. Phil Trans Roy Soc Lond B 327:171–186, 1990
5. David G: Biology and pathology of the pericellular heparan sulphate proteoglycans. Biochem Soc Trans 19:816–820, 1991
6. Lopez-Casillas, Cheifetz S, Doody J, et al: Structure and expression of the membrane proteoglycan betaglycan, a component of the TGF–β receptor system. Cell 67:785–795, 1991
7. Avraham S, Stevens RL, Nicodemus CF, et al: Molecular cloning of a cDNA that encodes the peptide core of a mouse mast cell secretory granule proteoglycan and comparison with the analogous rat and human cDNA. Proc Natl Acad Sci USA 86:3763–3767, 1989
8. Marcum JA, Rosenberg RD: Anticoagulantly active heparan sulfate proteoglycan and the vascular endothelium. Semin Throb Hemostasis 13:464–474, 1987
9. Noonan DM, Fulle A, Valente P, et al: The complete sequence of perlecan, a basement membrane heparan sulfate proteoglycan, reveals extensive similarity with laminin A chain, low density lipoprotein-receptor, and the neural cell adhesion molecule. J Biol Chem 266:22939–22947, 1991
10. Doege KJ, Sasaki M, Kimura T, et al: Complete coding sequence and deduced primary structure of the human cartilage large aggregating proteoglycan, aggrecan: Human-specific repeats, and additional alternatively spliced forms. J Biol Chem 266:894–902, 1991
11. Zimmerman DR, Ruoslahti E: Multiple domains of the large fibroblast proteoglycan, versican. EMBO J 8:2975–2981, 1989
12. Neame PJ, Christner JE, Baker JR: The primary structure of link protein from rat chondrosarcoma proteoglycan aggregate. J Biol Chem 261:3519–3535, 1986
13. Culty M, Miyake K, Kincade PW, et al: The hyaluronate receptor is a member of the CD44 (H-CAM) family of cell surface glycoproteins. J Cell Biol 111:2765–2774, 1990
14. Quentin E, Gladen A, Rodén L, et al: A genetic defect in the biosynthesis of dermatan sulfate proteoglycan: Galactosyltransferase 1 deficiency in fibroblasts from a patient with a progeroid syndrome. Proc Natl Acad Sci USA 87:1342–1346, 1990
15. Fisher LW, Termine JD, Young MF: Deduced protein sequence of bone small proteoglycan I (biglycan) shows homology with proteoglycan II (decorin) and several nonconnective tissue proteins in a variety of species. J Biol Chem 264:4571–4576, 1989
16. Oldberg A, Antonsson P, Lindblom K, et al: A collagen-binding 59-kd protein (fibromodulin) is structurally related to the small interstitial proteoglycans PG-S1 and PG-S2 (decorin). EMBO J 8:2601–2604, 1989
17. Shaw LM, Olsen BR: FACIT collagen: Diverse molecular bridges in extracellular matrices. Trends Biochem Sci 16:191–194, 1991
18. Rizkalla G, Reiner A, Bogoch E, et al: Studies of the articular cartilage proteoglycan aggrecan in health and osteoarthritis: Evidence for molecular heterogeneity and extensive molecular changes in disease. J Clin Invest, 90:2268–2277, 1992
19. Poole AR: Cartilage in health and disease, Arthritis and Allied Conditions, A Textbook of Rheumatology. Edited by McCarty D, Koopman W. Philadelphia, Lea and Febiger, 12th ed, 279–333, 1993
20. Kolibas LM, Goldberg RL: Effects of cytokines and anti-arthritic drugs on glycosaminoglycan synthesis by bovine articular chondrocytes. Agents Action 27:245–249, 1989
21. Leroux J-Y, Poole AR, Webber C, et al: Characterization of proteoglycan-reactive T cell lines and hybridomas from mice with proteoglycan-induced arthritis. J Immunol 148:2090–2096, 1992
22. Caterson B, Mahmoodian F, Sorrell JM, et al: Modulation of native chondroitin sulphate structure in tissue development and in disease. J Cell Sci 97:411–417, 1990

4. THE ROLE OF IMMUNOLOGIC MECHANISMS IN THE PATHOGENESIS OF RHEUMATIC DISEASE

THE IMMUNE SYSTEM—NONSPECIFIC AND SPECIFIC

The immune system evolved to defend the body against foreign organisms and to maintain the sterility of the internal milieu. Although the most remarkable features of vertebrate immunity are the specificity and memory of the immune response, significant defense also derives from nonspecific mechanisms. These include the mucosal barriers, complement (particularly the alternative pathway, discussed in Chapter 7C), natural killer (NK) cells, preformed "natural" antibodies, and the activity of mononuclear and polymorphonuclear phagocytes.

Parts of the nonspecific immune system contribute to the pathogenesis of the inflammatory processes characteristic of most of the rheumatic diseases. In addition, inherited deficiencies of single complement components are associated with greatly increased risks for certain autoimmune diseases (1). Certain aspects of these systems may be important in the basic etiology of autoimmunity, although the mechanisms are not at present understood.

The specificity and the memory of the specific immune system provide two important advantages over the nonspecific immune system. First, the specific system learns to distinguish self from non-self. In this way, the highly efficient effector agents, antibodies, and cytotoxic T cells, can target external invaders without causing self damage. Second, these same features permit an immune response to focus on a specific antigenic attack by increasing production of the most efficient effector cells. It is probable that defects in self/non-self discrimination by the specific immune system are related to the basic causes of autoimmune diseases.

Structure and Development

The adult human immune system consists mostly of lymphocytes and mononuclear phagocytes. The latter are widely distributed in tissues. Lymphoid cells, in contrast, are primarily concentrated in the central lymphoid organs (spleen, bone marrow, thymus, and lymph nodes), although many lymphocytes recirculate through the lymphatics and peripheral blood. In humans, the bulk of immunoglobulin is produced in the bone marrow, while the spleen is the next most important site of antibody synthesis (2).

During fetal development, hematopoietic stem cells emerge from the yolk sac and populate the bone marrow, spleen, and liver, where differentiation into lymphoid and myeloid cells occurs. Later, the bone marrow becomes the major source of lymphoid and mononuclear phagocyte precursors. The thymus also plays a critical and complex role in the development and differentiation of T cells. Such cells originate in the bone marrow, but they usually pass through the thymus in order to acquire immunocompetence. Mature T lymphocytes are responsible for cell-mediated immunity and regulation of both humoral and cellular immunity. They can be readily distinguished from B lymphocytes by the presence of specific cell surface markers, such as CD2, CD3, CD4, CD8, and CD11, and by the absence of surface or cytoplasmic immunoglobulin (3). During their maturation in the thymus, some aspects of self-tolerance are established, and the specificity of the T cell repertoire becomes skewed toward recognition of foreign antigens in conjunction with self major histocompatibility complex (MHC) determinants. While this process may continue in adult life, the thymus is clearly of greatest importance during fetal and early neonatal T cell development.

B cells, on the other hand, develop independently of the thymus, although they are also derived from bone-marrow. B cell developmental pathways can be followed by observing the expression of cell surface markers, such as surface Ig, CD19, and class II MHC, and sequential rearrangement and expression of the genes coding for the H and L chains of immunoglobulin (4).

A central concept for the understanding of the immune system is the process of clonal selection. Individual lymphocytes are precommitted in their immune specificity before interaction with antigen. The biochemical basis for this precommitment is the selection for surface expression of a single antigen receptor from a vast number of possibilities determined by germline genes that undergo rearrangement and other somatic modifications. Upon interaction with antigen, clones of precommitted, receptor-bearing lymphocytes can undergo rapid expansion and differentiation, producing large numbers of specific B or T cells in a short time. This clonal growth depends not only on the interaction of the preexisting antigen receptor with antigen, but also on additional signals from other immunoregulatory lymphocytes, such as T helper cells, which recognize antigen by their surface receptors.

THE SPECIFIC IMMUNE RESPONSE

A *specific* immune response can be generated by both the cellular and humoral immune systems. Cellular immune responses are independent of immunoglobulin and are primarily directed by T lymphocytes. Humoral immunity depends on antibody molecules secreted by lymphocytes of the B cell lineage. Although the two systems overlap and interact, the dichotomy is useful. The cellular and humoral responses each depend on clonal expansion of specific precursor lymphocytes. The molecular mechanisms for generating the antigen receptors on T cells and B cells by selective utilization of a large repertoire of receptor genes are similar. In addition, nucleotide sequence homology suggests that the genes for the T cell receptor and for immunoglobulin molecules share a common evolutionary origin, and that other molecules important in the immune system, such as the MHC determinants and CD8, also belong to this "supergene family" (5).

Antigen Processing

In order to elicit an immune response, antigen must first come into contact with antigen-presenting cells (APC). Protein antigens undergo a highly organized process of enzymatic degradation and transport, which results in their reduction to simple peptides expressed on the cell surface bound to MHC determinants (6). As a rule, peptides derived from proteins synthesized within the cell associate with class I MHC molecules as they are transported to the cell surface (7). In contrast, the antigenic peptides bound to class II MHC molecules are generally derived from exogenous proteins that are ingested and then degraded in lysosomes. They then bind to intracellular class II MHC molecules in a post-Golgi compartment and are transported to the cell membrane (8). B lymphocytes are particularly efficient at processing and presenting antigens (9), since their antigen receptors can specifically trap and focus antigen. B cells express abundant class I and class II MHC determinants. The presentation of antigen by the B cell to the helper T cell efficiently directs the helper function of that T cell back onto the B cell, which will, in turn, be driven to antibody production. Other APC are also of importance in the

immune response, especially those with restricted tissue distribution, such as dendritic cells in the skin and lymph nodes and tissue-specific macrophages such as Kupffer cells in the liver.

The recognition by T cells of peptide antigen on APC is restricted by polymorphic molecules of the MHC (10). The specificity of this restriction results from the interactions of differentiating T cells with the MHC determinants of the host environment, mostly within the thymus. This "learning" process involves negative selection against those T cells that strongly react with self-MHC or with self-MHC plus non-MHC autoantigens (repertoire deletion). At the same time, T cells specific for potential foreign antigens in the context of self-MHC are positively selected (repertoire skewing). T cells that fail to go through this positive and negative intrathymic selection undergo programmed death. The resultant repertoire of T cells does not respond to self-MHC alone or to self-MHC plus self-peptide, but will recognize foreign antigens plus self-MHC. The molecular basis of this restricted recognition is the specificity of the T cell receptor for MHC plus antigen complexes.

The complex of MHC and antigen that is recognized by the T cell receptor is composed of the processed antigen, in the form of a peptide of limited length, associated with the MHC molecule on the surface of the APC. X-ray crystallographic studies have demonstrated a groove on the surface of class I and class II MHC molecules, in which antigenic peptides reside. Class I MHC molecules bind peptides of ~9 amino acid length (11); class II molecules accommodate peptides of 10–34 amino acids (12). The non-MHC-coded invariant chain stabilizes newly synthesized intracellular class II molecules that have not yet combined with peptides (13). Class I and class II MHC molecules isolated from cells not specifically challenged with antigen are nearly all associated with peptides derived from self proteins: class I binds peptides from cytosolic and nuclear proteins; while class II mainly binds peptides derived from membrane proteins, including other MHC molecules.

The selective association of certain MHC alleles with antigen-derived peptides may be related to the phenomenon of MHC-linked immune response (IR) gene effects (14). Some animal strains respond better than others to a certain immunogen. The responsible genes usually map to the MHC locus. This IR gene effect is highly specific for a given genotype and antigen; that is, a certain MHC type may confer responsiveness to antigens A, B, and C, while another genotype may respond well to C, D, and E. Several explanations for IR gene action can be offered. A responder phenotype MHC moiety may bind the immunogenic peptide of an antigen, while the corresponding non-responder MHC proteins may fail to bind. Alternatively, IR gene phenomena may be due to MHC-determined selection of the T cell repertoire, to the intervention of specific suppressor cells, or to the action of transporter or proteolytic enzyme genes also found in the MHC (15,16). Such IR gene effects may be related to the linkage of many autoimmune diseases to certain MHC alleles, particularly class II alleles.

The MHC-restricted interaction between the APC and the T cell delivers an activation signal to the T cell through its receptor. In addition, the APC produces a number of soluble molecules (cytokines) that also affect T cell functions, including IL–1, which also has effects beyond the immune system (17,18). APC-produced IL–1 can interact with IL–1 receptors on these same cells and activate them so that they can, in turn, provide stimulatory signals to T cells. Interleukin–1 may also interact directly with the T cells (19,20).

T Cells

In a T cell-dependent antibody response, CD4$^+$ T helper cells react with antigen associated with class II MHC determinants on the surface of the APC. On most T cells, the receptor that mediates this recognition is a complex of proteins consisting of two ~45 kDa peptides (alpha and beta), each of which contains variable and constant regions (21), and a complex of invariable proteins collectively designated CD3 (22). An important minor population of T cells instead expresses a distinct receptor with polymorphic chains termed gamma and delta, also in association

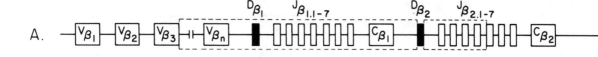

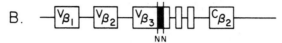

*Fig. 4–1. Organization and rearrangement of the genes for the beta chain of the human T-cell receptor. **A**. Germline configuration. **B**. Possible somatic rearrangement that utilizes the Vβ3 gene, Dβ2 element, Jβ2.5 element, and Cβ2 constant region gene. The portions of DNA enclosed in the dashed boxes in A are deleted during the process of somatic rearrangement in order to produce the complete T-cell receptor gene shown in B. The N regions marked are short sequences of nucleotides added at the junctions between the variable region and the D region, and between the D region and the J region.*

with CD3 (23). γ–δ T cells appear to serve important functions in defense of the gut mucosa and female genital tract. The α, β, γ, and δ chains undergo the special somatic rearrangements characteristic of the genes coding for the T cell and B cell antigen receptors. The genetic organization of the β chain is shown in Fig. 4–1. Multiple variable (V) regions are encoded 5′ to several short D region genes, followed by two constant region genes with separate J elements. During the development of an individual T cell, one variable region gene joins with one D and one J region gene by irreversible recombination events. The V–D and D–J joining positions can be somewhat variable, and non-genomic nucleotides can be added at these junctions, such that additional variability is created. The final VDJ product is transcribed into messenger RNA, along with one of the constant regions, and provides the template for the translation of the β chain of the T cell receptor. It is the process of selection of a particular V gene, D gene, and J gene; the precise joining of these elements; and the addition of a small number of nucleotides at the junctional points that determine the final sequence of the expressed β chain. This sequence, in conjunction with a similarly determined α chain sequence, then forms the T-cell receptor gene and determines its antigen and MHC specificity. Similar principles apply to the organization of the α, γ, and δ T cell receptor genes. The variety of available V, D, and J genes, along with the multiple combinatorial arrangements of their utilization; a similar set of possibilities for the α chain; and the possibility of pairing different α and β chains, all result in an enormous potential variability in the T cell receptor.

The activation of T cells by interaction of the receptor with specific antigen on the APC is augmented by auxiliary molecules such as CD4, CD8, and LFA–1. Other T cell molecules, such as CD2 (which interacts with LFA–3) and CD28 (which interacts with the B-cell-specific B7 protein), are critical to T cell activation and are called co-stimulator molecules (20). Normally, the initial activation of T cells involves crosslinking of the T cell receptor complex. In the presence of co-stimulation, this leads to stimulation of the phosphatidylinositol pathway (24). Multiple tyrosine kinases play a key role in receptor-mediated T cell activation (25); these events are mediated through the cytoplasmic components of CD3 (26). Activated T cells express receptors for the lymphokine interleukin–2 (IL–2), a 30 kDa protein required for further proliferation (27). Some CD4⁺ T cells are also capable of synthesizing IL–2, thereby supplying their own receptors with ligand and permitting so-called autocrine growth; other T lymphocytes must rely on IL–2 produced by other T cells. In addition, some activated T cells express receptors for interleukin–4 (IL–4, BSF–1), which functions like IL–2 in promoting growth of T and B cells (28).

Activated T cells produce other bioactive molecules with potent effects on the immune response (29). Among the most important are those which act on macrophages, such as macrophage migration inhibition factor (MIF), which causes the localization and activation of macrophages (30). Such recruited macrophages are different from the resting macrophages that may have initially ingested antigen. These activated cells have enhanced rates of phagocytosis, and are much more potent killers and inactivators

of microorganisms. They contribute to the typical acute lesion of delayed type hypersensitivity and are capable of forming epithelioid cells and giant cells characteristic of granulomata.

Some antigens, such as mycobacteria and fungi, elicit a purely cellular immune response. Most antigens, however, elicit a mixture of cellular and humoral reactivity. This usually requires the collaboration of CD4⁺ T cells with B lymphocytes. T cell help is most efficiently delivered by cell-to-cell contact mediated through the recognition of antigen presented in the context of class II MHC molecules on the surface of the B cell. In addition, helper T cells produce lymphokines capable of stimulating B cells in an antigen-nonspecific manner. T helper cells can be classified into two categories, based on the pattern of their lymphokine production (31). T$_{H1}$ cells produce IL–2, interferon–γ (IFN–γ), and granulocyte–monocyte colony stimulating factor (GM–CSF). T$_{H2}$ cells, by contrast, produce IL–4, IL–5, IL–6, and IL–10. Both T$_{H1}$ and T$_{H2}$ cells produce the hematopoietic growth factor interleukin–3 (IL–3) (32). In general, T$_{H1}$ cells promote delayed hypersensitivity reactions, while T$_{H2}$ cells stimulate production of IgG and IgE. Interferon–γ has important antiviral activity and induces NK cells. Interleukin–3 and GM–CSF are important in controlling the production of mast cells and phagocytic cells, thus contributing to the intensity of the overall immune response. In addition to these cytokines, a large number of additional factors (some exclusively T-cell derived, others of more general origin) exert positive and negative effects on the immune response.

The other major class of human T cell bears the cell surface protein CD8. Except for a subpopulation within the thymus, CD4⁺ T cells and CD8⁺ T cells constitute mutually exclusive subsets. CD8⁺ cells mediate MHC-restricted T cell killing. This phenomenon requires cell-to-cell contact through the T cell receptor and results in the lysis of target cells by a mechanism that may involve the exocytosis of proteins stored in cytoplasmic granules as well as apoptosis (programmed death) of the target cell. CD8⁺ cells have specificity for peptide antigens in conjunction with class I MHC products, the HLA–A, B, and C antigens. They constitute a critical defense against viruses and other intracellular organisms.

T suppressor cells in humans also bear CD8 (33). The difficulty in isolating such cells by present cloning techniques has impeded progress in understanding them, but they may serve important regulatory functions in the immune response. In some cases they have been shown to function through the elaboration of the cytokine TGF–β.

B Cells and Immunoglobulins

The B cell lineage derives from bone marrow precursors without undergoing differentiation in the thymus. In birds, the bursa of Fabricius is required for B cell development (hence the name B cell or bursal-derived cell), but no mammalian equivalent has been described. B cells are found in all the lymphoid organs, particularly in human tonsils, and in the germinal centers of lymph nodes and spleen. They express surface immunoglobulin Fc receptors (CDW 32), class II MHC molecules, and other

Table 4–1. *Human immunoglobulin classes (heavy chain isotypes)*

	IgM	IgD	IgG1	IgG2	IgG3	IgG4	IgA1	IgA2	IgE
H chain	μ	δ	$\gamma 1$	$\gamma 2$	$\gamma 3$	$\gamma 4$	$\alpha 1$	$\alpha 2$	ϵ
Molecular weight (kD)	900	180	150	150	150	150	160–350	160–350	190
Serum concentration (mg %)	100	3	900	300	100	50	300	50	0.001
Complement fixation by classical pathway	+++	–	++	+	+++	–	–	–	–
Placental transfer	–	–	+	+	+	+	–	–	–
Plasma half life (days)	5	3	21	20	7	21	6	6	2
$(H_2L_2)_n$, n=	5	1	1	1	1	1	1,2	1,2	1
Number of domains per heavy chain	5	5	4	4	4	4	4	4	5
Carbohydrate (%)	12	12	3	3	3	3	9	9	12

determinants recognized by monoclonal antibodies (CD19, CD20).

The major function of the B cell is to produce antibodies. B cells also are efficient at presentation to T cells of the antigens for which they are specific. For a B cell to fulfill its functions, it needs to be activated (34). The resting B cell bears surface immunoglobulin (usually IgM and IgD) as its antigen-specific receptor. Several additional invariable peptide chains are expressed in conjunction with the receptor and presumably mediate transmembrane signal transduction (35). When such a cell is appropriately stimulated, it undergoes differentiation and proliferation, which result in cells that initially are more effective at specific antigen presentation and eventually secrete large quantities of immunoglobulin with the same specificity, but not necessarily the same isotype, as the precursor's surface receptor. Some of these immunoglobulin-producing cells have a plasma cell morphology, although some still resemble lymphocytes. Activation of B cells can occur in several ways. Responses to so-called "T-dependent" antigens require interaction with helper T cells, mediated through CD40 or other B cell costimulatory surface molecules. An additional signal that is generally required for B cell activation is provided by antigen, particularly if the antigen can cross-link the B cell surface receptors. This may explain why antigens that have multiple repeating determinants, such as bacterial polysaccharides, can activate B cells in the absence of T cell help (T-independent antigens). Certain substances, such as lipopolysaccharide or pokeweed mitogen, or even viruses such as Epstein–Barr, can activate B cells in an antigen-nonspecific manner. The heterogeneous antibody response to such substances is called polyclonal activation. B cells can be found in tissues in different stages of activation, such that the requirements for differentiation into antibody-producing cells may vary depending on the previous experience of the individual cells. B cells also can be divided into different subsets based on surface markers such as CD5, although the functional significance of these divisions is not yet clear.

The principal product of the fully differentiated, activated B cell is immunoglobulin. The immunoglobulins are a group of glycoproteins that can be divided into nine principal classes or isotypes (Table 4–1). Each of these classes has a similar molecular structure (Fig. 4–2). The basic subunit consists of a multimer of two identical heavy chains of molecular weight 50,000–75,000, combined with two identical light chains of molecular weight 25,000. The light chains themselves exist in two classes, kappa and lambda, either of which can associate with any of the heavy-chain isotypes. The approximate 100 N-terminal amino acids of both the heavy and light chains comprise the variable region, and the remainder of the molecule is termed the constant region. The constant region itself is organized in domains of approximately 100 amino acids. The number of these constant domains varies from one for the light chains to five for the μ, δ, or ϵ heavy chains. The domains are folded into compact globular configurations. In a single molecule, adjacent heavy-chain domains can interact noncovalently or through disulfide bonds, as do heavy and light chain variable regions and the constant domain of the light chain and the first constant domain of the heavy chain (Fig. 4–2). The IgG and IgE molecules always exist as combinations of two heavy chains and two light chains (H_2L_2). Most IgM molecules and many IgA molecules have the H_2L_2 subunit aggregated into multimers (($H_2L_2)_5$ for IgM) through inter-subunit disulfide bonds and association with an additional polypeptide chain called

the J chain. When the IgA molecules are secreted through epithelial surfaces, they are associated with another peptide chain called the secretory fragment.

The constant region of the immunoglobulin molecules of a particular isotype is generally homogeneous, although there are allelic genetic variants, referred to as immunoglobulin allotypes. Many of the physiologic functions of the immunoglobulins, such as complement fixation by IgM, IgG1, IgG2, and IgG3, or binding to mast cells by IgE and IgG4, are mediated through one or more of the constant domains. The variable region, on the other hand, is responsible for specific binding to antigen. As its name implies, it differs from antibody to antibody, such that the variable regions present in the serum of a normal individual at a given time are heterogeneous and may represent millions of possibilities. Any given clone (progeny of a single mature B cell) of antibody-forming cells makes immunoglobulins with the same basic variable region. Large quantities of a single monoclonal immunoglobulin can be seen in individuals with multiple myeloma or related lymphoproliferative diseases. Individual clones of B cells can also be selected and propagated experimentally by hybridoma technology.

Within the variable region of the heavy and light chains, three subregions called hypervariable regions or complementarity-determining regions show even greater variation from molecule to molecule. The amino acid sequences between such regions are known as frameworks and are less variable. The hypervariable regions of the heavy chain, combined with the hypervariable regions of the light chain, form a pocket or cleft on the surface of the immunoglobulin molecule. This cleft is generally the site of interaction with antigen. This interaction with antigen is noncovalent but can be quite strong, so that for physiologic purposes it is sometimes irreversible. The antigen seen by antibody is usually in its native, soluble form and is not complexed with self-MHC determinants.

The variable regions of the B cell receptor immunoglobulin

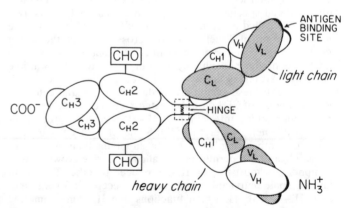

Fig. 4–2. The structure of an IgG molecule. Two identical heavy chains and two identical light chains are joined together by noncovalent and disulfide interactions as shown. Additional disulfide bonds may also exist between the C_H1 domain of the heavy chain and the C_L domain of the light chain. The hinge regions between the C_H2 and C_H1 domains are cross-linked by several disulfide bonds. Carbohydrate (CHO) is bound to the C_H2 domain. Antibodies of other isotypes have basically similar structures, although they may have different numbers of domains in the heavy chain, different placement of disulfide bonds and carbohydrates, and may be complexed into multimers of the basic H_2L_2 subunit.

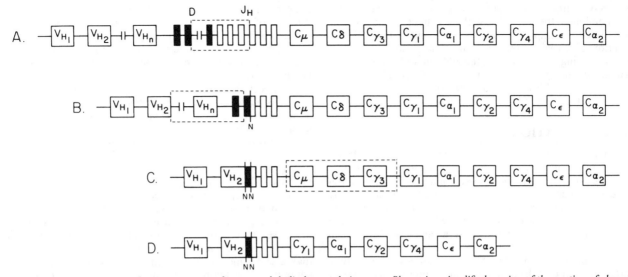

Fig. 4–3. *Genetic organization and rearrangement of immunoglobulin heavy chain genes. Shown is a simplified version of the portion of chromosome 14 containing the immunoglobulin heavy chain variable region and constant region genes. A. Genomic organization, found in all cells except committed B cells. B. Initial rearrangement produces the D-J joining, which results from deletion of the DNA enclosed in the dashed box in A. The junction between D and J regions includes additional random nucleotides constituting an N region. Two nucleotides can also be added from the non-coding DNA strand, resulting in a P region. C. The next step in rearrangement is V–D–J joining, which results from the deletion of the DNA enclosed in dashed box in B. A B cell expressing the rearranged gene shown in C might express IgM with the V$_{H2}$ variable region. D. Such a B cell could then undergo an isotype switch by deleting the DNA shown in the dashed box in C to express IgG1 with the same V$_{H2}$ variable region.*

molecules are the same as those expressed on the immunoglobulin molecules eventually secreted by such a B cell or its progeny. Since the binding avidity or strength of interaction of this immunoglobulin receptor with antigen determines whether a B cell will be stimulated, B cells with higher avidity receptors for antigen will be selectively activated. Consequently, as an immune response matures, antibodies of higher and higher avidity are produced. The overall avidity of antigen–antibody interactions is governed by the affinity of the antigen for the antibody-combining sites, but it also depends on the valency of interaction. The IgG molecules are divalent (two heavy/light-chain pair-determined combining sites per molecule), while the multimeric immunoglobulins, such as IgM, have even higher potential valencies.

The immunoglobulin molecule itself may function as an antigen. It is relatively easy to raise anti-immunoglobulin antibodies by immunizing one species with the immunoglobulins of another species. Such antibodies generally react with the constant regions of the immunizing immunoglobulins, and they can be isotype-specific. Anti-constant region autoantibodies have clinical importance, as discussed in Chapter 8B. The variable regions of immunoglobulins may also serve as antigens. When antibodies are directed to determinants that depend on the specific structure of a given variable region, they are called anti-idiotypes (36). Not only are such anti-idiotypes useful in identifying immunoglobulin variable region genes, but they may play an important role in normal immunoregulation.

Major advances in the understanding of the basis of immunoglobulin variable region diversity and immunoglobulin gene organization have occurred over the last 10 years. The genes for kappa and lambda light chains are found on separate chromosomes (chromosome 2 for kappa, chromosome 22 for lambda). All of the heavy chain genes are found in a small region of chromosome 14. The association of relatively few constant region-determined isotypes with multiple variable regions is accomplished by utilizing different genes for the variable and constant regions (Fig. 4–3). The heavy chain genetic locus is organized in a manner analogous to that of the T cell receptor beta chain. Multiple (about 200) variable region genes are represented by families of closely related genes. At 3' on the chromosome to the variable regions are about nine D region genes, followed by six functional J region genes. Further 3' are the constant region genes. The variable region genes code for approximately 100 amino acids, the D region for 0–5 amino acids, and the J region approximately five amino acids. As a given B cell

develops, it first recombines a single D region with a single J region segment. It subsequently rearranges the DJ pair with one variable region gene. Although in fetal development 3' variable regions may be preferentially used, for the most part the rearrangement process appears to be random. The rearrangements usually occur by removing the DNA between the chosen gene segments and splicing of those segments together. The D and J genes help determine the third hypervariable region of the heavy chain. The rearrangement of these genes can occur in various ways, often including the addition of several extra nucleotides (N region and P region), which further diversifies the third hypervariable region. Once a heavy chain variable region gene is appropriately rearranged, the B cell can then rearrange a light chain gene in a similar manner. The kappa and lambda light chains each have their own individual sets of variable region, J, and constant region genes. Abortive rearrangements, which are incapable of producing a messenger RNA that codes for a complete translatable heavy or light chain, are common. An individual B cell will eventually utilize only a single heavy chain and a single light chain variable region gene, although it may switch light chains if the one initially selected results in an autoreactive specificity (receptor editing). Consequently, a B cell clone expresses a homogenous (monoclonal) immunoglobulin.

The rearranged immunoglobulin genes are transcribed in such a way that they are initially expressed as a membrane form of IgM and IgD, which can be inserted onto the B cell's surface as the antigen receptor (37). As the B cell differentiates, it can switch to express constant regions 3' to μ and δ, for example, IgG3. It usually does this by recognition of specific genomic switch regions and splicing out the intervening constant regions at the DNA level.

An additional mechanism that contributes to immunoglobulin variable region diversity is somatic hypermutation. After stimulation by antigen, B cells pass through a developmental phase during which a high rate of DNA mutation is focused on the rearranged variable region gene segment. Base-pair changes that result in antibody peptide chains with enhanced antigen binding cause positive selection of the resultant higher affinity B cells. An ongoing antibody response therefore matures by becoming increasingly dominated by a small number of B cell clones, and the members of those clones accumulate replacement mutations affecting particularly their complementarity-determining regions.

The overall potential for variable region diversity, and therefore for antigen-binding possibilities, is great (38). First, multiple variable region genes exist for both the heavy chains and the light chains. Second, in an H_2L_2 pair, heavy chain variable regions may be combined theoretically with any light chain variable regions, thereby multiplying the possible combinations. Third, the selection of D regions (heavy chains only) and J regions, as well as the splicing variability and the addition of N and P region amino acids, create at least another order of magnitude of potential diversity in the third hypervariable region. Fourth, somatic mutation introduces still further variability.

IMMUNOREGULATION

The immune system is regulated at a number of different levels in order to maintain normal physiologic homeostasis. Initially, the system's non-responsiveness to self antigens is learned. Response to an exogenous antigen by T cells and B cells has already been described. The interactions that occur ensure that immunoreactivity to an invading microorganism will be enhanced at the appropriate time and in the most useful anatomic site. Such responses must also be down-regulated, if they are not to exhaust the organism or to develop malignant or autoimmune potential.

The requirement that the immune system ignore a vast array of self molecules to which it is constantly exposed, and yet be prepared to respond vigorously to an even larger repertoire of potential exogenous antigens, is met by learned immunoregulatory control mechanisms capable of maintaining a fine balance in each individual. For the most part, nonreactivity to self is a result of *immune tolerance*, which is the lack of response to a specific antigen based on prior exposure (39). Genetic diversity within a species demands that tolerance be a learned phenomenon. Because each individual expresses multiple self-antigenic determinants, which may differ from those of other individuals, the genes that determine immune reactivity (the T cell receptor and immunoglobulin variable regions) could not efficiently delete autoreactivity on a germline genetic basis without leaving extensive gaps in the potential repertoire for recognition of foreign antigens. Instead, self reactivity is controlled as part of the development of each individual immune system. In this way, pathogenic autoimmunity is avoided. The failure of such immunoregulation may lead to the self reactivity characteristic of many of the rheumatic diseases.

Tolerance can be induced by several mechanisms. T cells are more easily tolerized than B cells in experimental systems, and this probably holds true for self antigens. For both T cells and B cells, tolerance can result from deletion of those cells bearing antigen receptors that recognize self components (40). Self-reactive cells can also be inactivated (anergized), a process sometimes accompanied by changes in surface phenotype (41). T suppressor cells supply negative signals that prevent responses by some potentially autoreactive cells, although the cellular and molecular mechanisms utilized by such cells remain controversial. Finally, certain self antigens are normally hidden from the immune system and provoke no reactivity as long as they remain so.

The avoidance of autoimmunity is not absolute. Certain kinds of autoantibodies are routinely seen after infectious processes, for example anti-lymphocyte antibodies, and these normally do not lead to pathologic consequences. In addition, some $CD4^+$ T cells recognize self class II antigens (the so-called autologous mixed lymphocyte reaction). Self reactivity to autologous immunoglobulin idiotype is also a normal physiologic response and may in itself be an important form of immunoregulation. A certain degree of autoreactivity thus normally occurs and must be controlled to prevent autoimmune disease.

The mechanisms of immune regulation have been best studied for exogenous antigens. A key factor is antigen. The immune response generally does not begin until the organism has been appropriately exposed to exogenous antigen. The subsequent removal of this antigen through normal physiologic degradation by both immune and non-immune mechanisms leads to a diminution of the ongoing response, because the differentiative and proliferative potential of activated T cells and B cells is limited in the absence of an ongoing antigenic stimulus. Another important factor in immunoregulation is antibody. In general, the administration of specific antibody at the time of immunization with

antigen suppresses the potential immune response. Likewise, the removal of endogenous antibody during an ongoing immune response causes an increase in antibody production. A potentially important exception to the down-regulatory effect of antibody is that certain subclasses of IgG, such as IgG2a in the mouse, can be specifically stimulatory rather than inhibitory (42). This may have important immunopathologic consequences.

T cells play a major role in orchestrating the immune response. T helper cells are of critical importance for responses to many antigens, as already described. Likewise, the immune response is probably down-regulated by T suppressor cells, which may act on other T cells or on B cells directly. The cytokines produced by one T cell subset may inhibit another. For example, T_{H1} cells produce IFN-γ, which downregulates T_{H2} cells, while T_{H2} cells produce IL-10, which downregulates T_{H1} cells.

Much of immunoregulation is specific. Cells or factors that control one immune response will generally not affect parallel responses to different antigens. This specificity results in part from antigen recognition by regulatory cells. Specific regulation may also be mediated through recognition of idiotype. In fact, some investigators have postulated that the components of the immune system are linked through extensive self recognition of individual idiotypes to form a network that functions even without antigen stimulation (43). Whether or not this is true, it is still probable that individual immune systems recognize the idiotypic determinants of their own immunoglobulins and T cells. This anti-idiotype reactivity occurs both through anti-idiotypic antibodies and idiotype-recognizing T cells. Such recognition has been clearly shown in experimental situations to have an important potential for controlling immune responses. For example, pre-administration of anti-idiotype antibodies to a mouse can prevent that mouse from producing idiotype-bearing antibodies (44), even though such antibodies would normally be made following challenge with antigen. The production of antibodies during the course of a normal immune response may likewise engender anti-idiotypic antibodies with the potential of down-regulating the response in a specific manner. So far, the evidence is only suggestive that such physiologic idiotype control actually occurs (45).

Although the fine tuning of the immune system and the distinction between self and non-self are achieved mainly through mechanisms of specific immunoregulation, a number of influences can also affect immune reactivity in a non-antigen specific manner. For example, the immune reactivity to a given antigen can liberate cytokines that are not antigen specific and therefore can influence an irrelevant parallel response, such as by favoring the development of T_{H1} over T_{H2} cells, or vice versa. In addition, several endocrine hormones are known to have profound effects on the immune system. For example, corticosteroids can inhibit immune responses. Certain cell types have effects on the immune system without antigen specificity. Macrophages activated by such influences as lipopolysaccharide are nonspecifically immunosuppressive. Natural killer cells, a subset of lymphocytes without classical antigen specificity, can in some circumstances be immunosuppressive. Additionally, environmental influences, including drug ingestion and nutrition, can affect the immune system. Certain drugs, such as cytotoxic agents, are immunosuppressive, because they preferentially affect proliferating cells. Protein and calorie malnutrition is immunosuppressive in itself; however, specific nutritional deficiencies, particularly of heavy metals such as zinc, can have profound effects on the immune system, at least in experimental animals (46).

IMMUNOPATHOLOGY

The immune system protects the individual against invasion by agents that are perceived as foreign. On the other hand, in many human diseases, the immune system can be injurious to the organism. In some cases, this immunopathology is an unavoidable by-product of the immune system's attempts to attack a chronic infectious agent. In conditions such as tuberculosis or leprosy, the destructive effects of the invading organism are magnified by an intense immune reaction. The treatment of such diseases, of course, is to destroy the invading organism, although in some cases a short-term down-regulation of the immune system with corticosteroids is of benefit. In conditions such as sarcoidosis, histologic and epidemiologic evidence suggests an immune reaction to an external insult; however, since the agent has not been identified, corticosteroids alone are sometimes used for therapy. It is possible that the synovial immune infiltrates that are important in the pathology of inflammatory arthritis such as rheumatoid arthritis, Reiter's syndrome, or ankylosing spondylitis, are also directed toward as yet unidentified infectious agents.

Immune injury can also result from the inappropriate targeting by the immune system of self-components. The differentiation between self and non-self depends on the ability of the immune system to learn specificities. Certain types of self-recognition are part of normal physiology, including anti-idiotype immunoregulation and MHC recognition by T cells. Abnormal autoimmunity, on the other hand, occurs in a variety of rheumatic diseases and probably plays important immunopathologic roles in many of them. In human conditions, the best studied and most convincing demonstrations of pathologic autoimmunity are for autoantibodies. However, sites of ongoing tissue inflammation in autoimmune diseases, such as systemic lupus erythematosus (SLE), Sjogren's syndrome and rheumatoid arthritis, are heavily infiltrated with T lymphocytes, which suggests that cell-mediated autoimmunity may also play an important role (47). Unfortunately, it has thus far been impossible to show convincingly that these T lymphocytes exhibit specific autoreactivity. Nevertheless, the recent demonstration of specific immunopathologic T cell autoreactivity in several animal models of organ-specific autoimmune disease strongly suggests that similar mechanisms occur in human disease.

The development of pathologic autoimmunity represents, therefore, a failure of the normal immunoregulation of the immune system. Several potential mechanisms could result in autoimmunity, although most of these possibilities have yet to be demonstrated in human disease.

Hidden antigen. Some autologous antigens are anatomically confined and not exposed to the immune system. If tissue injury should cause these antigens to escape from their anatomic seclusion, active immunization may occur, which would result in further tissue injury and more release of antigen. Such a mechanism may pertain in sympathetic ophthalmitis, which occurs in the contralateral eye after injury to a single eye.

Molecular mimicry. Infection with a microorganism may generate an appropriate immune response that cross-reacts with autologous body constituents, perhaps on the basis of homologous segments of host and parasite protein sequences. Such a mechanism probably occurs in rheumatic fever. In this condition, the immune reaction to streptococci cross-reacts with heart antigens, at least at an antibody level (48). Whether these cross-reactive antibodies directly cause cardiac manifestations of rheumatic fever has not been proven.

Cross-reactive antigen. Immunization with a related foreign antigen may bypass T cell tolerance and stimulate a response to an autologous antigen. Immunizing a mouse with a heterologous thyroglobulin, for example, elicits an anti-thyroglobulin response. This response recognizes the foreign thyroglobulin and also murine thyroglobulin, and causes an autoimmune thyroiditis (49). Since thyroglobulin-reactive B cells have been demonstrated in intact normal animals, it is probable that the T cell help generated against the foreign determinants on the heterologous protein causes this response by permitting the self-reactive B cells to be activated to produce autoantibody. Curiously, such activated B cells may then in turn stimulate T cells that recognize the autologous antigens (50).

Altered determinants. If autologous antigens are denatured so that new epitopes are presented to the immune system, an immune response may occur that could also recognize the native autologous antigen.

Change in valence. The induction of tolerance requires a certain threshold avidity of interaction between antigen and the immune receptors of the lymphocytes being tolerized. Cells bearing receptors of lower affinity would therefore remain in a nontolerant state. If the antigen in question is aggregated such that it presents its determinants in a multivalent fashion, the effective avidity of interaction with immune receptors could be greatly increased, and low-affinity B cells would be activated. This effect of valence may be particularly important in generation of rheumatoid factors.

Adjuvant. The administration of certain chemicals or biologic substances with antigen enhances immune responses (51). For example, the injection of an autoantigen, such as myelin basic protein in complete Freund's adjuvant (a mixture of oil and killed tubercle bacilli), can induce an autoimmune reaction with pathologic consequences (experimental allergic encephalomyelitis).

Anti-idiotype. Although the self-recognition of idiotype may play a role in normal immunoregulation, in other cases the idiotypic network can lead to destructive autoimmunity (52). This mechanism has been demonstrated experimentally in rabbits. Immunization of one rabbit with an acetylcholine analog results in antibodies to this material. Since this analog is also recognized by the acetylcholine receptor, the combining site of some of the antibodies resembles the active site of the acetylcholine receptor. If these anti-acetylcholine analog antibodies are then used to immunize a second rabbit, anti-idiotype antibodies are generated, some of which recognize those first antibodies resembling the acetylcholine receptor. Therefore, these anti-idiotypes are themselves directed at the acetylcholine receptor and produce the pathologic effects of myasthenia gravis (53).

Immune complexes. In some special cases, immune complexes may provoke an autoimmune reaction. This effect probably explains the generation of rheumatoid factors in mice during the course of a normal secondary immune response (54). Immune complexes consisting of foreign antigen and specific antibody are readily recognized by B cells that express rheumatoid factor specificity, because of the increased affinity of interaction due to the multivalence of the immunoglobulin determinants in the immune complex. These rheumatoid-factor-specific B cells may then ingest the entire immune complex and present the foreign antigen in conjunction with their own class II molecules to T helper cells directed against the foreign antigen. These T cells will thereby provide help for rheumatoid factor production.

Nonspecific bypass of immunoregulation. Several mechanisms can provide abnormal help to B cells and thereby simultaneously activate a number of autoantibody specificities. Such mechanisms may be applicable to diseases characterized by generalized autoimmunity, such as SLE.

1) Loss of suppressor cells. Since suppressor cells down-regulate the immune response, a general loss or malfunction of such cells might be predicted to cause abnormal autoimmunity. Although decreases in circulating suppressor cells have been found in certain autoimmune conditions, the significance of this finding remains to be shown.

2) Abnormal help. If T helper cells interacted with B cells in an abnormal way, they could stimulate a large subset of such cells, including those that could produce autoantibodies. Such a mechanism occurs in experimental chronic graft-versus-host reaction in inbred mice (55). In this model, injected T cells recognize the class II antigens expressed on the host B cells and stimulate them to produce the spectrum of autoantibodies characteristic of SLE.

3) Polyclonal activation. Polyclonal activators stimulate B cells in a way that bypasses the requirement for specific T cell help. In experimental models, the chronic injection of an activator such as lipopolysaccharide induces some autoantibodies (56).

4) Failure of tolerance mechanisms. If a biochemical pathway necessary for tolerance induction is defective, autoreactive cells will survive inappropriately. In *lpr* mice, for example, a mutation in an apoptosis receptor gene results in abnormal T cells and B cells that create systemic autoimmunity (57).

Autoimmune Disorders

Autoimmune syndromes can be categorized as induced versus spontaneous or as generalized (systemic) versus organ-specific. Induced autoimmunity occurs when an exogenous insult initiates the disease. An example of this is the induction of experimental allergic encephalomyelitis in mice or rats by the injection of myelin basic protein in complete Freund's adjuvant. Spontaneous autoimmunity occurs without any intervention. Examples of this are found in the inbred autoimmune mouse strains (MRL/ Mp-lpr/lpr, NZB, BXSB, and others), in which most animals spontaneously develop an SLE-like syndrome with a variety of autoantibodies and severe immunopathologic effects (57). In these animals, the disease appears to be genetically determined, with no necessary involvement of environmental agents. In human diseases, certain presumed autoimmune diseases are clearly induced by an external stimulus, such as rheumatic fever following streptococcal infection. In other conditions, such as SLE and related connective tissue diseases, no convincing evidence has implicated an external environmental agent, but the possibility has not been eliminated.

Categorizing autoimmune diseases as organ-specific versus generalized depends on the extent of the pathologic manifestations. Organ-specific diseases include thyroiditis, allergic encephalomyelitis, diabetes mellitus, and blistering dermatologic conditions such as bullous pemphigoid. In such disorders, a single organ system is affected and autoantibodies or T cell reactivity is directed at antigens specific for that organ system. Generalized autoimmune diseases are characterized by a wide spectrum of autoreactivity. The most extreme example is SLE, in which dozens of different autoantibody specificities have been defined. In these systemic conditions, the pathologic manifestations involve multiple organ systems, and therefore the clinical consequences are correspondingly varied. In addition, the existence of a variety of autoantibodies implies that the abnormalities of immunoregulation that generate systemic autoimmunity are probably different from those that produce organ-specific autoimmunity.

Classically, immunopathologic mechanisms have been characterized by the effectors of immune injury. The divisions in this paradigm are:

Type I, IgE-mediated. Antibodies of the IgE class can bind to basophils or tissue mast cells by a high-affinity Fc receptor. If such antibodies are cross-linked by binding to antigen, which is generally an external allergen, the mast cell is stimulated to release its basophilic granules, which contain vasoactive substances such as histamine, bradykinin, serotonin, and slow-reacting substance of anaphylaxis, as well as eosinophil chemotactic factor. This type of injury is most important in clinical allergy such as asthma or allergic rhinitis. Whether type I injury plays a role in the autoimmune rheumatic diseases remains to be shown, although IgE autoantibodies, including rheumatoid factors and antinuclear antibodies, have been found (58).

Type II, Antibody-mediated effects on cells. If autoantibodies bind to their antigen in the appropriate manner, complement can be activated with consequent additional inflammatory effects (see Chapter 7C). In addition, the antibody coated cells can bind to Fc receptors. This can result in phagocytosis or in cell killing through antibody-mediated cellular cytotoxicity. Such mechanisms probably occur in some kinds of autoimmune hemolytic anemia and in Goodpasture's disease. Autoantibodies to cell surface receptors can either block (insulin-resultant diabetes) or abnormally stimulate (Graves' disease) receptor-mediated functions.

Type III, Immune complexes (59). When soluble antigen and antibody form multimolecular complexes, the possibilities for fixing complement and binding to cellular receptors are greatly increased. The classical experimental model for such immune complex mediated injury is bovine serum albumin (BSA) induced serum sickness in rabbits. In the acute disease, a large quantity of the foreign protein (BSA) is injected intravenously. After four or five days, anti-BSA antibodies appear and complex with the BSA remaining in the circulation. Such immune complexes then deposit in the kidneys and vessels, resulting in an acute immune injury. Serum sickness after administration of large quantities of exogenous antigen such as horse serum is the clearest human counterpart of such a condition. Certain of the immunopathologic manifestations of other human conditions, such as SLE, resemble immune complex mediated injury, and immune complexes between autoantigens and autoantibodies are surely present in these conditions. It remains to be shown, however, whether such immune complexes in circulating form have direct immunopathologic consequences.

Type IV, Cellular reactivity. T cells can injure tissue containing foreign antigen or bearing autoantigens. CD4$^+$ T cells secrete lymphokines that attract and activate other inflammatory cells. CD8$^+$ T cells can be directly cytotoxic.

Robert A. Eisenberg, MD
Philip L. Cohen, MD

1. Agnello V: Lupus diseases associated with hereditary and acquired deficiencies of complement. Springer Semin Immunopathol 9:161–178, 1986
2. McMillan R, Longmire RL, Yelenosky R, et al: Immunoglobulin synthesis by human lymphoid tissues: Normal bone marrow as a major site of IgG production. J Immunol 109:1386–1394, 1972
3. Romain PL, Schlossman SF: Human T lymphocyte subsets: Functional heterogeneity and surface recognition structures. J Clin Invest 74:1559–1565, 1984
4. Alt FW, Blackwell TK, De Pinho RA, et al: Regulation of genome rearrangement events during lymphocyte differentiation. Immunol Rev 89:5–30, 1986
5. Hood L, Kronenberg M, Hunkapiller T: T cell antigen receptors and the immunoglobulin supergene family. Cell 40:225–229, 1985
6. Braciale TJ, Braciale VL: Antigen presentation: Structural themes and functional variations. Immunol Today 12:124–129, 1991
7. Townsend A, Bodmer H: Antigen recognition by class I-restricted T lymphocytes. Ann Rev Immunol 7:601–624, 1989
8. Harding CV, Unanue ER, Slot JW, et al: Functional and ultrastructural evidence for intracellular formation of major histocompatibility complex class II-peptide complexes during antigen presentation. Proc Natl Acad Sci USA 87:5553–5557, 1990
9. Chesnut RW, Grey HM: Antigen presentation by B cells and its significance in T-B interaction. Adv Immunol 39:51–94, 1986
10. Schwartz RH: T-lymphocyte recognition of antigen in association with gene products of the major histocompatibility complex. Ann Rev Immunol 3:237–261, 1985
11. Madden DR, Gorga JC, Strominger JL, et al: The structure of HLA-B27 nonamer self-peptides bound in an extended conformation. Nature 353:321–329, 1991
12. Rudensky AY, Preston–Hurlburt P, Hong SC, et al: Sequence analysis of peptides bound to MHC class II molecules. Nature 353:622–627, 1991
13. Teyton L, O'Sullivan D, Dickson PW, et al: Invariant chain distinguishes between the exogenous and endogenous antigen presentation pathways. Nature 348:39–44, 1990
14. Paul WE: Immune response genes. Immunogenetics, edited by Paul WE. Raven Press, New York, NY, 1984
15. Spies T, Bresnahan M, Bahram S, et al: A gene in the human major histocompatibility class II region controlling the class I antigen presentation pathway. Nature 348:744–747, 1990
16. Brown MG, Driscoll J, Monaco JJ: Structural and serological similarity of MHC-linked LMP and proteosome (multicatalytic proteinase) complexes. Nature 353:355–357, 1991
17. Dinarello CA, Savage N: Interleukin–1 and its receptor. Crit Rev Immunol 9:1–20, 1989
18. Platanias LC, Vogelzang NJ: Interleukin–1: Biology, pathophysiology, and clinical prospects. Am J Med 89:621–629, 1990
19. Mueller DL, Jenkins MK, Schwartz RH: Clonal expansion versus functional clonal inactivation: A costimulatory signalling pathway determines the outcome of T cell antigen receptor occupancy. Ann Rev Immunol 7:445–480, 1990
20. Geppert TD, Davis LS, Wacholtz MC, et al: Accessory cell signals involved in T-cell activation. Immunol Rev 117:5–66, 1990
21. Acuto O, Reinherz EL: The human T-cell receptor. New Eng J Med 312:1100–1111, 1985
22. Oettgen HC, Terhorst C: The T-cell receptor-T3 complex and T-lymphocyte activation. Human Immunol 18:187–204, 1987
23. Spits H: Human T cell receptor gamma delta+ T cells. Semin Immunol 3:119–129, 1991
24. Desai DM, Newton ME, Kodlecek T, et al: Stimulation of the phosphotidylinositol pathway can induce T-cell activation. Nature 348:66–69, 1990
25. Klausner RD, Samelson LE: T cell antigen receptor activation pathway: The tyrosine kinase connection. Cell 62:875–878, 1991
26. Letourneur F, Klausner RD: Activation of T cells by a tyrosine kinase activation domain in the cytoplasmic tail of CD3e. Science 255:79–82, 1992
27. Waldmann TA: The interleukin–2 receptor. J Biol Chem 266:2681–2684, 1991
28. Paul WE, Ohara J: B-cell stimulatory factor-I/interleukin–4. Ann Rev Immunol 5:429–459, 1987
29. Arai K, Lee R, Miyajma A, et al: Cytokines: Coordinators of immune and inflammatory responses. Ann Rev Biochem 59:783–836, 1990
30. Petit JF, Lemaire G, eds: Macrophage activation. Ann Inst Pasteur/Immunol 137C:191–249, 1986
31. Mosmann TR, Cherivinski H, Bond MW, et al: Two types of murine helper T cell clones. I. Definition according to profiles of lymphokine activities and secreted proteins. J Immunol 136:2348–2357, 1986
32. Ihle JN, Weinstein Y: Immunological regulation of hematopoietic/lymphoid stem cell differentiation by interleukin–3. Adv Immunol 39:1–50, 1986
33. Rich RR, Elmasry MN, Fox EJ: Human suppressor T cells: Induction, differentiation, and regulatory functions. Human Immunol 17:369–387, 1986
34. Clark EA, Pane PJL: Regulation of human B-cell activation and adhesion. Annu Rev Immunol 9:97–128, 1991
35. Reth N, Hombach J, Wienands J, et al: Control of B-cell activation. Immunol Today 12:196–201, 1991

36. Burdette S, Schwartz RS: Current concepts: Immunology. Idiotypes and idiotypic networks. New Engl J Med 317:219–224, 1987

37. Rogers J, Wall R: Immunoglobulin RNA rearrangements in B lymphocyte differentiation. Adv Immunol 35:39–59, 1984

38. Perlmutter RM, Crews ST, Douglas R, et al: The generation of diversity in phosphorylcholine-binding antibodies. Adv Immunol 35:1–37, 1984

39. Miller JFAP, Morahan G, Allison J: Immunological tolerance: New approaches using transgenic mice. Immunol Today 10:53–57, 1989

40. Kappler JW, Roehm N, Marrack P: T cell tolerance by clonal elimination in the thymus. Cell 49:273–280, 1987

41. Goodnow CC, Crosbie J, Adelstein S, et al: Altered immunoglobulin expression and functional silencing of self-reactive B lymphocytes in transgenic mice. Nature 334:676–682, 1988

42. Coulie PG, Van Snick J: Enhancement of IgG anti-carrier responses by IgG2 anti-hapten antibodies in mice. Eur J Immunol 15:793–798, 1985

43. Jerne NK: Towards a network theory of the immune system. Ann Inst Pasteur/Immunol 125C:373–389, 1974

44. Sacks DL, Kelsoe GH, Sachs DH: Induction of immune responses with anti-idiotypic antibodies: Implications for the induction of protective immunity. Springer Semin Immunopathol 6:79–97, 1983

45. Ortiz–Ortiz L, Weigle WO, Parks DE: Deregulation of idiotype expression: Induction of tolerance in an anti-idiotypic response. J Exp Med 156:898–911, 1982

46. Fraker PJ, Gershwin ME, Good RA, et al: Inter-relationships between zinc and immune function. Fed Proc 45:1474–1479, 1986

47. Fox RI, Howell FV, Bone RC, et al: Primary Sjogren syndrome: Clinical and immunological features. Semin Arthritis Rheum 14:77–105, 1987

48. Dale JB, Beachey EH: Epitopes of streptococcal M proteins shared with cardiac myosin. J Exp Med 162:583–591, 1985

49. Weigle WO: Analysis of autoimmunity through experimental models of thyroiditis and allergic encephalomyelitis. Adv Immunol 30:159–273, 1980

50. Lin RH, Mamula MJ, Hardin JA, et al: Induction of autoreactive B cells allows priming of autoreactive T cells. J Exp Med 173:1433–1439, 1991

51. Warren HS, Vogel FR, Chedid LA: Current status of immunological adjuvants. Ann Rev Immunol 4:369–388, 1986

52. Plotz PH: Autoantibodies are anti-idiotype antibodies to antiviral antibodies. Lancet 2:824–826, 1983

53. Wassermann NH, Penn AS, Freimuth PI, et al: Anti-idiotypic route to anti-acetylcholine receptor antibodies and experimental myasthenia gravis. Proc Natl Acad Sci USA 79:4810–4814, 1982

54. Coulie PG, Van Snick J: Rheumatoid factor (RF) production during anamnestic immune responses in the mouse. III. Activation of RF precursor cells is induced by their interaction with immune complexes and carrier-specific helper T cells. J Exp Med 161:88–97, 1985

55. Gleichmann E, Pals ST, Rolink AG, et al: Graft-versus-host reactions: Clues to the etiopathology of a spectrum of immunological diseases. Immunol Today 5:324–332, 1984

56. Izui S, Eisenberg RA, Dixon FJ: IgM rheumatoid factors in mice injected with bacterial lipopolysaccharides. J Immunol 122:2096–2102, 1979

57. Cohen PL, Eisenberg RA: *Lpr* and *gld*: Single gene models of systemic autoimmunity and lymphoproliferative disease. Annu Rev Immunol 9:243–270, 1991

58. Zuraw BL, O'Hair CH, Vaughan JH, et al: Immunoglobulin E-rheumatoid factor in the serum of patients with rheumatoid arthritis, asthma, and other diseases. J Clin Invest 68:1610–1613, 1981

59. Williams RC: Immune complexes in clinical and experimental medicine. Harvard University Press, Cambridge, Mass., 1980

5. IMMUNOGENETICS

The immune response of each person is nearly unique, as is evident in their particular response to certain epitopes of antigens or allergens, their rejection of allografts, and their susceptibility to develop different rheumatic diseases that have an immune pathogenesis. This individuality of the immune response is primarily determined by genetic variations in the class I and II major histocompatibility complex (MHC) molecules or, as they are alternatively designated, the HLA molecules.

ROLE OF HLA MOLECULES IN INFLUENCING HOW ANTIGENS ARE RECOGNIZED AND IN DETERMINING SUSCEPTIBILITY TO RHEUMATIC DISEASE

Unlike the immunoglobulin (Ig) molecules on B cells that directly bind antigenic fragments, the clonotypic T cell antigen receptor only complexes to antigen fragments after the fragments have been bound to class I or class II MHC molecules. In this trimolecular interaction, much of the surface of the T cell antigen receptor also binds to part of the MHC molecule forming a context of "self" MHC in which the antigen is recognized. The phenomenon of *MHC restriction* results from the specificity of this interaction, because the clonally expanded group of T cells is restricted to seeing the same antigen in the context of the same MHC molecule. Because of this trimolecular interaction of antigen, MHC molecule, and T cell receptor, the different allelic forms of the HLA molecules significantly influence the recognition properties of a person's immune system in two ways. First, the differences in amino acid sequence of allelic forms of MHC molecules cause selective binding of one or another of the amino acid side chains of an antigenic fragment. This is known as the process of *determinant selection*. Thus, antigenic peptides (typically processed to a length of 8–9 amino acids) that bind effectively to one allelic form of a class I MHC molecule may not bind to another allelic form of the class I MHC molecule as a function of different complementary interactions between amino acid side chains of the peptide and those forming pockets and binding regions in the antigen binding cleft of the particular MHC molecule. The second way different MHC molecules influence immune responsiveness is by determining the T cell receptor repertoire. During the formation of the T cell repertoire before birth, MHC molecules select T cell clones bearing certain T cell antigen receptors from the nearly limitless number of clonal receptors that are randomly generated. This positive and negative selection

process explains the restriction of the immune response to self-MHC molecules and also accounts for tolerance of self, largely through the presentation of fragments of autologous antigens on self MHC molecules during early ontogeny. Random selective events in the formation of the T-cell repertoire are likely to be one of the reasons why identical twins are not 100% concordant for autoimmune diseases (1). As an important consequence of the tolerance process, T cells that might otherwise play a role in host defense but are reactive to self antigens presented in the context of an individual's particular polymorphic MHC molecule might be deleted, forming "holes" in the recognition properties of the T cell repertoire that vary from individual to individual.

Determining an individual's MHC genes by HLA typing is a simple way to gauge the role of genetically determined influences on immune recognition. Diseases may develop through a determinant selection mechanism in which particular self peptides have an amino acid sequence that would fit into the peptide binding cleft of a certain type of HLA molecule in such a way as to trigger T cell clones into an immune recognition event that bypasses tolerance. Molecular mimicry between an antigen and a self-component might induce such a bypass. Alternatively, diseases may develop through a "hole" formed during T cell repertoire generation. The immune system could exhibit a selective impairment in the ability to recognize specific antigenic peptides which might, for example, be critically involved in effectively eliminating a pathogen. Equipping nearly every person with a slightly different immune system selected by their HLA molecules appears to be a mechanism to avoid presenting a pathogen with a relatively fixed immune defense system common to all members of a species, thus creating a static target for the pathogen's evolution. Autoimmune disease can be thought of as a consequence of this requirement.

CLASS I GENES

A summary of genetic terminology appears in Table 5–1. The human MHC is situated on the short arm of chromosome 6 and encodes two somewhat similar varieties or classes of molecules, termed *class I* or *class II*, that share a close evolutionary relationship with both Ig and T cell receptor molecules (Fig. 5–1 and 5–2; Table 5–2). Class I molecules are present on virtually all nucleated cells. They are functionally specialized to combine with the CD8 molecule found on most cytotoxic T cells, and the T cell repertoire of CD8 T cells is selected to recognize antigens

Table 5–1. Genetic terminology

Term	Definition
Alleles	Alternative forms of genes arising by mutation and other mechanisms found in the population.
Allotype	The genetically determined alternative forms of the same molecule (allomorph) that characterize different people.
Dominance, Recessivity	The consequences of the outcome of an interaction among various gene products at the level of expression.
Gene	The unit of genetic information.
Genotypes	The various genes under consideration in an individual.
Haplotype	A group of linked genes located on an extended region of a single chromosome of either maternal or paternal origin.
Ia molecule	Generic term for class II MHC molecules. DR, DQ, and DP are three molecularly distinct kinds of class II or I2 molecules that are independently expressed.
Isotype	Distinguishable but homologous non-alternative forms of molecules encoded by different genes derived from an original primitive gene. Isotype differs from allotype in that all members of the species have each of these homologous molecules.
Locus	The segment of chromosome that contains a particular gene.
Penetrance	The extent to which, for example, a potentially dominant gene is actually expressed as a dominant trait as a reflection of the totality of the other genes in the individual.
Phenotype	The expression of the genotype as gene products and their resultant interaction.
Polymorphism	The presence of alleles at a frequency higher than can be accounted for by mutation, implying some positive selections.
Region	The general portion of the chromosome that contains two or more genes with related origins or functions.

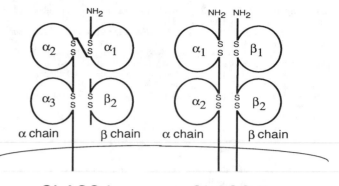

CLASS I   CLASS II

Fig. 5–2.   Class I and II molecules have a generally similar organization of their domains with two significant exceptions. In class II molecules the antigen binding superdomain is composed of the symmetric contribution of one domain from the α-chain (α1) and one from the β-chain (β1). In the class I molecule this superdomain is formed from one chain (α1 and α2 domains). In class I molecules the shortened β-chain (β2 microglobulin) forms a domain without a membrane spanning C-terminus.

presented in the context of MHC class I molecules. Class I molecules are "charged" during their synthesis by antigen fragments that usually arise endogenously from the cytoplasm of the cell. Accordingly, they alert the CD8 lineage cytotoxic T cells to the presence of virus-infected or otherwise altered body cells, providing immune surveillance. This mechanism eliminates cells supporting viral replication or undergoing certain types of virally driven neoplastic transformation.

The largest region of the MHC contains the class I genes that are arranged over about 1800 kb of DNA. The HLA–A locus is quite removed from that of HLA–B and HLA–C. There are several additional class I loci that have less well understood functions (Fig. 5–3). The class I molecule consists of a heavy or α chain, approximately 43,000 d in mass, with three extracellular

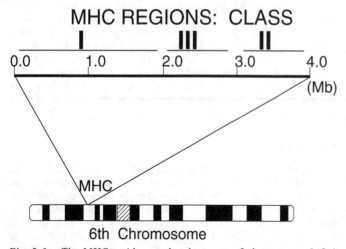

MHC REGIONS: CLASS

I   III   II

0.0   1.0   2.0   3.0   4.0

(Mb)

MHC

6th Chromosome

Fig. 5–1.   The MHC resides on the short arm of chromosome 6. It is divided into three main regions that are composed of nearly four million nucleotide base pairs.

domains, a transmembrane segment, and a small intracellular region (Fig. 5–2). The extracellular domains somewhat loosely bind a β2 microglobulin chain that consists of one domain. β2 microglobulin is essentially invariant and is not encoded by a gene in the MHC. The first two α chain domains combine to form the familiar basket-like structure in which antigenic fragments are presented (Fig. 5–4). This figure depicts the peptide backbone without amino acid side chains. The coiled sides of the antigen binding cleft are α-helices with amino acid side chains that either extend upward toward the T cell receptor or inwards into the antigen binding cleft. The residues comprising the floor of the cleft form a β-pleated sheet that contacts only the antigenic peptide and not the T cell receptor. HLA–A, HLA–B, and HLA–C loci encode the three different principal isotypes of the class I molecule. Each differs in certain characteristic amino acids from the other, but they exhibit the same overall organization and structure, resulting in the potential for six different MHC class I gene products on the surface of each nucleated cell.

The genes of these three loci in the population have undergone extensive mutations and other types of alterations resulting in a segregant series of alleles that encode the different HLA class I types or *allomorphs* (Table 5–3). The location of polymorphic amino acid residues that define the different allelic products are shown as numbers in circles in Fig. 5–4. There are several regions in the α chain that are located in the antigen binding cleft where polymorphic amino acid residues specified by the particular allele form hydrophilic or hydrophobic pockets in which the amino acid side chains of antigenic peptide bind with high or low affinity. The peptide antigen is typically 8–9 amino acids long, is usually oriented with its aminoterminus to the left, and is irregularly situated in the binding groove with some side chains extending upward toward the T cell receptor (2).

The nomenclature of this polymorphic system is based on a classification of serologically defined differences that were originally laboriously identified using human typing alloantisera. In the older literature, either A, B, or C and a number of up to two digits was used to designate the HLA type of a person. Some of these serologic classifications, such as those including HLA–B27, HLA–B7, and HLA–B42, were sufficiently similar to be designated *cross reacting antigen groups*. As molecular methods were applied to the HLA genes more recently it was found that often one serologic specificity was encoded by more than one allele defined at the level of nucleotide sequence (3–5). Two additional numbers, assigned in order of their discovery, are appended to the serologically defined number to identify the allelic forms. This results in a four-number code beginning at 0101 that defines the system of alleles for each locus. The locus is designated along with the allele, for example, B1*2701. Particular groups of alleles are characterized by the fact that they encode similar pockets, suggesting that they share the property

Table 5–2. *Comparison of the two classes of cell surface glycoproteins encoded by genes of the major histocompatibility complex*

	Class I	Class II
Terminology of molecules	HLA-A, B, C	Ia, DR, DQ, DP
Expression	Essentially all cells mature RBC, trophoblast, early embryonic tissue	Certain cells of immune system: B lymphocyte, monocyte, dendritic cell. Activated T cells plus various other cell types
Structure		
α chain	44 kDa	34 kDa
β chain	11.5 kDa	29 kDa
Membrane Relationship		
α chain	intrinsic	intrinsic
β chain	extrinsic	intrinsic
Location of polymorphism		
α chain	α1 and α2 domains	α1 domains of DQ and DP
β chain		β1 domains of DR, DQ and DP
Site of gene		
α chain	chromosome 6	chromosome 6
β chain	chromosome 15	chromosome 6
Number of expressed loci		
α chain	3 (HLA-A, B, C)	1 DR, 1 DQ, 1 DP
β chain	1	2 or 1 DR, 1 DQ, 1 DP
Nature of antigen bound	cytoplasmic e.g. viral capsid	soluble protein e.g. tetanus toxoid, bacterial exoenzyme
Antigen processing	proteasome	cathepsins
Location of MHC antigen charging	endoplasmic reticulum	endosome
Size of bound peptide	9 (8–13)	15 (13–25)
N and C terminus specificity	Yes	No
Phenotype of T cell recognizing antigen	CD8	CD4
TCR usage	Vα Vβ	Vα Vβ
Consequence of T cell recognition	killing of target cell bearing antigen	antigen specific T cell help, delayed hypersensitivity

of binding specific side chains. For example, there are six alleles of HLA-B27 designated B1*2701–B1*2706. There is some evidence that the B1*2703 allele is not associated with the usual HLA–B27-related diseases. Each allelic pocket has a negatively charged glutamic acid at position 45 at the end of a hydrophilic pocket that appears to be uniquely able to bind an antigenic peptide with a positively charged amino acid residue side chain in the fourth position. Access to this pocket is controlled in part by the amino acid cysteine found at position 67 (6).

CLASS II GENES

The second group of MHC molecules, designated as class II, or sometimes generically as "DR", is involved in the presentation of peptide antigen to CD4 lineage T cells and is normally found on monocytes, B cells, and other antigen-presenting cells (Fig. 5–2; Table 5–2). Following release of cytokines during inflammatory responses, they may be induced on a wide variety of other cell types. Unlike class I molecules, class II molecules are charged by peptide antigenic fragments that are present in lysosomal compartments, usually arriving there through phagocytosis or other pathways of receptor-mediated endocytosis. Typically, exogenous soluble antigens such as those resulting from bacterial infections are presented by class II molecules. Recognition of antigen fragments in the context of class II molecules is made by clonally specific T cell receptors on CD4 lineage T cells and

results in either the induction of T helper function for antibody production or delayed hypersensitivity responses.

Class II molecules have the same general conformation as class I molecules, but are composed of two similar chains, the heavier of which is designated α, and the lighter β, (Fig. 5–2). The α and β chains are both encoded in the MHC. Each chain consists of two principal extracellular domains, a short connecting piece, a transmembrane region, and a small intracellular region. Each first domain of the α and β chains is folded in mirror symmetry so that they fit together to form a superdomain for binding antigenic fragments. This superdomain is quite similar in its conformation to that of MHC class I molecules (Fig. 5–5).

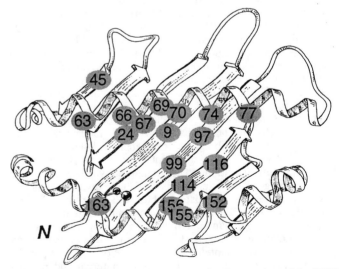

Fig. 5–4. *A representation of the antigen-binding portion of the MHC class I molecule illustrating the locations of the polymorphic amino acid residues that distinguish each of the allelic products. Certain of these are located on the floor of the molecule which is composed of β-pleated sheets, while others are situated on the α-helical margins of the antigen binding cleft. They interact to form a series of pockets and sites that specifically interact with the particular amino acid side chains and backbone of the fragments of peptide antigens.*

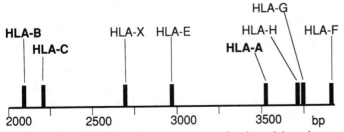

Fig. 5–3. *The MHC class I region consists of at least 8 homologous genes, of which HLA–A, HLA–B and HLA–C are the best understood. There are a large number of alternative gene forms (alleles) for each of these loci that specify different amino acid residues.*

Table 5–3. *A short example of the relationship between MHC locus, allele, and serologic specificity*

HLA Locus * Allele	Serology Specificity
A*0101	A1
A*0201	A2
A*0202	A2
.	.
.	.
.	.
A*7401	A74(AW19)
B*0701	B7
B*0702	B7
B*0703	B703
B*0801	B8
.	.
.	.
.	.
B*7801	B78
Cw*0101	Cw1
.	.
.	.
.	.
Cw*1401	—
DRA*0101	—
DRA*0201	—
DRB1*0101	DR1(Dw1)
DRB1*0102	DR1(Dw20)
DRB1*0103	DR1(DwBON)
.	.
.	.
.	.
DRB1*1001	DR10
.	.
.	.

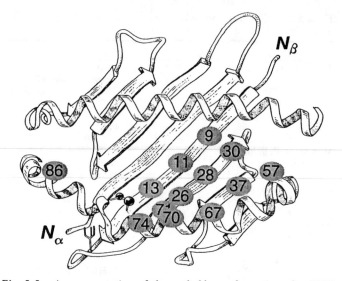

Fig. 5–5. *A representation of the probable conformation of a MHC class II DR molecule. It illustrates the overall similarity to the class I molecule. In the instance of the DR molecule the α-chain is without alternative alleles that involve potential differences in antigen binding. The polymorphism of the DRβ-chain is confined to three main diversity or "hypervariable" regions. The first two are situated on the floor of the antigen binding cleft and comprise residues 9, 11, and 13; and 26, 28, 30, and 37. The third diversity region includes polymorphic residues at position 67, 70, 71, and 74 as well as 85 and 86.*

preferential interactions with peptide antigen side chains, although the peptide is typically longer than that found in MHC class I molecules.

The relationship between serologic specificities, locus, and these variants is shown in Table 5–3. In the older nomenclature, the serologic specificities were simply numbered DR1, DR2, and so on. For many years, molecularly distinct forms of class II molecules that bore sufficiently similar serologically detectable specificities to be placed into the same serologic type were recognized by T cell-based typing, such as in mixed leukocyte typing reactions. This gave rise to a parallel classification of Dw, as opposed to DR, determinants, now largely of historic interest. For example, the serologic specificity HLA–DR4 included several T cell defined specificities such as Dw4, Dw10, Dw14, and Dw15. These latter specificities are encoded by various alleles, the more common of which are designated respectively DRB1*0401, *0402, *0403, and *0404, with several alleles now known to encode specificities that were not recognized as different using T cell-defined approaches.

Another complication in the nomenclature of class II molecules is that most individuals have two types of DRβ chain gene products usually designated DRβ1 and DRβ2, when referring to

The class II region contains the genes encoding both chains of the MHC class II molecules. These are designated by a three-letter name beginning with D and ending with A or B, according to whether they encode α or β chains. The middle letter refers to one of the six MHC class II isotypes recognized at the gene level that are designated by the letters M through R. The best studied of these are DRA and DRB encoding the DR molecules, DQA and DQB encoding DQ molecules, and DPA and DPB encoding DP molecules. The region from DPB2 to DRA covers nearly 750 kilobases (Fig. 5–6). Between the DMB and DOB loci there is an intriguing cluster of genes currently termed RING-12, -4, -9, -10, and -11, or TAP-1, TAP-2, which are involved in antigen transport and processing.

The three main isotypes of the class II molecule, DR, DQ, and DP are encoded by specific pairs of A and B locus genes. These are located in three subregions designated HLA–DR, HLA–DQ, and HLA–DP. To a varying extent these α- and β-chain genes have undergone mutations to create alternative gene forms. The DRA$_α$ chain gene, for example, is essentially invariant while the DRB$_β$ chain gene is the most variable, with more than 50 alleles currently recognized. Combinatorial assembly of α and β chains from the same region and polymorphism of each of the loci gives rise to as many as 10 different molecules capable of binding and presenting different peptides on the surface of a class II positive cell in a person, when contributions of maternal and paternal genes are considered. As with the class I molecules, the regions of polymorphism that define the different allelic forms are grouped in diversity regions, three per chain. For example, Fig. 5–5 illustrates polymorphic residues 9, 11, and 13 forming the first diversity region; 26, 28, 30, and 37 forming the second region; and 67, 70, 71, 74, and 86 forming the third diversity region of the DR β-chain. These side chains also appear to form pockets for

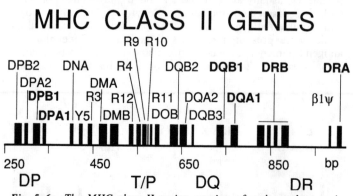

Fig. 5–6. *The MHC class II region consists of at least three main regions that are generally homologous to one another, the DR, DQ and DP regions. These are separated by a region containing genes involved in peptide processing and transport. Each region consists of at least one gene locus specifying an α-chain and a β-chain which preferentially combine. There are a large number of alternative gene forms (alleles) for each of these loci that specify different amino acid residues.*

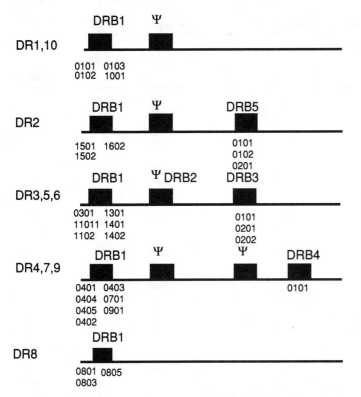

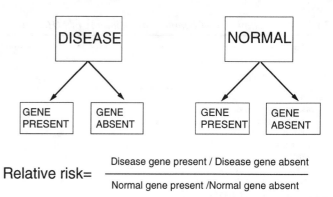

$$\text{Relative risk} = \frac{\text{Disease gene present / Disease gene absent}}{\text{Normal gene present / Normal gene absent}}$$

Fig. 5–8. *Calculation of the odds ratio, or the relative risk, which measures the likelihood of developing an illness given the presence of a particular allele.*

Fig. 5–7. *The five principal ways in which the DR β-chain region is organized in persons of different DR type. DR1, 8, and 10 haplotypes only contain a locus that encodes a single β-chain, while the other haplotypes specify two different β-chains. Note, for example, that the DR4 haplotype contains the DRB4 locus which encodes a chain that bears the DR53 specificity. The homologous locus on the DR5 haplotype which encodes a chain bearing the DR52 specificity is located at a different place, and the genes encoding these two specificities are not alleles.*

their protein forms (Fig. 5–7). The DRβ₁ product is always encoded by a gene at the locus designated DRB1. The gene encoding the DRβ₂ product differs according to the DR haplotype, being DRB3 for DR3, 5, w6, and 8; DRB4 for DR4, 7, and 9; DRB5 for DR2. There are no functional genes encoding a second DR molecule in DR1, DR8, and DR10 haplotypes. The DRB4 locus encodes a molecule bearing the DR53 serologic specificity, the DRB5 encodes a molecule with the DR51 specificity, and DRB3 encodes a molecule bearing the DR52 specificity. This accounts for the association of DR53 with DR4, DR7, and DR9; and DR52 with DR3, DR5, and DR6.

HOW HLA ALLELES ARE DETERMINED

Until recently nearly all HLA or "tissue" typing was performed at the serologic level using human alloantisera as the primary reagent. The use of alloantisera served the needs of histocompatibility typing for use in transplantation reasonably well. It did not, however, adequately approach some regions of hypervariability that appear to be of critical importance in determining disease susceptibility. Currently, typing for HLA class II alleles and, indeed, most alleles of the MHC is performed at the DNA level. The development of the polymerase chain reaction (PCR) has greatly facilitated this task, and quite often samples of DNA expanded by PCR are probed by labelled oligonucleotides specific for regions of sequence in given alleles. Binding to the DNA amplified by the PCR reaction occurs only with identity or near identity of probe and target DNA sequences, permitting delineation of the allele.

DISEASE ASSOCIATIONS

The degree of association between a marker allele and a disease is usually determined in a case control experimental design by the relative risk (Fig. 5–8) and a test of statistical significance

of this association. The standard χ^2 statistic or an exact probability calculation is usually used to determine statistical significance, which is independent of the magnitude of the relative risk. There is no association, for example, between the presence of the allele and the occurrence of the disease when the relative risk ratio has a value of one. A positive association results in an increasing positive number, reflecting the odds of developing the illness if the particular allele is present. A negative association, or protection from acquiring the disease, is either represented as a fraction or the reciprocal of this fraction preceded by a negative sign. Table 5–4 summarizes some MHC class I and II allelic associations with rheumatic diseases (7).

The percentage of patients expressing the marker is also of major importance. A significant association with a marker present in only a portion of patients may mean that the disease is heterogeneous with only one form associated with an MHC determinant. There are more complex statistics such as the attributable risk that take into account the proportion of those with disease that have the genetic marker. When large numbers of clinical traits and alleles are studied, it is likely that associations will be observed where none should exist simply as a result of chance. For example, a level of significance of p=.05 means that there is 1 chance in 20 of observing these results by chance alone. Accordingly, if the null hypothesis is that there is no association with any HLA marker, then the calculated probability must be reduced by correcting the number of independent alleles and clinical measurements that are examined (the Bonferroni correction).

ETHNICITY AND DISEASE ASSOCIATIONS

The frequency of the serologically defined HLA specificities, and especially those of the molecularly defined alleles, vary greatly among different ethnic groups. These differences require that, when the association of the presence of an allele or marker with a particular disease is studied, every effort should be made to avoid drawing the control population from a different ethnic subgroup. For example, the haplotype HLA–A1–B8–DR3 is primarily found among European Caucasians from north of the Alps where it is also closely associated with susceptibility for systemic lupus erythematosus. Another example is the observation that rheumatoid arthritis (RA) was associated with HLA–DR4 among northern European Caucasians but not those from the eastern Mediterranean, such as Jewish people or Asian Indians. Further research revealed that RA is associated with the HLA–DRB1*0401 but not the DRB1*0402 allele (Fig. 5–7). Since the former allele is the most common of those encoding the DR4 serologic specificity among northern European Caucasians, RA is strongly associated with DR4 in this ethnic group. In contrast, the most common allele encoding DR4 among those in eastern Mediterranean regions such as Israel, or further east in the Indian subcontinent, is HLA–DRB1*0402, and as a consequence, RA was not found to be significantly associated with DR4 in studies involving these ethnic groups. In both of these ethnic groups, however, RA susceptibility was associated with HLA–DR1. Mo-

Table 5–4. Summary of common associations of MHC alleles with rheumatic diseases (see also Chapter 20A)

| Disease | Class I Alleles | | | |
	HLA Allele	Relative Risk	Patients %Pos	Control %Pos
Seronegative Spondylarthropathy				
Ankylosing spondylitis	B27	69.1	89	9
Pauciarticular peripheral arthritis	B27	15.6	69	9
Isolated sacroiliitis	B27	20.4	62	9
Reiter's syndrome	B27	37.1	80	9
Reactive arthritis				
Salmonella species	B27	35.5	85	10
Shigella flexoeri	B27	28.7	85	14
Campylobacter jejuni	B27	13.8	71	14
Yersinia species	B27	21.4	77	11
Inflammatory bowel disease ankylosing spondylitis	B27	10.2	52	10
Psoriatic arthritis				
Axial arthropathy	B13	3.9	16	5
Axial arthropathy	Bw16	7.8	26	5
Axial arthropathy	B17	2.2	13	7
Axial arthropathy	B27	10.8	47	8
Axial arthropathy	B38	10.3	23	3
Peripheral arthropathy	B13	2.4	12	7
Peripheral arthropathy	Bw16	2.1	10	7
Peripheral arthropathy	B17	5.1	25	7
Peripheral arthropathy	B27	2.0	14	10
Peripheral arthropathy	B38	5.5	15	3
Behcet's Syndrome "East"	B5(W51)	7.2	69	23
"West"	B5(W51)	3.8	31	12
Whipple's Disease	B27	4.6	30	8

lecular analysis revealed that the third diversity region of the DRB1*0401 allele was nearly identical to that of the DRB1*0101 (DR1) allele but markedly different from the DRB1*0402 allele. This is an example of *trans allelic* disease association that has been used to map RA susceptibility to a sequence or motif of shared amino acids or shared epitopes encoded by several alleles including DRB1*0401, DRB1*0404, DRB1*0101, DRB1*0601, and DRB1*1001 that otherwise might not appear related at the serologic level, but which share a motif of nucleotides that encode similar amino acids from position 67–86 (8). The presence of one allele bearing this shared motif accounts for susceptibility to RA. Whether a person inherits one or two of these alleles appears to influence disease severity. A person homozygous for DRB1*0401 alleles has an increased risk for more severe disease (9).

Robert J. Winchester, MD

1. Shen HH, Winchester RJ: Susceptibility genetics of systemic lupus erythematosus. Springer Semin Immunopathol 9:143–159, 1986
2. Madden DR, Gorga JC, Strominger JL, et al: The three-dimensional structure of HLA-B27 at 2.1 Å resolution suggests a general mechanism for tight peptide binding to MHC. Cell 70:1035–1048, 1992
3. Bodmer JG, Marsh SG, Albert ED, et al: Nomenclature for factors of the HLA system, 1991. Tissue Antigens 39:161–173, 1992
4. Bodmer JG, Marsh SG, Parham P, et al: Nomenclature for factors of the HLA system, 1989. Tissue Antigens 35:1–8, 1990
5. Bodmer JG, Marsh SG, Albert ED, et al: Nomenclature for factors of the HLA system, 1990. Tissue Antigens 37:97–104, 1991
6. Buxton SE, Benjamin RJ, Clayberger C, et al: Anchoring pockets in human histocompatibility complex leukocyte antigen (HLA) class I molecules: analysis of the conserved B ("45") pocket of HLA–B27. J Exp Med 175:809–820, 1992
7. Tiwari JL, Terasaki PI: HLA and Disease Associations. New York, Springer Verlag, 1985
8. Winchester R, Dwyer E, Rose S: The genetic basis of rheumatoid arthritis: the shared epitope hypothesis. Rheum Dis Clin North Am 18:761–783, 1992
9. Weyand CM, Hicok KC, Conn DL: The influence of HLA–DRB1 genes on disease severity in rheumatoid arthritis. Ann Intern Med 117:801–806, 1992

6. MOLECULAR MECHANISMS UNDERLYING AUTOANTIBODY EXPRESSION

Autoantibodies are a hallmark of essentially all autoimmune diseases. As discussed in Chapter 8, laboratory measurement of certain autoantibodies may be helpful to the diagnostician because of the characteristic patterns of autoantibody specificities observed in individual rheumatic diseases. In other instances, the presence of a particular autoantibody may be of prognostic value, such as anti-native DNA in systemic lupus erythematosus (SLE) and rheumatoid factor (RF) in rheumatoid arthritis (RA). Also, changes in the level over time may correlate with changes in clinical status, such as anti-native DNA in SLE. While compelling evidence implicates particular autoantibodies in disease pathogenesis, the role of the vast majority of autoantibody specificities in disease either remains unclear or of dubious pathogenetic significance.

Interest in delineating the mechanisms underlying autoimmune

responses has been stimulated by several considerations: 1) understanding of such responses is critical in ultimately determining how the immune system distinguishes self from non-self; 2) the availability of powerful new molecular biology techniques enables researchers to address mechanisms of autoimmune responses; 3) anticipation that elucidation of mechanisms underlying autoimmune responses will facilitate understanding of the pathogenesis of the associated diseases; and 4) the likelihood that such insights will lead to improved therapeutic approaches for these diseases.

Studies of animal models of autoimmune diseases including adjuvant arthritis, experimental allergic encephalomyelitis, spontaneous diabetes, and collagen-induced arthritis have defined critical autoimmune responses involved in disease pathogenesis. These studies facilitated the development of interventions capable of specifically blocking the relevant autoimmune response and ameliorating the disease. Optimally, the design of such interventions requires precise delineation of the self peptide(s) responsible for the induction or perpetuation of the response, the major histocompatibility complex (MHC) alleles housing the relevant peptides for presentation to the autoreactive T cell and the nature of the T cell receptors (TCR) expressed on the responding T cells capable of inducing the disease. In turn, the activated T cell may cooperate with relevant B cells in the presence of the autoantigen, culminating in the expresstion of autoantibodies directed against the autoantigen.

In the case of human rheumatic diseases, there is little detailed knowledge concerning the nature of the putative disease-initiating trimolecular complex (antigen peptide, MHC allele accommodating the peptide, and responding TCR heterodimer). On the other hand, progress has been made in elucidating the molecular characteristics of some human autoantibodies and defining their target epitopes. Ultimately, such knowledge should aid in identification of autoreactive T cells presumably driving the anti-self B cell response in rheumatic disease.

DEVELOPMENTALLY REGULATED V REGION GENES AND NATURAL AUTOANTIBODIES

During the first half of this century, it was widely accepted that antibody responses directed against self, a phenomenon termed *horror autotoxicus* by Erlich and Morgenroth, did not occur in healthy individuals. Burnet subsequently argued that:
"It is axiomatic that no immunological reaction takes place against the normal constituents of the body; no other situation is conceivable in health, and the variety of serious diseases which arise when this role is transgressed merely underlines its importance" (1).

However, the notion that self-reactive B cells are deleted from the normal repertoire was subsequently refuted by evidence that autoantibodies often occur in sera from healthy humans and several animal species (2). These so called *natural autoantibodies* characteristically are IgM isotype, exhibit reactivity with multiple antigens (both self and foreign), and are preferentially but not exclusively elaborated by CD5$^+$ B cells. Surprisingly, an appreciable fraction of peripheral blood B cell clones rescued from healthy adult peripheral blood following Epstein–Barr transformation or heterohybridization secrete antibodies reactive with at least two self antigens, including human IgG, single stranded DNA, native DNA, cytoskeletal proteins, thyroglobulin, histones, actin, and cardiolipin.

Natural autoantibodies elaborated by cloned B cells from healthy individuals are generally encoded by germline variable (V) region genes with little or no somatic mutation: V_H, D_H, and J_H gene segments for heavy chains; V_L and J_L for light chains. Unexpectedly, the responsible germline V_H genes are commonly drawn from a small set of V_H genes preferentially expressed by B cells early in fetal development (3,4). The propensity of these developmentally regulated V region genes to encode polyspecific antibodies prompted speculation that these highly conserved V genes form an initial functional B cell network that shapes the ensuing B cell repertoire (5). Moreover, the characteristic broad reactivity of antibodies encoded by these genes may serve as a highly flexible recognition system permitting responses to a variety of potentially harmful exogenous organisms commonly encountered in the environment.

Evidence that the expression of natural autoantibodies reflects somatic selection of particular H and L chain V region elements, in contrast to random pairing, further argues for the functional significance of these antibodies in the early B cell repertoire (6).

MARKERS OF V REGION GENES ASSOCIATED WITH AUTOANTIBODIES

The pioneering studies of Henry Kunkel and colleagues established that paraproteins with RF activity could be separated into distinct groups based on expression of shared variable region epitopes, designated *idiotypes* (7). The initial serologic reagents (anti-idiotypes) used in the studies were polyclonal antibodies raised in laboratory animals and therefore contained multiple individual antibody specificities. More precise serologic characterization of autoantibody V region determinants has been achieved by the use of monoclonal antibodies (mAbs) recognizing structurally defined idiotypes. In the case of RF paraproteins, several mAbs have been generated that recognize cross-reactive idiotypes (CRI) expressed by a significant fraction of these RF. Both H and L chain CRI have been defined using this approach.

In some cases, it has been possible to relate CRI recognized by mAbs to particular germline V region genes. For example, the mAbs 17.109 and 6B6.6 recognize CRIs that are encoded by distinct V_κ germline genes designated Humkv 325 (8) and Humkv 328 (9), respectively. Both of these CRIs are also expressed on some non-RF paraproteins, but at lower frequencies.

Frequently, CRI cannot be ascribed to a particular germline V region element. In some cases this is explained by the fact that the recognized determinant (idiotype) is generated by interaction between H and L chain V regions, called *combinatorial idiotypes*. Indeed, radiographic diffraction analysis has clearly shown that an anti-idiotypic mAb may interact with residues residing in both V_H and V_L structures of the idiotype-bearing antibody (10). Alternatively, some CRI are expressed by several V region genes, which may reflect the presence of a framework determinant shared by several V region genes or the presence of an epitope shared by otherwise unrelated V region genes.

GENETIC ORIGINS OF DISEASE-ASSOCIATED AUTOANTIBODIES

Two approaches have been used to investigate the genetic origin of autoantibodies expressed in autoimmune diseases: serologic analysis of expressed autoantibody using mAbs directed against structurally defined CRI, and sequence analysis of autoantibodies elaborated by cloned B cells from patients with autoimmune diseases. The serologic approach is hindered by the limited number of mAbs available that identify germline gene-encoded CRI. Nonetheless, this approach has provided evidence that at least some disease-associated autoantibodies are encoded by identical germline V genes as their paraprotein (or natural autoantibody) counterparts. For instance, sera from most patients with RA contain RF expressing the 17.109 or 6B6.6 CRI; however, these CRI(+) RF constitute a negligible fraction of the total RF (11). These observations are in striking contrast to the dominance of these idiotypes among RF paraproteins (12) and suggest either that germline Humkv 325 and Humkv 328 (or closely related genes) encode only a small proportion of RF in RA or that extensive somatic mutation occurs such that these germline gene-encoded CRI are no longer expressed.

The alternative approach of rescuing autoantibody-producing B cell clones from patients with autoimmune disease offers the advantage of permitting direct determination of the autoantibody V region sequences. However, drawbacks include the technical demands of B cell cloning, hybridization, or both, and concerns regarding the precise relationship of these cloned B cells to plasma cells responsible for autoantibody production in vivo. Early studies utilizing this approach indicate that multiple V_H and V_L genes are capable of encoding RF and polyreactive autoantibodies in RA (13). In general the sequences of these IgM autoantibody V regions exhibited minimal somatic mutation suggesting they are part of the normal B cell repertoire. To assess more fully the role of antigen selection in human autoantibody production in disease, it will be necessary to examine IgG and IgA autoantibody V region sequences also. B cell clones secreting IgG autoantibodies exhibiting V region mutation patterns consistent with antigen selection have been rescued from patients with SLE (anti-DNA) (14) and RA (RF) (15).

The initial molecular studies of human autoantibodies expressed in autoimmune disease do not yet permit firm conclusions regarding the mechanisms involved in their induction, (that is, polyclonal activation versus antigen selection). However, analyses of autoantibody V region sequences obtained from spontaneously autoimmune mice indicate a dominant role for antigen selection. Indeed, most of the RF expressed in a single autoimmune MRL/lpr mouse derives from a single B cell precursor (16).

In summary, the origin of autoantibodies expressed in autoimmune disease has not yet been precisely delineated. At least a portion of these disease-associated autoantibodies derive from identical germline genes responsible for encoding natural autoantibodies and paraproteins with autoantibody activity. In studies of autoimmune animal models the autoantibody response is antigen-driven, whereas insufficient data exists regarding this issue in man.

AUTOANTIGEN TARGETS OF AUTOANTIBODIES

Considerable progress has been made in the characterization of the autoantigens recognized by autoantibodies in several human autoimmune diseases. Indeed, in many instances the autoantibodies have served as important tools in the identification and subsequent cloning of their respective autoantigen targets. These studies have provided clues concerning the mechanisms underlying the induction of these autoantibodies. For example, the fact that intracellular autoantigens targeted in a particular disease generally colocalize within the cell provides strong, albeit circumstantial, evidence that these autoantibody responses are driven by subcellular particles or organelles containing several associated molecules (17). For instance, anti-Sm autoantibodies, characteristically present in some patients with SLE, recognize several core proteins contained in a small RNA–protein complex involved in pre-mRNA splicing. Similarly, a subset of patients with a limited form of systemic sclerosis commonly express anticentromere autoantibodies (ACA) that bind to several protein constituents in this organelle.

Many autoantibodies exhibit broad cross-reactivity with homologous target antigens from different animal and plant species. For instance, tissue sections from mice are commonly used to detect human antinuclear antibodies, and extracts of calf thymus are often used as a source of nuclear antigens for clinical laboratory assays of certain human autoantibodies. Such observations indicate that autoantibodies recognize highly conserved rather than unique or altered self epitopes. The capacity of several autoantibodies to inhibit function of their respective autoantigen targets reflects the dependence of these functions on highly conserved portions of the molecules bound by these autoantibodies. On the other hand, experimentally induced antibodies raised by immunization of animals with purified intracellular antigens preferentially react with epitopes divergent from self (non-conserved) and generally do not inhibit functional activity of the immunogen.

MHC MOLECULES AND EXPRESSION OF AUTOANTIBODIES

The apparent association of certain autoimmune diseases such as SLE, Sjogren's syndrome, and systemic sclerosis with particular MHC class II molecules has been recognized for several years (see Chapter 5). In general these associations have been weak and not always reproducible. Major histocompatibility complex analyses of subsets of these diseases characterized by the expression of certain autoantibody specificities have been more informative. Using techniques of restriction fragment length polymorphism, oligonucleotide DNA typing, and nucleotide sequencing of MHC genes, it has been possible to correlate the presence of several autoantibodies with particular MHC class II sequences. For instance, expression of ACA in systemic sclerosis strongly correlates with a sequence motif in the second hypervariable region of HLA–DQB1 chains (18). Similarly, other MHC class II variable region sequences have been related to the expression of anti-Ro (SS–A), anti-La (SS–B), anti-histidyl tRNA synthetase, anti-Sm, lupus anticoagulant, and anti-native DNA.

Since the primary function of MHC class II molecules is to present processed antigen-derived peptides to $CD4^+$ T helper cells, these data are consistent with the view that T cells participate in the induction or perpetuation of autoantibody responses and that the configuration of the MHC class II peptide binding site determines whether a given autoantigen can be effectively presented to responding T helper cells.

T CELLS AND AUTOANTIBODY RESPONSE

Efforts to identify T cells reactive with self antigens have been hampered by technical problems in devising suitable methods for their detection; nonetheless, autoreactive T cells clearly also occur in healthy individuals. Increased numbers of autoreactive T cells may occur in certain autoimmune diseases. For example, T cells reactive with myelin basic protein, a major candidate as a target autoantigen in multiple sclerosis (MS), occur in both healthy adults and patients with MS; however, they are more prevalent in the blood and cerebrospinal fluid of MS patients in relapse than either healthy individuals or MS patients in remission (19,20).

That T cells participate in the induction of autoantibody responses seems clear; however, the precise nature of these cells remains elusive. With regard to anti-DNA responses, a subpopulation of T helper cells expressing anionic residues in their TCR β-chain V–D–J junctional regions are required for the expression of nephritogenic anti-DNA antibodies in autoimmune mice (21). Presumably, these T helper cells recognize a cationic autoantigen-derived peptide presented by the anti-DNA producing B cells. In the case of RF responses, autoreactive T cells may not be required. By virtue of their surface immunoglobulin, RF B cells are capable of binding IgG-containing immune complexes and subsequently processing and presenting the antigens residing in the complex. Thus, RF B cells can present any antigen contained within an immune complex and can be triggered by T cells specific for the processed antigen.

TOLERANCE AND AUTOANTIBODY RESPONSES

The existence of autoreactive T and B cells in healthy individuals argues strongly that regulatory mechanisms ordinarily prevent activation of these cells. Studies in transgenic animal models have indicated that self-reactive T and B cells are extensively deleted during development. Residual self-reactive cells escaping into the periphery are either deleted following antigen exposure or rendered functionally inactive.

The mechanisms underlying induction of autoantibodies in disease likely involve a breakdown of normal tolerance mechanisms. Inactive autoreactive B cells can be induced to express autoantibodies by polyclonal activators such as lipopolysaccharide. In addition, fundamental defects in tolerance maintenance, both at the level of thymic deletion of self-reactive T cells and in peripheral inactivation, have been observed in spontaneously autoimmune mice. In the MRL/lpr mouse, this is at least partially attributable to a defect in the Fas gene that appears responsible for self-destruction, and perhaps peripheral tolerance, of self-reactive immune cells (22). Other molecular defects will likely be identified that influence tolerance induction and maintenance and thereby confer enhanced susceptibility to autoimmune diseases.

William J. Koopman, MD

1. Burnet FM: The Clonal Selection Theory of Acquired Immunity. London, Cambridge University Press, 1949
2. Avrameas S: Natural autoantibodies: from 'horror autotoxicus' to 'gnothi seauton'. Immunol Today 12(5):154–159, 1991
3. Schroeder HW Jr, Hillson JL, Perlmutter RM: Early restriction of the human antibody repertoire. Science 238:791–793, 1987
4. Sanz I, Casali P, Thomas JW, et al: Nucleotide sequences of eight human natural autoantibody V_H regions reveals apparent restricted use of V_H families. J Immunol 142:4054–4061, 1989
5. Coutinho A, Grandien A, Faro-Rivas J, et al: Idiotypes, ballots and networks. Ins Pasteur Immunol 139:599–607, 1988
6. Martin T, Duffy SF, Carson DA, et al: Evidence for somatic selection of natural autoantibodies. J Exp Med 175:983–991, 1973
7. Kunkel HG, Agnello V, Joslin GS, et al: Cross-idiotypic specificity among monoclonal IgM proteins with anti-gamma globulin activity. J Exp Med 137:331–342, 1973
8. Radoux V, Chen PP, Sorge JA, et al: A conserved human germline V_κ gene directly encodes rheumatoid factor light chains. J Exp Med 164:2119–2124, 1986
9. Chen PP, Robbins DL, Jirik FR, et al: Isolation and characterization of a light chain variable region for human rheumatoid factors. J Exp Med 166:1900–1905, 1987

10. Bentley GA, Boulot G, Riottot MM, et al: Three-dimensional structure of an idiotype-anti-idiotype complex. Nature 348:254–257, 1990

11. Koopman WJ, Schrohenloher RE, Carson DA: Dissociation of expression of two rheumatoid factor cross-reactive κ L chain idiotypes in rheumatoid arthritis. J Immunol 144:3468–3472, 1990

12. Crowley JJ, Goldfien RD, Schrohenloher RE, et al: Incidence of three cross-reactive idiotypes on human rheumatoid factor proteins. J Immunol 140:3411–3418, 1988

13. Pascual V, Kimberly V, Randen I, et al: IgM rheumatoid factors in patients with rheumatoid arthritis derive from a diverse array of germline genes and display little evidence of somatic mutation. J Rheum 19(suppl 32):50–53, 1992

14. Van Es JH, Gmelig Meyling FJH, van de Akker WRM, et al: Somatic mutations in the variable regions of a human IgG anti-double-stranded DNA auto-antibody suggest a role for antigen in the induction of SLE. J Exp Med 173:461–470, 1991

15. Olee T, Lu EW, Huang D-F, et al: Genetic analysis of self-associating immunoglobulin G rheumatoid factors from two rheumatoid synovia implicates an antigen-driven response. J Exp Med 175:831–842, 1992

16. Shlomchik MJ, Marshak-Rothstein A, Wolfowicz CB, et al: The role of clonal selection and somatic mutation in autoimmunity. Nature 328:805–811, 1987

17. Tan EM: Autoantibodies in pathology and cell biology. Cell 67:841–842, 1991

18. Reveille JD, Owerbach D, Goldstein R, et al: Association of polar amino acids at position 26 of the HLA-DQB1 first domain with the anticentromere auto-antibody response in systemic sclerosis (Scleroderma). J Clin Invest 89:1208–1213, 1992

19. Lisak RP, Zweiman B: In vitro cell-mediated immunity of cerebrospinal-fluid lymphocytes to myelin basic protein in primary demyelinating diseases. New Engl J Med 297:850–853, 1977

20. Allegretta M, Nicklas JA, Sriram S, et al: T cells responsive to myelin basic protein in patients with multiple sclerosis. Science 247:718–721, 1990

21. Adams S, Leblanc P, Datta SK: Junctional region sequences of T-cell receptor β-chain genes expressed by pathogeneic anti-DNA autoantibody-inducing helper T cells from lupus mice: Possible selection by cationic autoantigens. Proc Natl Acad Sci USA 88:11271–11275, 1991

22. Watanabe-Fukunaga R, Brannan CI, Copeland NB, et al: Lymphoproliferation disorder in mice explained by defects in Fas antigen that mediates apoptosis. Nature 356:314–317, 1992

7. MEDIATORS OF INFLAMMATION
A. Cellular Constituents of Inflammation

Three types of highly specialized cells—polymorphonuclear leukocytes, monocyte-macrophages, and platelets—play a central role in host defense, the normal immune response, and in hemostasis. These cells are also the major participants in the development of acute, subacute, and chronic immunologically-mediated tissue injury. This chapter reviews some of the functions of these important cells and the mediators they release in the inflammatory process. Lymphocytes are discussed in Chapter 4.

POLYMORPHONUCLEAR LEUKOCYTES: NEUTROPHILS

The chief function of polymorphonuclear leukocytes is phagocytosis and destruction of microorganisms. Neutrophils, however, also mediate many of the key events that unfold at sites of acute, subacute, and at times chronic inflammation. For example, the following experimental models of immunologic tissue damage have shown a common dependence on the neutrophil: the Arthus reaction; necrotizing arteritis of experimental serum sickness in rabbits; proteinuria due to acute nephrotoxic vasculitis in rabbits and rats; and intraarticular reverse, passive Arthus reaction-induced arthritis in rabbits; as well as the local and generalized Shwartzman phenomenon (1).

Neutrophil responses following exposure to such stimuli as C5a, immune complexes, and interleukin–8 (IL–8) include adherence, chemotaxis, phagocytosis, and, following phagocytosis, intracellular killing. The neutrophil membrane has surface receptors capable of binding to C3b, iC3b, and C5a complement components as well as the Fc portion of immunoglobulins G and M (IgG and IgM). In autoimmune diseases, immune complexes and activated complement components engage these surface receptors, and thereby induce the secretion of inflammatory mediators (for example, proteolytic enzymes and superoxide anion), resulting in tissue injury (Fig. 7A–1).

Three major classes of Fc receptors have been described on phagocytic cells (2). FcRI, the high affinity receptor for monomeric IgG, is found mainly on mononuclear cells. Both neutrophils and mononuclear cells have two low affinity receptors—FcRII and FcRIII—that bind immune complexes with greater affinity than monomeric IgG. FcRII, with a molecular weight of approximately 40 kDa, is also present on B cells and platelets. Engagement of this receptor on phagocytic cells induces superoxide anion generation and degranulation. FcRIII also prefers multimeric IgG, has a molecular weight of 50 to 70 kDa and is present on neutrophils, macrophages, platelets, and some T cells. FcRIII is linked to the external plasma membrane by phosphatidylinositol. These phospholipid-linked receptors are mobile within the plane of the membrane and accumulate at the interface between the phagocyte and an immunoglobulin-coated surface.

Neutrophil Aggregation and Adhesion to Vascular Endothelium

Phagocytic cells also express receptors for C3b (designated CR1) and its inactivated cleavage product iC3b (designated CR3, also called Mac–1, CD11b/CD18) (3). On the surface of phagocytes, both CR1 and CR3 play important roles in clearing particles, such as opsonized bacteria, to which C3b or iC3b are bound (Fig. 7A–1). This clearance mechanism is also essential for removing immune complexes containing C3b and iC3b (4). In addition to its role as a receptor for iC3b, CR3 is the major neutrophil adhesion molecule responsible for the capacity of the neutrophil to adhere to vascular endothelium and to other neutrophils (5). The adhesion of activated neutrophils to vascular endothelium is one of the initial events in the inflammatory process. Adhesion depends in part on the activation of surface glycoproteins known as β_2 integrins, which are heterodimers consisting of a common beta sub-unit (CD18) and distinct alpha sub-units. CD11a/CD18 is known as LFA–1, CD11b/CD18 as Mac–1 or CR3, and CD11c/CD18 as GP150/95. Intercellular adhesion molecule–1 (ICAM–1), expressed on resting and activated endothelial cells, has been identified as a ligand for the CD18 integrins (6). Interaction between CD18 and ICAM–1 mediates both the adhesion of neutrophils to vascular endothelium and their egress to the extravascular space. The initial rolling of

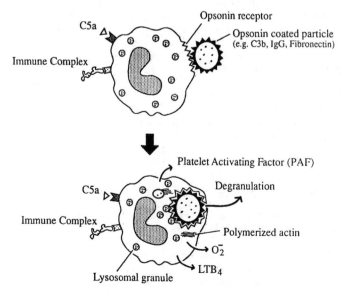

Fig. 7A–1. *Release of mediators of inflammation from activated phagocytes.*

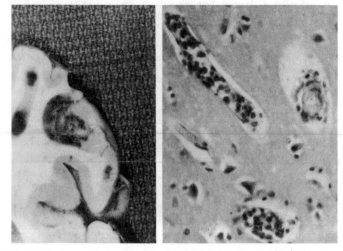

Fig. 7A-2. *In a patient who died with CNS lupus, cerebral infarcts were subtended by vessels occluded by leukocyte thrombi, similar to those observed in a Shwartzman reaction (1,5). (Photo courtesy of Dr. Nelson Torre, Buffalo, NY).*

activated neutrophils on endothelium, a prerequisite for CD18-dependent adhesion under conditions of flow, is mediated by a separate molecular interaction: that between the selectin, endothelial leukocyte adhesion molecule (ELAM-1, E-Selectin), and a carbohydrate ligand, sialyl-Le^x, on the neutrophil (6-8). In conditions characterized by the excessive intravascular activation of complement, the exposure of circulating neutrophils to C5a promotes both neutrophil–neutrophil aggregation and neutrophil–endothelial adhesion, which lead to the occlusion of small blood vessels with leukothrombi. Such clinical conditions, which represent human equivalents of the generalized Shwartzman phenomenon, include endotoxic shock and a recently described syndrome of hypoxemia—cerebritis observed in systemic lupus erythematosus (SLE) (5,9) (Fig. 7A-2).

Phagocytosis

When a neutrophil makes contact with a suitable particle, the particle is ingested in a process called phagocytosis. At the point of contact, neutrophils invaginate their surface membranes and engulf the particle, resulting in an intracellular vacuole called a *phagosome*, which pinches off from the cell's surface and is internalized within the cell (Fig. 7A-1). Neutrophils contain two morphologically distinct granules (specific and azurophilic) that contain proteases, which under normal circumstances are sequestered within the granule and the phagosome, presenting no threat to the host. However, the extracellular release of granule contents may promote inflammation and damage at tissue sites.

Phagocytosis is not necessary for neutrophil degranulation, which may be provoked by soluble stimuli (for example, C5a, IL-8) as shown in Fig. 7A-1. Degranulation is augmented when neutrophils encounter stimuli deposited on surfaces. Lysosomal release unfolds by a process of reverse endocytosis, or what has been called "frustrated phagocytosis." This exuberant release of lysosomal enzymes from neutrophils may be relevant to the pathogenesis of tissue injury in diseases characterized by the deposition of immune complexes on cell surfaces or on such extracellular surfaces as vascular basement membranes or articular cartilage.

Oxidative Metabolism

When phagocytic leukocytes are activated, molecular oxygen consumption by the leukocyte is increased. The majority of this oxygen is transformed directly into superoxide anion radicals. Stimulated neutrophils also produce hydrogen peroxide, hydroxyl radicals, and possibly, singlet oxygen. Oxygen-derived free radicals are significant mediators of inflammation causing tissue injury and irreversible modification of macromolecules (Table 7A-1).

Table 7A-1. *Potential effects of oxygen-free radicals (adapted from reference 10)*

On cells
  Killing of microbes (e.g., viruses, bacteria, fungi, protozoa)
  Injury of tumor cells
  Stimulation of secretion by platelets, mast cells, endothelial cells, glomerular cells
  Mutagenesis of bacteria and mammalian cells
  Tumor promotion and carcinogenesis
On extracellular products
  Generation of chemotactic lipids from arachidonate
  Activation of leukocyte collagenase, gelatinase
  Inactivation of chemotactic leukotrienes, chemotactic peptides, α-1-antiprotease, met-enkephalin, leukocyte hydrolases, bacterial toxins

MONOCYTES/MACROPHAGES

Macrophages are tissue phagocytes derived from circulating monocytes that release a broad inventory of inflammatory mediators. In addition, through their role in antigen presentation and cytokine secretion, macrophages modulate the function of T and B cells. Macrophages are present in large numbers not only in chronic inflammatory tissues, but also under normal conditions in pulmonary alveoli, juxtaglomerular and perivascular spaces, bony trabeculae, and renal tubules. Due to their abundance, wide distribution, and motility, macrophages exert broad effects on both the immune and inflammatory response.

Macrophages as Secretory Cells in Inflammation

Macrophages secrete up to 100 substances, ranging from free radicals such as superoxide anion, to macromolecules such as fibronectin (10). Some products are secreted in response to inflammatory stimuli while others are constitutively released (Table 7A-2). For example, plasminogen activator, which converts plasminogen to plasmin, is secreted at low levels by monocytes or nonstimulated macrophages, and is augmented by inflammatory stimuli. Plasmin not only degrades fibrin, it also activates complement components, C1 and C3. Activated macrophages produce plasminogen activator in two forms, a soluble form released into the extracellular medium and a cell-associated form.

Collagenase is another neutral protease constitutively secreted

Table 7A-2. *Secretory products of mononuclear phagocytes (adapted from reference 10)*

Polypeptide hormones
  Interleukin 1-α and 1-β (collectively, IL-1)
  Tumor necrosis factor-α (cachectin, TNF)
  Interferon-α
  Interferon-γ (confirmation needed)
  Platelet-derived growth factor(s)
  Transforming growth factor-β
  β-Endorphin
  Neutrophil-activating factor/interleukin-8
Complement (C) components
  Classical path: C1, C4, C2, C3, C5
  Alternative path: factor B, factor D, properdin
  Inhibitors: C3b inactivator, β-1H
Coagulation factors
  Intrinsic path: IX, X, V, prothrombin
  Extrinsic path: VII
  Surface activities: tissue factor, prothrombinase
  Prothrombolytic activity: plasminogen activator inhibitors, plasmin inhibitors
Bioactive lipids
  Cyclooxygenase products: prostaglandin E$_2$ (PGE$_2$), prostaglandin F$_{2\alpha}$, prostacyclin, thromboxane
  Lipoxygenase products: monohydroxyeicosatetraenoic acids, dihydroxyeicosatetraenoic acids, leukotrienes B4, C, D, E
  Platelet-activating factors (1 O-alkyl-2-acetyl-*sn*-glyceryl-3-phosphorylcholine)
Reactive oxygen intermediates (e.g., superoxide anion)
Reactive nitrogen intermediates (e.g., nitric oxide)

Table 7A–3. *Platelet constituents with inflammatory potential (adapted from reference 14)*

Alpha granule	Dense granule	Other
Fibronectin	Serotonin	Thromboxane A$_2$
Fibrinogen	Adenosine diphosphate	12-hydroxytetraenoic
Thrombospondin	Calcium	acid
von Willebrand factor		
Plasminogen		
α_2-Plasmin inhibitor		
Platelet-derived growth factor		
Platelet factor 4		
Tumor growth factors α and β		
Factors D and H		

^{a} TXA$_2$, thromboxane A$_2$; ADP, adenosine diphosphate; 12-HETE, 12-hydroxytetraenoic acid; PDGF, platelet-derived growth factor; PF4; TGF, transforming growth factor.

at low levels by nonactivated macrophages; stimulation with interleukin-1 (IL–1) and endotoxin augments secretion. In such chronic inflammatory sites as the rheumatoid synovium, collagen may be partially degraded by macrophage-secreted collagenases. Lysozyme, a cationic protein that hydrolyzes the glucose linkages in bacterial cell walls, is also a macrophage secretory product.

Monocytes and macrophages exhibit a procoagulant activity when stimulated by exposure to immune complexes, endotoxin, IL–1, or C3b-coated particles (11). The procoagulant products include tissue factor, factor X activator, prothrombin activator, and vitamin K-dependent clotting factors II, VII, IX, and X. Monocytes in rheumatic disease patients display a higher procoagulant-producing activity than normal, perhaps as a result of exposure to cytokines and cleavage products of complement. Increased procoagulant activity may contribute to fibrin deposition at sites of inflammation. Whether such increased procoagulant activity observed in these conditions also promotes a hypercoagulable state, such as observed in SLE, remains unknown.

Fibronectin is both synthesized and released by activated macrophages. This molecule, which binds to the β_1 class of integrins, mediates some types of cellular adhesion: fibroblasts to substrata, for example. It is chemotactic for fibroblasts, and activated macrophages can stimulate fibrogenesis at sites of inflammation.

As shown in Table 7A-2, macrophages also secrete a variety of polypeptide hormones that regulate immune function and inflammation as well as wound healing and repair (12). Macrophages, for example, produce three cytokines IL–1α, IL–1β and TNF–α, which not only have overlapping functions, but are also capable of inducing each others' release by the macrophages themselves (10). Macrophages also produce the cytokine neutrophil-activating peptide–1/IL–8, which is a potent neutrophil chemo-attractant. The production of IL–8, induced by IL–1α, IL–1β, and TNF–α has been described in a variety of tissues, including alveolar macrophages, renal mesangial cells, and psoriatic skin lesions (13).

Monocytes and macrophages are additionally significant sources of lipid mediators of inflammation. For example, macrophages metabolize arachidonic acid via cyclooxygenase to stable prostaglandins such as PGE–2 and via the lipoxygenase enzyme to leukotrienes B$_4$, C, D and E. Leukotriene B$_4$ is a potent

Table 7A-4. *Adhesive molecules and their counterreceptors (adapted from ref 7)*

Endothelium	Leukocyte
P-selectin*	L-selectin (also other glycoproteins)
E-selectin	Sialylated Lewis X glycoproteins
ICAM-1	β_2-integrins (CD11a,b,c/CD18)†
VCAM-1	VLA-4

*P-selectin is also expressed on platelets
†The counterreceptor for CD11b/CD18 in homotypic adhesion of neutrophils (aggregation) is unknown

chemo-attractant for macrophages and neutrophils identified in rheumatoid and gouty synovial effusions. An additional lipid-derived chemo-attractant generated by neutrophils, monocytes, and macrophages is platelet activating factor.

Macrophages are also among the cellular sources of reactive nitrogen intermediates such as nitric oxide. Nitric oxide, although originally identified as a product of endothelial cells which accounts for "endothelium derived relaxation factor" activity, is now appreciated to be a highly reactive molecule with diverse biological functions (14). The exposure of macrophages to cytokines (eg., IL-1β, interferon gamma) markedly increases nitric oxide production. Nitric oxide produced by activated macrophages contributes to their cytotoxicity to tumor cells, intracellular bacteria and protozoans. Extracellular activities of nitric oxide which may be important in the inflammatory response include vasodilation, inhibition of platelet aggregation, inhibition of neutrophil superoxide anion production and inhibition of T cell proliferation.

PLATELETS

Platelets, derived from marrow megakaryocytes, are involved in hemostasis, wound healing, and cellular responses to injury (15,16). In primitive organisms, a single cell type served both leukocyte and platelet functions. In higher organisms, platelets have retained some properties of inflammatory cells. For example, platelets release inflammatory mediators upon activation and aggregation; they are activated by phlogistic agents such as complement activation products; they play a role in animal models of inflammatory disease; and they have been identified at tissue injury sites in human inflammatory diseases. Platelet activation at sites of tissue injury is achieved by such hemostatic factors as thrombin, adenosine diphosphate, arachidonate derivates, and exposed subendothelial collagen. There is evidence for platelet activation in some immunologically mediated diseases such as asthma, cold urticaria, systemic sclerosis, and SLE (17–19).

At sites of inflammation activated platelets release a variety of

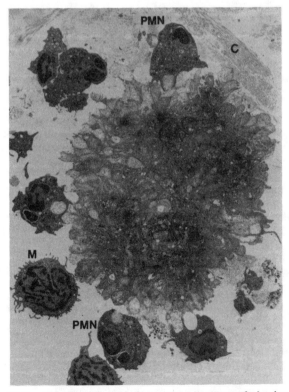

Fig. 7A–3. *Platelet aggregate formed upon contact of platelets with collagen (C) during addition of collagen to a mixture of platelets and leukocytes. The platelets are mostly degranulated, and the aggregate is beginning to be digested by polymorphonuclear neutrophils (PMN) which, however, have not been incorporated into the platelet aggregate. (M) Monocyte (photograph by D. Zucker-Franklin, from reference 14).*

both protein and lipid-derived mediators with inflammatory potential (Table 7A–3). Stimuli that activate platelet adhesion and degranulation also trigger the release of arachidonic acid from the membrane. This initiates the synthesis of thromboxane A_2 (TxA_2), which promotes platelet aggregation and vasoconstriction, and 12–hydroxytetraenoic acid (12–HETE) which activates neutrophils and macrophages.

Proteins released from alpha and dense granules also promote local inflammation. Two that are secreted in large amounts from alpha granules are platelet factor 4 and β–thromboglobulin. These molecules have chemo-attractant properties and activate both mononuclear and polymorphonuclear phagocytes. In addition, thrombospondin, a 450 kDa trimeric glycoprotein is secreted by platelets and endothelial cells at sites of inflammation. There is evidence that thrombospondin plays an important role in neutrophil adherence to blood vessel walls, which is independent from a CD11/CD18 mechanism. Dense granules release ADP, which activates platelet fibrinogen binding sites of the integrin gpIIb/IIIa and serotonin, a potent vasoconstrictor.

Finally, platelets express two surface adhesion promoting molecules (Table 7A–4). First, gpIIb/IIIa, which promotes platelet aggregation, is a member of the β_3 integrin family that binds fibrinogen, fibronectin, vitronection, and von Willebrand Factor (20). Second, P-selectin (GMP–140), a member of the selectin family of adhesion molecules, is a membrane glycoprotein located in the alpha granules of platelets and Weibel–Palade bodies of endothelium. When these cells are activated by agents such as thrombin, P-selectin is rapidly translocated to the plasma membrane where it functions as a receptor for neutrophils and monocytes (Fig. 7A–3). Expression of P-selectin on activated platelets may therefore facilitate recruitment of neutrophils and monocytes to sites of thrombosis or inflammation (7).

Steven B. Abramson, MD

1. Stetson CA: Similarities in the mechanisms determining the Arthus and Shwartzman phenomena. J Exp Med 94:347–358, 1951

2. Unkeless JC: Function and heterogeneity of human Fc receptors for immunoglobulin G. J Clin Invest 83:355–361, 1989

3. Ross GD, Medof ME: Membrane complement receptors specific for bound fragments of C3. Adv Immunol 37:217–267, 1985

4. Schifferli JA, Ng YC, Peters DK: The role of complement and its receptor in the elimination of immune complexes. N Eng J Med 315:488–495, 1986

5. Philips MR, Abramson SB, Weissmann G: Neutrophil adhesion and autoimmune vascular injury. Clin Aspects Autoimmun 3:6–15, 1989

6. Yong K, Khwaja A: Leucocyte cellular adhesion molecules. Blood Rev 4:211–225, 1990

7. Cronstein B, Weissman G: The adhesion molecules of inflammation. Arthritis Rheum 36:147–157, 1993

8. Lawrence MB, Springer TA: Leukocytes roll on a selection of physiologic flow rates: Distinction from and prerequisite for adhesion through integrins. Cell 65:859–873, 1991

9. Abramson SB, Dobro J, Eberle MA, et al: The syndrome of acute reversible hypoxemia of systemic lupus erythematosus. Ann Int Med 114:941–947, 1991

10. Nathan CF: Secretory products of macrophages. J Clin Invest 79:319–326, 1987

11. Wharram BL, Fitting K, Kunkel SL, et al: Tissue factor expression in endothelial cell/monocyte co-cultures stimulated by lipopolysaccharide and/or aggregated IgG: Mechanisms of cell-cell communication. J Immunol 146:1437–1445, 1991

12. Schultz G, Rotater DS: EGF and TGF-alpha in wound healing and repair. J Cell Biol 45:346–352, 1991

13. Kusner DJ, Luebbers EL, Nowinski RJ: Cytokine- and LPS-induced synthesis of interleukin-8 from human mesangial cells. Kidney-Int 39:1240–1248, 1991

14. Stamler JS, Singel DJ, Loscalzo J: Biochemistry of nitric oxide and its redox-activated forms. Science 258:1898–1902, 1992

15. Weksler BB: Platelets, Inflammation, Basic Principles and Clinical Correlates. Edited by Gallin JI, Goldstein M, Snyderman R. New York, Raven Press, 1988, pp 543

16. Skaer RJ: Platelet degranulation, Platelets in Biology and Pathology, Vol 2. Edited by Gordon JL. Amsterdam, Elsevier, 1981, pp 321

17. Krauer KA: Platelet activation during antigen-induced airway reactions in asthmatic subjects. N Eng J Med 304:1404–1406, 1981

18. Grandel KE, Farr RS, Wanderer AA, et al: Association of platelet activating factor with primary acquired cold urticaria. N Eng J Med 313:405–409, 1985

19. Ginsberg MH: Role of platelets in inflammation and rheumatic disease. Adv Inflamm Res 2:53–71, 1986

20. Pytela R, Pierschbacher M, Ginsberg M, et al: Platelet membrane glycoprotein IIb/IIIa: Member of a family of Arg-Gly-Asp-specific adhesion receptors. Science 231:1559–1562, 1986

B. Growth Factors and Cytokines in the Rheumatic Diseases

Cytokines are small molecular weight proteins that mediate communication between cells. The generic term *cytokines* includes colony stimulating factors (CSFs), growth factors, interleukins (ILs), and interferons (IFNs). The terminology of these molecules is confusing because it is largely on a historical basis and not functional. For example, some interleukins primarily serve to regulate cell growth and differentiation, whereas some growth factors have other major properties.

Cytokines carry out their functions largely in the immediate pericellular environment either in an autocrine fashion, influencing the same cell that produced the cytokine, or in a paracrine fashion, influencing adjacent cells. Cytokines bind to specific plasma membrane receptors on target cells. Secondary messenger pathways or other intracellular mechanisms are subsequently activated that lead to alterations in gene transcription and production of proteins.

Cytokines are mediator molecules in normal biologic processes. These physiologic functions include growth and differentiation of hematopoietic, lymphoid, and mesenchymal cells as well as orchestration of host defense mechanisms. Multiple cytokines operate as a network in a redundant, overlapping, and synergistic fashion. However, the cytokine network is largely self-regulating. Pathophysiologic consequences may result from the unregulated action or inappropriate production of particular cytokines.

This chapter will review information about cytokines using arbitrary groupings based on primary functions. These categorizations include CSFs, growth and differentiation factors, immunoregulatory cytokines and pro-inflammatory cytokines (Table 7B–1). The relevance of each cytokine to the function of lymphoid and inflammatory cells, particularly their possible role in rheumatic diseases, will also be emphasized. Lastly, the self-regulatory nature of the cytokine network will be discussed in a review of mechanisms of inhibition of cytokine effects.

COLONY-STIMULATING FACTORS

The CSFs, and related molecules, function primarily as hematopoietic growth factors (1). However, this group of cytokines also exerts profound effects on mature lymphocytes, neutrophils, monocytes, and macrophages, possibly giving them a significant role in rheumatic diseases.

Granulocyte–macrophage colony stimulating factor (GM–CSF) and interleukin–3 (IL–3) potentiate the growth of numerous early bone marrow precursor cells, whereas erythropoietin solely influences erythroid precursor cells. Both of these factors are preceded in their actions by other stem cell growth and differentiation factors. Also, these effects of GM-CSF and IL-3 are enhanced by the presence of interleukins–1 and –6. In contrast, granulocyte colony stimulating factor (G–CSF) influences the growth and function of mature neutrophils while macrophage colony stimulating factor (M–CSF) serves the same role for monocytes and macrophages. Monocytes, fibroblasts, and endothelial cells all produce GM–CSF, G–CSF, and M–CSF. Lymphocytes also produce GM–CSF.

In addition to its effects as a growth factor, GM–CSF influences the function of mature cells of the granulocytic and monocytic lineages. It primes neutrophils, eosinophils, and basophils

Colony-stimulating factors (CSFs)
GM–CSF (granulocyte–macrophage CSF)
G–CSF (granulocyte CSF)
M–CSF (macrophage CSF or CSF–1)
IL–3 (interleukin–3)
Erythropoietin
Growth and differentiation factors
PDGF (platelet-derived growth factor)
EGF (epidermal growth factor)
FGF (fibroblast growth factor)
TGF–β (transforming growth factor–beta)
Immunoregulatory cytokines
IL–2 (interleukin–2)
IL–4 (interleukin–4)
IL–5 (interleukin–5)
IL–7 (interleukin–7)
IL–9 (interleukin–9)
IL–10 (interleukin–10)
IL–11 (interleukin–11)
IFN–γ (interferon–gamma)
Pro-inflammatory cytokines
TNF–α (tumor necrosis factor–alpha)
IL–1 (interleukin–1)
IL–6 (interleukin–6)
IL–8 (interleukin–8)

to respond to triggering agents with enhanced chemotaxis, oxygen radical production, and phagocytosis. Also, GM–CSF enhances eosinophil cytotoxicity and stimulates basophil release of histamine. These multiple effects of GM–CSF probably serve to heighten the inflammatory response in acute rheumatic diseases.

Granulocyte–macrophage colony stimulating factor also influences diverse functions of monocytes and macrophages leading to enhanced ability of these cells to present antigen and induce an immune response. These functions include increased expression of membrane-bound IL–1α and of class II major histocompatibility complex (MHC) molecules. In addition, monocytes differentiated in the presence of GM–CSF produce more IL–1 receptor antagonist (IL–1ra), thereby promoting inhibition of IL–1 effects. These properties of GM–CSF illustrate an essential principle of cytokine biology: a single cytokine may simultaneously exhibit both activating and suppressive effects.

The possible role of GM–CSF in rheumatic diseases is best illustrated in rheumatoid arthritis (RA). This is the only human disease in which both GM–CSF protein and mRNA have been localized in the damaged tissue. GM–CSF is also present in rheumatoid synovial fluids. The enhanced expression of class II MHC molecules observed on rheumatoid synovial tissue macrophages may be secondary to the effects of GM–CSF.

Furthermore, IL–1 and tumor necrosis factor α (TNF–α) enhance production of GM–CSF by monocytes, fibroblasts, and endothelial cells. Some investigators believe that chronic inflammation and tissue destruction in certain patients with RA may result from a cytokine-mediated self-perpetuating cycle without a significant component of continuous T cell activation.

GROWTH AND DIFFERENTIATION FACTORS

The major property of a number of cytokines is growth enhancement of specific cell types. These cytokines include platelet-derived growth factor (PDGF), epidermal growth factor (EGF), fibroblast growth factor (FGF), and transforming growth factor β (TGF–β). Other cytokines also are growth-promoting, such as the CSFs and many of the interleukins.

Platelet-derived growth factor is primarily a product of platelets but also is produced by macrophages, endothelial cells, and other cells (2). There are three different forms of PDGF and two different PDGF receptors. The biologic properties exhibited by PDGF vary with both the form synthesized by a particular cell and the predominant receptor expressed on a target cell. Epidermal growth factor is found throughout the body and is a potent angiogenic factor, as is FGF (3). Two main forms of FGF exist, although many structural variants have been described (4). Both

EGF and FGF induce the growth and proliferation of a variety of mesenchymal and epithelial cells.

The marked proliferation of synovial fibroblasts that occurs in the rheumatoid synovium is probably secondary to the effects of PDGF, EGF, and FGF. In addition, the greatly enhanced growth of new capillaries that characterizes rheumatoid synovitis is likely due to EGF and FGF. These growth factors are all present in synovial fluids of RA patients and are produced by synovial macrophages. Tissue fibrosis present in other diseases, such as systemic sclerosis, may also be due, in part, to PDGF, EGF, and FGF.

The last and most important growth factor to be discussed, TGF–β, exhibits both potent pro and antiinflammatory effects (5). While TGF–β exhibits multiple biologic properties, those most important to rheumatic diseases include recruitment of monocytes into tissues, dampening of lymphocyte and macrophage functions, and stimulation of tissue fibrosis. More than any other cytokine, TGF–β exemplifies the apparent paradox of simultaneously enhancing inflammatory responses and promoting repair.

Transforming growth factor-β is the major member of a family of molecules that may serve important roles in embryogenesis of mesenchymal tissues. It is released in a latent form and must be activated in tissues, presumably by proteases. Many cells in the adult contain mRNA for TGF–β but macrophages and platelets are the main sources of protein. When released, TGF–β exists in a latent form and must be activated in tissues, presumably by proteases.

Depending on the co-presence of other cytokines, TGF–β may either enhance or inhibit growth and differentiation in fibroblasts. For example, TGF–β and EGF together suppress growth of particular types of fibroblasts, whereas the combination of PDGF and TGF–β stimulates growth. The enhancing effects of TGF–β on cell growth may be mediated through induction of PDGF production. Collagen and fibronectin production in fibroblasts is induced by TGF–β; however, IFN–γ and TNF–α both oppose this effect on collagen synthesis. In the presence of PDGF, EGF, and FGF, TGF–β also inhibits fibroblast production of collagenase and other neutral proteases while enhancing production of inhibitors of these enzymes.

Transforming growth factor-β is thought to be responsible, at least in part, for tissue fibrosis in a variety of human diseases including systemic sclerosis, pulmonary fibrosis, and chronic glomerulonephritis. Infiltrating monocytes in skin and organ lesions in scleroderma contain TGF–β mRNA. Transforming growth factor-β protein has been localized in the skin lesions adjacent to fibroblasts and areas of fibrosis. The observation that IFN–γ inhibits TGF–β-induced collagen production by fibroblasts in vitro has prompted clinical trials of therapy with IFN–γ in systemic sclerosis patients.

Lastly, TGF–β exhibits potent effects on both monocytes and lymphocytes. It is the strongest known chemotactic agent for monocytes. In addition, TGF–β enhances expression of Fc receptor III on these cells but may block production of cytokines. Transforming growth factor-β can promote inflammation; injection of TGF–β into rat joints leads to an influx of monocytes with swelling, redness, and eventual hyperplasia of synovial fibroblasts. However, the net effects of TGF–β on macrophage function are suppressive, including a decrease in HLA–DR expression and a diminution in H_2O_2 production. Overall, TGF–β is thought to recruit monocytes into an acutely inflamed tissue, contribute to fibroblast proliferation, and promote fibrosis.

Transforming growth factor-β exhibits immunosuppressive effects on B cells, T cells, and NK cells. It inhibits IL–1-induced T cell proliferation as well as B cell growth and immunoglobulin production after stimulation by IL–2 and IL–4. Interferon-γ-induced NK cell function is opposed by TGF–β. The immunosuppression present in streptococcal cell wall-induced arthritis in rats is thought to be secondary to TGF–β and a similar situation may occur in the joints of patients with RA.

Thus, growth and differentiation factors may be responsible primarily for fibroblast proliferation and angiogenesis in many human chronic inflammatory diseases. In addition, TGF–β also may be involved in enhancing acute inflammatory events. These net biologic effects are secondary to multiple cytokines acting in both synergistic and opposing fashions. In addition, the state of differentiation of potential target cells for growth factors influences the resultant biologic response.

IMMUNOREGULATORY CYTOKINES

Interleukins 2, 4, 5, 7, 9, 10, and 11, and IFN-γ are all produced by T lymphocyte subsets during an immune response and exert effects primarily on that response. Also, IL-4, IL-10, and IFN-γ have important effects on monocytes and macrophages.

Macrophage presentation of processed antigen peptides bound to a class II MHC molecule stimulates IL-2 production by CD4+ helper T cells. Then, IL-2 binds to a specific two-chain receptor on target cells in the immediate microenvironment. Interleukin-2 induces a clonal expansion of T cells, enhances B cell growth, augments NK cell function, and activates macrophages.

In patients with autoimmune diseases, IL-2 production was originally thought to be deficient (6). However, these observations may represent an in vitro artifact, and IL-2 production actually may be excessive in these diseases in vivo. The administration of monoclonal antibodies to the IL-2 receptor ameliorates collagen-induced arthritis or lupus in mice. This observation argues for the probable importance of IL-2-driven T cell responses in the counterpart human diseases of RA and systemic lupus erythematosus (SLE).

Soluble IL-2 receptors are found in the circulation of many patients with autoimmune, chronic inflammatory, or neoplastic diseases (7). These receptors are probably released by activated T cells and their circulating levels correlate with clinical disease activity in some diseases, including SLE and RA.

Interleukin-4 is produced by a subset of T cells during the immune response and exhibits potent effects on multiple other cells (8). It also is elaborated by mast cells. Interleukin-4 exerts a major influence on B cells through enhancing IgG1 and IgE production, inducing the expression of Fc receptors for IgE, and stimulating the expression of class II MHC molecules. In addition, IL-4 influences T cell function by acting as a growth factor for varied types of T cells and inducing activity of cytotoxic T cells.

Interleukin-4 exhibits both stimulatory and suppressive effects on mononuclear phagocytes, again illustrating the principle that a single cytokine may predispose to mixed consequences. By inducing the expression of class II MHC molecules, IL-4 enhances the ability of these cells to present antigen. Paradoxically, IL-4 directly inhibits monocyte production of IL-1, IL-6, and TNF-α at the level of transcription; these effects of IL-4 are potentially quite antiinflammatory. In addition, IL-4 alters the pattern of expression of adhesion molecules on endothelial cells resulting in decreased neutrophil attachment but enhanced lymphocyte migration into tissues. Although not yet directly proven, IL-4 may influence the function of many immune and inflammatory cells in rheumatic diseases.

Interleukins 5, 7, 9, and 11 also function primarily as growth and differentiation factors. Interleukin-5 is produced by T cells and enhances the immune response through effects on both T and B cells. It increases IL-2 receptor expression on these cells and promotes antibody secretion by B cells. In addition, IL-5 is the most active cytokine on eosinophils, inducing chemotaxis, enhancing growth, and stimulating superoxide production.

Interleukins 7, 9, and 11 are primarily growth factors for T lymphocytes. Interleukins 7 and 11 are synthesized by bone marrow stromal cells and exhibit additional effects on B cells and hematopoietic cells. Recent studies also have shown that IL-7 is a requisite factor for IL-1-induced thymocyte proliferation. These cytokines influence the function of other cells in addition to T lymphocytes. Interleukin-9 induces proliferation of mast cells; IL-11 synergizes with IL-3 in effects on megakaryocytes; IL-11 induces the hepatic synthesis of acute phase proteins along with IL-1 and IL-6; and IL-11 enhances antigen-specific B cell responses.

Unlike IL-2, interleukins 5, 7, 9, and 11 have not been directly incriminated in pathophysiologic events in rheumatic diseases.

However, these cytokines are indirectly involved through their effects on T lymphocytes and other cells.

Interleukin-10 differs from other immunoregulatory cytokines in displaying primarily an inhibitory profile of effects. It is produced by a T cell subset, B cells, and mast cells. Together, IL-10 and IL-4 enhance mast cell survival, and IL-10 synergizes with IL-2 and IL-4 in induction of thymocyte proliferation. In addition, IL-10 alone induces class II MHC expression on B cells. However, the most important effect of IL-10 may be inhibition of cytokine production by T cells and monocytes (9). This potent effect is seen at low IL-10 concentrations in vitro, suggesting that IL-10 may be a significant regulator of cytokine production in vivo. Whether therapeutic administration of IL-10 will block production of inflammatory cytokines in rheumatic diseases remains to be examined.

Interferon-γ is produced simultaneously with IL-2 by antigen-stimulated T cells (10). A major function of IFN-γ is to enhance antigen presentation by stimulating the expression of MHC class I and II molecules on macrophages, endothelial cells, fibroblasts, and other more tissue-specific cells. Interferon-γ also is a potent activator of macrophages, cytotoxic T cells, and NK cells. It stimulates antibody production by B cells but, paradoxically, opposes the effects of IL-4 on these cells. This is an example of self-regulation of the cytokine network through opposing effects, discussed in more detail below.

Interferon-γ may be relevant to many human autoimmune diseases, particularly SLE and RA. The poor production of IFN-γ by SLE T cells in vitro, and weak response to IFN-γ, may reflect cells exhausted by intense IFN-γ effects in vivo, similar to IL-2. In the rheumatoid joint, IFN-γ could antagonize the stimulatory effects of TNF-α on many functions of synovial fibroblasts. However, IFN-γ production is probably deficient in the rheumatoid synovium, predisposing to unregulated TNF-α effects. The administration of IFN-γ to patients with RA appears to offer, at best, moderate benefit.

Thus, the immunoregulatory cytokines may be important in rheumatic diseases both for their effects on immune cells and on macrophages. The possible manipulation of this group of cytokines for therapeutic advantage has yet to be completely explored.

PRO-INFLAMMATORY CYTOKINES

The last group of cytokines to be discussed in this chapter includes TNF-α and interleukins 1, 6, and 8. Their functions in normal physiology remain unclear. In contrast, their possible role as inadvertent mediators of inflammation and tissue necrosis continues to grow. Tumor necrosis factor-α and IL-1 are usually produced together and may act separately or together in different diseases. Clarifying the independent contribution of TNF-α and IL-1 to pathophysiologic events is made more difficult by the fact that each cytokine can induce production of itself and of the other.

Tumor necrosis factor-α and -β are related molecules that share the same receptors on plasma membranes of target cells (11). However, TNF-α is the more important factor and TNF-β, or lymphotoxin, will not be discussed further. Structurally, TNF-α resembles a transmembrane molecule, and 1% to 2% of TNF-α produced resides in the plasma membrane. Tumor necrosis factor-α is produced by monocytes, macrophages, lymphocytes, and a variety of transformed cell lines. Its production is stimulated by endotoxin, viruses and other cytokines.

Two different TNF-α receptors are present on a variety of target cells. The extracellular portions of both TNF-α receptors can be cleaved, probably by proteases, releasing soluble receptors. These soluble TNF receptors will be discussed below as possible regulators of extracellular TNF-α effects.

Tumor necrosis factor-α exhibits many biologic properties relevant to rheumatic diseases. Along with IL-1, TNF-α induces collagenase and PGE_2 production in synovial fibroblasts. Tumor necrosis factor-α is present in rheumatoid synovial tissues and may be an important inducer of IL-1 in this disease. Also, TNF-α may induce muscle breakdown and has been associated with the cachexia of congestive heart failure and of other chronic diseases. In addition, TNF–α may play pathophysiologic roles in sepsis and in the acute respiratory distress syndrome.

Interleukin–1 is a family of three known molecules; IL–1α and IL–1β bind to the same receptors and produce the same biologic responses (12). The third member of the IL–1 family, IL–1 receptor antagonist (IL–1ra), will be discussed in the next section. IL–1α and IL–1β are primarily products of monocytes and macrophages, but they may also be produced by endothelial cells, epithelial cells, fibroblasts, activated T cells, and multiple other cells. In humans, IL–1β is the major extracellular product, and IL–1α remains primarily membrane-bound.

Two different IL–1 receptors exist; type I IL–1 receptors are present on T cells, endothelial cells and fibroblasts while type II IL–1 receptors exist on B cells, monocytes, and neutrophils (13). Target cells are exquisitely sensitive to small concentrations of IL–1 as occupancy of only 1% to 2% of available receptors stimulates complete biologic responses in a cell. The expression of IL–1 receptors can be down-regulated by TGF–β, partially explaining the immunosuppressive properties of this cytokine.

Interleukin–1 exhibits both systemic and local biologic effects in acute and chronic inflammatory diseases. Systemic effects of IL–1 include fever, muscle breakdown and, along with IL–6 and IL–11, induction of synthesis of acute phase proteins in the liver. Local effects of IL–1 can be best summarized by describing its purported role in RA (14). Early in this disease process, IL–1 may enhance expression of adhesion molecules on endothelial cells and induce chemotaxis of neutrophils, monocytes, and lymphocytes. Furthermore, IL–1 may contribute to tissue destruction in the rheumatoid joint through inducing PGE$_2$ and collagenase production by synovial fibroblasts and by chondrocytes present in the articular cartilage. Interleukin–1 may exert similar effects on fibroblasts in immune and inflammatory diseases of other organs, producing tissue damage in lungs, kidneys, or other organs.

Interleukins 6 and 8 also play important roles in acute inflammatory diseases. Interleukin–6 is produced by many cells, including synovial cells stimulated by IL–1 or TNF–α. The major functions of IL–6 probably are to induce hepatic synthesis of acute phase proteins and to enhance immunoglobulin synthesis by B cells (15). High levels of IL–6 are present in inflammatory synovial fluids. In the rheumatoid synovium, IL–6 is present in fibroblasts. However, in this disease process IL–6 does not induce collagenase and PGE$_2$ production by synovial fibroblasts. It may actually enhance synthesis of a collagenase inhibitor. Interleukin–6 may be primarily responsible for the hypergammaglobulinemia that characterizes many chronic inflammatory diseases.

Interleukin–8 is one member of a family of chemotactic peptides (16). Tumor necrosis factor–α and IL–1 stimulate IL–8 production by monocytes, macrophages, endothelial cells, fibroblasts, and other cells. Interleukin–8 is an extremely potent chemotactic factor for neutrophils and may be responsible for attracting these cells into the joint in RA, gout, and other forms of inflammatory arthritis. In addition, IL–8 enhances other neutrophil functions, including expression of adhesion molecules, generation of oxygen radicals, and release of lysosomal enzymes. Thus, IL–8 may contribute to rheumatic diseases by recruiting neutrophils into sites of acute inflammation and by activating these cells into an enhanced destructive profile.

REGULATION OF CYTOKINE EFFECTS

The cytokine network functions in a self-regulatory fashion. Five different mechanisms that regulate the actions of cytokines will be discussed in this section: specific receptor antagonists, soluble cytokine receptors, opposing actions of different cytokines, antibodies to cytokines, and protein binding of cytokines.

Because of the probable central role that IL–1 plays in acute and chronic inflammatory diseases, it is thought that a specific mechanism must exist to block the effects of IL–1. Several "IL–1 inhibitors" have been described as biologic activities in the supernatants of cultured cells or in human plasma, urine, or synovial fluids. Most of these activities have not been further characterized and probably represent nonspecific inhibitors of IL–1.

A specific receptor antagonist of IL–1, termed IL–1ra, was originally described in the supernatants of monocytes cultured on adherent IgG and in the urine of febrile patients (17). The cDNA has been cloned and recombinant IL–1ra is now being studied in experimental models of disease in animals and in human diseases. Interleukin–1 receptor antagonist is structurally related to IL–1 and binds to both types of human IL–1 receptors on a variety of target cells without inducing discernable biologic responses. This represents the first known naturally-occurring molecule that functions as a specific receptor antagonist.

A secreted form of IL–1ra is produced by monocytes, macrophages, and neutrophils. An intracellular variant of IL–1ra, which lacks the structural characteristics that lead to secretion, is produced by keratinocytes and other epithelial cells. Alveolar and synovial macrophages produce little IL–1β but synthesize large amounts of IL–1ra, particularly under the influence of GM-CSF. Thus, IL–1ra is a major product of tissue macrophages and may offer significant antagonism to IL–1 in the pericellular microenvironment in inflammatory tissues.

Interleukin–1 receptor antagonist has been extensively evaluated in vitro and in vivo, and it blocks the inflammatory effects of IL–1 in every system evaluated (18). Most importantly, IL–1ra does not affect normal T or B cell responses in vitro or in vivo, suggesting that IL–1 is not required for these responses. This molecule has shown beneficial effects in many animal or in vitro models of human disease including septic shock, RA, graft-vs-host disease, inflammatory bowel disease, chronic myelogenous leukemia, diabetes mellitus, and asthma. Currently, IL–1ra is being evaluated as a therapeutic agent in most of these human diseases. This represents the first example of a therapeutic intervention in human diseases that specifically blocks the effects of a single cytokine.

Soluble cytokine receptors represent another possible mechanism to interfere with the action of cytokines in vivo through binding cytokines in solution and blocking their interaction with target cells (19). A truncated form of the IL–1 receptor has been genetically engineered and is currently being evaluated as a therapeutic agent in human diseases. Soluble IL–2 receptors bind IL–2 too weakly to interfere with its action but occur naturally and are markers of activity in autoimmune, inflammatory, or neoplastic diseases. Soluble IL–4 receptors also occur naturally and may serve to transport IL–4 from sites of synthesis to target cells without preventing biologic activity of IL–4. When IL–6 binds to soluble IL–6 receptors, this complex actually activates target cells. Both types of TNF receptors occur in soluble forms and may be effective in blocking TNF effects in vitro and in vivo. Other soluble cytokine receptors have been described, but their in vivo relevance remains unclear.

Numerous examples have been presented throughout this chapter of the opposing action of different cytokines. Tumor growth factor–β has some opposing effects to IL–1 and TNF–α, while some effects of TGF–β are opposed by IFN–γ and TNF–α. Lastly, both IL–4 and IL–10 block monocyte production of IL–1, TNF–α, IL–6 and other cytokines. Whether these opposing biologic effects of cytokines can be utilized in the treatment of human diseases has not yet been determined.

Antibodies to many cytokines have been described in the serum of normal individuals, including antibodies to IL–1α (but not IL–1β), TNF–α, and IL–6 (20). These antibodies appear to block the biologic effects of some cytokines, but their in vivo relevance has not been established. Multiple cytokines bind to α_2-macroglobulin in circulation; however, many of these cytokines still retain partial or full biologic activities. Thus, protein binding of cytokines as a mechanism to inhibit the effects of cytokines in vivo has not been proven.

William P. Arend, MD

1. Metcalf D: Control of granulocytes and macrophages: Molecular, cellular, and clinical aspects. Science 254:529–533, 1991
2. Raines EW, Bowen-Pope DF, Ross R: Platelet-derived growth factors, Peptide Growth Factors, and Their Receptors I. Edited by MB Sporn, AB Roberts. Berlin, Springer-Verlag, 1990, pp 173–368
3. Carpenter C, Wahl MI: The epidermal growth factor family, Peptide Growth Factors and Their Receptors I. Edited by MB Sporn, AB Roberts. Berlin, Springer-Verlag, 1990, pp 69–171
4. Baird A, Pöhlen P: Fibroblast growth factors, Peptide Growth Factors and

Their Receptors I. Edited by MB Sporn, AB Roberts. Berlin, Springer-Verlag, 1990, pp 369–418

5. Roberts AB, Sporn MB: The transforming growth factors-βs, Peptide Growth Factors and Their Receptors I. Edited by MB Sporn, AB Roberts. Berlin, Springer-Verlag, 1990, pp 419–472

6. Kroemer G, Wick G: The role of interleukin–2 in autoimmunity. Immunol Today 10:246–251, 1989

7. Rubin LA, Nelson DL: The soluble IL–2 receptor: Biology, function, and clinical application. Ann Int Med 113:619–627, 1990

8. Paul WE: Interleukin–4: A prototypic immunoregulatory lymphokine. Blood 77:1859–1870, 1991

9. de Waal Malefyt R, Abrams J, Bennett B, et al: Interleukin–10 (IL–10) inhibits cytokine synthesis by human monocytes: An autoregulatory role of IL–10 produced by monocytes. J Exp Med 174:1209–1220, 1991

10. Vilček J: Interferons, Peptide Growth Factors and Their Receptors II. Edited by MB Sporn, AB Roberts. Berlin, Springer-Verlag, 1990, pp 3–38

11. Jäättelä M: Biologic activities and mechanisms of action of tumor necrosis factor-α/cachectin. Lab Invest 64:724–742, 1991

12. Dinarello CA: Interleukin–1 and its biologically related cytokines. Adv Immunol 44:153–205, 1989

13. Dower SK, Sims JE: Molecular characterization of cytokine receptors. Ann Rheum Dis 49:452–459, 1990

14. Arend WP, Dayer JM: Cytokines and cytokine inhibitors or antagonists in rheumatoid arthritis. Arthritis Rheum 33:305–315, 1990

15. Hirano T, Abira S, Taga T, et al: Biological and clinical aspects of interleukin–6. Immunol Today 11:443–449, 1990

16. Baggiolini M, Walz A, Kunkel SL: Neutrophil-activating peptide–1/interleukin–8: A novel cytokine that activates neutrophils. J Clin Invest 84:1045–1049, 1989

17. Arend WP: Interleukin–1 receptor antagonist: A new member of the interleukin–1 family. J Clin Invest 88:1445–1451, 1991

18. Dinarello CA, Thompson RC: Blocking IL–1: Interleukin–1 receptor antagonist in vivo and in vitro. Immunol Today 12:404–410, 1991

19. Fernandez-Botran R: Soluble cytokine receptors: Their role in immunoregulation. FASEB J 5:2567–2574, 1991

20. Bendtzen K, Svenson M, Jonsson V, et al: Autoantibodies to cytokines–friends or foes? Immunol Today 11:167–169, 1990

C. The Complement System

The name *complement* was originally given to the heat-labile substance in normal serum that was required to "complete" the killing of gram-negative bacteria by specific antibody. The *complement system* now comprises 14 plasma proteins that interact in a cascade sequence to mediate a variety of inflammatory effects besides bacteriolysis (1–5), as well as six plasma proteins and five membrane proteins (6) that regulate this cascade. In addition to its important role in host defense, the complement system also mediates immunologically-induced tissue damage in rheumatic diseases. Activation of the system leads to lowered levels of complement proteins, making measurements of plasma levels useful in the diagnosis and management of patients with these diseases. Congenital deficiencies of complement proteins increase the risk for developing rheumatic disease and impair host defenses, leading to systemic sepsis and septic arthritis.

PATHWAYS FOR COMPLEMENT ACTIVATION

Two separate pathways, the classical and the alternative, recognize activating agents and lead to the generation of two enzymes with identical specificity. These both cleave the third complement component, C3, releasing the 8 kDa activation peptide C3a and generating metastable C3b that binds covalently to the activating agent or adjacent cell membranes. Both pathways also lead to cleavage of C5 and assembly of the membrane attack complex from the terminal sequence (C5b–9).

The *classical pathway* is activated by immune complexes containing IgG or IgM antibody (Fig. 7C–1). The first component (C1) exists in serum as a calcium-dependent complex of one molecule of C1q with two molecules each of C1r and C1s. The C1q subunit has six globular heads that recognize sites on the Fc portions of immunoglobulins and probably other activators of the classic pathway, including lipopolysaccharide, porins from gram-negative bacteria, and ligand-bound C-reactive protein. The binding of two or more globular recognition heads of C1q to an activator converts C1r to an active protease that cleaves and activates both itself and C1s. The natural substrates of active C1s are C4 and C2. Both are cleaved, releasing activation peptides, while the major fragments are incorporated into a magnesium-dependent enzyme complex, C4b2b, the classical pathway C3 convertase. Like C3b, C4b is also metastable and forms amide or ester bonds with nearby cell surface proteins or carbohydrates. An α-2 neuraminoglycoprotein present in normal serum, the C1 inhibitor, complexes with both C1s and C1r, and irreversibly blocks the activities of these proteases, thereby preventing further activation of C1s and the cleavage of C4 and C2.

Activation of the *alternative pathway* does not require antibody. It is triggered by polysaccharides such as those found in the cell walls of yeasts and bacteria (Fig. 7C–2). In a reaction that is strikingly similar to that of the classical pathway, four factors participate in the formation of the alternative pathway convertase. Factor $\bar{D}$, C3, and Factor B are the homologues of C1s, C4, and C2, respectively. Just as cleavage of C4 to C4b reveals a site for interaction with C2, cleavage of C3 to C3b permits its participation in a complex with Factor B. Cleavage of C3b-bound B by Factor $\bar{D}$ yields C3bBb. An extra protein, properdin, serves to stabilize the magnesium-dependent complex enzyme C3 convertase, C3bBb, which is identical to C4b2b in its capacity to cleave C3 and C5 and to initiate the terminal sequence. Amplification of the alternative pathway occurs when C3b, the product of the cleavage reaction catalyzed by C3bBb, complexes with additional B, permitting cleavage by $\bar{D}$ and the formation of more C3bBb.

Regulation of complement activation involves control of the classical and alternative pathway C3 convertases by: 1) acceler-

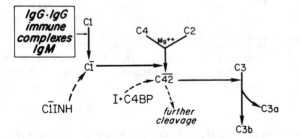

Fig. 7C–1. The classical activation pathway. *Immune complexes containing either IgG or IgM convert the first component (C1) from its precursor form to an active protease. Activated C1 cleaves the fourth (C4) and second (C2) components, forming from them the complex enzyme C42 that cleaves the third (C3) component into C3a and C3b. C1 inhibitor (C1INH) blocks the effect of C1. In the presence of C4-binding protein (C4BP), Factor I (I) inactivates C4b by cleaving it to C4c and C4d.*

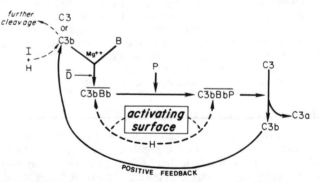

Fig. 7C–2. The alternative pathway. *Either C3b or native C3 that has been altered by hydrolysis of an internal thioester bond interacts with Factor B (B), which is subsequently cleaved by Factor $\bar{D}$ (D) forming C3bBb. This enzyme is stabilized by combining with properdin (P) to form C3bBbP. C3b, the major fragment of C3, interacts with additional Factor B, generating additional C3bBb and creating a positive feedback loop. The loop is controlled by Factor H (H) which accelerates the decay of C3bBb and by Factor I (I) which in the presence of H, further degrades C3b to iC3b. Surfaces that activate the alternative pathway provide a microenvironment inimical to the action of Factor H.*

Table 7C–1. *C3/C4 receptors*

Receptor	Molecular Structure	Ligand	Cell Type	Function
CR1 (CD35)	190–280 kDa Variable number of tandem short consensus repeats (SCR)	C3b C4b	Erythrocyte Neutrophils	Immune complex clearance Enhanced phagocytosis
		iC3b	Monocytes B lymphocytes T lymphocytes Follicular dendritic cells	Immune complex binding Antigen localization
CR2 (CD21)	145 kD, 15 SCR	iC3b (C3dg, C3d)	B lymphocytes	B cell activation (part of CD19 complex)
			Follicular dendritic cells	Antigen localization, lymphocyte memory
CR3 (CD11b/CD18)	α:150 kD β:95 kD Member of integrin family	EB Virus iC3b	Neutrophils Monocytes	Mediates viral infection Enhanced phagocytosis Adhesion to endothelium

ating the decay of the C3 convertases and 2) proteolytic cleavage by factor I of the C4b and C3b subunits of the convertases. The latter reaction requires binding of a cofactor protein to C4b or C3b. Decay of C4b2b is accelerated by: 1) decay-accelerating factor (DAF), a protein anchored by a glycolipid bond to the membranes of many different cell types, 2) C4-binding protein (C4BP), a 560 kDa plasma protein, and 3) complement receptor type 1 (CR1), a membrane glycoprotein present on most peripheral blood cells. Decay of C3bBb is accelerated by DAF and CR1, as well as Factor H, a plasma protein that functions in the alternative pathway in a fashion homologous with C4BP in the classical pathway. Cofactors for the cleavage of C4b by Factor I include membrane cofactor protein (MCP, which is present on a wide variety of cells), CR1, and C4BP. Cofactors for the cleavage of C3b are MCP, CR1, and Factor H. All of the proteins involved in convertase regulation are encoded in a gene cluster on the long arm of chromosome 1. They all contain common short consensus repeats of approximately 60 amino acids, suggesting that they arose from a common ancestor by gene duplication and rearrangement. Short consensus repeats are also found in C1r, C1s, C2, Factor B, C6, and C7.

THE MEMBRANE ATTACK COMPLEX

Binding of C3b to C4b2b forms a trimolecular complex that efficiently cleaves C5. Binding of a second C3b molecule to C3bBb has the same effect. Cleavage of C5 yields an activation peptide, C5a, and the major fragment, C5b. Activated C5b combines with C6 to form C5b6, which reacts with C7. Binding of the nascent complex of C5b67 to cell membranes is the first step in assembling the membrane attack complex (MAC). The complex formed by components up through C8, C5b–8, is capable of membrane damage, but formation of a stable transmembrane channel requires the binding of multiple molecules of C9 that polymerize to form the mature MAC. C9 is homologous both in amino acid sequence and function to perforin, the pore-forming protein of cytotoxic T lymphocytes. The C5b–C9 complex is inserted through the lipid bilayer of the cell membrane, with hydrophobic residues on the exterior in contact with the lipid bilayer, forming a lesion or hole that leads to osmotic lysis and cell death. A wide variety of cells, including viruses, bacteria, protozoa, tumor cells, "innocent bystander" erythrocytes, and platelets are susceptible to MAC-induced damage, although some nucleated cells repair such damage and manage to remain alive. Action of the MAC is regulated by the glycolipid-anchored membrane proteins Homologous Restriction Factor and Membrane Inhibitor of Reactive Lysis (CD59). Both of these proteins function most efficiently on MACs formed from plasma proteins of the same species as the cells on which they are located, thereby protecting host cells from lysis as innocent bystanders during complement activation. Vitronectin, or S-Protein, prevents the insertion of the C5b67 complex into the lipid bilayer of cell membranes and probably also protects host cells from lysis.

BIOLOGIC CONSEQUENCES OF COMPLEMENT ACTIVATION

The activation peptides, C4a, C3a, and C5a are *anaphylatoxins* that trigger degranulation of mast cells and basophils. The mediators that are subsequently released promote increased vascular permeability, smooth muscle contraction, and local edema. These peptides also possess smooth muscle contractile activity independent of histamine release. The activities are blocked by removal of the N-terminal arginine by carboxypeptidase N, a magnesium-dependent enzyme, which also has been termed the anaphylatoxin inactivator. C5a is responsible for most of the chemotactic activity that appears in plasma after activation of the complement system. It attracts neutrophils, eosinophils, and monocytes and also releases lysosomal enzymes from polymorphonuclear neutrophils (PMNs) into phagocytic vacuoles or the surrounding medium.

The biologic activities of C3b and its degradation products iC3b and C3dg are governed by the types of cells bearing the *receptors* to which they bind (Table 7C–1). In addition to its function as a regulator of complement activation mentioned above, CR1 on the membranes of erythrocytes promotes the clearance of immune complexes by binding and transporting them to the liver and spleen where they are removed from the circulation. CR1 on PMNs and monocytes enhances the phagocytosis of C3b-coated particles by these cells. Recombinant soluble CR1, lacking transmembrane and cytoplasmic domains, inhibits both alternative and classical pathway activation and reduces tissue injury in the rat model of reperfusion injury in ischemic myocardium. CR2, the receptor for C3d and C3dg, is present on B lymphocytes in a membrane complex that also contains CD19, a member of the immunoglobulin superfamily, as well as three other proteins of 130, 50, and 20 kDa (6). Interaction of this complex with polymeric C3dg results in transmembrane signalling and priming of B cells for proliferation induced by anti–IgM. The Epstein–Barr virus binds to the same domains of CR2 as do C3d and C3dg, and achieves infection of B cells via this route. CR3, a member of the integrin family of adhesion molecules, specifically binds iC3b on PMNs and monocytes and promotes the phagocytosis of iC3b-coated particles by these cells. CR3 also promotes the attachment of PMNs and monocytes to endothelium via direct interaction that does not involve complement proteins.

GENETICS AND DEFICIENCIES

With the exception of properdin, which is X-linked, the synthesis of complement proteins is encoded by genes inherited in an autosomal codominant fashion. Congenital deficiency is the consequence of an inherited null allele, which codes for nonsynthesis of the protein and is allelic with the normal structural gene. A single null allele usually results in approximately one-half normal plasma levels of the protein; inheritance of two null alleles results in complete deficiency. The genes for C2, Factor B, and C4 are located on the short arm of chromosome 6, in the major histocompatibility complex between the HLA–D/DR and HLA–B loci

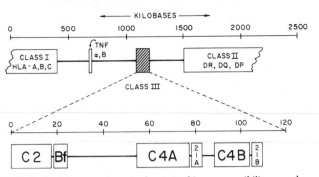

COMPLEMENT LOCI WITHIN THE MAJOR HISTOCOMPATIBILITY COMPLEX

Fig. 7C–3. Complement genes in the major histocompatibility complex on the short arm of chromosome 6.

(Fig. 7C–3). Inheritance of C4 is complicated by the existence of two adjacent loci, C4A and C4B. Individuals homozygous for null alleles in both loci (C4AQ0, BQ0/C4AQ0, BQ0) are rare, but those with one, two, or three null alleles and C4 levels in serum equal to three-fourths, one-half, or one-fourth of the normal mean occur more frequently.

Complete or homozygous deficiencies of the classical pathway proteins, C1, C4, and C2, are frequently associated with rheumatic disease, including a syndrome resembling systemic lupus erythematosus (SLE), vasculitis, glomerulonephritis, and polymyositis. C2 deficiency is the most common, the frequency of C2Q0 being about 1%. More than one-half of Caucasians with SLE have one C4AQ0 allele, and 10% to 15% are homozygous C4A deficient. The C4AQ0 gene is usually found as part of a "supratype" containing HLA–B8 and DR3. Impaired processing of immune complexes may account for the association of classical pathway deficiencies with rheumatic diseases.

Homozygous deficiencies of components of the MAC predispose to recurrent sepsis with *Neisseria gonorrhoeae* or *N. meningitidis*. Failure of deficient serum to form a functional MAC for bacteriolysis of Neisserial organisms has been demonstrated in vitro.

MEASUREMENT

The *total hemolytic complement activity* (also called the CH50 assay) is a useful screening procedure for detecting homozygous deficiency of a complement protein, but does not reliably detect heterozygous deficiency states. Because complement activity is heat labile, considerable care is required in proper collection and handling of specimens to preserve this activity. *Immunoassays* measure the complement protein as antigen, without regard to

whether or not it is active, so that special handling or processing of plasma samples is not required. Assays for C4 and C3 are widely available clinically. Detection by enzyme-linked immunosorbant assay (ELISA) of cleavage products of complement reactions, such as C4a, C3a, C5a, Bb, C3c, or C3dg may provide a more sensitive index of complement activation during disease than a fall in the concentration of a particular component in plasma. Antibodies to neoantigens that arise during the formation of the membrane attack complex have been used in ELISAs to measure concentrations of C5b–9 (or more correctly SC5b–9, since the S-protein is present in the spent serum complex) in plasma and other biologic fluids.

CLINICAL SIGNIFICANCE

Elevations of complement levels are due to increased synthesis and occur as part of the acute-phase response. Elevations in levels of total hemolytic activity, C3, and C4 in plasma occur regularly during the active phase of virtually all rheumatic diseases including rheumatoid arthritis (RA), SLE, dermatopolymyositis, systemic sclerosis, rheumatic fever, Reiter's syndrome, ankylosing spondylitis, and temporal arteritis. In diseases in which elevated levels are frequent, a level at the lower limit of normal may be inappropriate and indicate in vivo complement activation. Other conditions in which elevated levels have been observed include acute viral hepatitis, myocardial infarction, cancer, diabetes, pregnancy, sarcoidosis, amyloidosis, thyroiditis, inflammatory bowel disease, typhoid fever, and pneumococcal pneumonia.

Any disease associated with circulating immune complexes is likely to lead to acquired hypocomplementemia, including SLE, RA, subacute bacterial endocarditis, hepatitis B surface antigenemia, pneumococcal infection, gram-negative sepsis, viremias such as measles, or recurrent parasitemias such as malaria. Essential mixed cryoglobulinemia, a disease characterized by arthritis or arthralgias, cutaneous vasculitis, and nephritis, is invariably accompanied by profound hypocomplementemia due to classic pathway activation by the immune complexes that occur in this disease.

Shaun Ruddy, MD

1. Moxley G, Ruddy S: Immune complexes and complement. In: Textbook of Rheumatology, 4th ed. Edited by Kelley WN, Harris ED Jr, Ruddy S, Sledge CB. Philadelphia, WB Saunders, 1993, pp 188–200
2. Frank MM: Complement in the pathophysiology of human disease. N Engl J Med 316:1525–1530, 1987
3. Atkinson JP: The Complement System. In: Immunology. Kalamazoo, MI. The Upjohn Company, 1991, pp 111–131
4. Whaley K: Methods in Complement for Clinical Immunologists. New York, NY, Churchill Livingstone, 1985
5. Muller-Eberhard HJ: Molecular organization and function of the complement system. Annu Rev Biochem 57:321–339, 1988
6. Ahearn JM, Fearon DT: Structure and function of the complement receptors, CR1 (CD35), and CR2 (CD21). Adv Immunol 46:183–120, 1989

D. Proteinases and Their Inhibitors

The destruction of normal tissue structures, replacement of these structures by inflammatory and fibrotic tissue, and finally, loss of function are key elements of rheumatic diseases. This chapter considers the proteolytic events responsible for inflammation and connective tissue remodeling, and the cellular and molecular mechanisms controlling these processes.

EXTRACELLULAR MATRIX-DEGRADING PROTEINASES

Proteinases are important mediators of the degradation of the extracellular matrix (ECM) during inflammation. There are four classes of proteinases, two active at acid pH (aspartic and cysteine proteinases), and two active at neutral pH (serine and metalloproteinases) (Tables 7D–1 and 7D–2). The proteinases are

derived from many cell types, including neutrophils, monocytes, macrophages, and fibroblasts.

Aspartic Proteinases

Most intracellular protein digestion in mammalian cells occurs at acid pH in lysosomes. The most prominent lysosomal proteinase acting at acid pH is cathepsin D, an enzyme belonging to the same multigene family as pepsin and renin (1). Cathepsin D is found in the lysosomes of most cells, including fibroblasts; however, its activity is higher in phagocytic cells, such as macrophages, and is increased by connective tissue activation. Under inflammatory conditions, and during periods of rapid ECM destruction, cathepsin D is secreted extracellularly by macrophages and connective tissue cells, mostly as the proenzyme.

Table 7D–1. *Proteinases of connective tissues*

Class	Examples	Location	pH range	Protein inhibitors
Aspartic			3–6	
	Cathepsin D	lysosomes, extracellular		α_2-macroglobulin
Cysteine			3–7	
	Cathepsin B	lysosomes, extracellular		α_2-macroglobulin
	Cathepsin L	lysosomes, extracellular		α_1-cysteine proteinase inhibitor
Serine			6–10	
	Plasmin	extracellular		α_2-macroglobulin, protease nexin-1, α_2-antiplasmin
	Kallikrein	extracellular		
	Thrombin	extracellular		protease nexin-1
	Urokinase-type plasminogen activator	extracellular, cell surface		protease nexin-1, plasminogen activator inhibitor-1, plasminogen activator inhibitor-2
	Tissue-type plasminogen activator	extracellular, cell surface		plasminogen activator inhibitor-1
	PMN elastase	granules, extracellular		α_1-proteinase inhibitor
	Cathepsin G	granules, extracellular		α_1-cysteine proteinase inhibitor
	Mast cell chymase	granules, extracellular		α_1-cysteine proteinase inhibitor
	Mast cell tryptase	granules, extracellular		Aprotinin
	Granzymes	granules, extracellular		
Metallo			6–9	
	Collagenase	extracellular		α_2-macroglobulin, TIMP-1, TIMP-2
	Stromelysin-1, -2	extracellular		α_2-macroglobulin, TIMP-1, TIMP-2
	PMN collagenase	granules, extracellular		α_2-macroglobulin, TIMP-1, TIMP-2
	Metalloelastase	extracellular		α_2-macroglobulin, TIMP-1, TIMP-2
	Gelatinase B (92 kDa)	granules, extracellular		α_2-macroglobulin, TIMP-1, TIMP-2
	Gelatinase A (72 kDa)	extracellular		α_2-macroglobulin, TIMP-1, TIMP-2
	Matrilysin-1	extracellular		α_2-macroglobulin, TIMP-1, TIMP-2

Modified from reference 1. TIMP = tissue inhibitors of metalloproteinases.

Cysteine Proteinases

Cysteine proteinases have been associated with inflammatory reactions and with osteoclasts of bone. Cathepsin B and cathepsin L are the best-known lysosomal cysteine proteinases. These enzymes are related to each other and, evolutionarily, to papain, and have catalytic sites that require cysteine and histidine residues (1). The lysosomal cysteine proteinases are naturally inhibited by α_2-macroglobulin and by protein inhibitors of the cystatin family, such as the plasma protein α_1-cysteine proteinase inhibitor (1). In human tissues, the cysteine proteinases with greatest activity against collagen and proteoglycan are cathepsins L and N. Cysteine proteinases are also inactivated by thiol-blocking reagents in general, but more selective inhibitors usable in biologic systems include leupeptin, E-64 and certain chloromethanes.

Serine Proteinases

These proteinases, with a catalytically essential serine residue at their active site, are most active at about neutral pH. Their physiologic importance is reflected by the fact that serine proteinase inhibitors represent 10% of all plasma protein. The serine proteinases include many of the proteins of the coagulation, fibrinolytic, complement, and kinin cascade in the plasma, such as thrombin, plasmin, Cls, Clr, and kallikrein, as well as trypsin, chymotrypsin, and elastase from the exocrine pancreas. Plasmin and the plasminogen activators, plasma kallikrein, the tissue kallikreins and the serine proteinases from the granules of the polymorphonuclear leukocytes (PMN), T-cells and mast cells likely play a role in tissue degradation.

Plasminogen activators. Two distinct genes for plasminogen activators, the tissue-type plasminogen activator (tPA), made

Table 7D–2. *Proteinase susceptibility of extracellular matrix proteins*

Matrix protein	Proteinases
Cartilage:	
Cartilage proteoglycans	Stromelysin-1, -2, matrilysin, metalloelastase, plasmin, mast cell chymase, cathepsin G, PMN elastase, cathepsin B, cathepsin L
Collagen type II	Collagenases
Collagen type IX	Stromelysin-1
Collagen type X	Collagenase, 72 kDa gelatinase
Collagen type XI	92 kDa gelatinase
Interstitial connective tissue:	
Collagen type I	Collagenase, PMN collagenase, cathepsins B, L, N
Collagen type III	Collagenase, plasmin
Collagen type V	92 kDa gelatinase, 72 kDa gelatinase
Collagen type VII	Collagenase, 92 kDa gelatinase, 72 kDa gelatinase
Fibronectin	Stromelysin, cathepsin G, uPA, plasmin, PMN elastase, metalloelastase, stromelysin, cathepsin L, 72 kDa and 92 kDa gelatinases
Elastin	PMN elastase, macrophage elastase, 72 kDa gelatinase, stromelysin, cathepsin D
Basement membrane:	
Collagen type IV	Stromelysin, 72 kDa gelatinase, 92 kDa gelatinase, plasmin, PMN elastase, mast cell chymase
Heparan sulfate proteoglycans	Mast cell chymase, PMN elastase
Laminin	Plasmin, stromelysin, PMN elastase, gelatinases
Entactin	Stromelysin
Denatured collagen	92 kDa gelatinase, 72 kDa gelatinase, PMN elastase, cathepsin B, cathepsin L

Modified from references 1,2.

largely by endothelial cells, and the urokinase-type plasminogen activator (uPA), contribute to the activation of plasminogen, the zymogen of plasmin (1). Plasminogen activators are secreted proteinases produced by macrophages, fibroblasts, synovial cells, endothelial cells, and PMN. Both proenzyme and active forms of uPA bind tightly to the surface of macrophages and fibroblasts via a specific receptor. uPA is inhibited by protease nexin-1, an inhibitor produced by fibroblasts that also inhibits plasmin and thrombin. Both uPA and tPA are inhibited by plasminogen activator inhibitors-1 and -2 made by fibroblasts, macrophages, and endothelial cells; uPA is also inhibited by aprotinin, a 7 kDa inhibitor from mast cells.

Polymorphonuclear leukocyte elastase. The PMN elastase is present in the azurophil granules of PMN and monocytes as a precursor containing two additional amino acid residues (GlyGlu) compared to the active form, as is true for cathepsin G as well (1). It degrades cartilage proteoglycans by removing the hyaluronic acid-binding region, and then fragmenting the glycosaminoglycan attachment region. Elastin, the cross-linked structural protein important for the elastic strength of the arterial walls, lung, joint capsule, and skin, is degraded by PMN elastase. The PMN elastase also actively degrades fibronectin, laminin, and type IV collagen of basement membranes, making it a proteinase that is highly destructive to ECM. Extracellular activity of PMN elastase is controlled by α_1-proteinase inhibitor and α_2-macroglobulin.

Cathepsin G. Cathepsin G, a chymotrypsin enzyme of PMN, is structurally related to the chymases of mast cell granules. The action of cathepsin G on cartilage proteoglycan is somewhat more restricted than that of PMN elastase, and the enzyme has little or no action on elastin or type I collagen (1). Cathepsin G is effective in solubilizing collagen from cartilage and may generate physiologically active products from complement components. Physiological inhibitors of cathepsin G include the plasma proteins α_1-antichymotrypsin, α_1-proteinase inhibitor, and α_2-macroglobulin. Cathepsin G is an activator of metalloproteinases.

Metalloproteinases

The enzymes that are most important in the degradation of the ECM macromolecules in connective tissues are the matrix metalloproteinases (MMP), which are zinc-dependent enzymes. The MMP gene family (reviewed in 1–7) consists of eight well-characterized members in human tissues that have been cloned and show sequence conservation. The primary sequence of metalloproteinases consists of activation, catalytic, zinc-binding, and hemopexin/vitronectin homology domains (1–7). Their catalytic activity is inhibited by zinc-chelating agents such as 1,10 phenanthroline. All family members are inhibited by tissue inhibitors of metalloproteinases (TIMP).

Collagenases. There are three distinct collagenases, enzymes that are able to cleave the triple helical backbone of fibrillar collagens. Interstitial collagenase (also called matrix metalloproteinase [MMP]-1) is specific for collagen as substrate and cleaves all three chains of the triple helix at one susceptible point, between residues 775 and 776 of the α_1 (I) chain. The bonds cleaved are between residues of glycine and isoleucine of collagen types I, II, and III (2). Collagenase also cleaves type VII and VIII collagens and makes two cleavages in collagen type X, but does not degrade basement membrane collagen type IV, or types V or VI collagen. Interstitial collagenase is produced by a wide variety of cells, including macrophages, fibroblasts, synovial cells, chondrocytes, and endothelial cells (7).

Polymorphonuclear leukocytes elaborate a collagenase that has a different but closely related sequence to the collagenase produced by cells of tissues such as the synovium (8). The PMN collagenase (also called MMP-8), of about 75 kDa, is stored in the specific granules of PMN and secreted in response to appropriate stimuli (1). This collagenase degrades type I collagen more readily than type III collagen and prefers collagen in solution to fibrillar collagen. The PMN collagenase occurs in much smaller amounts in the cells than elastase and cathepsin G. Its significance in collagen degradation remains to be determined.

Osteoblasts and osteosarcoma cells from rat and mouse express a collagenase that degrades triple helical collagens, but has a sequence as distinct from interstitial and PMN collagenases as it is from stromelysin (9). Its role in collagen turnover has yet to be evaluated.

Collagenase and the other mammalian metalloproteinases are commonly found in culture and tissues in inactive proenzyme form. The procollagenases of 53 and 57 kDa are activated by a multienzyme cascade and a cysteine switch mechanism to active forms of about 45 kDa (2,7).

The majority of the inhibitory and rheumatoid synovial fluid capacity of plasma for collagenase is due to α_2-macroglobulin. α_2-macroglobulin reacts more slowly with PMN collagenase than with interstitial collagenase from other cells (1,7). Although plasma concentrations of metalloproteinase appear to be controlled by α_2-macroglobulin, the major tissue inhibitor is TIMP-1 of about 28 kDa. TIMP, unlike α_2-macroglobulin, can enter interstitial spaces such as cartilage matrix. It forms tight complexes with all members of the matrix metalloproteinases family. A second member of the TIMP family, TIMP-2, also inhibits collagenase (10).

Stromelysin. There are three distinct stromelysin genes in man. Stromelysin-1 (also called proteoglycanase, MMP-3, transin, and neutral proteinase) is the major metalloproteinase, other than collagenase, and it is produced as a proenzyme of about 51 kDa that is activated to forms of 41 kDa and further degraded to active enzymes of 21–25 kDa. Stromelysin has a wide variety of connective tissue and plasma protein substrates, including proteoglycans, collagen types IV, V, VII, and IX, denatured type I collagen, laminin, fibronectin, elastin, α_1-proteinase inhibitor, immunoglobulins, and substance P. In addition, it has a significant function in the multienzyme cascade involved in activating procollagenase (2,11).

Stromelysin-1 is inhibited by α_2-macroglobulin and TIMP. It is produced by the same range of cells as interstitial collagenase. Although it is frequently synthesized and secreted coordinately with collagenase, it is clear in human fibroblasts, chondrocytes, and macrophages that collagenase and stromelysin-1 may be regulated independently.

A second enzyme closely related to stromelysin, called stromelysin-2 (also called MMP-10, transin-2), with sequence identity of nearly 80%, has been cloned and characterized (1–7). It has nearly identical substrate specificity as stromelysin-1, but very distinct regulation with predominant expression in epithelial cells. Its role in inflammatory diseases is unknown.

A new member of the metalloproteinase family, stromelysin-3, has recently been cloned as a stromal gene induced in human breast carcinoma (12). It exhibits the same size class and general domain structure of stromelysins and collagenases, although it is distantly related to both (about 40% sequence identity). Because it is also expressed in human embryonic fibroblasts after treatment with growth factors or phorbol esters, it may have significance in inflammatory diseases, although its substrates are not yet known.

Metalloelastase. Stimulated macrophages secrete a 21 kDa metalloproteinase that degrades elastin, proteoglycan, type IV collagen, fibronectin, and also serpin serine proteinase inhibitors, including α_1-proteinase inhibitor (1). The proenzyme form of the elastase is about 50 kDa and is related to stromelysin and collagenase. If this enzyme is produced by the macrophage-like cells of the synovial lining, it may contribute to tissue damage.

72 kDa gelatinase. A gelatin-degrading proteinase of 72 kDa (also called gelatinase A, MMP-2, type IV collagenase) that is secreted by many cells in culture (including fibroblasts) has been characterized as an enzyme that degrades type IV collagen (1–5). The 72 kDa gelatinase shows sequence homology with collagenase and stromelysin, and even more so with the 92 kDa gelatinase (1–7). The difference in size compared to collagenase is due to an additional domain homologous with the collagen-binding domain of fibronectin, inserted next to the zinc-binding pocket of the active site. It too requires proteolytic cleavage for activation and is inhibited by TIMP-1 and TIMP-2. The 72 kDa gelatinase in proenzyme form binds one molecule of TIMP-2 (10). A second molecule is required to inhibit the activated enzyme. The TIMP-2 bound to the proenzyme may stabilize it against autoactivation.

In addition to denatured collagen and type IV collagen, it has significant proteolytic activity against fibronectin and collagen types V, VII and X, but not against collagen types I and VI (1–7).

92 kDa gelatinase. The 92 kDa gelatinase (also called gelatinase B, type IV collagenase, type V collagenase, MMP-9, invadolysin) is a major secretion product of stimulated PMNs and macrophages (1–7). In PMN, this gelatinase is present in specific granules. It is related to the 72 kDa gelatinase in sequence, and is characterized by a domain closely related to the collagen-binding sequence of fibronectin. It also has a sequence homologous to the nonhelical C-terminal domain of $\alpha2(V)$ collagen.

Like other metalloproteinases, the 92 kDa gelatinase is a proenzyme that requires limited proteolytic cleavage for activation. However, the plasminogen activator/plasmin cascade does not activate this enzyme. The active forms of this gelatinase cleave denatured collagens, fibronectin, elastin and collagen types IV, V, VII, and XI (1–5). It is inhibited by TIMP-1 and, in parallel with 72 kDa gelatinase and TIMP-2, the proenzyme form of the 92 kDa enzyme binds one molecule of TIMP-1, requiring a second molecule for inhibition of the activated form. It does not cross-react immunologically with the 72 kDa gelatinase.

Matrilysin. Matrilysin (also known as Pump-1, punctuated metalloproteinase, small uterine metalloproteinase, MMP-7) was initially described as a truncated cDNA with the proenzyme activation, catalytic, and zinc-binding sequences of metalloproteinases, but lacking the hemopexin domain found in all other members of the family (1–5). It has been shown to have a substrate specificity like that of stromelysin, degrading fibronectin, proteoglycans and gelatin. It also is a co-activator of collagenase. It is expressed in involuting uterus and certain tumors and is induced in fibroblasts by concanavalin A.

CONTROL OF PROTEINASE GENE EXPRESSION

Two major mechanisms exist for regulating ECM degradation. In cells such as PMN and mast cells, the enzymes are present in granules and are released upon stimulation. For metalloproteinases the major control is at the level of gene regulation. Many cells secrete little, if any, metalloproteinase unless appropriately triggered. Factors involved in the stimulation or suppression of metalloproteinase activity in tissue or cell culture are well described and appear to act directly on the enzyme-producing cells (Table 7D–3).

Collagenase and stromelysin are expressed by cells cultured from a variety of cells and tissues (1). Synovial fibroblasts can be induced in culture to express collagenase and stromelysin transcripts, and collagenase and stromelysin mRNA and protein can be readily demonstrated in rheumatoid synovium by in situ methods (13,14). In fact, higher amounts of stromelysin-1 mRNA and protein have been found in patients with rheumatoid arthritis than in osteoarthritis patients (15). The rather broad tissue specificity and potentially high expression levels of metalloproteinases, in contrast to the low or undetectable collagen turnover rates observed in the normal organism, suggest a complex control

of metalloproteinase activity in vivo, which is partially achieved at the level of proteinase gene expression.

Collagenase and stromelysin expression increase during fibroblast aging and in response to stress in culture. With increasing age, stromelysin can be extracted from human cartilage (16). Osteoarthritic cartilage contains degraded type II collagen around chondrocytes and fragments of cartilage link protein that can be attributed to stromelysin action (17,18).

The fragments of fibronectin produced by plasmin and metalloproteinases may also amplify metalloproteinase expression by acting as agonistic ligands for the fibronectin receptor (19). This may play an important role in osteoarthritis because of the increase in fibronectin in cartilage.

EXTRACELLULAR REGULATION OF MATRIX DEGRADATION

One of the key factors in our understanding of connective tissue catabolism is the regulation of the activity of proteinases. Degradation of collagen is likely to be rate-limiting in most cases of ECM degradation. For collagens, one mechanism of regulation is the variation in susceptibility to collagenases by the genetic type of collagen in the tissue, as well as the degree of cross-linking of the collagen. Other proteinases may also be involved in the breakdown of collagen in vivo by removing proteoglycans and glycoproteins surrounding collagen fibrils, by breaking collagen cross-links before the action of collagenase, and by further degrading the products of the initial collagen cleavage. A second mechanism involved in the local control of metalloproteinase activity is that of inhibitors and activators. Metalloproteinase inhibitors, as well as proenzyme forms and putative activators, have been found in association with connective tissue. In particular, bone has the highest concentration of TIMP-1, and cartilage has high concentrations of TIMP-2 (6).

CONTROL OF PROTEINASE ACTIVATION

Most proteinases are present in tissues as proenzymes. The activation of the cysteine and serine tissue proteinases such as uPA and PMN elastase is not well understood.

It has been appreciated for many years that metalloproteinase activation occurs by multiple pathways (2). There is a pathway involving initial cleavage by a proteinase such as trypsin (for collagenase) between amino acid residues 81 and 82, followed by a concentration-independent autocatalysis. Collagenase is activated in the absence of stromelysin; however, stromelysin-1 and -2, matrilysin, or small forms of collagenase are required for the full activation of procollagenase by trypsin (11). Stromelysin is activated by the proteinases that activate collagenase, as well as by mast cell tryptase, PMN elastase, and cathepsin G. In vivo, the generation of plasmin by uPA or tPA is likely to be a significant activation mechanism for collagenase and stromelysin (6). The mechanism of activation of the 72 kDa and 92 kDa gelatinases in vivo is unknown. Plasmin does not activate these en-

Table 7D–3. *Regulation of metalloproteinase expression*

Stimulatory factors	Inhibitory factors
Cell-matrix interactions via integrins, fibronectin fragments, soluble collagen, tenascin, SPARC	TGF-β
Proteinases	Glucocorticoids
Growth factors (epidermal growth factor, platelet-derived growth factor, fibroblast growth factor, transforming growth factor-α, nerve growth factor, relaxin)	Retinoids
Cytokines (interleukins-1α, -1β, and -6, tumor necrosis factor-α)	Hormones (estrogens, progesterone)
Parathyroid hormone	Increased production of endogenous inhibitors
1,25-dihydroxy vitamin D	Autocrine inhibitory factor
Serum amyloid A	Interferon-γ
β_2-Microglobulin	Indomethacin
Transformation (*src, ras*)	Transformation (T-antigen, Ela)
Cell aging	Inducers of TIMP expression
Phagocytosis, formation of multinucleate giant cells	
Prostaglandin E	
Phorbol diester tumor promoters	

Modified from reference 1.

zymes (20); however, neutrophil serine proteinases cathepsin G and elastase can activate the 72 kDa gelatinase. There are also data indicating that an activating system for the 72 kDa gelatinase is membrane associated (21). TIMP-2 also regulates activation of the 72 kDa gelatinase by controlling autocatalytic activation (22).

The degradation of ECM macromolecules is mediated by the availability of active proteolytic enzymes in the face of large amounts of proteinase inhibitors from plasma and local tissue sources. These inhibitors control cascade activation reactions and limit proteolysis to areas where the enzyme-inhibitor balance is in favor of the enzyme. Tissues like cartilage that are resistant to degradation and invasion by synovial pannus and blood vessels are rich in inhibitors such as TIMP-1 and TIMP-2 (23). The regulatory mechanisms involved in ECM degradation are complicated and involve a fine balance between proteolytic enyzme and inhibitor activity (1,6). Growth regulatory peptide factors such as TGF-β, PDGF, and cytokines are regulators of ECM synthesis, proteinase, and inhibitor expression. Their precise role in the fine control of matrix degradation remains to be elucidated.

Zena Werb, PhD
A. Huttenlocher, MD

1. Werb Z, Alexander CM: Proteinases and matrix degradation. Chapter 14. *In:* Textbook of Rheumatology, 4th edition. Edited by WN Kelley, ED Harris, Jr, S Ruddy, and CB Sledge. WB Saunders Co., Philadelphia, PA. 248–268, 1992
2. Birkedal-Hansen H, Moore WGI, Bodden MD, et al: Crit Rev Oral Biol Med 4:197–250, 1993
3. Matrisian LM: Metalloproteinases and their inhibitors in matrix remodeling. Trends Genet 6:121–125, 1990
4. Matrisian LM, Hogan BL: Growth factor-regulated proteases and extracellular matrix remodeling during mammalian development. Curr Top Dev Biol 24:219–259, 1990
5. Alexander CM, Werb Z: Curr Opin Cell Biol 1:974–982, 1989
6. Alexander C, Werb Z: In: Hay ED, ed. Cell Biology of Extracellular Matrix, ed. 2. New York: Plenum, 255–302, 1991
7. Werb Z: In: Kuettner KE, Schleyerbach R, Peyron JG, Hascall VC, eds. Articular Cartilage and Osteoarthritis. New York: Raven, 295–304, 1991
8. Hasty KA, Pourmotabbed TF, Goldberg GI, Thompson JP, et al: J Biol Chem 265:11421–11424, 1990
9. Quinn CO, Scott DK, Brinckerhoff CE, at al: J Biol Chem 265:22342–22347, 1990
10. Stetler-Stevenson WG, Krutzsch HC, Liotta LA: J Biol Chem 264:17374–17378, 1989
11. Murphy G, Cockett MI, Stephens PE, Smith BJ, et al: Biochem J 248:265–268, 1987
12. Basset P, Bellocq JP, Wolf C, et al: Nature 348:699–704, 1990
13. McCachren SS, Haynes BF, Niedel JE: J Clin Immunol 10:19–27, 1990
14. Woolley DE, Crossley MJ, Evanston JM: Arthritis Rheum, 20:1231–1239, 1977
15. Case JP, Sano H, Lafyatis R, et al: J Clin Invest 84:1731–1740, 1989
16. Gunja-Smith Z, Nagase H, Woessner JF Jr: Biochem J 258:115–119, 1989
17. Dodge GR, Poole AR: J Clin Invest 83:647–661, 1989
18. Nguyen Q, Murphy G, Roughley PJ, Mort JS: Biochem J 259:61–67, 1989
19. Werb Z, Tremble P, Behrendtsen O, Crowley E, et al: J Cell Biol 109:877–889, 1989
20. Behrendtsen O, Alexander CM, Werb Z: Development 114:447–456, 1992
21. Ward RV, Atkinson SJ, Slocombe PM, Docherty AJP, et al: Biochim Biophys Acta 1079:242–246, 1991
22. Howard E, Bullen E, Banda MJ: Regulation of the autoactivation of human 72 kDa progelatinase by tissue inhibitor of metalloproteinases-2. J Biol Chem 266:13064–13069, 1991
23. Moses MA, Sudhalter J, Langer R: Identification of an inhibitor of neovascularization from cartilage. Science 248:1408–1410, 1990

E. Lipid Mediators, Active Oxygen, Amines, Nitric Oxide, Kinins, and Clotting Factors

The coordination of vascular and cellular responses and other processes that are required for inflammation to occur depends on a number of active mediators which are derived either from the plasma, migrating inflammatory cells, or resident cells comprising the local vasculature or other tissues at sites of inflammation. Several of the more important groups of inflammatory mediators are described briefly in this chapter. Other important mediators include complement components, proteases, and cytokines, and these groups of compounds are each discussed elsewhere.

ARACHIDONIC ACID METABOLITES

A large number of biologically active metabolites are derived from the reactions of oxygen with arachidonic acid. These include the cyclooxygenase products, prostaglandins and thromboxanes, and lipoxygenase products including the leukotrienes (1–3). Arachidonic acid is an abundant polyunsaturated fatty acid in nearly all tissues. It is primarily found in ester linkage in the sn-2 or middle carbon of the glycerol portion of phospholipids. Before arachidonic acid can be metabolized, it must be released by phospholipases. There are two classes of phospholipases that account for most of the arachidonic acid, which is hydrolyzed. Phospholipase A_2 hydrolyzes arachidonic acid from the ester group at the sn-2 position producing arachidonic acid and lysophospholipids (4). A second route for arachidonic acid release is the hydrolysis of the glycerophosphate bond at the sn-3 carbon by phospholipase C. This reaction produces the phosphphosphoryl base and diacylglycerols. Subsequently, lipases cleave arachidonic acids and other fatty acids from diacylglycerol.

Cyclooxygenases are lipoxygenases that catalyze the addition of molecular oxygen to arachidonic acid to form initially the endoperoxide intermediate prostaglandin G_2 (Fig. 7E–1). The same enzyme also possesses peroxidase activity, which catalyzes a reduction of the 15-hydroperoxy group of PGG_2 to form the 15-hydroxy compound, PGH_2. This endoperoxide (PGH_2) may then react with a number of enzymes sometimes called isomerases to become one of the prostaglandins or thromb-

anes. The prostaglandins are characterized by a 5-membered ring, which determines the type of prostaglandin. In addition, PGH_2 can be converted to a 6-membered ring, thromboxane A_2. These compounds differ markedly in spite of the similarities in structure. For example, thromboxane A_2 is a powerful vasoconstrictor and causes platelet aggregation, whereas prostacyclin, or PGI_2, causes vasodilation and opposes platelet aggregation.

Two prostaglandins, PGE_2 and PGI_2, are mediators of vascular phases of inflammation. They are both potent vasodilators. In addition, they act synergistically with certain other vasoactive mediators, such as histamine and kinins, to increase vascular permeability. Prostaglandins E_2 and I_2 also stimulate osteoclastic bone resorption suggesting that bone erosion in chronic inflammatory diseases may be mediated, at least in part, by prostaglandins produced by inflamed tissues. In addition to their vascular effects, PGE_2 and PGI_2 have many other effects on cells and tissues. They elevate levels of cyclic 3', 5'-adenosine monophosphate (cyclic AMP) in cells, and many of their biologic effects may be related to elevations of cyclic AMP.

In addition to pro-inflammatory effects, PGE_2 and probably PGI_2 as well, may have antiinflammatory effects. Both T cell activation and interleukin–2 formation as well as the proliferation and maturation of B cells may be inhibited by exposure to PGE_2. In addition, several investigators have documented that PGE_2 may inhibit the secretion of inflammatory mediators by cells. This is especially prominent in the case of the synthesis of leukotrienes, which may be actively inhibited both in vitro and in vivo. Finally, it has been shown that administration of the E prostaglandins or their derivatives suppress experimental inflammation in several model systems, although pharmacologic doses are often required. It is not well established whether endogenous production of PGE_2 acts as a suppressing agent in these pathologic models.

Lipoxygenases other than cyclooxygenases also catalyze the addition of molecular oxygen to specific double bonds in polyunsaturated fatty acids, primarily arachidonic acid (3). The most important lipoxygenases are named for the position in the arachidonic acid molecule to which oxygen is added. The 5-lipoxy-

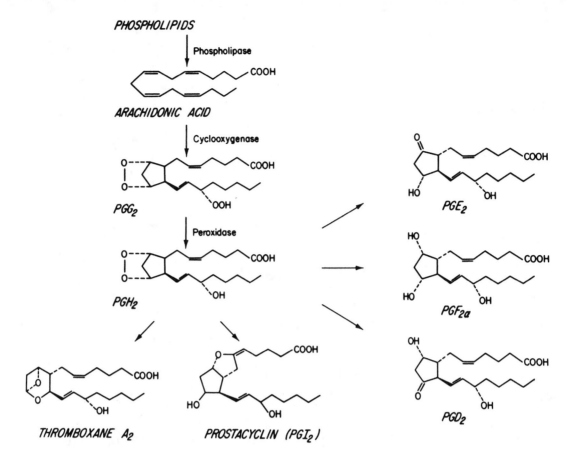

Fig. 7E–1. *The synthesis of prostaglandins and thromboxane A₂ (from Reference 2, with permission).*

genase leads to the formation of leukotrienes as illustrated in Fig. 7E–2. The addition of oxygen to the 5 position of arachidonic acid forms 5-hydroperoxyeicosatetraenoic acid (5-HPETE). The same enzyme catalyzes the cyclization of the hydroperoxy compound to form cyclic 5,6 epoxide, LTA₄. The LTA₄ intermediate undergoes two important reactions to form two different classes of leukotrienes. In the first, the LTA₄ hydrolase reaction converts LTA₄ to the stereospecific dihydroxy derivative, LTB₄. Alternatively, LTA₄ may react with glutathione to form LTC₄, which is further metabolized to LTD₄ and LTE₄ by elimination of a gamma glutamyl residue and, subsequently, a glycine residue. The three compounds, LTC₄, LTD₄, and LTE₄ are collectively called the *sulfidopeptide leukotrienes*, compounds that account for the activity of the previously recognized slow-reacting substance of anaphylaxis, an important mediator of immediate hypersensitivity reactions.

Products of the 5-lipoxygenase pathway are important mediators of inflammation. LTB₄ is a potent chemoattractant for leukocytes. It promotes the adherence of leukocytes to endothelial cells, and also activates secretion of active oxygen species and degradative enzymes from neutrophils. In contrast, the sulfidopeptide leukotrienes LTC₄, LTD₄, and LTE₄ contract smooth muscle in vascular, respiratory, and intestinal tissues. They cause vasoconstriction, but they increase microvascular permeability. They are important mediators of bronchial asthma because of their ability to induce bronchoconstriction and their ability to increase the flow of bronchial mucus. Other organs may also be affected by these compounds. For example, the sulfidopeptide leukotrienes stimulate mesangial cell contraction and exert a negative inotropic and an arrhythmogenic effect on the heart. In addition to the leukotrienes, the lipoxygenases can also produce hydroperoxy derivatives of arachidonic acid, many of which have biologic activity that has not been characterized in detail. Finally, the combined action of the 5 and 15 lipoxygenases produces triple lipoxygenation of the lipoxins (Fig. 7E–3). These compounds are produced by neutrophils and by neutrophils interacting with certain other cells. Lipoxins have counter-regulatory properties. They tend to produce vasodilatation and are weakly chemotactic. Recent evidence indicates that lipoxin A₄

may also be involved in intracellular signaling through its capacity to activate protein kinase C. In addition, the lipoxins inhibit human natural killer cell cytotoxicity.

Regulation of Eicosanoid Synthesis

A large number of factors are capable of stimulating the synthesis of eicosanoids, but the mechanisms by which these agents augment eicosanoid synthesis are not well understood. It is generally accepted that stimulation of eicosanoid synthesis requires stimulation of phospholipase activity to provide adequate quantities of free arachidonic acid for cyclooxygenase and lipoxygenase, because quantities of free arachidonic acid existing in resting cells are low (4–6). In addition, the stimulation of prostaglandin synthesis by interleukin–1 is accompanied by the induction of synthesis of the enzyme cyclooxygenase, suggesting that the synthesis of new enzyme may account for the enhanced production of prostaglandins in interleukin-1-stimulated cells (7).

The mechanism of inhibition of cyclooxygenase activity most familiar to physicians is inhibition by the nonsteroidal antiinflammatory drugs (NSAIDs) (1,2). Vane and colleagues proposed that the major therapeutic action of aspirin and other NSAIDs may be accounted for by the inhibition of the enzyme cyclooxygenase. In part, this is based on reasonably good correlations between the relative antiinflammatory potencies of different NSAIDs and their potencies as cyclooxygenase inhibitors. In addition, many toxic effects of NSAIDs can also be accounted for reasonably by cyclooxygenase inhibition. For example, the tendency of NSAIDs to cause erosive gastritis may be related to elimination of the cytoprotective effects of PGE₂ in the gastric mucosa. While other pharmacologic effects of NSAIDs may also be important for their activity, cyclooxygenase inhibition appears to be one prominent mechanism of action of these agents.

Glucocorticoids also inhibit the synthesis of prostaglandins and leukotrienes, but the mechanism of action differs from that of NSAIDs. Glucocorticoids appear to inhibit release of free arachidonic acid from phospholipids (1,2). Several laboratories have provided evidence that glucocorticoids induce the synthesis of proteins called *lipocortins*, which in turn inhibit the hydrolysis of

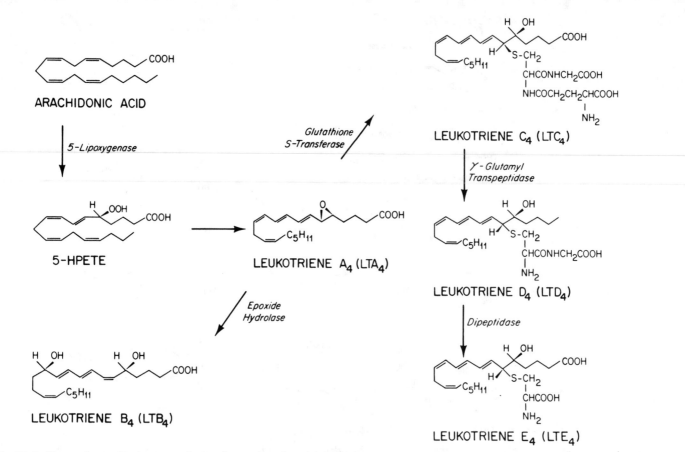

Fig. 7E–2. *The synthesis of leukotrienes (from reference 2, with permission).*

arachidonic acid from phospholipids (5). At least one of the lipocortins is similar to cytoskeletal proteins called calpactins; these proteins inhibit the reactions of phospholipases by complexing with phospholipids, rendering them ineffective as substrates for phospholipases (6). Other lipocortins apparently inhibit phospholipases directly (5). Glucocorticoids also may inhibit prostaglandin synthesis by inhibiting the synthesis of the enzyme, cyclooxygenase (8). Glucocorticoids inhibit the formation of both cyclooxygenase and lipoxygenase products in some systems, while NSAIDs lack any important activity on lipoxygenases. In fact, under some conditions, NSAIDs may augment leukotriene synthesis (2).

The prostaglandins are ubiquitous; one or more of these compounds are produced by all cells with the exception of erythrocytes. Lipoxygenase products are more restricted, and leukotrienes are only produced by inflammatory cells, including

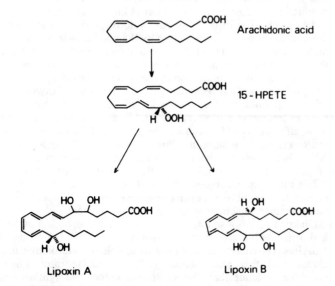

Lipoxin A

Lipoxin B

Fig. 7E–3. *The synthesis of lipoxins (from reference 2, with permission).*

neutrophils, monocyte–macrophages, mast cells, basophils and eosinophils. Eicosanoids act locally either on the cells from which they are produced or on neighboring cells (autocrine or paracrine effects, respectively). The eicosanoids are labile in tissues, either because of chemical instability, such as the endoperoxide prostaglandins, prostacyclin and thromboxane A_2, or because of rapid enzymatic degradation such as occurs with PGE_2 and the leukotrienes.

PLATELET ACTIVATING FACTOR

Platelet activating factor is the only phospholipid with potent biologic activities (9). It belongs to the class of ether phospholipids, having an O-alkyl ether residue in the sn–1 position of the glycerol moiety. Platelet activating factor is produced by neutrophils, macrophages, and to some extent, platelets. It causes platelet aggregation as the name implies, but in addition, it has a wide range of other biologic activities including chemotaxis, aggregation, and granule secretion by neutrophils and macrophages; and smooth muscle contraction in the gut and lung. It induces microvascular permeability and is considered to be a mediator of immediate hypersensitivity reactions.

ACTIVATED FORMS OF OXYGEN

Molecular oxygen is activated to form free radicals and other species that are important for host defense against microorganisms (10). In addition, active oxygen may react with several components of tissues including lipids, proteins, and other components resulting in tissue injury during inflammatory reactions. Molecular oxygen has a unique electron structure related to many of its biologic properties. Unlike most stable molecules, molecular oxygen has two unpaired electrons in its outer orbitals. In its fully reduced state with a −2 valence, as it exists in water and most stable organic molecules, each oxygen molecule may be considered to have gained four electrons. Reactive oxygen species are formed by partial reduction. Addition of a single electron to molecular oxygen yields superoxide anion and reduction by two electrons yields peroxide anion. Other reactive species are derived from superoxide and hydrogen peroxide and oxygen may also undergo electron rearrangement to form singlet oxygen, as described below.

Phagocytosis of bacteria, crystals or other particulate matter by neutrophils and macrophages is accompanied by a burst of oxygen consumption and by the production of several reactive oxygen species. The first reduction is due to a pyridine nucleotide linked oxidase, which reduces oxygen to the oxygen free radical, superoxide anion:

$$2 O_2 + NAD(P)H \xrightarrow{\text{oxidase}} 2 O_2^- + NAD(P)^+ + H^+$$

Superoxide is converted to hydrogen peroxide (H_2O_2) by the enzyme superoxide dismutase:

$$2 O_2^- + 2H^+ \xrightarrow{\text{superoxide dismutase}} H_2O_2 + O_2$$

Formation of H_2O_2 in neutrophils probably cannot account for the bacteriocidal activity of these cells. The most important bacteriocidal agent in neutrophils appears to be hypochlorous acid, HOCl, formed from H_2O_2 by the enzyme, myeloperoxidase. Macrophages lack this enzyme and probably utilize other reactive oxygen species for bacterial killing.

Superoxide anion (O_2^-) and hydrogen peroxide (H_2O_2) form the reactive hydroxyl radical ($OH^.$) in the Haber–Weiss reaction:

$$O_2^- + H_2O_2 \rightarrow O_2 + OH^. + OH^-$$

This reaction may actually result from two steps catalyzed by ionic iron. First, superoxide ion reduces ferric ion to ferrous ion, following which hydrogen peroxide is then reduced to form hydroxyl radical by ferrous ion:

$$O_2^- + Fe^{3+} \rightarrow O_2 + Fe^{2+}$$

$$Fe^{2+} + H_2O_2 \rightarrow Fe^{3+} + OH^. + OH^-$$

Hydroxyl radical and another form of oxygen, singlet oxygen, are highly reactive oxygen species and are able to induce lipid peroxidation, polypeptide chain cleavage, and many other reactions. Oxygen in its stable ground state with two unpaired electrons in outer orbitals is referred to as a triplet state due to its electromagnetic behavior (11). This triplet structure stabilizes oxygen, because in order to be reduced by a two-electron donor, the donor electrons must also have parallel spins, or in molecular orbital terms, each electron must have the same spin quantum number. The electronic structure of singlet oxygen differs from that of the triplet state by having all electrons paired, leaving vacant the antibonding orbital that has a single unpaired electron within the triplet molecule. Singlet oxygen is formed in many reactions such as the enzymatic degradation of lipid peroxides, including the formation of PGH_2 from PGG_2 (Fig. 7E–1), and by the one-electron oxidation of superoxide anion by heavy metal anion-containing catalysts. The antiinflammatory activity of gold compounds and carotenoids has been postulated to be due in part to quenching singlet oxygen or converting it to its ground state, triplet oxygen (12).

VASOACTIVE AMINES AND NITRIC OXIDE

Three low-molecular weight amines are potentially important inflammatory mediators: histamine, serotonin, and adenosine (10). Histamine is the decarboxylation product of the amino acid, histidine. It is stored in mast cell granules and is released on mast cell activation by substances such as IgE immunoglobulin, which promotes immediate hypersensitivity reactions. The biologic effects of histamine are mediated through its interactions with specific receptors. Histamine produces vasodilation and enhanced permeability of post-capillary venules. It produces bronchoconstriction and enhances the flow of bronchial mucus. Serotonin or 5-hydroxytryptamine is stored in dense body granules of platelets. It is a vasoconstrictor, but it enhances microvascular

permeability. Serotonin also promotes fibrosis by enhancing collagen synthesis by fibroblasts. Adenosine is a nucleotide generated during mast cell activation from the breakdown of adenosine triphosphate (ATP) (13). It inhibits platelet aggregation and modulates the activation of inflammatory cells in different ways through interaction with two different surface receptors. Studies of neutrophils have demonstrated that at low adenosine concentrations, occupancy of the A1 receptor enhances phagocytosis of immune complexes through Fc receptors and superoxide formation, whereas at high adenosine concentrations, occupancy of the A2 receptors by adenosine inhibits Fc receptor-mediated phagocytosis and superoxide formation.

In recent years a simple nitrogenous compound, nitric oxide (NO) has emerged as a pleiotropic mediator affecting several organ systems (14). Nitric oxide is synthesized by the enzyme, nitric oxide synthetase, from the amino acid arginine. Nitric oxide is derived from the guanidinium group of arginine in the presence of molecular oxygen and several cofactors including NADPH and flavoproteins. Nitric oxide synthetases have been purified and characterized from brain, endothelial cells, and macrophages. Some of these enzymes are constitutive and are dependent on Ca^{++} and calmodulin, while others are induced by certain stimuli and are independent of Ca^{++}. The effects of nitric oxide are mediated by the activation of guanylyl cyclases through nitrosation of the heme component of this enzyme. The biologic effects attributed to nitric oxide are probably due to several reactive derivatives of this compound, including other oxides of nitrogen, nitrosamines, nitrosothiols, and S-nitrosylated proteins.

In the central nervous system, nitric oxide modifies synaptic transmission and mediates neuronal responses to excitatory amino acids. Nitric oxide may act as a neurotransmitter for some peripheral neurons. In the vasculature, nitric oxide causes vasodilation and accounts, at least in part, for the activity of endothelial-derived relaxing factor. In the kidney, the microcirculation may be regulated by nitric oxide, leading to control of intravascular volume and pressure, as well as renin release. Finally, the cytotoxicity of macrophages for tumor cells and pathogenic microorganisms has been attributed to the synthesis of nitric oxide by macrophages. Nitric oxide may exert its toxic effects on tumor cells through inactivation of the heme component of the enzyme, ribonucleotide reductase.

Potential therapeutic interventions related to nitric oxide have centered on the smooth muscle relaxing effects of this agent in disorders such as pulmonary hypertension and myocardial ischemia. Nitric oxide represents a new form of intercellular signalling through covalent interactions with key molecules that have appropriate redox potentials. This mediator may resemble active oxygen molecules in its ability to activate or inhibit certain enzymes or regulatory proteins (14).

KININS AND RELATED PROTEINS

The so-called contact system consists of a group of four proteins that circulate in the plasma in inactive forms. These are activated to provide a host defense system (15). The contact system consists of Hageman factor (also called coagulation factor XII), prekallikrein, high molecular weight kininogen (HMWK), and coagulation factor XI (plasma thromboplastin antecedent). Thus, the contact system is closely related to the coagulation system. The contact system is activated by contact with negatively charged surfaces, which may be found in a variety of substances. Organic and inorganic materials that have been shown to activate the contact system include monosodium urate crystals, collagen, vascular basement membranes, and glycosaminoglycans. Activation is initiated by Hageman factor binding to negatively charged surfaces via positively charged amino acids near the amino terminal end of the factor. Binding may be accompanied by limited cleavage of Hageman factor to form active Hageman factor. This activation is accelerated by binding of bimolecular complexes containing both prekallikrein and HMWK and Factor XI and HMWK. The active fragment of Hageman factor, HFa, then cleaves prekallikrein to release the active enzyme, kallikrein, and also cleaves Factor XI to produce

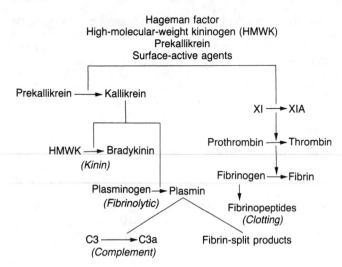

Hageman factor
High-molecular-weight kininogen (HMWK)
Prekallikrein
Surface-active agents

Prekallikrein → Kallikrein

XI → XIA

HMWK → Bradykinin
(Kinin)

Prothrombin → Thrombin

Fibrinogen → Fibrin

Plasminogen → Plasmin
(Fibrinolytic)

Fibrinopeptides
(Clotting)

C3 → C3a
(Complement)

Fibrin-split products

Fig. 7E–4. The contact system (modified from Reference 10).

active Factor XIa. Factor XIa and kallikrein are capable of cleaving HMWK to release bradykinin (Fig. 7E–4).

Components of the contact system may function in several ways as mediators of inflammation. Active Hageman factor may increase vascular permeability and when infused, causes hypotension. Bradykinin, a nonapeptide, causes vasodilatation, increases vascular permeability, and produces hypotension. Moreover, bradykinin produces pain and induces leukocyte margination in blood vessels. It is inactivated by kininases, one of which (kininase II) is a dipeptidase that is identical to angiotensin converting enzyme and cleaves the two carboxy terminal amino acids.

THE CLOTTING SYSTEM

As noted above, the contact and clotting systems are intimately related (10). The activation of Hageman factor is the initial step in both of these systems. The end-product of the clotting pathway, fibrin, is a component of many inflammatory reactions. The fibrinolytic system may also be considered a component of the clotting system and plays an important role in inflammation. Fibrinopeptides, which are cleaved from fibrin by the fibrinolytic system (primarily plasmin), possess chemotactic activity and increase vascular permeability. The enzyme plasmin in addition to lysing fibrin clots is capable of activating Hageman factor and cleaving the C3 component of complement. Thus, components of the complement, kinin, and clotting pathways interact with each other to facilitate inflammation.

Dwight R. Robinson, MD

1. Needleman P, Turk J, Jakschik BA, et al: Arachidonic acid metabolism. Ann Rev Biochem 55:69–102, 1986
2. Robinson DR: Lipid mediators of inflammation, Rheumatic Disease Clinics of North America. Edited by Zvaifler N. Philadelphia, Penn. W.B. Saunders Company, 385–405, 1987
3. Samuelsson B, Dahlen S–E, Lindgren JA, et al: Leukotrienes and lipoxins: Structures, biosynthesis, and biological effects. Science 237:1171–1176, 1987
4. Scott DL, White SP, Otwinowski Z, et al: Interfacial catalysis: The mechanism of phospholipase A₂. Science 250:1541–1546, 1990
5. Cirino G, Peers SH, Flower RJ, et al: Human recombinant lipocortin 1 has acute local anti-inflammatory properties in the rat paw edema test. Proc Natl Acad Sci USA 86:3428–3432, 1989
6. Davidson FF, Dennis EA, Powell M, et al: Inhibition of phospholipase A₂ by "lipocortins" and calpactins. An effect on binding to substrate phospholipids. J Biol Chem 262:1698–1705, 1987
7. Maier JAM, Hla T, Maciag T: Cyclooxygenase is an immediate-early gene induced by interleukin-1 in human endothelial cells. J Biol Chem 265:10805–10808, 1990
8. Fu J–Y, Masferrer JL, Seibert K, et al: The induction and suppression of prostaglandin H₂ synthase (cyclooxygenase) in human monocytes. J Biol Chem 265:16737–16740, 1990
9. Hanahan DJ: Platelet activating factor: A biologically active phosphoglyceride. Ann Rev Biochem 55:483–509, 1986
10. Cotran RS, Kumar V, Robbins SL: Inflammation and repair, Robbins Pathologic Basis of Disease, 4th ed. Edited by Cotran RS, Kumar V, Robbins SL. Philadelphia, Penn. W.B. Saunders Company, 39–86, 1989
11. Naqui A, Chance B: Reactive oxygen intermediates in biochemistry. Ann Rev Biochem 55:137–166, 1986
12. Corey EJ, Mehrotra MM, Khan AU. Antiarthritic gold compounds effectively quench electronically excited singlet oxygen. Science 236:68, 1987
13. Salmon JE, Cronstein BN: Fcg Receptor-mediated functions in neutrophils are modulated by adenosine receptor occupancy. A1 receptors are stimulatory and A2 receptors are inhibitory. J Immunol 145:2235–2240, 1990
14. Nathan C: Nitric oxide as a secretory product of mammalian cells. FASEB J 6:3051–3064, 1992
15. Kozin F, Cochrane CG: Plasma Contact Activation, Textbook of Rheumatology, 3rd ed. Edited by: Kelley WN, Harris Jr. ED, Ruddy S, Sledge CB, Philadelphia, Penn., W.B. Saunders Company, 266–284, 1989

8. EVALUATION OF THE PATIENT
A. History and Physical Examination

A thorough history and physical examination remain the cornerstones of evaluating patients with rheumatic diseases, despite many advances in laboratory testing and radiologic imaging. Skills in these techniques are important since most patients have a variety of non-musculoskeletal manifestations of their illness and many rheumatic diseases are systemic in nature. Patients also may have other illnesses that must be taken into consideration when evaluating their rheumatic disease. Special expertise must be developed in evaluating articular and periarticular structures (1–4). More than 100 articular and nonarticular diseases cause what a patient reports as joint pain. A physician cannot always make a precise diagnosis on the first visit, and must often wait for further examinations, tests, or for nonspecific findings to evolve into a more definite diagnosis. Careful attention to detail is requisite to the proper evaluation and care plan for these patients. The findings should be systemically recorded so that the patients' response to therapy and progress of disease can be followed over time. Functional evaluation and health status measurements are available through a variety of instruments (5). These outcomes are ultimately the most important measurement tools in evaluating treatment.

Table 8A–1. Patterns of some articular symptoms

Intermittent	Migratory	Additive
Intermittent hydrarthrosis (Non-inflammatory)	Gonococcal arthritis	Rheumatoid arthritis
Palindromic rheumatism (Inflammatory)	Rheumatic fever	Osteoarthritis
Gout	Gout	Spondylarthropathies
Pseudogout	(during individual episode)	Gout
Reiter's syndrome (longer duration episodes)		
Behcet's disease		
Early rheumatoid arthritis (occasionally)		

HISTORY

The patient with a rheumatic illness may give a chief complaint of joint pain (Table 8A–1), or may instead report a systemic complaint; joint symptoms may sometimes be absent. If a patient complains about a single joint, one must inquire about other articular symptoms, past and present. The patient may not consider the spine or sacroiliac articulation to be joints, and the examiner must ask specifically for such information.

The examiner must try to determine if there was an initiating event. The patient should be asked about any recent inoculation, viral or bacterial illness, new medication, trauma, or other possible contributing factors. Also, the patient should be asked if there was a prodrome to the current illness and if there have been previous episodes. In addition, the date of onset and the type of progression should be determined. Monarticular disease suggests concern about infection, trauma, and crystal-induced arthritis. Polyarticular disease can be organized by the distribution of joint manifestations (see physical examination), the type of progression, and the accompanying extraarticular manifestations. Inflammatory disease is suggested by morning stiffness of greater than 1 hour (a similar "gel" phenomenon occurs with sitting or resting), swelling, fever, and systemic fatigue.

Pain may be described as focal or diffuse and by quality, as well as by radiation (dermatome). Patients also may be asked to identify the intensity of pain on a visual analog or verbal description scale. This quantitative approach allows the physician to follow the response to therapy. The physician should also determine if pain is worse with activity or rest and what other interventions make it better or worse. Weakness should be classified as true muscular weakness or apparent weakness secondary to pain.

Patients should also be closely questioned about their activities of daily living and function. In some, there may be excellent function despite pain and deformity; in others, because of multiple reasons (psychologic and systemic disease), there may be poor function with minimum articular involvement. Other psychosocial aspects of their life, including sexuality, should be ascertained as these may lead to diagnostic clues and aspects needing concern in management.

A full review of systems will detect clues to many of the rheumatic diseases. Once a specific disease is suggested, the examiner should inquire about systemic features of such a disease. A family history is very useful to determine if there is a genetic linkage for diseases such as rheumatoid arthritis (RA), systemic lupus erythematosus (SLE), spondylarthropathy, osteoarthritis (OA), or gout. Finally, a detailed history of medications including doses, timing, efficacy, and adverse effects should be obtained.

PHYSICAL EXAMINATION

The physical examination is divided into the general evaluation and the musculoskeletal assessment. A full general examination is essential. As in the history, part of the general examination should focus on organ systems that may have pathology related to the rheumatic disease, or can show an important concomitant illness or complications that will affect or modify treatment.

Usually after the vital signs are taken (hypertension is a notorious asymptomatic feature of several rheumatic diseases), the first organ examined is the integument, including the hair and nails. Skin changes associated with some rheumatic diseases are delineated in Table 8A–2. Obviously, the patient's clothing must be removed, including shoes and stockings. Special attention must be given to the scalp, oral mucosa, genital areas, and nails. The search for nodules, tophi, telangiectasia, vasculitic changes, ulceration, embolic lesions, psoriasis, and onycholysis is valuable.

Special emphasis on given areas will depend on symptoms and diseases under consideration. For example, in juvenile rheumatoid arthritis (JRA), chronic iridocyclitis may be silent and cause blindness. Children with JRA should have regular ocular examination by an ophthalmologist. Oral ulcers or nasal erosions can be relatively asymptomatic in Reiter's syndrome and SLE respectively. In an older patient with proximal muscle soreness, the temporal arteries should be palpated to find if temporal arteries should be pursued.

Chest expansion (measured by the difference between full inspiration and expiration at the nipple line) may be compromised by thoracic spine arthritis, an early asymptomatic physical finding in ankylosing spondylitis. It also may be affected by chronic lower airway disease. Interstitial lung disease, pulmonary infiltrates, and pleural effusions are found in systemic sclerosis, SLE, and RA and may produce associated physical findings. Cardiac abnormalities are often nonspecific. Valvular insufficiency (aortic and mitral) may complicate spondylarthropathies, and pericarditis may complicate autoimmune diseases. Likewise, arrhythmias

Table 8A–2. *Examples of some integumentary changes suggesting underlying rheumatic disease*

Lesion	Disease
Alopecia	Systemic lupus erythematosus
Nail pitting	Psoriatic arthritis
Onycholysis	Psoriatic arthritis
	Reiter's syndrome
Keratoderma blennorrhagica	Reiter's syndrome
Leg ulcers	Rheumatoid vasculitis, Felty's syndrome
Buccal or genital ulcers	SLE, Reiter's syndrome
	Behcet's disease
Palpable purpura	Vasculitis
Nodules	RA, gout, amyloid, sarcoidosis, multicentric reticulohistocytosis
Petechiae	SLE, ITP
Raynaud's phenomenon	SLE, systemic sclerosis, limited cutaneous scleroderma
Nocturnal febrile macular rash	JRA, adult onset Stills disease
Erythema nodosum	Sarcoidosis, inflammatory bowel disease
Sun sensitivity malar rash (trunk)	SLE
Rash over knuckles (Gottron's papule)	Dermatomyositis
Calcinosis	Dermatomyositis, systemic sclerosis, limited cutaneous scleroderma, apatite arthropathy
Hemorrhagic pustules	Gonococcal arthritis
Livedo reticularis	Antiphospholipid syndrome

are seen when the conduction system is involved with vascular abnormalities or fibrosis. A careful neurologic examination should focus on central, peripheral, and psychologic examinations that could suggest SLE or vasculitis.

Joint Evaluation

The core of rheumatologic diagnosis is a proper musculoskeletal examination. Each joint should be examined, not just the sources of major complaints. Assess each joint for warmth, redness, and effusion; synovial thickening; deformity; range of motion; pain on motion; tenderness on palpation; and function.

Pain and tenderness should be localized, if possible, to the precise muscle, joint, tendon, bone, or bursa involved. Soft swelling around the joint may be due to fluid or synovial proliferation. Bony prominences are due to osteophytes or subluxation. Compare joints for bilateral symmetry and perform an orderly exam beginning from head to foot, with the spine being examined later. Observe the patient's gait and ability to dress and undress, to arise from a seated position, and to get on the examining table. The examination will usually occur first in the seated, then the supine and prone position, and finally standing. The first determination that is made is to differentiate intraarticular from extraarticular abnormalities (Table 8A–3).

Small Joints

The temporomandibular (TM), sternoclavicular (SC), sternomanubrial (SM), and acromioclavicular (AC) joints are often

Table 8A–3. *Intraarticular vs. extraarticular disease*

	Intraarticular	Extraarticular
Range of Motion	Pain on active, as well as passive motion	Pain more on active and specific motion, unless severe inflammation
Tenderness	Parallel to joint surface, Diffuse around circumference of joint	Localized over bony prominence along tendons or ligaments perpendicular to joint surfaces
Pain Description	Generalized hard to pinpoint specific area, "Deep, Inside", "Poorly localized"	Precisely localized, Superficial

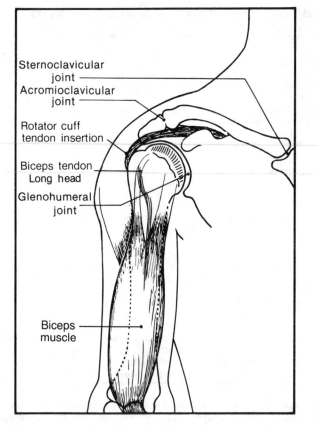

Fig. 8A–1. *Anterior view of the shoulder, showing areas of tenderness that suggest local pathology.*

should be fixed and the arm lifted laterally until the scapula rotates (90°). With active motion the scapula begins to rotate at 60°. Internal and external rotation is measured with the elbow flexed at 90°. For a functional examination, have patients reach behind their head with both arms and reach behind the back touching the opposite scapula as well. Observe any difficulty in performing these tasks.

Elbow

The elbow is a relatively simple hinge joint. It should be examined for rheumatoid nodules, tophi, and olecranon bursitis. Palpate for synovitis in the fossa lateral to the olecranon. Pain localized over the epicondyles suggests epicondylitis (tennis and golf elbows). Normal flexion is between 150° and 160°. Extension is normally 0°. Loss of full extension can be an early sign of synovitis. Hyperextension greater than 5° suggests hypermobility. The elbow participates along with the wrist in supination and pronation of the forearm.

Wrist and Hand

Eight carpal bones articulate proximally with the radius and ulna and distally with the metacarpals. Synovitis may be seen dorsally or on the volar surface. Soft tissue or bony proliferation in the wrist may entrap the median nerve causing carpal tunnel syndrome. Symptoms of dysesthesia over the thumb, index, long, and radial half of the ring fingers may be brought on by flexing the wrist (Phalen's sign) or tapping over the median nerve (Tinel's sign). Look for thenar muscle atrophy. Ulnar subluxation due to rupture of the radial ulnar ligament and wrist subluxation should be noted. Synovial cysts (ganglia) can be differentiated from solid tissue here and elsewhere by their fluctuance and occasionally by transillumination. Flexion of the wrist from 80° to 90° and extension for 60° to 70° is normal. Loss of motion may be an early sign of synovitis. Side to side (ulnar–radial) motion is around 10° and 20° respectively. Grasping the thumb in a fist and moving the wrist in an ulnar direction pulls the thumb abductors which is a test for De Quervain's disease, a stenosing tenosynovitis of the thumb extensors and abductors. Patients with extreme hypermobility such as in Ehlers–Danlos syndrome can flex the wrist so that the thumb is able to approximate the volar surface of the forearm. Dupuytren's contractures over the palm are nodular contractures of the flexor retinaculum.

The metacarpophalangeal (MCP) joints are frequently involved with synovitis in RA and other inflammatory synovitis. Bony degenerative changes suggest trauma or metabolic arthropathy in the MCPs. With synovitis, subluxation and ulnar drift of the digits occur at MCPs. If there is rupture of an extensor tendon in the wrist or hand, the affected finger cannot be extended. Proximal interphalangeal (PIP) and distal interphalangeal (DIP) joints may be involved in synovitis or in bony proliferation. In the latter situation the PIP enlargement is called a *Bouchard's* and the DIP, a *Heberden's node*. Finger joint circumference can be measured with a tape or ring sizing device. Synovitis leads to tendon laxity and slippage. When hyperextension of the PIP occurs, the deformity is called a *swan neck*, and DIP hyperextension with PIP flexion is called a *boutonniere deformity*. The ROM of hand joints may be measured or more grossly estimated by first making a fist and then extending the hand. Hand function should be observed. Grip strength can be measured with a blood pressure cuff. The balloon is rolled in three equal parts, surrounded by the rest of the cuff, and inflated to 20mm Hg. The patient then squeezes the cuff and the pressure is read.

Hip

The localization of tenderness or pain is important in establishing the origin of the symptom. Lateral tenderness over the trochanter is usually trochanteric bursitis. Posterior pain may emanate from the sacroiliac joint, lumbar spine, or the ischial bursa. True hip pain is usually anterior in the groin.

To test hip flexion with a patient supine, bend the knee while supporting the leg and bringing the knee up toward the chest. Hip

inappropriately ignored. Temporomandibular joints are located anterior to the external auditory canal. Swelling and pain on palpation is located anterior to the tragus. Crepitation and motion disorders may be palpated directly over the joint, or by inserting both index fingers in the external auditory canal, gently pulling forward while the patient opens and closes the mouth. Malocclusion should be noted and the inter-incisor distance may be measured. The SC and AC joints are located by tracing the clavicle medially and laterally to the articulations. Swelling may occur and crepitus may be felt on motion. Acromioclavicular motion may be assessed by pulling the forearm down, while SC motion occurs when shrugging the shoulders. The sternomanubrial joint is located adjacent to the second rib and does not normally move; however, it may be tender or swollen.

Shoulder

The shoulder is a modified ball and socket joint formed by the head of the humerus and the glenoid fossa of the scapula (Fig. 8A–1). Pain over the lateral portion may be due to the subdeltoid (subacromial) bursa, and anterior pain along the long head of the biceps is often due to bicipital tendinitis. Effusions, when seen, usually bulge anteriorly. Palpation of the shoulder and surrounding structures should be followed by range of motion (ROM). First, the examiner should determine if the rotator cuff is injured. Tendons involved in the cuff include those of the supraspinatus, infraspinatus, teres minor, and subscapularis. Tenderness may occur over the anterior portion of the humeral head with the shoulder extended to expose the only palpable attachment of the cuff. The patient with a total rupture of the cuff cannot initiate abduction of the shoulder without hunching the shoulder until the deltoids can continue the motion, or may not be able to maintain the arm in abduction (drop arm test). The ROM is measured in a plane relative to the midline of the body in this and all joints. Forward flexion occurs when the examiner passively, or the patient actively, moves the arm forward over the head. The patient should be able to move through a 180° arc. Extension is a backward motion of 30° to 60°. To abduct the arm the scapula flexion is normally between 120° and 130°. While the hip is fully flexed and the pelvis is stabilized, check the opposite hip for flexion contracture (Thomas test). Make sure that the contracture is coming from the hip rather than from a flexed knee inhibiting the extremity from lying flat on the examining table. Extension of the hip may be further tested with the patient supine dropping the leg over the side of the table, or while the patient is prone or standing. Abduction is measured by moving the leg laterally while keeping one hand on the opposite pelvic rim. The limit of abduction is when the pelvis begins to rotate at 45° to 70°. Compare one side to the other. One may measure intramalleolar distance with both hips abducted. Adduction moves the leg across the midline and to the opposite side at 20° to 30°. Rotation is best measured with the knee and hip flexed 90°. Rotating the heel medially causes external hip rotation (40° to 60°) and outwardly internal rotation (10° to 40°). A quick estimation of hip movement is done by placing the heel next to the medial portion of the opposite knee and slowly moving the knee laterally towards the surface of the table (Patrick's test). Flexing both knees 90° and performing the same procedure, one may measure the distance between the knees (Fabere's test). This can be compared on subsequent visits.

Posteriorly, the sacroiliac (SI) joint should be palpated or percussed. Compression of the pelvis with the subject lying on his side may cause pain to be referred to an abnormal SI joint.

Knee

Palpate the knee for swelling and effusion. Small effusions may be detected by pushing the fluid out of the medial portion of the knee and then stroking the lateral side, causing the fluid to bulge medially once again (bulge sign) (Fig. 8A–2). Larger amounts of fluid will cause the patella to be ballottable and a bulge sign will not be possible.

Inspect the knees for valgus (knock knee) and varus (bow leg) deformities. Swelling directly over the patella may be a prepatellar bursitis while actual synovitis of the knee is more diffuse. Posterior swelling in the popliteal area may be a popliteal (Baker's) cyst or rarely an aneurism. Also check the muscles above the knee for quadriceps atrophy. Tenderness over the medial portion of the tibia below the knee may be caused by an anserine bursitis, or at the joint space by medial collateral ligament or meniscus damage. While flexing and extending the knee, feel for crepitation which suggests cartilaginous loss. Extension to 0° is normal; greater than −5° would be defined as hyperextension (genu recurvatum); flexion contractures also occur and are significant if they are greater than 3° to 5°. Full flexion should be

approximately 140°. Collateral ligament instability is measured by flexing the knee approximately 100°, grasping the femoral condyle in one hand and rocking the distal leg back and forth with the other hand. Cruciate instability may be tested with the knee flexed 90° while pulling the leg forward. If motion is detected (positive drawer sign), the cruciate is lax or not entirely intact. Other special tests are available for minuscule injuries.

Ankle and Foot

The ankle consists of two joints. The tibiotalar or true ankle joint moves to dorsi and plantar-flex the foot (20° and 45° to 50° respectively). The subtalar joint causes medial (inversion) and lateral (eversion) of the rear-foot. Tenderness may be palpated over the joint space adjacent to either malleolus. Synovitis may be noted anywhere over the joint and must be differentiated from peripheral edema by its localization to the joint, usual absence of pitting, and by pain related to motion. The ankle also should be viewed while the patient is bearing weight to look for rear-foot valgus or other abnormalities. Valgus causes the patient to be prone to pes planus (flat feet) by unlocking the mid-foot and, thus, the arch.

When inspecting the mid-foot, note any soft tissue abnormalities or osteophytic spurs. The forefoot may show lateral deviation of the great toe (hallux valgus) and hammertoe or cock up deformity. Feel the plantar surfaces of the foot for metatarsal subluxation and calluses, both often symptomatic. Pain and tenderness may be felt, particularly at the plantar fascial and achilles attachment, and over the joints. Test for mid-foot motion by turning the forefoot while stabilizing the calcaneus. Also place the individual toe joints through their ROM. Observe the patient's shoes for abnormal wear patterns and observe the gait as well.

Spine

The spine may be observed in the seated and prone positions; however, it is best to examine alignment while the patient is standing. Pelvic and shoulder tilt suggest abnormal curvature due to leg length abnormalities or spinal curvature (scoliosis-rotational; list-lateral bending). Observe for accentuation of thoracic kyphosis or lumbar lordosis. Palpate the paraspinal musculature for tenderness and spasm and percuss the spinous processes.

Cervical spine motion includes lateral bending (45°), rotation (60° to 80°), extension (50° to 60°) and flexion (45°). The thoracic spine, along with the lumbar spine, participates in rotation of the upper trunk. Also, the examiner may measure the occiput to wall

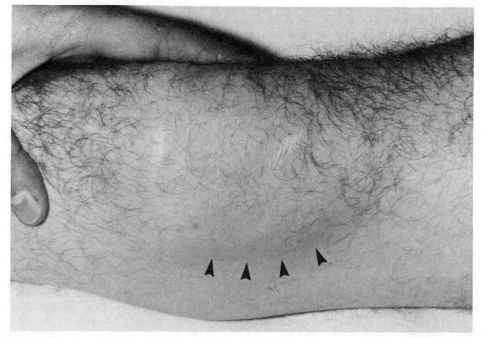

Fig. 8A–2. The "bulge" sign for demonstrating small knee effusions. After fluid has been compressed away from the medial aspect, gentle pressure over the lateral aspect moves fluid back into this area, creating a visible bulge (arrows).

distance with the patient erect. This will show changes of increased thoracic kyphosis as well as fixed cervical and lumbar spine flexion.

The lumbar spine normally has a lordosis. This should reverse when the patient flexes and tries to touch the floor. Finger-to-floor distance may change over time due to changes in hip function, posture, and lumbar mobility. The modified Schöber test (see Chapter 20B) requires a measurement of 15 cm to be marked over the lumbar area with the patient erect. The patient then is asked to try and touch the floor. The marked distance is remeasured and should increase to at least 20 cm as the lordosis reverses. Less change suggests structural spine disease or muscle spasm. The lumbar spine extends and bends laterally as well. The neurologic examination is part of a careful spine evaluation. Sensory, motor, and reflex abnormalities can be associated with

spinal root impingement. The straight leg raising test may be useful in bringing out this irritation.

Eric P. Gall, MD

1. Gall EP, Gooden MA: Examination of the Musculoskeletal system, 2nd Ed. Tucson, AZ, University of Arizona Biomedical Communications Publisher, 1983, pp 1–32
2. Hoppenfeld S: Physical Examination of the Spine and Extremities. New York, Appelton Century Croft, 1976, pp 1–276
3. Polley HF, Hunder GC: Rheumatologic Interviewing and Physical Examination of the Joints. New York, WB Saunders Co, 1978, pp 1–286
4. American Rheumatism Association Glossary Committee. Dictionary of the Rheumatic Diseases, Volume 1: Signs and Symptoms. New York, Contact Associates International Ltd. 1982, pp 1–95
5. American College of Rheumatology Glossary Committee. Dictionary of the Rheumatic Diseases, Volume III: Health Status Measurement. New York, Contact Associates International Ltd., 1988, pp 1–65

B. *Laboratory Evaluation of Rheumatic Diseases*

LABORATORY EVALUATION STRATEGY

The laboratory evaluation of patients with rheumatic complaints is often informative but rarely definitive. An elevated serum uric acid is not gout; 20% of patients with acute gout have a normal serum uric acid. In a sizeable subset of persons with rheumatoid arthritis (RA), the rheumatoid factor may be negative. Also, many other conditions and healthy individuals may have a positive rheumatoid factor. Discussion of the specific laboratory features of rheumatic disorders will follow in individual chapters. This chapter outlines a strategy for the use of common laboratory tests in the diagnosis and management of rheumatic disorders (1).

Ideally, diagnostic tests should change treatment, that is, they should make a diagnosis indicating specific rather than symptomatic treatment, help in estimating prognosis, or define response to treatment. Laboratory evaluation in the differential diagnosis of rheumatic complaints is most useful when there is strong clinical suspicion of a specific disorder as suggested by a constellation of signs and symptoms; occasionally to exclude a condition; or to aid prognosis. In systemic illnesses, testing is performed to define the extent of disease or detect other organ systems that may be involved.

Four characteristics of diagnostic tests can help determine their usefulness in evaluating patients (2). These are sensitivity, specificity, predictive value positive, and predictive value negative. Sensitivity is the likelihood of a positive test result in a person with a disease. This is also termed the true positive rate of a diagnostic test. Specificity is the likelihood of a negative test in a patient without disease and is also the true negative rate of a test. The predictive value positive of a test is the probability of a disease if the test is positive; likewise the predictive value negative of a test is the probability of a disease being absent if the test is negative. It is possible to calculate the predictive value of a specific test by Bayes' Theorem, an equation that utilizes the prevalence of the disease in the population (the pre-test probability of a disease in a given population), and the test's sensitivity and specificity. The prevalence is frequently not known. The relationship is such that the test is most helpful in increasing diagnostic certainty in a given patient when the pre-test likelihood as judged by the clinician is moderate.

ACUTE PHASE REACTANTS

Acute phase reactants are a heterogeneous group of proteins synthesized in the liver that are rapidly induced in the presence of inflammation or tissue necrosis and that appear to parallel chronic inflammation. They include the coagulation proteins–fibrinogen and prothrombin; transport proteins such as haptoglobin, transferrin and ceruloplasmin; complement components such as C3 and C4; protease inhibitors; and miscellaneous proteins such as albumin, fibronectin, C reactive protein (CRP), and serum amyloid-A related protein. The tests most commonly used

clinically are the erythrocyte sedimentation rate (ESR) and the CRP. C reactive protein levels respond more rapidly than the ESR to changes in inflammatory activity, and thus CRP is probably a more sensitive measure of inflammation. However, the ESR takes only 1 hour and minimum equipment whereas the CRP takes a day to perform and requires an enzyme-linked immunosorbent assay (ELISA) or radioimmunodiffusion equipment. The ESR can be high or low in the absence of pathology. The ESR increases with age and anemia and is higher in women than in men. A rough rule of thumb is that the age-adjusted upper limit of normal for an ESR is the age divided by 2 for men. For women, it is the age plus 10 divided by 2.

The ESR is important in the diagnosis of giant cell arteritis and polymyalgia rheumatica as it is included among the criteria for the clinical diagnosis of these disorders. However, up to 10% of patients with these two diseases may have a normal ESR.

A normal ESR does not reduce the probability of crystal-induced or septic arthritis enough to preclude the necessity for other tests such as synovial fluid analysis, and the ESR is not helpful in monitoring disease activity in such patients. The ESR is generally elevated in systemic vasculitis, but is often normal in patients with primary central nervous system angiitis, Henoch-Schönlein purpura, lymphomatoid granulomatosis, and thromboangiitis obliterans.

The ESR is useful for monitoring the disease activity of patients with RA and PMR/GCA but less useful in patients with systemic lupus erythematosus (SLE), and spondylarthropathies (3).

AUTOANTIBODIES

Autoantibodies, immunoglobulins directed against autologous intracellular, cell surface, and extracellular antigens, are seen in a number of rheumatic diseases. The intracellular antigens include nuclear components (anti-nuclear antibodies or ANA) or cytoplasmic components (anti-neutrophilic cytoplasmic antibodies, or ANCA). Antibodies to cell surface antigens react with a variety of antigens including HLA molecules. Other antibodies may react with plasma components such as coagulation factors (lupus anticoagulant).

Autoantibodies are detected by a variety of techniques including indirect immunofluorescence, enzyme immunocytochemistry, passive hemagglutination, particle agglutination, immunodiffusion, counter immunoelectrophoresis (CIE), radioimmunoassay (RIA), and ELISA. When autoantibodies are directed against cellular or insoluble extracellular components, indirect immunofluorescence is the method most widely used to screen body fluids for the presence of these antibodies. Autoantibodies directed against soluble components such as coagulation factors, DNA, nuclear protein, and components of complement are assayed by immunodiffusion, CIE, RIA, or ELISA.

The sensitivity of techniques varies considerably. At present there is no standardization of either the assay method or the units

Table 8B–1. *Antinuclear antibodies in rheumatic disease (4)*

Disease**	Antinuclear antibody			Precipitin panel				
	ANA	pattern*	Titer	anti-dsDNA	anti-Sm	anti-RNP	anti-Ro (SSA)	anti-La (SSB)
SLE	95–99%	P,D,S,N	50% > 1:640	20–30%	30%	30–50%	30%	15%
Sjogren's	75%	D,S	low	<5%	0%	15%	50%	25%
RA	15–35%	D	10% > 1:640	<5%	0%	10%	10%	5%
Scleroderma	60–90%	S,N,D	often high	0%	0%	30%	5%	1%
DILE	100%	D,S	may be high	0%	<5%	<5%	<5%	0%
MCTD	95–99%	S,D	may be high	0%	0%	95%	<5%	<5%
normal	<5%	D	rarely > 1:80	0%	0%	<5%	<5%	rare

* P = peripheral, D = diffuse, S = speckled, N = nucleolar, presented in order of decreasing frequency.
** SLE = systemic lupus erythematosus; RA = rheumatoid arthritis; DILE = drug-induced lupus erythematosus; MCTD = mixed connective tissue disease.

in which they are reported. Comparison from one laboratory to another, therefore, is problematic. The detection of many auto-antibodies requires sophisticated immunochemistry available primarily in research centers. Autoantibodies are present in a small proportion of the normal population, albeit usually in low titer. It is important, therefore, not to assign a rheumatic diagnosis based solely on autoantibody findings.

Antinuclear antibodies (ANA)

Testing for ANA is useful primarily in the evaluation of suspected SLE, as the test is highly sensitive in this disease. Furthermore, certain ANA subsets such as Sm and double stranded (dsDNA) are highly specific for SLE. The predictive value of ANA is highest when the titer and pattern are considered in the context of other specific autoantibodies and the clinical presentation. In SLE, the ANA is positive in at least 95% of patients; thus, a negative test argues strongly against the diagnosis. The pattern of the ANA (diffuse, peripheral, speckled, or nucleolar) correlates with the specific antigen against which the antibody is targeted (4) (Table 8B–1). For example, anti–dsDNA antibodies generally produce a peripheral staining ANA, while anti–Ro antibodies produce a speckled ANA. While some of these may add to the specificity of the test, they possess variable, and often limited, sensitivity. When SLE is highly suspected but the ANA is negative, anti–Ro antibody and a CH50 should be ordered as some "ANA-negative" SLE will be anti–Ro positive and others will be complement deficient (5,6).

The ANA's most important limitation is its lack of specificity. Other rheumatic disorders such as systemic sclerosis, Sjogren's syndrome and RA are also associated with a positive ANA, although the sensitivity of the test in these diseases is much lower than in SLE (Table 8B–1). Patients without rheumatic disease, including the healthy aged, patients with infectious illness, or those taking certain medications (procainamide, hydralazine, phenytoin), may also test positive for ANA. Anti–Sm and anti–dsDNA antibodies are highly specific (though not highly sensitive) for SLE and are subject to variability depending on the laboratory and technique.

The prevalence of these conditions in the population for whom the ANA is ordered affects the utility of the test. For example, if the ANA is routinely ordered in elderly patients with a fever of unknown origin, but no other features to suggest SLE, more false-positive than true-positive results will likely be observed. While false-positive ANAs tend to be in low titer, a significant proportion will be of medium to high titer; furthermore, SLE patients have low titer ANAs in a sizeable minority of cases. Thus, the ANA should be ordered only when the pre-test probability is appreciable and the result must be interpreted in light of its titer and specific autoantibody profile (7,8). Variability among laboratories as noted above can be appreciable with ANA and anti–dsDNA tests accounting for some occurrences in normal persons.

Rheumatoid Factor (RF)

Rheumatoid factors are antibodies directed against the Fc portion of immunoglobulin G (IgG). These autoantibodies appear to be synthesized in response to immunoglobulins that have been confirmationally altered after reaction with an antigen. The most common rheumatoid factor is an IgM antibody to IgG. Traditional techniques to detect rheumatoid factor include agglutination of IgG sensitized sheep red blood cells or latex particles coated with human IgG. Results are expressed as the dilution titer at which reactivity is eliminated. Refinements using radioimmunoassays, ELISA, and nephelometric techniques have improved quantitation, reliability, and perhaps sensitivity and specificity.

Rheumatoid factor is among the most frequently ordered tests in the evaluation of patients with arthralgia or suspected rheumatic disease, but its clinical utility may be limited (9,10). The test is positive in approximately 75% to 90% of patients with RA (sensitivity = 0.75–0.90), but such estimates are derived from highly selected populations such as rheumatology practices or studies establishing criteria for the disease, and are therefore subject to referral bias (11,12). Other rheumatic diseases may be accompanied by a positive RF, but the sensitivity in most of these is even lower. The assay technique and titer of the RF may alter the sensitivity, but use of a more sensitive assay or setting a lower titer as a cutoff for a positive test will produce lower specificity.

The RF is a test with low specificity in non-referral settings or in the general population. A variety of nonrheumatic diseases are associated with a positive RF. In the patient with a fever and arthralgia, endocarditis may be a more likely cause of a positive RF than RA. Other rheumatic diseases such as Sjogren's syndrome, SLE, and cryoglobulinemia may have clinical features in common with RA and may also have elevated titers of RF. The high specificity reported in referral outpatient rheumatology practices may not be observed in patients with weak clinical indications for the test or a high prevalence of confounding diseases. For patients over the age of 75, the reported prevalence of false-positive RFs ranges from 2% to 25% (11,13).

The practice of repeated testing and of ordering a rheumatic disease panel of laboratory tests should be avoided, because they increase the likelihood of false positive test results, especially in populations with a low prevalence of rheumatic illness (14). One situation in which repeated testing may be useful is monitoring Sjogren's syndrome, in which the disappearance of a previously positive RF may herald the onset of a hypogammaglobulinemic state associated with lymphoma (15).

Given the modest sensitivity and specificity of the RF test, the pre-test probability, as estimated by the clinician, in large part determines its usefulness. Even with generous estimates of sensitivity and specificity, the number of false-positive test results is often greater than true-positive results, and therefore the RF should only be ordered in patients with a moderate likelihood of RA. A positive test result may not affect initial management, even when the RF is a true-positive. However, some clinicians may prescribe a second-line agent sooner in seropositive RA patients. Population-based screening studies suggest that among asymptomatic patients, a positive RF may place the individual at increased risk to develop RA (16), but the RF performs poorly as a screening test due to the high frequency of false-positive results.

COMPLEMENT

The complement cascade is a series of over 20 biologically active proteins and inhibitors produced in the liver that comprise 2% to 3% of the total plasma protein concentration (see Chapter 7C). Complement activated by the classical pathway is responsible for the lysis of cells coated with antibody directed against cell surface antigens. Complement may be assayed by techniques that measure the presence of the component or its function. The best screening test for a complement abnormality is the CH50, which is a functional assay of the entire classical pathway. A low level suggests either consumption of complement or a deficiency of one or more components. Complement activation is generally triggered by exposure of the host to a foreign protein, especially when bound to host antibody (immune complex disease). While the foreign protein is usually unknown in patients with suspected or known rheumatic disease, low complement in such patients may be an indicator of consumption of these proteins.

Conditions characterized by immune-complex formation and hypocomplementemia include SLE (especially with nephritis), idiopathic membranoproliferative glomerulonephritis (GN), cryogobulinemia, chronic infections causing GN or vasculitis, post-streptococcal GN, generalized vasculitis, and serum sickness (17). In SLE nephritis, serial measurement of complement may prove useful in monitoring patients, as complement levels may decrease just before or concomitant with disease flare, and return to normal over weeks to months when disease activity diminishes. The correlation of lupus disease activity with complement levels is variable between patients, however, and thus complement should be considered in the context of the clinical picture.

Hereditary complement deficiency may cause hypocomplementemia and in some instances (especially C2 or C1 component deficiency), SLE or SLE-like illness has been described, often in the setting of a negative ANA (6). Thus, for ANA-negative patients in whom the clinical suspicion of SLE is high, a CH50 and a C2 level should be performed along with the anti–Ro antibody. Conditions associated with reduced complement without known immune complex formation include atheromatous embolization, hemolytic uremic syndrome, septic shock, liver failure, severe malnutrition, pancreatitis, severe burns, malaria with hemolysis, and some cases of porphyria.

CIRCULATING IMMUNE COMPLEXES

Circulating immune complexes consisting of an antigen, an antibody, and complement components are believed to play an important role in the pathogenesis of systemic rheumatic diseases such as SLE and vasculitis. Occasionally, low levels of immune complexes may be detected in normal individuals. High concentrations of circulating immune complexes can be seen in active systemic rheumatic diseases, vasculitis, infectious diseases, and some malignancies. In most of these conditions a clear-cut pathogenic role for the complexes has not been established. Similarly, the clinical utility of this test is unclear. Assays for immune complexes include the Raji cell assay, Clq-binding, Clq-precipitin assays, or RIA.

IMMUNOCHEMICAL TESTS

Many rheumatic diseases are thought to be the result of abnormalities of the immune system and have abnormalities of cellular and humoral immunity. However, analysis of lymphocyte phenotypes or electrophoresis of serum proteins are useful only in limited clinical contexts, such as suspected HIV infection, myeloma, or cryoglobulinemia. Otherwise the information obtained is usually non-specific and adds little diagnostic information.

HLA–B27

The strong association between the HLA–B27 allele and the spondylarthropathies makes this genetic marker a potentially useful test in evaluating patients with musculoskeletal symptoms. The diagnostic sensitivity of this test is approximately 95% in ankylosing spondylitis, 80% in Reiter's syndrome, 50% in symptomatic spondylitis associated with inflammatory bowel disease, and 70% in patients with spondylitis and psoriasis. Moreover, patients without rheumatic symptoms who are HLA–B27 positive have an increased relative risk (though low absolute risk) for the development of these associated spondylitides compared with those who are HLA–B27 negative.

The background prevalence of this genetic marker (approximately 6% to 10% in Caucasian populations) and the fact that only a small minority of HLA–B27 positive individuals will ever develop a spondylarthropathy limit the utility of the test. For example, even with a sensitivity of 95% and specificity of 94% for ankylosing spondylitis, a patient with a pre-test likelihood of 10% has only a 64% chance of having the disease if the test is positive; thus more than one-third of such patients would have false-positive results. When ordered for patients with low back pain not strongly suggestive of an inflammatory disorder, the test yields more false-positives than true-positive results. In confusing cases, a positive HLA–B27 may provide "soft" evidence that a spondylitis is present; however, significant misclassification will occur if the test is relied on too heavily (18). Perhaps the most useful application of this test lies in research into the pathogenesis of the spondyloarthropathies.

ASSESSING ORGAN DAMAGE OR INVOLVEMENT

In patients with systemic rheumatic disorders, extraarticular involvement is often the rule even in the absence of signs or symptoms. The agents used in their treatment may have systemic toxicity as well. Such involvement can be deduced by appropriate laboratory testing, such as renal or liver function tests, blood counts, muscle enzymes, or urinalysis. For selected patients, more elaborate testing may be indicated, such as a 24-hour urine collection for protein and creatinine clearance, lumbar puncture, or ANCA measurement, depending on the suspicion of specific organ systems involved and diagnoses under consideration.

Robert H. Shmerling, MD
Matthew H. Liang, MD, MPH

1. ARA Glossary Committee, Dictionary of the Rheumatic Diseases: Vol II: Diagnostic Testing. Contact Associates Int. Ltd., NY 1985
2. McNeil BJ, Keeler E, Adelstein SJ: Primer on certain elements of medical decision making. NEJM 293:211–5, 1975
3. Sox HC, Jr., Liang MH: The erythrocyte sedimentation rate: Guidelines for rational use. Annals Int Med 104:515–23, 1986
4. McCarty GA: Autoantibodies and their relation to rheumatic diseases. Med Clin NA 70:237–61, 1986
5. Atkinson JP: Complement deficiency: Predisposing factor to autoimmune syndromes. Am J Med 85:45–47, 1988
6. Maddison PJ, Provost TT, Reichlin M: Serologic findings in patients with "ANA-negative" systemic lupus erythematosus. Medicine (Baltimore) 60:87–94, 1981
7. Juby A, Johnston C, Davis P: Specificity, sensitivity, and diagnostic predictive value of selected laboratory generated autoantibody profiles in patients with connective tissue diseases. J Rheumatol 18:354–358, 1991
8. Richardson B, Epstein WV: Utility of the fluorescent antinuclear antibody test in a single patient. Ann Int Med 95:333–338, 1981
9. Shmerling RH, Delbanco TL: The Rheumatoid Factor: An analysis of clinical utility. AmJMed 91:528–534, 1991
10. Lichtenstein MJ, Pincus T: Rheumatoid arthritis identified in population based cross-sectional studies: Low prevalence of rheumatoid factor. J Rheum 18:989–993, 1991
11. Wolfe F, Cathey MA, Roberts FK: The latex test revisited: Rheumatoid factor testing in 8,287 rheumatic disease patients. Arthritis Rheum 34:951–960, 1991
12. Arnett FC, Edworthy SM, Bloch DA, et al: The American Rheumatism Association 1987 revised criteria for the classification of rheumatoid arthritis. Arthritis Rheum 31:315–324, 1988
13. Litwin SD, Singer JM: Studies of the incidence and significance of antigamma globulin factors in the aging. Arthritis Rheum 8:538–580, 1965
14. Lichtenstein MJ, Pincus T: How useful are combinations of blood tests in "rheumatic panels" in the diagnosis of rheumatic disease? J Gen Intern Med 3:435–442, 1988
15. Anderson LG, Talal N: The spectrum of benign to malignant lymphoproliferation in Sjogren's syndrome. Clin Exp Immunol 10:199–221, 1972
16. Aho K, Heliovaara M, Maatela J, et al: Rheumatoid factors antedating clinical rheumatoid arthritis. J Rheumatol 18:1282–1284, 1991
17. Hebert LA, Cosio FG, Neff JC: Diagnostic significance of hypocomplementemia. Kid Int 39:811–821, 1991
18. Hawkins BR, Dawkins RL, Christiansen FT, et al: Use of the B27 test in the diagnosis of ankylosing spondylitis: A statistical evaluation. Arth Rheum 24:743–746, 1981

C. Arthrocentesis, Synovial Fluid Analysis, and Synovial Biopsy

Examination of synovial fluid is often called the most useful test in rheumatology—a "liquid biopsy of the joint." Much has been written about its clinical use (1–3). However, outside of its use by subspecialists and in teaching centers, this examination appears to be infrequently performed. One reason may be the lack of generally accepted guidelines for what constitutes an appropriate routine synovial fluid analysis. Some recommendations offer a rather long list of chemical, immunologic, and microbiologic studies that have been borrowed from routine tests on other body fluids and which can cost several hundred dollars. Some of these tests have played important roles in our understanding of the physiology and pathophysiology of the joint. Most, however, have been inadequately tested or are otherwise inappropriate for general clinical use. As it happens, much of the most useful information can be provided by the least expensive tests, so it is usually best to perform those portions of synovial fluid analysis that will give reasonable incremental information. Another potential reason for underuse is that many clinical laboratories lack the experience and proficiency to perform some components of synovial fluid analysis (4).

Synovial fluid analysis provides the physician and scientist with unique and valuable information about what is going on inside joints. It alters diagnosis and affects subsequent treatment decisions (5,6). Together with the medical history, physical examination, and plain roentgenograms, synovial fluid analysis is a fundamental part of the clinical data base. As with the study of urine, the microscopic analysis of synovial fluid is best performed by the individual most familiar with the patient. Technical competence and the ability to interpret the results of analysis are acquired skills that will reward the physician and the patient. With experience and familiarity gained from practice and the judicious selection of tests, the practitioner will allow synovial fluid analysis the best chance of living up to its reputation as the most valuable test in rheumatology.

ARTHROCENTESIS

Indications

There are a few disorders for which synovial fluid analysis is diagnostic, providing information that is usually not available any other way. Chief among these are infectious arthritis and crystal-induced arthritis. In fact, some would argue that the only proper way to confirm these diagnoses is through synovial fluid analysis. There are a few additional forms of arthritis in which synovial fluid analysis can be diagnostic, or strongly supporting, but not necessarily in the routine clinical laboratory. Synovial fluid analysis can suggest or confirm a diagnosis of diseases as disparate as amyloidosis, hypothyroidism, ochronosis, hemochromatosis, systemic lupus erytrematosus (SLE), or even simple edema. The presence of a grossly bloody fluid should trigger consideration of a number of disorders. (See Table 8C–1).

Perhaps the most frequent question asked of synovial fluid analysis is to differentiate between inflammatory and noninflammatory arthritis (7). This seemingly trivial distinction is not always as easy to make clinically as might be believed. A traditional rule of thumb is that "noninflammatory" arthritis has a total white blood cell (WBC) less than 2000 mm³. Thus, one should not uncritically accept a diagnosis of simple osteoarthritis (OA) in which the WBC is greater than, nor a diagnosis of active rheumatoid arthritis (RA) in a given joint with a WBC count less than, this threshold value.

The coexistence of two or more types of arthritis in a single patient or even in a single joint is not uncommon. Making the correct diagnosis in these situations is virtually impossible unless synovial fluid analysis is performed. Rheumatoid arthritis, either active or in complete remission, may coexist with crystal-in-

Table 8C–1. Conditions associated with hemarthrosis

Trauma with or without fracture
Coagulation disorders
  Hemophilia
  von Willebrand's disease
  Therapeutic anticoagulation
  Other bleeding disorders
Thrombocytopenia
Essential thrombocytosis
Scurvy
Hemangioma or A-V malformation
Pigmented villonodular synovitis
Tumor (metastatic or local)
Ehlers Danlos syndrome
Pseudoxanthoma elasticum
Sickle cell disease
Postsurgical
Munchausen's syndrome
Preexisting arthritis with any of above
Idiopathic

duced arthritis, hemarthrosis, infectious arthritis, or secondary degenerative change. Rheumatoid arthritis frequently occurs in individuals who already have primary OA. Up to 7% of all patients with gout also have chondrocalcinosis. Hemarthrosis and bacterial infection usually occur in joints already damaged by another form of arthritis. Joints previously involved by inflammatory disease of any type can develop secondary degenerative change. Even experienced clinicians have difficulty sorting out these problems without synovial fluid analysis.

One of the most important reasons to perform synovial fluid analysis is to rule out bacterial infection in severely inflamed joints. There is no other sufficiently reliable way to differentiate septic arthritis from acute crystal-induced arthritis, or for that matter from severe flares of idiopathic inflammatory arthritis. Although clinical information may favor another diagnosis, failure to aspirate a severely inflamed joint risks delaying the diagnosis of septic arthritis. In this regard, the results of synovial fluid analysis dictate the pace of diagnostic and therapeutic evaluation. Thus, a WBC greater than 100,000 mm³ demands that the physician make decisions swiftly because of the high possibility of infectious arthritis and the potential for joint destruction. If the clinical picture is otherwise unthreatening, a WBC below 50,000 mm³ would permit a more measured approach.

Arthrocentesis may be therapeutic as well as diagnostic. For tense effusions in which the intraarticular pressure is high, removal of fluid will relieve symptoms and at least theoretically decrease joint damage (8). Removal of the products of inflammation is an important part of the treatment of infectious arthritis, and may be beneficial in other forms of arthritis as well.

There are more reasons for doing than for not doing arthrocentesis. Diagnostic arthrocentesis is indicated for all significant undiagnosed arthritis, certainly for arthritis that alters the ability of the patient to function. Even if the physician is convinced of the diagnosis, arthrocentesis is indicated, especially before embarking on long-term treatment with expensive or toxic modalities. For example, many physicians would not commit a patient to lifelong urate lowering drugs without demonstration of urate crystals in fluid (or tophi). Similarly, it is desirable to confirm the absence of urate or calcium pyrophosphate dihydrate (CPPD) crystals before committing a patient to second-line agents for suspected RA. Even the most experienced physicians make diagnostic errors; inexperienced ones make them frequently. For acute or severe inflammatory mono- or oligoarticular arthritis, arthrocentesis is highly recommended, even in a patient with chronic arthritis. A useful rule of thumb is that if it occurs to the examiner that arthrocentesis might be indicated, it probably is! Do not waste time thinking of reasons not to perform this procedure in a safe and timely way.

Technique

There are too many patients with arthritis for arthrocentesis to be performed only by rheumatologists or orthopedic surgeons. Operators who have received initial supervised instruction can be qualified to handle frequently involved and easily aspirated joints such as the knee. For less frequently aspirated joints, the assistance of an experienced physician is advised. Experience and detailed knowledge of the relevant anatomy is necessary to minimize discomfort and tissue damage, as well as to permit a sound judgment of whether a nonproductive aspiration is due to absence of effusion or failure to enter the joint.

Joints may have more than one route of entry. The preferred route usually involves the shortest distance through tissue, and avoids any skin lesions or superficial infections, major vessels, tendons, or nerves. There are several good illustrated references available that provide step-by-step guidelines (9). Although space does not permit identification of all approaches here, a brief outline of the usual routes follows. For the shoulder this may be an anterior approach just lateral to the coracoid process (Fig. 8C–1). An alternate approach is posteriorly, 1 in. below the posterior-lateral pole of the acromium process. The elbow is entered laterally through the groove between the olecranon process and the lateral epicondyle (Fig. 8C–2). The wrist is aspirated at its dorsal surface at the radiocarpal joint (Fig. 8C–3). The metacarpophalangeal and proximal interphalangeal joints are best approached from their dorso-lateral surface. The hip can be aspirated anteriorly without fluoroscopy, but is best left to those with training and experience. The knee joint is entered from either a lateral or medial approach at the superior third of the patella, into the groove between the patella and the femur (Fig. 8C–4). The ankle is entered anywhere anterior to the malleoli where the joint space can be identified, avoiding the dorsalis pedis artery or major tendons (Fig. 8C–5).

A few decades ago arthrocentesis was performed in operating rooms, but today it is considered an office procedure. The patient and the physician should be in comfortable positions. Drapes are not generally necessary. Synovial fluid may be biologically hazardous, and the operator should wear gloves and observe other standard precautions. Great care must be taken with used needles. They should not be recapped, and alternatives should be used to avoid transferring fluid in syringes with needles still attached.

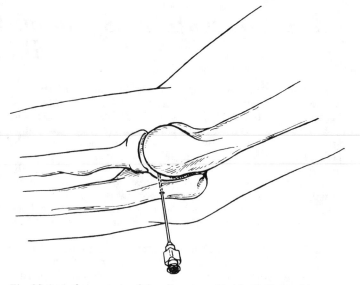

Fig. 8C–2. *Arthrocentesis of the elbow (provided by D Neustadt).*

The joint should be moved through its range of motion to resuspend its contents. Landmarks may be difficult to identify in a swollen and tender joint. Comparison with a normal joint on the other side can be helpful. The skin should be cleaned of obvious dirt with soap and water. It is not usually necessary to shave the skin. A brief scrub with an alcohol pad, followed by an application of an iodine preparation provides adequate protection. If so desired, the skin can be marked before cleaning, or an impression made with a closed retractable pen. It is important not to touch the skin at the injection site after cleaning. To avoid losing anatomical landmarks, it is best to keep one hand on the joint near the injection site to help orient the operator, to position or distract the joint, and to steady the syringe. It is a mistake to clean a vast area and then try to aspirate without such "hands on" orientation.

The skin can be infiltrated with xylocaine to decrease the pain of penetration. However, this increases the materials necessary, prolongs the procedure, and can in itself be painful. Infiltration

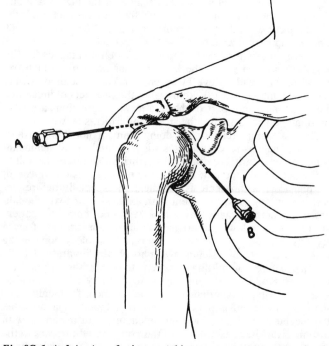

Fig. 8C–1. A, *Injection of subacromial bursa or supraspinatus tendon;* **B,** *anterior approach for injection of glenohumeral joint (provided by D Neustadt).*

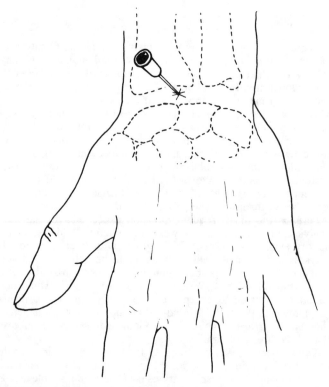

Fig. 8C–3. *Arthrocentesis of the wrist; radial approach (provided by D Neustadt).*

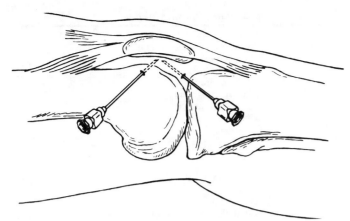

Fig. 8C–4. *Arthrocentesis of the knee; medial approach (provided by D Neustadt).*

into the deeper, pain-sensitive structures of the capsule or periosteum increases the risk of injecting anesthetic into the joint space and interfering with the results of the analysis. Reactions to xylocaine are unusual, but the patient should be asked if they have received the agent before. A simple alternative is to freeze the skin with a spray of ethyl chloride or fluori-methane. This reduces the "needle bite" and is sufficient for virtually all patients.

It is a mistake to select a small needle with the intention of sparing the patient pain. Viscous fluid full of particulate material flows with difficulty, if at all, through needles smaller than 20 gauge. The use of a larger needle shortens the procedure and is usually less painful overall. In general, use an 18- or 19-gauge needle for the knee, and 20-gauge needle for smaller joints. The size of the syringe should correlate with the estimated volume of the effusion. Large plastic syringes are hard to manipulate with one hand and can cause unnecessary pain. Break the initial resistance or "bead" of the syringe before insertion to prevent

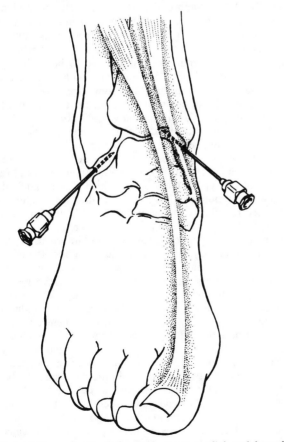

Fig. 8C–5. *Arthrocentesis of the ankle joint; medial and lateral approaches (provided by D Neustadt).*

sudden, painful movement of the needle. Stretch the skin slightly, penetrate it deftly, aspirate gently, and advance the needle until fluid appears in the syringe. If bone is encountered before fluid, the needle may be partially withdrawn and advanced in a more promising direction. Lateral traction on the skin and deeper tissues should be avoided. If after a few passes no fluid is obtained, the operator will need to decide whether no effusion was actually present, or whether another site or operator would be more productive. In the knee, pressure with the hand against the other side of the joint or in the infra patellar space can push effusions towards the needle and facilitate aspiration.

Fluid may stop flowing into the syringe because of inadvertent movement of the needle or tissue encroachment onto the needle as the size of the joint space decreases. A slight adjustment of the needle is in order if it seems that there is still fluid remaining. At other times the needle will be obstructed. In this event, if there is no resistance, a very small volume can be reinjected and may reestablish flow. For diagnostic aspirations, however, it is not necessary to aspirate all the fluid. An entire synovial fluid analysis with culture can be performed on from 1–5 cc of fluid. It is better not to try to switch syringes in the middle of the procedure. This opens the sterile path and increases the possibility of contamination. Removing the needle may take considerable physical force and cause pain to the patient. If a new syringe is to be used for more complete aspiration or for an injection of steroids, use a hemostat or other grasping device to hold the needle hub.

Complications

There are probably no absolute contraindications to diagnostic arthrocentesis, particularly if septic arthritis is suspected. Relative contraindications include infections of the skin or subcutaneous tissue over the joint or significant bleeding diathesis. The most serious potential complication is iatrogenic infection of a previously sterile joint, but it is a rare event. It has been estimated that infection occurs in less than 1 in 10,000 instances of diagnostic arthrocentesis. The likelihood of unsuspected infectious arthritis must be many times greater than this. The risk of infection can be minimized by not puncturing the skin through obvious cutaneous infections or existing skin lesions.

There is often some bleeding at the puncture site following the procedure and presumably this occurs within the joint as well. Rarely does this become a problem, although the operator should note if the initial fluid appearing in the syringe was bloody or not so that the significance of a grossly bloody fluid can be judged. When the needle is withdrawn, pressure on the puncture site will spare the patient a painful bruise and is especially important if serial aspirations are necessary. In anticoagulated patients who develop acute arthritis, anticoagulation itself is not a contraindication. Patients with known serious coagulation disorders have major complications of recurrent hemarthrosis. If diagnostic or therapeutic aspiration is necessary, it can be most safely done after prophylactic treatment with the appropriate coagulation factors.

A potential but unquantifiable complication is the possibility of direct injury to cartilage by the needle. Such injuries will not heal and can serve as a nidus for further degenerative change, particularly if they are in a weight-bearing area of the joint. This possibility can be minimized by not moving the needle from side to side; by selecting an aspiration site that will minimize contact with cartilage; by aspirating as the needle is advanced so that penetration is not deeper than necessary; and by not trying to get every last drop of fluid.

An occasional patient will have a vasovagal episode during or following the procedure. It is best to have the patient reclining and to take care when first getting up. It is important to explain the reasons for the procedure and the theoretical risks. Put things into perspective for the patient by explaining that the chances of unsuspected infection or treatable disease outweigh the very small risk of infection, bleeding, or even pain. Local custom or comfort level may require the use of a signed consent form, but not all physicians use one.

SYNOVIAL FLUID TESTS OF PROVEN VALUE

In the past, synovial fluids have been classified into groups (Groups I, II, III, IV, and so on) depending on the gross appearance, WBC count, differential cell count, protein, glucose, mucin clot, viscosity, or other parameters. The groups have been variously called normal, noninflammatory, inflammatory, septic, or hemorrhagic. These classifications have suffered from variable terminology and a lack of uniform criteria for inclusion into any one group. Classification into groups has limited diagnostic usefulness as fluids from a single disease may fall into any group. The crucial and correct message from these older classifications is that it is important to differentiate inflammatory arthritis from noninflammatory arthritis, to attempt to identify the cause of the inflammation, and to exercise greater vigilance for infectious arthritis when the WBC count is high or the fluid otherwise looks purulent.

The operator begins the gross inspection of the fluid at the time of aspiration by noting whether any blood in the syringe appeared during the aspiration, or whether the fluid was uniformly bloody, indicating prior hemarthrosis. There is rarely any indication to perform a red blood cell count. The fluid should then be transferred to a glass tube anticoagulated with liquid ethylenediaminetetra-acetate (EDTA) or heparin for subsequent inspection, WBC counts, or microscopic and polarized light examination. Powdered anticoagulants of any kind should not be used because undissolved crystals will hinder subsequent examination for crystals of diagnostic significance. When transferring the fluid from the aspirating syringe to a sterile vacuum tube, a new sterile needle should be used. In no event should a needle used for injection of microcrystalline steroids be used to transfer fluid as this will introduce innumerable crystals into the fluid and compromise the ability to identify intraarticular crystals. Such crystals will be phagocytosed within minutes by synovial cells. It is best to do the analysis on the same day that the fluid is aspirated as cell count and morphology will change. Pathologic crystals will be easily identifiable at least for a few days, facilitating consultation and examination by experts although artefactual crystals may appear over time (10).

Normal and "noninflammatory" fluids are a transparent straw or yellow color depending on the amount of albumin–bilirubin present. The color will be stronger in a jaundiced patient. Edema produces a relatively colorless fluid because of its low protein. A commonly used test is to determine if newsprint can be read through the glass tube containing the fluid. Inflammatory fluid will usually be translucent or opaque, so that newsprint cannot be read through the tube. The color will range from yellow to yellow-green depending on the amounts of protein, cells, or other debris present. The more inflammatory the fluid, the more opaque or purulent its appearance. Do not assume that cloudiness is always the result of leukocytes. Fluids can be cloudy or opaque because of crystals or other particulates as described below. Furthermore, there is no discrete gross appearance that separates infected from noninfected fluid.

The examiner should record the appearance of any unusual material seen visually or microscopically. Fragments of material (floaters) can be extracted for subsequent inspection (3). Such material can provide information of diagnostic usefulness and is a good starting place to look for crystals in patients with suspected gout or chondrocalcinosis. The list of interesting and potentially important particulates found in synovial fluid is long (Table 8C-2).

Leukocyte Counts

All fluids removed for diagnostic purposes should have total WBC and differential counts. The degree of elevation of the WBC count indicates the severity of the inflammation present, suggests the likelihood of bacterial infection, and may help estimate the rate of potential joint destruction. The absolute cell count is the major discriminating factor between an inflammatory and noninflammatory fluid. Fluids with a WBC count less than 2,000 mm^3 are traditionally considered noninflammatory although they can

Table 8C–2. *Particulates in synovial fluid*

Cells
Fibrin strands and clumps
Rice bodies
Collagen fibrils
Cartilage fragments
Synovial fragments
Adipose tissue cores from needle
Crystals
   Monosodium urate monohydrate
   Calcium pyrophosphate dihydrate
   Apatite
   Cholesterol
   Calcium Oxalate
   Other
Bacteria and fungi
Lipid globules and crystals
Amyloid fibrils
Immune complexes
Metal and plastic wear fragments
Parasites
Unrecognizable "junk"

be seen in some patients with systemic inflammatory diseases such as SLE or systemic sclerosis, and even in intercurrent crystal-induced arthritis (7,11). Most uncomplicated osteoarthritic joint fluids actually have leukocyte counts well under 1000/mm^3. It is important to recognize that there are many disorders other than OA or mechanical conditions that have noninflammatory fluids as defined by the WBC count. These include sickle cell disease, hypertrophic pulmonary osteoarthropathy, hypothyroidism, and amyloidosis.

Fluids with a cell count of more than 100,000 mm^3 may properly be considered septic until proven otherwise. Even the demonstration of crystals in such a highly inflammatory fluid does not rule out coexisting infection. Dealing with fluids that have WBC counts between 50,000 mm^3 and 100,000 mm^3 is more difficult (12). Some septic fluids will be in this range, or even lower, especially in the compromised host or partly treated patient. Gonococcal or tuberculosis infections do not cause very high WBC counts. To further complicate matters, fluids from patients with crystal-induced, or idiopathic inflammatory arthritis, such as RA or Reiter's syndrome, will commonly be in this intermediate range or even higher. Patients with such high WBC counts need to be observed carefully and sometimes even treated empirically pending culture results. A repeat aspiration 12 to 24 hours later may clarify things. Many studies of synovial fluid are comprised mostly of knee fluids. Smaller joints have higher WBC counts for the same diseases.

The differential leukocyte count adds additional information. Although many different types of normal and abnormal resident or transient cell types have been described in synovial fluid, there is probably no routine clinical reason to differentiate further than among neutrophils and mononuclear cells. When for one reason or another there is insufficient fluid to be sent for cell counts, the differential count alone can provide useful information. A noninflammatory fluid generally has considerably less than 50% neutrophils, while inflammatory fluids usually have a higher percentage. Infected fluids generally have greater than 95% neutrophils, while rheumatoid fluids usually have less than 90%, even when the absolute cell count is very high. Many crystal-induced effusions also have a very high proportion of neutrophils. As an example of how the differential count might be weighted, a total WBC count of 20,000 with 98% neutrophils and without other known cause should still make the physician consider septic arthritis. This scenario may occur in the compromised host.

The presence of lupus erythematosus cells in freshly smeared synovial fluid strongly suggests the presence of SLE, although in theory such cells can form in other diseases. Reiter's cells (large histiocytes that have ingested neutrophils or other cells) were originally described in that disorder, but also occur in other conditions.

Culture

Very turbid fluids, or those in which septic arthritis is considered for other reasons, should be sent for culture. It is probably better to err on the side of caution in culturing fluids, but it is not advisable to send all fluids for culture. Laboratory or handling contaminants do occur and will cause unneeded confusion in a patient with a low probability of infection. If the results of the WBC count or differential are truly a surprise, the joint can be re-aspirated promptly for culture. If the synovial fluid removed prior to a therapeutic injection of steroids looks unusually turbid, it is better to send the fluid for cell count and culture before injection. Although it is not necessary to send fluids routinely for fungal or tuberculosis cultures, refractory monarthritis or oligoarthritis are important indications for such cultures. In gonococcal disease, the majority of joint fluid cultures are probably bacteriologically sterile although bacterial antigens or products may be found.

Gram stains of synovial fluid should be done if there is a likelihood of infection. Staining synovial fluids presents technical difficulties different from other materials. Many fluids are so spectacularly positive that little experience is required in interpretation. However, precipitated stain, pyknotic extracellular or intracellular nuclear material, and debris can create traps for the unwary. False-positive reports do occur.

Wet Preparation

All fluids should be examined under a coverslip by routine microscopy for cells and particulate material. A polarizing light microscope provides the gold standard for crystal identification (13); unfortunately, one may not be immediately available. The helpfulness of a simple light microscope should not be underestimated (14). Unless crystals are very few, they can be seen with regular light and at least a preliminary crystal identification can be attempted based on shape. This is usually done prior to the polarized light examination. In fact, refractile CPPD crystals can be more easily seen in a good light microscope than a poor polarizing one. Cell numbers can also be estimated on the wet preparation and other particulate material such as lipid droplets noted (Table 8C–2). Rheumatoid arthritis cells, or ragocytes, are neutrophils with refractile peripheral inclusions that contain immune complexes and complement. They were originally described in RA, but are nonspecific. Sickled red cells indicate the presence of the hemoglobinopathy in either the homozygous or heterozygous state.

In general however, there is no substitute for definitive polarized light examination. Proper polarized light microscopy requires a high quality, well maintained microscope as well as an experienced observer. Unfortunately at this time, many routine hospital or clinical laboratories are not adequately equipped with either resource, and appropriate training is lacking in the schools of medical technology (4). The CPPD crystals are more likely to be missed.

Monosodium urate crystals are needle shaped or long with blunt ends. They are strongly birefringent—brilliantly bright against the dark background between the polarizing plates. The direction of the birefringence (what might be said to be the direction of rotation of light) is negative by convention and requires an interposed first-order red compensatating plate for determination (2). The CPPD crystals are more weakly birefringent in a positive direction of rotation. Fortunately, CPPD crystals are quite refractile. Crystals have the same diagnostic significance whether they are intracellular or extracellular but are in general easier to find and less likely to be confused with artifacts when they are intracellular.

The number of different crystals associated with human disease is increasing and includes calcium oxalate in renal failure (15), crystals of protein in dysproteinemic states, cholesterol in chronic inflammatory effusions, and apatites. Apatites are nonbirefringent and therefore not detected by polarized light. When present in large amounts, as in calcific tendinitis, they can be seen as amorphous particulates. Smaller amounts can be detected by characteristic appearance in electron micrographs or by

chemical analysis. These research methods are not yet appropriate for clinical use and the significance of apatite in effusions such as in OA is not fully understood. A new syndrome has been described of acute arthritis associated with brightly birefringent intracellular spherular inclusions that appear to be lipid in nature (16). This syndrome is not rare, but still poorly understood.

Tests of No, Limited, or Uncertain Clinical Value

Glucose and Lactate. Measurement of synovial fluid glucose, and more recently lactic acid, was previously considered traditional, particularly to make a diagnosis of septic arthritis. In severely inflamed joints, such as most septic joints, the glucose is very low and the lactic acid is high. The alterations in these metabolites reflect an increase in consumption of glucose by the cells of the joint cavity and synovial tissues, a decrease in effective circulation to the joint, and represent a switch to anaerobic metabolism. These changes in joint physiology reflect the degree of inflammation in the joint, and not its etiology. In those cases of severe intraarticular inflammation for which the physician needs the most help in ruling against infection, glucose and lactate measurements are the least helpful. Low or absent glucose can be observed in RA or crystal-induced arthritis (17). If glucose measurements are made, it is important to use specimen tubes containing fluoride, as leukocytes will convert glucose into lactate in vitro. Although initial clinical studies were performed on fasting patients to allow comparison with serum levels, deferring arthrocentesis for this purpose is not advisable if infection is suspected.

Viscosity. Description of fluid viscosity is a time-honored test, and this property actually gave synovial fluid its name. The easiest way to estimate viscosity is to allow a few drops of fluid to drip from the aspirating needle. A long "string" implies high viscosity, and an absent or short string implies low viscosity. The implied justification for estimating viscosity is to differentiate between inflammatory (low viscosity) and noninflammatory fluids. However, when quantitative methods of measuring viscosity are used, the test fails even this simple request. If the string sign is extremely long, consideration should be given to hypothyroidism or SLE.

Synovial fluid is a biologic fluid and has all the potential biohazards of other body fluids. Do not estimate viscosity by manipulating a drop between the fingers as suggested by older, published photographs.

Mucin clot. The mucin clot test estimates the density and friability of the precipitate that forms when synovial fluid is placed in dilute acetic acid. A good or excellent clot implies high molecular weight hyaluronic acid and normal hyaluronate–protein interactions. A fair or poor clot implies inflammatory arthritis. Unfortunately, there are no standard criteria for the performance of the test, and its endpoints are very subjective. There are more accurate and objective ways of determining whether a fluid is inflammatory. Once one of the diagnostic criteria for RA, the best use of the mucin clot test today is with bloody or other fluids where there is some doubt as to its anatomic origin. The presence of a mucin clot implies that it is synovial fluid. This property of synovial fluid to coagulate in acid underlies the reason that dilution of fluid for WBC counts must be done in saline and not the usual acid diluant used for blood.

Protein. The custom of measuring protein concentration in synovial fluid analysis originated from use of this test in evaluating pleural or peritoneal fluids. While low protein may be useful to differentiate between transudates and exudates in pleural fluid, the equivalent of a joint transudate (edema) is infrequently seen. There is no useful difference in total protein among any of the major groups of arthritis, including RA and degenerative arthritis. Thus, use of total protein measurement in synovial fluid analysis is not recommended. The rarely encountered true transudate will be recognized by the clinical setting and by the colorless nature of the joint fluid.

Immunologic tests. Because most synovial fluid immunoglobulin is derived from plasma, any patient with a positive result of a serologic test in blood is likely to have a positive result in synovial fluid. Theoretically, patients who are seronegative in blood could have a positive result in joint fluid as a result of local synthesis of immunoglobulin. While there may be some research interest in this potential, it is rarely if ever demonstrated and has no current clinical role. Because of viscosity and other chemical differences, chemical or immunologic protocols appropriate for serum or plasma may not necessarily be applied to synovial fluid without modification.

Measurement of immune complexes and complement proteins in joint tissues and fluids has played an important research role. Low complement activity and proteins are frequent in RA because of activation by immune complexes. Low levels are seen, however, in some patients with crystal-induced arthritis or even infection. Levels are low in most fluids from SLE, but there is no evidence of complement activation in these fluids to explain this finding. High levels of complement have been described in Reiter's syndrome and some psoriatic arthritis but when corrected for total protein or globulin content, this difference disappears. The literature is filled with reports on measurement of a host of biochemical substances and immunologic or inflammatory mediators. These include keratan sulfate and other macromolecules of cartilage, a variety of degradative and other enzymes, and several of the cytokines. Despite much that has been published about these tests, there is no convincing reason to perform them in a clinical setting.

SYNOVIAL BIOPSY

The connective tissue lining the joint cavity, the synovial membrane, can be biopsied at open arthrotomy, under direct vision with arthroscopy, or blindly through closed needle biopsy. In truth, pieces of tissue large enough to examine are commonly found in routine synovial fluid aspirations. Closed needle biopsy with a Parker–Pearson, or other needle has been the method by which rheumatologists could obtain tissue for diagnostic or research purposes (18). This approach has the advantage of being minimally traumatic and less expensive, but the disadvantage of providing small fragments blindly. The knee lends itself to this approach most easily, although other large joints can be biopsied.

Biopsy under arthroscopic observation yields larger and more obviously involved tissue fragments, but is still limited to those joints amenable to arthroscopy. Arthroscopy is more expensive but provides additional diagnostic and therapeutic approaches. As arthroscopy becomes generally available in local communities, closed needle biopsy for clinical purposes is much less frequently performed. Despite the availability of computed tomography and magnetic resonance imaging scans, for some joints and circumstances there will be no substitute for open surgical biopsy of synovium or bone.

Some rheumatologists are learning to perform diagnostic and even operative arthroscopy (19,20) (see Chapter 8D). Needle arthroscopes are available that make arthroscopy even less traumatic and potentially increase the number of joints amenable to study. Biopsy can be performed through separate incisions in the skin, but can be taken under direct vision. The utility, indications, and role in either research or clinical medicine of these new tools remains to be defined.

It is difficult to set forth a simple set of guidelines for synovial biopsy. It is usually performed in the setting of chronic nontraumatic synovitis limited to a single or very few joints, when a diagnosis is necessary but not possible even after synovial fluid analysis and culture. This will be an infrequent occasion in most rheumatologic practices, and certainly in general medical ones. These are usually more difficult cases, and consultation with experienced or specialist physicians may be advisable. The most common indication is to look for tuberculosis or fungal infections in susceptible patients. Culture of tissue may be positive even when synovial fluid culture and smears are not. Pathologic examination may show granulomata or fungal organisms. Synovial biopsy generally is not necessary for diagnosis of the usual bacterial pathogens.

Chronic sarcoidosis is another disease in which demonstration of granulomata in synovium can provide a diagnosis. Biopsy can play an important role in pigmented villonodular synovitis, multiple synovial chondromatosus, and plant thorn or other foreign body synovitis. The infrequent primary or metastatic tumor provides another indication for biopsy, but this is usually in the hands of the operative orthopedist.

Hemochromatosis, ochronosis, and amyloidosis are examples of diseases with distinctive synovial pathology, but synovial fluid analysis, clinical diagnosis, and non-invasive testing are often sufficient for diagnosis. Indeed, the synovium in many diseases has characteristic findings, but biopsy for clinical purposes is rarely necessary. In systemic sclerosis and polymyositis, the synovial lining cells are covered with a dense layer of fibrin. The counterpart in the synovial fluid is an abundance of fibrin strands and tangles. In amyloidosis involving the joints, the synovial lining cells are covered with a layer of amyloid. Pure amyloid material can be observed in the synovial fluid, and may be stained with congo red to assist with the diagnosis. The original American Rheumatism Association (now the American College of Rheumatology) criteria for RA included compatible synovial pathology, but the changes of thickening of the synovial cell layer, increased vascularity, fibrin deposition, lymphoid follicles, and infiltration with a variety of chronic inflammatory cells are not specific for that disease. Current research shows a broad correlation of pathologic changes with intensity of the rheumatoid disease and overall prognosis, but these are not useful enough to guide management of individual patients. The research importance of synovial biopsy, however, coupled with other physiologic, biochemical and immunological studies remains unquestioned.

Peter Hasselbacher, MD

1. Schumacher HR, Reginato AJ: Atlas of Synovial Fluid Analysis and Crystal Identification. Philadelphia, Penn., Lea & Febiger, 1991
2. Gatter RA, Schumacher HR: A Practical Handbook of Joint Fluid Analysis, 2d ed. Philadelphia, Penn., Lea & Febiger, 1991
3. Hasselbacher P: Synovial fluid analysis, Rheumatoid Arthritis: Etiology, Diagnosis, Management. Edited by Utsinger P, Zvaifler N, Ehrlich G. Philadelphia, Penn., JB Lippincott, 1985, pp 193–208
4. Hasselbacher P: Variation in synovial fluid analysis by hospital laboratories. Arthritis Rheum 30:637–642, 1987
5. Eisenberg JM, Schumacher HR, Davidson PK, et al: Usefulness of synovial fluid analysis in the evaluation of joint effusions. Arch Intern Med 144:715–719, 1984
6. Freemont AJ, Denton J, Chuck A, et al: Diagnostic value of synovial fluid microscopy: A reassessment and rationalisation. Ann Rheum Dis 50:101–107, 1991
7. Louthrenoo W, Sieck M, Clayburne G, et al: Supravital staining of cells in noninflammatory synovial fluids: Analysis of the effect of crystals on cell populations. J Rheumatol 18:409–413, 1991
8. James MJ, Cleland LG, Rofe AM, et al: Intraarticular pressure and the relationship between synovial perfusion and metabolic demand. J Rheumatol 17: 521–527, 1990
9. Steinbrocker O, Neustadt D: Aspiration and Injection Therapy in Arthritis and Musculoskeletal Disorders. Hagerstown, Harper and Row, 1972
10. Kerolous G, Clayburne G, Schumacher HR: Is it mandatory to examine synovial fluids promptly after arthrocentesis? Arthritis Rheum 32:271–278, 1989
11. Pascual E: Persistence of monosodium urate crystals and low-grade inflammation in the synovial fluid of patients with untreated gout. Arthritis Rheum 34: 141–145, 1991
12. Krey P, Bailen D: Synovial fluid leukocytosis: A study of extremes. Am J Med 67:436, 1979
13. Gordon C, Swan A, Dieppe P: Detection of crystals in synovial fluids by light microscopy: Sensitivity and reliability. Ann Rheum Dis 48:737–742, 1989
14. Pascual E, Tovar J, Ruiz MT: The ordinary light microscope: An appropriate tool for provisional detection and identification of crystals in synovial fluid. Ann Rheum Dis 48:983–985, 1989
15. Reginato AJ, Ferreiro SJ, Barbazan AC, et al: Arthropathy and cutaneous calcinosis in hemodialysis oxalosis. Arthritis Rheum 29:1387–1396, 1986
16. Gardner GC, Terkeltaub RA: Acute monoarthritis associated with intracellular positively birefringent Maltese cross appearing spherules. J Rheumatol 16: 394–396, 1989
17. Wheeler AP, Graham BS: Pseudogout presenting with low synovial fluid glucose: Identification of crystals by gram stain. Am J Med Sci 289:68–69, 1985
18. Schumacher HR: Needle biopsy of the synovial membrane: Experience with the Parker–Pearson technique. N Engl J Med 286:416–419, 1972
19. Arnold W: Arthroscopy in the diagnosis and therapy of arthritis. Hosp Practice 27:43–53, 1992
20. Arnold W, Kalunin K: Arthroscopic synovectomy by rheumatologists: Time for a new look. Arthritis Rheum 32:109–111, 1989

D. Arthroscopy

Fathers of arthroscopy explored the utility of this procedure as long ago as the 1920s. In the 1930s, the German rheumatologist Vaupel was interested in following the course of arthritis and proposed the use of arthroscopy. Unfortunately, limited optics and photographic systems frustrated these early arthroscopic pioneers.

For the most part, arthroscopy was not utilized until the 1960s, when Watanabe performed the first partial meniscus removal and heralded the way for wide usage. Subsequently, arthroscopy has primarily been used by orthopedists for diagnostic and therapeutic interventions. Over the last 30 years, there has been continued improvement in optical systems, which has allowed for further miniaturization and for the development of small-calibre "needle" arthroscopes.

The first arthroscopes were bulky lens systems that required the operator to look directly into the lens. This was often associated with equipment contamination and occasional retinal burns. Subsequent systems utilized a videocamera in place of the eyepiece and transmitted the image to a monitor, resulting in clearer images and safer operation.

Most recently, fiber optic technology has resulted in the development of arthroscopes composed of optical fibers. These fibers lead off the examination table to a camera, which captures the image electronically and transfers it for display on a monitor. Using this technology, arthroscopes as small as 0.5 to 1.9 mm in diameter have been developed, making them quite convenient for use in an outpatient setting while only sacrificing visualization to a small but generally acceptable degree. The procedure may be performed in a clean examination room using local anesthesia. Clearly, such equipment brings arthroscopy within the realm of both the rheumatologist and the orthopedist. Many joints, including those as small as the temporomandibular or interphalangeal joints, are accessible with this equipment. Careful attention to sterile techniques has kept this procedure safe, with few reported complications.

Despite 30 years of clinical use, the indications for arthroscopy are still being defined, but can be conveniently categorized as diagnostic, research, and therapeutic options. Diagnostically, arthroscopic evaluation provides the opportunity to observe small surface structures, including cartilage lesions, menisci, and ligaments in a manner unparalleled by any other procedure (Fig. 8D–1 and 8D–2). Clearly such a procedure has utility in the abnormal joint that defies diagnosis by other means. Perhaps the most obvious use of the arthroscope is as a research tool. Surface visualization may turn out to be a way to sensitively monitor therapeutic interventions, provided that there is adequate reproducibility (1). In addition, the opportunity to safely and conveniently remove large quantities of synovium provides a unique

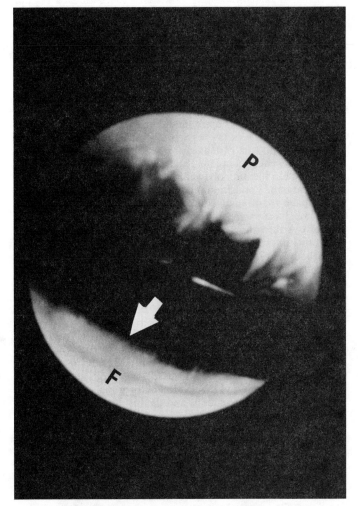

*Fig. 8D–2. Osteoarthritis: the inferior surface of the patella (**P**) is frayed and irregular. The femoral intercondylar groove (**F**) is ulcerated with a remnant of cartilage (**arrow**) (courtesy of Dr RD Altman).*

opportunity to study tissue from all stages of disease progression and to monitor the response to interventions.

The role of arthroscopy as a therapeutic tool is perhaps the least clear. Long utilized to repair internal derangements in individuals with otherwise healthy joints, the role in the individual with underlying joint disease is less certain. During the procedure, the joint is vigorously lavaged, and many patients have reported lasting pain relief following the procedure (2). In the patient with septic arthritis, arthroscopy provides a mechanism to salvage a joint that has not responded to antibiotics and closed needle drainage. Anecdotal experience with the outpatient needle arthroscope indicates that it may also have a role in synovectomy in patients with resistant inflammatory arthritis.

The procedure is generally very well tolerated. A tourniquet is not required, so that many of the complications previously attributed to the tourniquet are no longer seen. In a review of nearly 600 patients undergoing outpatient arthroscopy, there were only eight adverse events directly associated with the procedure, all of which responded to conservative therapy (3). There were no intraarticular infections.

Warren D. Blackburn, Jr, MD

1. Fife RS, Brandt KD, Braunstein EM, et al: Relationship between arthroscopic evidence of cartilage damage and radiographic evidence of joint space narrowing in early osteoarthritis of the knee. Arthritis Rheum 34:377–382, 1991

2. Ike RW, Arnold WJ, Rothschild EW, et al: Tidal irrigation versus conservative medical management in patients with osteoarthritis of the knee: a prospective randomized study. J Rheumatol 19:772–779, 1992

3. Huff JP, Sequeira W, Harris CA, Blackburn WD, Moreland LW: Survey of physicians doing office based arthroscopy. Arthritis Rheum 35(suppl):S292, 1992

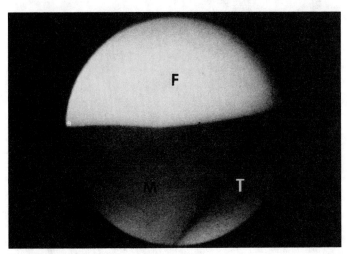

*Fig. 8D–1. Normal arthroscopic findings at the knee demonstrate the femoral condyle (**F**), tibial plateau (**T**), and meniscus (**M**) (courtesy of Dr RD Altman).*

E. Imaging Techniques in the Assessment of Rheumatic Diseases

Each imaging modality offers special advantages in specific situations, but there is significant overlap in the information each can provide. The current high cost of medical care dictates the need to utilize an imaging algorithm that is cost effective. This chapter will address the advantages of various imaging modalities related to specific problems of the musculoskeletal system.

Conventional radiography should be the first examination performed, because it is the least costly, provides the best spatial resolution, and usually defines the general nature of the problem (1). The presence, character, and distribution of bone erosions, soft tissue calcification or swelling, subluxation or malalignment, periosteal bone apposition, and changes in the interosseous cartilage space are often evident. Furthermore, the plain radiograph provides a baseline for future reference in monitoring response to therapy. Arthrography, with single or double contrast, provides additional information about the integrity of intraarticular structures, joint bodies, and synovial cysts (1). Linear or polydirectional tomography can provide spatial localization and reduces the problem of obscuration by overlying structures.

Computed tomography (CT) affords excellent anatomic localization of bone and soft tissue structures by directly imaging in the axial projection (2–4). The digital nature of the data allows flexibility in choosing window and level settings, as well as application of digital filters to optimize tissue contrast. The administration of intravenous or intraarticular contrast may further enhance the ability to image soft tissue or osseous structures (2). Image reconstruction in the sagittal and coronal planes is possible, but requires thin sections and the resultant image quality is inferior to those obtained by other more direct imaging techniques. Depending on the articular site, direct sagittal and coronal imaging may also be possible (3). Contrast resolution, or sensitivity to small radiographic density differences, is much better than with conventional radiography, but spatial resolution is somewhat less than with radiography.

Magnetic resonance imaging (MRI) characterizes tissue according to its morphologic appearance and physical properties. Each specific tissue type is associated with an image signal intensity determined by the number of "mobile" hydrogen atoms, and two physical parameters, called T1 and T2. Conventional spin-echo techniques emphasize T1 and T2-weighting, these being the most important factors affecting tissue contrast. A set of intermediate or "spin-density" images is often obtained as part of the T2-weighted pulse sequence. The spin-density images contain anatomic information similar to T1-weighting, but with slight enhancement of high water content structures, such as joint effusions. The tissue components of the musculoskeletal system are ideally suited for examination by MRI because of the wide range of contrast they normally exhibit (Table 8E-1). Marrow appears as high signal intensity or bright on T1-weighting and darker on T2-weighting, while cortical bone appears dark on all pulse sequences (5–7). The exceptional contrast resolution of MRI results in an increased sensitivity to pathologic processes that have altered both signal characteristics and morphology (2,5,8,9). Thus, MRI is particularly well suited for evaluating cartilaginous and ligamentous structures and changes in the bone marrow. The capability to directly obtain multiplanar images, the

Table 8E–2. *Normal sonographic appearances of tissues*

Tissue	Features
Tendons	Very bright (echogenic)
	Linear (anisotropic)
Bone	Very echogenic reflector (specular reflector)
Muscle	Moderately dark (hypoechoic) containing multiple fine linear echogenic bands (perimysial connective tissue)
Fibrocartilage	Echogenic
Hyaline Cartilage	Hypoechoic
Simple Fluid	Homogeneously dark (anechoic)
Complex Fluid	Dark with internal echoes or septations present

use of non-ionizing radiation, and the maintenance of relatively good spatial resolution, are major advantages.

Ultrasonography (US) is particularly useful for evaluating soft tissue structures, especially those that contain fluid (10). Lesions that are superficial in relation to the body surface are more easily evaluated than deep-seated lesions. It is more operator-dependent than the other imaging modalities and in experienced hands, can be quite effective in identifying and characterizing joint effusions and lesions of tendons, ligaments, and skeletal muscle. Imaging in "real-time" allows performance of provocative maneuvers, such as flexion-extension, that may enhance the appearance of a pathologic process (10). The normal sonographic appearances of various tissues are summarized in Table 8E-2. Simple fluid appears homogeneously dark (anechoic), while structures such as tendons appear bright (echogenic) and linearly oriented (anisotropic) (Fig. 8E-1). Ultrasound has recently been shown to have great potential for evaluating the presence of minimal surface irregularities of articular cartilage as seen in osteoarthritis (11).

Scintigraphy is an excellent screening tool that stresses functional rather than morphologic abnormalities. The distribution of a radiopharmaceutical is a function of local blood flow, vascular permeability, and tissue extraction which, in the case of diphosphonate complexes with ^{99m}Tc, relates to the rate of new bone formation. Although this technique is more sensitive than conventional radiography in the detection of musculoskeletal lesions, it is nonspecific and may show lesions that are not clinically important. In the case of infectious lesions, improved

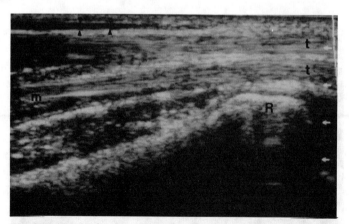

Fig. 8E–1. *Normal appearance of tendons on ultrasound. Sonogram obtained in the sagittal plane over the right wrist demonstrating superficial and deep flexor tendons (t). The underlying bright reflector depicts the cortical margin of the distal radius (R). The musculotendinous junctions (m) show the transition between linear echogenic (bright) tendon and hypoechoic (dark) muscle. A thin fluid collection (arrowheads) is present superficial to these tendons in the subcutaneous tissues.*

Table 8E–1. *Normal MRI signal characteristics*

Tissue	T1	T2
Cortical Bone	Low	Low
Muscle	Intermediate	Intermediate
Tendon/Ligament	Low	Low
Fibrocartilage (Menisci)	Low	Low
Hyaline Cartilage (Articular)	Low	High
Fat (SQ, Marrow)	High	Intermediate
Fluid (Effusion)	Low/Intermediate	High

specificity may be obtained with the addition of gallium (^{67}Ga citrate) or indium-labeled leukocyte (^{111}In-WBC) scans (1,12,13). Single photon emission tomography utilizes a tomographic approach to scintigraphy and in this respect is analogous to CT. It provides better anatomic detail and improved contrast enhancement relative to conventional scintigraphy. A significant advantage of scintigraphy is that it allows for screening of the entire skeleton in a single examination with moderate cost.

SPECIFIC ABNORMALITIES

Joint Effusion

The presence of excess joint fluid is usually nonspecific, often reflecting traumatic, inflammatory, or infectious etiologies (1). It can be due to increased levels of physical activity or the result of a preexisting intraarticular lesion such as osteoid osteoma. Many types of synovial inflammation may be causative. Radiologic diagnosis depends on secondary signs, such as displacement of adjacent fat tissue and widening of the joint space; the latter is particularly common in children. Computed tomography, ultrasound, and magnetic resonance imaging allow direct visualization of joint fluid.

Although MRI is extremely sensitive to the detection of fluid, ultrasound is an easy means of diagnosing and characterizing joint effusion and also provides direct guidance for the aspiration of such effusions (10). Small amounts of intraarticular fluid are evident sonographically as anechoic or hypoechoic (Table 8E–2) material distending the joint capsule (Fig. 8E–2). This application has been particularly useful in the hip, but may be applied to the shoulder, elbow, knee, and ankle (10). Complex fluid manifests itself as debris or septations within the collection. Although the sonographic appearance is often nonspecific, in the appropriate clinical setting, the nature of this material may be surmised, for example blood or pus. The high relative contrast of fluid on MRI, particularly on T2-weighting, makes this an excellent modality to detect even very small amounts of intraarticular fluid. Magnetic resonance imaging may provide additional information as to the nature of the fluid, as well as its relationship to other coexistent abnormalities (1,9,14). Edema or inflammation of tissue may be confused with joint fluid on MRI or CT, because they have a similar appearance with both modalities. This problem is often resolved if intravenous contrast is administered (Fig. 8E–3) at the time of examination (15).

Synovial or Synovial-like Proliferations

Synovial hyperplasia and inflammation occur in association with many forms of arthritis (1). Scintigraphy can detect affected joints with greater sensitivity than plain radiography because of increased bone turnover and alterations in blood flow (Fig. 8E–4). However, the character and distribution of the inflammatory

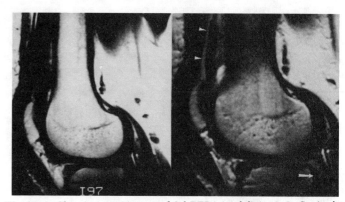

Fig. 8E–3. *Chronic synovitis: use of Gd-DTPA (gadolinium).* **L,** *Sagittal T1-weighted image through the medial knee joint shows low signal intensity material in the suprapatellar pouch.* **R,** *Following administration of Gd-DTPA, enhancement of a thickened synovial membrane (**arrowheads**) is apparent outlining the suprapatellar bursa, as well as synovial tissue posteriorly (**arrow**). Several areas of enhancement are present in the infrapatellar fat, likely reflecting underlying hyperemia and inflammation. The apparent difference in marrow signal intensity is artificial, relating to window/level settings used for photography.*

tissue within the affected joint are better assessed with CT, MRI, or US (1,10,15–17).

The multiplanar imaging capability and excellent tissue contrast inherent in MRI make it the most effective method of evaluating disease extent and activity, particularly when combined with intravenous contrast (gadolinium chelates); the latter enhances the acute inflammatory tissue and thickened synovial membrane (Fig. 8E–3) (15,16). Similar enhancement may be seen with CT using intravenous contrast but without the same degree of tissue differentiation. Areas of fibrosis, hemorrhage, or both may be distinguished based on their characteristic appearance on MRI. For example, hemosiderin deposition and fibrosis typically show a low signal on T2-weighting, but synovium itself is of intermediate-to-high signal intensity. The presence of methemoglobin, representative of subacute hemorrhage, is indicated by areas of high signal intensity on T1 and T2-weighted images (16,18). Amyloid deposition in soft tissues is associated with low-to-intermediate signal intensity on all pulse sequences (Fig. 8E–5). These soft tissue deposits are often lobular in configuration and contiguous with bone erosions seen on plain film (17). In amyloid deposition, displacement of adjacent soft tissue structures, such as the flexor tendons of the wrist, may be evident. Synovial inflammation on grayscale ultrasound appears as nodular hypoechoic soft tissue masses within a distended joint capsule and is often associated with a complex effusion (10). However, this appearance is nonspecific and would be difficult to distin-

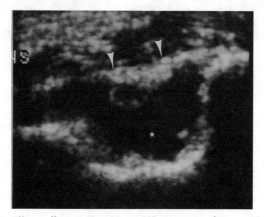

Fig. 8E–2. *Elbow effusion. Transverse US scan over the posterior joint space of the right elbow in a patient with calcium pyrophosphate deposition disease easily delineates the excess joint fluid (*) and displacement of the posterior capsule (arrowheads).*

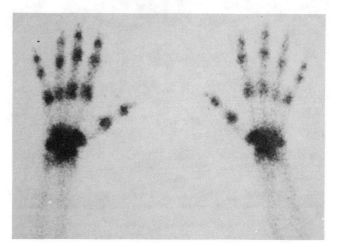

Fig. 8E–4. *Distribution of disease activity in rheumatoid arthritis. Delayed image of the hands from ^{99m}Tc-MDP scintigraphy showing distribution of active disease in a patient with rheumatoid arthritis.*

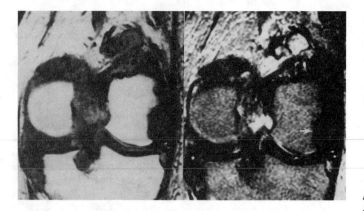

Fig. 8E–5. Dialysis-related amyloid arthropathy. Coronal spin-density (**L**) and T2-weighted (**R**) images of the right knee depicts nodular soft tissue which is low-to-intermediate signal intensity about both condyles, replacing the fat adjacent to the lateral meniscus (*), and contiguous with erosions (**arrows**) in the medial femoral condyle and tibial plateau. Spotty areas of joint fluid and marrow edema are evident.

guish from synovial changes secondary to hemorrhage or infection.

Articular Surface

The subchondral bone on the roentgenogram is best evaluated with a beam tangent to the articular surface. Visualization of the cartilaginous structures additionally requires introduction of intraarticular contrast material (arthrography) (1). Arthrography is often sufficient to characterize and follow abnormalities in a variety of joints. Certain complex joints and joints obscured by overlying bone may not be easily evaluated with plain roentgenograms. In such joints complete evaluation of the articular surfaces, surrounding soft tissues, effusion, and adjacent cortical and cancellous bone requires a tomographic imaging technique. Linear and polytomography provide spatial localization but poor spatial resolution.

Ultrasound is of limited value in these complex joints, the major limitation being limited acoustic access. Hyaline cartilage (Table 8E–2) appears as a hypoechoic band over the subjacent cortical bone. It is usually evident over portions of the femoral condyles, humeral and femoral heads, radial head, and capitellum (10). Areas of cartilage thinning or destruction may be evident, but assessment of cartilage thickness is not precise because of limited spatial resolution, variations in speed-of-sound, and the effect of adjacent soft tissues, such as synovial inflammation, that can obscure the cartilage surface. On the other hand, pre-

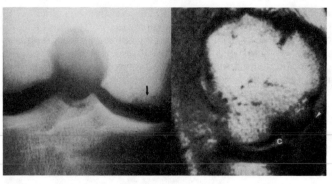

Fig. 8E–7. Osteochondritis dissecans. **L**, Notch view of the right knee shows an irregular ovoid osteochondral body (**arrow**) in the posterior medial femoral condyle. **R**, Sagittal T1-weighted image of the knee indicates that the fragment is partially dislodged into the thinned overlying articular cartilage (**c**), which is disrupted posteriorly (**arrowhead**).

liminary evidence suggests that ultrasound may be able to detect some of the earliest changes in cartilage in osteoarthritis (11). Fibrocartilage (Table 8E–2) appears echogenic and is seen to a limited extent in the knee, shoulder, and possibly the wrist. However, ultrasound has thus far not been useful in the detection of abnormalities of fibrocartilaginous structures in these joints.

Magnetic resonance imaging and computed tomography provide the best overall assessment of articular surfaces. Areas of focal cartilage deficiency, cortical erosions, subchondral cysts, and post-traumatic and or ischemic osteochondral defects are well depicted by either technique (1,2,7,8,14,19). In CT-arthrography the articular cartilage appears as a radiolucent band outlined by a thin layer of contrast material—and air on double-contrast examination—imaged in the axial plane (2). Magnetic

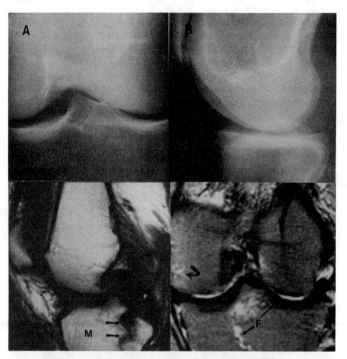

Fig. 8E–8. Occult tibial plateau fracture on MR. Frontal (**A**) and lateral (**B**) roentgenograms of the left knee in a patient with a history of seronegative arthritis and previously treated septic arthritis. Following treatment, the patient continued to complain of posterior knee pain. **C**, Sagittal T1-weighted spin-echo image of the knee shows an irregular low signal intensity area (**arrows**) originating from the articular surface with surrounding normal fatty marrow (**M**). **P** denotes the posterior cruciate ligament. **D**, Coronal T2-weighted image of the left knee. Homogeneous high signal intensity, corresponding to fluid, is present within the joint and within the serpentine abnormality in the proximal tibia (**F with arrows**). The latter denotes a radiographically occult subarticular fracture. Spotty high signal intensity in the medial femoral condyle indicates a small area of marrow edema (**curved arrow**).

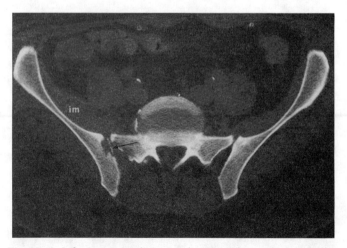

Fig. 8E–6. Infectious sacroiliitis. Axial computed tomogram with photography optimized to display bone, shows widening and destruction of the right SI joint. CT exquisitely demonstrates the erosive changes and sequestrum (**arrow**). Asymmetric enlargement of the right iliacus muscle (**im**) is secondary to involvement by adjacent inflammatory reaction.

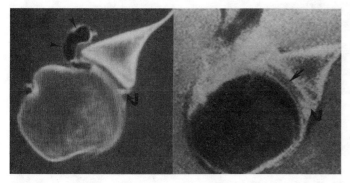

Fig. 8E–9. *Posterior labral tear.* **L,** *Axial CT through the right shoulder in external rotation following double-contrast arthrogram. Anterior capsule (**arrowheads**) is distended, and intact anterior labrum is evident. A linear collection of contrast material is present within a posterior labral tear (**curved arrow**).* **R,** *Reverse image from an axial T1-weighted scan of the right shoulder in the same patient. Linear increased signal intensity (**dark line**) (retouched) in the otherwise low signal intensity posterior labrum depicts the same tear (**curved arrow**). Hyaline cartilage is evident as intermediate signal intensity (**straight arrow**) in the glenohumeral joint.*

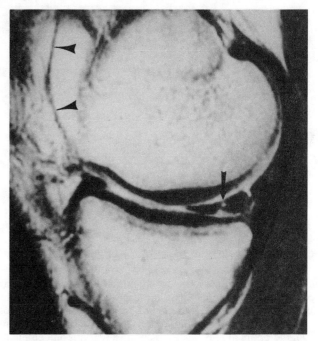

Fig. 8E–11. *Meniscal tear. Sagittal spin-density image through the medial left knee joint depicts a complex posterior horn tear (**arrow**). A moderate amount of fluid in the suprapatella pouch and medial plica (**arrowheads**) is evident.*

resonance imaging directly images the articular cartilage and allows greater flexibility in choosing the image plane without requiring repositioning of the patient in the scanner. Alterations in the biochemical composition of cartilage cause changes in its T1 and T2 relaxation times, and, hence, its appearance on spin-echo imaging. Furthermore, newer scan techniques allow acquisition of sections as thin as 1.5 mm, thereby reducing volume averaging artifacts often observed in conventional spin-echo images.

Computed tomography can detect subtle cortical erosions (Fig. 8E–6), the presence of calcification, bone production, or ankylosis (1,3). Similarly, thin-section CT can clearly define subtle lesions such as the nidus of an intraarticular osteoid osteoma or the site and type of fusion in tarsal coalition (3,4). Unlike CT, MRI is limited because fibrous tissue, dense bone, and calcification have similar appearances on all pulse sequences with standard spin-echo imaging; however, abnormalities in the adjacent marrow are best appreciated with MRI (see below). Osteochondritis dissecans or other forms of osteochondral fractures (Figs. 8E–7, 8E–8) are well assessed by either CT-arthrography or MRI. The latter is the technique of choice in osteochondritis

dissecans, because the integrity of the overlying articular cartilage can be evaluated as well as the presence of fluid around the fragment and subjacent reactive marrow edema or granulation tissue. These are important features in evaluating the stability of the osteochondral fragment (7,14).

The role of scintigraphy in evaluating joint abnormalities relates to its ability to detect areas of hyperemia typical of acute synovitis. This modality easily addresses the distribution of lesions and activity of disease (Fig. 8E–4). The use of the 3-phase bone scan or SPECT allows distinction between soft tissue abnormalities and those primarily within bone. Scintigraphy is helpful in determining the stability of osteochondral fragments on the basis of high levels of activity at the lesional site, denoting an unstable fragment (14).

Internal Joint Derangement

This category includes intraarticular abnormalities of ligaments and fibrocartilaginous structures, and secondary osteochondral bodies. Since visualization of detailed internal joint anatomy is required, scintigraphy and ultrasonography have no significant role. Because of the high contrast produced by air and iodinated

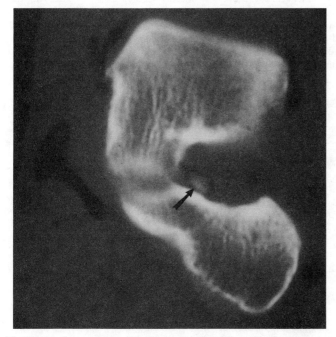

Fig. 8E–10. *Intraarticular joint body. Coronal CT readily demonstrates a small joint body (**arrow**) situated centrally in the subtalar joint. This was not definitely evident on initial plain films following contrast administration.*

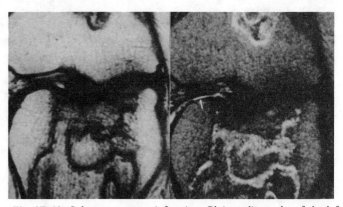

Fig. 8E–12. *Subacute marrow infarction. Plain radiographs of the left knee showed no abnormality.* **L,** *T1-weighted coronal image of the same knee depicts serpentine low signal intensity areas in marrow space. On T2-weighting (**R**), contiguous high signal intensity is present corresponding to granulation tissue. A small joint effusion is present (**arrow**).*

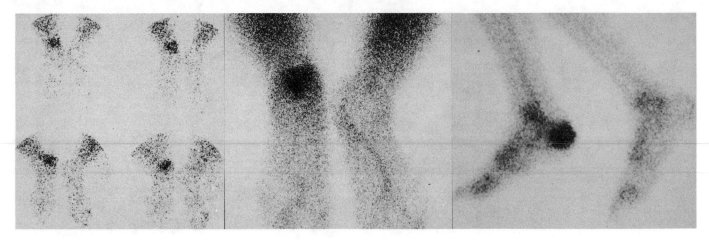

Fig. 8E–13. *Calcaneal osteomyelitis. 3-phase bone scan with 4 images from the flow phase (**L**), immediate blood pool (**center**) and delayed (**R**) images depicting abnormal tracer activity in the left calcaneus corresponding to an area of osteomyelitis.*

contrast material within a distended joint, CT-arthrography is an excellent technique to evaluate the capsular mechanism and labrum (Fig. 8E–9) of the glenohumeral joint (1,2). Such evaluation is enhanced by acquiring thin sections (3–5 mm), post-processing the data to optimally visualize air-contrast margins and obtaining axial images in both internal and external rotation. Similarly, CT-arthrography may be applied to the elbow, wrist, hip, and ankle (Fig. 8E–10). In comparison, spin-echo imaging takes advantage of inherent contrast between fibrocartilage and hyaline cartilage (Table 8E–1), and allows greater flexibility in choosing the image plane. In addition to the rotator cuff, periarticular soft tissues, and bony structures, MRI demonstrates the capsular mechanism in a near-comparable fashion to CT (2) (Fig. 8E–9), particularly when combined with intraarticular administration of gadolinium.

The knee is best assessed with MRI because of its complex internal anatomy, axial orientation, and predilection for harboring multiple concomitant abnormalities (6,7,9,14). Meniscal tears (Fig. 8E–11) appear as increased intrameniscal signal intensity extending to the articular surface with or without associated contour abnormalities and fragmentation (6). High levels of sensitivity and specificity for the diagnosis of meniscal tears may be achieved. Similar diagnostic capabilities apply to the cruciate and collateral ligaments, as well as adjacent tendons. Ligament and tendon disruptions are discerned as abnormal signal intensity with associated areas of discontinuity. A localized mass may be present corresponding to an area of hemorrhage or edema (5,6). Loose bodies have a variable appearance depending on whether they are cartilaginous, calcified or ossific. The latter appear corticated with normal internal marrow signal. Magnetic resonance

imaging has been particularly useful as an indicator of structural abnormalities that are not detectable easily with other imaging modalities (Fig. 8E–8) or arthroscopy (e.g. bone bruise and insufficiency fracture, see below).

These applications of MRI can be extended to other joints, although these joints have been less extensively studied than the knee (5,19). Wrist MRI has received recent attention with regard to imaging of the intercarpal ligaments. Apart from the triangular fibrocartilage complex, perforations of the intercarpal ligaments may be difficult to appreciate without a coexisting joint effusion or addition of an intraarticular contrast agent. In the assessment of carpal instability, the role of MRI is yet to be clearly defined (19). If abnormal soft tissue masses are suspected, as in amyloid or ganglion cysts, MRI, CT, and ultrasound may be of value (9,17). The presence of bone erosion, infarction or fracture is better assessed with either CT or MRI than with ultrasound or scintigraphy.

Marrow Abnormalities

Patients with rheumatic disorders are frequently at risk for the development of bone pain. Plain films may show spotty areas of demineralization and indistinctness or sclerosis of the subchondral bone. Possible etiologies for this pain include bone contusions, fractures, infarction, infection, or possibly underlying malignancy (1). Scintigraphy is a sensitive but generally nonspecific method to detect these abnormalities, unless combined with additional agents that may improve specificity (12,13). Magnetic resonance imaging is particularly sensitive to the presence of marrow abnormalities that may occur in association with joint

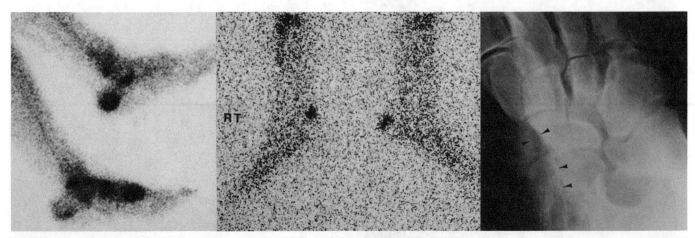

Fig. 8E–14. *Use of 111-In-labeled leukocytes to improve specificity.* **L**, *Delayed image of the feet from a 3-phase bone scan in a patient with diabetes mellitus. This shows markedly abnormal tracer uptake in the right calcaneus and left midfoot.* **C**, *24-hour image following administration of 111-In-labeled leukocytes fails to show concordant activity in abnormal areas present in ^{99m}Tc-scintigraphy effectively excluding osteomyelitis in these locations (**RT** denotes right side).* **R**, *Oblique view of the left foot shows fractures of the talus and navicular bones (**arrowheads**), without significant osteoporosis, typical of neuropathic joint disease.*

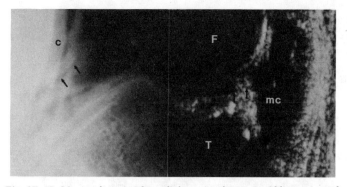

Fig. 8E–15. *Meniscal cyst with medial meniscal tear.* **L**, *Oblique view of the medial joint compartment from a double-contrast arthrogram of the knee. Both the articular cartilage (**c**) over the medial femoral condyle and medial meniscus are outlined by air and contrast material. A horizontal lucency (retouched) in the medial meniscus (**arrows**) illustrates a horizontal tear.* **R**, *Coronal US image over the posteromedial joint space.* **F** *and* **T** *denote femoral condyle and tibial plateau, respectively. The medial capsule is displaced laterally by a complex-fluid collection. In this case, a thin hypoechoic line (**arrows**) depicts the horizontal tear communicating with the associated meniscal cyst (**mc**).*

pathology. The presence of marrow edema or inflammation is a nonspecific finding, which may be seen with active arthritis, either inflammatory or infectious, as well as trauma. In trauma, localized areas of high signal intensity on T2-weighted images within the bone marrow, termed "bone bruises", presumably relate to trabecular microfractures with corresponding edema and hemorrhage. Fractures, whether due to direct trauma or insufficiency, are apparent as linear low signal areas on T1-weighted images with variable appearance on T2-weighting, depending on whether fluid extends into the fracture (Fig. 8E–8). Adjacent marrow edema is almost invariably present (7). Insufficiency fractures may cause pain. They may not be apparent on plain films. When these are axially oriented, CT sometimes does not demonstrate the fracture. Abnormal activity will be present at the fracture site on scintigraphy, and MRI can easily document the fracture with coronal or sagittal imaging.

Marrow infarction (Fig. 8E–12) can occur as a sequel to a number of conditions, such as SLE, Gaucher's disease, and steroid usage. The MRI appearances of subacute and chronic marrow infarction are virtually pathognomonic regardless of location and can precede changes on plain film, CT, or scintigraphy (8). Circumscribed, serpentine areas of low signal, corresponding to reactive new bone formation, are bordered by high signal areas, reflecting granulation tissue, on T2-weighted images. These central areas may show progressively lower signal intensity on all pulse-sequences as fibrosis or sclerosis appear. It has been shown that alterations in marrow signal intensity due to

edema and inflammation may be seen within the first week (20). As noted, however, marrow edema alone is nonspecific and may be seen in other entities such as migratory transient osteoporosis, frequently seen in the hip. The appearance of localized osteopenia on plain radiographs with marrow edema on MRI may be confused with early bone infarction. This condition is self-limited and subsequent imaging, including roentgenography, will return to normal. Scintigraphy is almost as sensitive as MRI in the detection of early marrow infarction, appearing as areas of diminished tracer activity in the acute phase (1). In the subacute or chronic phases, increased bone metabolism results in increased uptake of radionuclide, but this appearance is nonspecific.

Septic arthritis and osteomyelitis are common complications in patients with underlying rheumatic disorders, particularly rheumatoid arthritis. Scintigraphic techniques provide localization (Fig. 8E–13), and when combined with plain film analysis, may be sufficient for diagnosis. Separation of cellulitis from osteomyelitis can be made on 3-phase bone scan, and additional spatial localization can be provided with SPECT. The distribution of abnormal activity may indicate whether the infection is localized to the joint or marrow space. Additional specificity is gained with the use of gallium (^{67}Ga citrate) or indium-labeled leukocyte (^{111}In–WBC) scans (Fig. 8E–14) (12,13). False positives occur in the setting of superimposed active arthritis, whereas false negatives can occur if there has been prior antibiotic therapy (12). When plain film findings are equivocal and there is high clinical suspicion of an abnormality, MRI or CT may exquisitely demonstrate the underlying pathology (1). Magnetic resonance imaging is extremely sensitive in detecting marrow edema/inflammation, particularly if combined with fat suppression or intravenous contrast (gadolinium) (13,15). Likewise, the presence of associated soft tissue abscess and inflammatory masses can be well demonstrated. Computed tomography (Fig. 8E–6), on the other hand, better depicts bone changes such as sequestra, subtle erosions, and sinus tracts.

The presence of circumscribed loss of high marrow signal with abrupt transition on T1-weighted images, with or without accompanying destructive changes on plain radiographs, is compatible with underlying primary or metastatic neoplasm. This may be associated with endosteal scalloping, cortical disruption, and an abnormal soft tissue mass. The extent of marrow and soft tissue abnormality is best appreciated on MRI, while CT allows better depiction of cortical destruction and dystrophic calcification.

Periarticular Abnormalities

Ultrasound provides a readily accessible modality to evaluate many abnormalities of the periarticular soft tissues. Abnormal fluid collections, including synovial cysts, ganglion cysts, meniscal cysts, bursitis, and those due to infectious or hemorrhagic etiology are easily evaluated with sonography (Fig. 8E–15) (10).

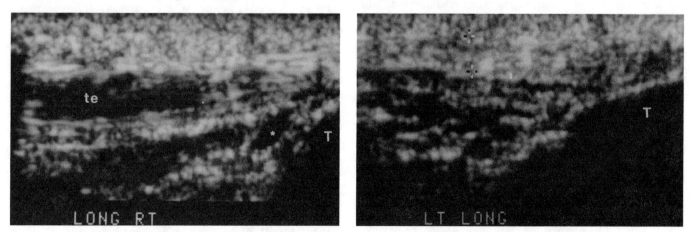

Fig. 8E–16. *Patella tendinitis. Longitudinal sonograms over the right (**L**) and left (**R**) patella tendons. The abnormal right patella tendon (**te**) is enlarged and hypoechoic centrally. A small amount of fluid distends the infrapatella bursa (***). The normal left patella tendon is included for comparison. The curvilinear reflector on the right of each image corresponds to the proximal anterior tibial cortex (**T**).*

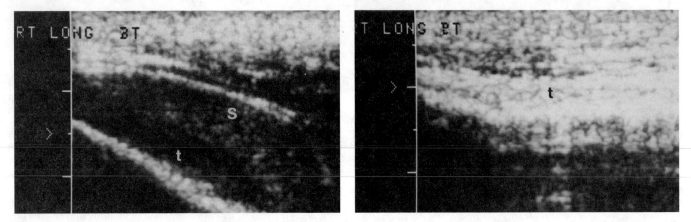

*Fig. 8E–17. Ultrasound in follow-up. Patient with tenosynovitis involving the right rotator cuff. **L**, Sagittal US over the long head of the biceps tendon (**t**) depicts an ill-defined hypoechoic tendon and adjacent inflamed synovium (**S**) with marked distension of the tendon sheath. **R**, Follow-up sonogram obtained 6 months after intraarticular steroids indicates a normal appearing tendon (**t**) with resolution of the adjacent inflammatory response.*

Associated findings such as meniscal tears, or fluid in typical locations such as the bursae, aid in diagnosis. With regard to the popliteal space, aneurysms may be suspected clinically as a palpable, pulsatile mass. A specific diagnosis can often be made using pulsed-Doppler or color-flow imaging that differentiates arterial and transmitted pulsation. Scintigraphy can depict areas of abnormal blood flow or tracer activity and is, therefore, a valuable overall screening technique (1,13). This technique may also be specific as when it utilizes Indium-labeled leukocytes to show a soft tissue abscess (12).

Linearly oriented, superficial tendons (Fig. 8E–1), such as the Achilles tendon, patella tendon, and tendons in the wrist, may be seen with the current generation of high frequency linear transducers (7.5–10 MHz) (10). Areas of focal or diffuse thickening, contour deformities, discontinuities, surrounding fluid collections, localized or diffuse calcification, and areas of internal hypoechogenicity denote tendon pathology (Figs. 8E–16, 8E–17). Similar diagnostic criteria may be applied to ligaments that are normally echogenic linear structures. Sonographic examination may be used to obtain follow-up of traumatic and inflammatory lesions (Fig. 8E–17), as well as to perform provocative maneuvers that may accentuate tendon pathology. In certain joints, such as the shoulder, the complexity of the anatomy and inherent tendon curvature require that stricter criteria be applied to diagnose tendon lesions. Sonographic examination can, nevertheless, be useful with sensitivity and specificity as high as 90% for the diagnosis of such abnormalities (10). The diagnostic accuracy of sonography depends heavily on the skill and expertise of the sonographer. Solid masses in periarticular locations, such as neurofibromas, can present as painful lesions. These can likewise be depicted as homogeneous masses with varying internal echo characteristics on grayscale imaging. Their relationship to adjacent joint, tendons, and nerves may be determined.

Magnetic resonance imaging, and to a lesser extent CT, provide better depiction of all these lesions, in view of the improved anatomic detail and tissue contrast compared to ultrasonography. The relationship of these abnormalities to the adjacent joints and soft tissues as well as to other coexistent lesions is more readily demonstrated. On MRI, edema or inflammation within tendons appear as increased signal intensity superimposed on the otherwise low signal intensity background (Table 8E–1) (5). Multiplanar imaging enables muscles, tendons, and ligaments to be seen in long axis. Both CT and MRI allow better depiction of associated avulsive lesions that may accompany traumatic tendon and ligamentous injuries (1). When there is a question of additional abnormalities or when deeply situated joints are being evaluated, MRI and CT are the modalities of choice. For example, both of these modalities allow demonstration of secondary abnormalities in adjacent structures such as nerve entrapment; two examples are compression of median and posterior tibial nerves in carpal and tarsal tunnel syndromes, respectively.

SUMMARY

A rational approach to imaging depends on identifying the specific clinical problem to be solved and a consideration of the advantages and cost-effectiveness of the available modalities. Scintigraphy, US, CT, and MRI can be used to evaluate a wide variety of pathologic entities, thereby providing valuable information complementary to roentgenography. Scintigraphy is a very sensitive, but relatively nonspecific, screening tool. It requires an intravenous injection, several hours to complete the examination, and is of moderate cost. Computed tomography is excellent for evaluating lesions that involve complex bony structures, and it provides contrast resolution that is superior to radiography with only slight loss in spatial resolution. It is performed in less than one hour, is not uncomfortable, but is expensive. Magnetic resonance imaging is of value for lesions that affect soft tissues, cartilage, and marrow. It is the most costly of these modalities, and imaging time takes approximately 30 minutes to one hour depending on various factors. It can be uncomfortable, because the patient is required to remain immobile during the scanning procedure. Claustrophobic patients can be adversely affected due to narrow scanner diameter. Ultrasonography is readily available, relatively inexpensive, and is performed usually in less than 30 minutes. It is useful in evaluating the soft tissues, especially fluid collections, and does not involve patient discomfort. It is also useful to detect and characterize lesions in muscles and tendons, but is dependent on the skill and experience of the operator.

Ronald S. Adler, PhD, MD
William Martel, MD

1. Resnick D: Common disorders of synovium-lined joints: Pathogenesis, imaging abnormalities, and complications. AJR 151:1079–1093, 1988
2. Kieft GJ, Bloem JL, Rozing PM, et al: MR imaging of recurrent anterior dislocation of the shoulder: Comparison with CT arthrography. AJR 150:1083–1087, 1988
3. Pineda C, Resnick D, Greenway G: Diagnosis of tarsal coalition with computed tomography. Clin Orthop 208:282–288, 1986
4. Schlesinger AE, Hernandez RJ. Intracapsular osteoid osteoma of the proximal femur: Findings on plain film and CT. AJR 154:1241–1244, 1990
5. Rosenberg ZS, Cheung Y, Jahsso MH, et al: Rupture of the posterior tibial tendon: CT and MR imaging with surgical correlation. Radiology 169:229–235, 1988
6. Mink JH, Levy T, Crues III JV: Tears of the anterior cruciate ligament and menisci of the knee: MR imaging evaluation. Radiology 167:769–774, 1988
7. Mink JH, Deutsch AL: Occult cartilage and bone injuries of the knee: Detection, classification, and assessment with MR imaging. Radiology 170:823–829, 1989
8. Mitchell MD, Kundel HL, Steinberg ME, et al: Avascular necrosis of the hip: Comparison of MR, CT, and scintigraphy. AJR 147:67–71, 1986
9. Burk DL, Dalinka MK, Kanal E, et al: Meniscal and ganglion cysts of the knee: MR evaluation. AJR 150:331–336, 1988
10. Kaplan PA, Matamoros A, Jr., Anderson JC: Sonography of the musculoskeletal system. AJR 155:237–245, 1990
11. Adler RS, Dedrick DK, Laing TJ, et al: Quantitative assessment of cartilage surface roughness in osteoarthritis using high frequency ultrasound. Ultrasound Med Biol 18:51–58, 1992
12. Schemwecker DS. Osteomyelitis: Diagnosis with In-111-labeled leukocytes. Radiology 171:141–146, 1989
13. Beltran J, McGhee RB, Shaffer PB, et al: Experimental infections of the

musculoskeletal system: Evaluation with MR imaging and TC-99m MDP and Ga-67 scintigraphy. Radiology 167:167–172, 1988

14. Mesgarzadeh M, Sapega AA, Bonakdarpour A, et al: Osteochondritis dissecans: Analysis of mechanical stability with radiography, scintigraphy, and MR imaging. Radiology 165:775–780, 1987

15. Reiser MF, Bongartz GP, Erlemann R, et al: Gadolinium-DTPA in rheumatoid arthritis and related diseases: First results with dynamic magnetic resonance imaging. Skeletal Radiol 18:591–597, 1989

16. Beltran J, Candill JL, Hesman LA, et al: Rheumatoid arthritis: MR imaging manifestations. Radiology 165:153–157, 1987

17. Cobby MJ, Adler RS, Swartz R, et al: Dialysis-related amyloid arthropathy: MR findings in four patients. AJR 157:1023–1027, 1991

18. Gomori JM, Grossman RI: Mechanisms responsible for the MR appearance and evolution of intracranial hemorrhage. Radiographics 8:427–440, 1988

19. Kang HS, Kindynis P, Brahme SK, et al: Triangular fibrocartilage and intercarpal ligaments of the wrist: MR imaging: Cadaveric study with gross pathologic and histologic correlation. Radiology 181:401–404, 1991

20. Brody AS, Strong M, Babikian G, et al: Avascular necrosis: Early MR imaging and histologic findings in a canine model. AJR 157:341–345, 1991

F. Health Status Assessment

Health status assessment is central to two key elements of rheumatic disease patient care: problem identification and outcome measurement. Problem identification is a necessary step in developing targeted and effective approaches to therapy. Problem identification based on health status assessment is particularly valuable because it focuses on issues that are of greatest concern to patients. Similarly, approaches to outcome measurement that incorporate health status assessments address the most important goals of patients, physicians, and payors. In the past decade, substantial research in rheumatology has focused on the development and application of improved methods for health status assessment.

Health status assessment involves two major elements: the measurement of organic impairments that produce physical signs and symptoms, and the measurement of functional disabilities that produce difficulties in the performance of tasks or roles (1). The measures that are most pertinent for assessing signs and symptoms may be different for each rheumatic disease. For example, joint tenderness count and morning stiffness are traditionally used to assess patients with rheumatoid arthritis (RA), while skin score and dyspnea are more relevant health status assessments for patients with systemic sclerosis (2). Specific chapters of this text provide information on the measures that are most often used to assess signs and symptoms in individual rheumatic diseases. In some assessment approaches, these measures are combined into a multi-item index designed to provide a comprehensive assessment of health status, disease activity, or both (3,4).

Pain is a nearly universal problem for individuals with arthritis and related diseases, and thus pain must be a principal component of any symptom assessment in rheumatology. Pain may be measured in a valid and reliable way by observation of pain behaviors such as wincing with movement, but most pain assessments are based on patient self-report (5). The visual analog scale is the simplest and most widely used approach. It typically consists of a 10 cm horizontal line that is labeled "no pain" at one end and "extreme pain" at the other. The patient is instructed to mark a point on the line that best indicates his or her level of arthritis pain over a particular interval of time such as a day or a week. Pain level is then measured as the distance from the "no pain" end. Pain may also be assessed by a single item adjectival pain scale or by a multi-item adjectival scale that asks about specific aspects of pain such as severity, frequency, and causation. Multi-item pain scales are available in short (4 item) and long (78 item) versions, and may be general or disease-specific in content.

The second major element of health status assessment in the rheumatic diseases involves the measurement of functional status, including physical, psychological, and social function. Psychological function is typically assessed in terms of affective domains such as depression and anxiety, while social function is usually measured in terms of social interactions and social support. Although assessment of health status in these domains is inherently subjective, numerous studies have shown that both psychological and social function can be measured reliably and validly using well-designed and relatively simple questionnaires. Mental abilities are also part of the broad concept of functional status, and may be relevant to health status assessment in selected rheumatic diseases. A variety of instruments, ranging from short mini-mental questionnaires to complex neuropsychiatric batteries, have been developed to measure this aspect of functional status.

Physical ability is the most important element of function for the vast majority of patients with rheumatic diseases. Multiple aspects of physical function are relevant, including lower extremity function, upper extremity function, personal care, recreation, and occupation. Lower extremity function involves such activities as walking, climbing stairs, and moving about the community. Upper extremity function includes hand activities such as opening a door and turning a key, plus arm activities such as reaching and carrying. Personal care involves basic activities of daily living such as eating and grooming. Recreation deals with the performance of preferred leisure time activities, while occupation relates to an individual's ability to perform his or her usual work, including house and school work. Although it is not exclusively based on physical function, sexual function may be an important health status problem for many rheumatic disease patients and may be addressed as well.

Physical function needs to be assessed in enough detail to provide useful information for problem identification and outcome assessment. The traditional four-category classification of functional status does not provide this level of detail (6). Although this approach has recently been revised and refined to emphasize the distinction between self care, vocational, and avocational activities (7), it is primarily useful for classification of subjects in population and clinical studies and not useful for problem identification or outcome measurement in individual patients.

Grip strength and walk time are two traditional measures that have been used to assess functional ability in the upper and lower extremities respectively. Unfortunately, while these two approaches are simple to perform, observable, and quantifiable, they are not particularly good measures of function. Recent studies have documented their poor reliability. Grip strength measurement produces variable results, because the instruments used, particularly the sewn sphygmomanometer bag, are not standardized. Walk time measurements vary greatly due to differences in technique, distance, and examiner exhortation.

A simple and practical way to assess both the sign/symptom and functional disability components of health status in patients with rheumatic diseases is to use one of the questionnaires that have been designed for this purpose (8). These questionnaires, which have been developed, tested, and refined during the past decade, generally incorporate multiple dimensions of health status, and they are designed to be completed by patients without the need for professional involvement. The health status of rheumatic disease patients can now be reliably and validly assessed using general questionnaires such as the Sickness Impact Profile and SF36, or by using arthritis-specific questionnaires such as the Arthritis Impact Measurement Scales, the Health Assessment Questionnaire, the Functional Status Questionnaire, the McMaster–Toronto Arthritis Questionnaire, and others. Many of these questionnaires are available in Spanish and other translations.

Second generation versions of these rheumatic disease health status questionnaires have been developed in an attempt to broaden content and improve sensitivity (9). Shorter versions of these questionnaires, some of which contain as few as eight items, have also been developed. These short questionnaires take only a few minutes to complete and are simple and practical enough to be used routinely for patient assessment in the office setting (10). The shorter questionnaires provide less detail for problem identification and are likely to be somewhat less sensitive as outcome measures. On balance, however, they represent an important new approach to health status assessment in the rheumatic diseases.

Questionnaire-based health status assessments should not stand alone as an approach to either problem identification or outcome assessment. For example, once a problem with lower extremity function has been identified, a more detailed assessment of the problem needs to be made before a specific functional diagnosis and treatment plan can be developed. Quite often the detailed evaluation and treatment of functional disability and pain problems should involve specialists such as physical therapists, occupational therapists, and physiatrists who can help develop more focused treatment plans. These professionals may employ other, more detailed assessment approaches in order to identify the underlying physical basis for the patient's functional disability and pain.

To produce a more sensitive and comprehensive estimate of therapeutic outcome, health status assessments should be used in conjunction with other relevant and proven measures of patient status such as joint tenderness count and physician global assessment. For example, a committee of the American College of Rheumatology has suggested that three health status-oriented measures of outcome (pain, physical function, and patient global assessment) be combined with three disease-activity measures of outcome (joint tenderness count, joint swelling count, and physician global assessment) to assess the results of RA clinical trials in a comprehensive, sensitive, and standardized way (11). Recent studies indicate that even the disease activity elements in such a comprehensive outcome assessment battery can be collected by means of a well-designed self-assessment questionnaire (12).

Robert F. Meenan, MD, MPH, MBA

1. Guccione AA, Jette AM: Multidimensional assessment of functional limitations in patients with rheumatoid arthritis. Arthritis Care Res 3:44–52, 1990
2. American Rheumatism Association Glossary Committee: Dictionary of the Rheumatic Diseases Volume I: Signs and Symptoms. Atlanta, American Rheumatism Association, 1982
3. Smythe HA, Helewa A, Goldsmith CH: Selection and combination of outcome measures. J Rheum 9:770–774, 1982
4. Liang MH, Socher SA, Larson MG, et al: Reliability and validity of six systems for the clinical assessment of disease activity in systemic lupus erythematosus. Arthritis Rheum 32:1107–1118, 1989
5. American College of Rheumatology Glossary Committee: Dictionary of the Rheumatic Diseases Volume III: Health Status Measurement. Atlanta, American College of Rheumatology, 1988
6. Steinbrocker O, Traeger CH, Batterman RC: Therapeutic criteria in rheumatoid arthritis. JAMA 140:659–662, 1949
7. Hochberg MC, Chang RW, Dwosh I, et al: The American College of Rheumatology 1991 revised criteria for the classification of global functional status in rheumatoid arthritis. Arthritis Rheum 35:498–502, 1992
8. Bell MJ, Bombardier C, Tugwell P: Measurement of functional status, quality of life, and utility in rheumatoid arthritis. Arthritis Rheum 33:591–601, 1990
9. Meenan RF, Mason JH, Anderson JJ, et al: AIMS2: The content and properties of a revised and expanded Arthritis Impact Measurement Scales health status questionnaire. Arthritis Rheum 35:1–10, 1992
10. Wolfe F, Pincus T: Standard self-report questionnaires in routine clinical and research practice: An opportunity for patients and rheumatologists. J Rheum 18:643–646, 1991
11. Felson DT, Anderson JJ, Boers M, et al: The American College of Rheumatology Core Set of Disease Activity Measures to be used in rheumatoid arthritis clinical trials. Arthritis Rheum 36:729–740, 1993
12. Mason JH, Anderson JJ, Meenan RF, et al: The Rapid Assessment of Disease Activity in Rheumatology (RADAR) Questionnaire: Validy and sensitivity to change of a patient self-report measure of joint count and clinical status. Arthritis Rheum 35:156–162, 1992

9. CLASSIFICATION OF THE RHEUMATIC DISEASES

Classification of the various rheumatic diseases considered in this *Primer* is hampered by the lack of a firm etiologic basis for most diseases. Thus, working classifications used in individual practices, disease discussions, and investigations are often dynamic as our understanding evolves.

The classification published here is one that was developed by Decker and the glossary subcommittee of the American College of Rheumatology (ACR, formerly American Rheumatism Association) Committee on Rheumatologic practice in 1983 (1). This is the only official revision of the tentative ARA classification of 1964 (2). Previous editions of the *Primer* have included arbitrary revisions by the current and past editors, and many textbooks provide their own modified classifications. Because there have been so many different approaches, we now return to the most recent official classification. Individual chapters in the *Primer* can serve as a reference for some of the newer concepts and how they may fit into the classification scheme. "Splitters" looking for subsets of interest will also be best served by reviewing individual chapters (4).

The 1983 classification was occasioned by plans for the World Health Organization to revise the 9th edition of the International Classification of Diseases (ICD). Such a revision of ICD has not yet appeared; we indicate ICD9 codes in our classification when available for interest.

Concepts in the classification reflect mostly clinical presentations; therefore, many diseases are left in the miscellaneous category. Different classifications may well be found useful for various working research groups. The impact of a diagnosis on healthcare needs and on function will need to be determined if diagnostic codes are used to guide compensation (5).

Classification criteria for a number of the rheumatic diseases have been developed by ACR committees. These appear in the appendices. The useful criteria for spondylarthropathies developed by Amor et al (3) are not given in the appendix but are referenced in Chapter 20.

An example of the need to revise preliminary classifications as information accumulates is provided by the whole concept of interactions of infection with rheumatic disease. In the 1983 classification, Lyme disease was identified as an infectious spirochaetal disease, but syphilis was not listed. The organism triggering Whipples disease has now been identified, so this can be switched into the diseases of known cause. The possibly too-inclusive and imprecise term, *reactive arthritis*, incorporated rheumatic fever, subacute bacterial endocarditis, post meningococcal arthritis and post dysenteric disease which must certainly involve very different mechanisms; and Reiter's syndrome was left under "Arthritis associated with Spondylitis".

It seems certain that the various pressures from health care policy, clinical practice and research will lead to new approaches to classification. Some of the important considerations have been recently reviewed (6).

H. Ralph Schumacher, Jr., MD

1. Decker JL and the Glossary Subcommittee of the ARA Committee on Rheumatologic Practice: Arthritis Rheum 26:1029–1032, 1983
2. Blumberg BS, Bunim JJ, Calkins E, et al: Nomenclature and classification of arthritis and rheumatism (tentative) accepted by the American Rheumatism Association. Bull Rheum Dis 14:339–340, 1964
3. Amor B, Dougados M, Mijiyawa M: Criteres de Classification des Spondylarthropathies; Rev Rheum 57:85–89, 1990
4. Sellick K, Littlejohn G, Wallace C, et al: Identifying subclasses of patients with rheumatoid arthritis through cluster analysis. J Rheumatol 17:1613–1619, 1990
5. Calkins DR, Rubinstein LV, Clearly PD: Failure of physicians to recognize functional disability in ambulatory patients. Ann Intern Med 114:451–454, 1991
6. Schumacher HR: Taxonomy and classification. In: Klippel J, Dieppe P (Eds) Rheumatology. London: Mosby, 1994

Table 9–1. ARA nomenclature and classification of arthritis and rheumatism (1983)*

	ICD9CM** Code
I. Diffuse Connective Tissue Diseases	
A. Rheumatoid arthritis	714.0
1. IgM rheumatoid factor positive	nc
2. IgM rheumatoid factor negative	nc
B. Juvenile arthritis	714.30
1. Systemic onset	714.2
2. Polyarthritic onset	714.30
a. IgM rheumatoid factor positive	nc
b. IgM rheumatoid factor negative	nc
3. Oligoarthritis onset (pauciarticular)	714.32
a. Associated with chronic uveitis and antinuclear antibody	nc
b. Associated with HLA-B27	nc
c. IgM rheumatoid factor positive	nc
C. Lupus erythematosus	
1. Discoid lupus erythematosus	695.4
2. Systemic lupus erythematosus	710.0
3. Drug-related lupus erythematosus	995.2
D. Scleroderma	710.1
1. Localized	701.0
a. Morphea	701.0
b. Linear	701.0
2. Systemic sclerosis	710.1
a. Diffuse scleroderma	710.1
b. CREST syndrome (i.e., calcinosis, Raynaud's, esophageal dysfunction, sclerodactyly, and telangiectasia)	710.1
3. Chemical (or drug) induced	995.2
E. Diffuse fasciitis with or without eosinophilia	729.4
F. Polymyositis	
1. Polymyositis	710.4
2. Dermatomyositis	710.3
3. Polymyositis or dermatomyositis associated with malignancy	710.4
4. Childhood polymyositis or dermatomyositis associated with vasculopathy	nc
G. Necrotizing vasculitis and other forms of vasculopathy	447.6
1. Polyarteritis nodosa	446.0
a. Associated with hepatitis B virus	446.0
b. Not associated with hepatitis B virus	446.0
2. Allergic granulomatosis (i.e., Churg-Strauss, polyarteritis nodosa with lung involvement)	446.0
3. Hypersensitivity angiitis	446.2
a. Serum sickness	999.5
i. Antigen known	999.5
ii. Antigen unknown	999.5
b. Henoch-Schonlein purpura	287.0
c. Mixed cryoglobulinemia	273.2
i. Associated with hepatitis B virus	273.2
ii. Not associated with hepatitis B virus	273.2
d. Associated with malignancy	446.2
e. Hypocomplementemic vasculitis	nc
4. Granulomatous arteritis	nc
a. Wegener's granulomatosis	446.4
b. Giant cell (or temporal) arteritis with or without polymyalgia rheumatica	446.5
c. Takayasu's arteritis	446.7
5. Kawasaki disease (i.e., mucocutaneous lymph node syndrome) including infantile polyarteritis	446.1
6. Behcet's disease	136.1
H. Sjögren's syndrome	710.2
1. Primary	710.2
2. Secondary, associated with other connective tissue disease	710.2
I. Overlap syndromes	nc
1. Mixed connective tissue disease	nc
2. Others	nc
J. Other	
1. Polymyalgia rheumatica (see also giant cell arteritis, G.4.b.)	725
2. Relapsing panniculitis (i.e., Weber-Christian disease)	729.30
3. Relapsing polychondritis	nc
4. Lymphomatoid granulomatosis	nc
5. Erythema nodosum	695.2
II. Arthritis Associated with Spondylitis (i.e., Spondylarthritis)	720
A. Ankylosing spondylitis	720.0
B. Reiter's syndrome	099.3
C. Psoriatic arthritis	696.0
1. Predominant distal interphalangeal involvement	nc
2. Oligoarticular	nc
3. Polyarticular	nc
4. Arthritis mutilans	nc
5. Spondylitis	696.0
D. Arthritis associated with inflammatory bowel disease	716.9
1. Peripheral arthritis	716.9
2. Spondylitis	720.9

	ICD9CM** Code
III. Osteoarthritis (i.e., Osteoarthrosis, Degenerative Joint Disease)	715.0
A. Primary	715.0
1. Peripheral	715.1
2. Spinal	721.9
B. Secondary	715.2
1. Congenital or developmental defects	715.2
2. Metabolic disease	715.2
3. Trauma	715.2
4. Other articular disorders	715.2
IV. Rheumatic Syndromes Associated with Infectious Agents	
A. Direct	
1. Bacterial	711.0
a. Gram-positive cocci	711.0
b. Gram-negative cocci	711.0
c. Gram-negative rods	711.0
d. Mycobacteria	031.9
e. Spirochetes	104.9
i. Lyme disease	nc
2. Viral	711.5
3. Fungal	711.6
4. Parasitic	711.8
5. Suspected infectious cause	nc
a. Whipple's disease	040.2
B. Reactive	
1. Bacterial	nc
a. Acute rheumatic fever	390
b. Subacute bacterial endocarditis	421.0
c. With intestinal bypass surgery	nc
d. Post-dysenteric (e.g., due to Shigella, Yersinia, or Campylobacter)	711.3
e. After other infections (e.g., due to Meningococcus)	nc
2. Viral	nc
3. Post-immunization	nc
4. Other classes of infectious agents	nc
V. Metabolic and Endocrine Diseases Associated with Rheumatic States	
A. Crystal-associated conditions	
1. Monosodium urate monohydrate (gout)	274.0
a. Inherited hyperuricemia	790.6
i. Hypoxanthine-guanine-phosphoribosyltransferase deficiency (Lesch-Nyhan syndrome)	277.2
ii. Increased phosphoribosyl-transferase synthetase activity	nc
iii. Associated with other disorders (e.g., sickle cell disease)	274.0
iv. Idiopathic	274.0
b. Acquired hyperuricemia	790.6
i. Drug-related	790.6
ii. Saturnine gout	790.6
iii. Due to renal insufficiency	790.6
2. Calcium pyrophosphate dihydrate (pseudogout, chondrocalcinosis)	712.2
a. Familial	nc
b. Associated with metabolic diseases (e.g., hyperparathyroidism)	712.2
c. Idiopathic	nc
3. Basic calcium phosphates (e.g., hydroxyapatite)	nc
B. Other biochemical abnormalities	277
1. Amyloidosis	277.3
a. Immunocyte dyscrasia (primary) AL protein	nc
b. Reactive systemic (secondary) AA protein	nc
c. Other	nc
2. Hemophilia	286.0
3. Other inborn errors of metabolism	
a. Connective tissue	
i. Marfan syndrome	759.8
ii. Ehlers-Danlos syndrome	756.83
iii. Pseudoxanthoma elasticum	757.3
iv. Homocystinuria	270.4
v. Osteogenesis imperfecta	756.51
vi. Hypophosphatasia	275.3
vii. Homogentisic acid oxidase deficiency (i.e., alkaptonuria, ochronosis)	270.2
viii. Mucopolysaccharidosis (e.g., Hurler, Hunter)	277.5
b. Hyperlipidemias	272
c. Hemoglobinopathies	282.6
d. Glucocerebrosidase deficiency (i.e., Gaucher's)	272.7
e. Galactosidase deficiency (i.e., Fabry)	272.7
f. Acid ceramidase deficiency (i.e., Farber)	272.8
4. Endocrine disease	
a. Diabetes mellitus	250.0
b. Acromegaly	253.0
c. Hyperparathyroidism	252.0
d. Hyperthyroidism	242.9
e. Hypothyroidism	244.9

	ICD9CM** Code
5. Immunodeficiency disease	
a. Hypogammaglobulinemia (e.g., Bruton)	279.04
b. IgA deficiency	279.01
c. Complement deficiency	279.8
d. Adenosine deaminase deficiency	nc
e. Purine nucleoside phosphorylase deficiency	nc
C. Hereditary disorders	
1. Familial Mediterranean fever	277.3
2. Arthrogryposis multiplex congenita	754.89
3. Hypermobility syndromes, not otherwise specified	728.5
4. Myositis ossificans progressiva	728.11
VI. Neoplasms	
A. Primary	
1. Benign (e.g., ganglion, osteochondromatosis)	213
2. Malignant (e.g., synovial sarcoma, hemangiosarcoma)	171
B. Secondary	
1. Leukemia	208
2. Multiple myeloma	203.0
3. Metastatic malignant tumors	198.89
VII. Neurovascular Disorders	
A. Charcot joint	713.5
B. Compression syndrome	
1. Peripheral entrapment (e.g., carpal tunnel)	355.9
2. Radiculopathy	729.2
3. Spinal stenosis	724.0
C. Reflex sympathetic dystrophy	337.0
D. Erythromelalgia	443.89
E. Raynaud's phenomenon or disease	443.0
VIII. Bone and Cartilage Disorders	
A. Osteoporosis	
1. Generalized	733.00
2. Regional	nc
B. Osteomalacia	268.2
C. Hypertrophic osteoarthropathy	731.2
D. Diffuse idiopathic skeletal hyperostosis (i.e., Forestier's disease)	nc
E. Paget's disease of bone (i.e., osteitis deformans)	731.0
F. Osteolysis or chondrolysis	nc
G. Avascular necrosis (Osteonecrosis)	
1. Osteochondritis dissecans	732.7
2. Associated with other conditions (e.g., alcoholism, hypercortisonism)	733.4
3. Caisson disease	993.3
4. Epiphysitis (e.g., Osgood-Schlatter)	732.9
5. Idiopathic	733.4
H. Costochondritis (i.e., Tietze)	733.6
I. Osteitis condensans ilii, osteitis pubis, or localized osteitis	733.5
J. Congenital dysplasia of hip	754.3
K. Chondromalacia patellae	717.7
L. Biomechanical or anatomic abnormalities	
1. Scoliosis/kyphosis	737.30
2. Pronated feet	736.7
3. Leg-length discrepancy	736.81
4. Genu varus or valgus	736.42
5. Pes cavus or planus	736.73
IX. Extraarticular Disorders	
A. Juxtaarticular lesions	nc
1. Bursitis (e.g., subdeltoid)	727.3
2. Tendon lesions (e.g., de Quervain)	727.9
3. Enthesopathy (e.g., epicondylitis)	726.90
4. Cysts (e.g., popliteal [Baker])	727.40
B. Intervertebral disc disorder	722
C. Low back pain, idiopathic	724.2
D. Miscellaneous pain syndromes	
1. Generalized (i.e., fibrositis fibromyalgia)	729.0
2. Psychogenic rheumatism	306.0
3. Regional pain syndromes	
a. Facial pain with temporomandibular joint dysfunction	524.6
b. Cervical pain	723.1
c. Wry neck (i.e., torticollis)	723.5
d. Cervicobrachial pain	723.3
e. Coccydynia	724.79
f. Metatarsalgia	726.70
X. Miscellaneous Disorders Associated with Articular Manifestations	
A. Palindromic rheumatism	719.3
B. Intermittent hydrarthrosis	719.3
C. Drug-related rheumatic syndromes (excluding drug-related lupus erythematosus; see I.C.3)	995.2
D. Multicentric reticulohistiocytosis	272.8
E. Villonodular synovitis	719.2
F. Sarcoidosis	135

	ICD9CM** Code
G. Vitamin C deficiency	267
H. Pancreatic disease	577
I. Chronic active hepatitis	571.49
J. Musculoskeletal trauma	
1. Internal derangement	717
2. Loose body	718.1

*Arthritis Rheum 26:1029–1032, 1983
**International Classification of Diseases, 9th Revision, Clinical Modification
nc = no code

10. RHEUMATOID ARTHRITIS
A. Epidemiology, Pathology, and Pathogenesis

Rheumatoid arthritis (RA) is a systemic autoimmune disorder of unknown etiology (1,2). Its major distinctive feature is chronic, symmetric, and erosive synovitis of peripheral joints. The majority of patients also have elevated titers of serum rheumatoid factors. The severity of the joint disease may fluctuate over time, but the most common outcome of established disease is progressive development of various degrees of joint destruction, deformity, and disability. Associated nonarticular manifestations may include subcutaneous nodules, vasculitis, pericarditis, pulmonary nodules or interstitial fibrosis, mononeuritis multiplex, episcleritis or, less commonly, scleritis. Sjogren's and Felty's syndromes commonly occur in association with RA.

EPIDEMIOLOGY

Estimates of the prevalence of RA are dependent on the criteria used to define the illness. This is a difficult problem, because there is no established etiologic agent or unique clinical or laboratory feature that can be used to define the disease. Diagnosis is based, therefore, on the presence or absence of combinations of clinical and laboratory abnormalities. These assessments, unfortunately, are subject to measurement variation. Until very recently, the most widely used definition of RA for studies of prevalence has been the 1958 American Rheumatism Association criteria (2,3). Estimates of prevalence, based on this set of criteria, indicate that between 1% and 2% of the adult population in every part of the world is affected with definite or classic RA. A modified definition of RA (see Appendix 1), now called the 1987 Revised Criteria for the Classification of Rheumatoid Arthritis, was published in 1988 (4). These criteria distinguish RA from other conditions with a specificity of 89% and sensitivity between 91% and 94%. The conditions most often confused with RA are systemic lupus erythematosus, psoriatic arthritis, and rheumatoid factor negative spondylarthropathies. Although the 1987 criteria have not been utilized as extensively as the 1958 criteria, the revised criteria appear to generate similar estimates of prevalence.

The prevalence of RA increases with age for both males and females. A US National Health Examination Survey (1960–1962) found a prevalence of 0.3% in adults under age 35 and a prevalence of over 10% in persons over age 65. The prevalence is clearly higher in females than males, but the ratio varies widely between studies. The overall ratio appears to be about 2.5 to 1 (3).

Unfortunately, prevalence studies have not provided solid insights into the etiology or pathogenesis of RA. Incidence surveys of RA, on the other hand, have generated some provocative observations regarding sex hormones as predisposing factors. For example, during the years 1987–1989 a prospective case-control study of newly diagnosed RA in women ages 18–64, who were members of a health maintenance organization in Seattle, found an overall incidence rate of 23.9 cases per 100,000 person-years (5). This rate is 44.7% lower than the incidence rate measured in 1950–1974 in Rochester. The greatest difference in inci-

dence rates between these two studies was in the 30–59 year age group, with no differences in the youngest age group and smaller differences in the older age group. These observations are consistent with other studies suggesting that oral contraceptives decrease the risk of RA (5). These data do not exclude the possibility that other reproductive factors influence the development of RA. For example, several studies have indicated that nulliparity is a risk factor for RA. It is also well known that pregnancy is associated with remissions of RA, and exacerbations are common in the postpartum period. Symptom onset at menopause is also common (6). The important point is that the neuroendocrine hormones play a role in determining susceptibility and severity of RA, but the exact mechanisms involved are unclear.

In addition to age- and sex-related predisposing factors, a number of other factors, including socioeconomic status, education, and psychosocial stress, have been suggested to play predisposing roles (3). Decreasing socioeconomic status is associated with increasing prevalence in men, and poorer outcomes in both men and women. Prevalence in men, but not women, decreases with higher education levels. Significant psychosocial stress has also been suggested as a factor that may be important in pathogenesis. Race, residence location, and climate, on the other hand, have not been shown to be significant factors in determining the development of RA (3).

A number of lines of evidence suggest that genetic factors other than gender play a role in development of RA. In one study of monozygotic and dizygotic twins, the concordance rate for RA was 34% in the monozygotic twins and only 3% in the dizygotic twins, an 11-fold increase in risk. In another study, the risk, particularly for high grade erosive disease, was increased 30-fold in the monozygotic twins. These data indicate that genetic factors are clearly operative, but they also indicate that disease penetrance is low and that environmental factors determine about 65% to 70% of the risk of developing RA (3).

The specific genetic loci that predispose to the development of RA are incompletely defined, but the available data indicate that the major histocompatibility complex (MHC) on chromosome 6 encodes important disease predisposing genes. A majority of patients with RA have the class II MHC alleles DR4 (also called DRB10401), DR1 (also called DRB10101), or both. Specific class I MHC alleles have not been linked to susceptibility. Detailed study of the structure of DR4 and DR1 molecules has better defined the basis for their association with RA. Class II MHC molecules consist of two chains, an alpha and a beta chain. The HLA–DR genes on chromosome 6 contain only one form of DR alpha but encode multiple polymorphic or allelic forms of DR beta. The inheritance of DR beta genes, therefore, determines allelic variation in the DR molecules. HLA–DR4 consists of at least five subtypes: Dw4, Dw10, Dw13, Dw14, and Dw15. Most of the variability in these subtypes is in a segment containing amino acids 70–74, which is in a region of the molecule called the third hypervariable domain. DR1, Dw14, and Dw15 have the same amino acid sequences in this region and are highly associated with RA susceptibility. Dw4 differs by one amino acid, a leucine to arginine, and is also highly associated with RA susceptibility. Dw10, on the other hand, differs by two amino acids in this segment and is not associated with susceptibility to RA.

These observations form the basis for the suggestion that *shared epitopes* or conformationally equivalent structures in the DR beta chains determine susceptibility to RA (2, 7). These MHC molecules may also play a role in determining severity of disease. Since class II molecules are involved in the presentation of antigens to CD4-positive T cells, a reasonable speculation is that RA-associated DR polypeptides regulate the immune response, or possibly an absence of an appropriate immune response, to an environmental etiologic agent.

ETIOLOGY

The primary cause of RA is unknown. In fact, it is possible that there is no single primary cause of RA (1,2,8). Many investigators have speculated that the clinical syndrome we define as RA may be induced, in genetically predisposed individuals, by many different arthritogenic agents. Bacteria and viruses remain the focus of suspicion, but convincing support for their etiologic role has been extraordinarily difficult to generate. Candidate viruses include human T cell lymphotropic virus Type-1 and other retroviruses, Epstein–Barr virus and other herpes viruses, rubella virus, and parvoviruses. Candidate bacteria include mycoplasma, mycobacteria, and various enteric organisms (1,2,8). It should be pointed out that failure to culture an organism from a joint does not exclude its involvement in RA, because it has become increasingly clear that dead whole bacteria, cell walls, toxins, and other components of a microorganism have the capacity to induce chronic inflammatory joint disease. For example, cell wall peptidoglycans from many bacteria induce severe, chronic, destructive arthritis resembling RA in genetically prone experimental animals.

Investigations of RA etiology have increasingly become intertwined with questions about the interrelationships of infectious agents, genetics, and autoimmunity. For example, it has been suggested that the third hypervariable regions of the beta chains of HLA–DR1 and DR4 influence susceptibility to disease by controlling the binding of arthritogenic peptides; that they trigger disease by expanding or deleting particular T cell populations; or both. Of note, the susceptibility sequence in the third hypervariable domain of the beta chain of HLA–DRDw4 is mimicked by at least two proteins from microorganisms that affect most people, namely Epstein–Barr virus Gp110 and *E. coli* heat shock protein dnaJ (9).

Patients with RA shed more Epstein–Barr virus in throat washings than do control subjects. They also have increased frequencies of B cells infected with the virus and have a diminished cytotoxic T-cell response to the virus (2). It is tempting to speculate that these abnormalities are related to the observation that Epstein–Barr virus Gp110 shares a six amino-acid sequence with the third hypervariable region of HLA–DRDw4. This stretch of amino acids constitutes a T cell recognition site or epitope in humans (8,9).

Heat shock proteins have been implicated in arthritis in both experimental animals and humans (2,8,9). These are major bacterial antigens, and antibodies and T cells reactive with heat shock proteins are abundant in patients with RA. Bacterial heat shock proteins are also highly homologous with human heat shock proteins. The *E. coli* heat shock protein dnaJ also has homology to the third hypervariable region of the beta chain of HLA–DRDw4 (9). This observation is interesting, because some of the human heat shock protein genes are located in the major histocompatibility complex. One hypothesis for the abnormalities in RA is that an immune response to a heat shock protein from an infectious agent is amplified and perpetuated because of molecular mimicry between heat shock proteins and MHC susceptibility sequences. At the very least, these observations indicate that the subjects of infectious agents, immunogenetics, and autoimmunity are very complex and highly overlapping.

Rheumatoid Factors

Rheumatoid factors are the prototypic forms of autoantibodies. These immunoglobulins react with the Fc portion of IgG molecules (2,10). The usual serologic tests employed in the clinical laboratory detect IgM rheumatoid factors, although it is well established that rheumatoid factors may be formed in any of the immunoglobulin subclasses. The major issues relative to rheumatoid factors are: 1) what is their biologic role in RA and normal physiology, and 2) what induces and regulates their synthesis?

Rheumatoid factors are detected in about 3% of apparently healthy persons, and the prevalence increases with age. Some individuals may have serum rheumatoid factors before the development of clinical arthritis. Moreover, rheumatoid factors are frequently observed in a variety of other conditions. Studies in experimental animals suggest that elevated production of rheumatoid factors develops in situations that generate sustained hypergammaglobulinemia such as chronic infections (10). They may play an important role in host defense by enhancing the clearance of small antigen–antibody complexes from the circulation or other fluids or by enhancing the killing of microorganisms. Conversely, they may augment deleterious inflammation by facilitating complement or inflammatory cell activation, or by altering the size or localization of immune complexes. The available data suggest that rheumatoid factors may play a role in amplifying rheumatoid inflammation but that they are not a primary triggering or etiologic factor.

Considerable investigation has been devoted to understanding the genes that encode rheumatoid factors (11). It is now clear that genes encoding kappa light chains of rheumatoid factors show limited heterogeneity. In addition, certain polymorphisms of variable and constant regions of the kappa light chain are associated with increased risk of RA. Provocative but complex data on heavy chain variable and constant region polymorphisms have also been published, indicating that immunoglobulin genes, in addition to the MHC, influence disease susceptibility to RA.

PATHOLOGY

Although data are limited, the initial pathologic event in RA appears to be activation and/or injury of synovial microvascular endothelial cells, which suggests that the disease triggering or etiologic agent is carried to the synovium by way of the bloodstream (12,13). The endothelial cells are swollen, and gaps appear between cells. The lumens of these blood vessels are typically occluded with platelet, leukocyte, and fibrin thrombi, and plasma exudation is prominent as indicated by the development of edema in the subsynovial lining tissue and an effusion in the joint cavity. The cells in the superficial lining cell layer that are exposed to the joint cavity are activated, and their numbers are increased. Polymorphonuclear leukocytes also appear in small numbers in this superficial layer of the synovium and are often the predominant cell type in the synovial joint effusion. Mononuclear cells, by contrast, accumulate initially around the abnormal blood vessels just beneath the lining cell layer and in the deeper sublining synovial tissues.

This constellation of pathologic processes appears to continue throughout the disease course but fluctuates in severity. As expected, the abnormalities are most severe during disease flares. Thus, microvascular endothelial cell activation, and/or injury appears to be a fundamental abnormality in RA. In some patients, isolated parts or all of the synovium develop such severe microvascular abnormalities that tissue ischemia and infarction are the result (14). In these circumstances, a bland, fibrin-rich synovial stroma, which is relatively devoid of inflammatory cells, is usually observed on histopathology.

As the disease progresses to more chronic stages, the synovium becomes massively hypertrophic and edematous, and innumerable villous projections of synovial tissue protrude into the joint cavity (1). The lining cell layer, which is normally no more than 1 to 3 cells thick, typically increases to a depth of 5 to 10 cells. The thickened lining layer is composed predominantly of macrophage-like cells, apparently recruited to the joint, and smaller numbers of proliferating fibroblast-like synoviocytes

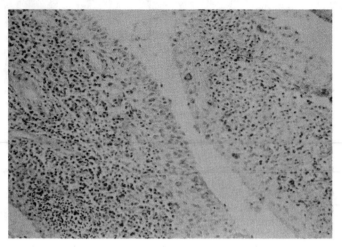

Fig. 10A–1. Knee synovitis. The multilayered synovial lining is composed of hyperplastic, hypertrophic synoviocytes with occasional multinucleated giant cells. The enlarged villi are diffusely infiltrated by lymphocytes and plasma cells. Moderate capillary proliferation is seen (from the Revised Clinical Slide Collection on the Rheumatic Diseases).

(Fig. 10A–1). The sublining layer is infiltrated with nodular collections of mononuclear cells, particularly around abnormal blood vessels. Primarily CD4-positive T lymphocytes predominant in the focal aggregates, and plasma cells usually form a mantle around the periphery of the nodule. Between nodules are more diffuse collections of mononuclear cells consisting of macrophages, T cells, B cells, and plasma cells. Many of the B cells and plasma cells produce rheumatoid factors. Immature B and T cells, or blast cells, are more common in the diffuse collections of mononuclear cells.

Most of the cells in the hyperplastic sublining synovial stromal connective tissues, however, are not infiltrating inflammatory cells. Most of these cells are highly activated and invasive fibroblast-like cells and new blood vessels (1,2,14). The synovial inflammatory process is accompanied by massive tumor-like proliferation and activation of the connective tissue stroma. These abnormal cells actively invade and destroy the periarticular bone and cartilage at the margins of joints where synovium and bone are attached. This highly proliferative and invasive granulation tissue is often referred to as *pannus* (Fig. 10A–2). As the disease progresses, periarticular bone and cartilage are progressively eroded and destroyed, and the joint capsule is distended or ruptured. In addition, subchondral bone is progressively lost, in part as a result of increased osteoclastic activity. The result of

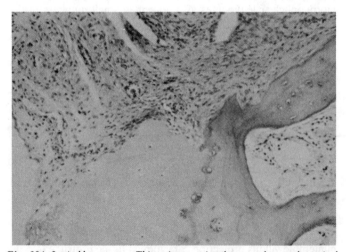

Fig. 10A–2. Ankle pannus. This microscopic photograph reveals typical pannus formation. Fibrovascular tissue protrudes from the inflamed synovium to the articular cartilage. A portion of the fibrous tissue extends over the surface of the cartilage, which shows death of chondrocytes and loss of basophilia of the matrix. Note the inflammatory exudate in the subchondral bone (from the Revised Clinical Slide Collection on the Rheumatic Diseases).

this multifaceted process is usually continuous pain, progressive deformity, and disability. Abnormal biomechanical factors in the joints also contribute to the process.

PATHOGENESIS

Although the etiology of RA is unknown, substantial progress has been made in understanding the molecular and cellular aspects of pathogenesis. Some of the these topics are briefly addressed below.

Neutrophils and Mediators in Synovial Fluid. Neutrophil accumulation in RA synovial fluids is a characteristic event (1,2). These cells are attracted to the fluid by a number of chemotactic substances, including the C5a component of complement, leukotriene B4, platelet activating factor, and interleukin–8, which are abundant in RA joint fluids. The activation of neutrophils in the joints results in the release of proteinases, prostaglandins, leukotrienes, and reactive oxidants. All of these substances contribute directly to joint inflammation and injury.

Complement activation is prominent in RA joint fluid. The formation of immune complexes containing rheumatoid factors is widely considered to be the major factor that drives complement activation. Complement activation parallels activation of the kinin, coagulation, and fibrinolysis pathways, which all contribute to the intense inflammatory process. For example, plasmin is formed from plasminogen by the action of plasminogen activator, and plasmin is a potent activator of metalloproteinases such as collagenase and transin/stromelysin. Collagenase and transin/stromelysin are largely responsible for the degradation of collagen and proteoglycan in the joint.

Endothelial Cells and Inflammatory Cell Homing. Endothelial cells form the interface between the blood and the extravascular space (2). These cells are not simply a passive barrier but are active participants in the inflammatory process. In RA, they regulate the coagulation, fibrinolysis, and the exudation of fluid and solutes from the vascular space. In addition, they play a critical role in facilitating the recruitment of specific inflammatory cells into the inflammatory site. In response to specific cytokines such as interleukin–1 (IL–1), tumor necrosis factor (TNF), and interferon gamma (IFN–γ), endothelial cells express specific homing molecules on their surface called *vascular adhesion molecules*. These receptor molecules bind cell surface ligands on various types of inflammatory leukocytes. The adherence of inflammatory cells to the endothelial cell surface is the first step in their infiltration into the synovial tissue. Interrupting this binding step is an attractive approach, at least in theory, for therapeutic intervention.

Macrophages and Cytokines. Macrophages are major components of the infiltrating mononuclear cell population in the rheumatoid synovium (2,15). They are recruited to the joint in response to a variety of chemotactic factors and migrate through blood vessel walls after adhering to the endothelium. Macrophages in the synovium are highly activated. The activating signals include phagocytosis of foreign materials, binding of immune complexes or complement fragments, or stimulation by various cytokines such as IFN–γ, colony stimulating factor for granulocytes and monocytes, and interleukin–2. In addition to their phagocytic functions, activated macrophages produce an extensive list of inflammatory mediators, including cytokines such as IL–1α and IL–β, TNF–α, platelet-derived growth factors (PDGF), heparin binding (fibroblast) growth factors (FGF), and transforming growth factors (TGF). These cytokines regulate the behavior of other cells in the rheumatoid joint. For example, IL–1α, IL1–β, and TNF–α are the major stimulators of prostaglandin, collagenase, and transin/stromelysin production by synovial fibroblast-like cells and chondrocytes. Interleukin–1 is a major stimulator of IL–6 production by fibroblast-like cells. Interleukin–6 regulates B lymphocyte function and the biosynthesis of hepatic acute phase proteins such as C-reactive protein. Platelet-derived growth factor and the heparin binding growth factors are potent stimulators of fibroblast-like cell proliferation (16). Transforming growth factor–β, which is produced by and affects many cells, has both proinflammatory and antiinflammatory effects in the rheumatoid joint (17). Large amounts of macrophage-derived cytokines are usually present in synovial tissues and fluids from active joints. In contrast, T lymphocyte-derived cytokines, such as IL–2, IL–3, and IFN–γ, are usually very difficult to detect. Some investigators have interpreted these findings to mean rheumatoid synovitis is largely driven by activated macrophages (15). Others suspect that both macrophages and T cells are critically involved in pathogenesis of RA, but macrophage activation results in the production of substances that inhibit T lymphocyte activation and cytokine production. Indeed, TGF–β is an example of an inhibitor with these properties. A latent form of this factor is abundant in rheumatoid synovial tissues and fluids (17).

Effector T Lymphocytes. T lymphocytes are major regulators of the immune response and are thought to be important in the initiation and perpetuation of RA (2). The synovial infiltrate contains considerable numbers of T cells, a small fraction of which express activation markers such as the interleukin–2 receptor (IL–2R). Therapies that block T cell activation, such as treatment with cyclosporine A, significantly ameliorate RA in many patients. Interestingly, T cells isolated from RA synovial tissue by in vitro cultivation preferentially react with the cells expressing the HLA–DRβ associated sequence of Glu-Leu-Arg-Ala-Ala in the third hypervariable region, irrespective of DR subtype. This suggests that T cells with restricted heterogeneity play a role in RA. Other studies, in support of this observation, indicate that T cell receptor (TCR) patterns with restricted heterogeneity are present in the synovial T cell populations. In fact, the majority of the activated T cells use a limited number of the possible TCR beta chain variable regions, namely $V_\beta 3$, $V_\beta 14$, and $V_\beta 17$ (18). This observation suggests that T cells bearing these specific T cell receptors are selectively retained in the synovium. Moreover, these three TCR V_β subtypes exhibit high sequence homology in the amino acid segments that are binding sites for some types of superantigens; in particular a superantigen derived from *Mycoplasma arthritidis*. Superantigens are products of certain bacteria and viruses that activate large numbers of T cells by virtue of relatively nonrestricted binding to MHC molecules and T cell receptors. Collectively, these data suggest that a superantigen, possibly structurally related to *M. arthritidis* mitogen, may play an important role in RA.

Mechanisms of Bone and Cartilage Erosion. Rheumatoid synovium is characterized by massive tumor-like expansion of the number of stromal connective tissue cells, primarily fibroblast-like cells and new blood vessels (16,17). The fibroblast-like cells in the rheumatoid joint are phenotypically immature and highly activated. Both in vivo and in vitro characteristics of these cells indicate that they behave very much like transformed cells. For example, these cells express activation markers, such as the protooncogenes c-fos and c-jun and metalloproteinases such as collagenase and transin/stromelysin, at levels found in invasive tumor cells. These cells are not malignant but are stimulated by factors such as PDGF, FGF (16), IL–1, and TNF to express the abnormal invasive phenotype. The importance of these cells is emphasized by the fact that they are the predominant cell type at sites of bone erosion by synovium.

Angiogenesis or the development of a network of new blood vessels is another essential element of the massive hyperplasia of the synovium, because it provides the vascular support for this tissue (2,14,16). The neovascularization appears to be driven by growth factors such as FGF–1 and FGF–2, which are abundant in these tissues (16). Activated synovial macrophages and fibroblast-like cells produce these cytokines. Activated endothelial cells are also found at sites of bone erosion by synovium and are abundant sources of mediators that are critical to destruction of bone and cartilage. Like fibroblast-like cells and macrophages, they also produce metalloproteinases such as collagenase and transin/stromelysin, which are clearly involved in the breakdown of extracellular matrix proteins in the joint (19).

Chondrocyte and extracellular cartilage matrix loss is also an active process in RA (2). In response to cytokines such as IL–1, chondrocytes synthesize collagenase and transin/stromelysin, which degrade the extracellular type II collagen and proteoglycans of cartilage. In addition, synthesis of collagen and proteoglycans by chondrocytes decreases. This loss of cartilage may be accelerated by the precipitation of rheumatoid factor containing immune complexes in the superficial layers of the cartilage, stimulating further invasive pannus formation. The net result is progressive thinning and loss of cartilage over the entire surface of the joint. Osteoclasts in the subchondral bone are also active participants in joint destruction. These cells increase in number and activity very early in the disease process, and are largely responsible for the subchondral osteopenia. The stimulus for increased osteoclastic activity is not fully understood, but prostanglandin E_2 appears to play an important role.

The Peripheral Nervous System and Inflammatory Response. In addition to numerous mediators that are produced locally by various cells in the RA synovium, it has become increasingly clear that neuropeptides are also released into the inflammatory site (2). These factors are produced in the spinal cord and sympathetic ganglia and delivered to the joint by sensory afferent and sympathetic efferent nerves. They clearly play an important role modulating the inflammatory response. Substance P is an important example (20). This neuropeptide activates macrophages and stimulates synovial fibroblast-like cells to produce prostaglandins and metalloproteinases. Studies in experimental animals demonstrate that blocking the release of substance P can dramatically inhibit the development of inflammation. It is strongly suspected that nervous system innervation plays a critical role in determining the severity and distribution of joint inflammation in RA. Our understanding of the role of the peripheral nervous system in RA should increase rapidly in the near future.

Ronald L. Wilder, MD, PhD

1. Rheumatoid arthritis, Etiology, Diagnosis and Treatment. Edited by PD Utsinger, NJ Zvaifler, GE Ehrlich. Philadelphia, JB Lippincott Co., 1985, pp 1–934
2. Harris ED Jr: Mechanisms of disease: Rheumatoid arthritis-pathophysiology and implications for therapy. NEJM 322:1277–1289, 1990
3. Mitchell DM. Epidemiology, Rheumatoid Arthritis, Etiology, Diagnosis and Treatment. Edited by PD Utsinger, NJ Zvaifler, GE Ehrlich. Philadelphia. JB Lippincott Co., 1985, pp 133–150
4. Arnett FC, Edworthy SM, Bloch DA, et al. The American Rheumatism Association 1987 revised criteria for the classification of rheumatoid arthritis. Arthritis Rheum 31:315–324, 1988
5. Dugowson CE, Koepsell TD, Voigt LF, et al. Rheumatoid arthritis in women: Incidence rate in group health cooperative, Seattle, Washington, 1987–1989. Arthritis Rheum 34:1502–1507, 1991
6. Goemaere S, Ackerman C, Goethals K, et al. Onset of symptoms of rheumatoid arthritis in relation to age, sex, and menopausal transition. J Rheumatol 17:1620–1622, 1990
7. Walport MJ, Ollier WER, Silman AJ: Immunogenetics of rheumatoid arthritis and the Arthritis and Rheumatism Council's National Repository. Br J Rheumatol 31:701–705, 1992
8. Moreland LW, Koopman WJ. Infection as a cause of arthritis. Curr Opin Rheumatol 3:639–649, 1991
9. Tuckwell JE, Esparza L, Carson DA, et al. The susceptibility sequence to rheumatoid arthritis is a cross-reactive B cell epitope shared by the *Escherichia coli* heat shock protein dnaj and the histocompatibility leukocyte antigen DRB10401 molecule. J Clin Invest 89:327–331, 1992
10. Koopman WJ, Schrohenloher RE. Rheumatoid factor, Rheumatoid Arthritis. Etiology, Diagnosis and Therapy. Edited by PD Utsinger, NJ Zvaifler, GE Ehrlich. Philadelphia, JB Lippincott Co., 1985, pp 217–241
11. Olsen NJ, Chen PP. Immunogenetics of autoantibodies and autoimmune diseases. Curr Opin Rheumatol 3:391–397, 1991
12. Kulka JP, Bocking D, Ropes MW, et al: Early joint lesions of rheumatoid arthritis. Arch Pathol 59:129–150, 1955
13. Schumacher HR: Synovial membrane and fluid morphologic alterations in early rheumatoid arthritis: Microvascular injury and virus-like particles. Ann NY Acad Sci 256:39–64, 1975
14. Stevens CR, Blake DR, Merry P, et al: A comparative study by morphometry of the microvasculature in normal and rheumatoid synovium. Arthritis Rheum 34:1508–1513, 1991
15. Firestein, GS. The immunopathogenesis of rheumatoid arthritis. Curr Opin Rheumatol 3:398–406, 1991
16. Remmers EF, Sano H, Wilder RL: Platelet-derived growth factors and heparin-binding (fibroblast) growth factors in the synovial tissue pathology of rheumatoid arthritis. Sem Arthritis Rheum 21:191–199, 1991
17. Wilder RL, Lafyatis R, Roberts AB, et al: Transforming growth factor-beta in rheumatoid arthritis. Ann NY Acad Sci 593:197–207, 1990
18. Howell, MD, Diveley JP, Lundeen KA, et al: Limited T-cell receptor beta-chain heterogeneity among interleukin–2 receptor-positive synovial T cells suggests a role for superantigen in rheumatoid arthritis. Proc Natl Acad Sci USA 88:10921–10925, 1991
19. Case JP, Lafyatis R, Remmers EF, et al: Transin/stromelysin expression in rheumatoid synovium: A transformation-associated metalloproteinase secreted by phenotypically invasive synoviocytes. Am J Pathol 135:1055–1064, 1989
20. Lotz M, Carson DA, Vaughan JH. Substance P activation of rheumatoid synoviocytes: Neural pathway in pathogenesis of arthritis. Science 235:893–895, 1987

B. Clinical Features and Laboratory

Rheumatoid arthritis (RA) is a clinical syndrome of unknown cause with varying features both between individual patients but also from time to time in the same patient. The diagnosis is essentially one of exclusion during the early weeks of the disease although characteristic features such as a symmetric sterile synovitis with typical serologic features strongly suggest RA. The destructive erosion of the cartilage and bone by the chronic and persistent synovitis will not become apparent radiographically for at least several months and more likely for over a year. The American College of Rheumatology (ACR) established criteria for RA in 1958, which were revised in 1987 (see Appendix 1). These criteria were established to assure uniformity for clinical trials and epidemiologic studies of the disease. They are not intended to be used in clinical practice for establishing the diagnosis in a specific patient.

DIAGNOSIS

Although the disease may be dominated in some patients by extraarticular manifestations, the single process essential for a diagnosis is identifying the presence of an inflammatory synovitis. This may be documented by: 1) The demonstration of a synovial fluid leucocytosis (WBC>2,000/mm^3), 2) Histologic demonstration of a chronic synovitis, or 3) Radiologic evidence of characteristic erosions.

Synovial biopsies are seldom performed or required for the clinical management of RA, and radiographic changes are not apparent early in the disease course when the diagnosis is in doubt. Consequently, establishing a diagnosis of synovitis is made by other means. Diagnosis should not be made solely on the basis of tenderness over the joint on physical exam. The presence of unequivocal evidence of synovial inflammation is required. If a palpable effusion is detected, it is useful to aspirate the joint in order to document a synovial fluid leucocytosis confirming the inflammatory nature of the process and to exclude the presence of crystals. The presence of a deformity is not always sufficient evidence to document the existence of synovitis. When the deformity occurs in a non-weight bearing joint such as the elbow or wrist, however, the physician may usually conclude, in the absence of a history of unique trauma such as a prior intra-articular fracture, that the deformity has resulted from synovitis.

Another diagnostic feature is the evolution of the disease process in a pattern consistent with RA. By definition RA cannot be diagnosed until the condition has been present for at least several weeks. In addition, many of the extraarticular features of the disease, the characteristic symmetry of inflammation, and the typical serologic findings may not be evident in the first month or two of the disease. Therefore, the diagnosis of RA is usually presumptive early in its course.

Other conditions causing synovitis must be excluded. Although this can often be done on initial evaluation, certain conditions such as systemic lupus erythematosus (SLE), or psoriatic arthritis may initially be indistinguishable from RA and only eventually evolve into another specific diagnosis. In these syndromes it is usually the development of extraarticular phenomena rather than the unique features of the associated synovitis that allows the physician to make a more specific diagnosis.

LABORATORY

There is no laboratory test, histologic, or radiographic finding that conclusively indicates a definitive diagnosis of RA.

Rheumatoid Factor. Rheumatoid factor is found in the serum of about 85% of patients with RA (1). The detection of the factor in patients with RA is of clinical value, because its presence tends to correlate with severe and unremitting disease, nodules, and extraarticular lesions of RA. In a population of patients with RA disease severity loosely correlates with the titer of rheumatoid factor. In a given patient, however, the titer is of little prognostic value and, moreover, serial titers of the rheumatoid factor are of

Table 10B–1. *Selected diseases associated with elevated serum rheumatoid factors*

Chronic bacterial infections
  Subacute bacterial endocarditis
  Leprosy
  Tuberculosis
  Syphilis
  Lyme Disease
Viral diseases
  Rubella
  Cytomegalovirus
  Infectious Mononucleosis
  Influenza
Parasitic diseases
Chronic inflammatory disease of uncertain etiology
  Sarcoidosis
  Periodontal disease
  Pulmonary interstitial disease
  Liver disease
Mixed cryoglobulinemia
Hypergammaglobulinemic purpura

From Koopman WJ and Schrohenloher RE (ref 10 from Chapter 10A) with modifications.

no value in following the disease process. Therefore, when an individual is known to be rheumatoid factor positive there is no purpose in repeating the test at a later date. A small percentage of patients who are rheumatoid factor negative early in the course of the disease will become positive as the disease progresses and assume the prognosis and features associated with rheumatoid factor positive RA. Also, rheumatoid factor can occur in other diseases, including several inflammatory disorders associated with synovitis (Table 10B–1).

Erythrocyte Sedimentation Rate and C-Reactive Protein. The erythrocyte sedimentation rate (ESR) is a measurement of the rate at which red blood cells will settle and is related to several factors in the serum (see Chapter 8B). In RA, the rate generally varies according to the degree of inflammation, and the range varies greatly from patient to patient. A rare patient with active inflammatory RA will have a normal ESR. However, it is sometimes a useful parameter for quantifying and comparing the level of inflammatory activity in the course of a given patient's illness. The C-reactive protein (CRP) is one of the acute phase reactants and may also be used to monitor the level of inflammation.

Other Laboratory Indicators. Other laboratory abnormalities observed in rheumatoid arthritis include hypergammaglobulinemia, anemia, occasional hypocomplementemia, thrombocytosis, and eosinophilia. These all occur more often in patients with more severe disease.

INITIAL PRESENTATION

The most common mode of onset is the insidious development of symptoms over a period of several weeks (2). Explosive acute polyarticular onset taking place over several days can be seen, but the appearance of an acute disabling monarticular arthritis as the initial manifestation is rare. Isolated less severe attacks of monarticular synovitis may occur with periods of complete remission before evolving into classic RA (3). These attacks, known as palindromic arthritis, usually last from three to five days. The initial presentation of RA often lacks the characteristic symmetry seen as the disease progresses to a more chronic state.

ARTICULAR MANIFESTATIONS

The articular manifestations of RA can be placed in two categories: reversible signs and symptoms related to inflammatory synovitis, and irreversible structural damage brought on by synovitis. This concept is used not only in staging disease and determining prognosis but also in selecting both medical and

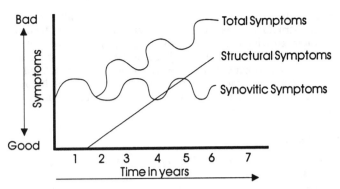

Fig. 10B–1. *Symptomatic course of rheumatoid arthritis.*

surgical therapy. It is often wise for a physician involved in the management of a patient with RA to ask: "What would the situation be in this patient if all active synovitis were eradicated?"

Structural damage in the typical patient usually begins sometime between the first and second year of the disease (4). Although the synovitis tends to follow a sine wave pattern of activity, structural damage progresses as a linear function of the amount of prior synovitis. This concept is shown in Figure 10B–1, which describes in a simplified form the clinical course of RA. Those remitting in the first year or so of the disease, before structural damage has occurred, will become virtually free of disease symptoms. However, those whose synovitis remits later in the course of the disease after structural damage has occurred will only experience partial benefit.

DEVELOPMENT OF JOINT DEFORMITIES

Joint deformities in RA may occur from several different mechanisms all related to synovitis and pannus formation, the resulting cartilage destruction, and the patient's attempt to avoid the pain of the process by posturing the joint in the least painful position. These mechanisms are described below.

Joint Immobilization. Any joint, normal or abnormal, subjected to prolonged immobilization will lose motion, both active and passive, as a result of tendon shortening and articular capsule constriction. Damage to the cartilage or the bone is not required and radiographs may be normal. The amount of motion lost and the resulting deformity may be related exclusively to the immobilization and is sometimes overcome by reinstituting motion or prevented by maintaining motion during the disease process. Some joints, such as the knee or ankle, that are put through a full range of motion in the normal activities of walking and arising from a chair seldom lose motion early in the course of an inflammatory arthritis. Joints whose motion is less critical to essential function, such as the shoulder, wrist and elbow, will often develop deformities early, because patients tend to splint the joint in an attempt to alleviate pain. The posture adopted is characteristically one in which the volume of the joint cavity is maximal so that the intraarticular pressure and resulting pain will be decreased.

Muscle Spasm and Shortening. Muscles and tendons that pass through or adjacent to an inflamed joint tend to develop spasm and shorten. This phenomenon is easiest to observe in the intrinsic muscles of the hand when they pass along the metacarpophalangeal (MCP) joint and in the anterior peroneal muscles as they pass over the talonavicular joint in the arch of the foot. Characteristic deformities of MCP flexion and tarsal pronation result, which may completely revert to normal when inflammation remits.

Bone and Cartilage Destruction. The ultimate destruction of the joint by the synovitis will denude the surface of cartilage and erode the bone leading to deformity by creating incongruous articular surfaces and occasionally bony blockade. Once the cartilage has disappeared, the opposing bones may fuse if immobilized.

Ligamentous Laxity. Ligaments that normally stabilize the joint may be weakened or severed by the erosive properties of persistent synovitis and pannus formation, which has the ability to lyse collagen in both tendons and ligaments in addition to cartilage. This will create instability in some joints. Also, most characteristically in the MCP joints, subluxations occur that are related to alterations of the lines of force of tendons that pull along an altered axis of rotation. The common development of ulnar deviation in RA is related to this mechanism.

Altered Tendon Function. The tenosynovium lining the tendon sheath is commonly inflamed in RA. Deformities may result from immobility related both to thickened or obstructing tendon sheath nodules and to tendon rupture, which is characteristically abrupt in onset. The pathognomonic abnormality of tendon dysfunction on physical exam is a discrepancy between active and passive motion.

STRUCTURAL VS SYNOVITIC SYMPTOMS

If RA persists and progresses, the patient will accumulate manifestations of the disease related to structural damage in addition to those related to the ongoing synovitis. It is critical to distinguish these two because the clinical management is different. Synovitis is a potentially reversible condition and is dealt with pharmacologically and by other nonsurgical means. The clinician follows its manifestations and orchestrates intervention based on fluctuations in symptoms and physical findings related to the presence and the severity of the synovitis. Structural damage to the articular surface characterized by cartilage loss and erosion of periarticular bone is an irreversible process, and its development is the end result of the inflammatory process. The management of this complication is either to live with it by emphasizing mechanical measures to control symptoms or to consider reconstructive surgery. Clinical features related to the activity and presence of synovitis are described below.

Morning Stiffness. Common in all the systemic inflammatory rheumatic disorders, morning stiffness is an almost universal feature of active RA. In contrast to the rather brief (5–10 minutes) period of gelling seen in osteoarthritis and sometimes in normal individuals, the morning stiffness of RA is prolonged, often lasting in excess of one hour. This phenomenon seems to depend on the prolonged immobilization of sleep and is not related to the hour of the day or periods of sunlight. Its duration also tends to correlate with the level of inflammation and will disappear when a remission occurs. For this reason, documenting the presence and length of morning stiffness is part of the data base used in following the disease. A question such as: "How long does it take, once you have gotten up until you're as good as you'll be?" can be used.

The Observation of Active Synovitis. This may be a subtle and often subjective clinical observation. The appearance of warm, swollen, obviously inflamed joints is usually seen only in the most active phases of inflammatory synovitis. In addition, these observations are usually restricted to superficial joints with an easily distensible capsule such as the knee and, occasionally, the wrist or proximal interphalangeal (PIP) joints. Joints that are deeply buried such as the hip will rarely present with a tense effusion apparent on physical exam. Joints such as the ankle are relatively nondistensible, because their capsules are restricted by multiple tendons and retinaculae. The ankle, therefore, may not appear swollen on physical exam or, if swollen, may be difficult to distinguish from edema or cellulitis.

Another factor to consider in evaluating the level of active inflammation in a joint in a patient with RA is the altered histopathology seen in chronic versus early rheumatoid synovitis. As the process continues, the vascularity of the synovitis decreases as granulation tissue and fibrosis develop. The resultant immobility of the joint brought on by the disease process further reduces the synovial vascularity, and the degree of obvious inflammation apparent on physical exam is significantly reduced. This leads to the faulty clinical concept of "burned-out" rheumatoid arthritis, a term sometimes mistakenly used to describe patients with long-standing RA who do not have warm, dramatically inflamed joints. Further observation of these patients reveals that they continue to experience prolonged morning stiffness, generalized malaise, and are easily fatigued; demonstrate laboratory evidence of anemia and an elevated sedimentation rate; and, most important, demonstrate progressive joint destruction on serial radiographs and physical exams over time. Rheumatoid arthritis rarely spontaneously remits after the first year (5).

The clinical features related to structural damage are marked by progressive deterioration both functionally and anatomically. Structural damage to the joint is irreversible and additive. Pain may be more related to motion or position. Objective evidence of cartilage destruction consists of either radiographic evidence of total loss of joint space or the demonstration on examination of *bone-on-bone crepitus*. This finding consists of detecting by palpation of a high-pitched screeching crepitus that occurs when denuded articular surfaces rub together. Nothing else makes this sound.

Another technique that may be used to document that the symptoms in a specific joint are related to irreversible structural damage is to demonstrate that the symptoms fail to respond to the most aggressive antiinflammatory therapy. Occasionally, depository corticosteroids may be injected into a joint presumed to be destroyed by persistent synovitis. The failure of the joint to benefit from this maneuver is good evidence that future attempts at antiinflammatory therapy are unlikely to provide benefit thus confirming the opinion that symptoms are predominantly structural.

MANIFESTATIONS IN SPECIFIC JOINTS

Principles regarding the role of synovitis and its ability to create joint deformities and destruction are applicable to all joints. Certain unique aspects are, however, pertinent to specific joints.

Cervical Spine

Although RA of the thoracic and lumbar spine is exceptionally rare, involvement of the cervical spine is frequent (Fig. 10B–2). The inflammatory process involves diarthrodial joints and is not palpable or visible to the examiner. Clinical manifestations of early disease consist primarily of neck stiffness that is perceived through the entire arc of motion; generalized motion loss also develops. Tenosynovitis of the transverse ligament of C1, which stabilizes the odontoid process of C2, may produce significant C1–C2 instability. Myelopathy may develop either by erosion into the odontoid process, by creating laxity, or by rupture of the ligament allowing pressure on the cord. Instability related to disease of the apophyseal joints may also contribute to laxity. Clinical evaluation of patients with RA should always include a careful neurologic exam. When neck pain develops it is important to define the syndrome as being accompanied or not with neuro-

logic features. Perhaps because it is not predominantly a weight-bearing structure, neck pain without neurologic features tends to be nonprogressive and usually will improve symptomatically despite radiographic evidence of joint destruction. On the other hand, the development of a significant myelopathy related to cervical spine instability is not universally accompanied by neck pain. Frequently, the course of neck pain and neurologic symptoms are not synchronous.

Shoulders

Because the shoulder capsule lies beneath the muscular rotator cuff, the presence of an effusion is frequently undetected on physical exam. When present, it is easiest to palpate and observe anteriorly. More frequently, only motion loss is observed. This occurs almost universally when the shoulder is inflamed. The patient will unconsciously restrict shoulder motion, because the fundamental activities of daily living do not require the extremes of shoulder motion. This process results in motion loss which, in the absence of a preventive exercise program, can develop rapidly into a "frozen shoulder syndrome". At this point the patient's symptoms are usually much more severe at night when the gyrations occurring during sleep stretch the tightened joint capsule. Although shoulder involvement is more common than hip involvement in patients with RA, the need for reconstructive surgery of the hip far exceeds that of the shoulder (6). This may be related to the fact that the shoulder is both a relatively unconstrained and nonweight-bearing joint.

Elbow

The elbow is one of the easiest of all joints in which to detect inflammation. Being a superficial joint, synovitis is evident by palpating fullness and thickening laterally between the olecranon and lateral epicondyle posterior to the radial–humeral joint. Flexion deformities develop early in RA. The ulnar nerve passes posterior–medially to the elbow, and compressive neuropathies may develop at this site related to the synovitis. Symptoms include sensory loss or paresthesia over the 4th and 5th fingers, weakness in the *flexor digiti quinti* or both. When structural symptoms develop, the physician should distinguish symptoms of radial–humeral disease accentuated by pronation–supination from those related to ulnar–humeral disease brought on by flexion–extension.

Hand

In virtually all patients with RA, the wrist, MCP and PIP joints are affected while the distal interphalangeal (DIP) joints are most often but not always spared. Ulnar deviation at the MCP joints often is associated with radial deviation at the wrists. *Swan-neck deformities* (Fig. 10B–3) can develop as can the boutonniere

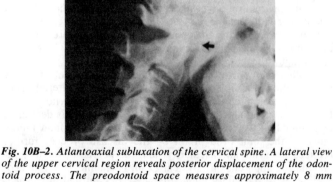

Fig. 10B–2. *Atlantoaxial subluxation of the cervical spine. A lateral view of the upper cervical region reveals posterior displacement of the odontoid process. The preodontoid space measures approximately 8 mm (arrow). Normally this measurement should not exceed 2.5–3 mm in the adult. In the child, 4–5 mm may be within normal limits. Measurement is made at the base of the anterior aspect of the dens with the neck in flexion. The film should be taken in flexion and extension in order to document abnormal motion (from the Revised Clinical Slide Collection on the Rheumatic Diseases).*

Fig. 10B–3. *"Swan-neck" deformities are present in the second and third fingers of this patient with RA. Deformity results from contracture of the interosseous and flexor muscles and tendons, resulting in a flexion contracture of the metacarpophalangeal joint, hyperextension of the proximal interphalangeal joint, and flexion of the distal interphalangeal joint (from the Revised Clinical Slide Collection on the Rheumatic Diseases).*

deformity with flexion at the PIP and hyperextension at the DIP joints. In addition to symptoms related to joint synovitis, RA is also associated with pain or dysfunction related to compression of a peripheral nerve entrapped in a confined area by synovitis. This most commonly occurs in the carpal tunnel of the wrist. Many patients with early RA will have neuropathic symptoms consistent with carpal tunnel syndrome. If the disease progresses, distention of the retinaculum of the wrist occurs, the capsule is given room to expand, and symptoms related to the compressive neuropathy may improve. The ulnar nerve passes through Guyon's canal, and ulnar nerve paresthesias of the same pathophysiology may occur, although less frequently than the carpal tunnel syndrome. Because the muscle body of the *flexor digiti quinti* lies between the elbow and the wrist, a Guyon's canal syndrome may be distinguished from the entrapment neuropathy at the elbow by the absence of weakness of the fifth finger when flexed against resistance.

In RA, tenosynovitis may often accompany synovitis. An additional cause of tendon dysfunction is the formation of rheumatoid nodules along tendon sheaths. In both situations nodular thickening may be palpated along the flexor tendons of the palm. This process may cause obstructive symptoms described as "locking and catching" as the nodule slides along its sheath. It also may lead to tendon rupture if the inflammatory tenosynovitis erodes through the tendon. This most commonly occurs in the *extensor pollicus longus* that extends the DIP joint of the thumb. Another cause of tendon rupture occurring in the wrist is the *attrition rupture* seen characteristically in the extensor tendons of the 3rd, 4th and 5th fingers. This rupture is due to the abrasion of the tendons as they course dorsal to an ulnar styloid that has been eroded down to jagged bone. The ulnar styloid then acts as a saw that destroys the tendons. All tendon ruptures present with a history of abrupt, usually painless, loss of a highly specific function. The characteristic discrepancy between active and passive motion is seen on physical exam.

Hip

Although commonly involved in RA, the early manifestations of hip disease often are not apparent, even to a skilled examiner. The joint is located deep within the pelvis so that evidence of palpable distention or synovial thickening are absent. In addition, early involvement is often asymptomatic, although subtle reductions of range of motion may be observed. The initial dysfunction is usually difficulty in putting on one's shoes and socks on the affected side. When symptoms do develop they characteristically occur in the groin or the thigh but also may be felt in the low back or knee. If cartilage destruction does occur, its symptoms may accelerate more rapidly than in other joints.

Knee

Effusions and synovial thickening of the knee are usually easily detected on examination. Joint aspiration, when indicated, may be easily done. Posterior herniation of the capsule creating a Baker's cyst may be associated with dissection or rupture into the calf and a picture suggestive of thrombophlebitis. However, the characteristic history, the lack of evidence of engorgement of collateral venous channels, and a distinct border of edema below the knee distinguish this syndrome from thrombophlebitis. Ultrasonography will readily define a Baker's cyst, but may be negative when a rupture or dissection has occurred. Arthrography, with a film taken after a brief period of exercise to the calf musculature, may be required to demonstrate a herniation.

Foot and Ankle

Because these are weight-bearing structures, lower extremity joint involvement leads to greater dysfunction and pain than will occur in the upper extremities. In descending order of frequency, RA characteristically affects the metatarsophalangeal, talonavicular, and ankle joints. Metatarsophalangeal (MTP) arthritis leads to cock-up deformities and subluxations of the MTP heads on the sole. Dysfunction may be related to the interruption of the normal flowing transmission of forces across the metatarsal heads in normal gait. This is important when considering surgical reconstruction of the foot, because surgery that removes painful prominences on the sole often only allows the next most painful prominence to bear weight and does nothing to restore the normal flow of forces across the MTP joints.

The surface of the talonavicular joint lies dorsally and medially on the proximal tarsal arch under the distal body and tendons of the anterior tibial musculature. Inflammation of this joint causes the adjacent muscles to go into spasm, with resultant pronation and eversion of the foot, a deformity characteristic of talonavicular inflammation. Less common in RA is involvement of the ankle joint. The tarsal tunnel, posterior and inferior to the medial malleolus, contains the posterior tibial nerve that is often compressed by synovitis. This may lead to a neuropathy manifested by burning paresthesias felt on the sole of the foot, which is made worse by standing or walking (7).

EXTRAARTICULAR MANIFESTATIONS

Rheumatoid arthritis is a systemic disease, and most individuals with the condition experience some extraarticular manifestations such as generalized malaise or fatigue. Significant inflammation of other organ systems, however, is predominantly limited to those individuals with the disease who have rheumatoid factor in their serum. Other risk factors that generally correlate with the development of extraarticular manifestations are the presence of rheumatoid nodules, the generalized severity of the articular process, and probably, the MHC class II DR B1 allele 0401 (8).

Skin Manifestations

The rheumatoid nodule is characteristic of RA and seen at some time in up to 25% to 50% of patients in some populations. Rheumatoid factor is found in virtually all patients with nodules. The nodules tend to develop in crops during active phases of the disease and form subcutaneously, in bursae and along tendon sheaths. Although they have been described in almost every region, and may occur in the viscera, the usual location is over pressure points such as the olecranons, the extensor surface of the forearm, the Achilles tendons, and even the ischial area (Fig. 10B-4). The development of the lesion can be gradual or abrupt but is often associated with some signs of inflammation. A nodule biopsy may be required if the diagnosis is unclear or if gout is suspected and the aspirate is negative for crystals. Over time nodules can either disappear or involute.

Vasculitic lesions are frequently seen in RA. Some suggest that the earliest abnormality observed in the formation of a rheumatoid nodule is a venulitis. Other patterns of dermal venulitis may be seen, occasionally with histologic evidence of leucocytoclastic vasculitis and a clinical appearance of small nail-fold infarcts or palpable purpura (Fig. 10B–5). The presence of such lesions does not necessarily imply a coexistent systemic vasculitis, but the

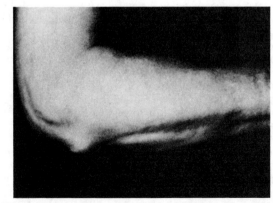

Fig. 10B–4. A large subcutaneous nodule is located on the extensor surface of the forearm near the elbow (from the Revised Clinical Slide Collection on the Rheumatic Diseases).

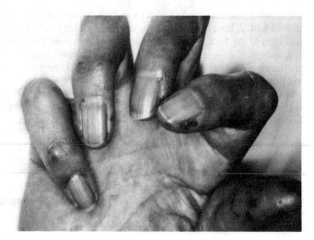

Fig. 10B–5. Splinter hemorrhages and necrotic areas at the fingertips and around the nails may be caused by vasculitis and occlusion of terminal arteries, resulting in subsequent skin infarction (from the Revised Clinical Slide Collection on the Rheumatic Diseases).

patient should be meticulously examined for evidence of involvement of other organ systems, most importantly neurologic dysfunction. The presence of ischemic ulcers is a dermatologic evidence of arteritis, but more frequently implies systemic involvement.

Drugs used to treat RA can also create abnormalities of the skin. Ecchymoses can occur as a consequence of either platelet dysfunction related to nonsteroidal use or capillary fragility related to the use of steroids. Petechiae may be a manifestation of thrombocytopenia secondary to gold, penicillamine, or sulfasalazine. Chrysiasis, a cyanotic hue with a predilection to be most apparent on the forehead, is a manifestation of chronic gold administration and the deposit of the metal in the skin.

Ocular Manifestations

Symptomatic keratoconjunctivitis sicca as a manifestation of associated Sjogren's syndrome is common. Patients may be unaware of its presence, and the history should actively be elicited because prophylactic measures are of value. Episodes of episcleritis are common and usually run a benign self-limited course. Scleritis, however, has a more morbid prognosis. Inflammation, which histologically resembles the formation of a rheumatoid nodule, may erode through the sclera into the choroid creating *scleromalacia perforans* with associated significant damage and visual loss.

Respiratory Manifestations

Inflammation of the cricoarytenoid joint is a common finding in RA. Its symptoms are usually episodic consisting of laryngeal pain, dysphonia and occasionally pain on swallowing, all of which may be accentuated in the morning (9). Laryngeal obstruction rarely occurs but may be seen in the few hours following extubation for endotracheal anesthesia.

Histologic evidence of interstitial lung disease is present to some extent in the majority of autopsies done on patients with RA. Its pathologic features are nonspecific and cannot be distinguished from interstitial lung disease of other sterile inflammatory etiologies. The prevalence of clinical symptoms in RA patients is significantly less, in part related to the restrictions on physical exertion brought on by the articular aspects of the disease (10). However, the mortality from pulmonary disease in RA is twice that of the general population (11). The prevalence of radiographic abnormalities lies somewhere between the two features mentioned above and consists of interstitial fibrosis with a predilection for basal involvement. Bronchiolitis obliterans may also occur. Solitary or multiple nodules may develop in the lung parenchyma and occasionally cavitation of these lesions can be identified on chest computed tomography. Rarely, a subpleural

nodule may rupture creating a bronchopleural fistula, which can progress to either a pneumothorax or empyema.

Interstitial lung disease with a histologic picture and clinical course identical to that seen in RA alone has been described in association with penicillamine or gold therapy for RA. The significance of this observation is uncertain.

Inflammatory pleural disease with nonspecific histology is seen often in autopsied RA patients. Symptomatic pleurisy can occur as can small pleural effusions seen incidently on chest X-rays. The characteristic laboratory finding in a pleural fluid due to rheumatoid pleuritis is a markedly low glucose level. Other laboratory parameters are consistent with an exudative process.

Cardiac Manifestations

Evidence of inflammatory pericarditis is found in close to 50% of autopsied patients with RA, and pericardial abnormalities or evidence of an effusion are seen in a similar percentage of asymptomatic patients with RA undergoing echocardiography (12). Symptomatic pericarditis manifested either by pain or altered cardiovascular physiology is rare. Episodes of pericarditis can occur at any time during the course of the disease but usually develop at the same time as a generalized flare. An occasional patient may progress to chronic constrictive pericarditis manifested by peripheral edema and signs of right-side heart failure (13). Inflammatory lesions similar to rheumatoid nodules may develop involving both the myocardium and the valves. Clinical manifestations include valvular dysfunction, embolic phenomena, conduction defects, and perhaps myocardiopathy. Aortitis has been described involving segments of the entire aorta and associated with both aortic insufficiency related to dilation of the aortic root and aneurysmal rupture (14).

Gastrointestinal Manifestations

There are no specific gastrointestinal abnormalities related to RA, with the exception of xerostomia seen in patients with associated Sjogren's syndrome and ischemic complications of rheumatoid vasculitis. On the other hand, gastritis or peptic ulcer disease is the major complication of nonsteroidal therapy and is a significant cause of morbidity and mortality in RA.

Renal Manifestations

In contrast to SLE, glomerular disease is absent or rare in RA (15). If proteinuria develops, it is usually either related to a drug toxicity (gold or penicillamine) or secondary to amyloidosis. Interstitial renal disease may occur in Sjogren's syndrome but in RA it is related more often to the use of nonsteroidal antiinflammatory drugs, acetaminophen, or other analgesics. Papillary necrosis may occur as a result of this process.

Neurologic Manifestations

Neurologic complications are frequently seen in RA and usually are subtle in their presentation so that the distinction between articular and neuropathic lesions is difficult (16). Their pathogenesis is fundamentally related to one of three mechanisms described below.

Myelopathies Related to Cervical Spine Instability. This most commonly occurs at C1–C2 in conjunction with a failure to stabilize the odontoid related either to destruction of the transverse ligament of C1 or a destruction of the odontoid itself. A *step-off* subluxation related to apophyseal joint destruction may also occur, most commonly at C4–C5 or C5–C6. Lateral radiographs taken in flexion and extension are required to demonstrate the instability. Magnetic resonance imaging is then used to further define the precise anatomy of the region and document the presence of cord compression. Symptoms of myelopathy due to RA are typically gradual in onset and often unrelated to either the development or accentuation of neck pain. When neck pain does occur, it frequently radiates over the occiput in the distribution of the C1–C3 nerve roots. *L'hermitte's sign*, the sudden development of tingling paresthesias that descends the thoraco–lumbar spine in conjunction with cervical spine flexion, may occur. The most common symptoms associated with a cervical myelopathy are the development over weeks to months of bilateral sensory paresthesias of the hands and motor weakness occurring in a patient with long-standing destructive RA. Physical exam may demonstrate pathologic reflexes such as Babinski's or Hoffman's, and deep tendon reflexes are hyperactive. Patients with long-standing RA usually have hypoactive reflexes related to joint contracture, disuse atrophy, and a mild peripheral neuropathy, which may accompany the disease; therefore, the observation of hyperreflexia should alert the clinician to the presence of a presumed myelopathy.

Entrapment Neuropathies. When a peripheral nerve passes through a compartment also occupied by synovium or tendon sheath, the potential for compression by synovitis or tenosynovitis exists. Symptoms are related to fluctuations in the activity of the synovitis and also the posture assumed by the joint. Nerves that are frequently compressed in addition to those previously described are the posterior interosseous nerve in the antecubital fossa, the femoral nerve anterior to the hip joint, the peroneal nerve adjacent to the fibular head, and the interdigital nerve at the MTP joint. Compression syndromes of these nerves may be confirmed by neurophysiologic studies.

Ischemic Neuropathies Related to Vasculitis. The syndrome of *mononeuritis multiplex*, is marked by the abrupt onset of a persistent peripheral neuropathy unaltered by either change in posture or reductions in synovial inflammation. Concurrent evidence of rheumatoid vasculitis is often seen. Neurophysiologic studies reveal an axonal lesion and frequently demonstrate multiple clinically inapparent mononeuropathies. A sural nerve or muscle biopsy may confirm the diagnosis.

Hematological Manifestations

A hypochromic–microcytic anemia with a low iron and low or normal iron-binding capacity that meets the criteria of an anemia of chronic disease is an almost universal accompaniment of active RA. Because most patients with the disease are taking ulcerogenic antiinflammatory agents and may have coexistent positive stool exams for occult blood, distinguishing this anemia from an iron-deficiency anemia is difficult. This is compounded by the failure of such patients to vigorously respond to iron therapy with a brisk reticulocytosis when iron deficiency is an underlying cause. Ferritin levels also fail to distinguish the two. Only an examination of the bone marrow for iron stores will provide a definitive answer. The clinician must generally restrict more aggressive diagnostic gastrointestinal or hematologic evaluation to those patients whose pattern of gastrointestinal symptoms, degree of anemia, or documented loss of blood by stool exam seems to require such studies.

Felty's syndrome was originally described as the combination of RA, splenomegaly, leucopenia, and leg ulcers. Subsequent observations have shown an association with lymphadenopathy, thrombocytopenia, and the HLA–DR4 haplotype (17). Felty's syndrome is most common with severe, nodule-forming RA, but the synovitis may be less active when the patient is neutropenic. Hypersplenism appears to explain a portion of cases. Leukopenia is selective involving neutrophils. The "large granular lymphocyte" syndrome has recently been described and shares many of the features of Felty's syndrome (18). The hematologic features are not exclusively seen in RA and may represent a process that permits RA to develop rather than resulting from the disease itself. Thrombocytopenia may be seen either as a result of marrow suppression due to immunosuppressive or cytotoxic therapy, or related to an autoimmune process with gold, penicillamine, or sulfasalazine therapy.

COURSE AND PROGNOSIS

The prognosis of RA is uncertain (19), due to the prolonged nature of the disease, its inherent variability, and the difficulty in defining the milder or subclinical forms of the disease. Many patients never see a physician about their condition, let alone consult a rheumatologist or present to a medical center. In addition, the diagnosis of RA often is not included on the death certificate.

Criteria for remission have been established. The frequency of its occurence is affected both by therapy and patient selection. An epidemiologic study searching for the prevalence of RA in a given population was unable to substantiate this diagnosis in well over half of the patients originally diagnosed with the disease when they were reexamined several years later (20). On the other hand, Short and Bauer, in their classic monograph on the clinical picture of RA in patients treated only with salicylates and simple orthopedic measures, found that only 10% of patients would undergo a clinical remission in over a decade of follow-up (21). This observation is similar to that of Ragan who described a similar low rate of spontaneous remission and also noted that most remissions that occurred did so in the first two years of the disease (5). Both studies focused on patients seeking medical care from rheumatologists. Their experience seems to more closely parallel current clinical observations. Factors that predict a more severe and persistent course are the presence of rheumatoid factor, nodules, and the HLA–DR4 haplotype (22). In patients who fail to undergo a spontaneous remission, the prognosis in regard to joint destruction seems to depend on the severity of the synovial inflammation.

Evidence exists that close to 90% of the joints ultimately involved in a given patient are involved on clinical exam during the first year of the disease (6). Therefore, a patient who has had RA for several years may be assured, given the worst case scenario, which joints will or will not be involved over the course of the disease.

Some studies done over the last decade have reported increased mortality rates in patients with RA and have shown that patients with severe forms of the disease die 10 to 15 years earlier than expected. The causes of death, which were disproportionately high compared to the U.S. population, were infections, pulmonary and renal disease, and gastrointestinal bleeding (11).

DATA BASES USED IN FOLLOWING PATIENTS WITH RHEUMATOID ARTHRITIS

Criteria (see Appendices 1 and 2) have been established by the American College of Rheumatology for the diagnosis of RA, the classification of severity using roentgenographic criteria, functional class, and the definition of a remission. These criteria were developed for the standardization of epidemiologic and clinical investigations and were not designed for the management of individual patients. However, they are useful both as a frame of reference and in describing clinical phenomena.

In the management of an individual patient, the clinician attempts to determine the precise etiology of the patient's pain and dysfunction, evaluate the extent to which inflammatory synovitis and structural damage play a role in the articular symptoms, consider the potential options for both medical and surgical therapy, and provide guidance to the patient in dealing with the psychological, social, and economic consequences of the entire process.

Ronald J. Anderson, MD

1. Singer JM, Plotz CM: The latex fixation test: application to the serological diagnosis of rheumatoid arthritis. Am J Med 21:888, 1956

2. Fleming A, Benn RT, Corbett M, et al: Early rheumatoid disease: patterns of joint involvement. Ann Rheum Dis 35:361, 1976

3. Schumacher HR: Palindromic onset of rheumatoid arthritis. Arth Rheum 25:361, 1982

4. van der Heijde DM, van Riel PL, van Leeuwen MA, et al: Prognostic factors for radiographic damage and physical disability in early rheumatoid arthritis: a prospective study of 147 patients. Br J Rheumatol 31:519–525, 1992

5. Ragan C, Farrington E: The clinical features of rheumatoid arthritis. Prognostic Indices JAMA 2:16, 1959

6. Roberts WN, Daltroy LH, Anderson RJ: Stability of normal joint findings in persistent classical rheumatoid arthritis. Arth Rheum 31:267, 1988

7. McGuigan L, Burke D, Fleming A: Tarsal tunnel syndrome and peripheral neuropathy in rheumatoid disease. Ann Rheum Dis 42:128, 1983

8. Weyand CM, Hicok KC, Conn DL, et al: The influence of HLA–DR B1 genes on disease severity in rheumatoid arthritis. Ann Intern Med 117:801–806, 1992

9. Bienenstock H, Ehrlich GE, Freyberg RH: Rheumatoid arthritis of the cricoarytenoid joint: A clinicopathologal study. Arth Rheum 6:48, 1963

10. Walker WC, Wright V: Pulmonary lesions and rheumatoid arthritis. Ann Rheum Dis 28:252, 1969
11. Pincus T, Callahan LF: Early mortality in RA predicted by poor clinical status. Bull Rheum Dis 41:4, 1992.
12. John JT Jr, Hough A, Sergent JS: Pericardial disease in rheumatoid arthritis. Am J Med 66:385, 1979
13. Franco AE, Levine HD, Hall AP: Rheumatoid pericarditis: report of 17 cases diagnosed clinically. Ann Intern Med 77:837, 1972
14. Gravallese EM, Corson JM, Coblyn JS, et al: Rheumatoid aortitis: a rarely recognized but clinically significant entity. Medicine: 68 (2):95, 1989
15. Boers M, Dijkmans AC, Breedveld FC, et al: Subclinical renal dysfunction in rheumatoid arthritis. Arth Rheum 33:95–101, 1990
16. Nakano KK, Schoene WC, Baher RA, et al: The cervical myelopathy associated with rheumatoid arthritis. Am Neuro Assoc 3:144, 1978

17. Dinant HJ, Muller WH, Vandenberg-Loonen, et al: HLA–Drw4 in Felty's syndrome. Arth Rheum 23:1336, 1980
18. Barton JC, Prasthofer EF, Egan ML, et al: Rheumatoid arthritis associated with expanded populations of granular lymphocytes. Ann Int Med 104:314, 1986
19. Harris ED. Rheumatoid arthritis. Pathophysiology and implications for therapy. N Engl J Med 322:1277–89, 1990
20. O'Sullivan JB, Cathcart ES: The prevalence of rheumatoid arthritis. Follow-up evaluation of the effect of criteria on rates in Sudbury, Mass. Ann Int Med 76:573, 1972
21. Short CL, Bauer W, Reynolds WE: Rheumatoid arthritis, Harvard University Press, 1957
22. Van Zeben D, Hazes JM, Zwinderman AH, et al: Association of HLA–DR4 with a more progressive disease course in patients with rheumatoid arthritis: results of a follow-up study. Arth Rheum 34:822, 1991

C. Treatment

Because of the potential impact of rheumatoid arthritis (RA), therapy for the disease has become more aggressive. The aim of present therapy is to provide pain relief, to decrease joint inflammation, and more importantly, to maintain or restore joint function and prevent bone and cartilage destruction. While some of the existing therapies are considered to be disease-modifying, this modification of the natural course is difficult to prove in scientific studies. The current approach to treatment is to interrupt the complex inflammatory process.

The basic treatment program consists of patient education, balance between rest and exercise (often with physical and occupational therapy), and the use of aspirin or other nonsteroidal antiinflammatory drugs (NSAIDs).

Appropriate and early education can improve patient motivation and compliance and can also provide encouragement when a potentially disabling diagnosis is discussed. The patient needs to be informed as to aggravating activities, medication toxicities, possible systemic manifestations, and the potential need for close follow-up.

The value of rest in RA patients would appear intuitive, but the evidence for its benefit is largely anecdotal. However, fatigue is a prominent manifestation and 8 to 10 hours of bedrest at night and an hour rest in the afternoon can improve the patient's sense of well-being and reduce fatigue. Prolonged bed rest does not appear to provide any particular benefit; in fact, it can even worsen contractures and promote muscle atrophy. Patients should be encouraged to participate in reasonable activity.

Although there is a paucity of data to document the efficacy of physical therapy in RA, these measures continue to be a part of the treatment program (1). The goal of exercise is to maintain or improve muscle tone, prevent or correct deformities, and maintain or increase joint mobility and function. Regular range-of-motion exercises help to preserve joint motion in patients who tend to limit normal motion in painful and swollen joints. These therapies can usually be taught to the patient and/or the family, and they can be done at home. Occupational therapy can assist patients in adapting the activities of daily living to the limitations of the disease and can supply splints and assistive devices to aid in self-care. Rehabilitative therapies are described in more detail in Chapter 60.

Available medications for RA treatment have been shown to be more effective than placebo. These agents can be considered in two groups: those that have potential for symptomatic relief and those that may have potential to modify the disease. The latter are often referred to as slow-acting antirheumatic drugs (SAARDs) or disease-modifying antirheumatic drugs. These SAARDs do seem to have the promise of greater impact on the disease process and may modify the natural course.

SYMPTOMATIC MEDICAL THERAPY

The symptomatic medications include aspirin, other NSAIDs, and the glucocorticoids. These agents are generally prescribed as baseline therapy in every newly diagnosed patient with RA unless contraindicated. In appropriate dosage, these agents can decrease pain and swelling but are not capable of preventing cartilage destruction or bone erosion. They provide relief of pain and swelling that can promote better function in the activities of daily living and facilitate the exercises necessary for good health and maintenance of joint motion and muscle strength.

NSAIDs

All NSAIDs are inhibitors of the enzyme cyclooxygenase, which catalyzes the conversion of arachidonic acid to prostaglandins, prostacyclin, and thromboxanes (see Chapter 55). However, NSAID inhibition of cyclooxygenase is variable and the degree of inhibition is not predictive of clinical response, suggesting that other mechanisms of action are likely. While aspirin has been the standard of therapy for many years, numerous NSAIDs have been developed that have efficacy similar to aspirin but with a lower risk of gastrointestinal toxicity. The mechanism of action of these agents differs from that of aspirin in that the inhibition of cyclooxygenase is competitive while that of aspirin is irreversible. Although controlled studies have not shown any particular NSAID to be more effective than aspirin or any other NSAID, individual patient response can be quite variable and response to a given drug will vary from patient to patient (2). An adequate trial at maximum dosage of at least two weeks duration appears to be the most appropriate and accurate procedure to assess the benefit of any single agent in a specific patient.

Aspirin has often been the first choice for initial treatment of RA. It is relatively inexpensive and is antiinflammatory in therapeutic doses ranging from 3,900 mg to 6,500 mg/day divided into three or four doses. A serum steady state is attained after five to seven days of therapy and the desired serum salicylate level is 20–30 mg/dL (3). Because of the pharmacokinetics of high dose aspirin, small increases or decreases in the dose can result in large changes in serum concentrations. Serum salicylate levels are indicated in elderly patients and children, as well as in patients with tinnitus on unusually low doses, patients on unusually high doses, and patients using enteric-coated preparations that may have variable absorption.

Aspirin is not tolerated in therapeutic doses in a significant number of patients (3). Rare hypersensitivity reactions such as asthma, nasal polyps, angioedema, and urticaria can be seen, but the most frequently observed side effects are tinnitus or gastropathy (gastritis, gastric ulceration, and bleeding). Occult blood loss can also occur. Misoprostol, an oral prostaglandin analog, may be indicated in high risk patients on aspirin or NSAIDs in an attempt to reduce the risk of gastric ulceration. Aspirin has been implicated in a transient and reversible decrease in renal function and can also result in elevation of hepatic transaminases or even clinical hepatitis. Aspirin irreversibly acetylates platelets, interfering with platelet aggregation and prolonging bleeding time.

Non-acetylated or buffered salicylates induce fewer gastric symptoms but are more expensive. Enteric-coated aspirin preparations can reduce local gastrointestinal effects but still inhibit prostaglandins. Also, some formulations can be erratically absorbed in individual patients.

The non-aspirin NSAIDs were developed to decrease the risk of gastrointestinal ulceration and bleeding. While the chemical composition varies among these compounds, the efficacy and toxicity seem to be remarkably similar. These NSAIDs may be better tolerated than aspirin; however, they are expensive and gastrointestinal toxicity similar to that seen with aspirin, including bleeding, can occur (2). Hypersensitivity reactions similar to those seen with aspirin can also occur with other NSAIDs and cross-reactivity to NSAIDs in patients with aspirin sensitivity has been described. NSAIDs can also precipitate transient increases in serum creatinine, interstitial nephritis, or nephrosis similar to aspirin (2). Mild and transient elevations of transaminases also occur with NSAIDs. Toxic hepatitis is an infrequent occurrence. The inhibition of platelet cyclooxygenase by NSAIDs is reversible and persists only while the drug is present. Previous aspirin allergy recommends caution in implementing NSAID therapy since similar reactions may occur with NSAIDs.

Specific NSAIDs may have certain more frequent adverse reactions. For example, indomethacin and tolmetin are known to produce headache, dizziness, and confusion. Toxic amblyopia and aseptic meningitis have been reported as rare complications of ibuprofen. The physician should be familiar with the specific toxicities of any NSAID prescribed (see Chapter 55). There is no good evidence to suggest that the combination of two NSAIDs (or aspirin and another NSAID) is preferable to a single drug, and combinations may increase the potential for adverse effects.

Selection of a particular NSAID is based on many factors. Cost is always a consideration. Aspirin is usually the cheapest medication for RA. Generic substitutes are also usually less expensive. Availability may also dictate selection since some hospitals and insurance programs may limit choices. The personal experience of the prescribing physician is important since the physician should be familiar with the possible positive and negative effects of the drug. Lastly, compliance can be an issue, and studies suggest that a once or twice a day regimen has better compliance than more frequent dosing (4).

Corticosteroids

Glucocorticoids have both antiinflammatory and immunosuppressive effects but have not been shown to have disease modification potential (see Chapter 55). This issue remains controversial (5), and the exact mechanism of action has not been identified. Because of the adverse effects of long-term corticosteroids, these agents are avoided, if possible, in the routine treatment of RA. Use of these drugs is indicated for life-threatening complications of RA such as vasculitis. Low dose corticosteroids (≤10 mg daily prednisone or equivalent) are sometimes useful for individuals who are unable to work or care for themselves, but the steroid should be tapered or discontinued as soon as possible. These agents are also used to temporarily bridge the time between onset of therapy with a slow-acting second-line agent and the onset of effect or to permit a patient to exercise to maintain or improve joint function. However, tapering and completely discontinuing corticosteroids in RA patients takes time and is often unsuccessful.

Adverse effects of glucocorticoids are diverse and dependent on the agent, dose, and duration of therapy. In the low doses most frequently employed in treating RA, skin thinning and ecchymoses as well as a Cushingoid appearance may occur, but the most significant toxicity is a steroid-induced osteopenia that is superimposed on the osteoporosis inherent to RA.

Intraarticular steroids may be helpful when one or two joints flare out of proportion to the general disease (see Chapter 58). It is important that joint infection be excluded before steroids are injected.

SAARDS

Patients who do not respond adequately to symptomatic therapy or who have aggressive disease become candidates for SAARD therapy. There is a trend toward earlier use of these

Table 10C–1. *Current and potential slow-acting antirheumatic drugs for RA*

Drugs approved by FDA for use in RA
auranofin
azathioprine
gold salts
hydroxychoroquine
methotrexate
penicillamine
Drugs approved for other diseases, but not RA
chlorambucil
cyclophosphamide
cyclosporine
sulfasalazine
Some other experimental procedures and drugs (not inclusive)
fish oil, plant oils
total nodal irradiation
apheresis
biologics (see Chapter 57)

agents in an attempt to control the inflammatory process as early as possible in hopes that this will reduce joint destruction (6). While these second-line agents are sometimes referred to as disease-modifying antirheumatic drugs (DMARDS), true disease modification is difficult to document. Many feel that these agents may have a favorable impact on the natural disease course. These medications are generally slow-acting and require several months of use before response is seen. Various SAARDs also have significant toxicity and require close monitoring by a physician experienced in using them (see Chapter 56).

Table 10C–1 lists many of the second-line agents currently in use or under investigation. Those approved by the U.S. Food and Drug Administration for use in RA are listed first. Other agents or procedures should be considered experimental and should only be employed under clinical protocol.

The mechanism of action of SAARDs is generally not known. Many were first used empirically or because of theoretical considerations that would suggest efficacy. All of the approved or commonly used SAARDs have demonstrated efficacy in placebo-controlled trials (7).

While no consensus exists as to which SAARDs should be used in what order, most rheumatologists would agree that treatment must be individualized and that the initial use of less toxic therapies is preferred except in patients with fulminant progressive disease or life-threatening complications such as vasculitis. Table 10C–2 lists one classification by toxicity. The first group labelled as "Safer" includes agents whose toxicity is not only less frequent but also milder in degree of severity. The third group, labelled as "Very Toxic," consists of two agents with proven efficacy but which have oncogenic potential that makes them much less desirable unless all other approaches have been exhausted.

The toxicity of these drugs makes close clinical and laboratory monitoring mandatory, but specific toxicities vary from agent to agent. The SAARDs also are delayed in onset of action and several months of therapy are required before improvement is expected. The length of time needed varies depending on the drug. The treating physician should be aware of the potential and toxicity of any SAARD before beginning treatment.

While direct comparisons of SAARDs usually fail to demonstrate significant differences, clinical experience of most rheumatologists suggests that methotrexate may be the most effective treatment at least for control of symptoms and that injectable

Table 10C–2. *A classification of disease modifying antirheumatic drugs by toxicity*

Safer	More Toxic	Very Toxic
auranofin	azathioprine	chlorambucil
hydroxychloroquine	cyclosporine	cyclophosphamide
sulfasalazine	gold salts	
	methotrexate	
	penicillamine	

gold is still valuable. The SAARDs are often not effective or tolerated for long periods of time, although methotrexate may be an exception. One study demonstrated that the median time to discontinue therapy for parenteral gold, auranofin, hydroxychloroquine, or penicillamine was two years or less but was 4.25 years for methotrexate (8). Others have shown that about 25% of patients on most SAARDs continue the medication for more than two years (9) while about 50% of patients on methotrexate still continue therapy after two years (10). One caution is the relatively brief experience with chronic methotrexate treatment in RA patients and the potential for serious hepatic or pulmonary toxicity.

New approaches to therapy are still being sought (11). Combination SAARD therapy has been advocated but most of the controlled studies of two drug combinations have failed to demonstrate an advantage over single drug therapy (12). More aggressive approaches have also been encouraged (13) but must be considered experimental until data is acquired.

Auranofin. Auranofin is an oral gold preparation that is given in a dose of 6 mg/day. A maximum dose of 9 mg/day may be given, but abdominal discomfort and diarrhea make many patients intolerant of this dose. While many feel that the oral medication is less effective than injectable gold, direct comparisons in controlled trials fail to reveal significant difference in efficacy. However, toxicity is less common and less severe with the oral drug (14). Improvement is not expected for about three months, and a six month trial of the medication is recommended. Patients should have a complete blood count and urinalysis at least monthly while taking this medication.

Azathioprine. Azathioprine is an oral cytotoxic purine analog that is usually employed in a dose of 1.25–1.5 mg/kg/day but may be increased to 2.0–2.5 mg/kg/day after three months if clinical response is not adequate. Again, response is usually delayed for several months, and a six month trial is recommended. As with all cytotoxic medications, the potential for severe side effects exists and the drug requires careful monitoring, including monthly blood counts and quarterly liver function tests. Concomitant use of allopurinol increases toxicity by competitively inhibiting the degradation of azathioprine and should be avoided. If allopurinol is necessary, appropriate dose adjustments must be made. Renal excretion is a major route of elimination of azathioprine and its active metabolites. Dosages should be reduced when renal impairment is present.

Chlorambucil. An alkylating agent, chlorambucil should be reserved for treatment of life-threatening complications of RA such as systemic vasculitis or disease refractory to all other treatments. Beneficial effects may be seen in one to two months. The usual dose is 2–6 mg/day with 4 mg/day the usual starting dose. Laboratory monitoring requires a complete blood count and urinalysis at least monthly.

Cyclophosphamide. Cyclophosphamide is an alkylating agent with similar properties to chlorambucil. The usual starting dose is 75–100 mg/day, but the dose can be increased to 150 mg/day if no marrow suppression is seen. Patients taking cyclophosphamide should be cautioned to maintain a good urine flow by adequate hydration (six to eight glasses of water a day), because cyclophosphamide can result in a hemorrhagic cystitis that can lead to bladder fibrosis. Adequate monitoring requires a complete blood count and urinalysis at least monthly.

Cyclosporin. Cyclosporin is an immunomodulator that is used extensively to suppress rejection in organ transplantation. Although it is still an experimental drug in the treatment of RA, it appears to have a benefit in RA that may be limited by nephrotoxicity (15). Use of this medication should be limited to those familiar with it. It is usually instituted in a dose no greater than 5 mg/kg/day with close monitoring of renal function. The dose is manipulated to keep the serum creatinine within 25% of the baseline pretreatment measurement.

Parenteral Gold Salts. Gold salts have been used in the treatment of RA for about 60 years, and their efficacy has become the standard against which other treatment programs are compared. Two parenteral preparations are used in this country, gold sodium thiomalate and aurothioglucose. These compounds are given by deep intramuscular injection at weekly intervals. Improvement in the disease is not expected for at least eight weeks. A test dose of 10 mg is first given and is often followed by a second dose of 25 mg the next week. Injections of 50 mg are then given weekly until a total cumulative dose of 1 g is reached or until toxicity occurs. If no improvement in disease activity has been observed, many rheumatologists will discontinue therapy while others will continue to a total dose of 2 g. The dosing interval is increased to two weeks if a favorable response is observed, and eventually lengthened to three or four weeks as tolerated. Exacerbations of disease activity will often respond to a reinstitution of weekly injections. Monitoring therapy with a urinalysis and a complete blood count with platelet count prior to each injection is mandatory.

Hydroxychloroquine. Hydroxychloroquine is an antimalarial compound that has milder toxicity, but is felt by some to be less effective than parenteral gold. The usual dose is 400 mg/day, which may be given in a single daily dose. Response is often delayed for several months and a trial of six months is indicated. The dose can often be decreased to 200 mg/day after 6 to 12 months of treatment. A baseline ophthalmologic slitlamp examination with interval examinations every three to six months can detect early retinal changes and minimize the chance of permanent visual impairment.

Methotrexate. Methotrexate is a folic acid antagonist. Experience with the drug in RA is relatively limited, and long-term toxicity is not yet clear (16). It can be given orally or by injection, and the usual starting dose is 7.5 mg/week either as a single dose or divided over 24 hours. Clinical response is generally seen in six to eight weeks. The dosage can be increased to 15 mg/week. Doses of more than this have been suggested for refractory patients, but such doses are not well studied in RA patients and are not generally recommended. Concomitant therapy with sulfa-containing antibiotics or the presence of HIV infection are contraindications to methotrexate use. Alcohol consumption, gross obesity, and diabetes may be aggravating factors to hepatic toxicity. While taking the drug, patients should have a complete blood count monthly and liver enzyme studies every two to three months. Liver biopsy remains controversial but many physicians recommend a liver biopsy after 1.5–2 g of cumulative methotrexate or every two to three years. Persistent elevations of transaminase enzymes or significant hypoalbuminemia may indicate the need for liver biopsy.

Penicillamine. Penicillamine is an analog of the amino acid cysteine and is a chelator of heavy metals. It is about as effective as parenteral gold or azathioprine, but has considerable toxicity. Penicillamine is initiated in a dose of 250 mg/day taken on an empty stomach—one hour prior to and two hours after eating. The dose is increased by 125–250 mg/day every one to two months. The usual maintenance dose is 750 mg/day. A variety of autoimmune syndromes are associated with penicillamine toxicity, including myasthenia gravis, polymyositis, pemphigus, and Goodpasture's syndrome (17). Monitoring therapy with a monthly urinalysis and a complete blood count with platelet count is recommended.

Sulfasalazine. Sulfasalazine is frequently used, particularly in the United Kingdom. It may have comparable efficacy to parenteral gold with less toxicity. Doses of 2–3 g/day are usually employed with benefit occurring in about three months. A six month trial is warranted.

APPROACH TO THERAPY

Traditionally, a pyramid approach to therapy of RA has been useful (Figure 10C–1). The foundation of the pyramid consists of education, rest, exercise, and social services, including sex counseling and marital and family advising, combined with basic antiinflammatory therapy with salicylates or other NSAIDs. The pyramid is buttressed on one side by the use of mechanical measures such as physical therapy and occupational therapy (including ambulation assistive devices and splints) and orthopedic surgery. The latter has greatly added to the functional ability of patients through reconstructive surgery and joint replacement surgery. The other side consists of temporary measures of help

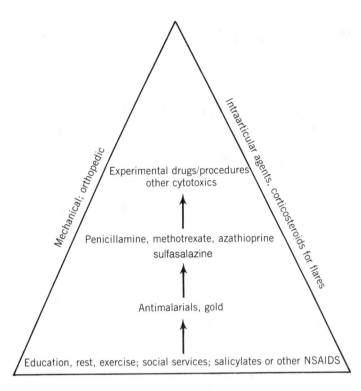

Fig. 10C-1. Treatment pyramid for rheumatoid arthritis.

such as oral or parenteral corticosteroids for general flares or intraarticular steroid injections for local flares.

Within the pyramid, additional therapies may be added to the foundation. The exact timing and order of added drugs is exceedingly variable from physician to physician, and there is no solid data to suggest which method is preferable. Much is based on the individual experience and inclination of the treating physician. SAARD therapy generally should not be delayed until erosions occur. This may be too late for any optimal effect. Earlier treatment is generally started in the presence of predictors of poor prognosis such as extraarticular disease, nodules, rheumatoid factor, and greater numbers of involved joints. As mentioned above, in the absence of severe, fulminant or life-threatening disease, less toxic drugs should be used first. These might include auranofin or hydroxychloroquine. The next level of drug therapy would include azathioprine, parenteral gold salts, methotrexate, sulfasalazine, or penicillamine. The last tier of therapy would be the cytotoxic drugs (chlorambucil and cyclophosphamide) or experimental agents or procedures.

There has been recent criticism of the pyramid approach (13,18). Some have suggested a reverse approach with the initiation of multiple medications and the gradual removal of treatments until the foundation therapy is reached. This treatment plan is similar to the approach oncologists use in malignancy. It has not been tested in controlled clinical trials, but it has many advocates and some anecdotal support.

MANAGEMENT OF COMPLICATIONS

Vasculitis. A necrotizing vasculitis can occur in RA patients with severe, nodular, and longstanding disease. The vasculitis can cause significant morbidity and be life-threatening. While scientific confirmation is still pending, aggressive treatment with high-dose corticosteroids is accepted as indicated therapy. Penicillamine may have benefit in less severe forms of vasculitis, while cyclophosphamide is indicated in severe disease.

Felty's Syndrome. This rare complication of severe seropositive RA consists of splenomegaly, granulocytopenia, leg ulcers, and recurrent infection. Splenectomy has only a variable affect

on leukopenia. There have been reports of improvement from SAARD therapy, particularly gold, methotrexate, and penicillamine. High-dose corticosteroids or lithium carbonate may provide short-term benefit with increases in neutrophil counts (19).

Atlantoaxial Subluxation. Disruption of the odontoid transverse cruciate ligament by synovial inflammation can lead to instability of the cervical atlantoaxial joint. Conservative treatment with cervical collars is indicated for patients with nonprogressive and mild neurologic symptoms, but surgical intervention is necessary for intractable pain or progressive neurologic disease.

Synovial Cysts. The most common synovial cyst is a popliteal cyst resulting from chronic knee effusions. Intraarticular steroids and rest are often effective but synovectomy may be required.

Rheumatoid Nodules. There is no effective treatment for subcutaneous nodules. Intralesional injections may provide temporary benefit. Surgical removal may help temporarily, but the nodules may recur. Surgery is generally indicated for infected nodules or nodules that mechanically interfere with usual activities. One study suggested that methotrexate may decrease nodules in some patients (20), but the experience of most rheumatologists is that methotrexate can more often lead to increased numbers of nodules.

Rheumatoid Lung Disease. Treatment of interstitial lung disease is generally futile. If therapy is to be useful, it needs to be instituted during the inflammatory stage and not after fibrosis has occurred. Gallium lung scans have been controversial as an indicator of inflammation. One approach is to obtain pulmonary blood gases and diffusion capacities followed by a three-month period of high-dose corticosteroids. If repeat pulmonary studies demonstrate improvement, continue the treatment; but if repeat studies are unchanged, taper and discontinue the corticosteroids.

H. James Williams, MD

1. Navarro AH: Physical therapy in the management of rheumatoid arthritis. Clin Rheumatol 1:125–130, 1983
2. Brooks PM, Day RO: Nonsteroidal antiinflammatory drugs—differences and similarities. New Engl J Med 324:1716–1725, 1991
3. Dromgoole SH, Furst DE, Paulus HE: Rational approaches to the use of salicylates in the treatment of rheumatoid arthritis. Semin Arthritis Rheum 11:257–283, 1981
4. Eisen SA, Miller DK, Woodward RS, et al: The effect of prescribed daily dose frequency on patient medication compliance. Arch Intern Med 150:1881–1884, 1990
5. Weiss MM: Corticosteroids in rheumatoid arthritis. Semin Arthritis Rheum 19:9–21, 1989
6. Klippel JH: Winning the battle, losing the war? Another editorial about rheumatoid arthritis. J Rheumatol 17:1118–1122, 1990
7. Furst DE: Rational use of disease-modifying antirheumatic drugs. Drugs 39:19–37, 1990
8. Wolfe F, Hawley DJ, Cathey MA: Termination of slow acting antirheumatic therapy in rheumatoid arthritis: a 14-year prospective evaluation of 1017 consecutive starts. J Rheumatol 17:994–1002, 1990
9. Situnayake RD, Grindulis KA, McConkey B: Longterm treatment of rheumatoid arthritis with sulfasalazine, gold, or penicillamine: a comparison using life table methods. Ann Rheum Dis 46:177–183, 1987
10. Fehlauer SC, Carson CW, Cannon GW: Two year follow up of treatment of rheumatoid arthritis with methotrexate: clinical experience in 124 patients. J Rheumatol 16:307–312, 1989
11. Klippel JH, Strober S, Wofsy D: New therapies for the rheumatic diseases. Bulletin Rheum Dis 38:1–8, 1989
12. Paulus HE: The use of combinations of disease-modifying antirheumatic agents in rheumatoid arthritis. Arthritis Rheum 33:113–120, 1990
13. Wilske KR, Healey LA: Remodeling the pyramid—a concept whose time has come. J Rheumatol 16:565–567, 1989
14. Ward JR, Williams HJ, Egger MJ, et al: Comparison of auranofin, gold sodium thiomalate, and placebo in the treatment of rheumatoid arthritis: a controlled clinical trial. Arthritis Rheum 26:1303–1315, 1983
15. Wilder RL: Treatment of the patient with rheumatoid arthritis refractory to standard therapy. JAMA 259:2446–2449, 1988
16. Tugwell P, Bennett K, Gent M: Methotrexate in rheumatoid arthritis: indication, contraindications, efficacy, and safety. Annals Intern Med 107:358–366, 1987
17. Jaffe IA: D-penicillamine. Bull Rheum Dis 6:948–952, 1978
18. Bensen WG, Bensen W, Adachi JD, et al: Remodelling the pyramid: the therapeutic target of rheumatoid arthritis. J Rheumatol 17:987–989, 1990
19. Rosenstein ED, Kramer N: Felty's and pseudo-Felty's syndromes. Semin Arthritis Rheum 21:129–142, 1991
20. Williams HJ, Willkens RF, Samuelson CO Jr., et al: Comparison of low-dose oral pulse methotrexate and placebo in the treatment of rheumatoid arthritis. Arthritis Rheum 28:721–730, 1985

11. SYSTEMIC LUPUS ERYTHEMATOSUS
A. Epidemiology, Pathology, and Pathogenesis

Systemic lupus erythematosus (SLE) is a prototypic autoimmune disease characterized by the production of antibodies to components of the cell nucleus in association with a diverse array of clinical manifestations. Because of the marked variability in the presentation of this disease, investigation into pathogenesis has been directed to understanding both the mechanisms of autoimmunity as well as the basis of its clinical heterogeneity and fluctuating activity. Whether SLE represents a single pathologic entity with variable expression or a group of related conditions remains unknown, however.

EPIDEMIOLOGY

Systemic lupus erythematosus is primarily a disease of young women. Its peak incidence occurs between the ages of 15 and 40, with a female to male ratio of approximately 5:1. Disease onset may occur from infancy to advanced age, although in both the pediatric and older onset patients, the female to male ratio approximates 2:1. The dramatic age and sex relationship in the incidence of SLE has suggested the importance of the hormonal milieu in disease pathogenesis.

The assessment of SLE prevalence has changed over time related to the recognition of its diversity, the utilization of more sensitive diagnostic tests, and the study of outpatient as well as inpatient populations. In a general outpatient population, SLE affects approximately 1 in 2,000 individuals, although its prevalence varies by racial and ethnic groups. In the United States, black and Hispanic individuals have a higher frequency of disease than whites (1). The prevalence of SLE is also affected by socioeconomic status, although dissecting the contributions of demographic factors to disease occurrence is difficult because of their interrelation.

Systemic lupus erythematosus shows a strong familial aggregation with a much higher frequency among first-degree relatives of patients. In extended families, SLE may, moreover, coexist with other autoimmune conditions such as hemolytic anemia, thyroiditis, and idiopathic thrombocytopenia purpura (2). In approximately 25% to 50% of monozygotic twins and 5% of dizygotic twins, SLE occurs concordantly. Despite the influence of heredity, most cases of SLE appear to be sporadic.

IMMUNOPATHOLOGY

The pathologic findings of SLE occur throughout the body and are manifested by inflammation, blood vessel abnormalities that encompass both bland vasculopathy and vasculitis, and immune complex deposition. Of organs involved in SLE, the pathology of the kidney is the best characterized since kidney biopsies are commonly performed to assess the disease course. In the past, kidney biopsy was frequently used to verify diagnosis, providing pathologic specimens of early as well as late lesions for study.

The kidney in SLE, as assessed by light, electron, and immunofluorescence microscopy, displays to a varying extent increases in mesangial cells and mesangial matrix, inflammation, cellular proliferation, basement membrane abnormalities, and immune complex deposition. These deposits are comprised of immunoglobulin M, G, and A (IgM, IgG and IgA) antibodies as well as complement components. On electron microscopy, the deposits can be visualized in the mesangium as well as subendothelial and subepithelial sides of the glomerular basement membrane (Fig. 11A–1).

Pathologic findings in the kidney are classified according to two grading schemes that together provide information for clinical staging. The World Health Organization (WHO) system is based on the extent and location of proliferative changes within glomeruli as well as alterations in the basement membrane (see Chapter 11B). These patterns are not static and, when repeat biopsies are performed, transitions between categories can be observed. The

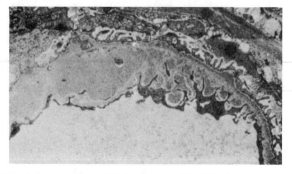

Fig. 11A–1. *Immune deposits in lupus nephritis. This electron micrograph illustrates large granular subendothelial immune deposits as well as smaller subepithelial and intramembranous deposits. Broadening and fusion of the foot processes are also present. (From the Revised Clinical Slide Collection on the Rheumatic Diseases)*

WHO classification scheme does not specify, however, the activity of lesions nor the presence of interstitial changes.

A second classification system is based on the signs of activity and chronicity (3). This system is especially useful in making treatment decisions, although it is based on nonspecific indicators of activity (Table 11A–1). With either scheme, lupus nephritis exhibits marked variability, differing in severity and pattern among patients, as illustrated in Fig. 11A–2. Whether these differences relate to the mechanisms of renal injury, the influence of therapy or intercurrent disease such as hypertension is unclear. Similarly, it is not certain that different patterns of nephritis in lupus patients are all stages of the same disease process rather than distinct clinical–pathologic subsets.

Like the kidney, the skin may be biopsied during the course of SLE, although the purpose is usually to substantiate diagnosis. Skin lesions in SLE demonstrate inflammation and degeneration at the dermal–epidermal junction with the basal or germinal layer being the primary site of injury. In these lesions, granular deposits of IgG as well as complement components can be demonstrated in a band-like pattern by immunofluorescence microscopy (Fig. 11A–3). Since both clinically involved and uninvolved skin show the characteristic band pattern, the IgG deposits may reflect the pervasiveness of immune complex deposition in SLE rather than a provocative factor. Necrotizing vasculitis involving small and medium sized vessels may also cause skin lesions.

Other organ systems affected by SLE are usually studied only at autopsy rather than during periods of active disease. Although these tissues may show nonspecific inflammation or vessel abnormalities, the pathologic findings are sometimes minimal, suggesting that mechanisms other than inflammation promote organ damage or dysfunction. For example, the central nervous system in SLE, despite its varied and dramatic clinical manifestations, may show only cortical microinfarcts and a bland vasculopathy with degenerative or proliferative changes; inflammation and necrosis indicative of vasculitis are only occasionally found. Furthermore, although the choroid plexus may contain IgG deposits,

Table 11A–1. *Histological classification of lupus nephritis*

Activity	Chronicity
1. Proliferative change	1. Sclerotic glomeruli
2. Necrosis/karyorrhexis	2. Fibrous crescents
3. Cellular crescents	3. Tubular atrophy
4. Leukocyte infiltration	4. Interstitial fibrosis
5. Hyaline thrombi	
6. Interstitial inflammation	

(Used with permission from reference 3.)

their presence is not directly correlated with clinical events and may only reflect incidental localization of immune complexes.

The heart in SLE may also show nonspecific foci of inflammation in the pericardium, myocardium, and endocardium, even in the absence of clinically significant manifestations. Verrucous endocarditis, known as Libman–Sacks endocarditis, is a classic pathologic finding of SLE and is manifested by vegetations (Fig. 11A–4). These lesions, most frequent at the mitral valve, consist of accumulations of immune complexes, inflammatory cells, fibrin, and necrotic debris.

Occlusive vasculopathy causes both venous and arterial thrombosis in SLE and is a common pathologic finding. Although coagulation is often a sequel of inflammation, autoantibodies to clotting system components may also directly trigger thrombotic events. The most notable serologic finding in patients with thrombosis is the presence of antibodies to phospholipid antigens including cardiolipin. These antibodies are part of the spectrum of SLE anticoagulants that are recognized by their interference with in vitro assays of clotting. The mechanisms by which these antibodies potentiate thrombosis in vivo is unknown (4).

Several other pathologic findings, prominent in SLE, have an uncertain relationship to inflammation. Patients with longstanding disease, including menstruating women lacking the other usual risk factors for cardiovascular disease, commonly develop atherosclerosis. It is unclear whether these lesions result from steroid-induced metabolic abnormalities, hypertension, or vascular changes caused by a chronic burden of immune complexes. Similarly, osteonecrosis as well as neurodegeneration in patients with chronic severe disease may arise from vasculopathy, drug side effects, or persistent immunologic insults. Periarterial fibrosis or "onion-skin" changes in the spleen has been considered pathognomonic of SLE.

IMMUNOPATHOGENESIS OF ANTINUCLEAR ANTIBODIES

The central immunologic disturbance in patients with SLE is autoantibody production. These antibodies are directed to a host of self molecules found in the nucleus and cytoplasm of cells as well as on their surface. In addition, SLE sera contain antibodies to soluble molecules such as IgG and coagulation factors. Because of the wide range of its antigenic targets, SLE is widely classified as a disease of generalized autoimmunity.

Among autoantibodies expressed in patient sera, those directed against components of the cell nucleus (antinuclear antibodies or ANA) are the most characteristic of SLE and are found in over 95% of patients (5). These antibodies bind DNA, RNA, and nuclear proteins as well as protein–nucleic acid complexes. Many of these autoantigenic molecules reside on particles, a feature shared with autoantigens in other rheumatic diseases. Cytoplasmic proteins associated with RNA are also prominent targets of autoreactivity in SLE. In general, these molecules play key roles in cell metabolism including cell division, RNA transcription, and RNA processing (Table 11A–2).

Although multiple ANA specificities occur in SLE, only two appear to be virtually unique to this disease. Antibodies to double-stranded DNA and an RNA–protein complex termed Sm are found essentially only in SLE patients and are included as serologic criteria in the classification of SLE (Appendix 3). Other ANA in SLE sera have a broader pattern of expression. Antibodies to the Ro (SS–A) and La (SS–B) antigens occur in SLE as well as Sjogren's syndrome. High titers of antibodies to RNP, a nuclear antigen structurally related to Sm, while very common in SLE, are also present in patients termed by some to have mixed connective tissue disease (see Chapter 16).

Among ANA in SLE, certain specificities frequently show concomitant expression and are called linked responses. These include antibodies to DNA and histones, antibodies to Sm and RNP, and antibodies to Ro and La. Since the target molecules in these sets are physically associated inside the cell, these findings suggest that ANA responses in SLE are directed to particles or complexes rather than isolated macromolecules.

Anti-DNA and anti-Sm antibodies show important differences in their patterns of expression and clinical associations. These antibodies are produced independently by patients, and while anti–DNA levels frequently fluctuate over time and may even disappear, anti–Sm levels remain more constant. It is of interest that the expression of anti–Sm varies significantly among racial and ethnic groups and appears much more common in black patients (6).

The anti–Sm and anti–DNA responses also differ in the nature of their target antigens. The Sm antigen is designated a snRNP (small nuclear ribonucleoprotein) and consists of a unique set of uridine-rich RNA molecules (U1, U2, U4, U5, U6) bound to a common group of core proteins as well as unique proteins specifically associated with the RNA molecules. Anti–DNA antibodies react to a conserved nucleic acid determinant widely present on DNA, whereas anti–Sm antibodies specifically target snRNP core proteins, (B, B′, D, and E) and not RNA. Similarly, anti–RNP antibodies bind to the proteins (A, C, and 70K) uniquely associated with U1 RNA.

Perhaps the most remarkable feature of the anti–DNA response is its association with immunopathologic events in SLE, in particular, glomerulonephritis. This role has been established by the correlation of serum levels of anti–DNA with periods of disease activity and the isolation of anti–DNA in enriched form from glomerular eluates of patients with active nephritis. The relationship between levels of anti–DNA and active renal disease is not invariable, however: some patients with active nephritis may lack serum anti–DNA while others with high levels of anti–DNA are clinically discordant and escape nephritis (7).

The occurrence of nephritis without anti–DNA may be explained by the pathogenicity of other autoantibody specificities. There is evidence that anti–Sm, anti–RNP, and anti–Ro autoantibodies among other ANA can have nephritogenic potential. Discrepancies between active nephritis and anti–DNA expression may also reflect problems in the serologic determinations. Some anti–DNA antibodies may be undetectable in the serum because of antigen binding, renal sequestration, or poor reactivity in commonly used clinical assays.

The converse situation of clinical quiescence despite serologic activity has suggested that only some anti–DNA provoke glomerulonephritis. Studies to delineate the basis of renal pathogenicity initially focused on the respective roles of antibodies to single-stranded (ss) DNA and double-stranded (ds) DNA. Anti–dsDNA antibodies are essentially exclusive to SLE, whereas anti–ssDNA antibodies have wider expression among inflammatory and infectious diseases. Both specificities frequently coexist in SLE, perhaps because many anti–DNA antibodies bind a common antigenic determinant present on both ss and dsDNA. In fact, sera binding only to dsDNA or ssDNA are rare in SLE. Since renal eluates show antibody activity to both DNA forms, it appears likely that, while the diagnostically important anti–dsDNA are pathogenic, antibodies with cross-reactive binding to ssDNA as well as antibodies only to ssDNA have a similar role.

Studies correlating immunochemical properties of anti–DNA antibodies with nephritis suggest several features that promote pathogenicity (Table 11A–3). Although assays to detect these properties have been developed, they are not used routinely for clinical monitoring. Indeed, most assays for anti–DNA are designed for their utility in diagnosis rather than for assessing disease activity.

In contrast to their role in nephritis, anti–DNA antibodies have not been clearly associated with other clinical events. Similarly, the pathogenicity of many other ANA found in SLE sera remains uncertain. The difficulties in ascertaining pathogenic ANA may relate to problems in quantifying disease activity and dissecting the contribution of individual autoantibodies in the presence of other specificities. Until recently, the assessment of most autoantibodies in SLE lacked quantitative immunoassays to detect fluctuations related to disease activity.

Although many ANA have never been adequately evaluated for pathogenicity, there is nevertheless evidence that certain autoantibodies other than anti–DNA have a clinical impact. Associations of other autoantibodies with disease events include antibodies to ribosomal P proteins (anti–P) with neuropsychiatric disease; antibodies to Ro with the neonatal lupus and subacute cutaneous lupus syndromes; antibodies to phospholipids with

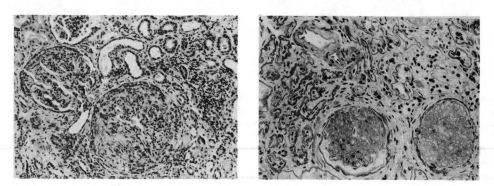

vascular thrombosis, thrombocytopenia, and recurrent abortion; and antibodies to blood cells and specific cytopenias.

Given the clinical diversity of SLE, the disease may be mediated by more than one autoantibody system and several immunopathogenic mechanisms. The contribution of ANA to these events has been difficult to understand, because the intracellular location of target antigens should protect them from antibody binding. Furthermore, these molecules are ubiquitous among cells and lack specificity for the tissues attacked in SLE. Thus, despite the essential role of these antigens in cell function, disruption of their activities by interaction with ANA does not appear to explain the tissue specificity observed in lupus.

Of clinical events in SLE, the mechanisms of nephritis have been most intensively studied because of the impact of kidney disease on morbidity and mortality. Clinical observations strongly suggest that SLE renal disease results from the deposition of immune complexes containing anti–DNA, since active nephritis is marked by elevation of anti–DNA levels with a corresponding depression of total hemolytic complement. The role of immune complexes in nephritis is substantiated by the finding of immunoglobulin and complement components in the kidney with localization to the region of the glomerular basement membrane. Since anti–DNA shows preferential renal deposition, these findings suggest that DNA–anti–DNA immune complexes are a major pathogenic species (8).

While renal injury in SLE may result from immune complexes, the composition, assembly, and trafficking of such complexes are poorly understood. Characterizing the constituents of circulating complexes has been difficult because of their low concentration; the amounts of DNA and anti–DNA in sera are miniscule. Using highly sensitive biochemical techniques, the nature of the DNA in complexes has been analyzed, however. This DNA exists as low molecular weight fragments and, while human in origin, shows a higher content of guanosine and cytosine residues than total cellular DNA. These findings have suggested that certain DNA regions have unusual antigenic properties that facilitate antibody interaction or immune complex formation. The identity

of other antigens in these complexes and the proportion of complexes that contain anti–DNA are not known, although these issues are important in understanding immunopathogenesis.

The formation of immune complexes in situ rather than within the circulation could also explain the paucity of DNA–anti–DNA complexes in serum. According to this mechanism, immune complexes would be assembled in the kidney on pieces of DNA adherent to the glomerular basement membrane. Like other charged antigens, DNA can bind to fixed sites on this structure, although this interaction may be further enhanced by the attachment of DNA to nuclear proteins. Once bound to the glomerulus, DNA could trap circulating anti–DNA to form complexes and activate complement.

Another mechanism by which anti–DNA antibodies may mediate nephritis is by direct interaction with glomerular antigens. Many anti–DNA antibodies are polyspecific and bind molecules other than DNA. Although differing in chemical composition, these molecules probably present a similar antigenic structure such as negative charge array. Among its polyspecific interactions, anti–DNA can bind heparan sulfate and laminin, two glomerular constituents. The binding of anti–DNA to these molecules could directly activate complement to incite local inflammatory damage. This binding could also anchor immune complexes to kidney sites whether they are formed in the circulation or in situ (9).

The pathogenesis of other SLE manifestations is less well understood, although immune complex deposition at relevant tissue sites has generally been considered a likely mechanism. Indeed, the frequent association of depressed complement levels and signs of vasculitis with active SLE suggests that immune complexes are important agents for initiating or exacerbating organ system damage. These considerations do not exclude the possibility that tissue injury in SLE results from either cell-mediated cytotoxicity or direct antibody attack on target tissues.

DETERMINANTS OF DISEASE SUSCEPTIBILITY

Studies of patients with SLE suggest that the disease is caused by genetically determined immune abnormalities that can be triggered by both exogenous and endogenous factors. While the predisposition to disease is hereditary, it is likely to be multigenic in origin and involve different sets of genes in different individu-

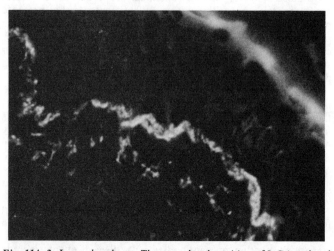

Fig. 11A–3. Lupus band test. The granular deposition of IgG in a band-like pattern is illustrated by immunfluorescence staining of skin from a patient with discoid lupus (from the Revised Clinical Slide Collection on the Rheumatic Diseases).

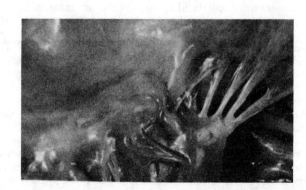

Fig. 11A–4. Libman–Sacks endocarditis. Verrucae are evident immediately below the insertions of the chordae tendinae to the mitral valve (from the Revised Clinical Slide Collection on the Rheumatic Diseases).

Table 11A–2. *Principal antinuclear antibodies in SLE*

Specificity	Target Antigen	Function	Frequency in SLE (%)
Native DNA	dsDNA	genetic information	40
Denatured DNA	ssDNA	genetic information	70
Histones	H1,H2A,H2B,H3,H4	nucleosome structure	70
Sm	snRNP proteins B,B',D,E	spliceosome component, RNA processing	30
U1RNP	snRNP proteins A,C,70K	spliceosome component, RNA processing	32
Ro (SS-A)	60 and 52 kDa proteins, complexed with Y1-Y5 RNA	unknown	35
La (SS-B)	48 kDa protein complexed with various small RNA	regulation of RNA polymerase 3 transcription	15
Ku	86 and 66 kDa proteins	DNA binding	3
PCNA/cyclin	36 kDa protein	auxillary protein of DNA polymerase d	10
Ribosomal RNP	38, 16, and 15 kDa phosphoproteins, associated with ribosomes	protein synthesis	10

(Used with permission in modified form from reference 5.)

als. This conclusion is supported by analysis of disease expression in identical and non-identical twins, extended families, and large populations surveyed for various genetic markers.

The analysis of genetic susceptibility is based primarily on the search for gene polymorphisms with an enhanced frequency in patients compared to control populations. Most of the markers tested involve genes for known immune response phenomena, on the assumptions that SLE results from an aberrant immune response to some antigen, whether self or foreign, and that the same genes regulate both normal and autoimmune responses.

Of genetic elements determining immune responses, the major histocompatibility complex (MHC) has been most intensively scrutinized for its contribution to human SLE. Population-based studies, using a variety of MHC gene markers, indicate that the susceptibility to SLE, like many other autoimmune diseases in man, involves class II gene polymorphisms. This association is consistent with the function of class II gene products. These molecules are found on the surface of antigen-presenting cells and form complexes with peptide fragments of processed antigens for recognition by T cells. Since sequence differences among class II molecules affect their peptide binding ability, polymorphisms of these molecules determine, at the level of antigen presentation, the generation of responses to specific antigens, presumably including self molecules (10).

An association of human leukocyte antigens (HLA) DR2 and DR3 (and recently defined subspecificities) with SLE is commonly observed, with these alleles producing a relative risk of disease of approximately 2–5. The magnitude of this effect is variable among population groups, however, with some studies failing to show an appreciable contribution of class II genes to disease susceptibility (11). Assessing these genetic relationships can be difficult, however, because class II alleles are differentially expressed in ethnic groups, including Caucasian nationalities. Unless control populations are carefully matched with patients, the interpretation of any association may be confounded by the effects of ethnicity.

The analysis of class II disease associations is also complicated by the existence of extended HLA haplotypes in which class II genes are in linkage disequilibrium with other potential susceptibility genes. Since the MHC is rich in genes for immune system elements, the association of disease with a class II marker does not denote a specific functional abnormality promoting pathogenesis. Indeed, a contribution of class II genes to SLE susceptibility has been difficult to conceptualize. These genes regulate responses in an antigen-specific manner whereas SLE is characterized by responses to a host of self antigens seemingly unrelated in sequence and structure.

In contrast to their uncertain role in disease susceptibility, class II genes appear to exert a more decisive influence on the production of specific ANA. The response to several SLE autoantigens has been associated with particular class II alleles as well as short amino acid sequences found in different class II specificities. These sequences are denoted as shared epitopes and may influence antigen specific responses by virtue of their location at contact points of class II molecules with processed peptides (12).

Among other MHC gene systems, inherited complement deficiencies show a powerful effect on disease susceptibility that is demonstrable among racial and ethnic groups. Complement components, in particular C4a and C4b, show striking genetic polymorphism, allowing identification of complotypes by serologic as well as molecular techniques. A deficiency of C4a molecules (null alleles) is usually attributable to gene deletions and occurs commonly. As many as 80% of SLE patients have null alleles irrespective of ethnic background, with homozygous C4a deficiency conferring a very high risk for SLE. Since C4a null alleles are part of an extended HLA haplotype with the markers HLA–B8 and DR3, the influence of these class I and class II alleles on disease susceptibility may reflect linkage disequilibrium with complement deficiency. Systemic lupus erythematosus is also associated with inherited deficiency of C1q, C1r/s, and C2 (13).

An association of SLE with inherited complement deficiency is perhaps unexpected because of the prominence of immune complex deposition and complement consumption in this disease. A decrease in complement activity could, however, promote disease susceptibility by impairing the neutralization and clearance of foreign antigen. With a burden of persistent antigen, the immune system would be excessively stimulated, allowing the emergence of autoreactivity. Since C4a and C4b differ in their interaction with antigens based on chemical composition, absence of either molecule would create only a selective deficiency state without jeopardizing overall host defenses. In contrast, deficiencies of late components of complement lead to bacterial infections rather than autoimmunity.

Immunoglobulin and T cell receptor (TCR) gene systems have also been investigated as possible susceptibility factors in SLE. These are both large multigene families that utilize a variety of genetic and somatic strategies to generate diversity among recognition structures. These include the construction of variable regions from smaller gene segments; nontemplate nucleotide additions at junctional regions; combinatorial diversity from polypeptide chain pairing; and in the case of immunoglobulins, variable region somatic mutations. These mutations accumulate as a response matures, leading to both higher affinity antibodies and novel specificities including antibodies to self (14). Given the enormous diversity inherent in the Ig and TCR systems, it seems unlikely that structural gene polymorphisms could promote autoimmunity by allowing the unique production of autoreactive B or T cells in the genetically predisposed individual.

Despite these theoretical considerations, an association of SLE with a polymorphism in the gene for the T cell α receptor chain has been demonstrated in population studies (15). Furthermore, the production of certain autoantibodies, including anti-Ro, appears linked to the β chain locus of the T cell receptor.

Table 11A–3. *Properties of pathogenic anti–DNA antibodies*

Quantity	Polyreactivity
Isotype	Cationic charge
Avidity	Idiotype
Ability to fix complement	Variable region sequences
Fine specificity for DNA	Disease induction in mice

These observations suggest that the array of TCR expressed by an individual is genetically constrained and could affect the generation of T cells that recognize self (16).

The contributions of Ig genes to a SLE diathesis is less clear, reflecting in part the difficulties in detecting inherited variants in this large multigene family. Informative markers for variable region gene polymorphisms have been limited, although studies of heavy chain allotypes suggest that SLE patients may preferentially express certain Gm markers. In addition to polymorphisms in the coding regions of antibody genes, gene deletions could cause immune system changes promoting autoimmunity. Thus, patients with both SLE and rheumatoid arthritis may lack a gene for a developmentally regulated heavy chain that can encode both anti–DNA and rheumatoid factors. The absence of this gene might distort the generation of the variable region gene repertoire during ontogeny creating a bias toward autoreactivity. In addition, a deficiency in rheumatoid factors, some of which serve a physiologic role in normal immunity, could impair host defense leading to antigen persistence and prolonged immune stimulation. This situation would be similar to a complement deficiency state (17).

Genetic studies suggest possible explanations for the clinical and serologic heterogeneity of patients with SLE. If conventional immune response genes also govern autoantibody production, the serologic profile of a patient would reflect the genotype and be predictable on the basis of MHC haplotype as well as TCR and Ig gene polymorphisms. Clinical disease manifestations would show similar hereditary influences to the extent that the production of the pathogenic antibodies is determined by these same polymorphic systems.

While suggesting an origin for the clinical heterogeneity of SLE, existing genetic studies have not yet explained the propensity of certain ethnic groups for SLE nor the variability in prognosis. The differences in disease prevalence and severity may nevertheless be genetically determined and, as the human genome is more extensively mapped, a susceptibility gene with differential expression in ethnic groups may be found. It remains possible, however, that the differences in disease course among ethnic groups relates solely to their environment and other social factors (18).

GENETICS OF MURINE LUPUS

Several strains of inbred mice with inherited lupus-like disease have now been described. These mice all display features of SLE such as ANA production, immune complex glomerulonephritis, lymphadenopathy, and abnormal B and T cell function mimicking the human situation. These strains differ in the expression of certain serologic and clinical findings such as anti–Sm, hemolytic anemia, and arthritis. Among these animals, disease is expressed with very high penetrance, although the occurrence of disease among males and females differs among strains. Because these mice were discovered fortuitously during breeding experiments with mice of various origins, the observations suggest that genes for SLE may be widely present among species (19).

Studies of murine lupus provide an important perspective on disease susceptibility because of the genetic manipulations possible in this species. Among various lupus strains described (NZB, NZB/NZW, MRL-lpr/lpr, BXSB and C3H-gld/gld), the development of a full-blown lupus syndrome requires multiple unlinked genes, some of which are present in otherwise normal mice. While single mutant genes (lpr, gld and Yaa) can accelerate disease and promote anti–DNA production, they must act in concert with other genes to induce nephritis. Mice expressing only mutant accelerating genes resemble patients with SLE who are serologically active but clinically quiescent. The number and linkage of the autosomal genes for nephritis in mice are not known.

In contrast to human SLE, the lupus strains lack a common MHC class I or II marker that can be identified as a susceptibility factor. Nevertheless, MHC molecules may contribute to pathogenesis as shown by formal genetic analysis of disease in New Zealand mice (NZB, NZB/NZW) as well the pattern of disease expression in congenic NZB mice with mutations in their class II

genes. Such mice have dramatically enhanced anti–DNA production as well as nephritis, suggesting that self antigen presentation may be influenced by the structure of the Class II molecules (20).

Among lupus mice, New Zealand strains have an MHC-linked deficiency in the expression of the proinflammatory cytokine tumor necrosis factor (TNF). This deficiency state, which has a counterpart in humans, may be pathogenic, because administration of TNF to mice with low endogenous production ameliorates disease. Finally, although a TCR gene polymorphism may contribute to disease in New Zealand mice, there is no evidence as yet that disease in any strain is linked to the Ig gene loci.

IMMUNE CELL DISTURBANCES IN SLE

Autoantibody production in SLE occurs in the setting of generalized immune cell abnormalities that involve the B cell, T cell, and monocyte lineages. These disturbances affect both the number and function of cells as manifested by the surface marker expression, state of activation, and response to stimulation. Since similar disturbances characterize other autoimmune and inflammatory diseases, they may represent a consequence of disease rather than a cause. However, the persistence of some abnormalities during inactive disease and expression of these abnormalities in unaffected relatives of SLE patients suggests their potential role as inherited susceptibility factors (21).

Although the origin of immunologic disturbances in patients is unclear, studies with lupus mice demonstrate that functional immune cell disturbances can be genetically determined and predate autoantibody production. The nature of these immunoregulatory disturbances and their linkage relationships differ among strains. In New Zealand mice, for example, both B and T cells are intrinsically abnormal. B cells hyperrespond to various stimuli whereas T cells resist tolerance induction. These disturbances result from different genes since they segregate independently in crosses with normal mice. In MRL-lpr/lpr mice, B and T cell disturbances are both the consequence of the lpr gene defect. The T cell abnormality is characterized by lymphoproliferation as well as aberrant signal transduction and cytokine production. The B cell abnormality is more subtle and is associated with enhanced autoantibody production in collaboration with lpr T cells.

Whatever their origin, these cellular immune disturbances appear to promote B cell hyperactivity leading to hyperglobulinemia, increased numbers of antibody-producing cells, and heightened responses to many antigens, both self and foreign. Generalized or polyclonal B cell activation appears sufficient to induce certain autoantibodies since the magnitude of these responses is proportional to the degree of hyperglobulinemia. The induction of anti–DNA by polyclonal activation also occurs in normal mice treated by the B cell mitogen lipopolysaccharide and reflects the presence of a large precursor population for so-called natural autoantibodies in the normal B cell repertoire. These IgM antibodies bind polyspecifically to both foreign and self antigens and are generally considered to be nonpathogenic. Their high frequency and conservation among species has suggested a physiologic role in normal immunity.

While nonspecific immune activation can provoke certain ANA responses, it does not appear to be the major mechanism for the induction of pathogenic autoantibodies, especially anti–DNA. Levels of these antibodies far exceed the extent of hyperglobulinemia. In addition, anti–DNA antibodies have features indicative of in vivo antigen selection by a receptor-driven mechanism, most significantly, variable region somatic mutations of the replacement type. These mutations can produce sequence changes in the complementarity determining regions of an antibody that increase DNA binding activity and specificity for dsDNA. The ability of DNA to drive autoantibody production in SLE contrasts with its poor immunogenicity when administered to normal animals. This discrepancy suggests that lupus patients either have a unique capacity to respond to DNA or, alternatively, are exposed to DNA in a much more potently immunogenic form during the course of disease.

The specificity of ANA directed to distinct nuclear proteins supports the hypothesis that these responses may be antigen driven. Many of these antigens have been cloned and sequenced by molecular genetic techniques providing novel reagents to map epitope structure. Using either cloned protein fragments or synthetic peptides as antigens, immunochemical studies have demonstrated that ANA bind multiple independent determinants found in different regions of these proteins. In this respect, ANA responses resemble responses to foreign antigens following immunization. Spontaneous ANA responses may differ from responses induced to these proteins in normal animals in their specificity for antigenic determinants of functional significance such as catalytic sites of enzymes, as well as their inability to bind to very short linear peptides. Whether these differences denote an important facet of immunoregulatory disturbances in SLE is not known.

The pattern of binding ANA minimizes the possibility that molecular mimicry is the exclusive etiology for autoimmunity in SLE. According to this mechanism, autoantibody production might be stimulated by a foreign antigen bearing an amino acid sequence or antigenic structure resembling a self molecule. This type of cross-reactivity has been hypothesized for many different autoimmune diseases. It has been suggested for SLE because of the sequence similarity between certain nuclear antigens and viral and bacterial products. Thus, the 70K RNP antigen shows a region of sequence homology with the p30^{gag} retrovirus protein, while the Ro protein has several sequence regions similar to a nucleocapsid protein of vesicular stomatitis virus. If SLE autoantibodies were to develop from molecular mimicry, however, they would be expected to bind self antigen only at sites of homology with foreign antigen rather than the entire molecule as has been observed. These arguments, while suggesting that self antigen rather than a mimic sustains the mature antibody response, do not eliminate the possibility that a cross-reactive response to a foreign antigen initiates ANA production (22).

Studies analyzing both the genetics of SLE as well as the pattern of ANA production both strongly suggest that T cells are important to disease pathogenesis. In the murine models of lupus, the depletion of helper T cells by monoclonal antibody treatment abrogates autoantibody production and clinical disease manifestations. The nature of the T cells helping ANA responses and the process of self antigen presentation, however, have not yet been elucidated. It is unclear whether self antigen is presented from endogenous sources or is first released from damaged or dying cells and then processed and presented by conventional antigen presenting cells. The mechanisms of T cell recognition of DNA is especially obscure, because models of antigen presentation by class II molecules are based on proteins and not nucleic acids. There is no evidence as yet that DNA, or any other nucleic acid, can associate with MHC molecules for presentation.

The mechanisms of T cell help in autoantibody responses may differ from conventional responses because of the physical nature of the antigens. Most SLE antigens exist as complexes or particles, such as nucleosomes, containing multiple protein and nucleic acid species. These structures bear repeating determinants that could promote their binding to B cells as well as other antigen presenting cells. In addition, the protein components themselves have features that could influence immunogenicity. These include a high charge content, local regions of positive and negative charge, a coiled structure, and repeating sequence motifs. Because these antigens may effectively trigger B cell activation by multivalent binding, T cell help for autoimmune responses could be delivered by nonspecifically activated T cells. Alternatively, T cell reactivity to these antigens could be elicited to only one protein on a complex, allowing a single T helper cell to collaborate with B cells for multiple protein and nucleic acid determinants. Table 11A–4 lists features of ANA responses indicative of antigen drive.

TRIGGERING EVENTS

Although inheritance may create a predisposition to SLE, the initiation of disease and its temporal variation in intensity likely result from environmental and other exogenous factors. Among these potential influences are the following: infectious agents that could both induce specific responses by molecular mimicry as well as perturb overall immunoregulation; stress, which can provoke neuroendocrine changes affecting immune cell function; diet, which can affect production of inflammatory mediators; toxins, including drugs, which could modify cellular responsiveness as well as the immunogenicity of self antigens; and physical agents such as sunlight, which can cause inflammation and tissue damage. The impingement of these factors on the predisposed individual is likely to be highly variable and could be a further explanation for disease heterogeneity as well its alternating periods of flare and remission.

David S. Pisetsky, MD, PhD

1. Fessel WJ: Systemic lupus erythematosus in the community: incidence, prevalence, outcome, and first symptoms; the high prevalence in black women. Arch Intern Med 134:1027–1035, 1974
2. Reveille JD, Bias WB, Winkelstein JA, et al: Familial systemic lupus erythematosus: immunogenetic studies in eight families. Medicine 62:21–35, 1983
3. Balow JE: Therapeutic trials in lupus nephritis. Nephron 27:171–176, 1981
4. Alarcon-Segovia D, Deleze M, Oria CV, et al: Antiphospholipid antibodies and the antiphospholipid syndrome in systemic lupus erythematosus: a prospective analysis of 500 consecutive patients. Medicine 68:353–365, 1989
5. Tan EM: Antinuclear antibodies: diagnostic markers for autoimmune diseases and probes for cell biology. Adv Immunol 44:93–151, 1989
6. Arnett FC, Hamilton RG, Roebber MG, et al: Increased frequencies of Sm and nRNP autoantibodies in American blacks compared to whites with systemic lupus erythematosus. J Rheum 15:1773–1776, 1988
7. Emlen W, Pisetsky DS, Taylor RP: Antibodies to DNA: a perspective. Arthritis Rheum 29:1417–1426, 1986
8. Fournie GJ: Circulating DNA and lupus nephritis. Kidney Internal 33:487–497, 1988
9. Sabbaga J, Pankewycz OG, Lufft V, et al: Cross-reactivity distinguishes serum and nephritogenic anti–DNA antibodies in human lupus from their natural counterparts in normal serum. J Autoimm 3:215–235, 1990
10. Todd JA, Acha-Orbea H, Bell JI, et al: A molecular basis for MHC class II—associated autoimmunity. Science 240:1003–1009, 1988
11. Howard PF, Hochberg MC, Bias WB, et al: Relationship between C4 null genes, HLA–D region antigens, and genetic susceptibility to systemic lupus erythematosus in Caucasian and Black Americans. Amer J Med 81:187–193, 1986
12. Reveille JD, Macleod MJ, Whittington K, et al: Specific amino acid residues in the second hypervariable region of HLA–DQA1 and DQB1 chain genes promote the Ro (SS–A)/LA (SS–B) autoantibody responses. J Immunol 146:3871–3876, 1991
13. Atkinson JP: Complement activation and complement receptors in systemic lupus erythematosus. Springer Semin Immunopathol 9:179–194, 1986
14. Davidson A, Shefner R, Livneh A, et al: The role of somatic mutation of immunoglobulin genes in autoimmunity. Ann Rev Immunol 5:85–108, 1987
15. Tebib JG, Alcocer-Varela J, Alarcon-Segovia D, et al: Association between a T cell receptor restriction fragment length polymorphism and systemic lupus erythematosus. J Clin Invest 86:1961–1967, 1990
16. Frank MB, McArthur R, Harley JB, et al: Anti-Ro (SSA) autoantibodies are associated with T cell receptor β genes in systemic lupus erythematosus patients. J Clin Invest 85:33–39, 1990
17. Yang P-M, Olsen NJ, Siminovitch KA, et al: Possible deletion of a developmentally regulated heavy-chain variable region gene in autoimmune diseases. Proc Natl Acad Sci USA 87:7907–7911, 1990
18. Liang MH, Partridge AJ, Daltroy LH, et al: Strategies for reducing excess morbidity and mortality in blacks with systemic lupus erythematosus. Arthritis Rheum 34:1187–1196, 1991
19. Smith HR, Steinberg AD: Autoimmunity—a perspective. Ann Rev Immunol 1:175–210, 1983
20. Chiang G-L, Bearer E, Ansari A, et al: The bm12 mutation and autoantibodies to dsDNA in NZB.H-2^{bm12} mice. J Immunol 145:94–101, 1990
21. Shoenfeld Y, Schwartz RS: Immunologic and genetic factors in autoimmune diseases. N Engl J Med 311:1019–1029, 1984
22. Query CC, Keene JD: A human autoimmune protein associated with U1 RNA contains a region of homology that is cross-reactive with retroviral p30^{gag} antigen. Cell 51:211–220, 1987

Table 11A–4. *Evidence for antigen drive in ANA responses*

IgG isotype
Levels disproportionate to hyperglobulinemia
High affinity antigen binding
Targeting of multiple epitopes
MHC association
Clonal restriction in individuals
Utilization of multiple variable region genes
Variable region somatic mutations
Elimination by anti-T cell reagents

B. Clinical Features

The frequencies of various clinical manifestations at presentation or at any time during the course of systemic lupus are shown in Table 11B–1. Constitutional complaints are common presenting features of SLE. The presence of malaise, overwhelming fatigue, fever, and weight loss are nonspecific manifestations that affect most patients at some time in their disease. However, the presence of these features does not help the physician diagnose the disease, or identify a flare, since they may just as likely represent the development of infection or of fibromyalgia. It is only with a high index of suspicion, a careful history and physical examination, and appropriate laboratory confirmation that the diagnosis will become obvious.

SKIN MANIFESTATIONS

The most recognized skin manifestation of SLE is the "butterfly" rash (Fig. 11B–1), commonly precipitated by exposure to sunlight. It usually presents acutely as an erythematous elevated lesion, pruritic or painful, in a malar distribution. Histologically the lesions may show only nonspecific inflammation, although the classic immune deposits at the dermal–epidermal junction may be seen by immunofluorescence. Other acute lesions include generalized erythema, which may or may not be photosensitive, and bullous lesions (1). The majority of patients with SLE demonstrate photosensitivity. In addition to the skin reaction, patients may develop exacerbation of their systemic disease with sun exposure.

Subacute cutaneous lupus erythematosus (SCLE) is a relatively distinct cutaneous lesion, which is nonfixed, nonscarring, exacerbating, and remitting (1). Lesions commonly occur in sun-exposed areas, may be generalized, and may evolve further into the papulosquamous variant, which mimics psoriasis or lichen planus. Alternatively, they may merge and form polycyclic or annular lesions that mimic erythema annulare centrifugum (Fig. 11B–2). Patients with SCLE commonly have antibody to Ro (SSA), which has also been demonstrated in the lesion.

Discoid lesions are chronic cutaneous lesions, which may occur in the absence of any systemic manifestations, or may be a manifestation of SLE. These lesions often begin as erythematous papules or plaques, with scaling that may become thick and adherent with a hypopigmented central area. They may produce scarring with central atrophy (Fig. 11B–3).

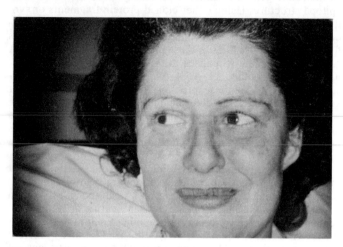

Fig. 11B–1. *Malar rash in a patient with SLE.*

Alopecia is a common feature of SLE. Hair loss may be diffuse or patchy. When associated with exacerbation of the disease, hair tends to regrow once the disease is under control. Alternatively, it may result from the extensive scarring of discoid lesions, in which case it may be permanent. Alopecia may also be drug-induced secondary to corticosteroids or cytotoxic drugs.

Mucous membrane lesions include mouth ulcers, vaginal ulcers, and nasal septal erosions. Panniculitis, urticarial lesions, and vasculitis may also be seen in SLE. Vasculitic lesions manifest as palpable purpura, nail-fold infarcts or digital ulcerations, splinter hemorrhages, pulp-space and palmar vasculitic lesions simulating Osler's nodes and Janeway spots. In addition, urticaria and livedo reticularis may represent a vasculitic process. There can occasionally be subcutaneous nodules similar to those seen in rheumatoid arthritis (RA).

MUSCULOSKELETAL MANIFESTATIONS

Arthralgias and arthritis constitute the most common presenting manifestations of SLE. Acute arthritis may involve any joint, but typically the small joints of the hands, wrists, and knees are involved. It may be migratory or persistent and chronic (2). Most cases are symmetric but a significant percent may have an asymmetric polyarthritis. Swelling is usually due to soft tissue thickening with effusions tending to be relatively small. Synovial fluid analysis generally reveals a mildly inflammatory fluid although leukocyte counts and PMN percentages may be high even without infection. There may be LE cells, or diminished complement levels. Unlike RA, the arthritis of SLE is typically not erosive or destructive of bone. However, joint deformities may occur. Ulnar deviation of the fingers, swan neck deformities, and sublux-

Table 11B–1. Frequency of lupus manifestations at onset and at any time during the course of lupus

Manifestations	Onset (108)*	Anytime (605)*
Constitutional	73%	84%
Arthritis	56%	63%
Arthralgia	77%	85%
Skin	57%	81%
Mucous membranes	18%	54%
Pleurisy	23%	37%
Lung	9%	17%
Pericarditis	20%	29%
Myocarditis	1%	4%
Raynaud's	33%	58%
Thrombophlebitis	2%	8%
Vasculitis	10%	37%
Renal	44%	77%
Nephrotic syndrome	5%	11%
Azotemia	3%	8%
CNS	24%	54%
Cytoid bodies	5%	5%
Gastrointestinal	22%	47%
Pancreatitis	1%	4%
Lymphadenopathy	25%	32%
Myositis	7%	5%

University of Toronto; frequency at onset based on 108 patients diagnosed at Lupus Clinic, and frequency at anytime for 605 patients registered prior to December, 1990.

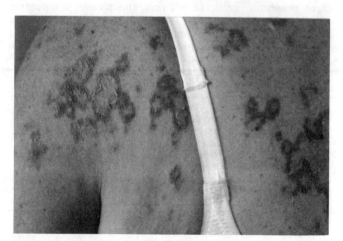

Fig. 11B–2. *Subacute cutaneous lupus lesions.*

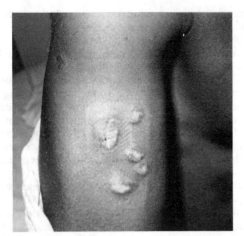

Fig. 11B–3. Discoid lupus lesions.

ations (Fig. 11B–4) are initially reversible but can become fixed. This pattern of nonerosive but deforming disease has been called *Jaccoud's arthritis*. Radiographic findings in such patients reveal no erosions even when severe subluxations are present. Occasionally one may see hook-like processes of the metacarpal heads late in the disease similar to those described in post-rheumatic fever Jaccoud's syndrome. Tenosynovitis and tendon ruptures may occur in patients with SLE.

Two complications of SLE or its treatment, septic arthritis and osteonecrosis, may confuse the diagnosis of acute synovitis in SLE. Septic arthritis is uncommon in SLE, despite the immunosuppressed state, but it should be suspected when one joint is inflamed out of proportion to all others. Patients with SLE may complain of muscle pain and weakness. True muscle inflammation may be seen in patients with SLE. However, the histologic features of myositis in SLE may not be as striking as those in idiopathic polymyositis/dermatomyositis. Patients with SLE may develop a drug-related myopathy secondary to corticosteroids or as a complication of antimalarials. In the differential diagnosis of musculoskeletal complaints in patients with SLE the possibility of secondary fibromyalgia must be considered (3).

RENAL MANIFESTATIONS

Specific symptoms referable to the kidney are not volunteered by the patient until there is advanced nephrotic syndrome or renal failure. The presence of proteinuria of more than 500 mg/24 hr (or more than 3+ on a dipstick if quantitative evaluation is not done), the presence of casts (including red blood cells, hemoglobin, granular, tubular, or mixed), the presence of hematuria (>5 rbc/high power field), or pyuria (>5 wbc/high power field), in the absence of infection, and the detection of an elevated serum

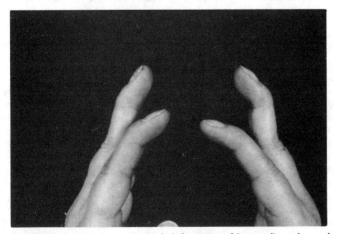

Fig. 11B–4. Correctable swan neck deformities of Jaccoud's arthropathy in a patient with SLE.

Table 11B–2. *WHO classification of lupus nephritis in 148 biopsies*

I. Normal glomeruli	12
a) Nil (by all techniques)	3
b) Normal by light but deposits on electron microscopy or immunofluorescence.	
II. Pure mesangial alterations (mesangiopathy)	62
a) Mesangial widening and/or mild hypercellularity	51
b) Moderate hypercellularity	11
III. A. Focal segmental glomerulonephritis	19
a) 'Active' necrotizing lesions	14
b) 'Active' and sclerosing lesions	5
III. B. Focal proliferative glomerulonephritis	3
a) 'Active' necrotizing lesions	1
b) 'Active' and sclerosing lesions	2
IV. Diffuse glomerulonephritis	37
a) Without segmental lesions	9
b) With 'active' necrotizing lesions	13
c) With 'active' and sclerosing lesions	14
d) With sclerosing lesions	1
V. Diffuse membranous glomerulonephritis	11
a) Pure membranous glomerulonephritis	2
b) Associated with lesions of category II	7
c) Associated with lesions of category III	0
d) Associated with lesions of category IV	2
VI. Advanced sclerosing glomerulonephritis	4

creatinine have been recognized as evidence for clinical renal disease.

A renal biopsy may provide a more accurate documentation of renal disease. Most SLE patients manifest some abnormality on renal biopsy, although in some cases it is only possible to document it with special techniques such as immunofluorescence or electron microscopy. In a study of clinical–morphologic features in 148 patients with SLE, only 3 patients with truly normal biopsies were found (4) (Table 11B–2). Mesangial alterations (WHO Class II) were most common, occurring in 62 biopsies. Twenty-two patients demonstrated focal (Class IIIA and B) glomerulonephritis, while 37 had diffuse proliferative glomerulonephritis (Class IV). In 11 patients, a predominantly membranous lesion was found (Class V), while 4 biopsies demonstrated advanced sclerosis (Class VI). Specific morphologic features seen on kidney biopsies have prognostic implications (5). The presence of chronic lesions is clearly associated with lower survival, both for the patient and the kidney (see Chapter 11A).

NEUROPSYCHIATRIC MANIFESTATIONS

Neuropsychiatric manifestations are common in SLE and may present in the context of active SLE elsewhere, or as an isolated event (6). There is a wide spectrum of clinical manifestations, which may be grouped into neurologic (including the central nervous system, cranial, and peripheral nerves) and psychiatric (including psychosis and severe depression). Many patients present with mixed neurologic and psychiatric manifestations.

Table 11B–3. *Neuropsychiatric manifestations at presentation and at any time during the course of SLE*

Manifestation	At presentation (108)	Any time (605)
Headache	15%	40%
Seizures	3%	14%
Cerebral vascular accidents	1%	7%
Cranial neuropathy	1%	6%
Peripheral neuropathy	4%	16%
Organic brain syndrome	7%	16%
Psychoneurosis	5%	22%
Psychosis	2%	6%

* University of Toronto; frequency at onset based on 108 patients diagnosed at Lupus Clinic, and frequency at anytime for 605 patients registered prior to December, 1990.

Patients may have more than one manifestation at a time, making their classification more difficult.

Intractable headaches that are unresponsive to narcotic analgesics are common features both at presentation and at follow-up (Table 11B–3). The headaches may be migrainous in type and may accompany other neuropsychiatric features. Seizures may be either focal or generalized. The occurrence of chorea (resembling Sydenham's chorea) in SLE has also been recognized, usually early in the course of the disease. Its association with the anticardiolipin antibody has recently been suggested. Cerebrovascular accidents and subarachnoid hemorrhage, like chorea, have been related to the anticardiolipin syndrome. Cranial neuropathies may present with visual defects, blindness, papilledema, nystagmus or ptosis, tinnitus and vertigo, or facial palsy.

The retinopathy seen in patients with SLE develops as a consequence of vasculitis and correlates with the presence of central nervous system involvement (7). Peripheral neuropathies may be motor, sensory (stocking glove distribution), mixed motor and sensory polyneuropathies, or mononeuritis multiplex. An acute ascending motor paralysis indistinguishable from Guillain–Barré has been reported. Transverse myelitis, presenting with lower extremity paralysis, sensory deficits, and loss of sphincter control has also been reported in SLE patients. Frank psychosis has long been recognized as a manifestation of SLE. The use of corticosteroids has been implicated in causing psychosis in some patients; however, stopping the drug in these patients, and demonstrating that the psychosis worsens, confirms its relationship to the disease process. Recently an association between SLE psychosis and anti-ribosomal P protein antibodies has been documented (8). The presence of anti-ribosomal P proteins may help distinguish true psychiatric features of SLE from drug-induced problems.

Organic brain syndrome in SLE is defined as a state of disturbed mental function with delirium, emotional inadequacy, impaired memory or concentration in the absence of drugs, infection, or a metabolic cause. The prevalence of cognitive impairment in SLE may be grossly underestimated. In a systematic study of neurocognitive function in SLE, more than 80% of the patients with neuropsychiatric involvement and 42% of the SLE patients who had never had neuropsychiatric manifestations demonstrated significant cognitive impairment, as compared with 17% of patients with RA and 14% of the controls (9).

The pathogenesis of central nervous system SLE is not well understood, but more than one mechanism must be operative to explain the wide spectrum of clinical findings. The most common finding in autopsy series is the presence of multiple microinfarcts. Noninflammatory thickening of small vessels by intimal proliferation, thrombotic occlusion of major vessels, and intracranial hemorrhage or embolism have also been seen. The pathologic findings do not always correlate with the clinical picture. A true vasculitis with inflammatory cell infiltrate and fibrinoid necrosis has rarely been demonstrated in brain pathology. However, support for vascular inflammation comes from studies showing enhanced cerebral blood flow during episodes of CNS activity. Autoantibodies that cross-react with neuronal membrane antigens and lymphocytotoxic antibodies have been found in both the serum and cerebrospinal fluid (CSF) of patients with SLE. These antibodies may be produced locally or pass through an immunologically damaged cerebral circulation or choroid plexus. Changes in antineuronal antibodies frequently parallel concurrent changes in anti–DNA antibodies and overall disease activity, as well as cognitive dysfunction. These antibodies may exert their effects by binding to molecules on neuronal membranes, preventing signal responses or propagation.

The diagnosis of neuropsychiatric SLE is primarily clinical. Exclusion of other possible etiologies such as sepsis, uremia, and severe hypertension is mandatory. Evidence of disease activity in other organs is helpful but not always present. Nonspecific CSF abnormalities such as elevated cell count, elevated protein, or reduced glucose may be present in one-third of the patients. Immune complexes have been detected in the CSF but have not been particularly helpful. Low levels of C4 and other complement components in the CSF of patients with neuropsychiatric disease have been reported. Elevations of IgG, IgA and/or IgM

have been described in patients with central nervous system SLE, and reflected CNS disease activity.

Electroencephalogram abnormalities are common in patients with neuropsychiatric SLE, but are nonspecific. Evoked potentials have been proposed as a sensitive measure of CNS involvement in SLE. Radionuclide scans have not been uniformly helpful; however, positron emission tomography showing areas of low attenuation that may represent areas of disturbed cerebral circulation and metabolism appear promising. Computed tomography (CT) findings such as evidence of cerebral infarction and hemorrhage may reflect specific pathologic processes. Cortical atrophy may be found in SLE, but does not necessarily reflect CNS disease. Magnetic resonance imaging (MRI) appears to be particularly useful in patients with diffuse presentations. The small focal areas of increased signal intensity on MRI, in both the cerebral white matter and the cortical grey matter, tend to disappear after therapy with corticosteroids. These lesions may therefore represent areas of local edema or inflammatory infiltrates that resolve with treatment. A more advanced technique, the ^{31}P nuclear magnetic resonance spectroscopy, may provide better demonstration of brain lesions in neuropsychiatric SLE (10).

SEROSITIS

Serositis in SLE is common and may present as pleurisy, pericarditis, or peritonitis (11). Pleural rubs are found less frequently than either clinical pleurisy or radiographic abnormalities. However, autopsy findings of pleural involvement are more common than clinical diagnoses. Pleural effusions are typically small, but can occasionally be massive. They are frequently bilateral. Pleural effusions are seen more frequently in older patients and in drug-induced SLE. When fluid is available for examination, it is usually an exudate and the glucose level is usually normal in contrast to RA, where it is low. The LE cells have been described in the pleural fluid. Antinuclear antibodies, immune complexes, and reduced levels of complement are also found. When pleural effusions are significant, other causes of effusion such as infection must be ruled out by thoracentesis before initiating therapy.

Pericarditis is the most common presentation of heart involvement in SLE, but it is less frequent than pleurisy as a feature of serositis (11). Clinical pericarditis has an incidence of 20% to 30% in most large series but may be found in over 60% of SLE patients at autopsy. The clinical diagnosis is frequently difficult and depends on a constellation of clinical findings including precordial chest pain and a pericardial rub. However, pericarditis may also be painless and clinically silent.

Posterior pericardial effusions may be found on echocardiography in patients who have no suspected history of pericarditis. Pericardial fluid has been examined only in a small number of cases in which leukocytosis with a high percent of neutrophils have been described. Glucose levels are significantly lower than in the serum, and several reports have documented reduced complement activity as well as elevated ANA levels and positive LE cells in the pericardial effusions. Although uncommon, constrictive pericarditis can occasionally develop in patients with pericardial involvement.

GASTROINTESTINAL MANIFESTATIONS

Gastrointestinal symptoms are common and are manifested by diffuse abdominal pain, anorexia, nausea, and occasionally vomiting. There are a number of possible etiologies for such symptoms including diffuse peritonitis, bowel vasculitis, pancreatitis, or inflammatory bowel disease. In the majority of such cases, peritoneal inflammation is the likely cause of the symptoms. Ascites may be associated with this peritonitis, and at autopsy evidence of peritoneal inflammation may be found. When ascites presents in conjunction with abdominal pain and active SLE elsewhere, it generally follows the course and response to treatment of the other SLE features. However, in a small number of patients, chronic ascites that is entirely asymptomatic may develop. Antibodies to double-stranded DNA may be found in the ascitic fluid in these patients. The peritoneum may be thickened with adhesions. When infection or malignancy is suspected, aspiration of ascitic fluid is necessary.

Patients with mesenteric vasculitis generally present with lower abdominal pain that may be insidious and intermittent over a period of weeks or months. Arteriography may reveal the presence of vasculitis. Rectal bleeding can occur and both small bowel and colonic ulcerations may be seen on colonoscopy. Intestinal perforations from mesenteric vasculitis have been described. If mesenteric vasculitis is suspected, intensive investigation should be undertaken and treatment instituted to abort perforation. However, if perforation is suspected or does occur, surgical intervention is necessary.

Inflammatory bowel disease has been reported in SLE. It may be difficult to distinguish this lesion from idiopathic inflammatory bowel disease. If due to SLE, other features of this illness are usually present.

Acute pancreatitis occurs in some patients with SLE. Presentation includes the typical symptoms of abdominal pain, nausea, and vomiting, as well as an elevated serum amylase. Although one may question whether the pancreatitis is due to SLE or corticosteroids, pancreatitis has been described in some patients not receiving these drugs. Elevated serum amylase levels have also been detected in patients without clinical signs of pancreatitis.

Hepatomegaly occurs commonly in SLE, but overt clinical liver disease is uncommon. Liver enzyme elevations have been associated with active SLE and the administration of nonsteroidal antiinflammatory medications, especially salicylates. Liver enzyme abnormalities return to normal when the disease is under control and the antiinflammatory medications are stopped.

PULMONARY MANIFESTATIONS

Pulmonary involvement in SLE may consist of pneumonitis, pulmonary hemorrhage, pulmonary embolism, pulmonary hypertension, and shrinking lung syndrome. Lupus pneumonitis may present as either an acute or chronic illness. The acute illness simulates infectious pneumonia and may present with symptoms of fever, dyspnea, cough, and occasionally hemoptysis. The pulmonary infiltrates are usually associated with other signs of active SLE and respond to corticosteroid administration. Acute pneumonitis must be differentiated from infection. When doubt persists, invasive investigation is indicated, including bronchoalveolar lavage. The chronic form of lupus pneumonitis presents as a diffuse interstitial lung disease and is characterized by dyspnea on exertion, nonproductive cough, and basilar rales. The pathophysiology of both of these forms of pulmonary involvement likely involves immune complex deposition in blood vessels and alveolar walls with or without associated vasculitis. In chronic lupus pneumonitis, the major clinical question is whether the pulmonary fibrosis has an active inflammatory component.

Pulmonary hemorrhage presenting with cough and hemoptysis or as a pulmonary infiltrate is an uncommon but serious feature of SLE (12). It is presumed to be due to pulmonary vasculitis. Other causes of hemorrhagic pneumonia, particularly viral pneumonia, must be considered in differential diagnosis.

Pulmonary involvement may also give rise to a syndrome of pulmonary hypertension similar to idiopathic pulmonary hypertension. In this syndrome, patients present with dyspnea and a clear chest radiograph. They are mildly hypoxic and have a restrictive pattern on pulmonary function testing. Raynaud's phenomenon is frequently present. Doppler studies and cardiac catheterization confirm pulmonary hypertension. The prognosis is generally grave. Secondary pulmonary hypertension must be ruled out by searching for sites of deep venous thrombosis and for multiple pulmonary emboli. When there is any doubt, pulmonary angiography should be performed, because a diagnosis of multiple pulmonary emboli might lead to potential life-saving therapy. One must also rule out the antiphospholipid antibody syndrome with intrapulmonary clotting.

CARDIAC MANIFESTATIONS

Cardiac involvement in SLE may consist of pericarditis as noted above, myocarditis, endocarditis, or coronary artery disease. Myocarditis is often suspected in patients who present with arrhythmias or conduction defects, unexplained cardiomegaly with or without congestive heart failure, or an unexplained tachycardia. Such patients usually have associated pericarditis and other features of active SLE. Congestive heart failure is a less common feature and is usually secondary to a combination of factors that may include myocarditis. However, associated hypertension and the use of corticosteroids are usually important contributing factors. The myocardial involvement may be more subtle in SLE. Abnormalities including reversible defects that suggest ischemia as well as persistent defects that indicate scarring. In patients with suspected myocarditis, endomyocardial biopsy may help confirm the diagnosis. The true incidence of endocarditis is very difficult to discern in SLE, since the majority of murmurs heard clinically are not associated with organic valvular disease. Endocarditis diagnosed on the basis of a murmur plus abnormal echocardiographic studies is infrequent. Nonbacterial verrucous vegetations described by Libman and Sacks are now much less common than they were in the pre-steroid era. Vegetations vary from mere valvular thickening detected by two-dimensional echocardiography to very large lesions causing significant valvular dysfunction. Valvular replacement has been required on occasion with significant mortality. Acute and subacute bacterial endocarditis may occur on previously involved valves. For this reason, prophylactic antibiotics for surgical procedures are advisable in patients with lupus endocarditis.

Coronary vasculitis is not common in SLE. When it occurs, it is usually associated with other features of active disease, in contradistinction to atherosclerotic coronary artery disease, which is usually associated with inactive SLE.

RETICULOENDOTHELIAL SYSTEM INVOLVEMENT

Splenomegaly is a common finding in patients with SLE. In addition, splenic atrophy, presumably secondary to infarction, and splenic lymphoma in patients with SLE have also been recognized.

Lymphadenopathy in single or multiple sites is recognized as a nonspecific feature of SLE. The nodes are usually soft, nontender, and variable in size. In some patients, there may be fluctuation of the lymphadenopathy with disease exacerbations. Pathologically, the lymph nodes demonstrate reactive hyperplasia.

LABORATORY FEATURES OF SLE

Hematologic Abnormalities

Cytopenias including anemia, leukopenia, lymphopenia, and thrombocytopenia are frequent manifestations of SLE. Anemia in SLE may have many different etiologies, including those secondary to chronic inflammatory disease, renal insufficiency, blood loss, or drugs. The most significant in acute SLE is autoimmune hemolytic anemia due to antibodies directed against red blood cell antigens. This form of hemolytic anemia is frequently associated with a positive Coombs' test, but occasionally hemolytic anemia in SLE is Coombs' negative. Similarly, one may find a positive Coombs' test in the absence of any evidence of hemolysis.

Leukopenia is a common finding in patients with SLE. The low white cell counts generally range between 2,500/mm³ and 4,000/mm³ and are often associated with active disease. Other causes for leukopenia, such as drugs and infection, must be considered. When the leukopenia is secondary to active SLE, the bone marrow is usually normal. The white blood count rarely falls below the levels of 1,500/mm³ in active SLE unless there is an additional cause. In some instances, when the total white count does reach these levels, patients will have high spiking fevers requiring significant doses of corticosteroids. Lymphocytopenia is usually associated with antibodies to lymphocytes and with active SLE.

Thrombocytopenia, as with anemia, requires that other etiologies such as infection or drugs be ruled out before ascribing the finding to SLE. Although antiplatelet antibodies are a frequent finding in SLE, they may not be associated with thrombocytopenia. Two distinct subsets of patients with thrombocytopenia have been identified in SLE (13). In one subset, the thrombocytopenia tends to be refractory and follows the course of acute SLE and its response to treatment. The second subset of patients usually presents with a platelet count of around 50,000/mm^3, without serious bleeding or active SLE elsewhere. Their thrombocytopenia need not be treated, but if the platelet count falls to a very low level, it is usually responsive to small doses of corticosteroids. Patients with refractory thrombocytopenia may require high doses of corticosteroids, cytotoxic drugs, or occasionally other modalities such as intravenous gammaglobulin. There are no good studies of the efficacy of these alternative forms of therapy. Unlike idiopathic thrombocytopenic purpura, splenectomy is rarely indicated in SLE, because the major problem is circulating autoantibodies. If this problem is not ameliorated, the condition will recur even after splenectomy.

A variety of clotting abnormalities have been reported in SLE (14), the most common being the SLE anticoagulant. Frequent laboratory accompaniments of this syndrome include a prolonged partial thromboplastin time with anticardiolipin antibody, and a false positive VDRL test for syphilis. The presence of these antibodies has been associated with specific manifestations such as thromboembolic phenomena and recurrent fetal loss.

A false-positive test for syphilis indicates a positive screening test (such as VDRL) but a negative TPI or an FTA–ABS test. The false-positive VDRL test may precede the onset of the other symptoms of SLE by many years.

The erythrocyte sedimentation rate (ESR) is frequently elevated in the course of active SLE, but it does not mirror disease activity. In remission, however, the ESR may remain elevated for long periods of time. A positive C-reactive protein test, at one time purported to be associated with infection in SLE, has not been proven to be a constant indicator of a superimposed infection.

Serologic Abnormalities

Complement levels measured as either total hemolytic complement or complement components C3 and C4 have been shown to be depressed in the serum of patients with SLE. These measures are often used to determine disease activity and are particularly useful when followed chronically to detect early changes in the disease. Tests to measure directly the presence of immune complexes in the serum are less useful in routine clinical monitoring.

Several of the autoantibodies that are seen in SLE are useful in diagnosis. These include antibodies to double-stranded DNA (dsDNA); anti–Sm, which are seen primarily in SLE; antihistone antibody, which is seen primarily in drug-induced lupus; and anti–Ro and La antibodies which are seen in patients with Sjogren's syndrome as well as in SLE patients.

Antibodies such as anti–DNA antibodies were initially felt to reflect disease activity in SLE, and therefore to be monitors of therapy. There are indeed a large number of patients who are clinically and serologically concordant. In these patients, flares of serology predict an impending flare in clinical disease. However, in many patients DNA antibodies are an imperfect predictor of clinical disease activity and elevated levels do not appear to consistently correlate with any clinical feature except renal disease (15). Elevated DNA antibody levels and low complement levels may persist for longer than one year prior to clinical disease flare. Thus, in any patient being seen for the first time, it is most appropriate to treat the clinical state and not laboratory abnormality. If observation confirms that these patients are in fact concordant, one might consider treating antibody changes. If these patients are discordant, then laboratory abnormalities should be followed but not treated.

A small minority of patients with SLE do not have antinuclear antibody or LE cells (so-called ANA-negative lupus). These patients have clinical evidence of SLE and tend to have more skin rash, photosensitivity, Raynaud's phenomenon, and serositis.

Some of these patients have subsequently been shown to have the anti–Ro/SSA antibody (16).

EVOLVING SPECTRUM OF SLE

The many different combinations of organ system involvement in SLE have been long recognized. Besides the traditional clinical manifestations resulting from inflammation, patients may present with signs and symptoms of SLE that may have a different underlying pathogenesis, different natural history, and require different therapeutic approaches. The most common of these presentations include latent lupus, drug-induced lupus, antiphospholipid antibody syndrome, and late-stage lupus.

Latent Lupus

Latent lupus describes a group of patients who present with a constellation of features suggestive of SLE, but who do not qualify by criteria or a rheumatologist's intuition as having classic SLE (17). These patients usually present with either one or two of the ACR classification criteria for SLE (see Appendix 3) and disease features not included among the criteria. These may include lymphadenopathy, fever, headache, nodules, Sjogren's syndrome, fatigue, neuropathy, less than two active joints, elevated partial thromboplastin time and gammaglobulin, elevated ESR, depressed complement, positive rheumatoid factor, or aspirin-induced hepatotoxicity. Many of these patients will persist with their constellation of signs and symptoms over many years without ever evolving into classic disease. They generally do not respond well to therapy and are best followed with symptomatic treatment. It is not clear that any of the presenting features of the illness are predictive for the small number of patients who will eventually evolve into classic SLE. Patients with latent lupus tend to have a milder form of disease and often do not present with central nervous system disease or renal disease. It would seem premature to include these patients in any large series of patients with SLE.

Drug-Induced Lupus

Drug-induced lupus may be diagnosed in a patient with no prior history suggestive of SLE, in whom the clinical and serologic manifestations of SLE appear while on the drug, and in whom improvement in clinical symptoms occurs quickly on stopping the drug with a more gradual resolution of serologic abnormalities (18). Drugs associated with this condition have been classified into three categories: 1) drugs in which proof of the association is definite and appropriate controlled, prospective studies have been performed, such as chlorpromazine, methyldopa, hydralazine, procainamide, and isoniazid 2) drugs that are only possibly associated, such as phenytoin, penicillamine, and quinidine, and finally, 3) drugs in which association is still questionable, represented by a wide variety of drugs including gold salts, a number of antibiotics, and griseofulvin.

The clinical features of drug-induced lupus are usually less severe than those of idiopathic SLE. The most commonly reported symptoms are fever, arthritis, and serositis. Central nervous system and renal involvement are rare. Laboratory testing reveals the presence of cytopenias, a positive LE prep, and positive ANA and rheumatoid factor tests. Antibodies to single stranded DNA are commonly found but antibodies to dsDNA are typically not present. In addition, complement levels are generally not depressed. Antihistone antibodies occur in over 90% of cases. However, antihistone antibodies are not specific, as they are also found in 20% to 30% of patients with idiopathic SLE.

Antiphospholipid Antibody Syndrome

The antiphospholipid syndrome describes the association of arterial and venous thrombosis, recurrent fetal loss, and immune thrombocytopenia with a variety of antibodies directed against cellular phospholipid components (see Chapter 12). This syndrome may be part of the spectrum of clinical manifestations seen

Table 11B–4. *Acute SLE features and late complications*

Acute Episodes	Chronic Morbidity
Glomerulonephritis	End-stage renal disease, dialysis, transplantation
Vasculitis	Atherosclerosis, venous syndromes, pulmonary emboli
Arthritis	Avascular necrosis
Cerebritis	Neuropsychological dysfunction
Pneumonitis and myopathy	Shrinking lung syndrome

in SLE (19), or it may occur as a primary form without other clinical features of SLE.

Late-Stage Lupus

Although the short-term prognosis in SLE has improved dramatically over the past three decades, the mortality rates in patients surviving more than 5 years and especially more than 10 years have not shown similar dramatic improvement. Patients with disease duration of greater than five years tend to die of causes other than active SLE (20). In such patients, mortality and morbidity are affected by long-term complications of SLE that result either from the disease itself or as a consequence of its therapy. These late complications of SLE are listed in Table 11B–4.

The nephropathy of late-stage lupus involves the development of end-stage renal disease after many months of stable renal function and in the absence of signs of multisystem SLE. In these patients, serologic abnormalities have generally converted to normal. At their presentation, the renal biopsies in these patients reveal glomerular hyalinization, vascular pathology, fibrinoid necrosis, and interstitial inflammation. The clinical problems that are present usually relate to severe hypertension and recurrent congestive heart failure.

Deaths occurring late in the course of SLE are often related to myocardial infarction and atherosclerosis in the absence of other evidence of active SLE. This complication generally occurs in premenopausal females, and has also been reported in adolescents. Thus far the complication has been reported primarily as atherosclerotic coronary artery disease with either angina or myocardial infarction, as peripheral vascular atherosclerotic disease with intermittent claudication, or as vascular insufficiency and gangrene. The atherosclerotic process may be severe enough to require angioplasty or bypass surgery to correct clinical symptoms.

Joint pain presenting in the later stages of SLE, especially localized to a very few areas such as the hips, may indicate the development of osteonecrosis. In most large series, osteonecrosis is recognized as an important cause of disability in late disease, occurring in about 10% of patients followed over a long period of time (20). Patients with osteonecrosis are generally in the younger age group and have an interval between diagnosis of SLE and osteonecrosis of about four years. The hip is the most commonly involved joint, although most joints have been reported to have been affected with osteonecrosis. One-half to two-thirds of patients with osteonecrosis will have multiple sites. Essentially all patients will have been on corticosteroids at some time during the course of their illness, although an occasional patient will not be on corticosteroids at the time of presentation with osteonecrosis. Since osteonecrosis is almost certainly not related to active SLE, the systemic disease may be active or inactive at the time of presentation. There is no general agreement as to the predictive role of any specific manifestation of SLE, such as Raynaud's phenomenon or vasculitis, in the subsequent development of osteonecrosis.

Diagnosis of osteonecrosis in patients presenting with focal pain can be difficult. Changes in routine radiographs may be late. Earlier diagnosis can be made using radionuclide bone scans or MRI scans to demonstrate bone abnormality.

In late-stage lupus, when there is no longer any evidence of active disease, and the patient is on low-dose or no corticosteroids, neurocognitive disabilities are a frequent complaint. Patients often present with decreased memory, decreased ability to do simple mathematical calculations, and increased speech disabilities. When such patients are submitted to a battery of neurocognitive tests, they are shown to have significant impairment (9,20). In addition, patients with SLE having neurologic investigation have been shown to demonstrate significant cortical atrophy on CT scanning. This has been shown both in patients with previous CNS disease due to SLE and in those without previous disease. It is also seen in those who have current neurocognitive symptoms and in those who do not. Thus, the neurocognitive disabilities that occur in late disease may be a feature of SLE in general, CNS disease of SLE in particular, related to the corticosteroids used to treat SLE, or a combination of these factors.

Patients may present in the late stages of SLE with the symptom of increasing dyspnea despite a normal chest examination. Chest radiographs may reveal elevated diaphragms but normal lung fields. Pulmonary function tests will usually reveal small lung volumes and a restrictive pattern. This syndrome, usually referred to as shrinking lung syndrome, is a result of altered respiratory mechanics either on the basis of impaired respiratory muscle or diaphragmatic function, or problems in the respiratory skeletal apparatus.

PREGNANCY AND SLE

Systemic lupus erythematosus does not interfere with conception. Fertility rates in patients with SLE have been reported to be the same as the general population. While a patient with SLE may conceive normally, chances of carrying a pregnancy through to term are reduced due to greater incidence of spontaneous abortion, prematurity, and intrauterine death. In all clinical series there are large numbers of therapeutic abortions, mostly for psychosocial reasons, but some because of concern about the effect of the pregnancy on the disease.

Early studies of SLE and pregnancy in the steroid era perpetuated the idea that pregnancy had an adverse effect on the clinical course of disease. However, recent studies have shown that the frequency of flares in pregnant patients with SLE is the same as in the nonpregnant state (21). Disease should, however, be controlled prior to conception.

Another issue that arises in patients with SLE who become pregnant is the differentiation between flares, particularly renal disease, and preeclampsia/eclampsia. The presence of other features of SLE, as well as laboratory abnormalities such as anti–DNA antibody or depressed complement levels, may favor the diagnosis of a flare.

Dafna D. Gladman, MD, FRCPC
Murray B. Urowitz, MD, FRCPC

1. Southeimer RD, Gilliam JN: Systemic lupus erythematosus and the skin. In: Systemic lupus erythematosus, 2nd ed. edited by Lahita RG. Churchill, Livingstone, New York, 1992, pp 657–681
2. Cronin ME: Musculoskeletal manifestations of systemic lupus erythematosus. Rheum Dis Clin North Am 14:99–116, 1988
3. Smythe H, Lee D, Rush P, Buskila D: Tender shins and steroid therapy. J Rheumatol 18:1568–1572, 1991
4. Gladman DD, Urowitz MB, Cole E, et al: Kidney biopsy in SLE. I. A clinical-morphologic evaluation. Quart J Med 73:1125–1153, 1989
5. Austin HA, Muenz LR, Joyce KM, et al: Diffuse proliferative lupus nephritis: identification of specific pathologic features affecting renal outcome. Kidney International 25:689–695, 1984
6. McCune WJ, Golbus J: Neuropsychiatric lupus. Rheum Dis Clin North Am 14:149–167, 1988
7. Stafford-Brady FJ, Urowitz MB, Gladman DD, et al: Lupus retinopathy: patterns, associations, and prognosis. Arthritis Rheum 31:1105–1110, 1988
8. Schneebaum AB, Singleton JD, West SG, et al: Association of psychiatric manifestations with antibodies to ribosomal P proteins in systemic lupus erythematosus. Am J Med 90:54–62, 1991
9. Carbotte RM, Denburg SD, Denburg JA: Prevalence of cognitive impairment in systemic lupus erythematosus. J Nerv Ment Dis 174:6:357–364, 1986
10. Griffey RH, Brown MS, Bankhurst AD, et al: Depletion of high-energy phosphates in the central nervous system of patient with systemic lupus erythematosus, as determined by phosphorus-31 nuclear magnetic resonance spectroscopy. Arthritis Rheum 33:827–833, 1990
11. Carette S: Cardiopulmonary manifestations of systemic lupus erythematosus. Rheum Dis Clin North Am 14:135–147, 1988
12. Schwab EP, Schumacher HR, Freundlich B, et al: Pulmonary alveolar hemorrhage in systemic lupus erythematosus. Semin Arthritis Rheum 23:8–15, 1993

13. Miller MH, Urowitz MB, Gladman DD: The significance of thrombocytopenia in systemic lupus erythematosus. Arthritis Rheum 26:1181–1186, 1983

14. Gladman DD, Urowitz MB, Tozman E, et al: Hemostatic abnormalities in systemic lupus erythematosus. Q J Med 52:424–433, 1983

15. Gladman DD, Urowitz MB, Keystone EC: Serologically active clinically quiescent systemic lupus erythematosus. Am J Med 66:210–215, 1979

16. Urowitz MB, Gladman DD: Anti-nuclear antibody negative lupus. Systemic lupus erythematosus. In: Systemic lupus erythematosus. Edited by Lahita RG. Churchill, Livingstone, New York, 1992: pp 561–568

17. Ganczarczyk L, Urowitz MB, Gladman DD: Latent lupus. J Rheumatol 16:475–478, 1989

18. Mongey AB, Hess EV: Drug-related lupus. Current Opinion Rheumatol 1:353–359, 1989

19. Love PE, Santaro SA: Antiphospholipid antibodies: anticardiolipin and the lupus anticoagulant in systemic lupus erythematosus (SLE) and non-SLE disorders. Ann Intern Med 112:682–698, 1990

20. Gladman DD, Urowitz MB: Morbidity in systemic lupus erythematosus. J Rheumatol 14(suppl 13):223–226, 1987

21. Urowitz MB, Gladman DD: Rheumatic disease in pregnancy. In: Medical complications during pregnancy, 3rd ed. Edited by Burrow GN, Ferris TF. W.B. Saunders Company, Philadelphia, 1988, pp. 499–525

C. Treatment

The management of systemic lupus erythematosus requires recognition that the disease is a chronic rheumatic syndrome with a relapsing and remitting clinical course. Treatment can be divided into two parts: A) principles of preventive disease management that apply to the chronic disease course and B) drug interventions aimed at exacerbations of the disease (flares). Advances in management of SLE have been a major factor in increased survival and reduced morbidity from the disease over the past several decades (1).

PRINCIPLES OF PREVENTIVE MANAGEMENT

Preventive practices include the assessment and detection of changes in disease activity as well as measures to reduce the likelihood of acute flares and minimize the risks of confounding illnesses.

Disease Activity and Severity

Decisions regarding SLE management are guided by the concepts of disease activity and severity. Activity refers to the contribution of inflammation to the clinical setting, and severity is the risk of morbidity or mortality from manifestations of the disease. Although in many patients determining whether disease is active and deciding if it is mild or severe and life-threatening is relatively easy, in others it is far more complicated. Typical examples of the latter include patients who have an elevated serum creatinine or who are grossly confused; in whom active lupus nephritis or central nervous system lupus is evident; who exhibit reversible effects of drug therapy such as corticosteroids or nonsteroidal agents; or for whom chronic scarring or atrophy of the kidneys or cerebral cortex must be distinguished.

Changes in disease activity should guide drug therapy. In the instance of patients with anemia or thrombocytopenia, proteinuria, or nephritis, objective laboratory measures may be followed. However, for many clinical manifestations, determinations of disease activity are more subjective and less easily quantitated. To provide a more reproducible and quantitative assessment of SLE activity, several standardized scoring systems have been developed (2). These global measures of SLE activity are valuable in clinical trials and in following the long-term course of individual patients.

Immunologic studies, particularly serum antibodies to double-stranded DNA and levels of complement, are often used as surrogate markers of disease activity. Patients with clinically active SLE typically have increased levels of anti–DNA antibodies and depressed complement levels. Resolution of these abnormalities has been shown to correlate with improvements in the clinical course of lupus nephritis (3). Recent additional immunologic studies of potential value in following disease activity include serum levels of complement split products (4) and serum levels of the soluble interleukin–2 receptor (5).

Prophylactic Measures

Many SLE patients are highly photosensitive and must be reminded of the importance of avoiding intense sun exposure. This includes giving practical advice such as wearing long-sleeved clothing and large brimmed hats, and going outdoors only during early morning or evening hours. Patients should be instructed in the liberal use of sun screens. Changes in the work setting may be required. Outdoor occupations may not be possible, and office workers may need to avoid sunlight from a window or even overhead fluorescent lights. Care also must be taken in the use of photosensitizing drugs, particularly antibiotics.

Infections are common in SLE patients. Because of this, prompt evaluation of unexplained fever is necessary, especially in patients at heightened risk of infection such as those with renal failure, ulcerative skin lesions, cardiac valvular abnormalities, or primary complement deficiencies. Similarly, patients after splenectomy or those treated with high doses of corticosteroids or immunosuppressive drugs are at increased risk of infection. Those at risk should be immunized with influenza vaccine yearly, and pneumococcal vaccine should be given to SLE patients following splenectomy. Antibiotic prophylaxis should be used for all dental and genitourinary procedures.

Birth control is important in female patients with active SLE, particularly nephritis, and as part of drug treatments in which pregnancy would be contraindicated such as cytotoxic or antimetabolite drugs. Pregnancy poses concerns of potential disease exacerbations in the mother and separate risks to the fetus. This requires more careful and frequent monitoring of disease activity than usual in the pregnant SLE patient. In addition, obstetrical care should be provided by a specialist trained in the management of high risk pregnancies.

Patient education and psychosocial interventions are an important aspect of disease management. Booklets specifically written for patients are often extremely helpful for this purpose and provide patients with basic information about the disease (6). In many hospitals and communities, SLE support groups have been organized. Besides the educational function provided by these groups, many patients benefit enormously by having the opportunity to interact with others with the disease. In particular, this type of forum often provides patients with necessary coping skills needed for dealing with a chronic illness.

DRUG THERAPIES

Agents that suppress inflammation or interfere with immune functions are used in primary drug management of SLE patients. It is important to recognize, however, the critical role of drugs in the treatment of comorbid conditions such as hypertension, infections, seizures, hyperlipidemia, and osteoporosis. These common medical complications in SLE patients account for considerable morbidity and mortality.

Nonsteroidal Antiinflammatory Drugs

Nonsteroidal antiinflammatory drugs (NSAIDs) are used for the treatment of musculoskeletal manifestations, serositis, and constitution signs such as fever and fatigue. They are often given before low-dose corticosteroids or antimalarials or in combination with corticosteroids in an effort to minimize dose-related side effects. The onset of action of NSAIDs is prompt with clinical improvement typically evident within days of beginning drug treatment. As with other rheumatic diseases, there is marked variability in patient responsiveness to individual NSAIDs, and brief trials of several different drugs may be needed to identify the single best agent. There is no reason to believe that one NSAID is superior to another and factors such as cost and how well the patient tolerates the drug are often important practical considerations.

Several adverse effects of NSAIDs, particularly renal and neurologic effects, are important since they may be easily confused with active SLE. Nonsteroidal drugs inhibit prostaglandin synthesis within the kidney and produce impairments of renal blood flow, glomerular filtration, and tubular function. A patient with lupus nephritis is particularly susceptible to these influences due to a heightened dependency on prostaglandins for maintenance of renal function. Rarely, NSAIDs have been shown to cause membranous nephropathy, acute interstitial nephritis, or acute tubular necrosis. Thus, in patients with SLE who present with loss of renal function or proteinuria, careful consideration should be given to the possibility of NSAID-induced nephropathy before ascribing the changes to active lupus nephritis. This should include questioning patients about nonprescription NSAID use. In patients who are being treated with NSAIDs, the drugs should be discontinued before proceeding with an evaluation or treatment. Renal abnormalities produced by NSAIDs, particularly impairments of renal function, are generally promptly and completely reversible.

Nonsteroidal drugs may cause various neuropsychiatric signs and symptoms such as headache, dizziness, confusion, and depression that may easily be confused with central nervous system SLE. An aseptic meningitis syndrome induced by several of the NSAIDs, particularly ibuprofen, has been described. The clinical presentation includes headache, meningismus, and fever. Pruritis, facial edema, and conjunctivitis may occur on occasion. Lymphocytosis, an elevated protein, and a sterile culture are findings in the cerebrospinal fluid. The syndrome promptly resolves with discontinuation of the nonsteroidal drug.

Corticosteroids

There are multiple uses for corticosteroids in SLE patients, including topical preparations for inflammatory rashes, intralesional injections for discoid lupus, low-dose oral therapy for mild active disease, and high-dose oral or bolus intravenous infusions for acute, severe manifestations (Table 11C–1) (7). The administration of corticosteroids typically results in prompt and complete resolution of most manifestations of SLE. In select patients with fulminant disease, corticosteroids can be lifesaving. The actual type of corticosteroid is of less importance than the dose; long-acting corticosteroids such as dexamethasone are generally avoided. Most physicians prefer to use prednisone since it is available in multiple strengths that facilitate dose changes. The dose of corticosteroids is based on the desire to minimize the risks of toxicities, yet assure that an adequate dose is given to control the disease. Oral therapy is generally begun as a single, daily dose taken in the morning. As a general rule, minor manifestations of lupus readily respond to prednisone doses of 0.5 mg/kg daily or less, whereas more serious disease manifestations require prednisone doses in the range of 1.0 mg/kg daily. There are probably very few indications for using oral prednisone in excess of these doses. In patients who fail to show improvement,

Table 11C–1. *The multiple uses of corticosteroids in SLE*

Indication	Corticosteroid Regimen
Cutaneous manifestations	Topical or intralesional corticosteroids
Minor disease activity	Prednisone (or equivalent) at a dose of <0.5 mg/kg in a single or divided daily dosage
Major disease activity	Oral: Prednisone (or equivalent) at a dose of 1 mg/kg in single or divided daily dosage; duration should not exceed 4 weeks
	IV bolus: Methylprednisolone (1 g or 15 mg/kg) over 30 minutes; dose often repeated for 3 consecutive days

Table 11C–2. *Dose guidelines for antimalarials in SLE*

	Daily Dose
4-Aminoquinoline Derivatives	
Hydroxychloroquine	200–400 mg*
Chloroquine	250 mg*
9-Aminocridine Derivative	
Quinacrine (Mepacrine)	100 mg*

* Dose needs to be reduced for patients weighing less than 45 kg; 5 to 7 mg/kg for hydroxychloroquine, 4 mg/kg for chloroquine, 1–2 mg/kg for quinacrine.

the dose of corticosteroids may either be increased or given in divided doses two or three times daily. The duration of high-dose corticosteroids (>0.5 mg/kg/day) should not exceed four weeks. Patients who fail to respond, who relapse with these doses of corticosteroids, or who develop unacceptable toxicities are candidates for other forms of aggressive therapy.

Once disease activity is judged to be under control, reductions of the corticosteroid dose should be undertaken. For patients on multiple daily dose regimens, the initial step should involve efforts to change the patient to a single morning dose regimen. With reductions of the corticosteroid dosage, patients need to be carefully monitored for signs of increasing disease activity. Many patients appear to have a corticosteroid threshold below which disease activity predictably develops. In patients with prolonged periods of disease remission, reduction and eventual discontinuation of the corticosteroid should be a goal of patient management. Intravenous methylprednisolone ("bolus therapy") is an alternative to high-dose oral corticosteroids.

Antimalarials

Antimalarial compounds, including both 4-aminoquinolines (hydroxychloroquine and chloroquine) and the 9-aminocridine derivative quinacrine, are widely used in the management of cutaneous, musculoskeletal, and constitutional features of SLE (Table 11C–2). Therapy is often initiated at twice the recommended maintenance dose, with reduction of the dose after four to six weeks once SLE activity has subsided. Antimalarials should be used with caution in SLE patients with glucose-6-phosphate dehydrogenase (G6PD) deficiency or in patients with liver disease.

Quinacrine and hydroxychloroquine are the best studied of the antimalarials; clinical experience with chloroquine is substantially less. Although some differences in onset of action and toxicities between quinacrine and hydroxychloroquine have been noted, the choice between these agents is largely a matter of physician preference. Improvements in cutaneous manifestations, including both discoid and erythematous, inflammatory lesions, can be remarkably rapid and often evident in a matter of days after starting therapy. In patients who fail to respond to a particular antimalarial, substitution or addition of an alternative antimalarial drug is often beneficial.

In general, there is a reluctance to completely discontinue antimalarials in stable SLE patients on long-term therapy, particularly those who have clearly benefitted from the drug. The discontinuation of antimalarials has been well documented to be associated with an increased risk of flares, including major exacerbations of the disease such as vasculitis, transverse myelitis, and nephropathy (8). This poses a particular dilemma in the SLE patient on antimalarials who wishes to become pregnant. Antimalarials cross the placenta and instances of congenital defects such as cleft palate, sensorineural hearing loss, and posterior column defects have been rarely reported. In general, antimalarials are considered to be contraindicated in pregnancy. The physician must decide whether the risk of disease flare from discontinuing the antimalarials exceeds the risks of drug-induced fetal abnormalities. The relative safety of antimalarials given during pregnancy has been noted in a small series of SLE patients (9).

The low doses of antimalarials used in patients with SLE are well tolerated and rarely need to be discontinued for an adverse reaction. Of the various toxicities associated with antimalarials, gastrointestinal intolerance, cutaneous eruptions, and nonspecific constitutional complaints are most frequent. Central nervous system toxicities have been rarely reported including headaches, emotional changes, psychosis, ataxia, and seizures. Antimalarials should be discontinued in patients with suspected neuropsychiatric manifestations from SLE. Long-term antimalarial therapy may cause a neuromyopathy, and assessment for muscle strength and reflexes should be done periodically. Although hematologic toxicities with antimalarials are distinctly uncommon, complete blood counts should be obtained occasionally.

Much of the concern regarding the use of antimalarials in SLE has focused on potential ocular toxicities (see Chapter 56). The risk of retinal toxicity in patients treated with low doses of antimalarials is extremely small. As a precaution, however, ophthalmologic examinations including visual acuity, slit-lamp, fundoscopic, and visual field testing should be performed prior to the start of therapy and every six months thereafter.

Methotrexate

Studies of the folate antagonist methotrexate in SLE are limited, but they suggest that methotrexate may be a reasonable alternative to antimalarials or low-dose corticosteroids. Weekly, low-dose oral methotrexate (7.5 mg–15 mg), similar to drug schedules used in rheumatoid arthritis, appears to be useful in the management of arthritis, skin rashes, serositis, or fever (10). Since methotrexate is eliminated by both glomerular filtration and active tubular secretion, reductions in drug dose are necessary in SLE patients with compromised renal function.

Diaminodiphenylsulfone

Diaminodiphenylsulfone (dapsone) has been used in the management of cutaneous manifestations of SLE including discoid, subacute cutaneous lupus, bullous, and lupus profundus lesions (11). Therapy is typically begun at 50 mg daily with gradual increases of the dose to a maximum of 150 mg daily. Hematologic side effects, in particular a dose-related hemolysis, are common and require careful monitoring. Patients with G6PD deficiency are at heightened risk for hematologic toxicities. Routine screening for G6PD deficiency prior to therapy is recommended. Methemoglobinemia with weakness, tachycardia, nausea, headache, and abdominal pain is a rare complication of therapy.

Azathioprine

The purine analogue azathioprine has been extensively studied in lupus nephritis and shown to reduce proteinuria, improve or stabilize renal function, and reduce mortality (12). In addition, azathioprine is widely used in the management of nonrenal lupus manifestations as a steroid-sparing agent.

The most common side effects of azathioprine are gastrointestinal intolerance and bone marrow toxicity. The onset of anemia or leukopenia may be abrupt; therefore, blood counts need to be monitored regularly during therapy. Bone marrow toxicity is generally reversible with reduction of the dose or discontinuation of the drug. Azathioprine can produce elevations of liver enzyme, particularly the pyruvic and glutamic oxaloacetic transaminases. Hepatocellular necrosis and mild biliary stasis have been seen on liver biopsy. Hepatotoxicity is thought to result from drug hypersensitivity and may be accompanied by fever, diffuse abdominal pain, diarrhea, and a maculopapular skin rash. Hepatic abnormalities are typically reversible upon discontinuation of the drug.

There is concern that azathioprine may increase the risk of malignancy, particularly of hematopoetic or lymphoreticular origin. Case reports of non-Hodgkin's lymphoma and leukemia and a fourfold increase in uterine cervical atypia have been documented in SLE patients treated with azathioprine (13,14).

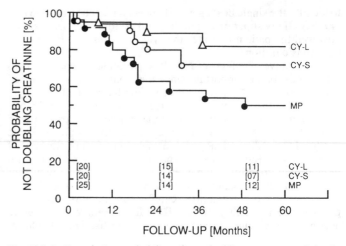

Fig. 11C–1. Cumulative probability of not doubling serum creatinine in patients with lupus nephritis treated with pulse methylprednisolone (MP), monthly intravenous cyclophosphamide for 6 months (CY-S) or cyclophosphamide given for total of 30 months (CY-L). CY-L significantly different from MP, p = 0.037. (From ref 16).

Alkylating Agents

Of the several different nitrogen mustard alkylating agents that have been used in SLE, cyclophosphamide has been the most studied. Both low-dose oral (1–4 mg/kg daily) and high dose intravenous schedules ($0.5–1.0 \text{ g/m}^2$) are used. Since cyclophosphamide is excreted by the kidneys, the dose must be reduced in patients with impairments of renal function. In randomized controlled trials in lupus nephritis, cyclophosphamide has been shown to retard progressive scarring within the kidney, prevent loss of renal function, and reduce the risk of end-stage renal failure requiring dialysis or renal transplantation (15,16) (Fig. 11C-1). The studies suggest that boluses of intravenous cyclophosphamide may be particularly beneficial. Intravenous cyclophosphamide has also been reported to be effective in the management of several other serious forms of the disease, including hematologic, central nervous system, and vascular manifestations (17–19).

The potential toxicities of cyclophosphamide are substantial. Gastrointestinal complications with nausea and vomiting are common and many patients require antiemetic therapy, particularly for high-dose, intravenous therapy. Alopecia may on occasion be severe and require the use of a wig; however, patients need to be reassured that the hair will regrow even with continued therapy. The drug must be given with caution in patients with leukopenia, and regular monitoring of white blood counts, hematocrit, and platelet counts are essential. Patients treated with cyclophosphamide are at heightened risk for infections and require careful evaluation for unexplained fever. Finally, cyclophosphamide is a well established teratogen, and tests to exclude pregnancy before starting therapy and effective birth control during therapy are essential.

Long-term cyclophosphamide therapy may produce damage to gonadal tissue and lead to ovarian failure and azospermia. In very young patients considerations should be given to the storage of ova or sperm prior to beginning therapy. In females, the risk of ovarian failure increases with patient age and is a nearly universal complication in patients treated with cyclophosphamide after the age of 30 years. The recovery of ovarian function or spermatogenesis is unpredictable.

Cyclophosphamide may damage the bladder mucosa to cause hemorrhagic cystitis, bladder fibrosis, and transitional and squamous cell carcinoma. A metabolite, acrolein, appears to be the irritant responsible for acute cystitis. Generous fluid intake to reduce concentrations of acrolein in the bladder is helpful in minimizing these complications. In addition, the sufhydryl mesna that binds acrolein should be considered in patients with known cyclophosphamide-induced bladder damage in whom continued drug administration is required. Patients treated with cyclophosphamide who develop evidence of reduced bladder capacity, such as frequency and small urinary volumes, should undergo complete cystometric evaluation. The findings of hematuria, particularly of new onset and after prolonged drug administration, should be assessed by urine cytology and cystoscopy for possible malignant changes of the bladder. Patients treated with prolonged courses of cyclophosphamide probably should be screened indefinitely for malignant changes in the bladder.

Malignancies of hematopoietic or lymphoreticular origin have been of particular concern in SLE patients treated with cyclophosphamide. Although the actual risks have not been clearly defined, it is generally accepted that they exceed the risks associated with the use of azathioprine.

Danazol

The attenuated androgen, danazol, has been shown to be useful in the management of lupus thrombocytopenia (20). The mechanism of action of the drug has not been defined but may involve the effects of endocrine changes (suppression of pituitary follicle stimulating hormone and luteinizing hormone) on immune or reticuloendothelial functions. Pregnancy, breast feeding, or unexplained vaginal bleeding are absolute contraindications to danazol therapy, and the drug must be used with caution in patients with liver or renal involvement. The major adverse reactions relate to hormonal changes induced by the drug, such as vaginitis, irregular menses including amenorrhea, virilization, and emotional lability. Drug effects on the liver require monitoring of liver chemistries. Hepatic tumors have been reported with long-term therapy.

INVESTIGATIONAL THERAPIES

Cyclosporin A

There have been very few clinical studies of the cytokine inhibitor cyclosporin A in patients with SLE (21). The side effects of hypertension and direct renal toxicity would appear to limit the usefulness of the drug in the management of SLE.

Immune Globulin

The principal indication for immune globulin in SLE is for the management of lupus thrombocytopenia (22). Therapy is associated with a prompt rise in the platelet count in the majority of patients, but the rate of relapse is high. The primary role of immune globulin in lupus thrombocytopenia may be for control of acute bleeding or to rapidly increase the platelet count to permit splenectomy or other surgery. In addition, immune globulins are often used in combination with other forms of slow-acting drug therapy such as immunosuppressives or danazol. Immune globulin has also been used in the investigational treatment of patients with lupus nephritis and cerebral vasculitis.

Intravenous immune globulin has a number of effects on immune function including the suppression of antibody formation, suppression of T lymphocyte proliferation, and reduction of natural killer cell activity. The mechanism of action may involve interference with Fc receptor function or interaction of antiidiotype antibodies with antibody-producing cells or secreted antibody. A number of different immune globulin preparations are available. Typical dose schedules used in investigational studies in SLE have ranged from 300 to 400 mg/kg/day given for five consecutive days, often followed by maintenance monthly therapy. The major contraindication is IgA deficiency, an occasional finding in SLE patients. Adverse reactions include fever, chills, myalgias, and abdominal or chest pain typically seen during or shortly after infusion. True anaphylactic reactions are very rare.

Plasma Exchange

Since immune complexes or pathologic antibodies in the serum of SLE patients are thought to mediate tissue inflammation, the removal of these immune factors by plasma exchange (plasma-pheresis) should theoretically be beneficial in disease management. Although concentrations of serum immunoglobulins, autoantibodies, and immune complexes may be reduced by plasma exchange, the changes are only transient with rapid recovery to abnormal levels once plasma exchange is stopped. To date, there is little evidence from randomized clinical studies to suggest that plasma exchange has a significant role in SLE management (23).

Total Lymphoid Irradiation

Fractionated radiotherapy to central lymphoid structures (total lymphoid irradiation or TLI) has been used experimentally in the treatment of a small group of patients with SLE (24). Total lymphoid irradiation produces a rather marked lymphopenia, with a preferential depletion of CD4 lymphocytes that may persist for several years or longer. This has been shown to lead to impairments of both cell-mediated immunity and T cell-dependent antibody production. In patients with lupus nephritis, reductions in proteinuria, increases in serum albumin, and improvements in renal function have been noted following TLI. Patients treated with TLI appear to be at increased risk for infectious complications and perhaps increases in the risks of acute leukemia and solid tumors and cardiovascular disease.

PREGNANCY

The management of SLE during pregnancy requires prompt control of flares. Therefore, careful monitoring of the patients with both clinical and laboratory assessment is mandatory. This monitoring should continue into the postpartum period. During pregnancy, salicylates are permitted but should be discontinued 7–10 days before delivery to avoid excessive bleeding. Prednisone in doses less than 60 mg/day is probably metabolized by the placenta and does not affect the fetus. Fluorinated steroids do cross the placenta and should not be used to treat maternal disease during pregnancy. On the other hand, such steroids are advised if placental transfer is desirable, such as in cases of fetal distress or the development of congenital heart block. The use of immunosuppressive therapy is generally avoided during pregnancy, although azathioprine is probably safe.

The mode of delivery is an obstetric decision. Breast feeding is not specifically contraindicated in patients with SLE, but may occasionally not be advisable because of the associated demands on the mother.

John H. Klippel, MD

1. Klippel JH: Systemic lupus erythematosus: treatment-related complications superimposed on chronic disease. JAMA 263:1812–1815, 1990
2. Liang MH, Socher SA, Larson MG, et al: Reliability and validity of six systems for the clinical assessment of disease activity in systemic lupus erythematosus. Arthritis Rheum 32:1107–1118, 1989
3. Laitman RS, Glicklich D, Sablay LB, et al: Effect of long-term normalization of serum complement levels on the course of lupus nephritis. Am J Med 87:132–138, 1989
4. Kerr LD, Adelsberg BR, Schulman P, et al: Factor B activation products in patients with systemic lupus erythematosus: a marker of severe disease activity. Arthritis Rheum 32:1406–1413, 1989
5. Campen DH, Horwitz DA, Quismorio FP, et al: Serum levels of interleukin-2 receptor and activity of rheumatic diseases characterized by immune activation. Arthritis Rheum 31:1358–1364, 1988
6. Rosinsky LJ, Wallace DJ: Lupus resource materials for patients, physicians, and medical personnel. In: Dubois' Lupus Erythematosus, 4th ed. Edited by Wallace DJ, Hahn BH. Philadelphia, Lea & Febiger, 1993, pp 629–633
7. Kimberly RP: Treatment: corticosteroids and anti-inflammatory drugs. Rheum Dis Clin N Amer 14:203–221, 1988
8. The Canadian Hydroxychloroquine Study Group: A randomized study of the effect of withdrawing hydroxychloroquine sulfate in systemic lupus erythematosus. N Engl J Med 324:150–154, 1991
9. Parke AL: Antimalarial drugs, systemic lupus erythematosus and pregnancy. J Rheumatol 15:607–610, 1988
10. Rothenberg RJ, Graziano FM, Grandone JT, et al: The use of methotrexate in steroid-resistant systemic lupus erythematosus. Arthritis Rheum 31:612–615, 1988
11. Holtman JH, Neustadt DH, Klein J, et al: Dapsone is an effective therapy for the skin lesions of subacute cutaneous lupus erythematosus and urticarial vasculitis in a patient with C2 deficiency. J Rheumatol 17:1222–1225, 1990
12. Felson DT, Anderson J: Evidence for the superiority of immunosuppressive drugs and prednisone over prednisone alone in lupus nephritis: results of a pooled analysis. N Engl J Med 311:1528–1533, 1984

13. Woolf AS, Conway G: Systemic lupus erythematosus and primary cerebral lymphoma. Postgrad Med J 63:569–572, 1987
14. Nyberg G, Eriksson O, Westberg NG: Increased incidence of cervical atypia in women with systemic lupus erythematosus treated with chemotherapy. Arthritis Rheum 24:648–650, 1981
15. Austin HA III, Klippel JH, Balow JE, et al: Therapy of lupus nephritis: controlled trial of prednisone and cytotoxic drugs. N Engl J Med 314:614–619, 1986
16. Boumpas DT, Austin HA, Vaughn EM, et al: Severe lupus nephritis: controlled trial of pulse methylprednisolone versus two different regimens of pulse cyclophosphamide. Lancet 340:741–744, 1992
17. McCune WJ, Golbus J, Zeldes W, et al: Clinical and immunologic effects of monthly administration on intravenous cyclophosphamide in severe systemic lupus erythematosus. N Engl J Med 318:1423–1431, 1988
18. Boumpas DT, Yamada H, Patronas NJ, et al: Pulse cyclophosphamide for severe neuropsychiatric lupus. Q J Med 296:975–984, 1991
19. Boumpas DT, Barez S, Klippel JH, et al: Intermittent cyclophosphamide for the treatment of autoimmune thrombocytopenia in systemic lupus erythematosus. Ann Intern Med 112:674–677, 1990
20. West SG, Johnson SC: Danazol for the treatment of refractory autoimmune thrombocytopenia in systemic lupus erythematosus. Ann Intern Med 108:703–706, 1988
21. Favre H, Miescher PA, Huang YP, et al: Ciclosporin in the treatment of lupus nephritis. Am J Nephrol 9 (Suppl 1):57–60, 1989
22. Maier WP, Gordon DS, Howard RF, et al: Intravenous immunoglobulin therapy in systemic lupus erythematosus-associated thrombocytopenia. Arthritis Rheum 33:1233–1239, 1990
23. Lewis EJ, Hunsicker LG, Lan SP, et al: A controlled trial of plasmapheresis therapy in severe lupus nephritis. N Engl J Med 326:1373–1379, 1992
24. Strober S, Field E, Hoppe RT, et al: Treatment of intractable lupus nephritis with total lymphoid irradiation. Ann Intern Med 102:450–458, 1985

12. ANTIPHOSPHOLIPID SYNDROME

Antiphospholipid syndrome (APS) is a disorder of recurrent vascular thrombosis, pregnancy wastage, and thrombocytopenia associated with a persistently positive lupus anticoagulant and/or moderate to high positive anticardiolipin test (Table 12–1) (1). Cardiac valvular vegetations, livedo reticularis, and Coombs positive hemolytic anemia (2) are seen in some patients. Some patients also have some features of systemic lupus erythematosus (SLE) or other systemic autoimmune disorders, while others have anticardiolipin antibodies in association with full-blown SLE. The term *primary antiphospholipid syndrome* has been proposed for patients with APS who do not have SLE or other systemic autoimmune disorders (2). Although this term may be useful in comparative studies, there is as yet no evidence to suggest that clinical or laboratory features of APS are different in the presence or absence of an associated systemic autoimmune disorder.

ETIOLOGY AND PATHOGENESIS

Factors that induce antiphospholipid (aPL) antibodies are unknown, nor is it certain why these antibodies are associated with thrombosis and pregnancy loss. Demonstration that immunization with bacteria or phospholipid binding proteins (3) can induce aPL antibodies suggests infection may play a role. Genetic factors may also be important (4).

Whether aPL antibodies are a direct cause of thrombosis and pregnancy loss has not been determined. Phospholipids on platelet or endothelial cell membranes play an integral role in catalyzing reactions of the clotting cascade and its inhibitory systems. Antiphospholipid antibodies might conceivably alter this catalytic process by interaction with phospholipids in cell membranes. Carreras et al first reported that these antibodies inhibit

prostacyclin release from endothelial cell membranes (5), but these findings have been contested by others (6). Alternatively, inhibition of protein C activation (7), inhibition of β_2 glycoprotein 1–phospholipid interactions (8), or antibody induced platelet activation (9) have all been proposed as mechanisms by which these antibodies can cause thrombosis.

CLINICAL FEATURES

Pregnancy Loss

The clinical presentation of patients with APS varies considerably. Some will have only recurrent pregnancy losses, often but not always in the late second or third trimester of gestation. Preeclampsia, intrauterine growth retardation, and "small for dates" babies are also frequent. Only some of these women have a history of thrombosis, thrombocytopenia, or features of SLE, but eliciting this history makes a diagnosis of APS more likely.

Thrombosis

Patients may present with signs and symptoms attributable to venous or arterial thrombosis. Swelling and pain may accompany venous thrombosis of a leg or arm. Renal vein thrombosis, the Budd–Chiari Syndrome, pulmonary embolism, Addison's disease, retinal or saggital vein thrombosis, as well as other presentations reflective of venous or arterial thrombosis at various sites have been described (10). Occlusion of the arterial circulation may lead to strokes, transient ischemia attacks, monocular blindness, myocardial infarction, gangrene of one or more extremities, or bowel infarction (2,10). Occlusion of arterioles and smaller vessels may result in renal insufficiency and dermal infarction (2,10).

Thrombotic events are often episodic and unpredictable. Occasionally patients present with acute, aggressive, widespread thrombosis (11) for which the term, *acute, disseminated vasculopathy–coagulopathy*, has been suggested (12). What triggers these events is unknown.

Other Features

Other clinical and laboratory features not attributable to thrombosis have been described (2). Cardiac valvular vegetations and valvular insufficiency (13), livedo reticularis, migraine headaches (14), thrombocytopenia, and Coombs positive hemolytic anemia (1,15) have been reported in many patients, although their true frequency has yet to be determined. Rare neurologic complications, such as chorea and transverse myelopathy, and a variety of skin lesions including ulcers have also been observed (2). Many of these features are not specific to APS and probably reflect an autoimmune diathesis to which APS may belong.

Table 12–1. *Clinical and laboratory features of antiphospholipid syndrome (1)*

Clinical	Laboratory
*Major Features	
Venous thrombosis	Lupus anticoagulant test
Arterial thrombosis	Anticardiolipin test (medium
Thrombocytopenia	to high positive, IgG, IgM or IgA)
Other (proposed) features	
Endocardial valvular vegetations	
Livedo reticularis	
Migraine headaches	
? Transverse myelopathy	
? Chorea	
? Leg ulcers	

* A diagnosis of the APS should be based on a history of one major clinical feature (preferably not explainable by any other predisposing condition) and a positive laboratory test (which has remained positive for several weeks to months).

DIFFERENTIAL DIAGNOSIS

Thrombosis and pregnancy loss can occur for many reasons. In addition, it should be borne in mind that positive aCL and lupus anticoagulant (LA) tests occur in many disorders and in many apparently normal individuals without ever being associated with thrombosis. Hence, concurrence of thrombosis (or pregnancy loss) and positive aCL or LA tests need not mean that APS is present. Unexplained recurrent thrombosis, cerebral or myocardial infarction without predisposing factors, venous thrombosis at unusual sites, and late second or third trimester pregnancy losses should prompt a search for APS, as should more than one of these events occurring in the same patient. Confirmation should rely on an unequivocally positive LA, or medium to high positive aCL test (preferably IgG isotype).

Other hypercoaguable states should be considered. These include protein C, protein S, or antithrombin III deficiency; dysfibrinogenemias; abnormalities of fibrinolysis; the nephrotic syndrome; malignancies; polycythemia vera; Behcet's syndrome; and paroxysmal nocturnal hemoglobinuria. In young patients with stroke, myocardial infarction, or peripheral gangrene, clinicians should exclude hyperlipidemias, diabetes, hypertension, vasculitis (medium or large vessel), sickle cell (HbSS) disease, homocystinuria, or Buerger's disease. Acute disseminated vasculopathy–coagulopathy occurring in APS should also prompt consideration of thrombotic thrombocytopenic purpura or diffuse intravascular coagulation.

Causes of pregnancy loss include fetal chromosomal abnormalities and anatomic anomalies of the maternal reproductive tract, as well as endocrine, infectious, autoimmune, drug induced, and other maternal disorders (16). Antiphospholipid syndrome probably accounts for only a small fraction of pregnancy losses, but this diagnosis should be considered in the appropriate clinical setting.

LABORATORY TESTS

The following criteria are required for a positive lupus anticoagulant test: 1.) prolonged partial thromboplastin time, Russell Viper Venom time, or kaolin clotting time; 2.) failure to correct the test by mixing patient plasma with normal plasma (suggesting a clotting inhibitor is present); 3.) normalization of the test with freeze-thawed platelets, or phospholipids (17).

Anticardiolipin tests utilize a standardized enzyme linked immunosorbent assay (ELISA) method (18). Isotypes are measured separately, and a level of positivity in GPL, MPL, or APL units for IgG, IgM, or IgA isotypes, respectively is reported. Most patients with APS have medium to high positive IgG aCL levels with or without other isotypes. There are occasional patients who have IgM aCL or IgA aCL antibodies alone. A serum protein, β_2 glycoprotein 1, has been demonstrated to enhance binding of aCL antibodies to cardiolipin (9). Whether β_2GP1 is the target antigen for aCL antibodies is controversial.

TREATMENT

Acute thrombotic complications of APS are managed no differently from thrombosis in other clinical settings. However, patients with APS appear more subject to recurrent thrombotic events. Hence, prolonged prophylaxis with warfarin in patients with histories of venous or arterial thrombosis, or aspirin with or without dipyridamole in those with arterial thrombosis is recommended. Prednisone, immunosuppressive agents, and anticoagulation are recommended acutely in patients with disseminated vasculopathy–coagulopathy, or in patients who get recurrent, life-threatening thrombosis despite prophylactic anticoagulation.

Management of women during pregnancy is controversial.

Several centers have reported successful pregnancy outcome with prednisone (doses of 20–60 mg/day) and low-dose aspirin 80–100 mg/day (19). Other centers have reported twice daily subcutaneous heparin (5,000–15,000 units) and low-dose aspirin to be equally effective (20). Subcutaneous heparin prophylaxis during pregnancy is recommended for women with APS who have a history of thrombosis. The use of 4- to 5-day pulses of intravenous gamma globulin (0.4 gm/kg/day) given monthly, plus daily low dose aspirin, has led to successful pregnancy outcome. Women with APS need to be monitored carefully during pregnancy, since preeclampsia, intrauterine growth retardation, and other obstetric complications are frequent.

PROGNOSIS

The prognosis of patients with APS is unknown. With the use of appropriate anticoagulants or aspirin, few patients appear to have recurrences of thrombosis. Aspirin prophylaxis in patients without a history of thrombosis is relatively safe and may be beneficial. Prognosis is guarded in patients with disseminated thrombosis or with thrombotic recurrences unresponsive to anticoagulation therapy.

E. Nigel Harris, MD

1. Harris EN: Syndrome of the Black Swan. Br J Rheumatol 26:324–326, 1987
2. Asherson RA: ''Primary'' Anti-Phospholipid Syndrome. In: Phospholipid Binding Antibodies. Edited by Harris EN, Exner T, Hughes GRV, Asherson RA. Boca Raton, Fla., CRC Press, 1991, pp 377–386
3. Sammaritano LR, Wen J, Elkon KB, et al: Induction of antiphospholipid antibodies by immunization with anticardiolipin cofactor. 90:1105–1109, 1992
4. Wilson WA, Perez MC, Michalski JP, et al: Cardiolipin antibodies and null alleles of C4 in black Americans with systemic lupus erythematosus. J Rheumatol 15:1768–1772, 1988
5. Carreras LO, Machin SJ, Deman R, et al: Arterial thrombosis, intrauterine death, and ''lupus anticoagulant'': detection of immunoglobulin interfering with prostacyclin formation. Lancet i:244–246, 1981
6. Hasselaar P, Derksen RHWM, Blokzijl L, et al: Thrombosis associated with antiphospholipid antibodies cannot be explained by effects on endothelial and platelet prostanoid synthesis. Thromb Haemostas 59:80–85, 1988
7. Cariou R, Tobelin G, Belluci S, et al: Effect of the lupus anticoagulant on antithrombogenic properties of endothelial cells—inhibition of thrombomodulin dependent protein C activation. Thromb Haemostas 60:54–58, 1985
8. McNeil HP, Hunt JE, Krilis SA: New aspects of anticardiolipin antibodies. Clin Exp Rheumatol 8:525–527, 1990
9. Khamashta MA, Harris EN, Gharavi AE, et al: Immune mechanisms for thrombosis: antiphospholipid binding to platelet membranes. Ann Rheum Dis 47: 849–854, 1988
10. Asherson RA, Cervera R: The antiphospholipid syndrome: a syndrome in evolution. Ann Rheum Dis 51:147–150, 1992
11. Greisman SG, Thayamparan RS, Goodwin TA, et al: Occlusive vasculopathy in systemic lupus erythematosus: association with anticardiolipin antibody. Arch Intern Med 151:389–392, 1991
12. Harris EN: An acute disseminated coagulopathy–vasculopathy associated with the Antiphospholipid Syndrome. Arch Intern Med 151:231–233, 1991
13. Chartash EK, Lans DM, Paget SA, et al: Aortic insufficiency and mitral regurgitation in patients with systemic lupus erythematosus and the antiphospholipid syndrome. Am J Med 86:407–412, 1989
14. Hughes GRV: Connective tissue disease and skin: the Prosser White oration. Clin Exp Dermatol 9:535–544, 1983
15. Deleze M, Alarcon-Segovia D, Oria C, et al: Hemocytopenia in systemic lupus erythematosus: Relationship to antiphospholipid antibodies. J Rheumatol 16:926–930, 1990
16. Pridham DD, Cook CL: Habitual abortion. In: Phospholipid Binding Antibodies. Edited by Harris EN, Exner T, Hughes GRV, Asherson RA. Boca Raton, Fla., CRC Press, 1991, pp 271–306
17. Triplett DA, Brandt JT: Lupus anticoagulants: misnomer, paradox, riddle, epiphenomenon. Hematol Pathol 2:121–143, 1988
18. Harris EN: Antiphospholipid antibodies (annotation). Br J Haematol 74:1–9, 1990
19. Pattison NS, Lubbe WF: Treatment of anti-phospholipid antibody mediated fetal loss: the case for corticosteroid therapy. In: Phospholipid Binding Antibodies. Edited by Harris EN, Exner T, Hughes GRV, Asherson RA. Boca Raton, Fla., CRC Press, 1991, pp 323–334
20. Cowchock FS: Alternative approaches to treatment of women with antiphospholipid antibodies and fetal loss. In: Phospholipid Binding Antibodies. Edited by Harris EN, Exner T, Hughes GRV, Asherson RA. Boca Raton, Fla., CRC Press, 1991, pp 347–354

13. SYSTEMIC SCLEROSIS AND RELATED SYNDROMES
A. Epidemiology, Pathology, and Pathogenesis

EPIDEMIOLOGY

Systemic sclerosis (SSc, scleroderma) is a connective tissue disease of unknown etiology characterized by fibrosis of the skin and visceral organs and accompanied by relatively specific antinuclear antibodies and microvascular disturbances (1). The disease is rare in childhood; incidence peaks in the fifth and sixth decades of life. Females are affected more commonly than males, and the female-to-male ratio varies with age, peaking at 15:1 during the childbearing years. Systemic sclerosis may be more frequent among black females. Familial cases have been reported but are rare (2).

Study of the epidemiology of SSc has been impeded by the lack of a specific diagnostic test and the relative rarity of the disease. It was not until 1980 that widely accepted criteria for the classification of SSc were developed (Appendix 4) (3). Furthermore, few studies have been designed to investigate cases occurring in a random sample of the general population. Instead, most epidemiologic studies have relied on information obtained from hospital records and death certificates, which probably underestimate the true incidence and prevalence of SSc. In such studies, prevalence has been reported to range from 0.1–13.8/100,000 (4). However, a recent study of a random sample of subjects from the general population of South Carolina reported the prevalence of SSc to be between 19–75/100,000, which is 1.4 to 5.4 times greater than the highest prevalence rate previously reported (5).

Although the current criteria for SSc have a high degree of sensitivity (97%) and specificity (98%) for definite SSc, many milder or atypical forms of the disease are likely to escape diagnosis using only these criteria. The inclusion of specific autoantibodies, such as anti-centromere or anti-topoisomerase I and the presence of microvascular abnormalities, which can be demonstrated by nailfold capillary microscopy (6), would likely increase estimates of the prevalence of SSc.

The epidemiology of SSc and related disorders must take into account potential exposure to a number of environmental agents. Occupational exposure to silica, vinyl chloride, or various organic solvents may give rise to scleroderma-like conditions (7). Two recent epidemics highlight the potential role that environmental agents may play in the pathogenesis of SSc and related conditions. The toxic oil syndrome affected 20,000 individuals in Spain who ingested adulterated rapeseed oil (8). The eosinophilia–myalgia syndrome, which closely resembled the toxic oil syndrome, affected at least 1,500 individuals in the United States who ingested chemically contaminated batches of L-tryptophan (9,10). These syndromes share a number of clinical and histologic features, and differ somewhat from idiopathic SSc. Nevertheless, the study of such syndromes may shed light on the etiology and pathogenesis of SSc. Certain host factors such as age and immunogenetic background may have played a role in determining susceptibility to or expression of such illnesses.

PATHOLOGY

Fibrosis of the skin and other organs, including the blood vessels, is the most consistent histopathologic feature of SSc. Marked increases in collagens and other extracellular matrix in the dermis is accompanied by thinning of the epidermis and loss of rete pegs (Fig. 13A–1). Lymphocytic and monocytic cell infiltrates are frequently present in the dermis, especially in early skin lesions. During the later atrophic phase, the skin may be relatively acellular. Mast cells and evidence of mast cell degranulation have been demonstrated in early skin lesions of SSc, as well as in related conditions such as toxic oil syndrome and graft-versus-host disease (11).

Vascular lesions occur in all organs affected by SSc. Micro-

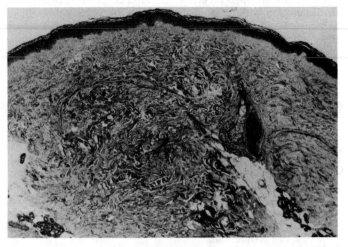

Fig. 13A–1. *Thinning of the epidermis with loss of rete pegs and marked increase in dermal thickness due to increased extracellular matrix.*

vascular disease is widespread and can be observed in vivo in the capillary bed of nailfold skin of nearly all patients with SSc (Fig. 13A–2). The degree of capillary destruction may help to classify the SSc as either diffuse or limited, which may have significant prognostic implications (12). Larger vessels may show intimal hyperplasia, which narrows and may obliterate the vessel lumen (Fig. 13A–3). Pathologic findings in specific tissues are described in Chapter 13B.

PATHOGENESIS OF SYSTEMIC SCLEROSIS

The generalized form of SSc involves a widespread disorder of the microvasculature resulting in exuberant, intense, and unregulated fibrosis. This may be viewed as unregulated wound healing and is the hallmark of scleroderma. Arteriolar and capillary lesions usually precede fibrosis and, when present in vital organs, determine the prognosis for the individual patient, which is principally dependent on the intensity and rapidity of involvement in the lungs, heart, gut, and kidneys. While the vascular lesions almost certainly contribute to the fibrotic reaction in poorly understood ways, evidence is also accumulating that the immune system either initiates or contributes substantially to the vascular process, the fibrosis, or both (13–15).

The Vascular Lesion

The presence of a distinctive, widespread vascular lesion characterized by endothelial abnormalities as well as an exuberant, proliferative reaction of the vascular intima was a factor in changing terminology from scleroderma to systemic sclerosis (16). More recently, the realization that the endothelium is abnormal in scleroderma arteries, arterioles, and capillaries, coupled with the improved ability to study endothelial cell function in vitro and in vivo, has led to the definition of several distinct endothelial cell-related abnormalities in SSc patients. These include elevated plasma levels of von Willebrand factor and decreased serum levels of angiotensin converting enzyme. These measurements could be used to monitor vascular integrity in patients. Therapy to correct the vascular problem is still in its infancy.

Perhaps more to the point, the serum of patients with diffuse SSc has a 50 kDa protein factor, which is cytotoxic to cultured endothelial cells, proteolytic in nature, and seems to derive from the granules of activated T or NK lymphocytes (granzyme one).

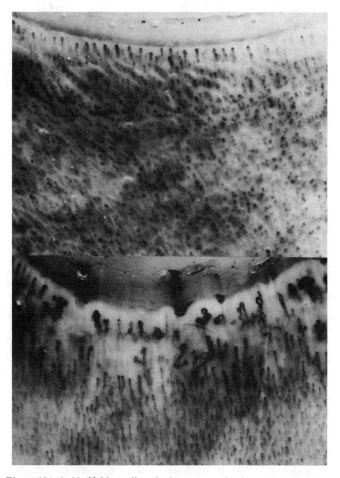

Figure 13A–2. Nailfold capillary bed in a normal subject (upper) and in a patient with systemic sclerosis (lower); the latter shows both enlarged capillaries and avascular areas, as well as capillary hemorrhages and staining of the cuticle (reprinted with permission from Dermatologica 168:73–77, 1984).

The Fibrotic Lesion

The relentless deposition of extracellular matrix in the intima of blood vessels, the pericapillary space, and the interstitium of skin is distinctive for SSc and distinguishes it from other autoimmune disorders. When cells from histologically involved lesions are cultured on tissue culture plastic, they display a constellation of abnormal characteristics conveniently termed the *scleroderma phenotype*, consisting of increased mRNA levels for collagens I, III, and VI, and fibronectin, and increased synthesis of gly-

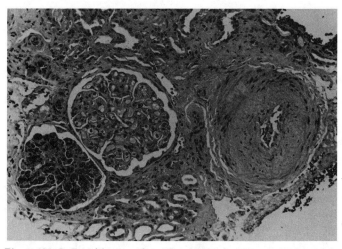

Figure 13A–3. Renal biopsy of an SSc patient showing minor abnormalities of the glomeruli but severe vascular disease with intimal hyperplasia of an arcuate artery.

cosaminoglycans. In addition, affected fibroblasts are hyporesponsive to platelet-derived growth factor (PDGF), and increase their expression of the PDGF alpha receptor after exposure to transforming growth factor beta (TGFβ). Moreover, SSc fibroblasts bind lymphocytes in increased numbers and express increased activity of the cell adhesion molecule, intercellular adhesion molecule 1 (ICAM–1). In culture, SSc fibroblasts are resistant to the induction of quiescence by serum deprivation, continuing to express immediate response genes such as *c-myc* and to undergo cell division for 8 to 16 hours after these activities have ceased in control cells. These in vitro phenomena persist for several cell divisions, suggesting an epigenetic alteration leading to a persistent activated state expressed as increased matrix secretion, exaggerated proliferation, and enhanced adhesion.

What triggers this activated state in SSc fibroblasts? If it is a soluble molecule, the best candidate is TGFβ, a ubiquitous growth factor that undergoes elaborate proteolytic posttranscriptional processing to form an active 25 kDa ligand. This ligand may interact with any or all of three "receptors": a beta glycan with no apparent signalling apparatus, a legitimate serine/threonine protein kinase, and the third yet a mystery. TGFβ induces its own transcriptional upregulation at the same time that it upregulates the message level of several extracellular matrix proteins, including collagen I, III, and VI, fibronectin, and proteoglycans. The best studied example, alpha one type I collagen, seems to be upregulated via a transcriptional protein activator called nuclear factor one. In addition, TGFβ seems to "prime" anchorage-dependent cells such as skin fibroblasts to express selective members of the PDGF family of major fibroblast mitogens. In particular, the scleroderma fibroblast is primed by TGFβ to increase its expression of the universal PDGF receptor (alpha), which transduces a signal after binding with the AA isoform of the PDGF ligand.

This receptor information has been gleaned from the study of nonimmortalized, nontransformed fibroblasts, because standard tissue culture cell lines that are immortal and transformed constitutively express abundant PDGFα receptors. It is remarkable how few alpha receptors are expressed on adult diploid fibroblasts until they are activated by stimuli such as TGFβ. This has led us to designate the PDGFα receptor as a profibrotic fibroblast receptor and to focus on its regulation as a means to control unregulated scarring in scleroderma and other fibrotic disorders. Because of its ubiquity, it may not be feasible to alter the expression of TGFβ receptors in vivo; PDGFα receptors, because of their rare occurrence, may be more appropriate to regulate.

The Immune Lesion

Scleroderma is considered a disorder of autoimmunity for good reason: autoantibodies of remarkable specificity abound in the sera of these patients (Table 13A–1). When, in the 1980s, a rapidly dividing human cell line from a laryngeal carcinoma

Table 13A–1. Autoantibodies in systemic sclerosis

Anticentromere antibodies
Antinuclear antibodies (speckled, nucleolar, other)
Antinucleolar antibodies
    RNA polymerase III
    Fibrillarin (U3 RNA protein complex)
    Nucleolar 4-65 RNA
    U2 RNA protein complex
Polymyositis/SSc overlay (Pm/Scl)
Antitopoisomerase I (formerly Scl-70)
Anticollagen type I (interstitial collagen, ubiquitous)
Anticollagen type IV (basement membrane structure)
Antilaminin (basement membrane attachment protein)
Antiribonucleoprotein (RNP)
Jo-1 (Anti-histidyl-transfer RNA [tRNA] synthetase)
SS-A(Ro), SS-B(La)
Ku
Anti Th (Nucleolar)

(HEp–2) was introduced as a substrate in the indirect immuno-fluorescence test to screen for antinuclear antibodies (ANA), the proportion of scleroderma patients—localized, limited, and diffuse—who tested positive for ANAs increased severalfold. Perhaps even more important, a new and distinctive ANA pattern, the anticentromere antibody, was distinguished from the several types of speckled ANA patterns. This realization spawned the discovery of several new auto-reactive specificities in scleroderma patients. These include multiple nucleolar components and several transfer RNA synthetases (most frequently associated with myositis in patients with overlapping connective tissue disease syndromes), as well as the nuclear housekeeping enzyme, topoisomerase I (formerly Scl–70) that tends to identify individuals with diffuse cutaneous disease. Some further preliminary correlations between disease and ANA patterns, including prognosis, have been made with, for example, anti-RNA polymerase III possibly indicating increased risk for renal crisis and anti-Th characterizing a small number of patients with limited disease. Despite these encouraging clinical applications of the HEp–2 ANA determination, the pathogenetic role or significance of these reactivities is not known. It is unclear how these autoantibodies arise and why they are selective for scleroderma and myositis, in contrast to systemic lupus erythematosus or other autoimmune disorders, for example. Several of these scleroderma-specific autoantibodies have been found to have strong immunogenetic associations, such as anti-topoisomerase–1 with HLA–DR5 and anti-PMScl with HLA–DR3.

In addition to these ANA patterns, several extracellular matrix proteins also seem to elicit autoimmune reactions in scleroderma. Antibodies to types I and IV collagens are present, and delayed hypersensitivity reactions to digested elastin epitopes and to the adhesion protein laminin have also been detected. These matrix components are present in the blood vessel wall and they may be a factor in the prominent vascular lesions of scleroderma.

A recent focus of several studies in scleroderma has been the preliminary delineation of T lymphocyte abnormalities. These tend to cluster around an exaggerated response by the CD4 positive, T-inducer lymphocyte subset prominent in several autoimmune disorders. These CD4 cells are responsive to interleukin–2 (IL–2); both IL–2 and soluble IL–2 receptors are increased in the serum of scleroderma patients. In addition, fractionated peripheral blood mononuclear cells from scleroderma patients can be shown to respond to exposure to type I collagen with increased production of IL–2 compared with control cells, providing further evidence that matrix antigens can propagate the autoimmune process.

On the basis of these observations, the extensive vascular lesions in scleroderma, characterized by endothelial activation/injury and intimal proliferation, could be explained by an initial cytolytic T lymphocyte attack on endothelial cells and the continued lesions explained by autoimmunity to vascular structural antigens, such as type IV collagen and laminin. This mosaic of immune, vascular, and fibrotic features occurring in the same patient in the same tissue may explain the therapeutic difficulties encountered in the treatment of the scleroderma patient.

E. Carwile LeRoy, MD
Richard M. Silver, MD

1. Silver RM, LeRoy EC. Systemic sclerosis (scleroderma). In Immunologic Diseases, 4th Ed. Edited by Samter M, Talmage DW, Frank MM, Austen KF, Claman HN. Boston, Mass., Little, Brown and Co., 1988, pp 1459–1499
2. McGregor AR, Watson A, Yunis E, et al: Familial clustering of scleroderma spectrum disease. Am J Med 84:1023–1032, 1988
3. Masi AT, Rodnan GP, Medsger TA Jr, et al: Preliminary criteria for the classification of systemic sclerosis (scleroderma). Arthritis Rheum 23:581–590, 1980
4. Tamaki T, Mori S, Takehara K: Epidemiological study of patients with systemic sclerosis in Tokyo. Arch Dermatol Res 283:366–371, 1991
5. Maricq HR, Weinrich MC, Keil JE, et al: Prevalence of scleroderma spectrum disorders in the general population of South Carolina. Arthritis Rheum 32:998–1006, 1989
6. Maricq HR: Widefield capillary microscopy. Technique and rating scale for abnormalities seen in scleroderma and related disorders. Arthritis Rheum 24:1159–1165, 1981
7. Owens GR, Medsger TA Jr: Systemic sclerosis secondary to occupational exposure. Am J Med 85:114–116, 1988
8. Toxic epidemic syndrome study group. Toxic epidemic syndrome, Spain, 1981. Lancet 2:697–702, 1982
9. Silver RM, Heyes MP, Maize JC, et al: Scleroderma, fasciitis, and eosinophilia associated with the ingestion of L-tryptophan. N Eng J Med 322:874–881, 1990
10. Belongia EA, Hedberg CW, Gleich GJ, et al: An investigation of the cause of the eosinophilia-myalgia syndrome associated with tryptophan use. N Eng J Med 323:357–365, 1990
11. Seibold JR, Giorno RC, Claman HN: Dermal mast cell degranulation in systemic sclerosis. Arthritis Rheum 33:1702–1709, 1990
12. Chen ZY, Silver RM, Ainsworth SK, et al: Association between fluorescent antinuclear antibodies, capillary patterns, and clinical features in scleroderma spectrum disorders. Am J Med 77:812–822, 1984
13. Smith EA, LeRoy EC: Etiology and pathogenesis of systemic sclerosis, Rheumatology, 1st Ed. Edited by Klippel J, Dieppe P. London, Mosby, 1994
14. LeRoy EC: Systemic sclerosis (scleroderma), Cecil's Textbook of Medicine, 19th Ed. Edited by Wyngaarden JB, Smith LH, Jr., Bennett KC. Philadelphia, Penn., W.B. Saunders Co., 1992, pp 1530–1535
15. LeRoy EC: A brief overview of the pathogenesis of scleroderma (systemic sclerosis). Ann Rheum Dis 51:286–288, 1992
16. Geotz RH: The pathology of progressive systemic sclerosis (generalized scleroderma) with special reference to changes in the viscera. Clin Proc 4:337, 1945

B. Clinical Features and Treatment

Systemic sclerosis (SSc) and its mimics may be classified according to the degree and extent of skin thickening (scleroderma), as shown in Table 13B–1. Patients with rapidly progressive, widespread skin thickening (*diffuse cutaneous involvement*) affecting the distal and often proximal extremities and trunk are at greater risk to develop early, serious visceral involvement. In contrast, individuals with *limited cutaneous involvement*, usually confined to the distal extremities of fingers and face, most frequently have a protracted interval of one or more decades before the appearance of certain characteristic visceral stigmata. This variant is sometimes termed the *CREST syndrome* (calcinosis, Raynaud's phenomenon, esophageal dysmotility, sclerodactyly, telangiectasia).

The major demographic, clinical, and laboratory differences between diffuse and limited scleroderma are shown in Table 13B–2. Either of these variants may coexist with typical features of another connective tissue disease (overlap syndrome), particularly systemic lupus erythematosus (SLE) or polymyositis/dermatomyositis.

CLINICAL FEATURES

In most patients, the first symptoms are Raynaud's phenomenon, swelling and puffiness of the fingers or hands, or polyarthralgias or polyarthritis involving the small joints of the hands. Convincing skin thickening generally follows these complaints by several months. Rarely, polymyositis, esophageal or small bowel disease, or pulmonary involvement may be the first abnormality recognized.

Raynaud's Phenomenon

Cold exposure and emotional stress may induce vasospasm, causing characteristic episodes of blanching or cyanosis of the digits. Bilateral involvement of the fingers, and sometimes the toes, is the rule. Infarction of tissue at the fingertips may lead to digital pitting scars or frank gangrene. In limited cutaneous disease, Raynaud's phenomenon is almost universally present, often antedating other evidence of SSc by years or even decades. In contrast, Raynaud's phenomenon is present at onset in only

Table 13B–1. *Classification of scleroderma and scleroderma-like syndromes*

I. Systemic sclerosis
   A. With diffuse skin thickening—symmetric, widespread thickening of skin affecting the distal and proximal extremities, face and trunk; rapid progression of skin changes; early appearance of visceral involvement (gastrointestinal tract, lungs, heart, kidneys)
   B. With limited skin thickening—symmetric skin involvement restricted to the distal extremities and face; slow progression of skin changes; late appearance of visceral involvement, including distinctive types such as pulmonary arterial hypertension and biliary cirrhosis; prominence of cutaneous telangiectasias and subcutaneous calcinosis (CREST syndrome)
   C. In overlap—either diffuse or limited skin thickening in association with features of one or more other connective tissue diseases (e.g., systemic lupus erythematosus, polymyositis-dermatomyositis).
II. Chemically-induced systemic sclerosis-like conditions
   A. Vinylchloride disease
   B. Bleomycin-induced fibrosis
   C. Trichloroethylene-induced fibrosis
III. Localized forms of scleroderma
   A. Morphea
   B. Linear scleroderma (includes ''en coup de sabre'')
   C. Diffuse fasciitis with eosinophilia (eosinophilic fasciitis)
IV. Chemically-induced localized forms of scleroderma
   A. Toxic oil syndrome
   B. Eosinophilia-myalgia syndrome
   C. Pentazocine-induced fibrosis
   D. Epoxy resin-induced fibrosis
   E. Scleroderma following autologous bone marrow transplantation (graft vs. host disease)
V. Diseases with skin changes resembling scleroderma (pseudoscleroderma)
   A. Edematous
      1. Scleredema adultorum of Buschke or associated with diabetes mellitus
      2. Scleromyxedema (papular mucinosis)
   B. Indurative and/or atrophic
      1. Lichen sclerosus et atrophicus
      2. Porphyria cutanea tarda
      3. Congenital porphyria
      4. Acromegaly
      5. Amyloidosis (primary and myeloma-associated)
      6. Phenylketonuria
      7. Carcinoid syndrome
      8. Localized lipoatrophy, including Gowers' panatrophy, lipoatrophy of ankles, orbicular lipoatrophy
      9. Congenital poikiloderma, including Rothmund's syndrome, Rothmund-Thompson syndrome
      10. Werner's syndrome
      11. Progeria
      12. Acrodermatitis chronica atrophicans
      13. POEMS syndrome
      14. Digital sclerosis of diabetes mellitus
      15. Infiltrating carcinomas

75% of patients with diffuse scleroderma; its absence is associated with an increased risk of subsequent renal involvement.

Raynaud's phenomenon is attributable to both vasospasm and structural disease of the blood vessels. Arterioles are most frequently affected, but digital arteries or even larger vessels are also abnormal. Variably severe intimal hyperplasia causes narrowing and occasionally obliteration of the lumen (1). A similar process (as noted in Fig. 13A–1) can be seen grossly in the nailbed and with wide-field nailfold capillary microscopy (2), leading to loss of capillaries and tortuosity and dilatation of the remaining vessels resulting in telangiectasias.

Skin

Bilateral symmetric swelling of the fingers and hands, and sometimes the feet, is often an early manifestation. After a few weeks to several months, edema is replaced by induration, resulting in thick, hard skin (Fig. 13B–1). Cutaneous sclerosis of both the digits and more proximal areas, such as the dorsum of hands, face, and trunk, is nearly pathognomonic of SSc and occurs only rarely in other conditions (3). In both variants, distal thickening is almost always more severe than proximal involvement. Accompanying changes include loss of normal skin folds, a shiny appearance, and hyper- and hypopigmentation.

In the diffuse cutaneous subtype, skin thickness spreads rapidly in a central direction and within months may affect the forearms, upper arms, face, and finally the trunk, particularly the upper anterior chest and abdomen. In contrast, patients with limited cutaneous disease most often have skin thickening only

Table 13B–2. *Comparison of features in patients with systemic sclerosis who have diffuse cutaneous involvement vs. those with limited cutaneous involvement*

	Diffuse (% patients)	Limited (% patients)
Demographic		
Age <40 at onset	35	50
Sex (female)	75	85
Duration of symptoms (years before first diagnosis)	3.0	8.5
Cumulative survival (10 years after first diagnosis)	55	75
Organ System Involvement		
Skin thickening	100	95
Telangiectasias	30	80
Calcinosis	5	45
Raynaud's phenomenon	85	95
Arthralgias or arthritis	80	60
Tendon friction rubs	65	5
Joint contractures	85	45
Myopathy	20	10
Esophageal hypomotility	75	75
Pulmonary fibrosis	35	35
Pulmonary hypertension	<1	10
Congestive heart failure	10	1
Renal crisis	15	1
Laboratory data		
Antinuclear antibody (any)	95	95
Anticentromere antibody	<5	50
Anti-topoisomerase I antibody	40	15

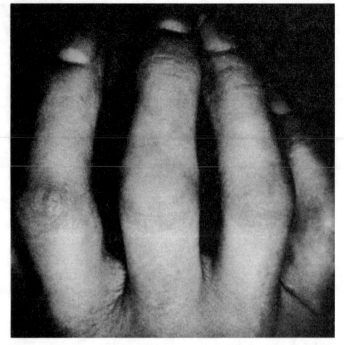

Figure 13B–1. Hand of an elderly woman with diffuse scleroderma. The fingers are puffy, the skin is indurated and normal skin folds are absent. There is some erythema over the proximal interphalangeal joints, and early flexion contractures are evident.

on the fingers or fingers and face, although sometimes hand and distal forearm involvement is found. In the latter circumstance, disease may remain stable for many years, without involvement of more proximal locations. A small subset (less than 2% of patients) does not develop skin thickness, but has characteristic visceral problems. This is referred to as *systemic sclerosis sine scleroderma*.

Physical examination is a more reliable method of establishing the diagnosis of scleroderma than skin biopsy. When obtained during the early indurative phase, a biopsy reveals a striking increase of compact collagen fibers in the reticular dermis. Small arterioles show subintimal hyperplasia and hyalinization. In at least 50% of patients, especially those with diffuse disease, focal collections of lymphocytes, nearly all of which are T cells, are identified in the deep dermis (4).

Once affected, skin in the diffuse cutaneous variant becomes increasingly thick for several years, but eventually softens to some degree in most patients. Improvement typically begins centrally. Thus, the last areas to become clinically involved are the first to show regression. After 5 to 10 years, atrophy of skin may occur. Thinning is particularly noted over the extensor surfaces of joints that have flexion contractures, such as the proximal interphalangeal joints and the elbows. Atrophy and mechanical stretching of skin are more important than ischemia in the development of ulcerations at these sites.

Numerous small macular punctate telangiectasias may appear after several years on the fingers, face, lips, and tongue. They are more frequently encountered in patients with limited cutaneous scleroderma, but also are found in the diffuse variant and may be quite striking during the second and third decades of disease. These lesions may contribute to confusion regarding patient classification. Persons with late-stage diffuse cutaneous disease, in whom skin thickness has regressed considerably, may have numerous telangiectasias and be misdiagnosed as having the limited cutaneous variant.

Subcutaneous calcinosis is a late-developing complication that is considerably more frequent in limited scleroderma (Table 13B–2). Sites of trauma are often affected, such as the fingers, forearms, elbows, and knees. Calcifications may vary from tiny punctate deposits to large masses ulcerating the overlying skin.

Joints and Tendons

Polyarthralgias affect both small and large joints and are especially frequent early in diffuse scleroderma; however, frank polyarthritis is unusual. When present, synovial effusions are small and have a white blood cell count less than 10,000/mm^3. Early in disease, synovial biopsies show mild chronic inflammatory cell infiltration (lymphocytes and plasma cells) and fibrin deposition, whereas later stages show fibrosis of the subsynovial connective tissue (5). Calcific deposits also may occur in joints.

Tenosynovial involvement is confirmed by the presence of carpal tunnel syndrome and by coarse, leathery friction rubs palpated during motion over the extensor and flexor tendons of the fingers, distal forearms, knees, ankles, and other sites (5). These rubs are found almost exclusively in patients with diffuse cutaneous disease. Their presence offers a clue to the subsequent development of widespread scleroderma long before it occurs. Flexion contractures are especially severe in individuals with diffuse cutaneous involvement.

Radiographic changes may be either articular or extraarticular. In most instances, disuse atrophy and osteopenia are the only abnormalities. Erosive arthritis, resembling rheumatoid disease, is seen in a few patients. Osteolysis is presumed due to hypovascularity, which causes bone resorption of the distal and, less commonly, the middle phalanges, sometimes resembling arthritis mutilans. Other affected sites include the distal radius and ulna, mandibular ramus, and superior portion of the posterior ribs ("notching").

Skeletal Muscle

Most patients with diffuse scleroderma have disuse atrophy of muscle due to limited joint motion secondary to skin, joint, or tendon involvement. However, two other forms of myopathy exist (6). The most frequent is a bland, nonprogressive process characterized by mild proximal weakness, minimal elevation of serum creatine kinase, and noninflammatory fibrotic replacement of myofibrils on muscle biopsy. In contrast, a few patients with overlap syndromes have impressive weakness and a classic inflammatory myopathy indistinguishable from polymyositis/dermatomyositis.

Intestinal Tract

Gastrointestinal involvement occurs in a majority of patients and differs little between the diffuse and limited cutaneous involvement subgroups. Distal esophageal motor dysfunction is the most common manifestation of internal involvement. Weakness and incoordination of esophageal smooth muscle lead to dysphagia, especially for solids. The lower esophageal sphincter musculature is similarly affected, resulting in reflux of gastric contents into the distal esophagus with peptic esophagitis, which may be complicated by ulcerations and stricture (Fig. 13B–2). Stricture is particularly common in longstanding limited cutaneous disease. A cine esophagram in the supine position demonstrates decreased motility in over 75% of patients with SSc, some of whom are asymptomatic. Peristaltic activity of the lower two-thirds of the esophagus is reduced or absent, and later the organ may be grossly dilated. A small, sliding hiatus hernia is often present.

Histologic changes are most prominent in the distal esophagus and include atrophy and fibrous replacement of the muscularis and increased collagen deposition in the lamina propria and submucosa. The myenteric plexuses appear to be intact, suggesting that involvement of esophageal smooth muscle is primary rather than secondary. Metaplastic changes in the distal esophageal mucosa (*Barrett's metaplasia*) predispose to the development of adenocarcinoma. Symptomatic gastric malfunction due to SSc is unusual. In contrast, the duodenum is frequently affected, leading to postprandial abdominal pain and bloating. Roentgenograms demonstrate evidence of duodenal atony and dilatation (*loop sign*). Rarely, iron malabsorption may result from extensive duodenal submucosal fibrosis.

Hypomotility of the jejunum and ileum is based on similar loss

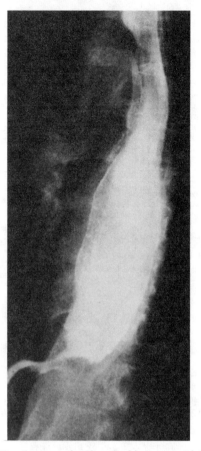

Figure 13B–2. *Esophagram of a 52-year old woman with limited scleroderma of 20 years duration who had increasing difficulty with gastroesophageal reflux symptoms and lower dysphagia. A long distal stricture is present with more proximal dilatation of the esophagus.*

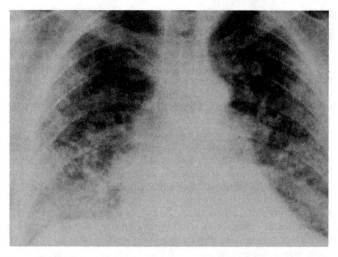

Figure 13B–3. *Bilateral basilar pulmonary interstitial fibrosis (from the Revised Clinical Slide Collection on the Rheumatic Diseases).*

of smooth muscle, but is far less common, affecting less than 20% of patients. However, intestinal malabsorption occurs in some of the latter patients because of improper mixing of lumenal contents and overgrowth of microorganisms that interfere with normal fat absorption, presumably as a result of bile salt deconjugation. Clinical clues to malabsorption include diarrhea, impressive weight loss, and intermittent episodes of marked abdominal distention, with or without painful episodes of "pseudoobstruction". Classic radiographic evidence of small bowel dilatation and hypomotility is uniformly present in such cases, the 72-hour fecal fat excretion is increased, and other biochemical markers of malabsorption are found, such as hypoalbuminemia and hypocalcemia.

Atrophy of the small intestinal mucosa and muscularis occasionally permits entry of air into the wall of the intestine (*pneumatosis intestinalis*), which can be identified radiographically. Dissection through the serosal layers produces benign, sterile intraperitoneal air. Conservative treatment rather than surgical intervention is indicated for this complication.

Patchy smooth muscle atrophy of the large intestine leads to the development of characteristic wide-mouthed diverticula, usually located along the antimesenteric border of the transverse or descending colon. These sacculations, which are unique to SSc, also have been reported in the small intestine. Colonic hypomotility may result in obstipation, and a few patients experience incontinence or rectal prolapse because of rectal sphincter incompetence.

Lungs

Clinical or radiographic evidence of pulmonary involvement develops in a majority of patients and is equally distributed between the diffuse and limited scleroderma groups. Parenchymal disease results in bibasilar linear or nodular interstitial fibrosis that can be demonstrated on chest roentgenograms (Fig. 13B–

3). In this circumstance, the most frequent pulmonary function abnormality is reduced diffusing capacity for carbon monoxide, followed by decline in vital capacity (restrictive lung disease). Despite these changes, many patients have no complaint of dyspnea. Although progression is variable, the few patients who become incapacitated usually have rapid reduction in forced vital capacity during the first several years of disease. The frequency and severity of interstitial fibrosis are increased in patients with serum antitopoisomerase I antibody and decreased in those with anticentromere antibody. Bronchoalveolar lavage has shown that some patients have an intense cellular response, especially by lymphocytes and macrophages, in the early stages of disease. Clinical evidence of pleural involvement is infrequent, consisting of pleuritic pain or friction rub. Autopsy evidence of chronic fibrous pleuritis, however, is common.

Isolated pulmonary arterial hypertension develops in a small proportion of patients, nearly all of whom have limited cutaneous involvement (7). This condition is heralded by rapidly progressive dyspnea and marked reduction of diffusing capacity (<50% of predicted normal), or early signs on echocardiography but it may escape detection for months or years until signs of advanced cor pulmonale appear. Other pulmonary function test results in these patients are normal or minimally abnormal, and there is seldom interstitial fibrosis on chest radiographs. Histologically, the small pulmonary arteries show intense subintimal hyperplasia without inflammation. The prognosis is poor despite the use of vasodilator therapy.

Heart

Clinical evidence of myocardial involvement is uncommon (less than 10%) and is restricted almost entirely to patients with diffuse scleroderma. In contrast, subtle evidence of left ventricular dysfunction is present in a high proportion of patients (8). The manifestations of myocardial disease include recalcitrant congestive heart failure and a variety of atrial and ventricular arrhythmias. The mortality rate is high. Patchy replacement of the myocardium and conducting system by fibrous tissue is the rule in such cases, but the vascular changes that occur in other organs are surprisingly infrequent in the heart. Myocarditis is rare and, when present, is associated with polymyositis affecting the proximal limb musculature. Acute pericarditis is also unusual, but echocardiographic and pathologic evidence of pericardial involvement, with effusion, is considerably more frequent. The right ventricle is secondarily affected by cor pulmonale in end-stage pulmonary disease of either the interstitial fibrosis or arterial hypertension type.

Kidneys

Renal involvement includes reduced creatinine clearance, hypertension, azotemia, and microscopic hematuria or proteinuria, but its symptomatic form is *scleroderma renal crisis*. In the past, this dramatic complication was the major cause of death in patients with diffuse cutaneous involvement. Renal crisis is rare in patients with limited cutaneous involvement. It affects approximately one-fourth of individuals with diffuse disease and typically occurs early (less than four years after onset) and during the phase of rapidly progressive skin thickening. Without warning, the patient develops malignant arterial hypertension with hyperreninemia and oliguric acute renal failure. Occasionally, there is accompanying hypertensive encephalopathy or acute congestive heart failure due to fluid overload. At presentation, urinalysis usually shows small amounts of protein and microscopic hematuria, and the serum creatinine may be normal or elevated. If not treated promptly, these patients have rapidly progressive renal insufficiency. Occasionally, the blood pressure remains normal; in these instances microangiopathic hemolytic anemia is generally prominent and thrombocytopenia is a feature.

The primary targets in renal crisis are arteries of arcuate and interlobular size, and arterioles. Angiographic examination reveals striking constriction of interlobular arteries and a sharp decrease in cortical blood flow. Severe mucoid subintimal hyperplasia is evident histologically, and blood vessel walls may undergo fibrinoid necrosis (9). An inflammatory component is lacking, and immunoglobulin deposition in vessel walls, although present, is unimpressive and similar to that found in like-sized vessels of patients with other forms of malignant hypertension.

Other Organs

Sjogren's syndrome has been confirmed in 20% or more of SSc patients and may be due to either lymphocytic infiltration or glandular fibrosis. Both lymphocytic inflammation (*Hashimoto's thyroiditis*) and fibrous replacement of the thyroid have been observed and are commonly associated with clinical evidence of hypothyroidism. Biliary cirrhosis is found in a few women with CREST syndrome, but hepatic involvement is otherwise rare. Trigeminal sensory neuropathy and other cranial neuropathies have been described, usually in association with limited cutaneous involvement.

LABORATORY FINDINGS

The typical patient with SSc has unremarkable results on routine laboratory tests. The erythrocyte sedimentation rate is generally normal or only slightly elevated. Anemia may result from peptic esophagitis, malabsorption, or renal involvement but is otherwise unusual. Mild hypergammaglobulinemia (IgG) and elevated serum rheumatoid factor are found in 25% of patients, especially in those with overlap syndromes. Nearly all patients with systemic sclerosis have serum antinuclear antibodies (Table 13A–1) (10). The specificities of a number of these autoantibodies have been identified (see Chapter 13A).

COURSE AND PROGNOSIS

The natural history of SSc varies considerably. Overall, the 10-year cumulative survival rate after first diagnosis is approximately 65%. Both death and disability are much more frequent early in the course of diffuse scleroderma, especially in patients with lung, heart, or kidney involvement. Pulmonary hypertension and intestinal malabsorption, however, are frequent causes of mortality in patients with the limited cutaneous variant.

TREATMENT

The evaluation of therapy in SSc has been a major challenge. The relative rarity of the disease makes it difficult to perform double-blind, controlled trials. Scleroderma has a wide spectrum of manifestations and severity as well as a variable course. Spontaneous improvement occurs frequently, rendering interpretation of the results of therapeutic intervention impossible without untreated comparison groups. Psychological aspects of disease and placebo responses to therapy are also important considerations. Only recently have objective measures been used to quantify disease changes. These techniques now include methods of mea-

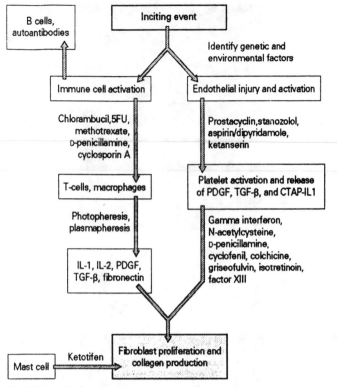

Fig. 13B–4. *Pathogenetic events in systemic sclerosis and location of possible sites where drugs might be useful for therapeutic intervention. Alteration of immune cell activation and function, prevention of endothelial cell injury and activation, and other mechanisms may interfere with the overproduction of collagen by fibroblasts.*

suring change in skin thickening (11), pulmonary function testing, cardiac contractility determination, and creatinine clearance, all of which may serve as useful endpoints.

The Search for Disease Modifying Agents

Many drugs are being studied in SSc, because there is no single agent that has been proven to be convincingly effective. Fig. 13B–4 summarizes the pathogenesis of SSc and potential sites of drug actions. Vascular abnormalities are prominent findings and thus are believed to be important in pathogenesis. Aspirin and dipyridamole, which alter platelet function, are not effective. Ketanserin, an experimental serotonin antagonist, did not result in improvement in skin thickening or internal organ damage, but did reduce the frequency and severity of Raynaud's phenomenon and promote the healing of digital ulcers. Iloprost, a prostacyclin analog, is a promising new agent for improving Raynaud's phenomenon and digital ulcers (12). Neither of the latter two drugs is approved for use.

Immune mechanisms such as lymphocytic infiltration, lymphokine stimulation of fibroblasts, and production of autoantibodies, have been considered potential sites for intervention in SSc. Unfortunately, the immunosuppressive agents chlorambucil (13) and 5-fluorouracil have failed to influence scleroderma features in double-blind controlled studies. Methotrexate and cyclosporin A (14) have been studied in several small series with promising results, but nephrotoxicity of the latter may be a limiting factor. Further studies of plasmapheresis and extracorporeal photopheresis are necessary. At present, several new drugs, including antithymocyte globulin, thymopentin, and FK 506 (antirejection transplant drug) are being examined as potentially effective therapy (15).

D-penicillamine, an immunomodulating agent that also interferes with cross-linking of collagen, is the most widely used drug in the treatment of scleroderma. A large retrospective study showed significant improvement in skin thickening after two years of therapy, and improved five-year survival in patients receiving 0.5–1.0 g/day compared with non-randomly selected untreated comparison patients (11). A reevaluation several years later confirmed these results. Gamma interferon, which suppresses fibroblast proliferation and collagen production in vitro (16), and colchicine, which affects procollagen transport and secretion by fibroblasts, have shown variable results. Ketotifen, a mast cell stabilizing agent, prevents skin fibrosis in the tight skin mouse, but a six-month double-blind study of 24 patients with SSc did not show any significant benefits.

Management of Affected Organ Systems

Raynaud's phenomenon is the most common symptom in SSc patients. Total abstinence from smoking, avoiding cold exposure, keeping the entire body warm, and biofeedback training (17) are usually effective for mild to moderate symptoms. When Raynaud's phenomenon becomes complicated by the occurrence of digital tip ulcers or when it interferes with daily activities, the use of vasodilators, particularly calcium channel blockers, is recommended. These drugs, especially nifedipine, which relaxes vascular smooth muscle, have been effective in decreasing the frequency and severity of Raynaud's phenomenon in double-blind studies (18). The slow-release preparation has improved tolerance with fewer patients experiencing hypotensive symptoms. Other agents, including prazosin and topical nitroglycerin, have also been useful in some patients.

Local management of digital tip ulcers includes soaking the affected fingers in antiseptic fluid such as half-strength hydrogen peroxide, air drying, and then covering only the ulcer with antibiotic ointment followed by a bandage. This occlusive type of dressing promotes wound healing and protects against trauma and infection. Commercial occlusive dressings are particularly helpful with larger noninfected ulcers. When an ulcer becomes infected, a trial of oral antistaphylococcal antibiotics should be given. For deeper infections, surgical debridement of devitalized tissue and intravenous antibiotics may be necessary. Local skin care includes avoiding excessive bathing, which dries skin, and using moisturizing creams containing glycerin. Pruritis is often a serious problem early in the course of diffuse disease. There is no effective treatment, but fortunately this complaint always disappears with time. Likewise, calcinosis cannot be prevented or dissolved despite initial encouraging reports about probenecid and warfarin. The inflammatory process associated with apatite crystal deposition may be controlled with a brief course of colchicine.

Joint and tendon sheath involvement is common. Treatment with nonsteroidal antiinflammatory drugs (NSAIDs) is helpful, but relief is often more difficult to achieve than in other connective tissue diseases. In early diffuse disease, tenosynovitis can be very painful, limiting joint movement. When NSAIDs are inadequate to control pain, low-dose corticosteroids (prednisone less than 10mg/day) or narcotic analgesics may be necessary for short courses. In addition to medication, early aggressive physical therapy with emphasis on stretching is important in preventing or minimizing contractures. Active and passive stretching exercises themselves can be quite painful and the use of adequate analgesia is required to optimize participation in an exercise program. Dynamic splinting has not been effective. Carpal tunnel symptoms, which often occur prior to the diagnosis of scleroderma, can be successfully treated with resting wrist splints and local steroid injections without requiring surgery. Overt myositis is treated with corticosteroids and sometimes requires the addition of immunosuppressive drugs, while the bland, fibrotic myopathy is best managed with strengthening and range-of-motion exercises alone.

Esophageal dysmotility most commonly causes heartburn and lower esophageal dysphagia. Instructions to elevate the head of the bed on four- to eight-inch blocks, eat small frequent meals in an upright position, abstain from nocturnal eating, and use frequent antacids may be adequate. However, the mainstay of therapy is histamine blockade. The newest and most potent agent is omeprazole, which completely eliminates heartburn in most patients (19); however, it has not currently been approved for chronic use. Calcium channel blockers and NSAIDs often aggravate reflux symptoms. Prokinetic drugs, such as metaclopramide, are used to stimulate esophageal muscle contraction but have limited effectiveness. Distal esophageal stricture is managed with periodic dilatations. Surgical procedures for reflux have not achieved general acceptance because of their high failure rate.

Primary small bowel involvement with delayed transit and bacterial overgrowth may result in abdominal distention or bloating, diarrhea, weight loss, and malabsorption. Broad-spectrum antibiotics such as ampicillin, tetracycline, metronidazole, or ciprofloxacin, given in tandem in two-week courses or continuously in low doses may produce a dramatic effect on these symptoms. Metaclopramide is less useful. Supplemental fat soluble vitamins and calcium are often required. Poor nutrition may require hyperalimentation. The first approach to patients with pseudo-obstruction should be conservative and includes nonsurgical decompression, nasogastric suction, bowel rest, and patience.

Pulmonary interstitial disease has become a major therapeutic problem in SSc. Fortunately, most patients have mild, nonprogressive involvement that does not require treatment. Attempts to reverse advanced, fixed fibrosis have been uniformly unsuccessful. In contrast, inflammatory alveolitis identified by bronchoaveolar lavage may be reversible. The use of corticosteroids, and more recently cyclophosphamide, has had variable success in altering the progression of lung disease in such patients. The best hope for patients with advanced pulmonary interstitial fibrosis today is a single or double lung transplant, but few have been performed.

Isolated pulmonary arterial hypertension without significant interstitial fibrosis has the worst prognosis of all scleroderma visceral problems. No therapy, including potent vasodilators, antiinflammatory agents, or immunosuppressive agents, has altered the progression or mortality of this complication, which is uniformly fatal within six months to five years. Most patients die from arrhythmias due to hypoxia, pulmonary arterial in situ thrombosis or cor pulmonale due to respiratory insufficiency. Supplemental oxygen, anticoagulation (to prevent pulmonary thromboembolism), and control of right heart failure are supportive measures available. Again, heart–lung or lung transplant is the only therapeutic option.

Pericarditis, congestive heart failure, and serious arrythmias are potential complications of SSc. All may be treated independent of scleroderma. Mild to moderate pericardial effusions and other asymptomatic cardiac abnormalities usually do not progress and require no treatment.

In previous decades, renal crisis was the most feared visceral complication of SSc. Renal failure was the rule since there was no effective pharmacologic method of managing malignant hypertension. With the introduction of angiotensin converting enzyme (ACE) inhibitors, which are capable of reversing underlying hyperreninemia and controlling hypertension, the outcome of renal crisis has dramatically changed. Patients now have an 80% survival at one year and 60% five-year survival in contrast to a 15% one-year survival without the use of ACE-inhibitors (20) (Fig. 13B–5). The key to successful treatment is early detection and rapid normalization of the blood pressure. ACE inhibitors are the most reliably effective agents, but other new and potent antihypertensives can also be used. In some cases renal failure ensues despite early and vigorous intervention. Even in those who progress to dialysis, approximately 50% continuing on ACE inhibitor therapy have enough improvement in renal function to discontinue dialysis after 6 to 18 months.

LOCALIZED FORMS OF SCLERODERMA

Circumscribed, patchy, or linear scleroderma without the typical serologic and visceral manifestations of systemic sclerosis is found in a heterogeneous group of conditions. These disorders should not be confused with limited cutaneous scleroderma, which is a form of systemic rather than localized disease. Localized scleroderma primarily affects children and young adults, mostly females.

Morphea

Morphea begins with one or more areas of erythematous or violaceous discoloration of the skin, which evolve to become

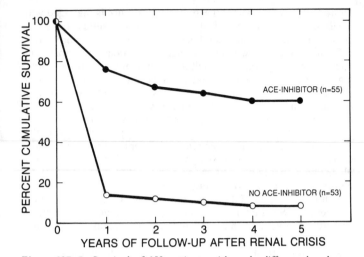

Figure 13B–5. *Survival of 152 patients with early diffuse scleroderma treated with D-penicillamine is significantly better than that of 80 untreated comparison patients.*

sclerotic and waxy or ivory-colored. During the active phase of disease, plaques may increase in size to several centimeters in diameter and are surrounded by a violaceous border of inflammation. Lesions may become widespread or confluent, in which case the term *generalized morphea* is used. After several months to two years, the vast majority of these lesions spontaneously soften. The major histologic changes consist of new collagen deposition in the dermis and septae of the subcutaneous tissue and inconsistently heavy, often intense, infiltration of lymphocytes, plasma cells, and histiocytes.

Linear Scleroderma

In the linear form of localized scleroderma, sclerotic lesions appear morphologically as linear streaks or bands, most commonly on the upper or lower extremities and less frequently on the trunk, forehead, or frontoparietal scalp (see Chapter 22). The latter, termed *en coup de sabre*, may result in disfiguring facial assymmetry with hemiatrophy. Linear scleroderma that crosses a joint may lead to a severe contracture and fibrotic distortion of the nearby neurovascular compartment. The inflammatory and fibrotic reaction may extend to the deep fascia, muscle and rarely, underlying bone (*melorheostosis*).

Considerable overlap exists between morphea and linear scleroderma, and both types of lesions coexist in many patients. During the active phase, laboratory features include a modest degree of peripheral eosinophilia, ANAs, especially anti-single-stranded DNA, and rheumatoid factor (21). A rare patient may develop an inflammatory, nondestructive arthropathy in a distribution characteristic of rheumatoid arthritis. No treatment has been consistently successful in localized scleroderma.

EOSINOPHILIC FASCIITIS

Diffuse fasciitis with eosinophilia is a disorder characterized by the appearance over days or weeks of tender swelling of the arms and legs that tends to spare the hands and feet (22). This evolves to brawny, corrugated induration, which may closely resemble SSc, except for the pattern of distribution and the tendency for retraction or "dimpling" of the subcutaneous tissue. Joint movement can be limited and the patient may become incapacitated. Raynaud's phenomenon is not expected, and these patients have normal nailfold capillaries (23), whereas greater than 90% of SSc patients show characteristic capillary abnormalities. Unaccustomed strenuous exertion may precipitate some cases.

Laboratory testing reveals a negative antinuclear antibody test, impressive eosinophilia, and hypergammaglobulinemia. The definitive diagnostic test is an "en bloc" biopsy of an involved area that includes contiguous tissue from the epidermis down to skeletal muscle, including the deep fascia, showing inflammation and sclerosis of the deep fascia, subcutis, and to a lesser extent,

the dermis. Mononuclear inflammatory cells are prominent and eosinophils are often, but not invariably, present. The typical visceral stigmata of systemic sclerosis are rarely encountered.

Eosinophilic fasciitis is usually treated with corticosteroids, although some patients note remarkable improvement after several months without treatment. Other treatments considered include hydroxychloroquine, penicillamine, and methotrexate, but none of these have been systematically evaluated. However, a disturbing number of patients with eosinophilic fasciitis develop a hematologic abnormality such as thrombocytopenia or aplastic anemia, which are rare in SSc.

EOSINOPHILIA-MYALGIA SYNDROME

The eosinophilia-myalgia syndrome (EMS) is a recently recognized disorder which results from ingestion of certain contaminated batches of L-tryptophan (24). Patients often have striking peripheral eosinophilia and incapacitating myalgias; they may also experience rashes, edema, fasciitis transient dyspnea, cutaneous thickening, neuropathies, myopathies, and cardiopulmonary and gastrointestinal involvement (25). Virtually all patients with EMS had consumed L-tryptophan, most often for treatment of insomnia. More than 12,500 cases were reported before L-tryptophan was withdrawn from the market.

There have been two concepts considered in the pathogenesis of EMS (26): product contamination and an aberration of tryptophan metabolism in susceptible individuals. Only a small percentage of the people who consumed L-tryptophan developed EMS, and only a few predisposing factors have been elucidated.

Persistent and incapacitating myalgias have been the predominant symptom of EMS. Muscle spasms can occur, frequently affecting the calf and abdominal muscles. The upper limbs, hands, jaw, neck, ocular muscles, and tongue may also be involved. Joint contractures, particularly in the elbows, were found in some patients (27). These tend to occur in patients with other features of fasciitis. Eosinophilia with leukocytosis is generally present during the first few weeks of the syndrome or until L-tryptophan is discontinued. Antinuclear antibody tests may be positive, but SSc-specific autoantibodies are absent.

Pains and muscle spasms may persist and remain an annoyance for years in many patients, occasionally affecting functional abilities, but generally more serious organ involvement has not developed after patients discontinue L-tryptophan. In contrast, patients with neurologic involvement, particularly ascending polyneuropathy, and other internal organ involvement tend to have a worse prognosis. As in eosinophilic fasciitis, active inflammatory disease disappears after several years and does not recur. Late-developing cognitive disturbances, such as memory loss and difficulty concentrating, have been reported.

The response to corticosteroids has been inconsistent (28). Patients who remain seriously ill do not appear to benefit from long-term corticosteroids. Methotrexate was thought to be effective in several patients. Isotretinoin, which under certain conditions can block collagen synthesis in vitro, may be of some benefit for the cutaneous thickening and flexion contractures. Medications have limited effectiveness for the myalgias and muscle cramps experienced by these patients.

Thomas A. Medsger, Jr., MD
Virginia Steen, MD

1. Rodnan GP, Myerowitz RL, Justh GO: Morphologic changes in the digital arteries of patients with progressive systemic sclerosis (scleroderma) and Raynaud's phenomenon. Medicine 59:393–408, 1980

2. Maricq HR: Comparison of quantitative and semiquantitative estimates of nailfold capillary abnormalities in scleroderma spectrum disorders. Microvasc Res 32:271–276, 1986

3. Masi AT, Rodnan GP, Medsger TA Jr., et al: Preliminary criteria for the classification of systemic sclerosis (scleroderma). Arthritis Rheum 23:581–590, 1980

4. Roumm AD, Whiteside TL, Medsger TA Jr., et al: Lymphocytes in the skin of patients with progressive systemic sclerosis: quantification, subtyping and clinical correlations. Arthritis Rheum 27:645–653, 1984

5. Schumacher HR: Joint involvement in progressive systemic sclerosis (scleroderma). Am J Clin Path 60:593–600, 1973

6. Clements PJ, Furst DE, Campion DS, et al: Muscle disease in progressive systemic sclerosis: diagnostic and therapeutic considerations. Arthritis Rheum 21:62–71, 1978

7. Stupi A, Steen VD, Medsger TA Jr, et al: Pulmonary hypertension (PHT) in

the CREST syndrome variant of progressive systemic sclerosis (PSS). Arthritis Rheum 29:515–524, 1986

8. Follansbee WP, Curtiss EI, Medsger TA Jr., et al: Physiologic abnormalities of cardiac function in progressive systemic sclerosis with diffuse scleroderma. N Engl J Med 310:142–148, 1984

9. Lapenas D, Rodnan GP, Cavallo T: Immunopathology of the renal vascular lesion of progressive systemic sclerosis (scleroderma). Amer J Pathol 91:243–258, 1978

10. Tan EM, Rodnan GP, Garcia I, et al: Diversity of anti-nuclear antibodies in progressive systemic sclerosis (scleroderma): anti-centromere antibody and its relationship to CREST syndrome. Arthritis Rheum 23:617–625, 1980

11. Steen VD, Medsger TA Jr., Rodnan GP: D-penicillamine therapy in progressive systemic sclerosis (scleroderma). Ann Intern Med 97:652–659, 1984

12. Constans T, Diot E, Lasfargues G, et al: Iloprost for scleroderma. Ann Intern Med 114:606, 1991

13. Furst DE, Clements PJ, Hillis S, et al: Immunosuppression with chlorambucil, versus placebo, for scleroderma. Results of a three-year parallel, randomized, double-blind study. Arthritis Rheum 32:584–593, 1989

14. Zachariae H, Halkier–Sorensen L, Heickendorff L, et al: Cyclosporin A treatment of systemic sclerosis. Br J Dermatol 122:677–681, 1990

15. Torres MA, Furst DE: Treatment of generalized systemic sclerosis. Rheum Dis Clin N America 16:217–241, 1990

16. Kahan A, Amor B, Menkes CJ, et al: Recombinant interferon-gamma in the treatment of systemic sclerosis. Amer J Med 87:273–277, 1989

17. Yocum DE, Hodes R, Sundstrom WR, et al: Use of biofeedback training in treatment of Raynaud's disease and phenomenon. J Rheumatol 12:90–93, 1985

18. Finch MB, Dawson J, Johnston GD: The peripheral vascular effects of nifedipine in Raynaud's syndrome associated with scleroderma: a double-blind crossover study. Clin Rheumatol 5:493–498, 1986

19. Olive A, Maddison PJ, Davis M: Treatment of oesophagitis in scleroderma with omeprazole. Br J Rheumatol 28:553, 1989

20. Steen VD, Costantino JP, Shapiro AP, et al: Outcome of renal crisis in systemic sclerosis: relation to availability of converting enzyme (ACE) inhibitors. Ann Intern Med 113:352–357, 1990

21. Falanga V, Medsger TA Jr., Reichlin M, et al: Linear scleroderma: clinical spectrum, prognosis, and laboratory abnormalities. Ann Intern Med 849–857, 1986

22. Shulman LE: Diffuse fasciitis with eosinophilia: a new syndrome. Arthritis Rheum 29S:205–215, 1977

23. Herson S, Brechignac S, Piette JC, et al: Capillary microscopy during eosinophilic fasciitis in 15 patients: distinction from systemic scleroderma. Am J Med 88:598–600, 1990

24. Hertzman PA, Blevins W, Mayer J, et al: Association of the eosinophilia-myalgia syndrome with the ingestion of L-tryptophan. N Engl J Med 13:864, 1990

25. Swygert LA, Maes EF, Sewell LE, et al: Eosinophilia-myalgia syndrome: results of national surveillance. JAMA 264:1698, 1990

26. Belongia EA, Hedberg CW, Gleich GJ, et al: An investigation of the cause of eosinophilic-myalgia syndrome associated with tryptophan use. N Engl J Med 323:357, 1990

27. Marchman HB, Gleason CB, Shaw JC: Upper extremity contractures in a patient with eosinophilic-myalgia syndrome. Arch Phys Med Rehabil 72:1029, 1991

28. Freundlich B, Werth VP, Rook AH, et al: L-Tryptophan ingestion associated with eosinophilic fasciitis but not progressive systemic sclerosis. Ann Intern Med 112:758, 1990

14. INFLAMMATORY AND METABOLIC MYOPATHIES

IDIOPATHIC INFLAMMATORY MYOPATHIES

Polymyositis and dermatomyositis are idiopathic inflammatory myopathies (IIM). Although they are recognized as distinct entities from other so-called connective tissue diseases, indistinguishable muscle inflammation may accompany any of these autoimmune diseases. Polymyositis and dermatomyositis are not common, with an annual incidence of 5 to 10 cases per million, but they have been increasingly recognized over the last two decades (1). They are more common in women than men in all age groups.

The clinical hallmark of these illnesses is proximal limb and neck weakness, sometimes associated with muscle pain. The laboratory hallmarks are elevated serum levels of creatine kinase, aldolase, lactic dehydrogenase, and the transaminases, and a more or less characteristic pattern on electromyography (EMG). Focal muscle necrosis, regeneration, and inflammation are characteristic pathologic findings. The presence of other features of connective tissue disease, such as autoantibodies, is common. Although polymyositis and dermatomyositis are considered primarily diseases of skeletal muscle, the heart, gastrointestinal tract, lungs, and other sites including joints may be involved.

Classification

Subdivision of these diseases is traditionally based on a combination of clinical and pathologic criteria and patient age (2). A useful classification scheme appears in Table 14–1. Recent observations that certain autoantibodies specific to myositis correlate with distinct clinical presentation, extraskeletal muscle man-

Table 14–1. Classification of idiopathic inflammatory myopathies

Type I:	Primary idiopathic polymyositis
Type II:	Primary idiopathic dermatomyositis
Type III:	Dermatomyositis or polymyositis associated with malignancy
Type IV:	Childhood dermatomyositis or polymyositis
Type V:	Polymyositis or dermatomyositis associated with another connective tissue disease
Type VI:	Inclusion body myositis
Type VII:	Miscellaneous—eosinophilic myositis, localized nodular myositis, and others

Table 14–2. Some syndromes associated with myositis-specific autoantibodies

Autoantibodies	Characteristic Clinical Features
Anti-Jo-1 and other anti-synthetases	Relatively acute onset; frequent interstitial lung disease, fever, Raynaud's phenomenon, arthritis, and "mechanic's hands". Moderate response to therapy, but persistent disease.
Anti-SRP	Very acute onset, often in Fall, severe weakness, no rash, palpitations, $♀>>♂$, poor response to therapy.
Anti-Mi-2	Relatively acute onset, classic dermatomyositis with V sign and shawl sign rashes, cuticular overgrowth, good response to therapy.

ifestations, course, prognosis, response to therapy, and genetic background suggest that these autoantibodies define discrete groups of patients (3). Table 14–2 lists the major myositis-specific autoantibodies and their associated distinguishing clinical features.

Inclusion body myositis (IBM) is an under-recognized entity within the idiopathic inflammatory myopathies. The diagnostic separation of IBM from the other inflammatory myopathies is based on the presence of characteristic cytoplasmic vacuoles in skeletal muscle in this disease. Patients with an insidious onset and slowly progressive, treatment-resistant polymyositis often are found to have IBM after repeated and directed evaluation of muscle biopsies.

Differential Diagnosis

The differential diagnosis of adult polymyositis and dermatomyositis includes an extensive list of conditions affecting muscle. Table 14–3 lists the diseases most commonly misdiagnosed as idiopathic myositis. A complete history of the illness, family history, physical examination, EMG, muscle biopsy, and laboratory tests will usually point to the correct diagnosis. A family history of a similar disease should lead the physician away from a diagnosis of polymyositis or dermatomyositis since they are less often familial than are the dystrophies. Similarly, if the symptoms and signs are closely related to muscular exertion or fasting, myositis is less likely than a genetic, metabolic disorder. These illnesses are discussed in more detail below.

Table 14–3. *Differential diagnosis of idiopathic inflammatory myopathy*

Neuromuscular disorders
  Genetic muscular dystrophies
  Spinal muscular atrophies
  Neuropathies: Guillain-Barré and other autoimmune
    polyneuropathies, diabetes mellitus, porphyria
  Myasthenia gravis and Eaton-Lambert syndrome
  Amyotrophic lateral sclerosis
  Myotonic dystrophy and other myotonias
  Familial periodic paralysis
Endocrine and electrolyte disorders
  Hypokalemia, hyper- or hypocalcemia, hypomagnesemia
  Hypothyroidism, hyperthyroidism
  Cushing's syndrome, Addison's disease
Metabolic myopathies
  Familial periodic paralysis
  Disorders of carbohydrate metabolism—McArdle's disease,
    phosphofructokinase deficiency, adult acid maltase deficiency and
    others
  Disorders of lipid metabolism—carnitine deficiency, carnitine
    palmitoyl transferase deficiency
  Disorders of purine metabolism—myoadenylate deaminase deficiency
  Mitochondrial myopathies
Toxic myopathies
  Alcohol
  Chloroquine and hydroxychloroquine
  Cocaine
  Colchicine
  Corticosteroids
  D-penicillamine
  Ipecac
  Lovastatin and other lipid-lowering agents
  Zidovudine
Infections
  Viral—influenza, EBV, HIV, coxsackievirus
  Bacterial—staphylococcus, streptococcus, clostridium
  Parasitic—toxoplasmosis, trichinosis, schistosomiasis, cysticercosis
Miscellaneous
  Polymyalgia rheumatica
  Vasculitis
  Eosinophilia myalgia syndrome
  Paraneoplastic syndrome

Etiology and Pathogenesis

The etiology and pathogenesis of the idiopathic inflammatory myopathies are not well defined, but a variety of causes and mechanisms have been implicated. A genetic predisposition is likely, as shown by an increased prevalence of certain histocompatibility antigens in some groups of patients with polymyositis or dermatomyositis. Whether drug-induced cases, IBM, or connective-tissue disease-associated or cancer-associated myositis have a similar genetic relationship is unknown. Familial aggregation of cases is rare.

Except in drug-induced and obviously virus-related cases, no etiologic factors have been clearly identified. A list of the most common drugs that cause myositis or myopathy is shown in Table 14–3. Several clues suggest that viral agents are responsible for some cases. In a few cases of IBM, evidence of viral involvement has been presented, but not confirmed (4). Crystalline arrays resembling picornaviruses have been identified in muscle in a few cases of polymyositis, and there is serologic evidence of recent coxsackievirus infection in some cases of both adult and childhood disease (5,6). However, a careful and sensitive search for candidate viral genomes was negative (7). Toxoplasmosis may present as an acute myositis, but some serologic evidence suggests that it may have a role in idiopathic myositis as well (8).

Autoimmune factors are felt to be important, because autoantibodies are present in most patients (3,9). Some of the autoantibodies found in myositis patients—including anti-Jo-1, anti-PL-7, anti-PL-12, anti-EJ, anti-OJ, anti-Mi-2, anti-MAS, anti-Fer, and anti-SRP—are specific to myositis (10); whereas others such as anti-Ro(SS-A), anti-La(SS-B), anti-RNP, anti-Sm, and related antinuclear antibodies, are found in other dis-

eases as well. As described below, the myositis-specific autoantibodies appear to define discrete groups of patients.

None of these antibodies is likely to be directly responsible for tissue damage since their target antigens are believed to be entirely intracellular, and furthermore, are not limited to muscle cells, but are found in all cells. Antibodies directed against muscle cells are not a specific feature of these illnesses. In both childhood and adult dermatomyositis, perivascular inflammation may be striking, and the so-called membrane attack complex of late complement components is found in vessel walls, suggesting that vascular injury within muscles and skin has a pathogenetic role (11). Vessel density in muscle is diminished in patients with dermatomyositis (12).

Although cellular immunity to muscle tissue has not been demonstrated unequivocally, careful analysis of biopsy specimens has shown that CD8$^+$ cytotoxic T lymphocytes are the predominant cells surrounding or invading muscle cells in affected tissue (13). Many of these T cells, as well as accompanying macrophages, express class II histocompatibility antigens on their surface, indicating that they are activated. In contrast, B cells, CD4$^+$ helper T cells, and natural killer cells are less abundant and more distant from the fiber damage in both polymyositis and IBM.

CLINICAL FEATURES

Symmetric proximal muscle weakness is the dominant feature of these diseases, although it is variable in its onset, progression, and severity. In some patients, symptoms appear suddenly, progress rapidly, and quickly result in a bedridden state, sometimes requiring ventilatory assistance and tube feeding. More typically, weakness, malaise, and weight loss develop insidiously over months or even years, with some patients either unable to identify the onset of the disease or unaware of their gradual disability. In a few patients, spontaneous remissions and exacerbations occur.

History

Patients most often first complain of hip girdle symptoms, including difficulty climbing stairs, getting into or out of a car, and rising from a chair without the use of their arms. Later symptoms involve the arms, with complaints of difficulty lifting objects from high places, putting on heavy clothes, and combing hair. Weakness of the anterior neck flexors, which occurs in about one-half of patients, can result in inability to raise the head from a pillow while in bed. Upon questioning, fewer than 50% of patients describe muscle pain and tenderness, about one-fifth report difficulty chewing or swallowing, and some complain of shortness of breath, joint pains, a tendency to fall, Raynaud's phenomenon, facial swelling, mild fever, muscle cramping, palpitations, and hoarseness or a nasal voice.

In IBM, there is an insidious onset of painless, bilateral yet asymmetric, proximal and distal weakness; slowly relentless progression; and relatively poor response to the standard therapies used for myositis. Falling episodes are common, often resulting in fractures. Patients with IBM are most often white men, and the disease is diagnosed in the fifth, sixth, or seventh decades.

Physical Examination

Proximal limb muscle weakness is detected by physical examination in most symptomatic patients. The weakness is usually symmetric and diffuse. Affected muscles are sometimes tender to palpation or atrophied. The patient's gait is often slow and waddling. Contractures, not usually seen at presentation, may develop as the disease progresses. Facial and ocular muscle weakness almost never occur, which distinguish myositis from myasthenia gravis and some inherited myopathies. Manual muscle testing and tests of functional abilities are useful supplements to a careful history and laboratory testing. They help provide an organized approach to following disease progression and therapeutic response over a long period.

In IBM, the clinical characteristics of a long-standing myopa-

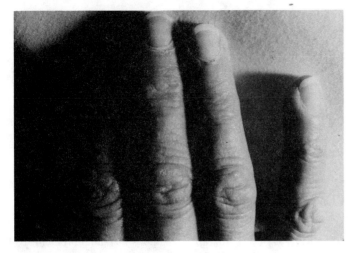

Fig. 14–1. Gottron's rash in a patient with dermatomyositis.

thy—profound weakness and focal muscle atrophy—are often evident on physical examination. There is more distal involvement than in dermatomyositis or polymyositis. Although weakness is usually bilateral in distribution, asymmetry is common. The legs are often more affected than the arms, and the anterior thigh is more frequently involved than the posterior thigh. Some patients also have a mild peripheral neuropathy with loss of deep tendon reflexes. This may be evident on electromyography, which is otherwise indistinguishable from that in other inflammatory myopathies. Extraskeletal muscle involvement of the lungs, joints, and heart, common in other inflammatory myopathies, is rare in patients with IBM.

In dermatomyositis, cutaneous manifestations can precede, follow, or develop concomitantly with muscle involvement, and their severity may vary independently. The only pathognomonic skin findings are Gottron's papules, which occur in approximately one-third of patients with dermatomyositis. These are violaceous, flat-topped papules overlying the dorsal surface of the interphalangeal joints of the hands. These areas can develop central atrophy, with telangiectasia and hypopigmentation. Gottron's sign or rash (see Fig. 14–1), a more common finding, consists of erythematous smooth or scaly patches, with or without associated edema, over the dorsal interphalangeal or metacarpophalangeal joints, elbows, knees, or medial malleoli. A similar erythema may overlie the extensor tendons of the hands, forearms, and arms. There is often a coexistent, sometimes photosensitive, dusky eruption on the face, especially in the malar and periorbital areas, on the V area of the neck (the so-called V sign), and over the shoulders and upper back (the shawl sign). The skin may show a characteristic speckled thinning with areas of hyperpigmentation and hypopigmentation known as *poikiloderma*. The heliotrope rash is dusky purple and occurs over the often-edematous upper eyelids, especially along the edges. Hyperemia and scaling, roughened skin may be present over the sides and tips of the fingers, a condition known as mechanic's hands. The nailbeds frequently show cuticular overgrowth, periungual erythema, and telangiectasia. Subcutaneous calcification, though more common and severe in childhood dermatomyositis, occasionally occurs in the adult myositis syndromes.

Cardiac involvement is not uncommon and contributes significantly to mortality. Nearly one-half of patients have dysrhythmias, congestive heart failure, or electrocardiographic evidence of conduction defects, ventricular hypertrophy, or pericarditis.

Pulmonary disease can result from weakness of the respiratory muscles, intrinsic lung pathology, or aspiration. Abnormal pulmonary function tests are found in about 50% of the patients. Depressed lung volumes, diffusing capacity, and arterial oxygenation are the primary findings. Interstitial pulmonary fibrosis is reportedly present in 5% to 10% of patients overall but is a common finding in a subgroup of patients with anti-synthetase autoantibodies (anti-Jo–1 and related specificities). Swallowing difficulties, nasal regurgitation, and esophageal dysphagia and reflux are common, especially in severe cases.

A mild nondestructive arthritis can be an early feature; arthropathy due to apatite deposition has also been seen.

Malignancy is found in a higher than expected proportion of patients with polymyositis and dermatomyositis. The relative risk was found to be 1.8 for men, and 1.7 for women with polymyositis; and 2.4 for men, and 3.4 for women with dermatomyositis in a carefully studied Scandanavian population (14). Coincident onset of the two diseases (within a year of one another) is somewhat less frequent. It is highest for dermatomyositis, with 10% having a malignancy diagnosed within the first year of the diagnosis of myositis. Of most importance to the practicing clinician, however, is how to approach the patient who presents with new onset of an inflammatory myopathy. Taking a thorough history, performing a careful physical examination including a rectal examination and pelvic in women, and doing basic laboratory tests, including those usually recommended for patients in that age group (for example, mammography or colonoscopy) will detect the great majority of malignancies present at the time of the diagnosis of myositis. This should be followed by a rigorous investigation of any abnormalities found. Extensive blind radiologic screening studies are probably not justified.

LABORATORY FINDINGS

Results of most routine laboratory tests are normal, with the exception of elevated serum levels of various muscle-associated enzymes. The transaminases, creatine kinase, lactate dehydrogenase, and/or aldolase activities are elevated in virtually all patients at some time during the course of their disease, and may be over 100 times the upper limit of normal. Serum enzyme activities within the normal range can be found, however, in a small proportion of patients at presentation, as well in patients without active muscle inflammation or in those who have lost considerable muscle mass. Myoglobinemia, myoglobinuria, and creatinuria, though seldom sought, are commonly present.

In IBM, the serum creatine kinase level is not usually elevated more than four or five times above the upper limit of normal. Autoantibodies including ANA and extractable nuclear antigen (ENA) antibodies do occur in IBM patients, but none of the myositis-specific autoantibodies, such as anti-Jo–1 antibodies, has yet been reported in IBM.

Electromyography and nerve conduction velocity studies are useful in establishing the diagnosis and excluding muscle diseases that result from denervation. The following are characteristic findings in the idiopathic inflammatory myopathies: 1) small-amplitude, short-duration, polyphasic motor-unit potentials; 2) spontaneous fibrillations, positive spike waves at rest, and increased irritability; 3) bizarre, high-frequency complex repetitive discharges; and 4) absence of neuropathy (except in IBM).

PATHOLOGY

Muscle biopsy is usually indicated to establish the diagnosis. Careful selection of the biopsy site and proper tissue processing are essential. The muscle to be biopsied should be moderately weak, without severe atrophy, and with no recent trauma (no recent intramuscular injections, or insertion of electromyographic needles). The quadriceps, deltoid and biceps muscles are most often selected because of their accessibility and frequent involvement. Tissue examination reveals focal or diffuse inflammatory infiltrates consisting primarily of lymphocytes and macrophages surrounding muscle fibers and small blood vessels. Muscle cells show features of degeneration and regeneration: variation in fiber size, fiber necrosis, and basophilia of some fibers with centralization of nuclei. Fiber atrophy is often most severe at the periphery of the muscle bundle, producing the characteristic perifascicular atrophy. Extensive interstitial fibrosis and fatty replacement are common in long-standing cases. Unfortunately, the pathology can be extremely focal, sometimes resulting in non-diagnostic biopsies. Magnetic resonance imaging (Fig. 14–2) can reveal muscle inflammation and may help to select the site to biopsy in difficult cases (15).

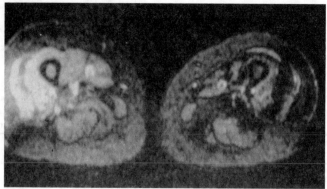

Fig. 14–2. Magnetic resonance image of the thighs of a patient with IBM. Inflamed muscle appears brighter than uninflamed muscle tissue. This image demonstrates several features often found in IBM: atrophy, especially in the anterior compartment; asymmetry of inflammation; and asymmetry of atrophy.

Inclusion body myositis has pathologic and immunologic findings similar to yet distinct from other inflammatory myopathies (16). The characteristic vacuoles or inclusions of IBM, rimmed with granular material, are best seen on frozen sections of skeletal muscle stained with Gomori's trichrome. On ultrastructural study there are typical nuclear and cytoplasmic filaments and membranous whorls. The muscle biopsy usually shows foci of chronic inflammatory cells without perifascicular atrophy, the capillaries are not abnormal, there is increased expression of the major histocompatibility (MHC) class I product on myocytes in close relation to inflammatory cells, and CD8[+] T lymphocytes infiltrate the muscle. Despite these findings and the apparently distinctive clinical course of patients with IBM, the boundary between IBM and the other inflammatory myopathies such as polymyositis remains uncertain, as does the boundary with non-inflammatory myopathies such as oculopharyngeal muscular dystrophy.

TREATMENT

High-dose daily oral corticosteroid therapy is the usual initial treatment for dermatomyositis and polymyositis (17). Retrospective studies comparing corticosteroid therapy with no therapy and high-dose with low-dose corticosteroid therapy showed no effect of treatment on survival. Steroids, however, decreased the inflammation, shortened the time to normalization of muscle enzymes, and reduced morbidity. Therapy is usually begun with prednisone (1–2 mg/kg/day) until strength improves and serum creatine kinase enzyme activity normalizes, which may take several months. The dosage is then reduced, preferably on alternate days. Many patients require maintenance therapy. Initial alternate-day therapy may reduce steroid-related complications, but has not been widely used. Clinical history and measurements of a patient's strength and functional abilities are the simplest routine tests to monitor disease activity. The level of serum creatine kinase or aldolase usually parallels clinical activity accurately, although elevated levels sometimes persist in periods of clinical inactivity. Conversely, active inflammation may be demonstrated on biopsy despite normal muscle enzyme activity.

Approximately three-fourths of patients exhibit good clinical response to steroids alone. Patients refractory to steroids or unable to tolerate high doses because of complications require the addition of an immunosuppressive agent. Methotrexate appears to be as effective orally as parenterally. The starting dose should be 7.5 mg/week, but doses of 25 mg/week or more may be needed. Azathioprine (50–150 mg/day), and oral cyclophosphamide and chlorambucil have all been reported to be of benefit.

Approximately 5% to 10% of patients do not respond to corticosteroids and immunosuppressive agents. Plasmapheresis and leukapheresis are ineffective in this population (18). Reports of treatment with oral steroids plus the combination of oral methotrexate and chlorambucil or cyclosporin A are promising, as is

intravenous gamma globulin therapy (19). Skin rash unresponsive to therapy effective for muscle involvement may respond to the addition of hydroxychloroquine. Because the rash may be photosensitive, sun screens are advisable.

Graded exercise after inflammation has subsided helps restore strength, and range-of-motion can be preserved with attentive physical therapy. Aggressive early exercise can cause rhabdomyolysis. No therapy has a proven record in improving interstitial pulmonary fibrosis or cardiac involvement.

PROGNOSIS

Earlier studies reported cumulative survival rates of approximately 50% at six to seven years from diagnosis. More recent studies report increased survival rates of 70% to 80%, possibly due to a combination of earlier diagnosis and improvement of general medical treatment. Morbidity from the illness and the complications of drug therapy remain a substantial problem. Patients over 45 years of age at onset, women, and blacks may have higher morbidity and mortality, as do those with heart or lung involvement. A long interval between the onset of weakness and the initiation of therapy adversely affects prognosis.

Since the description of IBM as a separate entity, the lack of improvement with therapies usually effective for the other idiopathic inflammatory myopathies has resulted in its characterization as a treatment-resistant form of polymyositis. There have been no published prospective therapeutic trials in IBM, but corticosteroids rarely result in improvement in strength. In patients with IBM, the long course of the illness before the patient ever sees a physician suggests that the destruction of muscle is slow. Atrophy from disease, disuse and corticosteroid-induced myopathy in varying proportions is distinctly more pronounced in IBM than in the other inflammatory myopathies. Thus, active inflammation probably contributes little to the current weakness. Some patients, however, may experience a halt in the progression of their weakness with therapy. With this in mind, reasonable goals are slowing the rate of myocyte destruction and progressive weakness. This limited goal, difficult to document in an individual patient, remains to be examined in a sufficiently long therapeutic study.

In rheumatoid arthritis and systemic lupus erythematosus, myositis is usually mild and often asymptomatic. In scleroderma and mixed connective tissue disease, it may be severe and dominate therapeutic decisions. The myositis of malignancy may respond during the treatment of the malignancy alone, although the rash is commonly refractory.

METABOLIC AND OTHER GENETIC MYOPATHIES

Many entities can cause signs and symptoms that closely mimic idiopathic myositis in adults and can lead to difficulty in diagnosis and therapy (20). Some of these disorders can be differentiated on the basis of the clinical setting in which they occur, others by laboratory and muscle biopsy findings. A few patients require biochemical or molecular characterization available only in a few referral centers. Most of these myopathies have been historically classified as either metabolic myopathies, including diseases associated with abnormal glycogen, lipid, or mitochondrial metabolism; or as muscular dystrophies, including syndromes characterized by progressive muscle weakness and atrophy, often in the setting of a sex-linked or familial pattern.

Glycogen storage diseases, which result from abnormal glycogen synthesis, degradation or glycolysis, lead to increased deposition of glycogen in muscle as demonstrated by periodic acid-Schiff (PAS)-positive vacuoles within myocytes. In addition to the critical role of the clinical history and exam, and diagnostic enzyme activity assays in fresh or frozen muscle specimens, the *ischemic forearm exercise test* is also useful in distinguishing among the various metabolic myopathies. This test is performed by obtaining a baseline blood sample for analysis of lactate and ammonia, and then inflating a sphygmomanometer cuff on the arm to at least 20 mm Hg above systolic pressure while the patient squeezes an object strenuously every 2 seconds for a period of 90 seconds. At this point, the cuff is deflated and repeated venous samples for lactate and ammonia are obtained 1, 3, and 5 minutes thereafter. Lactate and ammonia levels increase at least threefold from baseline in normals.

The major forms of glycogen storage disease confused with idiopathic myositis are as follows:

1) *Adult onset (partial) acid maltase deficiency*, an autosomal recessive disease, with exercise intolerance, frequent respiratory insufficiency, mildly elevated creatine kinase, gradually progressive limb-girdle weakness, a myopathic EMG, a normal ischemic forearm exercise test, and a vacuolar myopathy on biopsy;

2) *Myophosphorylase deficiency (McArdle disease)* with elevated creatine kinase, exercise-induced fatigue, myalgias, cramps, weakness, and occasional myoglobinuria, a "second wind phenomenon", and lack of a rise of venous lactate after the ischemic forearm exercise test; and

3) *Phosphofructokinase deficiency*, an autosomal recessive disease, with a similar clinical presentation and the same abnormality in the forearm ischemic exercise test as myophosphorylase deficiency, but with less "second wind phenomena," often with nausea and vomiting after exercise, and occasional hemolytic anemia.

Disorders of lipid metabolism and substrate transport across the mitochondrial membrane include *carnitine palmitoyl transferase (CPT) II deficiency* and *carnitine deficiency*, which are often autosomal recessive diseases that present as progressive limb and trunk weakness with intrafiber Oil red O-positive lipid droplets on muscle biopsy.

Mitochondrial myopathies are a group of very rare clinically diverse disorders characterized histopathologically by "ragged red fibers" (containing peripheral and intermyofibrillar accumulations of abnormal mitochondria) on modified Gomori's trichrome staining of frozen muscle biopsy sections, and defined biochemically by defects of mitochondrial metabolism involving electron transport enzymes.

Muscular dystrophies are a group of syndromes with mild to moderately elevated creatine kinase levels, myopathic EMGs, and occasional inflammatory biopsies that can make differentiation from idiopathic inflammatory myopathy difficult. The identification of the huge gene on the X chromosome encoding the ~425 kDa myocyte membrane protein dystrophin was a major recent advance allowing the molecular characterization of Duchenne dystrophy and Becker dystrophy. These disorders are caused by abnormal, diminished, or absent dystrophin. These X-linked juvenile-onset dystrophies can be confused with juvenile myositis.

Different genetic patterns, frequent spontaneous cases, and variable expression and penetrance of disease all contribute to the lack of understanding of the rare types and adult forms of muscular dystrophy. The forms sometimes confused with adult-onset idiopathic myositis include:

1) *Fascioscapulohumeral dystrophy* (~1 in 100,000 births)—an autosomal dominant disease with variable penetrance and expression and onset in adolescence to middle adult years. It often presents with facial, shoulder, and proximal arm weakness, sometimes as a flu-like syndrome with creatine kinase elevation up to five times normal and inflammatory changes on muscle biopsy closely mimicking idiopathic myositis. Some patients may be partially responsive to corticosteroids;

2) *Limb–girdle dystrophy*—an autosomal recessive disease

with progressive shoulder and pelvic weakness, but sparing of the facial muscles; and

3) *Myotonic dystrophies* (~13 cases per 100,000 births)—autosomal dominant diseases with adult onset characterized by delayed relaxation and stiffness of muscles (*myotonia*). Patients have facial weakness with ptosis, distal limb weakness, frequent systemic features (cardiac, respiratory and gastrointestinal involvement), excessive insertional activity on EMG, and ringed myofibers in 70% of cases. Phenytoin or quinine therapy may improve the myotonia.

Paul H. Plotz, MD
Richard L. Leff, MD
Frederick W. Miller, MD

1. Oddis CV, Conte CG, Steen VD, et al: Incidence of polymyositis-dermatomyositis: a 20-year study of hospital diagnosed cases in Allegheny County, PA 1963–1982. J Rheumatol 17:1329–1334, 1990

2. Bohan A, Peter JB, Bowman RL, et al: Computer-assisted analysis of 153 patients with polymyositis and dermatomyositis. Medicine (Baltimore) 56:255–286, 1977

3. Love LA, Leff RL, Fraser DD, et al: A new approach to the classification of idiopathic inflammatory myopathy: myositis-specific autoantibodies define useful homogeneous patient groups. Medicine (Baltimore) 70:360–374, 1991

4. Nishino H, Engel AG, Rima BK: Inclusion body myositis: the mumps virus hypothesis. Ann Neurol 25:260–264, 1989

5. Christensen ML, Pachman LM, Schneiderman R, et al: Prevalence of cox-sackie B virus antibodies in patients with juvenile dermatomyositis. Arthritis Rheum 29:1365–1370, 1986

6. Travers RL, Hughes GRV, Cambridge G, et al: Coxsackie B neutralization titres in polymyositis/dermatomyositis. Lancet 1:1268, 1977

7. Leff RL, Love LA, Miller FW, et al: Viruses in idiopathic inflammatory myopathies: absence of candidate viral genomes in muscle. Lancet 339:1192–1195, 1992

8. Magid SK, Kagen LJ: Serologic evidence for acute toxoplasmosis in polymyositis-dermatomyositis. Increased frequency of specific anti-toxoplasmosis IgM antibodies. Am J Med 75:313–320, 1983

9. Reichlin M, Arnett FC Jr: Multiplicity of antibodies in myositis sera. Arthritis Rheum 27:1150–1156, 1984

10. Targoff IN: Immune mechanisms in myositis. Curr Opin Rheumatol 2:882–888, 1990

11. Kissel JT, Mendell JR, Rammohan KW: Microvascular deposition of complement membrane attack complex in dermatomyositis. N Engl J Med 314:329–334, 1986

12. De Visser M, Emslie-Smith AM, Engel AG: Early ultrastructural alterations in adult dermatomyositis. Capillary abnormalities precede other structural changes in muscle. J Neurol Sci 94:181–192, 1989

13. Engel AG, Arahata K: Mononuclear cells in myopathies: quantitation of functionally distinct subsets, recognition of antigen-specific cell-mediated cytotoxicity in some diseases, and implications for the pathogenesis of the different inflammatory myopathies. Hum Pathol 17:704–721, 1986

14. Sigurgeirsson B, Lindelof B, Edhag O, et al: Risk of cancer in patients with dermatomyositis or polymyositis. A population-based study. N Engl J Med 326:363–367, 1992

15. Fraser DD, Frank JA, Dalakas M, et al: Magnetic resonance imaging in the idiopathic inflammatory myopathies. J Rheumatol 18:1693–1700, 1991

16. Lotz BP, Engel AG, Nishino H, et al: Inclusion body myositis. Observations in 40 patients. Brain 112:727–747, 1989

17. Oddis CV, Medsger TA: Current management of polymyositis and dermatomyositis. Drugs 37:382–390, 1989

18. Miller FW, Leitman SF, Cronin ME, et al: Controlled trial of plasma exchange and leukapheresis in polymyositis and dermatomyositis. N Engl J Med 326:1380–1384, 1992

19. Cherin P, Herson S, Wechsler B, et al: Efficacy of intravenous gammaglobulin therapy in chronic refractory polymyositis and dermatomyositis: an open study with 20 adult patients. Am J Med 91:162–168, 1991

20. Wortmann R: Metabolic diseases of muscle. Arthritis and Allied Conditions, 11th ed. Edited by Daniel J McCarty. Philadelphia, Lea & Febiger, 1989, pp 1778–1797

15. SJOGREN'S SYNDROME

Sjogren's syndrome is a chronic, slowly progressive inflammatory autoimmune exocrinopathy of unknown etiology (1–4). The typical clinical presentation of Sjogren's syndrome includes keratoconjunctivitis sicca and xerostomia, due to diminished lacrimal and salivary gland secretion. This autoimmune disease may evolve from an organ specific (exocrine glands) to a systemic (extraglandular) disorder affecting lungs, kidneys, blood vessels, and muscles, as well as a B cell lymphoproliferative disorder. These features are believed to be the consequence of overt immune system activation, manifested by various autoantibodies, and lymphocytic invasion of the exocrine glands and other affected organs. When not associated with other connective tissue diseases, the syndrome is designated primary Sjogren's syndrome. Secondary Sjogren's syndrome defines the disease complex in the presence of other autoimmune disorders, including rheumatoid arthritis (RA), systemic lupus erythematosus (SLE), systemic sclerosis, myositis, biliary cirrhosis, chronic hepatitis, cryoglobulinemia, vasculitis and thyroiditis.

CLINICAL PRESENTATION

Sjogren's syndrome is the second most common autoimmune rheumatic disorder, following RA (5). It progresses very slowly, with 8 to 10 years elapsing from the initial symptoms to the full-blown development of the syndrome. Although Sjogren's syndrome typically occurs in middle-aged women, the disease is known to appear in all ages and in men.

Glandular Manifestations

Most Sjogren's patients develop symptoms related to decreased lacrimal and salivary gland function. Patients with the primary syndrome usually complain of dry eyes, frequently experienced as a sandy feeling under the eyelids or a gritty sensation. In addition, symptoms include burning, accumulation of thick strands at the inner canthus, decreased tearing, redness, itching, eye fatigue, and increased sensitivity to light. These symptoms result from the destruction of corneal and bulbar conjunctival epithelium referred to as *keratoconjunctivitis sicca*. Enlargement of the lacrimal glands is uncommon.

Keratoconjunctivitis sicca is assessed by tear flow and composition. Tear flow is measured using the Schirmer test, while tear composition can be examined by tear break-up time or tear lysozyme content. The Schirmer test, commonly performed at the bedside, is considered positive when filter paper wetting of less than 5 mm occurs in 5 min and suggests clinically significant keratoconjunctivitis sicca. However, the predictive value is extremely limited, owing to the high percentage of false-positive and false-negative results. Integrity of the corneal and bulbar conjunctival epithelium is assessed using Rose Bengal staining and slit-lamp examination. Slit-lamp examination after Rose Bengal staining in Sjogren's patients is a more specific procedure and should reveal punctate corneal ulcerations and attached filaments of corneal epithelium indicating destruction of corneal and bulbar conjunctival epithelium.

Xerostomia is the other principal symptom of Sjogren's syndrome. Patients with oral dryness complain of a burning oral discomfort and difficulty in chewing and swallowing dry foods and increased adherence of food to buccal surfaces. Xerostomia is often associated with changes in the sense of taste and an inability to speak continuously for more than a few minutes. It may manifest with accelerated development of dental caries. The parotid or submandibular glands exhibit a firm, diffuse, nontender enlargement in most patients (Fig. 15–1). The oral mucosal

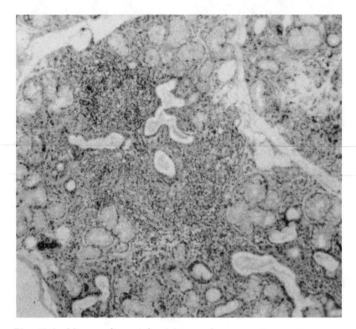

Fig. 15–2. *Minor salivary gland biopsy from a patient with primary Sjogren's syndrome demonstrates extensive focal lymphocytic infiltration and destruction of acinar tissue (original magnification, ×40).*

surfaces tend to be dry, sticky and often exhibit ulcerations. The tongue appears dry and red with atrophy of the filiform papillae.

Xerostomia can be documented by salivary flow measurements, parotid sialography, and salivary scintigraphy. Salivary flow measurements must be corrected for age, sex, time of day, and concomitant medications. Sialography, when performed with a hydrosoluble contrast media, appears to be a useful method. In addition, scintigraphy of the major salivary glands may be used to document xerostomia. This is a sensitive and noninvasive method based on the ability of salivary glands to take up technetium-sodium pertechnetate and secrete it into the oral cavity.

Abnormal salivary gland function is associated with well-defined histologic alterations including clustering of lymphocytic infiltrates. Salivary gland biopsy is used extensively. Focal sialadenitis is generally well-accepted as an important objective criterion for the diagnosis of Sjogren's syndrome. The histologic findings of the major salivary glands consist of clusters of lymphocytic infiltrates with acinar atrophy and hypertrophy of ductal epithelial and myoepithelial cells. Hence, biopsy permits histopathologic confirmation of the destructive lymphocyte infiltration. Salivary gland lesions are characterized by multiple aggregates of lymphocytes that replace the acinar tissue. Experience indicates that Sjogren's patients typically demonstrate more than one focus (an aggregate of more than 50 lymphoid cells) per 4 mm² of glandular tissue. Furthermore, there appears to be a relatively good correlation between histopathologic changes in minor and major salivary glands. Hence, minor gland biopsy is being used more often for diagnostic purposes. It should be noted, however, that biopsies of the minor glands lack the myoepithelial island configuration and tend to demonstrate only foci (Fig. 15–2).

Involvement of exocrine glands other than the lacrimal and salivary glands occurs less frequently. A decrease in mucous gland secretions of the upper and lower respiratory tree results in dry nose, throat, and trachea (*xerotrachea*). In addition, diminished secretion of the exocrine glands of the gastrointestinal tract (esophageal mucosal atrophy, atrophic gastritis, subclinical pancreatitis), the external genitalia, and the skin can be observed (Fig. 15–3).

Systemic Manifestations

Five to ten years after diagnosis, about one-half of primary Sjogren's syndrome patients present with organ involvement in extraglandular sites, including the lungs, kidneys, blood vessels, muscles, and the reticuloendothelial system (Table 15–1). On the

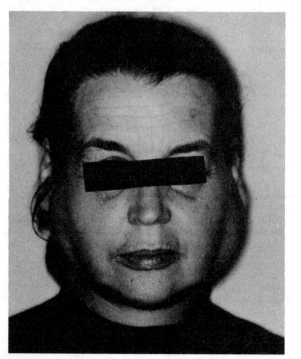

Fig. 15–1. *Primary Sjogren's syndrome patient with persistent, bilateral parotid gland enlargement.*

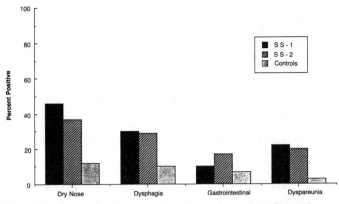

Fig. 15–3. *Other glandular manifestations observed in Sjogren's syndrome patients from a multicenter study for the diagnostic criteria for Sjogren's syndrome, Pisa, 1992. (626 cases; 19 European centers)*

other hand, extraglandular processes are rare in Sjogren's patients with RA. Common complaints include easy fatigue, low-grade fever, myalgias, arthralgias, and non-erosive arthritis. Raynaud's phenomenon occurs in 35% of primary Sjogren's syndrome patients and usually precedes sicca manifestations by several years.

Subclinical diffuse interstitial lung disease is the most common form of pulmonary involvement in primary Sjogren's syndrome patients. When clinically apparent, pulmonary involvement is mild and usually consists of lymphoid interstitial disease. Although over 30% of primary Sjogren's patients present subclinical interstitial lung disease, secondary Sjogren's patients with RA characteristically manifest more obstructive ventilatory defects. Pleurisy is rare in primary Sjogren's syndrome patients.

Renal involvement in primary Sjogren's patients may be latent or overt and includes interstitial nephritis clinically manifesting with hyposthenuria and renal tubular dysfunction, with or without acidosis and Fanconi's syndrome. Renal tubular acidosis may be silent or can manifest with hypokalemic paralysis and bouts of renal colic resulting from stones. Untreated acidosis leads to nephrocalcinosis. Membranous or membranoproliferative glomerulonephritis usually presents in conjunction with systemic vasculitis and cryoglobulinemia or as an overlap with SLE. Although both interstitial or glomerular lesions are clinically apparent in only about 10% of primary Sjogren's patients, about 30% of these patients have subclinical tubular dysfunction.

The most common manifestation of vasculitis in primary Sjogren's patients is palpable purpura. Systemic vasculitis affects small and medium-sized vessels, resulting in organ involvement such as the peripheral nervous system, lungs, kidneys, gastrointestinal tract, spleen, and salivary glands. Histologically, the patterns of vessel disease include leukoclastic and lymphocytic vasculitis, acute necrotizing angitis, and endarteritis obliterans involving small- and medium-sized arteries. The pathogenesis of vascular lesions is not clear, however, there is some evidence to suggest that terminal complement activation may play some role in the pathogenesis of vasculitic disorders, as well as central nervous system disorders.

It has been suggested that primary Sjogren's patients with

vasculitis may also present with multifocal, recurrent, and progressive central nervous system disease including hemiparesis, transverse myelopathy, hemisensory deficits, seizure, and movement disorders. Encephalopathy and aseptic meningitis, as well as multiple sclerosis, have been reported in these patients.

Myositis is an uncommon manifestation of Sjogren's syndrome. Muscle enzymes are elevated and muscle biopsy usually indicates lymphocytic infiltrates with little or no muscle necrosis.

About one-half of Sjogren's patients have subclinical thyroid disease. These patients present with antithyroid antibodies and signs of altered thyroid function as assessed by basal thyroid-stimulating hormone levels and the thyrotropin-releasing hormone stimulation test.

Lymphoma and Waldenstrom's macroglobulinemia are well-known manifestations of Sjogren's syndrome. Most lymphomas are of B cell origin, although some are pleomorphic, consisting of well-differentiated cells (immunocytomas), and in the majority of cases, lymphoproliferation remains confined to salivary and lacrimal tissue. Other parenchymal organs such as lungs, bone marrow and gastrointestinal tract may also be involved. Lymphomas may appear after several years of an apparently benign disease, may or may not be preceded by pseudolymphoma, and are observed more often in patients with systemic disease. Lymphomatous involvement of the major salivary glands should be suspected in patients who develop massive, firm, or persistent major salivary gland enlargement.

Immunology and Immunogenetics

The pathogenesis of Sjogren's syndrome remains elusive. Available evidence, however, suggests that these patients have an abnormal immunologic response to one or more unidentified antigens. Furthermore it has been hypothesized that these antigens may be viral antigens or virus-altered autoantigens. In this regard, it is of interest that patients who are HIV-positive demonstrate Sjogren's syndrome-like manifestations. (See Chapter 44). Finally, it appears that genetic makeup may play a critical role in determining an individual's susceptibility to the development of Sjogren's syndrome (6,7). The immunologic findings in Sjogren's syndrome are shown in Table 15–2.

The absolute number of the peripheral blood total lymphocytes, T cells as well as B cells, of patients with Sjogren's syndrome do not differ significantly from that observed in normal individuals.

Autoantibodies are common in patients with Sjogren's syndrome. Tests for antinuclear antibodies (ANA) are positive in about 90% of patients. Rheumatoid factor can be detected by the latex fixation test in approximately 60% of patients, and serum protein electrophoresis shows polyclonal hypergammaglobulinemia in 80% of the Sjogren's syndrome population. In some cases, hyperviscosity of the serum may be observed. Circulating cryoglobulins, consisting of a monoclonal rheumatoid factor and polyclonal immunoglobulins of IgG or IgA isotypes, are present in one-third of the patients, particularly those with systemic disease and autoantibodies. Patients with cryoglobulinemia usually present with depressed serum complement levels. Antibodies to small RNA protein complexes and particularly to La (SS–B), a nucleoprotein antigen, are found in 40% of patients with primary Sjogren's syndrome. Other nonspecific laboratory abnormalities commonly noted include: elevated erythrocyte sedimentation rates (ESR); mild normocytic anemia; and hypoalbuminemia (Table 15–3).

Lymphocytic infiltration of the exocrine glands leading to *au-*

Table 15–1. *Incidence of extraglandular manifestations in primary Sjogren's syndrome*

Clinical Manifestation	Percent
Arthralgias/Arthritis	60
Raynaud's phenomenon	35
Lymphadenopathy	14
Lung involvement	14
Vasculitis	11
Kidney involvement	9
Liver involvement	6
Lymphoma	6
Splenomegaly	3
Peripheral neuropathy	5
Myositis	1

Table 15–2. *Immunologic findings in Sjogren's syndrome*

Peripheral blood	Salivary glands
Polyclonal hypergammaglobulinemia	T-helper/inducer cells
Multiple autoantibodies	Activated B cells
Monoclonal immunoglobulins	HLA-DR$^+$ glandular epithelial cells
Deficient IL-2 production	Monoclonal B cell subset
Decreased NK cell function	Absence of NK cells

Table 15–3. *Laboratory findings in patients with primary Sjogren's syndrome*

Finding	Percent
ANA (>1:80)*	90
Rheumatoid factor (>1:40)#	60
Cryoglobulinemia	30
CRP (>8 mg/l)	5
Anemia (Hematocrit<30)	10
Leukopenia (WBC<3,500 cells/mm^3)	
Thrombocytopenia (PLT<10,000/mm^3)	
ESR (>25 mm/h)	60
anti–Ro (SSA)	55
anti–La (SSB)	40

* Hep-2 cells as substrate
# Latex fixation

toimmune exocrinopathy is one of the main autoimmune phenomena observed in Sjogren's syndrome. The application of monoclonal antibody technology has demonstrated that the T-helper cell (CD4 positive) is the predominant phenotype of the lymphoid cells infiltrating the labial minor salivary glands. Furthermore, it appears that the majority of these cells are helper/inducers and that the T cells present in these lesions are activated. B cells constitute approximately 20% of the total infiltrating population, while monocytes/macrophages and natural killer cells are rarely observed.

B cell activation is the most consistent immunoregulatory aberration in Sjogren's syndrome patients. It is the B cells infiltrating the salivary glands that synthesize large amounts of immunoglobulins with rheumatoid factor activity. Hence, it appears that the exocrine gland tissues in Sjogren's syndrome may be the major site of B lymphocyte activation.

A genetic predisposition to the development of Sjogren's syndrome has been indicated by HLA typing studies. These immunogenetic studies demonstrate an increased prevalence of HLA antigens B8, DR3, and DRW52 in primary Sjogren's syndrome patients as compared with the control population. Further analysis of HLA class II genes by molecular techniques revealed that Sjogren's syndrome patients, with anti-Ro (SSA) and/or anti-La (SSB) antibodies possess DQA_1/DQB_1 chains containing specific amino acid residues in the second hypervariable region (8). Furthermore, there appear to be different antigen frequencies between primary and secondary Sjogren's syndrome. HLA–DR4 is associated with secondary Sjogren's syndrome in the presence of RA, while DRW52 has been detected with a high frequency in both primary and secondary Sjogren's syndrome.

DIAGNOSIS AND DIFFERENTIAL DIAGNOSIS

Apart from Bloch et al (1), several sets of criteria from different study groups have been applied for the diagnosis of Sjogren's syndrome. Recently, preliminary criteria for the diagnosis of Sjogren's syndrome have been published after a prospective European multicenter concerted action (9). This study was based on the sensitivity and specificity of different parameters referred to ocular and oral symptoms, ocular signs and salivary gland involvement, histopathologic features and the presence of autoantibodies anti-Ro/SSA and anti-La/SSB (Table 15–4). The presence of 4 out of 6 items exhibited a high sensitivity and specificity, suggesting that these criteria may be used to establish a definitive diagnosis of primary Sjogren's syndrome.

The differential diagnosis of Sjogren's syndrome includes other conditions that may cause dry mouth or eyes or parotid salivary gland enlargement as shown in Table 15–5. Bacterial or viral sialadenitis may be confused with the parotitis seen in Sjogren's syndrome. In addition, HIV infection also appears to produce a similar clinical picture. However, these patients lack circulating antibodies to Ro (SS–A) or La (SS–B) nucleoprotein antigens characteristic of Sjogren's syndrome patients. The clinical features of Sjogren's syndrome may be mimicked not only by other diseases, such as amyloidosis, lipoproteinemias, and chronic graft versus host disease, but also by drugs with anticholinergic

Table 15–4. *Preliminary criteria for the classification of Sjogren's syndrome (modified from Reference 9).*

1. Ocular symptoms
    A positive response to at least 1 of the following 3 questions:
    (a) Have you had daily, persistent, troublesome dry eyes for more than 3 months?
    (b) Do you have a recurrent of sandy or gravel feeling in the eyes?
    (c) Do you use tear substitutes more than 3 times a day?
2. Oral symptoms
    A positive response to at least 1 of the following questions:
    (a) Have you had a daily feeling of dry mouth for more than 3 months?
    (b) Have you had recurrent or persistently swollen salivary glands as an adult?
    (c) Do you frequently drink liquids to aid in swallowing dry foods?
3. Ocular signs
    Objective evidence of ocular involvement determined on the basis of a positive result on at least 1 of the following 2 tests:
    (a) Schirmer-1 test (≤5 mm in 5 minutes)
    (b) Rose bengal score (≥4, according to the van Bijsterveld scoring system)
4. Salivary gland involvement
    Objective evidence of salivary gland involvement, determined on the basis of a positive result on at least 1 of the following 3 tests:
    (a) Salivary scintigraphy
    (b) Parotid sialography
    (c) Unstimulated salivary flow (≤1.5 ml in 15 minutes)
5. Histopathologic findings
    Focus score ≥1 on minor salivary gland biopsy
    (focus defined as an agglomeration of at least 50 mononuclear cells, focus score defined as the number of foci/4mm^2 of glandular tissue)
6. Autoantibodies
    Presence of at least 1 of the following autoantibodies in the serum:
    Antibodies to Ro (SS-A) or La (SS-B) antigens or antinuclear antibodies or rheumatoid factor.

A patient is considered as having probable Sjogren's syndrome if 3 of 6 criteria are present, and as definite if 4 of 6 criteria are present

effects. Infiltrative processes such as sarcoidosis may cause parotid gland enlargement and must be distinguished from Sjogren's syndrome by histologic means. Hence, biopsy of the minor salivary glands usually reveals noncaseating granulomas in sarcoidosis patients. These patients also lack autoantibodies.

TREATMENT

Sjogren's syndrome remains a fundamentally incurable disease. As yet, no therapeutic modality has been identified that can alter the course of the disease. Hence, treatment is aimed at symptomatic relief and limiting the damaging local effects of chronic xerostomia and keratoconjunctivitis sicca by substitution of the missing secretions (10).

The sicca complex is treated with fluid replacement supplied as often as necessary. To replace deficient tears, there are several readily available ophthalmic preparations. In severe cases, it may be necessary for patients to use these as often as every 30

Table 15–5. *Differential diagnosis of parotid gland enlargement*

Unilateral

Salivary gland neoplasm
Bacterial infection
Chronic sialadenitis

Bilateral

Viral infection
    (mumps, influenza, Epstein–Barr, Coxsackie A, cytomegalovirus, HIV)
Sjogren's syndrome
Sarcoidosis
Miscellaneous
    (diabetes mellitus, hyperlipoproteinemia, hepatic cirrhosis, chronic pancreatitis, acromegaly, gonadal hypofunction)
Recurrent parotitis of childhood

minutes. If corneal ulceration is present, eye-patching and boric acid ointment is recommended. Certain drugs that may further lacrimal and salivary hypofunction, such as diuretics, antihypertensive drugs and antidepressants, should be avoided.

Bromhexine given orally at high doses (48 mg/d) appears to improve sicca manifestations. Alocarpine use has been suggested. However, frequent ingestion of fluids, particularly with meals, is often the best solution.

Preliminary studies suggest that hydroxychloroquine, which is efficacious and safe in other autoimmune diseases, may be useful in treating Sjogren's patients. A dose of 200 mg/d partially corrects hypergammaglobulinemia, and decreases IgG antibodies to La/SS–B antigen. Furthermore, hydroxychloroquine treatment decreases the ESR and increases the hemoglobin levels. Although cyclosporine appears to help alleviate some of the dry mouth symptoms, in light of the potent side effects and the minimal therapeutic effects, it is not recommended for treating Sjogren's syndrome patients. Propionic acid gels may be used to treat vaginal dryness.

Corticosteroids or other immunosuppressive agents are indicated in treatment of extraglandular manifestations, particularly when renal or severe pulmonary involvement and systemic vasculitis has been defined.

Treatment of malignant lymphomas, depending upon the location, histology and extent of lymphoma, should include chemotherapy or radiotherapy.

Haralampos M. Moutsopoulos, MD

1. Bloch KJ, Buchanan WW, Wohl MJ, et al: Sjogren's syndrome: a clinical, pathological, and serological study of 62 cases. Medicine 44:187–231, 1965
2. Moutsopoulos HM, Chused TM, Mann DL, et al: Sjogren's syndrome (sicca syndrome): current issues. Ann Intern Med 92:212–226, 1980
3. Talal N, Moutsopoulos H, Kassan S, editors: Sjogren's Syndrome: Clinical and Immunological Aspects, Berlin, Springer–Verlag, 1987
4. Moutsopoulos HM, Manousakis MN: Immunopathogenesis of Sjogren's syndrome: "facts and fancy." Autoimmunity 5:17–24, 1989
5. Youinou P, Moutsopoulos HM, Pennec YL: Clinical features of Sjogren's syndrome. Curr Opinion Rheumatol 2:687–693, 1990
6. Moutsopoulos HM, Tzioufas AG, Talal N: Sjogren's syndrome: a model to study autoimmunity and lymphoid malignancy, Molecular Autoimmunity. Edited by Talal N, New York, NY, Academic Press, 1991, pp 319–340
7. Moutsopoulos HM, Youinou P: New developments in Sjogren's syndrome. Curr Opinion Rheumatol 3:815–822, 1991
8. Reveille JD, MacLeod MJ, Whittington K, et al: Specific amino acid residues in the second hypervariable region of HLA–DQA1 and DQB1 chain genes promote the Ro(SS-A)/La(SS-B) autoantibody responses. J Immunol 146:3871–3876, 1991
9. Vitali C, Bombardieri S, Moutsopoulos HM, et al: Preliminary criteria for the classification of Sjogren's syndrome. Arthritis Rheum 36:340–347, 1993
10. Moutsopoulos HM, Vlachoyiannopoulos PG: What would I do if I had Sjogren's syndrome? Rheumatol Rev 2:17–23, 1993

16. UNDIFFERENTIATED CONNECTIVE TISSUE SYNDROMES

The concept of undifferentiated connective tissue syndromes (UCTS) has grown from the recognition that the systemic rheumatic diseases have several properties that may make a specific diagnosis difficult (1,2).

Of most importance is the occurrence of several clinical features that are shared to a variable extent by rheumatoid arthritis (RA), systemic lupus erythematosus (SLE), systemic sclerosis (scleroderma), poly and dermatomyositis (PM and DM), and Sjogren's syndrome. These include Raynaud's phenomenon, polyarthritis, interstitial lung disease, pleuritis or pericarditis, and vasculitis. Patients who present with one or more of these features often do not satisfy criteria for any of the recognized systemic rheumatic diseases. In addition, evolution to a recognizable connective tissue disease may require years, may never occur, or the signs and symptoms may disappear removing the necessity for any disease designation.

In addition to the shared clinical features, serologic features are also shared to a variable extent by all of these diseases. Chief among these are the presence of antinuclear antibodies (ANA), measured by indirect immunofluorescence, and rheumatoid factors, autoantibodies directed to the Fc fragment of immunoglobulin G (IgG). This frequent sharing of clinical features and serologic findings makes early diagnosis difficult in a group of diseases for which no etiology has been established. Moreover, no definitive diagnostic tests exist in the absence of a cluster of clinical features that comprise the diagnostic features of the differentiated form of each of these diseases. In addition to these complexities, each of the systemic rheumatic diseases is extremely heterogeneous. It is very clear that especially for SLE, systemic sclerosis, PM, and DM, numerous subsets exist that can be classified on the basis of a combination of clinical characteristics and the recognition of specific autoantibodies directed to well-defined molecular target antigens.

Finally, there are numerous instances in which there is overlap with the presence of two or more diseases, which are more or less fully expressed. An example that has generated much controversy is the concept of mixed connective tissue disease (MCTD) in which there may be the presence of SLE, PM, DM, and systemic sclerosis in various combinations, in association with high titers of autoantibodies to the nRNP or U_1RNP antigen (3,4). There are, however, many known instances of overlap among and between these diseases unaccompanied by antibodies to U_1RNP. Conversely these specific antibodies occur to a variable extent with each of these diseases when they occur alone. Reports that antibodies to the 70 kDa polypeptide of the U_1RNP antigen are characteristic of MCTD have been confirmed, but these also occur in at least one-half of SLE patients with anti-U_1RNP precipitins who do not have overlap features (5).

RECOGNITION OF DIFFERENTIATED CONNECTIVE TISSUE DISEASES

A reasonable approach to clinical investigation in the systemic rheumatic diseases requires that criteria be established to classify patients for the purposes of clinical research. Patients with UCTS are generally not entered into such studies, because they do not satisfy criteria for a specific disease.

In the investigation of individual patients for clinical diagnosis, characteristic differentiated features are sought that comprise the disease picture for each of the systemic characteristic diseases. While these are discussed in detail in other chapters, a brief review is presented so that the specific clinical and serologic features of these diseases can be contrasted with the nonspecific clinical and serologic findings that lead to the designation of UCTS, a waystation for the numerous incomplete connective tissue syndromes that cannot be classified.

Systemic Lupus Erythematosus. In SLE, the "differentiated" features rarely seen in the other connective tissue diseases are glomerulonephritis, photosensitivity, characteristic skin rashes, central nervous system disease, and various cytopenias such as Coomb's positive hemolytic anemia, leukopenia, and thrombocytopenia. These are all very unusual in systemic sclerosis, RA, and PM/DM. Pleuropericarditis and peritonitis are most common in SLE but are seen to a variable extent in the other systemic rheumatic diseases. Serologically, antibodies to double stranded DNA, Sm, and ribosomal P proteins are seen almost exclusively in SLE, while precipitating antibodies to U_1RNP, Ro/SS–A and La/SS–B, which are present in aggregate in 85% of SLE patients, are present in other rheumatic diseases. Precipitating antibodies to Ro/SS–A and La/SS–B are seen more commonly in primary Sjogren's syndrome than in SLE. There are numerous combinations of these clinical findings in association with several defined autoantibodies that would definitively make the diagnosis of SLE.

Systemic Sclerosis. There is less heterogeneity in systemic sclerosis than in SLE, but the diagnosis depends strongly on the presence of thickened skin due to dermal collagen accumulation in a diffuse pattern, in which the thickening extends proximal to the wrists and also involves the trunk and face. Patients with diffuse skin involvement have an increased risk of sclerosis of the internal organs such as the heart, lungs, and bowel, as well as renal nephrosclerosis with malignant hypertension. Virtually all patients with systemic sclerosis have Raynaud's phenomenon, and a subset called limited cutaneous scleroderma exists, which has limited skin involvement restricted to the hands (sclerodactyly) and face, calcinosis, esophageal motility disturbances, and telangiectaesiae (CREST syndrome). Patients with limited skin disease may have various combinations of these findings (such as REST and RST) constituting limited forms of the syndrome.

There is also a family of antinuclear antibodies highly specific for systemic sclerosis, which include antibodies to various nucleolar antigens, Scl_{70} or topoisomerase I, and the centromere antigens. Antibodies to the centromere antigens correlate highly with the presence of the CREST or limited cutaneous variants. There is no serologic marker that occurs in the majority of patients with diffuse skin disease, although antibodies to topoisomerase I occur more frequently in diffuse disease than in limited skin disease or CREST (6).

Polymyositis/Dermatomyositis. In the differentiated forms of polymyositis and dermatomyositis, there is a family of disease specific autoantibodies many of which are disease specific and are associated with clinical subsets (see Chapter 14). Patients with PM and interstitial lung disease produce antibodies to a set of translation-related proteins that include Jo-1, PL-7, and PL-12, which are histidyl, threonyl and alanyl tRNA synthetases respectively, as well as the translation component KJ. Antibodies to signal recognition particle occur in patients with PM without interstitial lung disease, and antibodies to Mi_2, a nuclear protein complex, occur specifically in patients with DM. These antibodies have not been reported in the other connective tissue diseases to any significant extent even when sensitive tests are employed in their detection (7).

THE DIAGNOSTIC PROBLEM

Patients who do not clearly express the clinical features of any disease or have partial overlap of features of two or more diseases probably comprise 15% to 25% of tertiary referrals in patients with suspected systemic rheumatic diseases. An example of this conundrum is illustrated by the patients who present with Raynaud's phenomenon and no other clinical findings, a common clinical problem for rheumatologists. The first issue is whether the Raynaud's phenomenon is an isolated phenomenon or is the harbinger of a systemic rheumatic disease. Should a thorough laboratory and physical exam fail to reveal evidence of

a systemic rheumatic disease, a positive ANA test is useful since its presence indicates high risk (and absence low risk) for the development of a systemic rheumatic disease. If the positive ANA is anti-centromere antibody, it is likely that systemic sclerosis will develop in those patients. Prospective studies are in progress and, in the coming years, data will become available that will enable doctors to tell patients with isolated Raynaud's phenomenon and anti-centromere antibody what their risk and time frame are for the development of systemic sclerosis. Similarly, patients with Raynaud's phenomenon and any of the disease-specific autoantibodies are likely to develop the differentiated connective tissue disease associated with that particular autoantibody. Another common conundrum is the patient with an inflammatory polyarthritis without bone erosions and with or without a positive ANA, but no rheumatoid factor and no disease specific autoantibodies or other clinical findings which define the clinical syndrome.

Patients with any of the incompletely expressed rheumatic diseases accompanied by autoantibodies that are not diagnostic are best designated UCTS. Such patients are not well served by making a definitive diagnosis before the clinical data indicate the nature of the disease, because in many instances the disease remits permanently, or the undifferentiated nature of the malady may be long lasting or evolve slowly, requiring only that symptomatic therapy be given since the prognosis and course are unknown.

As our knowledge expands, etiologies, disease specific autoantibodies, or both which antedate clinical disease with certain disease specificity will be discovered. This type of knowledge should reduce the numbers of patients designated UCTS, but for the reasons cited, such a category serves as a constant reminder of our incomplete knowledge of the systemic rheumatic diseases. For the present, it is important to help the patient deal with uncertainty. Treatment can be directed at manifestations present, even without a firm diagnosis.

Morris Reichlin, MD

1. LeRoy EC, Maricq HR, Kahaleh MB: Undifferentiated connective tissue syndromes. Arthritis Rheum 23:341–343, 1980
2. Christian CL: Connective tissue disease: overlap syndromes. Rheumatology and Immunology, 2nd ed. Edited by Cohen A, Bennett JC. New York, NY, Grune & Stratton, 1986, pp 175–179
3. Sharp GC, Irwin WS, May CH, et al: Association of antibodies to ribonucleoprotein and Sm antigens with connective tissue disease, systemic lupus erythematosus, and other rheumatic diseases. N Engl J Med 295:1149–1154, 1976
4. Sharp GC, Irvin WS, Tan EM, et al: Mixed connective tissue disease—an apparently distinct rheumatic disease syndrome associated with a specific antibody to extractable nuclear antigen (ENA). Am J Med 52:148–159, 1972
5. Reichlin M, van Venrooij WJ: Autoantibodies to the URNP particles: relationship to clinical diagnosis and nephritis. Clin Exp Immunol 83:286–290, 1991
6. Reichlin M: Progressive Systemic Sclerosis in Systemic Autoimmunity. Edited by Bigazzi PL, Reichlin M. Marcel Dekker, New York, NY, 1991, pp 275–287
7. Targoff IN: Polymyositis in Systemic Autoimmunity. Edited by Bigazzi PL, Reichlin M. Marcel Dekker, New York, NY, 1991, pp 201–246

17. VASCULITIS
A. *Epidemiology, Pathology, and Pathogenesis*

EPIDEMIOLOGY

The vasculitides are a heterogenous group of clinical syndromes characterized by inflammation of blood vessels. Epidemiologic information on the different vasculitis syndromes is shown in Table 17A–1. (1–4). Studies of epidemiology have been complicated by the relative rarity of the vasculitic syndromes, discordant disease definitions, regional variations, and ethnic biases. The pattern of the age of onset is quite variable among the vasculitides. Although the mean age of onset of several of the primary vasculitic syndromes—including polyarteritis nodosa, allergic granulomatosis and angiitis, Wegener's granulomatosis, and hypersensitivity vasculitis—is in the fifth decade of life, these diseases can present at both extremes of age. Kawasaki disease

is seen almost exclusively in the pediatric population. The incidence of Henöch–Schönlein purpura (HSP) has a bimodal distribution. The majority of cases occur in pediatric populations between the ages of 4 and 7 years. In contrast, the mean age at onset of HSP in adults is 45. Thromboangiitis obliterans and Takayasu arteritis tend to affect young adults, while giant cell arteritis is generally limited to populations beyond the sixth decade of life.

PATHOLOGY

Vasculitis can involve any blood vessel in the body with considerable overlap in the pathologic processes in the major vasculitic syndromes (Table 17A–2) (2–5). With the possible exception

Table 17A–1. *Epidemiology of the major vasculitides**

Vasculitides	Incidence (per 100,000)	Mean Age (yr) at Onset	Sex (% males)	Geographic Association	Genetic Markers
Polyarteritis nodosa	1.8	48 ± 1.7	62%	none	none (HBsAg+)
Allergic granulomatosis and angiitis	rare[†]	50 ± 3.0	52–65%	—	—
Wegener's granulomatosis	rare[†]	45 ± 1.2	64%	—	HLA–B7, B8 DR2
Kawasaki disease (Japan)	rare[†]	1.0–1.5 (0.1–11)ǀ	60%		HLA–Bw22
Kawasaki disease (USA)	very rare[†]	2.9–3.8 (0.1–13)ǀ	60%	Japan	HLA–Bw51
Hypersensitivity vasculitis	less common[†]	47 ± 2.0	46%	—	—
Henoch-Schonlein purpura	14	4.5–17 (0.2–adult)ǀ	54%	—	—
Behcet's syndrome	variable[#]	27	66%	E. Mediterranean, Japan	HLA–B51, DRw52
Takayasu arteritis	0.26	26 + 1.2 (3–75)ǀ	14%	Orient	HLA–A10, B5 Bw52, DR2, DR4, MB1
Giant cell arteritis	15-30	69 + 0.5	20%	N. Europe	HLA–DR4
Thromboangiitis obliterans	rare[†]	33 (11–45)ǀ	80%	Far East, Middle East, Asia	HLA–A9, B5

* The data are summarized from references 1–4.

[†] Because of the relatively rarity of the vasculitides and variations in disease definition, precise data on disease incidence is unavailable.

[#] The frequency of Behcet's disease is variable. The prevalence of 1/1000 has been reported in Japan while a prevalence of 1/300,000 has been reported in USA.

ǀ Reports the range in onset of disease in years.

of the hypercellular occlusive thrombus seen in thromboangiitis obliterans, none of the pathologic processes seen with vasculitis are diagnostic for a specific vasculitic syndrome. In some cases, immunofluorescent studies may provide additional useful information. Both IgM and C_3 may be demonstrated in early hypersensitivity vasculitic lesions. The presence of IgA and C_3 in a small vessel vasculitic lesion is suggestive of HSP. The overlap seen between the pathologic changes in the vasculitides is especially evident in the kidney. Even though many of these diseases affect renal function, the histologic pattern of involvement is generally nonspecific; consequently, the renal biopsy may not differentiate between these syndromes. The major vasculitic syndromes are defined by clinicopathologic parameters. The publication of The American College of Rheumatology 1990 Criteria for the Classification of Vasculitis (1) emphasizes the importance of combining clinical information with pathologic findings in establishing the correct diagnosis.

Vasculitic lesions tend to be both focal and segmental. The lesions are focal in the sense that not all vessels of a similar size will be affected. The lesions are considered segmental because only certain portions, or segments, of an affected vessel may be involved. For example, serial sections through a temporal artery biopsy may go from a normal vessel to a site of severe involvement in a space of several millimeters. Moreover, the pattern of inflammation within the vessel wall is not always uniform. Early lesions in both polyarteritis nodosa and Takayasu arteritis may be limited to the media. The pattern of inflammation in Takayasu arteritis may be patchy rather than diffuse in nature. Finally, the entire circumference of the vessel may not be uniformly involved. Instead of involving the entire circumference, only a portion of the blood vessel wall may be involved producing a sectorial pattern of inflammation. The focal, segmental, and even sectorial nature of vasculitic lesions is an important consideration in evaluating diagnostic biopsies. Increasing the volume of evaluated tissue increases the likelihood of identifying an inflammatory lesion if present. For example, the need to obtain an adequate sized biopsy specimen and to do serial step sections on temporal artery biopsies has been emphasized (Fig. 17A–1).

PATHOGENESIS

Because the vasculitides are a group of different diseases, no single pathophysiologic process will account for clinical disease expression. Even within a specific vasculitic syndrome, one of several different initiating events may lead to a final common pathway resulting in a similar pattern of clinical disease expression. At present, we lack sufficient knowledge to classify the vasculitides based on pathophysiologic parameters. This lack of knowledge on the causes of vasculitis reflects, in part, the paucity of relevant animal models to study and the inherent difficulties in studying pathogenesis in clinical populations (6). The following mechanisms may have pathophysiologic relevance in at least some of the vasculitic syndromes.

Immune Complexes. The concept that immune complexes mediate inflammatory vessel disease is based on systematic studies of animal models of serum sickness and the Arthus reaction (2,7). The following elements must be present for the expression of vasculitis in animal models: 1) increased vascular permeability, 2) deposition of circulating (or the in situ precipitation of) immune complexes below the level of the vascular endothelium, 3) activation of complement, and 4) attraction of polymorphonuclear leukocytes (PMN) to the vessel wall. A variety of mechanisms might result in increased vascular permeability, including the release of platelet-activating factor or vasoactive amines from platelets, mast cells, or basophils. The relevance of these potential mediators in the clinical expression of immune complex mediated vasculitis has not been established.

In the serum sickness model of vasculitis, the nature of the soluble circulating immune complexes has been systematically evaluated. The immune complexes formed in slight antigen excess (greater than 19S in size) are associated with vascular deposition and the expression of vasculitis. The circulating immune complexes appear to be passively deposited in the vessel wall. Multiple immunoregulatory mechanisms may contribute to the presence of circulating immune complexes. The required parameters for tissue deposition include: 1) T cell, B cell, and monocyte mediated regulation of parameters effecting Ig responses, 2) binding of soluble immune complexes to complement receptor type I for transport to the mononuclear–phagocyte system (reticuloendothelial system), and 3) processing of immune complexes by the mononuclear–phagocyte system. Potential mechanisms for the in situ development of immune complexes in blood vessel walls have not been defined. Complement activation appears to be critical in the development of immune complex mediated vasculitis. The Fc piece from IgG or IgM activates the complement cascade through the first component of complement. The IgA-containing complexes seen in HSP may activate complement through the alternative pathway. Although the activated complement cascade can damage cells by the assembly of the membrane attack complex, this activity does not appear to be the principal role of complement in the pathogenesis of vasculitis. The activation of the complement cascade produces C3a, C5a, and C567,

*Table 17A–2. Pathologic parameters of the major vasculitides**

Vasculitides	Class of Vessel Involvement	Organ System Involvement	Vessel Wall Involvement	Histopathology of the Vessels†		Renal and [Other] Pathology
				cellular	other	
Polyarteritis nodosa	small and medium sized muscular arteries	viscera, muscle, testes, nerves, renal (not pulmonary arteries)	early lesion: media, full: transmural	early: PMN full: L,M,PMN less: Eos,Gr	fibrinoid necrosis, fibrin, thrombosis, ↓ internal elastic membrane, ↓ media, aneurysms	segmental necrotizing GN, crescents, arteritis
Allergic granulomatosis and angiitis	small and medium sized arteries, veins, venules	lungs, viscera, cardiac, renal nerves, muscle	transmural	early: Eos full: Eos,L,M,PMN, Gr,GC	less common: fibrinoid necrosis, thrombosis, aneurysms	focal segmental necrotizing GN, crescents, vasculitis, interstitial Eos infiltrate. [tissue Eos, necrotizing granuloma]
Wegener's granulomatosis	small arteries and veins; also larger arteries, arterioles, venules & capillaries	upper and lower respiratory, renal skin, eye, heart, nervous system	transmural	early: PMN full: L,M,PMN,Gr,GC less: Eos	fibrinoid necrosis, necrotizing granuloma, ↓ elastic membrane	focal segmental necrotizing GN, crescents; less common: vasculitis and interstitial nephritis. [lung necrosis; necrotizing granuloma]
Kawasaki disease	medium muscular arteries; rarely veins, large arteries	cardiac; also iliac, renal, internal mammillary	panarteritis	early: PMN,L,M full: L,M,H	thrombosis, aneurysm, endothelial proliferation, rare: fibrinoid necrosis	renal: none. [pericarditis, epicarditis, myocarditis, valvular involvement]
Hypersensitivity vasculitis	postcapillary venule, arteriole, venule; rare: small arteries, veins	skin; rare: viscera, heart, synovium	—	early: PMN; L,M full: PMN; L,M or PMN,L,M,Eos	leukocytoclasis, fibrin, fibrinoid necrosis, RBC extravasation	rare: interstitial nephritis, [rare: myocarditis, hepatitis]
Henoch-Schonlein purpura	precapillary arterioles, postcapillary venules, capillaries	skin, GI, renal synovium	—	early: PMN full: PMN,L,M rare: Eos	fibrinoid necrosis of arterioles, fibrin, RBC extravasation, thrombosis	proliferation of mesangial cells, increased matrix, epithelial crescents
Behcet's syndrome	small vessels; rare: large vessel vasa vasorum	oral, genital, other skin sites, eye, CNS, GI, synovium	—	early: ?PMN full: L,M	early: leukocytoclasis, less common: fibrin, thrombosis, RBC extravasation	rare: GN, immune complexes. [thrombophlebitis, pustular skin lesions with PMN]
Takayasu arteritis	large elastic arteries, selected muscular arteries	aorta and major branches (arch), pulmonary artery	early lesion: media, full: panarteritis	L,M,Gr, plasmacytoid rare: GC	↓ media, muscloelastic lamellae; dissection, aneurysm, fibrosis	renal: 2° ischemic and hypertensive changes. [rare: pericarditis, myocarditis]
Giant cell arteritis	large and medium muscular arteries; less common: aorta	extra-cranial arteries of head and neck; less common: any other artery	panarteritis dominant site: media	L,M,H,Gr,Gc, plasmacytoid less: PMN, Eos	↓ elastic membrane, intimal proliferation, aneurysm, dissection, rare: necrosis	renal: rare ischemic changes 2° to renal artery angiitis, [granulomatous hepatitis]
Thromboangiitis obliterans	intermediate and small arteries and veins	extremities: distal > proximal; very rare: head, cardiac, viscera	transmural	early: PMN full: L,M,H,PMN rare: GC	hypercellular occlusive thrombus, fibrosis, spares elastic membrane and vessel structure, no necrosis	renal: none

* Summarized from references 2–5.
† PMN-polymorphonuclear leukocytes, L-lymphocytes, M-monocyte, H-histiocytes, Eos-eosinophils, Gr-granuloma, GC-giant cells/multinucleated giant cells, "↓" represents damage or destruction.

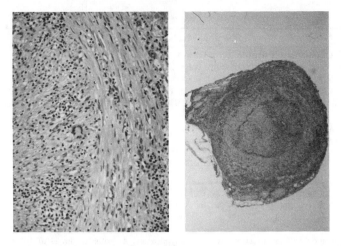

Fig. 17A–1. Giant cell arteritis. Photomicrograph of temporal artery biopsy. Low magnification on left shows thickening of the wall and an occluded lumen. High magnification on the right shows mononuclear cell infiltration and a multinucleated giant cell (courtesy of Dr. Gene Hunder).

which act as chemoattractants for PMNs and monocytes. Moreover, both PMNs and monocytes have cell surface complement receptors that further facilitate the development of an acute inflammatory response at the site of complement activation. The damage to the blood vessel wall appears to be mediated by PMNs and possibly by monocytes. These cells both have the capability to damage tissue by the release of degradative enzymes and oxidative products.

Indirect evidence suggests immune complex mediated mechanisms of vasculitis may be pertinent in hypersensitivity vasculitis, HSP, cryoglobulinemia, and the hepatitis B virus associated polyarteritis nodosa. Immunofluorescent studies in these diseases often demonstrate the presence of antigen (bacterial, mycobacterial, or viral), Ig and C_3 in biopsies of early vasculitic lesions. Currently, there is no convincing evidence that immune complex mediated mechanisms play a primary role in other vasculitides.

Antibodies. The role of antibodies, other than those present in immune complexes, in the development of vasculitis is less well defined. Antineutrophil cytoplasmic autoantibodies (ANCA) are present in patients with systemic necrotizing vasculitis, including Wegener's granulomatosis and polyarteritis nodosa (Fig. 17A–2). A subset of these autoantibodies (C–ANCA) bind to specially preserved PMNs with a diffuse cytoplasmic staining pattern. The C–ANCA binds to a serine proteinase (proteinase 3) found in the

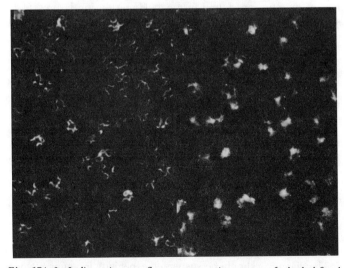

Fig. 17A–2. Indirect immunofluorescence microscopy of alcohol-fixed neutrophils demonstrating the staining pattern produced by cytoplasmic antineutrophil cytoplasmic autoantibodies (C-ANCA) on right and perinuclear antineutrophil cytoplasmic autoantibodies (P-ANCA) on left (courtesy of Dr. Gene Hunder).

primary granules of the PMN. The presence of C-ANCA is useful as a diagnostic tool and the levels of the antibody may correlate with disease activity. In vitro studies suggest a potential role for C-ANCA in the pathophysiology of necrotizing vasculitis (8). Under normal conditions the proteinase 3 is in an intracellular location and inaccessible to extracellular antibodies. However, granule constituents, including proteinase 3, may be expressed on the cell surface of both PMNs and monocytes following exposure to cytokines. The C-ANCA may interact with these activated cells stimulating respiratory burst activity and degranulation. Polymorphonuclear leukocytes that have been activated with cytokines and stimulated with C-ANCA have been shown in vitro to have the ability to damage endothelial cells. The role for this potential mechanism in the in vivo expression of necrotizing vasculitis requires additional investigation.

A potential causal role has been suggested for antibodies directed toward structures on the surface of endothelial cells (EC). Antiendothelial cell antibodies (AECA) have been demonstrated in a number of autoimmune and vasculitic diseases (9). Studies of AECA in vitro have demonstrated an ability to damage EC by both antibody-dependent cellular cytotoxicity and complement activation mechanisms. Serum from patients with acute Kawasaki syndrome has been shown to lyse cytokine activated allogenic EC in complement-dependent in vitro study systems (10,11). The significance of these observations in the clinical expression of arteritis in patients with Kawasaki syndrome requires further investigation.

Endothelial Cells. Because the endothelium serves as the interface between the intra- and extravascular compartments, these cells are involved in a wide variety of physiologic regulatory functions, such as vascular permeability, aggregation of vascular formed elements, adhesion of formed elements including platelets and leukocytes, regulation of cell trafficking into the extravascular compartment, and regulation of coagulation. These EC regulatory functions are mediated, in part, by a number of secreted substances such as prostaglandins, adenosine nucleotides, and platelet activating factor.

In addition to these functions, EC clearly have the potential to regulate and modify immune responses. The EC can secrete a number of cytokines that may regulate immune responses at the vascular level (12). In vitro EC secrete low levels of interleukins 1 and 6 (IL–1 and IL–6). A marked increase in the production of these cytokines can be demonstrated following stimulation. The EC can also be stimulated to secrete interleukin–8, interferon–α and –β, colony stimulating factor for granulocytes and monocytes, and granulocyte colony stimulating factor. These cytokines, locally secreted, could have a significant effect on vascular inflammatory responses. The EC can also express important cell-surface immunoregulatory molecules (12–14) (Table 17A–3). The low level of basal major histocompatibility complex (MHC) I expression on EC, which can be enhanced following a variety of stimuli, provides a potential ligand for cell-mediated cytotoxic responses. Although absent in the basal state, MHC II expression on EC surfaces can be stimulated by interferon–γ. Such MHC II expressing EC can effectively present antigen to $CD4^+$ T cells, thus stimulating a proliferative response. The ability of the EC to present antigen may play a central role in mechanisms of T cell mediated vasculitis. In addition, EC can express cell surface adhesion molecules (Table 17A–3). Such molecules play an important role in physiologic cell-to-cell interactions as they facilitate leukocyte egress from the intravascular space. The cell adhesion molecules may also play a role in the clinical expression of vasculitis. In the animal model of the Shwartzman reaction, the binding of the leukocyte adhesion molecule from the CD18 family of integrins to the intercellular adhesion molecule–1 (ICAM–1) on the EC plays a critical role in the expression of the vasculitis (13). Antibodies to either CD18 or ICAM–1 markedly inhibit the development of the vasculitis. Further investigation of adhesion molecules as a potential mechanism in the expression of the vasculitides is clearly warranted.

Lymphocytes. Although direct evidence for a primary lymphocyte mediated vasculitis in man is currently lacking, sensitized T cells are responsible for the expression of vasculitis in several

Table 17A–3. *Endothelial cells: potential immunoregulatory functions*

Parameter	Expression		Potential Mechanism
MHC I	Basal: +		Ligand to CD8 which is present on a subset of T cells and LGL. May serve as target for cell mediated cytotoxicity, regulation of T cells
	Induced: TNF, IFN-γ		
	IFN-α/β, infection		
MHC II	Basal: 0		Ligand to CD4 which is present on a subset of T cells. EC can present antigen in MHC restricted fashion with resulting T cell proliferation
	Induced: IFN-γ		
	? antigen		
LFA-3	Basal: +		Ligand to CD2 on T cells and LGL. May provide signal to T cell that results in augmented T cell IL-2 production
	Induced: ?		
ICAM-1	Basal: +		Ligand to CD18 family of leukocyte integrins which are present on lymphocytes, LGL, monocytes and activated macrophages and PMN
	Induced: IL-1, TNF		
	IFN-γ, bacterial endotoxins		

* The information is summarized from references (12–14). The abbreviations used in the table include: MHC-major histocompatibility complex, TNF-tumor necrosis factor, IFN-interferon, EC-endothelial cell, LFA-lymphocyte function associated, ICAM-intercellular adhesion molecule.

well-described murine models of autoimmunity (7). Lymphocytes from BALB/c mice, following in vitro sensitization with vascular smooth muscle cells, will cause a granulomatous vasculitis when injected into a syngeneic host. Lymphocytes also are important in the expression of vasculitis seen in several of the murine strains prone to develop autoimmune diseases. A primary role for lymphocyte mediated vasculitis is certainly a consideration in Takayasu arteritis and temporal arteritis. Mononuclear cells including lymphocytes comprise the primary infiltrating cell populations in these two vasculitic syndromes.

Thomas R. Cupps, MD

1. American College of Rheumatology Subcommittee on Classification of Vasculitis: The American College of Rheumatology 1990 Criteria for the Classification of Vasculitis. Arthritis Rheum 33:1065–1144, 1990
2. Cupps TR, Fauci AS: The Vasculitides. In: Major Problems in Internal Medicine. Edited by Smith LH. Philadelphia, WB Saunders 21:1–211, 1982
3. Fauci AS, Haynes BF, Katz P: The spectrum of vasculitis: clinical, pathologic, immunologic, and therapeutic considerations. Ann Intern Med 89:660–676, 1978
4. Systemic Vasculitides. Edited by Churg A, Churg J. New York, Igaku–Shoin, 1991, pp 1–389
5. Lie JT, Members and Consultants of the American College of Rheumatology Subcommittee on Classification of Vasculitis: Illustrated histopathologic classification criteria for selected vasculitis syndromes. Arthritis Rheum 33:1074–1087, 1990
6. Cupps TR: Infections and vasculitis: mechanisms considered. In: Systemic Vasculitis. Edited by LeRoy EC. New York, Marcel Dekker, (in press)
7. Reinisch CL, Moyer CF: Animal models of vasculitis. In: Systemic Vasculitides. Edited by Churg A, Churg J. New York, Igaku-Shoin, 1991, pp 31–40
8. Falk RJ, Terrell RS, Charles LA, et al: Anti-neutrophil cytoplasmic autoantibodies induce neutrophils to degranulate and produce oxygen radicals in vitro. Proc Natl Acad Sci USA 87:4115–4119, 1990
9. Brasile L, Kremer JM, Clarke JL, et al: Identification of an autoantibody to vascular endothelial cell-specific antigens in patients with systemic vasculitis. Am J Med 87:74–80, 1989
10. Leung DYM, Collins T, Lapiere La, et al: Immunoglobulin M antibodies present in the acute phase of Kawasaki syndrome lyse cultured vascular endothelial cells stimulated by gamma interferon. J Clin Invest 77:1428–1435, 1986
11. Leung DYM, Geha RS, Newburger JW, et al: Two monokines, interleukin–1 and tumor necrosis factor, render cultured endothelial cells susceptible to lysis by antibodies circulating during Kawasaki syndrome. J Exp Med 164:1058–1972, 1985
12. Huges CCW, Savage COS, Pober JS: The endothelial cell as a regulator of T–cell function. Immunol Reviews 117:85–102, 1990
13. Argenbright LW, Barton RW: Interactions of leukocyte integrins with intercellular adhesion molecule 1 in the production of inflammatory vascular injury in vivo. J Clin Invest 89:259–272, 1992
14. Springer TA, Dustin ML, Kishimoto TK, et al: The lymphocyte function-associated LFA-1, CD2, and LFA-3 molecules: cell adhesion receptors of the immune system. Ann Rev Immunol 5:223–252, 1987

B. Clinical and Laboratory Features

The clinical course in the different forms of systemic vasculitis may be brief or prolonged, benign or fatal (1,2). Considerable overlap exists among the vasculitis syndromes. When a patient is seen who has manifestations that overlap with more than one type of vasculitis or who does not easily fit into a specific category, the extent of involvement should be defined as carefully as possible and treatment decided accordingly.

TAKAYASU ARTERITIS

Clinical Manifestations

Takayasu arteritis, a chronic vasculitis of the aorta and its branches, is most common in young women of Asian descent (3,4). It seldom starts after the age of 40 years. The proximal aorta and its branches tend to be involved to the greatest degree, but any part of the aorta may be affected. In the early phases, nonspecific symptoms such as malaise and arthralgias are frequent. Mild synovitis is noted in about 20% of patients. Erythema nodosum-like vasculitis lesions may occur over the legs. The disease progresses at a variable rate; after weeks or months, manifestations of vascular insufficiency become apparent. These include cool extremities, headaches, dizziness, amaurosis, or diplopia. Angina pectoris may develop due to narrowing of coronary artery ostia secondary to aortitis. The blood pressure may become difficult to detect because of narrowing of the subclavian or more distal vessels. In the legs, claudication results from narrowing of the distal aorta or iliac vessels. Intra-abdominal and cerebral ischemia may develop due to narrowing of mesenteric or cervical vessels.

Asymmetrically reduced peripheral pulses are present in nearly all patients. Blood pressure differences of greater than 10 mm of mercury are found in most. Hypertension is present in 40% of patients secondary to renal artery stenosis, peripheral arterial obstruction, or rigidity of inflamed large vessels. Bruits may be audible over the carotid, subclavian, and other large arteries, and aortic valve insufficiency may be present due to aortic root dilation.

Laboratory Tests

A normochromic anemia, increased erythrocyte sedimentation rate, and thrombocytosis are present during the inflammatory phase of the disease. Hyperglobulinemia occurs occasionally. The electrocardiogram may reveal an ischemic pattern, and widening of the thoracic aorta may be detected on chest radiography. Arteriography shows smooth, tapered narrowings or occlusions or aneurysms of the aorta and its proximal branches (Fig. 17B–1).

Diagnosis

The diagnosis should be suspected especially in young women with a history of a systemic inflammatory illness, altered arterial pulses, or bruits over large arteries. The diagnosis generally is confirmed by arteriography. Digital subtraction angiography with intravenous dye injection provides less distinct resolution of the

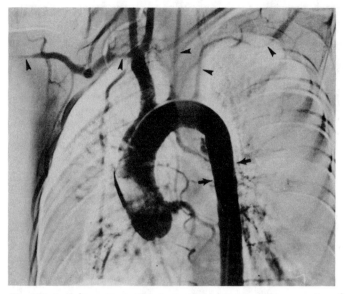

Fig. 17B–1. Takayasu arteritis. Aortogram showing slight narrowing of the descending aorta (arrows) and multiple narrowed segments of large thoracic and cervical arteries (arrow heads).

vessel wall outlines and a more restricted survey of the arterial tree but may be adequate in some cases. Computed tomography and magnetic resonance angiography (MRA) studies show luminal narrowing and mural thickening in vessels and may be useful to support initial arteriographic findings and in follow-up monitoring. Because of the size of the vessels affected, biopsies are rarely obtained. Takayasu arteritis tends to be chronic. The five-year survival rate has been reported to be over 90%.

The differential diagnosis includes carotid artery dissection that is usually localized, early arteriosclerosis in the setting of risk factors, heritable connective tissue disorders such as Ehlers–Danlos syndrome, and giant cell arteritis.

GIANT CELL ARTERITIS

Clinical Manifestations

Giant cell arteritis—also known as temporal arteritis or cranial arteritis—affects almost exclusively individuals over 50 years of age (5,6). It is more common in women. In the years following Horton's description in 1932, it was thought to be an unusual condition. Today it is recognized frequently, particularly in the northern portions of Europe and in the United States with populations of the same ethnic background. In these groups, it is one of the most frequent forms of vasculitis with incidence rates as high as 20 to 30 new cases annually per 100,000 persons over the age of 50 years. It affects the same population as the closely associated process of polymyalgia rheumatica (see Chapter 18).

The disease usually begins gradually and may be present for a number of weeks or months before its' recognition. At times, the onset is abrupt and flu-like. Early symptoms include malaise, fatigue, fever (sometimes as high as 40°C), weight loss, and polymyalgia rheumatica. Frequent manifestations related to vascular involvement include headaches, tenderness of the scalp, especially over the temporal arteries, jaw claudication (fatigue and discomfort in the muscles of mastication during chewing), visual loss, diplopia, aortic arch syndrome, and cough or sore throat.

The temporal arteries may be erythematous, thickened, and tender (Fig. 17B–2). Occasionally the occipital, facial, or postauricular arteries are similarly affected. Visual loss occurs in about 15% and may be an early symptom (7). This usually results from retinal ischemia secondary to involvement of the ophthalmic or posterior ciliary arteries. It is abrupt and painless. However, amaurosis fugax may precede permanent blindness. Permanent visual impairment varies from a partial deficit of one eye to complete bilateral blindness. In patients with visual manifesta-

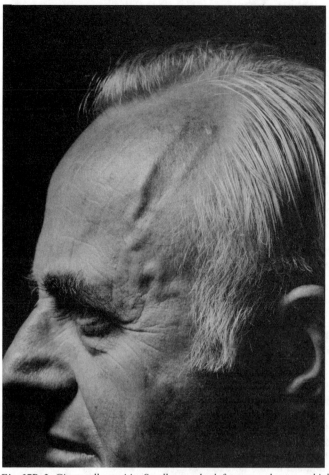

Fig. 17B–2. Giant cell arteritis. Swollen tender left temporal artery which is more prominent than seen in most cases. Pulsations were present on palpation but the wall was thickened when compared to the right side.

tions, the ophthalmologic examination may reveal ischemic optic neuropathy early, and optic atrophy after several weeks.

Involvement of the aortic arch and its branches occurs in approximately 10% of patients and may cause reduced blood pressure in one or both arms, arm claudication, or focal cerebral ischemia. Peripheral neuropathy occurs in a minority of patients; involvement of the skin, intracranial vessels, kidneys, or lungs rarely occurs.

Laboratory Tests

Blood tests reflect the underlying inflammatory processes. The erythrocyte sedimentation rate tends to be higher than in other vasculitides, averaging about 80–100 mm/hr (Westergren) in many series. Rarely, it may be normal, even when the disease is active. Other acute phase serum proteins are similarly elevated. Additional laboratory alterations include increased hepatic enzymes in 20% to 30%, and elevated levels of factor VIII and interleukin–6.

Diagnosis

Giant cell arteritis should be suspected in patients over 50 years of age who develop a new type of headache, jaw claudication, fever, or polymyalgia rheumatica. Careful examination may reveal a thickened or tender temporal artery, new carotid artery bruits, or bruits over the axillary or brachial arteries. Biopsy of the most abnormal segment of the temporal arteries should be performed to confirm the diagnosis even when manifestations seem relatively typical. If biopsy proof is not obtained, decisions regarding therapy may be more difficult after several months of corticosteroid therapy when drug side effects are prominent and the presence of earlier vasculitis seems less clear. If a temporal artery is clearly inflamed, only a short piece of the abnormal part of the artery needs to be biopsied. However, because involvement tends to be patchy, a 3–6 cm segment should be obtained when the physical findings are indeterminate. The biopsied arterial segment should be examined at multiple levels. If the first side is negative, consideration should be given to biopsying the other temporal artery also. A properly performed temporal artery biopsy will define the need for corticosteroid therapy in about 90% of cases.

Other forms of arteritis occasionally affect the temporal artery and cause clinical findings compatible with giant cell arteritis. These include Wegener's granulomatosis and polyarteritis nodosa. The histologic sections in such instances show acute or chronic arteritis. Takayasu's arteritis begins at an earlier age, less commonly involves branches of the external carotid artery and has not been demonstrated to involve the temporal artery. Occasionally amyloidosis affects temporal arteries or causes jaw or arm claudication.

POLYARTERITIS NODOSA

Clinical Features

Polyarteritis nodosa may affect any organ of the body, but skin, peripheral nerves, joints, intestinal tract, and kidneys are most commonly involved (8,9). The lungs are usually spared. The severity varies, but polyarteritis nodosa is a serious and often progressive and fatal illness. Vasculitis similar to polyarteritis nodosa may be an occasional secondary or associated manifestation of other diseases such as rheumatoid arthritis (RA) and systemic lupus erythematosus (SLE).

Polyarteritis nodosa is uncommon and estimates of its incidence in the general population have ranged from about 5 to 220 per million persons per year. The disease is twice as frequent in men. It may be observed in children and the elderly but is more common in middle age.

Onset of disease may be gradual or abrupt. Constitutional symptoms such as fever and malaise are usually present. Cutaneous manifestations include palpable purpura, infarctive ulcers of varying sizes, and livido reticularis. Joint pains are common; synovitis is less frequent.

Multiple mononeuropathies are the most typical neurologic manifestation and occur in one-half or more of all cases. Sharp sudden pain or paresthesias in the distribution of a peripheral nerve are often the first symptoms, followed by weakness of the muscles supplied by that nerve. Several nerves may become involved progressively resulting in a severe diffuse polyneuropathy.

Segmental necrotizing glomerulonephritis is the usual renal lesion. Renovascular hypertension may develop. Gastrointestinal ischemia causes abdominal pain and findings of an acute abdomen. Occasionally the cystic or appendiceal artery may be involved. Hematemesis or melena may result from vasculitis of the upper or lower gastrointestinal tract. Liver involvement causes elevated serum enzymes. Coronary arteritis may result in myocardial ischemia or congestive heart failure.

Laboratory Tests

As in most systemic vasculitides, tests show a normochromic, normocytic anemia, an elevated erythrocyte sedimentation rate and other acute phase reactants, neutrophilic leukocytosis, and thrombocytosis. Serum complement is usually normal, but may be reduced in patients with diffuse cutaneous or renal disease. Serum rheumatoid factor may be present in this latter group.

Hepatitis B surface antigen and antibody have been found in 15% or more of patients. This antigen may be present continuously or transiently. Hepatitis C and A also have been identified. Patients with hepatitis antigen or antibodies usually appear similar to those who are negative. Hepatic dysfunction is generally mild and does not parallel the severity or activity of the vasculitis. Urinalysis in those with glomerulonephritis shows red blood cells, red cell casts, and proteinuria.

Histologic examination of biopsy specimens reveals an acute

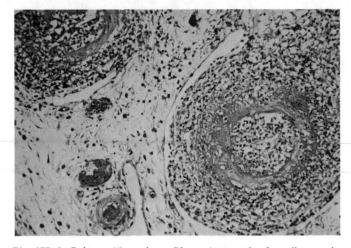

Fig. 17B–3. *Polyarteritis nodosa. Photomicrograph of small muscular artery showing acute inflammation, destruction of mural structures and fibrinoid necrosis.*

inflammatory infiltrate with polymorphonuclear leukocytes accompanied by a variable number of lymphocytes and eosinophils (4) (Fig. 17B–3). Fibroid necrosis is often present. Lesions in various stages of development may be present in the same specimen. Disruption of the elastic laminae results in arterial dilation or formation of an aneurysm.

Diagnosis

It is important to pursue the diagnosis aggressively and start therapy promptly to limit organ damage. Polyarteritis nodosa should be suspected in patients with unexplained fever, weight loss, fatigue, and multisystem findings. Evidence of vasculitis should be established whenever possible by biopsy of clinically involved tissue such as skin, sural nerve, muscle, and testes. Biopsy of the first two tissues generally yields small arteries and the latter two somewhat larger vessels. The chances of finding vasculitis in a biopsy of an organ without other evidence of involvement are lower. A kidney biopsy may be considered in patients with abnormal urinary sediment or proteinuria. This biopsy may document the presence of glomerulonephritis and, less commonly, will show vasculitis.

Mesenteric arteriograms may be helpful when abdominal pain or elevated hepatic enzymes are present and a biopsy site cannot be readily indentified. Typical angiographic changes include multiple arterial aneurysms and tapered narrowings and irregularities. However, similar changes may be present in other forms of vasculitis including Wegener's granulomatosis, Churg–Strauss syndrome, vasculitis in SLE, or other illnesses such as infective endocarditis, atrial myxoma, and noninflammatory connective tissue disorders such as fibromuscular dysplasia.

Prior to the use of corticosteroids, the five-year survival of polyarteritis was reported to be less than 15%. In recent years survival has improved; studies now indicate a five-year survival of 60% or more. The prognosis of polyarteritis nodosa is worse in older persons and those with more extensive visceral or central nervous system involvement. Most deaths caused by polyarteritis nodosa occur within the first year of the disease as a result of uncontrolled vasculitis or superimposed infections related to therapy.

CHURG–STRAUSS SYNDROME

Clinical Features

The Churg–Strauss syndrome, initially reported under the descriptive title allergic granulomatosis and angiitis, is an uncommon but distinct process (10,11). Involvement of the lungs helps distinguish it from polyarteritis nodosa. This condition occurs in patients with asthma or history of allergy. It usually develops in middle age and affects men more commonly than women. In many patients a phasic pattern is followed. Initially, an increase in allergic manifestations occurs, especially asthma, followed by eosinophilia, and finally vasculitis.

Fever, malaise, and weight loss are common early manifestations. As the vasculitis develops, asthma may become less prominent. Cutaneous findings include petechiae, purpura, or ulcerations. Chest discomfort or shortness of breath may result from pulmonary lesions. Peripheral neuropathy, usually multiple mononeuropathies, is common. Abdominal symptoms include diarrhea, pain, or a mass due to ischemia or infarction of abdominal organs. Glomerulonephritis tends to be less frequent and severe than in polyarteritis nodosa. Eosinophilic granulomatous involvement of the urinary tract or prostate is a unique feature of this syndrome.

Laboratory Tests

Eosinophilia is present in essentially all patients but resolves in response to treatment. Serum complement is usually normal. Renal function may diminish in those with glomerulonephritis. Urinalysis reveals proteinuria and red cell casts. Chest radiographs show patchy or nodular infiltrations or diffuse interstitial disease.

Biopsy of involved tissues shows angiitis and extramural necrotizing microgranulomas, usually with eosinophilic infiltrates (4). The vascular infiltration includes eosinophils and may be granulomatous or nongranulomatous. Veins may be affected as well as arteries.

Diagnosis

The syndrome should be suspected in patients with worsening asthma who develop fever and evidence of a systemic illness. The diagnosis should be confirmed by biopsy of involved tissues. Abdominal angiograms may show findings similar to those in polyarteritis nodosa.

The mortality rate appears to be less than in polyarteritis nodosa. Remission is seen in some cases. This syndrome also needs to be differentiated from Loffler's syndrome, hypersensitivity vasculitis, and Wegener's granulomatosis.

WEGENER'S GRANULOMATOSIS

Clinical Findings

Wegener's granulomatosis is an uncommon vasculitis that occurs in young or middle-aged adults and is slightly more common in men (12,13). It is often considered a triad of necrotizing granulomatous vasculitis of the tissues of the upper respiratory tract, the lower respiratory tract, and focal segmental glomerulonephritis. However, limited forms occur that may affect only one of these areas. Additional tissues also may be involved. Small arteries and veins are the predominant vessels affected.

Patients often present with nonspecific findings of fever, malaise, weight loss, arthralgias, myalgias, and chronic rhinitis or worsening sinusitis. Pain over the sinus areas and purulent or bloody nasal discharge are typical upper respiratory symptoms. Nasal or oral mucosal ulcerations are early findings. Destructive changes lead to a saddle nose deformity.

Pulmonary involvement may be asymptomatic or may cause chest pain, shortness of breath, bloody or purulent sputum, and hemorrhage. Tracheal lesions and especially subglottic involvement may produce stenosis. Eye symptoms include episcleritis, uveitis, and proptosis due to orbital granulomas. Cranial nerve deficits may be the result of granulomatous inflammation in or near the upper airways.

Peripheral neuropathy may occur as in other forms of vasculitis. Cutaneous findings include nodules, purpura, and ulcerations. Arthritis is less common and usually transient.

Laboratory Tests

Patients with renal involvement have proteinuria, urinary dimorphic red cells, and red cell casts. Chest radiographs show nodules and infiltrations that often cavitate.

Serum antibodies that react with cytoplasmic components of neutrophils are present in the majority of patients, especially in those with active multisystem disease (14). Approximately 80% of patients with Wegener's granulomatosis have C-ANCAs, but they are less frequent in limited forms and inactive disease. P-ANCAs are present in a minority of patients with Wegener's granulomatosis, but are more common in so-called pauci-immune necrotizing and crescentic glomerulonephritis, with or without an accompanying systemic vasculitis. ANCA are found in a minority of patients with polyarteritis nodosa and other forms of vasculitis.

Histologic examination of involved specimens shows a necrotizing granulomatous inflammatory process with involvement of small arteries and veins (5). In some inflammatory lesions, especially of the upper airway structures, vasculitis is not a prominent feature and it may not be found in biopsy specimens of limited size. Purpuric skin lesions may show leukocytoclastic vasculitis.

Diagnosis

The diagnosis should be suspected in patients with progressive upper or lower respiratory tract manifestations and nasal or oral ulcerations. The presence of serum C-ANCA makes the diagnosis likely. Biopsy of involved tissues to should be performed to confirm the diagnosis.

Septic processes, especially fungal and mycobacterial infections, should be excluded. Angiocentric T cell lymphomas (lymphomatoid granulomatosis) produce somewhat similar destructive lesions. Patients with Churg–Strauss syndrome may present with a similar triad of organ involvement.

VASCULITIS ASSOCIATED WITH RHEUMATIC DISEASES

Clinical Findings

Blood vessels are involved in many connective tissue disorders. Perivascular leukocyte cuffing without damage to the vessel or tissue ischemia is part of the disease processes but is not considered vasculitis by itself. Proliferation of the blood vessel intima (obliterative endarteritis) with little evidence of active inflammation may develop and cause tissue ischemia. This bland thickening of the intima is often seen in systemic sclerosis and results in ulcers or infarction of the distal finger pads. Somewhat similar changes may occur in rheumatoid arthritis and other connective tissue disorders producing dermal infarctions at the fingernail folds and elsewhere.

In a small proportion of cases of RA, SLE, and other connective tissue disorders, necrotizing vasculitis develops during the course of the disease. The vessels involved may be small, medium-sized muscular arteries or even larger arteries that show changes indistinguishable from polyarteritis nodosa. Large arteries show acute vasculitis. Immune complex processes are considered important in the vasculitis of connective tissue diseases.

Patients with RA who develop necrotizing vasculitis are more likely to be male, have erosive joint disease, rheumatoid nodules, and high titers of serum rheumatoid factor. At the time of active vasculitis, serum complement is reduced and immune complexes appear in the serum. Frequent manifestations include skin infarctions over the lower extremities and multiple mononeuropathies. Mesenteric ischemia may occur. Renal disease is absent.

Patients with SLE who develop necrotizing vasculitis are not as readily recognizable but usually have livedo reticularis, Raynaud's phenomenon, cutaneous lesions, and digital gangrene. Precipitating antibodies to DNA may be more common in this group.

Diagnosis

Vasculitis should be suspected in patients with a connective tissue disorder whose symptoms rapidly become worse (especially systemic symptoms such as fever), and who develop skin lesions, neuropathy, or abdominal pain.

Electromyograms help elucidate the type of neuropathy. Skin or nerve (sural) biopsies aid in documenting the presence of vasculitis. Mesenteric angiograms help clarify the nature of abdominal pain when present, gastrointestinal bleeding secondary to bowel ischemia, or both.

CENTRAL NERVOUS SYSTEM VASCULITIS

Clinical Features

Many forms of vasculitis affect the central nervous system; however, when vasculitis occurs without an associated disease, it is designated primary vasculitis of the central nervous system. This vasculitis is uncommon and only slightly more than 100 cases have been reported. It occurs at all ages with onset common between 40 and 50 years of age. It appears to be somewhat more frequent in men (15). Very little is known of its pathogenesis; however, about 25% of cases have been associated with lymphoreticular neoplasms and some also had herpes zoster infection. It has been associated also with human T lymphotrophic virus type III and human immunodeficiency virus (HIV) infection.

The course of primary central nervous system vasculitis is variable. It may be fatal within weeks or chronically progressive over one or more years. Early symptoms are confusion, headache, and progressive impairment of intellectual functioning. Focal neurologic deficits, seizures, and cranial nerve involvement occur frequently. In occasional instances, spinal cord vessels also become involved.

Laboratory Tests

The hemoglobin, leukocyte count, and erythrocyte sedimentation rate are likely to be normal. Cerebrospinal fluid may show an increased opening pressure, mild pleocytosis, and mild increased protein concentration. Examination of the head with MRI demonstrates multiple lesions. Cerebral angiograms typically show intermittent narrowing and dilation of small and medium-sized intracranial blood vessels. Vessels in one region such as the base of the brain may be affected more prominently. In other cases, generalized intracerebral involvement is present.

Diagnosis

Diagnosis is often difficult. This condition should be considered in patients who present with progressive headache, impaired mental function, and multifocal neurologic deficits especially in the presence of a history of herpes zoster infection, lymphoma, or illicit drug use. In these cases, angiograms should be performed and show smooth-walled tapered areas and aneurysms. However, angiograms are not always definitive. Arterial spasm (related to the procedure or intracranial hemorrhage) and other diseases may produce similar changes. Normal angiograms are rare in vasculitis of the central nervous system, but do not exclude the diagnosis.

Brain and leptomeningeal biopsy is not a simple procedure, but is definitive when positive. It should be considered when the diagnosis seems likely. Because the vessels are involved in a patchy distribution, the small biopsy specimens possible to obtain via burr holes may not include an involved artery. Cases diagnosed by angiograms alone constitute a less well-defined group.

Conditions that produce similar findings to central nervous system vasculitis include Cogan's syndrome (nonsyphilitic interstitial keratitis and vestibular dysfunction), Behcet's syndrome, SLE, polyarteritis nodosa, and antiphospholipid syndrome.

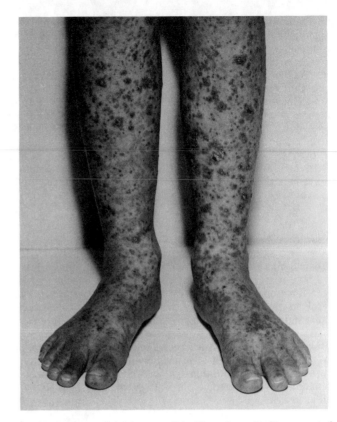

Fig. 17B–4. *Hypersensitivity vasculitis. Extensive palpable purpuric lesions over legs. Some lesions became confluent and superficial ulcerations developed.*

HYPERSENSITIVITY VASCULITIS

Clinical Findings

This category includes cases of vasculitis of small vessels, especially arterioles and venules, secondary to an immune response to exogenous substances (16). Reactions to drugs are the most common cause (17).

Onset is usually abrupt and occurs after exposure to the etiologic agent. Palpable purpura is the most common clinical manifestation (Fig. 17B–4). Cutaneous ulcerations may develop. Transient arthralgias are frequent. Systemic symptoms may be present. The severity of the illness varies considerably from a few scattered purpuric spots to an extensive, prolonged, systemic process.

Laboratory Findings

The laboratory alterations are usually nonspecific and may be limited in mild cases. The erythrocyte sedimentation rate is usually elevated. Serum complement, especially C4, may be reduced during the acute phase due to the immune complex nature of the process. Eosinophilia may be present.

Biopsy of cutaneous lesions shows leukocytoclastic vasculitis of arterioles and postcapillary venules with the presence of neutrophils, nuclear fragments secondary to karyorrhexis, perivascular hemorrhage, and fibrinoid deposits. Eosinophils are often present. In a minority of cases, lymphocytic infiltrations predominate. Microhematuria occurs, but renal failure is uncommon.

Diagnosis

Diagnosis is made by biopsy identifying the presence of cutaneous vasculitis and identification of a potential inciting agent. Manifestations usually appear abruptly. All lesions tend to be at approximately the same stage of development and generally resolve after a brief period of days or weeks.

The clinical definition of this syndrome has been difficult because a responsible agent cannot be identified in many patients who have compatible clinical and biopsy findings. Some cases may become chronic with persistent symptoms even though there is no apparent continuous exposure to a sensitizing substance. These observations raise questions about other possible pathogenetic mechanisms. Furthermore, clinical manifestations in hypersensitivity vasculitis are not distinctive, and similar clinical pictures may be associated with a variety of other disorders such as Henoch–Schonlein purpura (see Chapter 22C), rheumatic disorders, cryoglobulinemia, and infections. Cases of so-called microscopic polyarteritis nodosa and cutaneous polyarteritis nodosa may be difficult to distinguish from hypersensitivity vasculitis other than the chronic course in the former. Other less common forms of vasculitis such as hypocomplementemic urticarial vasculitis, and some infections such as bacterial endocarditis, need to be differentiated.

CRYOGLOBULINEMIA

Classification

Cryoglobulins are immunoglobulins that have the exceptional property of reversibly precipitating at reduced temperatures. Cryoglobulins are present in a variety of autoimmune, neoplastic, and infectious disorders. They may be grouped into two general categories (Table 17B–1).

Type I cryoglobulins consist of a single monoclonal protein and are generally associated with multiple myeloma, macroglobulinemia, and less common other neoplastic proliferations of lymphocytes. These cryoglobulins generally are readily detectable as monoclonal components on electrophoresis of serum. They often produce no symptoms but occasionally cause Raynaud's phenomenon, livedo reticularis, purpura, or ischemic ulcers due to hyperviscosity and plugging of small vessels in the acral parts of the body when cooled. Vasculitis is rare. In several large series of patients with cryoglobulinemia, monoclonal cryoproteins constitute about one-third of those encountered. The frequency of immunoglobulin types seen in this group is the same as the frequency of all immunoglobulins producing tumors (IgG is most frequent, IgM less often, and IgA least frequent).

Type II cryoglobulins consist of more than one class of immunoglobulin. They are common, constituting about two-thirds of the cryoglobulins seen in the Western world. Type II cryoglobulinemia appears as a primary disease (essential or primary mixed cryoglobulinemia) or a manifestation of some other underlying disease. Mixed cryoglobulins generally contain IgM molecules together with IgG, although other combinations are seen. One component, usually IgM, has antiglobulin activity (rheumatoid factor) and is the reason for the complex formation and the cryoprecipitation. They may also contain other antigens such as hepatitis B virus, other infecting agents, and nuclear and complement proteins. These cryoglobulins are more difficult to detect because they precipitate more slowly and tend to be present in small quantities (50–500 mg/dL).

Mixed cryoglobulins have been further subdivided into those in which one component is monoclonal, usually the IgM, and those in which all components are polyclonal. This division appears to have little clinical or prognostic significance in patients whose cryoglobulins are associated with nonmalignant disorders.

Pathophysiology of Mixed Cryoglobulinemia

The frequent association with chronic infections and the presence of infecting agent proteins in the cryoprecipitates have suggested that IgG antibodies complexed with an infecting agent (antigen) induce the production of IgM anti–antiglobulins. When infections resolve, the cryoglobulins and antiglobulins are no longer formed.

Mixed cryoglobulins have all the properties of an immune complex. They activate the complement sequence and when deposited in small peripheral blood vessels, cause the development of vasculitis through complement-mediated inflammation. It is uncertain why some patients have symptoms and others do not, and why there are differences in severity and organ involvement. Determining factors may be related to the nature of the antigen or antibody raised, the size of the complexes, the function of the reticuloendothelial system, the ability to activate complement, or endothelial cell immune complex interactions.

Clinical Features of Mixed Cryoglobulinemia

Cutaneous lesions are most common and include palpable purpura, urticaria, and ulcers. Other features include Raynaud's phenomenon, arthralgias, glomerulonephritis, peripheral neuropathy, hepatomegaly, splenomegaly, and lymphadenopathy. Thyroiditis, Sjögren's syndrome, pneumonitis, and pericarditis may be present.

The course may be mild or prolonged and is influenced by the specific organs involved or by an associated underlying disease if present. Progressive glomerulonephritis is often the most serious manifestation (18). In some patients with primary mixed cryoglobulinemia, cirrhosis or a lymphoproliferative disorder eventually develops.

Laboratory Tests in Mixed Cryoglobulinemia

Serum gammaglobulins are often elevated, rheumatoid factor is present, and complement levels are decreased. Hepatitis B virus frequently has been associated with mixed cryoglobulinemia (19). Hepatitis A and C, and other agents including Epstein–Barr virus, cytomegalovirus, and HIV are also found and suggest a viral-related pathogenesis.

Serum containing cryoglobulins becomes opalescent and forms a visible precipitate when incubated at 0–4°C. The quantity of cold-insoluble proteins can be determined either by means of a cryocrit or more accurately by isolating the cryoglobulin and measuring the amount of precipitate formed. Further characterization of the protein type can be carried out by immunoelectrophoresis or immunoglobulin quantitation. In searching for cryoglobulins, it is important to draw the blood in a warm syringe, allow it to clot, separate the serum at 37°, and then incubate the serum in the cold for several days.

Diagnosis

Serum should be tested for cryoglobulins in patients with vasculitis and those with connective tissue disorders, infections, and neoplasms, especially when cutaneous or renal involvement or evidence of vasculitis develops. Analysis of the cryoglobulin components may elucidate the nature of the disease and help in the decisions regarding therapy.

Gene G. Hunder, MD

Table 17B–1. *Clinical associations of cryoglobulinemia*

I. Monoclonal Cryoglobulins
    Multiple myeloma (IgG, IgA), macroglobulinemia (IgM), lymphoproliferative disorders, angioimmunoblastic lymphadenopathy
II. Mixed Cryoglobulins
    Essential mixed cryoglobulinemia
    Connective tissue diseases
        Systemic lupus erythematosus, rheumatoid arthritis, polyarteritis nodosa, Sjögren's syndrome, systemic sclerosis, etc.
    Infections
        Viral: Hepatitis A;B;C, infectious mononucleosis, cytomegalovirus
        Bacterial: subacute bacterial endocarditis, poststreptococcal glomerulonephritis, leprosy, syphilis, Lyme disease, intestinal bypass disorder
        Parasitic: schistosomiasis, echinococcosis, toxoplasmosis, malaria, kalar-azar
    Lymphoproliferative disease
        Macroglobulinemia, chronic lymphocytic leukemia, lymphoma, angioimmunoblastic lymphadenopathy
    Miscellaneous
        Chronic liver disease, proliferative glomerulonephritis, sarcoidosis

1. Systemic Vasculitides. Edited by Churg A, Churg J. New York, NY, Igaku-Shoin, 1991, pp 389
2. Systemic Vasculitis. The Biologic Basis. Edited by Leroy EC. New York, NY, Marcel Dekker, Inc., 1992, pp 583
3. Arend WP, Michel BA, Bloch DA, et al: The American College of Rheumatology 1990 criteria for the classification of Takayasu arteritis. Arthritis Rheum 33:1129–1136, 1990
4. Giordano JM, Leavitt RY, Hoffman G, Fauci AS: Experience with surgical treatment of Takayasu's disease. Surgery 1991;109:252–258.
5. Hunder GG, Bloch DA, Michel BA, et al: The American College of Rheumatology 1990 criteria for the classification of giant cell arteritis. Arthritis Rheum 33:1122–1128, 1990
6. Machado EBV, Michet CJ, Ballard DJ, et al: Trends in incidence and clinical presentation of temporal arteritis in Olmsted County, Minnesota, 1950–1985. Arthritis Rheum 31:745–749, 1988
7. Aiello PD, Trautmann JC, McPhee TJ, et al: Visual prognosis in giant cell arteritis. Submitted for publication in Ophthalmology
8. Lightfoot RW, Michel BA, Bloch DA, et al: The American College of Rheumatology 1990 criteria for the classification of polyarteritis nodosa. Arthritis Rheum 33:1088–1093, 1990
9. Guillevin L, Le Thi Huong Du, Godeau P, et al: Clinical findings and prognosis of polyarteritis nodosa and Churg–Strauss angiitis: a study in 165 patients. B J Rheumatol 27:258–264, 1988
10. Masi AT, Hunder GG, Lie JT, et al: The American College of Rheumatology 1990 criteria for the classification of Churg–Strauss syndrome (allergic granulomatosis and angiitis). Arthritis Rheum 33:1094–1100, 1990
11. Lanham JG, Elkon KB, Pusey CD, et al: Systemic vasculitis with asthma and eosinophilia: A clinical approach to the Churg–Strauss syndrome. Medicine (Baltimore) 63:65–81, 1984
12. Hoffman GS, Kerr GS, Leavitt RY, et al: Wegener Granulomatosis: an analysis of 158 patients. Ann Intern Med 116:488–498, 1992
13. Leavitt RY, Fauci AS, Bloch DA, et al: The American College of Rheumatology 1990 criteria for the classification of Wegener's granulomatosis. Arthritis Rheum 33:1101–1107, 1990
14. Jennette JC, Falk RJ: Disease associations and pathogenic role of antineutrophil cytoplasmic autoantibodies in vasculitis. Curr Opin Rheum 4:9–15, 1992
15. Moore PM: Diagnosis and management of isolated angiitis of the central nervous system. Neurology 39:167–173, 1989
16. Calabrese LH, Michel BA, Bloch DA, et al: The American College of Rheumatology 1990 criteria for the classification of hypersensitive vasculitis. Arthritis Rheum 33:1108–1113, 1990
17. Michel BA, Hunder GG, Bloch DA, et al: Hypersensitivity vasculitis and Henoch-Schonlein purpura. J Rheumatol 19:721–728, 1992
18. Sinico RA, Winerals CG, Sabadini E, et al: Identification of glomerular immune deposits in cryoglobulinemia glomerulonephritis. Kidney Int 34:109–116, 1988
19. Ferri C, Greco F Longombardo G, et al: Antibodies to hepatitis C in patients with mixed cryoglobulinemia. Arthritis Rheum 34:1606–1610, 1991

C. Treatment

The cornerstone for successful treatment of vasculitis is making an accurate diagnosis as quickly as possible, recognizing prognosis, and anticipating the effects of disease and treatment on other concurrent illnesses (1). It is important to recognize that the systemic vasculitides are uncommon, and that even major referral centers may encounter no more than 5 to 10 newly diagnosed patients with any one type of systemic vasculitis per year. Consequently almost all studies of treatment have been uncontrolled.

The severity of disease, anatomic distribution of involvement, rate of progression, and pre-existing conditions should determine the aggressiveness of immunosuppressive therapy rather than the specific diagnosis. With the exception of acute Kawasaki syndrome, in which salicylates and high dose intravenous immunoglobulin are indicated, all other forms of severe systemic vasculitis should begin therapy with high dose corticosteroids such as prednisone (1 mg/kg/day). Whether corticosteroids should be given as a single morning dose, in two or three split doses, or as a large intravenous "pulse" or "bolus" (such as methylprednisolone 1 gram), or whether a cytotoxic agent should be used at the onset requires consideration of details of each situation. For example, most patients with giant cell arteritis will dramatically improve after corticosteroid therapy alone, whereas most patients with generalized Wegener's granulomatosis and associated glomerulonephritis will progress to renal failure and death if not treated with a cytotoxic agent such as cyclophosphamide (2).

INITIAL THERAPEUTIC INTERVENTIONS

Takayasu Arteritis. Most patients with Takayasu arteritis readily respond to corticosteroid therapy and can be successfully tapered off this agent without disease relapse. However, some patients with clinically active disease will be steroid-resistant or not be able to stop treatment without relapse. Those individuals may improve and require lower doses of corticosteroids when daily cyclophosphamide (3) or weekly methotrexate is added (4,5). The most difficult management problems in Takayasu arteritis occur in those patients who have clinically silent progressive disease, as may occur even with a normal erythrocyte sedimentation rate. Active disease in asymptomatic individuals has been recognized by periodic arteriographic studies, which have revealed new sites of stenosis or aneurysm formation. Still other individuals who are clinically "silent", but require bypass surgery for old critically stenotic lesions, may provide histopathologic evidence of unsuspected active disease from tissue obtained at the origin and insertion of the surgical graft (6). In one vascular surgery study of 33 patients, preoperative signs of active inflammation were rarely found, but 22% of 41 vascular specimens had evidence of acute inflammation and 20% had signs of chronic inflammation, which was of less clear significance (6). These observations emphasize the importance of intraoperative biopsies in all patients with Takayasu arteritis undergoing vascular surgery. The finding of unsuspected active disease obligates corticosteroid therapy. It has been assumed, although not proven, that the likelihood of sustained graft patency would be enhanced by decreasing inflammation. Similar reasoning has been applied to recommendations for suppression of any suspicious signs of disease activity before surgery. These therapeutic goals are frustrated by the fact that inflammatory markers such as clinical features, erythrocyte sedimentation rate, or von Willebrand factor antigen are not sufficiently sensitive or specific to identify all patients with active disease.

The ideal goal of medical therapy to prevent permanent vascular morphologic changes is often not achieved. Vascular bypass procedures have been successful in diminishing morbidity and mortality in carefully selected patients with cerebral, coronary, peripheral ischemic vascular disease, and renal artery stenosis with hypertension (7). Less often dilatation of the aortic root may lead to severe aortic regurgitation, requiring an aortic graft and aortic valve replacement. The usual limitations of vascular surgery are further complicated by the possibility of active arteritis leading to graft occlusion at the origin or insertion. As many as 20% to 33% of bypass procedures will require revision at some time (7). Some unanswered questions affecting vascular surgery in Takayasu arteritis are: (A) Do the limitations in detecting active disease justify pre- and post-operative corticosteroid therapy for all patients? (B) Should patients with anatomically severe, but asymptomatic lesions have prophylactic surgery (e.g. bilateral common carotid occlusion), or should one temporize until ischemic symptoms occur? (C) Is there a difference in long-term graft patency comparing use of autologous vein or artery, to synthetic graft materials? (D) Does chronic anti-coagulation with anti-platelet agents or warfarin affect graft patency? (E) Does transluminal angioplasty have comparable success to by-pass surgery for some specific lesions?

Giant Cell Arteritis. Corticosteroids continue to be the most effective therapy for giant cell arteritis. Prednisone (1 mg/kg/day) will reduce symptoms within one to two days and often eliminate symptoms within a week. One month after clinical and laboratory parameters, particularly the ESR, have normalized, tapering can begin. Unfortunately the ESR does not always normalize even with disease control so it should not be relied on as the only measure. Occasional patients may either not achieve complete remission or not be able to be tapered off steroids. Cytotoxic or immunosuppressive agents have been recommended for such individuals by some authors, but the utility of these agents, as demonstrated in controlled comparative trials, has not been addressed.

Polyarteritis Nodosa. Untreated polyarteritis nodosa has been estimated to have a five year mortality rate in excess of 85% (8,9). Treatment with high dose corticosteroids has decreased this figure to about 30% to 45% (9–11). When corticosteroids have been used in conjunction with an immunosuppressive/cytotoxic agent (usually cyclophosphamide and less often azathioprine, about 2 mg/kg/day) five year mortality was reported to be 20% to 25% (9) and relapses were less frequent (11) than noted with only steroid therapy. Clinical features that have most adversely affected survival include intestinal ischemia, cardiac involvement, and renal insufficiency. A reasonable approach to treatment, in the setting of normal renal function and in the absence of critical organ ischemia, would be to initiate therapy with only corticosteroids. If improvement does not follow within days; if deterioration occurs; or if renal, cardiac, intestinal, or central nervous system disease becomes apparent; daily therapy with a cytotoxic agent should be added.

Churg–Strauss Syndrome. Churg–Strauss syndrome is much less common than polyarteritis nodosa, and consequently information about its therapy is even more anecdotal. It appears to be more responsive to corticosteroids. The same principles noted for polyarteritis nodosa would apply for adding a cytotoxic agent, but the need for such is less frequent.

Wegener's Granulomatosis. Untreated or inadequately treated full-blown Wegener's granulomatosis is associated with a mean survival time of five months. Treatment with corticosteroids alone increases mean survival time to about 12 months. Survival has been dramatically improved by aggressive combination therapy with prednisone and daily cyclophosphamide, as well as by recognition of milder more indolent forms of disease without renal involvement (about 20%). Although combined drug therapy has been life-saving for many patients, it has become clear that for limited indolent disease such treatment may have excessive risk. Palliation of limited disease is often achieved with only corticosteroid therapy, but disease progression and relapses frequently occur. In the setting of severe life-threatening disease, most would agree that corticosteroid and daily low dose cyclophosphamide (2 mg/kg and in extreme situations up to 4 mg/kg) remain the treatment of choice (2,12,13). However, even in this setting toxicity is distressing and has led to trials of high-dose intravenous (''pulse'') cyclophosphamide and studies of other antimetabolite agents such as methotrexate. Preliminary results indicate that pulse cyclophosphamide and corticosteroids may provide substantial initial improvement but is not as effective as daily low dose cyclophosphamide therapy in maintaining improvement (12,13). Attempts to identify less toxic therapies for mild disease include trials of daily trimethaprim-sulfamethoxazole (14–16). Further prospective controlled studies with this agent are required before it can be considered clearly effective.

Wegener's granulomatosis is an excellent example of the necessity for a multidisciplinary team approach to achieve the best possible outcome. Chronic otitis media may require tympanotomy and drainage tubes; hearing loss may progress to the need for hearing aids. Nasal and sinus disease may be complicated by chronic crusting, mucopurulent discharge, and secondary infection that may require daily irrigation and occasionally debridement or surgery. The development of subglottic stenosis may necessitate dilatation, resection, tracheostomy, or even extensive reconstructive surgery. Retroorbital pseudotumor and lacrimal duct obstruction may demand ophthalmic surgery as well as medical treatment. Finally, complications of aggressive immunosuppressive therapies such as infections or hemorrhagic cystitis from cyclophosphamide may require special expertise for management.

Central Nervous System Vasculitis. Patients with primary central nervous system vasculitis are generally treated with high-dose prednisone (1-2 mg/kg) for 4 to 6 weeks given in combination with oral cyclophosphamide (2 mg/kg). The prednisone should be tapered over a period of several months and the cyclophosphamide continued for at least 12 months after all signs of disease have resolved. Other forms of vasculitis involving the central nervous system, in particular postpartum cerebral angiopathy and benign angiopathy of the central nervous system, are treated with high-dose corticosteroids for several weeks with tapering over 4 to 6 months. A calcium channel blocker may be beneficial. Persistence or progression of symptoms in these patients necessitates a biopsy; if vasculitis is confirmed, cyclophosphamide should be added to the corticosteroid regimen (17).

Hypersensitivity Vasculitis. Because visceral involvement is less common and less severe and the prognosis is better than for polyarteritis nodosa, Wegener's granulomatosis, or Churg–Strauss syndrome, a more cautious therapeutic approach is advised. If illness is mild and a drug reaction is suspected, the likely causative medication should be discontinued. If the precipitant may have been a self-limiting or treatable infection, cautious follow-up with or without antibiotics may be adequate. However, in the setting of visceral ischemia or glomerulonephritis, it would be prudent to treat with daily corticosteroids. Persistent resolution of abnormalities should lead to a slow taper and discontinuation of steroids over four to eight weeks (1).

Cryoglobulinemia. In patients with secondary forms of cryoglobulinemic vasculitis such as malignancy, infections, or inflammatory disorders, treatment should be directed at the primary disease process. Treatment of patients with essential or viral-associated mixed cryoglobulinemia depends on the severity of the disease. In the typical patient with mild purpura and arthralgias, only symptomatic treatment is indicated. In patients with progressive renal disease or neuropathy a more aggressive therapeutic approach is indicated that may include high-dose corticosteroids, immunosuppressive agents, and plasmapheresis (18). It is not yet known if alpha interferon therapy of chronic hepatitis will affect the associated cryoglobulinemia.

CHRONIC THERAPY

Because most systemic vasculitides are not cured, realistic goals include diminishing morbidity from disease and treatment, while hoping that the underlying process will go into an extended treatment-induced remission or be self-limited. Examples of vasculitides that may be monophasic are the hypersensitivity vasculitides, Henoch–Schoenlein purpura, polyarteritis nodosa, and Takayasu's arteritis. However, many individuals with polyarteritis nodosa, Takayasu's arteritis, Wegener's granulomatosis, Churg–Strauss syndrome, Behcet's disease, and giant cell arteritis who achieve remission will later relapse. These patients do not possess any clinical or serologic markers that predict risk of recurrence. Thus, regardless of how well a patient with these disorders has fared over time, the physician is obligated to maintain surveillance. This is especially true for those processes that involve the kidney as a target organ. Renal recurrences may not be apparent until advanced renal injury has occurred.

The clinician embarking on corticosteroid therapy should consider effects of treatment on intravascular volume, blood pressure, glucose metabolism, and electrolyte balance. This is especially important in the elderly and in patients with preexisting hypertension, cardiac disease, and diabetes mellitus. When treatment is indicated for systemic vasculitis, high doses should be maintained until all manifestations of active disease have abated. Tapering prednisone should follow after about one month. The literature does not provide a consensus opinion about the subsequent strategy for tapering steroids. One approach involves the reduction of prednisone on an alternate day basis so that within two to three months (in the absence of relapse or exacerbations) a dose of about 1 mg/kg every other day is achieved. During the subsequent two to three months, tapering of the alternate day schedule continues until therapy is discontinued. Waxing and waning of disease may force alterations in these guidelines. The rationale for this approach has been recently reviewed (19). The immunologic defects induced by corticosteroids are dependent on dose, frequency, and duration of treatment. As each factor increases, the incidence of opportunistic infections and other side effects increases. The use of alternate day prednisone (single morning dose) is associated with less toxicity than daily treatment.

The relative indications for adding a cytotoxic agent are discussed above. However, in some vasculitides that respond to corticosteroids, relapses become so common that continuous prednisone therapy may begin to produce more morbidity than the underlying illness. Cytotoxic therapy should be considered in this setting for enhancing the likelihood of remission as well as for steroid-sparing effects. Cyclophosphamide has been the most thoroughly studied cytotoxic agent for treatment of vasculitis. In a recent review of its use in Wegener's granulomatosis over a period of 24 years, it was associated with cystitis (43%), bladder cancer (2.8%, 33 times higher than expected rate), lymphoma (1.5%, 11 times the expected rate), myelodysplasia (2%), infertility (>57% of women), and an increased frequency of infections, especially when used in conjunction with corticosteroids (2). Although such treatment may be life-saving, and may be the best-known means of achieving remission in severe systemic vasculitides, it may also cause substantial morbidity and even mortality. Its use requires close vigilance of bladder and bone marrow effects, titration of doses, high oral fluid intake to dilute cyclophosphamide-derived bladder toxins (such as acrolein) and urologic consultation for any sign of bladder toxicity. The latency from initial use of cyclophosphamide to detecting bladder cancer may be as brief as 7 months or as long as 10 to 15 years, even after medication had been discontinued (2).

Many investigators are currently studying alternative modes of cytotoxic therapy. However, even under the best of circumstances the effects of most such agents are too broadly immunosuppressive. The most promising opportunities for the future may be realized through a better understanding of cytokines and immunologically active cloned human proteins that are produced by genetic engineering.

Reports of effectiveness of intravenous immunoglobulin therapy in Kawasaki disease and idiopathic thrombocytopenic purpura have encouraged an open trial of the agent in patients with anti-neutrophil cytoplasmic antibody positive systemic vasculitis. Improvement was noted within three weeks in all seven patients (20). These encouraging results will need to be confirmed by others.

Gary S. Hoffman, MD

1. Hoffman GS, Kerr GS: Recognition of systemic vasculitis in the acutely ill patient. Management of Critically Ill Patients with Rheumatologic and Immunologic Diseases. Edited by Mandell BF, Marcel Dekker, Inc., in press
2. Hoffman GS, Kerr GS, Leavitt RY, et al: Wegener's granulomatosis: an analysis of 158 patients. Ann Intern Med 116:488–498, 1992
3. Shelhamer JH, Volkman DJ, Parillo JE, et al: Takayasu's arteritis and its therapy. Ann Intern Med 103:121–126, 1985
4. Hoffman GS, Leavitt RY, Kerr GS, et al: Treatment of Takayasu's arteritis with methotrexate. Arthritis Rheum 34(supple):S74, 1991
5. Liang GC, Nemickas R, Madayag M: Multiple percutaneous transluminal angioplasties and low dose pulse methotrexate for Takayasu's arteritis. J Rheumatol 16:1370–1373, 1989
6. Lagneau P, Michel JB, Vuong PN: Surgical treatment of Takayasu's disease. Ann Surg 205:157–166, 1987
7. Giordano JM, Leavitt RY, Hoffman GS, et al: Experience with surgical treatment of Takayasu's disease. Surgery 109:252–258, 1991
8. Frohnert PP, Sheps SG: Longterm follow-up study of polyarteritis nodosa. Am J Med 43:8–14, 1967
9. Leib ES, Restivo C, Paulus HE: Immunosuppressive and corticosteroid therapy of polyarteritis nodosa. Am J Med 67:941–947, 1979
10. Cohen RD, Conn DL, Ilstrup DM: Clinical features, prognosis and response to treatment in polyarteritis. Mayo Clin Proc 55:146–155, 1980
11. Guillevin L, Jarrousse B, Lok C, et al: Longterm followup after treatment of polyarteritis nodosa and Churg–Strauss angiitis with comparison of steroids, plasma exchange, and cyclophosphamide to steroids and plasma exchange. A prospective randomized trial of 71 patients. J Rheumatol 18:567–574, 1991
12. Hoffman GS, Leavitt RY, Fleisher TA, et al: Treatment of Wegener's granulomatosis with intermittent high-dose intravenous cyclophosphamide. Am J Med 89:403–410, 1990
13. Steppat D, Gross WL: Stage adapted treatment of Wegener's granulomatosis. Klin Wochenschr 67:666–671, 1989
14. DeRemee RA: The treatment of Wegener's granulomatosis with trimethoprim/sulfamethoxazole: illusion or vision? Arthritis Rheum 31:1068–1072, 1988
15. Israel HL: Sulfamethoxazole-trimethoprim therapy for Wegener's granulomatosis. Arch Intern Med 148:2293–2295, 1988
16. Leavitt RY, Hoffman GS, Fauci AS: Response: the role of trimethaprim/sulfamethoxazole in the treatment of Wegener's granulomatosis. Arthritis Rheum 31:1073–1074, 1988
17. Moore PM. Diagnosis and management of isolated angiitis of the central nervous system. Neurology 39:167–173, 1989.
18. Geltner D. Therapeutic approaches in mixed cryoglobulinemia. Springer Semin Immunopathol 10:103–113, 1988.
19. Hoffman GS, Fauci AS: Respiratory disease in patients treated with glucocorticoids. Respiratory Diseases in the Immunosuppressed Host. Edited by Shelhamer J, Pizzo PA, Parillo JE, Masur H. Philadelphia, JB Lippincott, 1991
20. Jayne DRW, Davies MJ, Fox CJV, et al: Treatment of systemic vasculitis with pooled intravenous immunoglobulin. Lancet 337:1137–1139, 1991

18. POLYMYALGIA RHEUMATICA

Polymyalgia rheumatica is a common syndrome of older patients, characterized by pain and stiffness in the neck, shoulders, or hips that persists for at least one month. The erythrocyte sedimentation rate is often elevated and symptoms respond dramatically to a small dose of prednisone.

The annual incidence has been estimated at 50/100,000 for persons over the age of 50 (1). The great majority of patients are Caucasian and the disease may be less common in the southern United States than in northern states and in Canada. The etiology is unknown.

CLINICAL PICTURE

Polymyalgia rarely occurs before age 50; the majority of patients are older than age 60. It is twice as common in women as in men. Patients complain of pain in the neck, shoulders, upper arms, lower back, and thighs. The onset may be abrupt; patients go to bed feeling well and are stiff and sore when they awaken the next day. Gelling and morning stiffness are pronounced. Patients may describe how difficult it is to get out of bed in the morning. Symptoms are usually symmetric, but at times the pain may appear in one shoulder, suggesting bursitis, and then gradually spread to other areas (2).

Physical examination reveals only tenderness and limited shoulder motions. Radiographs are normal. An elevated erythrocyte sedimentation rate is the only abnormal laboratory test; rheumatoid factor and antinuclear antibodies are not present. Polymyalgia rheumatica can occasionally occur with a normal sedimentation rate. In such patients, the diagnosis must be based on the typical history of proximal pain and stiffness, exclusion of other causes, and the response to treatment with prednisone.

Despite the name "polymyalgia", biopsies have shown that muscles are normal but nonspecific inflammation is present in synovial tissues of the shoulders (3). This demonstration of synovitis very likely explains the marked morning stiffness and gelling that are characteristic of the disease and also indicates why it is often difficult to separate polymyalgia from the onset of rheumatoid arthritis (RA) in older patients in whom rheumatoid factor is not present. In RA, the small joints of the hands and feet are more often involved, as opposed to the proximal distribution of polymyalgia. However, some patients with polymyalgia rheumatica may have mild synovitis of the wrists with swelling and carpal tunnel syndrome, or synovitis of the knee with effusions.

TREATMENT

Polymyalgia rheumatica responds rapidly and completely to a low dose of prednisone. If this response is not seen within a week, the diagnosis should be doubted. The usual starting dose is 10–20 mg/day, which can be tapered to a daily maintenance dose of 5–7.5 mg/day following the clinical response. Aspirin and other antiinflammatory drugs are much less effective. Methotrexate is effective for the rare patient who requires a higher dose of prednisone to control inflammation.

Long-term follow-up has shown that polymyalgia is not always the self-limited condition it was once thought to be. Some patients can discontinue prednisone after a year or two, but approximately one-third require prolonged treatment to control inflammation. Even in these patients who require prednisone for many years, no joint damage is seen. In patients who have stopped prednisone, recurrences are not rare and may occur after intervals as long as eight years. The recurrence may be similar to the initial episode of polymyalgia rheumatica. Alternatively, the synovitis may involve wrists and metacarpophalangeal joints and resemble seronegative RA. With either presentation, recurrences respond well to low-dose prednisone, and there is no joint destruction (4). Polymyalgia rheumatica is not statistically associated with neoplastic disease, seropositive rheumatoid arthritis, or with any disease other than giant cell arteritis (see Chapter 17).

ASSOCIATION WITH GIANT CELL ARTERITIS

It is evident that polymyalgia and giant cell arteritis are related, but the nature of the link between them is not known (5). The frequency of concurrence varies in different populations from as high as 50% in Scandinavia, approximately 20% in the northern United States, and less than 1% in Israel. They frequently occur in the same patient, although not necessarily at the same time; the interval between them may be as long as 10 years. In some patients with polymyalgia, giant cell arteritis is found on biopsy of an asymptomatic temporal artery. Clinically, they seem to be separate syndromes. Polymyalgia is a pain syndrome often with a nondestructive synovitis that may run a prolonged or recurring course. Giant cell arteritis is a vasculitis that may either precede, coincide with, or follow the appearance of polymyalgia. Many patients seem to have polymyalgia alone; these respond well to low dose prednisone and never develop clinical arteritis.

L. A. Healey, MD

1. Chuang TY, Hunder GG, Ilstrup DM, Kurland LT: Polymyalgia rheumatica: a 10-year epidemiologic and clinical study. Ann Intern Med 97:672–680, 1982
2. Fitzcharles MA, Esdaile JM: Atypical presentations of polymyalgia rheumatica. Arthritis Rheum 33:403–406, 1990
3. Chou C–T, Schumacher HR: Clinical and pathologic studies of synovitis in polymyalgia rheumatica. Arthritis Rheum 27:1107–1118, 1984
4. Healey LA: Polymyalgia rheumatica and seronegative rheumatoid arthritis may be the same entity. J Rheumatol 19:270–272, 1992
5. Healey LA: Relation of giant cell arteritis to polymyalgia rheumatica. Balliere's Clin Rheumatol 5:371–378, 1991

19. RELAPSING POLYCHONDRITIS

In 1923, Jaksch–Wartenhorst (1) described a patient with a systemic illness characterized by external ear swelling, nasal bridge collapse, fever, and arthritis. Biopsy of the nasal septal cartilage revealed an absence of cartilage and a hyperplastic mucosa. He described this as a degenerative disorder and wondered if a toxin in the liquor this brewer made may have been responsible for this entity. Pearson et al (2) first coined the term *relapsing polychondritis*, and described, in detail, the clinical features of several of their own patients along with those in the literature as examples of this recurring malady. Since then this disorder has been described in over 450 patients worldwide, occurring in all age groups, although it peaks in the fifth decade. The five-year survival is approximately 74%. The male:female ratio is equal (3). HLA–DR4 is increased compared to normal controls, although no DR4 subtype was predominant (4).

Relapsing polychondritis is a recurring inflammatory disorder of unknown etiology causing inflammatory reactions in the cartilaginous structures of the nose, ears, trachea, and joints. It is considered an autoimmune disorder. Over 30% of patients have an associated disorder, usually autoimmune or hematologic. These include systemic lupus erythematosus, Sjogren's syndrome, rheumatoid arthritis, systemic vasculitis syndromes, overlap connective tissue disorders, spondylarthropathies, dysmyelopoietic syndromes, Hodgkins disease, diabetes mellitus, and psoriasis vulgaris (5). The pathology shows destructive changes in the fibrocartilagenous junction by mononuclear cells (Fig. 19–1). These cells have been found to be CD4-positive lymphocytes (6). Evidence of local complement activation has been observed (7,8). Elevated levels of anticollagen antibodies and cell mediated immunity to cartilage components also have been described (9). Recently, preferential cellular and humoral immune responses to collagen types IX and XI have been reported (10). Auricular chondritis has been observed to occur spontaneously in a strain of rats as well as following immunization with type II collagen (11–13). These observations are consistent with the current thought that autoimmune mechanisms are involved in this disease.

OTORHINOLARYNGEAL DISEASE

One of the hallmarks of this disease and the presenting feature in 40% of the patients is acute painful swelling and redness of the external ear (Fig. 19–2). This may occur spontaneously or following minor injury. Even though the swelling is unilateral initially, most patients develop it bilaterally. Ultimately, 80% of the patients experience this symptom (Table 19–1). The lobule of the external ear is characteristically spared. Recurrent inflammatory episodes lead to destruction of the external ear cartilage resulting in either a soft, flopped ear or a firm, fibrotic, knobby ear. The nasal bridge may be similarly involved and can cause nasal bridge collapse. The external auditory canal may be stenosed by the inflammatory swelling and cause conductive deafness. About one-third of the patients experience vestibular or auditory abnor-

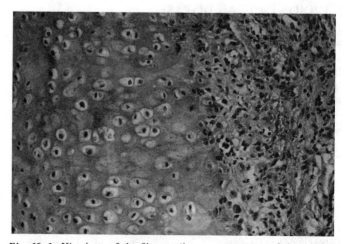

Fig. 19–1. *Histology of the fibrocartilagenous junction of the ear in a patient with relapsing polychondritis. Inflammatory mononuclear cells infiltrate this region with occasional polymorphonuclear leukocytes with damage to the cartilage (H and E stain, magnification × 200, courtesy of Dr LE Wold).*

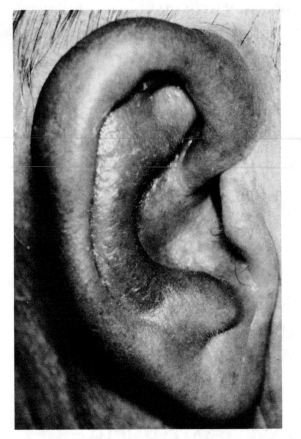

Fig. 19–2. *Acutely inflamed pinna of the ear with sparing of the noncartilageneous lobule.*

malities of varying degrees from vasculitis of the internal auditory artery (14).

RESPIRATORY DISEASE

Hoarseness, coughing, wheezing, and dyspnea are commonly observed. The severity of these depends on the severity of the inflammation of the tracheal cartilages. Tenderness of the thyroid cartilage and trachea can be a clue to this involvement. Narrowing of the trachea, either localized or generalized, leads to inability to clear the throat, choking spells and respiratory infections. These symptoms should be taken seriously because this is a potentially lethal complication. Respiratory symptoms of varying degree may be observed in up to 50% of the patients (14,15).

CARDIOVASCULAR DISEASE

Vasculitis of various types can be observed in about 10% of the patients. Small vessel involvement leading to a leukocytoclastic vasculitis, medium vessel disease of the polyarteritis variety, and large vessel disease of the Takayasu's arteritis variety occur. Signs and symptoms depend on the type of involvement as well as the associated disease. Inflammation of the root of the aorta

Table 19–1. *Clinical manifestations of relapsing polychondritis*

Frequency	Initial (%)	Total (%)
Auricular chondritis	40	85
Nasal cartilage	20	50
Hearing loss	9	30
Arthritis	35	50
Ocular	20	50
Laryngotracheal–bronchial	26	48
Laryngotracheal stricture	15	23
Systemic vasculitis	3	10
Valvular dysfunction	0	6

(Modified from ref. 14)

can cause aortic valve dysfunction including aortic incompetence. Myocarditis may manifest as arrhythmias or even heart block (14).

OCULAR SYMPTOMS

Ocular involvement is variable with both intra- and extraocular disease. Intraocular changes include iridocyclitis and retinal vasculitis; extraocular disease manifests as periorbital edema, extraocular muscle palsy, conjunctivitis, keratitis, scleritis, and episcleritis. Proptosis is observed rarely (14).

MUSCULOSKELETAL AND OTHER FEATURES

A seronegative episodic inflammatory oligo or polyarthritis can be observed in 30% to 75% of patients. This is generally non-erosive and nondeforming, and affects both the small and large joints. Articular cartilage damage can cause symmetric joint space narrowing, and costal cartilage damage may lead to a pectus excavatum deformity (16).

Segmental proliferative glomerulonephritis may be observed in approximately 10% of patients (17). Systemic features including fever, weight loss, and fatigue are commonly seen.

DIAGNOSIS

McAdam et al (18) proposed that the diagnosis of relapsing polychondritis require three or more of the following clinical criteria: 1) bilateral auricular chondritis, 2) nonerosive, seronegative inflammatory polyarthritis, 3) nasal chondritis, 4) ocular inflammation (conjunctivitis, keratitis, scleritis/episcleritis, uveitis), 5) respiratory tract chondritis (laryngeal and/or tracheal cartilages), and 6) cochlear and/or vestibular dysfunction (neurosensory hearing loss, tinnitus, and/or vertigo), and a compatible biopsy. The need for a biopsy has not been necessary in retrospective studies (3), and is often unnecessary in clinical practice since the diagnosis may be obvious in established patients. If, however, the history is recent and the clinical picture unclear or confusing, a biopsy (Fig. 19–1) may be essential to make a diagnosis.

As with other inflammatory diseases, anemia of chronic disease, elevated sedimentation rate, and hypergammaglobulinemia may occur. An abnormal urinalysis generally reflects renal involvement. Respiratory involvement is always a serious complication and may go undiagnosed until complications develop. Thus serious consideration should be given to obtaining pulmonary function tests, as well as inspiratory and expiratory flow volume curves in all patients (15). Radiologic assessment by tomography or computed tomography scan (3,18–21) has been helpful in delineating the inflammatory changes of the trachea and the bronchial tree as well as the presence of stricture(s), localized or diffuse. Other investigations depend on the associated disease.

When faced with a patient with early relapsing polychondritis, other diagnoses must be considered. Chondritis due to streptococcal infection, local fungal infections, syphilis, or leprosy should be kept in mind. Local trauma may cause inflammatory changes that mimic chondritis. Nasal cartilage damage leading to collapse of the bridge can occur from trauma, infections, and granulomatous diseases like Wegener's granulomatosis, as well as neoplastic diseases. Vasculitis of large and small blood vessels from other connective tissue diseases should be considered.

MANAGEMENT

The management of patients with relapsing polychondritis depends on the disease manifestations. If the patients have mild disease with fever, and ear cartilage, nasal cartilage inflammation, or both, with arthalgias, then nonsteroidal antiinflammatory drugs (NSAIDs) may be adequate. If however the symptoms are severe or resistant to NSAID therapy, low to moderate doses of corticosteroids may be necessary. Presence of respiratory symptoms, renal disease, or vasculitis require high dose corticosteroids. As the disease is better controlled the steroid dose can be reduced. Immunosuppressives may be necessary as steroid-sparing agents. Other drugs, such as dapsone and cyclosporine, have been reported to be helpful in small numbers of patients. There are reports of two patients treated with anti–CD4 monoclonal antibody (22, 23). Involvement of the trachea is a serious complication and necessitates aggressive management, including tracheostomy, use of stents if there is tracheal collapse, high dose corticosteroids and immunosuppressives (24). Infection from respiratory compromise and immunosuppressed state, as well as systemic vasculitis, have been increasingly common causes of death. Aortic valve disease can be successfully treated by surgery (25).

Harvinder S. Luthra, MD

1. Jaksch-Wartenhorst R: Polychondropathia. Wien. Arch. F. inn. Med. 6:93–100, 1923
2. Pearson CM, Kline HM, Newcomer VD: Relapsing polychondritis. N Eng J Med 263:51–58, 1960
3. Michet CJ, Jr, McKenna CH, Luthra HS, et al: Relapsing polychondritis: survival and predictive role of early disease manifestations. Ann Int Med 104:74–78, 1986
4. Lang B, Rothenfusser A, Lanchbury JS, et al: Susceptibility to relapsing polychondritis is associated with HLA–DR4. Arthritis Rheum 36:660–664, 1993
5. Luthra HS, Michet CJ Jr: Relapsing polychondritis. In: Rheumatology. Edited by Klippel JH, Dieppe P. London, Mosby, 1994
6. Riccieri V, Spadaro A, Taccari E, et al: A case of relapsing polychondritis: pathogenetic considerations. Clin Exp Rheum 6:95–96, 1988
7. Homma S, Matsumoto T, Abe H, et al: Relapsing polychondritis: pathological and immunological findings in an autopsy case. Acta Pathol Jpn 34:1137–1146, 1984
8. McKenna CH, Luthra HS, Jordan RE: Hypocomplementemic ear effusion in relapsing polychondritis. Mayo Clin Proc 51:495–497, 1976
9. Alsalameh S, Mollenhauer J, Scheuplein F, et al: Preferential cellular and humoral immune reactivities to native and denatured collagen types IX and XI in a patient with fatal relapsing polychondritis. J Rheumatol 20:1419–1424, 1993
10. Herman JH, Dennis MV: Immunopathologic studies in Relapsing Polychondritis. J Clin Invest 52:549–558, 1973
11. Cremer MA, Pitcock JA, Stuart JM, et al: Auricular chondritis in Rats. J Exp Med 154:535–540, 1981
12. McCune WJ, Schiller AL, Dynesius-Trentham RA, et al: Type II collagen-induced auricular chondritis. Arthritis Rheum 25:266–273, 1982
13. Prieur DJ, Young DM, Counts DF: Auricular chondritis in Fawn–Hooded rats: a spontaneous disorder resembling that induced by immunization with type II collagen. Amer J Path 116:69–76, 1984
14. Isaak BL, Liesegang TJ, Michet CJ Jr: Ocular and systemic findings in relapsing polychondritis. Ophthalmology 93:681–689, 1986
15. Krell WS, Staats BA, Hyatt RE: Pulmonary function in relapsing polychondritis. Am Rev Respir Dis 133:1120–1123, 1986
16. O'Hanlon M, McAdam LP, Bluestone R, et al: The arthropathy of relapsing polychondritis. Arthritis Rheum 19:191–194, 1976
17. Chang-Miller A, Okamura M, Torres VE, et al: Renal involvement in relapsing polychondritis. Medicine 66:202–217, 1987
18. McAdam LP, O'Hanlon MA, Bluestone R, et al: Relapsing polychondritis: prospective study of 23 patients and a review of the literature. Medicine 55:193–215, 1976
19. Booth A, Dieppe PA, Goddard PL, et al: The radiological manifestations of relapsing polychondritis. Clin Radiol 40:147–149, 1989
20. Mendelson DS, Som PM, Crane R, et al: Relapsing polychondritis studied by computed tomography. Radiology 157:489–490, 1985
21. Davis SD, Berkmen YM, King T: Peripheral bronchial involvement in relapsing polychondritis: demonstration by thin-section CT. Amer Jour Roentgen 153:953–954, 1989
22. van der Lubbe PA, Miltenburg AM, Breedveld FC: Anti-CD4 monoclonal antibody for relapsing polychondritis. Lancet 337:1349, 1991
23. Choy EH, Chikanza IC, Kingsley GH, et al: Chimaeric anti-CD4 monoclonal antibody for relapsing polychondritis. Lancet 338:450, 1991
24. Eng J, Sabanathan S: Airway complications of relapsing polychondritis. Ann Thorac Surg 51:686–692, 1991
25. Buckley LM, Ades PA: Progressive aortic valve inflammation occuring despite apparent remission of relapsing polychondritis. Arthritis Rheum 35:812–814, 1992

20. SERONEGATIVE SPONDYLARTHROPATHIES
A. Epidemiology, Pathology, and Pathogenesis

The seronegative spondylarthropathies are an interrelated group of multisystem inflammatory disorders. As rheumatic disorders, they affect the spine, peripheral joints, periarticular structures, or all three, and they are variably associated with characteristic extraarticular manifestations. The latter include acute or chronic gastrointestinal or genitourinary inflammation, sometimes due to bacterial infection; anterior ocular inflammation; psoriasiform skin and nail lesions; and, uncommonly, lesions of the aortic root, cardiac conduction system, and pulmonary apices (1,2). Most but not all of these disorders show an increased prevalence among individuals who have inherited the HLA–B27 gene.

Recognized diagnostic entities, terms, or concepts within the spondylarthropathies include ankylosing spondylitis (AS), reactive arthritis, Reiters syndrome, spondylitis and peripheral arthritis associated with psoriasis or inflammatory bowel disease, juvenile onset spondylarthropathy, and a variety of less easily classifiable disorders often termed undifferentiated spondylarthropathies (see Table 20A–1). Sets of diagnostic criteria for the various spondylarthropathies have been proposed during the past three decades, the most recent addition is criteria for the undifferentiated disorders, proposed by the European Spondyloarthropathy Study Group (3). In none of these diseases is the etiology or pathogenesis well understood. Any concept of their pathogenesis must explain, on the one hand, the striking association that most of the disorders share with HLA–B27, and on the other hand, the observation that B27 by itself seems neither universally necessary nor sufficient for the development of any of the individual diseases. The association of the various disorders with B27 is summarized in Table 20A–2.

PATHOLOGY

Sacroiliitis is the pathologic hallmark—and usually one of the earliest pathologic manifestations—of AS. The early lesion consists of subchondral granulation tissue that ultimately erodes the joint, which is then gradually replaced by fibrocartilage regeneration followed by ossification. The initial lesion in the spine consists of inflammatory granulation tissue at the junction of the annulus fibrosus of the intervertebral disc and the margin of vertebral bone. The outer annular fibers may eventually be replaced by bone, forming a syndesmophyte. Progression of this process leads to the *bamboo spine* observed radiographically. Other lesions in the spine include diffuse osteoporosis, erosion of vertebral bodies at the disc margin (Romanus lesion), "squaring" of vertebrae, and inflammation and destruction of the disc–bone border. Inflammatory arthritis of the apophyseal joints is common, with erosion progressing to bony ankylosis. Similar axial pathology can occur in the other spondylarthropathies as well, although with some differences that will be discussed under the individual syndromes.

The pathology of peripheral joint arthritis in AS can show synovial hyperplasia, lymphoid infiltration, and pannus formation, but the process lacks a number of features commonly seen in rheumatoid arthritis, including proliferation of synovial villi, fibrin deposits, and ulceration. Central cartilagenous erosion due to proliferation of subchondral granulation tissue is a common finding in AS. Similar synovial pathology can be seen in the other chronic spondylarthropathies, although Reiters syndrome typically shows many more polymorphonuclear neutrophils in early disease.

Enthesitis, inflammation at sites of tendinous or ligamentous attachment to bone, is another pathologic hallmark of the

Table 20A–1. *Comparison of ankylosing spondylitis and related disorders*

Characteristic	Ankylosing Spondylitis	Reactive Arthritis (Reiter's Syndrome)	Juvenile Spondylarthropathy	Psoriatic Arthropathy*	Enteropathic Arthropathy[†]
Usual age at onset	Young adult age <40	Young to middle age adult	Childhood onset, ages 8 to 18	Young to middle age adult	Young to middle age adult
Sex ratio	3 times more common in males	Predominantly males	Predominantly males	Equally distributed	Equally distributed
Usual type of onset	Gradual	Acute	Variable	Variable	Gradual
Sacroiliitis or spondylitis	Virtually 100%	<50%	<50%	≈20%	<20%
Symmetry of sacroiliitis	Symmetric	Asymmetric	Variable	Asymmetric	Symmetric
Peripheral joint involvement	≈25%	≈90%	≈90%	≈95%	Frequent
Eye involvement[‡]	25–30%	Common	20%	Occasional	Occasional
Cardiac involvement	1–4%	5–10%	Rare	Rare	Rare
Skin or nail involvement	None	Common	Uncommon	Virtually 100%	Uncommon
Role of infectious agents as triggers	Unknown	Yes	Unknown	Unknown	Unknown

* About 5–7% of patients with psoriasis develop arthritis, and psoriatic spondylitis accounts for about 5% of all patients with psoriatic arthritis.
[†] Associated with chronic inflammatory bowel disease.
[‡] Predominantly conjunctivitis in reactive arthritis & acute anterior uveitis in the other disorders listed above. (Adapted from Arnett Jr. FC, Khan MA, Willkens RF: A new look at ankylosing spondylitis. Patient Care, Nov. 30 1989, pp. 82–101.)
(From Ref. #2)

spondylarthropathies. In AS, it is especially common at sites localized around the spine and pelvis, where it may eventually undergo ossification. In the other spondylarthropathies, it is more common at peripheral sites, such as the calcaneal attachment of the Achilles tendon.

THE GENETIC EPIDEMIOLOGY OF HLA–B27

HLA–B27 is a serologically defined allele of the HLA–B locus, one of the three classical HLA loci encoding class I major histocompatibility (MHC) gene products (HLA–A, B, and C), which are 44 kDa molecules expressed on cell surfaces in noncovalent association with β2-microglobulin (β2m). At least seven allelic subtypes of B27 have been identified, designated B*2701 through B*2707 (5). B*2705 is the predominant subtype in most populations in which B27 is prevalent. Recent studies have suggested that B*2703 is the predominant subtype in West Africans (6). The prevalence of B27 in different racial groups is indicated in Table 20A–3.

Among the spondylarthropathies, AS has been the disorder most extensively studied in epidemiologic surveys. The estimated prevalence of AS in North American Caucasians is 0.1% to 0.2%. In large population surveys in Holland and Australia, 1% to 2% of adults inheriting HLA–B27 have been found to have AS. In contrast, in families of patients with AS, 10% to 20% of adult first degree relatives inheriting HLA–B27 have been found to have the disease. The concordance rate of AS in identical twins is estimated to be 60% or less. These epidemiologic findings indicate that both genetic and environmental factors play a role in

the pathogenesis of the disease, and that the genetic factors may include allelic genes in addition to HLA–B27, although to date no additional genes have been identified (7).

For many years it was debated whether HLA–B27 itself is a direct disease susceptibility factor, or alternatively, merely a marker for a disease gene in close linkage disequilibrium with HLA–B27. Currently, B27 itself is generally believed to be involved in disease pathogenesis. This is based on a large body of indirect evidence from clinical epidemiology and on the direct demonstration that transgenic rats expressing HLA–B*2705 spontaneously develop a broad spectrum of disease manifestations closely resembling human B27-associated disease. The propensity of the B27 molecule to induce disease thus presumably derives from one or more unique features of its structure. An analysis of the structure–function relationships of the B27 molecule and a detailed dissection of its unique features should therefore provide insight into its role in the pathogenesis of the spondylarthropathies.

It has not yet been established whether B27-related disease is associated preferentially with one or more of the B27 subtypes. An association with AS has been clearly shown for B*2702, B*2704, B*2705, probably B*2707, and possibly B*2706. B*2701 has been found in too few individuals to be amenable to population studies. As of this writing, no individuals with B*2703 and spondylarthropathy have been reported, and the suggestion has been made that this allele does not predispose to disease. If this suggestion withstands further scrutiny, it may have important implications for the molecular mechanism of the B27-disease association, since B*2703 differs from B*2705 by only one amino acid. B*2703 bears a histidine at position 59, whereas a tyrosine at this position is conserved in virtually all other mammalian MHC class I molecules that have been sequenced. Since substitutions at position 59 would be expected to alter the repertoire of

Table 20A–2. *HLA–B27 associations among the spondylarthropathies*

Disorder	B27 Frequency, %
Ankylosing spondylitis	90
With uveitis or aortitis	nearly 100
Reactive arthritis	
with sacroiliitis or uveitis	60–80
(Including Reiter's syndrome)	
Juvenile spondylarthropathy	80
Inflammatory bowel disease	not increased
With peripheral arthritis	not increased
With spondylitis	50
Psoriasis vulgaris	not increased
With peripheral arthritis	not increased
With spondylitis	50
Normal Caucasians	6–8

(Modified from references 1 and 4.)

Table 20A–3. *Racial distribution of the HLA–B27 subtypes*

Subtype	Racial Group	% of B27 Within Group
B*2701	Caucasians, ?others	rare
B*2702	Caucasians	10–15%
B*2703	Blacks (West Africa)	60–70%
B*2704	Orientals	50–90%
B*2705	Caucasians	85–90%
	Orientals	10–50%
	Blacks (West Africa)	30–40%
B*2706	Orientals	rare
B*2707	Unknown	—

(Modified from reference 4.)

peptides bound to the B27 molecule, the argument could be made that B27 functions in promoting disease by binding and presenting a critical peptide or set of peptides. However, since the alleles at other loci on B*2703-bearing HLA haplotypes most likely differ substantially from those of HLA haplotypes bearing other B27 subtypes, the absence of B*2703-associated disease might possibly be accounted for by other HLA-linked factors.

STRUCTURE AND FUNCTION OF HLA–B27

The x-ray crystallographic three-dimensional structure of three class I HLA molecules including HLA–B27 has been determined (8). The surface-expressed class I molecule consists of a complex of HLA-encoded heavy chain, β2m, and endogenously synthesized nonamer peptide. Under the current model, the complex is assembled during biosynthesis in the endoplasmic reticulum, such that the heavy chain α_1 and α_2 domains are folded to form a cleft in which the peptide is bound. The polymorphic residues along the antigen binding cleft form pockets that accommodate side chains of the bound peptide, and in this way a distinct spectrum of peptides binds each different class I allele. The peptides can be derived from either normal cellular constituents or intracellular infectious agents or tumors. The bound peptides are displayed along with the class I molecule itself on cell surfaces, where they can be recognized as either self or foreign by T lymphocytes.

The consensus B27 sequence shared by the different B27 subtypes (except B*2707, which lacks Asn97) contains a cluster of amino acids within the peptide-binding cleft, including two B27-unique residues Lys70 and Asn97, as well as His9, Thr24, Glu45, Cys67, Ala69, and Ala71 (9). No other known class I HLA sequence shares more than three of these residues with B27. These residues either form, or lie contiguous to, the so-called "B" or "45" pocket, which is formed by residues 9, 24, 45, and 67. This pocket constitutes a most distinctive feature of B27 structure (8). Strikingly, all peptides that have been shown to bind to B27 bear an arginine residue at position 2, and radiographic crystallography of B27 has shown that the side chain of this arginine residue fits snugly into the "45" pocket, forming hydrogen bonds with the surrounding B27 side chains (8,10). Whether B27-associated disease derives from a particular peptide or family of peptides binding to B27 is not yet known, but such a scenario seems probable.

MICROBES AND REACTIVE ARTHRITIS

Reactive arthritis has traditionally been considered a sterile inflammatory response to an infection remote from the site of inflammation. This concept was based on the failure of numerous investigators to culture the inciting organisms from inflamed joints. Recent studies have indicated that although viable organisms have not been convincingly demonstrated in the inflamed joints by cultures, bacteria-like structures, antigens and RNA derived from these organisms can indeed be detected, largely within intrasynovial cells, by immunofluorescence, electron microscopy and molecular hybridization (11). This phenomenon has been demonstrated for *Chlamydia trachomatis*, *Yersinia enterocolitica*, and *Salmonella typhimurium*. In the case of Yersinia, antigen could be detected within synovial cells even a decade or more after the acute attack. Thus, persistence of microbial antigens is likely to play an important role in the pathogenesis of the acute and chronic inflammation characteristic of reactive arthritis. How these antigens reach the joints, and possibly other sites of inflammation such as periarticular structures and the anterior ocular chamber, is not known.

Two other pieces of evidence suggest unusual persistence of the trigger agents themselves in patients with reactive arthritis. Individuals with reactive arthritis triggered by *Yersinia*, *Salmonella*, or *Chlamydia* infections show serum IgA responses against the triggering organisms that are much more persistent than do individuals with uncomplicated infections with these agents (12). Persistently elevated serum IgA levels are also characteristic of AS, although in this case there is no known triggering agent. Furthermore, recent therapeutic studies have suggested that pro-

Table 20A–4. *Evidence linking B27-associated disease with gastrointestinal inflammation*

Triggering of reactive arthritis by GI pathogens
Increased prevalence of AS in patients with inflammatory bowel disease
Increased prevalence of inflammatory bowel disease in family members of patients with AS
Acute GI inflammation occurring in the setting of venereally acquired reactive arthritis
Persistent elevation of IgA levels in AS and reactive arthritis
Presence of microscopic bowel inflammation in the majority of patients with B27-associated spondylarthropathies, even in the absence of arthropathy
Antigenic cross-reactivity between the HLA-B27 molecule and components of enteric bacteria
Triggering of inflammatory arthritis in rats by injection of peptidoglycan from normal bowel flora
High prevalence of early GI inflammation in transgenic rats expressing HLA-B27

longed therapy with long-acting tetracycline agents can ameliorate the course of *Chlamydia*-induced reactive arthritis, whereas conventional two-week courses have traditionally been considered ineffective (13).

How microbial antigens and antigenic stimulation can persist remains unclear. Whether expression of HLA–B27 contributes to the unusual microbial persistence, perhaps by modulation of a host response, or whether B27 participates in the inflammatory response, perhaps by presenting microbial antigens or infection-induced self antigens such as heat shock proteins to disease-inducing T lymphocytes, is not yet known. Several groups have derived T cell lines from the synovial fluid of patients with reactive arthritis that proliferate apparently specifically to preparations of organisms thought to have incited the arthritis, and in some cases to heat shock proteins (14). However, these T cells have generally been CD4+CD8−, and it has not been demonstrated that the B27 molecule is involved in restricting their specificity. Better understanding of these phenomena will help explain the pathogenesis of reactive arthritis and perhaps other B27-associated disease processes as well.

SPONDYLARTHROPATHIES AND THE INTESTINE

A large body of evidence, summarized in Table 20A–4, suggests an intimate association between the pathogenesis of the B27-associated diseases and intestinal bacteria or intestinal inflammation. Many important questions will need to be answered before the basis for this connection can be understood. Perhaps most fundamental is the question of whether some bowel-related process is a necessary precursor to the development of some or all of the spondylarthropathies. Furthermore, it is not yet known whether the usually mild and often asymptomatic inflammation seen in patients with B27-associated arthropathy (15) represents one end of the spectrum of Crohn's disease or ulcerative colitis, or whether it represents an altogether different process. Progress in understanding this link will undoubtedly help unravel the mystery of the pathogenesis of the spondylarthropathies.

HLA–B27 AND MOLECULAR MIMICRY

A few years after the association of B27 with the spondylarthropathies was established, it was hypothesized that the association might be explained by antigenic mimicry (molecular mimicry) between the B27 molecule and a triggering microorganism, most likely a gram-negative bacillus. Although it has never been explained how mimicry of a class I MHC molecule would lead to the anatomically localized disease seen in the spondylarthropathies, several investigators have sought and obtained evidence for the sharing of antigenic determinants between HLA–B27 and different bacterial products. Some early reports of mimicry and B27 were questionable, but in recent years it has been more convincingly demonstrated that some antibodies to bacteria known to trigger reactive arthritis can crossreact with B27, and vice-versa (16). In addition, amino acid homology between the polymorphic region of the B27 α1 domain and certain bacterial products has been documented. However, there is still little clinical or experimental evidence supporting the hypothesis that molecular mimicry plays a role in the pathogenesis of B27-associated disease, and the significance of these findings remains unclear.

TRANSGENIC ANIMALS EXPRESSING HLA–B27

Because HLA–B27 is a human gene, it has not been possible until recently to investigate its function in the context of an experimental animal model. The advance of transgenic technology in the mid-1980s made it possible to produce animals expressing HLA–B27, and mice transgenic for HLA–B27 were promptly bred by a number of laboratories. Disappointingly, attempts to reproduce the phenomena associated with reactive arthritis or AS in humans were unsuccessful in these mice. However, a different story emerged when the B27 gene was introduced into rats (17). Rats of the inbred Lewis and Fischer 344 strains expressing high levels of B27 and human β2m show striking spontaneous inflammatory abnormalities. These include peripheral and axial arthritis, gastrointestinal inflammation and diarrhea, psoriatic-like skin changes, and male genital and cardiac inflammation. Histologically, the joint, gut, skin, and heart lesions closely resemble the lesions seen in B27-associated disease in humans. These findings provide direct evidence for the participation of the HLA–B27 molecule in disease pathogenesis. The spontaneously occurring disease in these transgenic rats should prove useful in elucidating the pathogenetic role of HLA–B27, because it permits detailed cellular and molecular analysis and manipulation of the developing lesions in the various involved tissues.

The earliest and most consistent finding in the B27 transgenic rats is gastrointestinal inflammation, especially in the colon. Histologically, the intestinal lesions show a predominantly mononuclear cell infiltrate in the lamina propria. The lesions resemble those found in ileocolonoscopically obtained biopsies from patients with AS and reactive arthritis. These findings reinforce the significance of observations in humans that gastrointestinal and B27-associated articular inflammation are intimately related. Whether a B27-related process in the bowel proves to be a pathogenetic *sine qua non* for the spondylarthropathies, either in humans or in transgenic rats, remains to be determined.

SUMMARY

A large collection of observations has accumulated regarding the pathogenesis of the spondylarthropathies, and an experimentally validated model that integrates the available data seems attainable within the foreseeable future. The bacteria most strongly implicated in triggering reactive arthritis all have at least some capacity for surviving intracellularly. Inasmuch as MHC class I molecules are known to function by presenting intracellularly derived peptides, and B27 is known to bind a distinctive set of peptides, a model that includes the binding of one or more "pathogenic peptides" to B27 seems most attractive. However, MHC class I molecules with bound peptides can function either

in initiating immune responses or in selecting the T cell repertoire during T cell development in the thymus. It is not a foregone conclusion that susceptibility to disease brought about by peptide binding to B27 would necessarily involve an active immune response to the B27-peptide complex; deletion of a critical part of the T cell receptor repertoire might be involved. The documented persistence of microbial antigens in reactive arthritis synovium might argue for either a critical B27-restricted response or the absence of a critical response. As of this writing, B27-restricted CD8$^+$ T cells have not been directly implicated in B27 associated disease. Other mechanisms, such as presentation by class II MHC molecules of a B27-derived peptide, must still be considered.

Finally, perhaps the greatest enigma of the spondylarthropathies is their pathologic diversity. Any complete answer to the role of B27 must explain how the same molecule can predispose to the acute, microbially triggered asymmetric peripheral arthritis and extraarticular phenomena of reactive arthritis on the one hand, and to the insidious, progressive axial phenomena of AS on the other. It also must explain how virtually the same clinical manifestations can occur in the absence of B27. To investigators in this area, these questions loom as the challenge for the future.

Joel D. Taurog, MD

1. Calin A, ed. Spondylarthropathies. 1984, Grune & Stratton: Orlando FL.
2. Khan MA, ed. Ankylosing spondylitis and related spondyloarthropathies. Spine: State of the Art Reviews, 1990, Hanley & Belfus, Inc.: Philadelphia.
3. Dougados M, van der Linden S, Juhlin R, et al: The European Spondylarthropathy Study Group preliminary criteria for the classification of spondylarthropathy. Arthritis Rheum 34:1218–1227, 1991
4. Taurog JD, Lipsky PE: New approaches to the molecular analysis of the spondyloarthropathies. Concepts Immunopathol 8:222–237, 1992
5. Choo SY, Fan L-A, Hansen JA: A novel HLA–B27 allele maps B27 allospecificity to the region around position 70 in the α1 domain. J Immunol 147:174–180, 1991
6. Hill AV, Allsopp CE, Kwiatkowski D, et al: HLA class I typing by PCR: HLA–B27 and an African B27 subtype. Lancet 337:640–2, 1991
7. HLA–B27+ Spondyloarthropathies. Edited by Lipsky PE, Taurog JD. New York, Elsevier, 1991.
8. Madden DR, Gorga JC, Strominger JL, et al: The three-dimensional structure of HLA–B27 at 2.1 Å resolution suggests a general mechanism for tight peptide binding to MHC. Cell 70:1035–1048, 1992
9. Benjamin R, Parham P: Guilt by association: HLA–B27 and ankylosing spondylitis. Immunol Today 11:137–142, 1990
10. Jardetzky TS, Lane WS, Robinson RA, et al: Identification of self peptides bound to purified HLA–B27. Nature 353:326–329, 1991
11. Granfors K, Jalkanen S, von Essen R, et al: Yersinia antigens in synovial-fluid cells from patients with reactive arthritis. N Engl J Med 320:216–221, 1989
12. Reactive Arthritis. Edited by Toivanen A, Toivanen P. Boca Raton, FL, CRC Press, Inc., 1988
13. Lauhio A, Leirisalo-Repo M, Lähdevirta J, et al: Double-blind, placebo-controlled study of three-month treatment with lymecycline in reactive arthritis, with special reference to Chlamydia arthritis. Arthritis Rheum 34:6–14, 1991
14. Hermann E, Lohse AW, Van der Zee R, et al: Synovial fluid-derived Yersinia-reactive T cells responding to human 65-kDa heat-shock protein and heat-stressed antigen-presenting cells. Eur J Immunol 21:2139–2143, 1991
15. Mielants H, Veys EM, Goemaere S, et al: Gut inflammation in the spondyloarthropathies: clinical, radiologic, biologic and genetic features in relation to the type of histology. A prospective study. J Rheumatol 18:1542–1551, 1991
16. Williams KM, Raybourne RB: Demonstration of cross-reactivity between bacterial antigens and class I human leukocyte antigens by using monoclonal antibodies to Shigella flexneri. Infect Immun 58:1774–1781, 1990
17. Hammer RE, Maika SD, Richardson JA, et al: Spontaneous inflammatory disease in transgenic rats expressing HLA–B27 and human β2-m: an animal model of HLA–B27-associated human disorders. Cell 63:1099–1112, 1990

B. Ankylosing Spondylitis

Ankylosing spondylitis (AS) is a chronic systemic inflammatory rheumatic disorder that primarily affects the axial skeleton, with sacroiliac joint involvement (sacroiliitis) as its hallmark (1–4). Involvement of the limb joints other than hips and shoulders is uncommon. The name is derived from the Greek roots *ankylos* meaning "bent" (although now it has come to imply fusion or adhesions) and *spondylos* meaning spinal vertebra. The disease is strongly associated with HLA–

B27 and may show familial aggregation. The inflammatory process involves the synovial and cartilagenous joints, as well as the osseous attachments of tendons and ligaments, frequently resulting in fibrous and bony ankylosis. The disease may occur in association with reactive arthritis, (Reiter's syndrome), psoriasis, or chronic inflammatory bowel disease (secondary AS), but most patients have no evidence of these associated diseases.

Table 20B–1. *Clinical features of ankylosing spondylitis*

Skeletal	Extraskeletal
Axial arthritis, such as sacroiliitis and spondylitis	Eyes (acute iritis)
Arthritis of hip and shoulder joints	Heart and ascending aorta
Peripheral arthritis	Lung (apical fibrosis)
Others: enthesopathy, osteoporosis, spinal fracture, spondylodiscitis, pseudoarthrosis	Cauda equina syndrome
	Amyloidosis

CLINICAL MANIFESTATIONS

Clinical manifestations of the disease usually begin in late adolescence or early adulthood. Onset after age 40 is very uncommon. The disease has both skeletal and extraskeletal manifestations (Table 20B–1) and is three times more common in men than women. The clinical as well as the roentgenographic features seem to evolve more slowly in women. The diagnosis is based on clinical features. Often the best clues are offered by the patient's symptoms, family history, articular and extraarticular physical findings, and roentgenographic evidence of bilateral sacroiliitis. The first internationally accepted diagnostic criteria were proposed in Rome in 1961. They were revised five years later in New York to require roentgenographic evidence of sacroiliitis for the diagnosis. Further revision of these criteria have recently been proposed in light of the better understanding of the disease spectrum (5,6).

Skeletal Manifestations

The most common and characteristic early complaint is chronic low back pain of insidious onset, usually beginning in late adolescence or early adulthood. The pain is dull in character, difficult to localize, and felt deep in the gluteal or sacroiliac region (2,4). It may be unilateral or intermittent at first. However, within a few months it generally becomes persistent and bilateral, and the lower lumbar area becomes stiff and painful. Pain in the lumbar area, rather than the more typical buttock-ache, may be the initial symptom in some patients. The pain can be quite severe, and may be accentuated on maneuvers that cause a sudden twist of the back.

The second common early symptom is back stiffness, which is worse in the morning, and is eased by mild physical activity or a hot shower. Prolonged periods of inactivity worsen back pain and stiffness. The patient often experiences considerable difficulty in getting out of bed in the morning and may have to roll out sideways, trying not to flex or rotate the spine in order to minimize pain. At times the pain may awaken the patient from sleep. Some patients have difficulty sleeping well or find it necessary to wake up at night to move about or exercise for a few minutes before returning to bed (1,4).

Back symptoms may be absent or very mild in an occasional patient, while some may complain only of back stiffness, fleeting muscle aches, or musculotendinous tender spots. These symptoms may worsen on exposure to cold or dampness, and such patients may occasionally be misdiagnosed as having fibrositis.

Extraarticular or juxtaarticular bony tenderness may be an early feature of the disease, and can be a major or presenting complaint in some patients. It is due to enthesitis (inflammatory lesions of entheses) that results in tenderness of costosternal junctions, spinous processes, scapulae, iliac crests, greater trochanters, ischial tuberosities, tibial tubercles, or heels. Involvement of the thoracic spine, including the costovertebral and the costotransverse joints, and occurrence of enthesitis at costosternal areas and manubriosternal joints may cause chest pain that may be accentuated on coughing or sneezing. Some patients complain of inability to expand the chest fully on inspiration. Stiffness and pain in the cervical spine and tenderness of the spinous processes occur in early stages of the disease in some patients, but generally this tends to occur after some years.

Sometimes the first symptoms result from involvement of hips and shoulders. Accurate assessment of range of motion of these joints is important, because they are involved at some stage of the disease in one-third of the patients (1–4). Hip joint involvement as the presenting manifestation is relatively more common when the disease begins in childhood or adolescence (7). The reported frequency of hip joint involvement varies from 17% to 36%. It is usually bilateral, insidious in onset, and potentially more crippling than involvement of any other joint. Some degree of flexion contractures at the hip joints is not uncommon at later stages of the disease, giving rise to a characteristic, rigid gait with some flexion at the knees to maintain erect posture. Involvement of peripheral joints, other than hips and shoulders, is infrequent in primary AS. This involvement is rarely persistent or erosive, and tends to resolve without any residual joint deformity. For example, intermittent knee effusions may occasionally be the presenting manifestation of juvenile onset AS (7). Involvement of the temporomandibular joint with resultant pain and local tenderness may occur in about 10% of patients.

Mild constitutional symptoms such as anorexia, malaise, or mild fever may occur in some patients in early stages of their disease, and may be observed relatively more often among patients with juvenile onset (7).

A thorough physical examination, particularly of the axial skeleton, is critical in making an early diagnosis. Physical signs may be quite minimal in the early stages of the disease. However, there is often some limitation of motion of the lumbar spine, most easily recognized on hyperextension, lateral flexion, or rotation. Often there is associated spasm and soreness of the paraspinal muscles. The ability of a patient to touch the floor with fingertips, keeping the knees fully extended, should not be solely relied on for evaluation of spinal mobility, since a good range of motion of the hip joints can compensate for considerable loss of mobility of lumbar spine. The *Wright-Schöber test* is quite useful in detecting limitation of forward flexion of the lumbar spine. A gradual loss of the normal lumbar lordosis develops with progression of the disease.

Direct pressure over the inflamed sacroiliac joints frequently causes pain, but sometimes the sacroiliac pain may be elicited by pressure over both anterior iliac crests with the patient lying supine; maximal flexion of one hip and hyperextension of the other; maximal flexion, abduction, and external rotation of the hip joints; compression of the pelvis with the patient lying on the side; or direct pressure over the sacrum with the patient lying prone. These signs may be negative in some AS patients because the sacroiliac joints are surrounded by strong ligaments that may allow only minimal motion, or in late stages of the disease when inflammation is replaced by fibrosis and bony ankylosis.

Involvement of costovertebral and costotransverse joints results in restriction of chest expansion and breathing that becomes primarily diaphragmatic. The ventilatory lung function, however, is seldom markedly impaired. The entire spine becomes increasingly stiff after many years of disease progression, with continued flattening of lumbar spine and gentle thoracic kyphosis. Involvement of the cervical spine results in progressive limitation of neck motion and a forward cervical stoop that can be assessed by measuring the distance from occiput to wall with the patient standing with back against the wall. The chest becomes flattened, the breathing becomes primarily diaphragmatic, and the abdomen becomes protuberant. The diagnosis is readily apparent at this advanced stage because of the characteristic gait and posture and the way the patient sits or rises from the examining table.

Back pain and stiffness generally diminish over the years but some degree of inflammatory pain usually persists. Spinal ankylosis develops at a variable rate and pattern. Sometimes the disease remains confined to one part of the spine. Typical deformities tend to evolve after 10 or more years. In extreme cases, the entire spine may be fused in a flexed position, limiting the field of vision and making it difficult for some patients to look ahead as they walk.

Extraskeletal Manifestations

The most common extraskeletal involvement is acute anterior uveitis (acute iritis), which occurs in 25% to 30% of patients at some time in the course of their disease (8). The inflammation is typically unilateral and has an acute onset. Symptoms include pain, increased lacrimation, photophobia, and blurred vision. On examination there is circumcorneal congestion, and the iris is edematous and appears discolored compared to the contralateral side. The pupil is small but may become irregular, especially on pupillary dilatation, if posterior synechiae (adhesions) are formed. Slit-lamp examination of the eye shows copious exudate in the anterior chamber and small keratitic precipitates. An individual episode of uveitis usually subsides in four to eight weeks, but may recur in the same or the contralateral eye. Although many diseases are associated with uveitis, the possibility of AS or related spondylarthropathies should always be considered when a patient presents with acute nongranulomatous anterior uveitis.

Cardiovascular involvement is rare and includes ascending aortitis, aortic valve incompetence, and conduction abnormalities (9). Risk increases with age, duration of AS, and the presence of arthritis of peripheral joints (other than the hips and shoulders). The aortitis can range from chronic hemodynamically unimportant fibrosis to a relatively acute aortic and even mitral insufficiency with rapid deterioration of cardiac function. Aortic incompetence has been observed in 3.5% of patients who have had AS for 15 years and in 10% after 30 years (10). Cardiac conduction disturbances have occurred in 2.7% of those with disease of 15 years' duration and in 8.5% after 30 years. Complete heart block causing Stokes–Adam's attacks may supervene in some patients, necessitating implantation of cardiac pacemakers (9).

Lung parenchymal involvement is a rare and late extraskeletal manifestation and is characterized by a slowly progressive fibrosis of the upper lobes of the lungs that appears, on average, two decades after onset of the AS (11). It is usually bilateral and appears as linear or patchy opacities on chest radiograph, eventually becoming cystic. These cavities may subsequently be colonized by aspergillus with the formation of mycetoma. The patient may complain of cough, increasing dyspnea, and occasionally hemoptysis.

Neurologic involvement may occur, most often related to spinal fracture/dislocation, atlantoaxial subluxations, or cauda equina syndrome (1–3,12,13). The fracture usually occurs in the cervical spine; the resultant quadriplegia is the most dreaded complication, with a high mortality. Spontaneous anterior atlantoaxial subluxation is a well-recognized complication of AS. It occurs in about 2% of the patients and presents as occipital pain with or without signs of spinal cord compression. It is generally observed in the later stages of the disease, more commonly in those with peripheral joint involvement (12). Slowly progressive cauda equina syndrome is a rare but significant and under-diagnosed complication of longstanding AS, manifested clinically by a gradual onset of urinary and fecal incontinence, pain, and sensory loss in the sacral distribution, ("saddle anesthesia") impotence, and occasionally loss of ankle jerks (13).

There is a lack of convincing evidence for involvement of skeletal muscles. The marked muscle wasting seen in some patients with advanced disease results from disuse atrophy, although some ultrastructural changes and raised levels of serum creatine phosphokinase have been observed in patients (1,2). Amyloidosis (secondary) is a rare complication, especially in the United States (14); presence of proteinuria and progressive azotemia should raise the possibility of amyloidosis with renal involvement. IgA nephropathy can cause hematuria.

LABORATORY FINDINGS

There are no diagnostic or pathognomonic tests. An elevated erythrocyte sedimentation rate is seen in up to 75% of patients, and mild to moderate elevation of serum IgA concentration is also frequently observed (1,2,4). There is no association with rheumatoid factor and antinuclear antibodies, and the synovial fluid does not show distinctive features as compared to other inflammatory arthropathies. A mild normocytic normochromic anemia may be present in 15% of patients.

Biopsies of spinal lesions are virtually never done for diagnosis but peripheral joints may be aspirated or biopsied as part of diagnostic investigation in puzzling cases. Synovial tissue may show even more dramatic plasma cell infiltration than is seen in rheumatoid arthritis, but this and the mildly inflammatory joint fluid are nonspecific (15).

HLA–B27 typing can occasionally be used as an aid to the diagnosis of AS, but an overwhelming majority of patients can be diagnosed clinically on the basis of history, physical examination, and roentgenographic findings (16). It is not a routine, diagnostic, confirmatory, or screening test for AS in patients with back pain, even though the test in some ethnic and racial groups is highly sensitive for AS (90% sensitivity among caucasians). The clinical usefulness of a test depends on the setting in which it is performed (see Chapter 8B).

RADIOLOGIC FINDINGS

The characteristic radiographic changes of AS evolve over many years, and are primarily seen in the axial skeleton, especially in the sacroiliac, discovertebral, apophyseal, costovertebral, and costotransverse joints (1–4). Sacroiliitis is the earliest and most consistent finding. A simple anteroposterior roentgenogram is usually sufficient for its detection. The changes are bilateral and symmetric, and consist of blurring of the subchondral bone plate, followed by erosions resembling postage stamp serrations, and sclerosis of the adjacent bone (Fig. 20B–1). These changes are sometimes better visualized on Ferguson's view. They are first noted and are more prominent on the iliac side of the joint. Progression of the subchondral bone erosions can lead to "pseudo-widening" of the sacroiliac joint space, followed later by gradual narrowing due to interosseous bridging and ossification. After many years there may be complete bony ankylosis of the sacroiliac joints and resolution of the juxtaarticular bony sclerosis.

The inflammatory lesions in the vertebral column affect the superficial layers of the annulus fibrosus, at their attachment to the corners of vertebral bodies, resulting in reactive bone sclerosis, seen roentgenographically as highlighting of the corners, and subsequent bone resorption (erosions). This leads to "squaring" of the vertebral bodies and gradual ossification of the superficial layers of the annulus fibrosus, which form intervertebral bony "bridging" called *syndesmophytes* that often begin in the thoraco-lumbar and upper lumbar area (Fig. 20B–2). There are often concomitant inflammatory changes resulting in ankylosis of

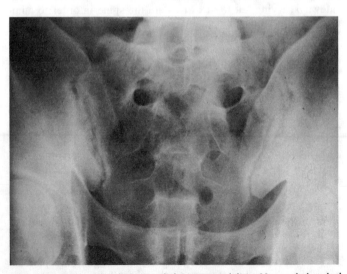

Fig. 20B–1. Early sacroiliitis in ankylosing spondylitis. Note subchondral bone resorption and irregularity of sacroiliac joint spaces. Increased sclerosis is present around the sacroiliac joints (from the Revised Clinical Slide Collection on the Rheumatic Diseases).

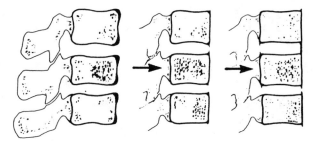

Fig. 20B–2. Schematic representation of the lateral view of lumbar spine showing progressive squaring and fusion of vertebral bodies anteriorly (syndesmophytes), and gradual fusion of the apophyseal joints posteriorly.

the apophyseal joints and ossification of the spinal ligaments, ultimately resulting in a virtually complete fusion of the vertebral column (bamboo spine) in patients with severe AS of long duration (1,3). Spinal osteoporosis is also frequently observed as a result of ankylosis and lack of spinal mobility. Bony erosions and osteitis ("whiskering") at sites of osseous attachments of tendons and ligaments are frequently seen, particularly at the ischial tuberosities, iliac crest, calcaneum, femoral trochanters, and spinous processes of the vertebrae.

Hip joint involvement leads to symmetric concentric joint space narrowing, irregularity of the subchondral bone plate with subchondral sclerosis, and osteophyte formation at the outer margin of the articular surface, including the acetabulum and the femoral head. It may result in bony ankylosis. Shoulder joint involvement causes concentric joint space narrowing, with erosions primarily at the superolateral aspect of the humeral head.

In patients with early disease in whom standard roentgenography of the sacroiliac joints may show normal or equivocal changes, computed tomography appears to be more sensitive but equally specific. However, it is rarely needed. Magnetic resonance imaging can produce excellent but costly imaging without ionizing radiation, and is especially useful in visualizing posterior lumbosacral arachnoid diverticuli associated with cauda equina syndrome (17,18). Quantitative radioactive scintigraphy may be too nonspecific to be useful in detecting early sacroiliitis (4).

DIFFERENTIAL DIAGNOSIS

The absence of a known etiology of AS provides a hurdle to its early disgnosis (2,4). The patient's clinical history and the clinical and roentgenographic findings are of obvious importance. Low back pain and stiffness are the most common presenting symptoms, although a variety of other presentations may antedate back symptoms. However, low back pain is an extremely common symptom in the general population, and is mostly due to mechanical, not inflammatory, causes. This pain is generally aggravated by activity and relieved by rest. There is no limitation of chest expansion or of lateral flexion of the lumbar spine, the erythrocyte sedimentation rate is frequently normal, and pelvic radiograph reveals absence of sacroiliitis.

Ankylosing hyperostosis (also called Forestier's disease or diffuse idiopathic skeletal hyperostosis) is a condition usually first seen at an older age, and characterized by thick, layered hyperostosis affecting the anterior longitudinal ligament and bony attachments of tendons and ligaments. It might be roentgenographically confused with advanced AS. Malignancies should always be considered in the differential diagnosis of back pain, both in young and old patients. Other causes of back pain include pelvic inflammatory diseases, septic discitis, septic sacroiliitis, Paget's disease, Scheuermann's disease, osteofluorosis, tuberculous spondylitis, chronic brucellosis, calcium pyrophosphate dihydrate deposition disease, ochronosis, axial osteomalacia, congenital kyphoscoliosis and hypoparathyroidism. Primary and secondary hyperparathyroidism can lead to irregularity of the sacroiliac joint surfaces, particularly on the iliac side, as a result of subchondral resorption and adjacent bony sclerosis. Narrowing and ankylosis of the joint space, however, do not occur. Sacroiliac joint changes resembling sacroiliitis, and even com-

plete fusion of these joints, can be observed in paraplegics and quadriplegics. Osteitis condensans ilii is most common in young women and produces bone sclerosis limited to the iliac side of the joint. Comparison of AS and related spondylarthropathies was summarized in Chapter 20A.

DISEASE COURSE

The course of AS is highly variable and characterized by spontaneous remissions and exacerbations, but it is generally favorable. Earlier studies suggesting a generally unremitting course primarily involved patients with severe disease studied in hospitals (10,19). In the last decade, a number of B27-positive individuals, not previously recognized as having AS, manifested clinical features that are often relatively mild or self-limited. As a result, our understanding of what ought to be encompassed in the diagnostic entity is undergoing evolution (5,6), and is reflected in the recently proposed criteria for spondylarthropathies (20).

Good functional capacity and the ability to work are maintained in most patients, even in cases of protracted disease (1,5,21). Although it is difficult to predict the prognosis for an individual patient, those with hip involvement or completely ankylosed cervical spine with kyphosis are more likely to be disabled. Fortunately, the results of total hip arthroplasty in recent years are very gratifying in preventing partial or total disability. Some studies have suggested a slightly reduced life expectancy of patients with AS, but because of the selection bias for severe disease inherent in those studies, patients with relatively milder disease will likely have normal life expectancy (1,2,4,5,10).

MANAGEMENT

There is currently no preventive measure or cure for AS, but most patients can be well managed (Table 20B–2). A concerned physician providing continuity of care can be most valuable. Patient education is crucial for successful management. The patient should thoroughly understand that although pain and stiffness can often be controlled by appropriate use of nonsteroidal antiinflammatory drugs (NSAIDs), regular therapeutic exercise to minimize and prevent deformity and disability is the single most important measure in medical management. The patient should walk erect, do back extension exercises regularly, and sleep on a firm mattress, without a pillow if possible. It is better to sleep on the back or in a prone position with an extended and stretched back, and avoid sleeping curled up on one side. The patient should stop or avoid cigarette smoking and do regular deep breathing exercises to preserve normal chest expansion. Swimming is the best overall form of exercise for patients with AS, and use of snorkel and face-mask can permit even those with considerable cervical flexion deformity to do freestyle swimming.

Aspirin seldom provides an adequate therapeutic response.

Phenylbutazone is probably the most effective NSAID for AS patients and offers good symptomatic relief. However, because of its potentially greater risk of bone marrow toxicity, other NSAIDs such as indomethacin, naproxen, diclofenac, or sulindac should be tried first. Other NSAIDs may be equally effective in AS, but they are not currently approved by the US Food and Drug Administration (FDA) for such clinical use.

Sulfasalazine may be effective for peripheral arthritis in some AS patients, and because of its efficacy in inflammatory bowel disease as well, it appears to be especially useful in enteropathic AS, with peripheral arthritis, or for those intolerant to NSAIDs (1). Oral corticosteroids have no therapeutic value in the long-term management of the musculoskeletal aspects of AS because of their potential for serious side effects, and they do not halt the progression of the disease. Recalcitrant enthesopathy and persistent synovitis may respond quite well to a local corticosteroid injection.

Acute anterior uveitis can be very well managed with dilatation of the pupil and use of corticosteroid eye drops (8). Systemic steroids or immunosuppressives may be needed for refractory iritis. Cardiac complications may require aortic valve replacement or pacemaker implantation (9). Apical pulmonary fibrosis is not easy to manage; surgical resection may rarely be required (11).

Radiotherapy has little role in the modern management of patients with AS because of the high risk of leukemia and aplastic anemia although the possibility is still raised in the most difficult cases. Splints, braces and corsets are generally not helpful in the management of AS.

Cervical spine involvement may lead to marked impairment of neck motion in all directions, but the atlanto-occipital and atlanto-axial joints do not usually become completely ankylosed, thus allowing some degree of rotatory or nodding movements of the head (1–3). Many patients have difficulty driving however, because of the impaired neck mobility. Special wide-view mirrors can be very helpful for such patients. Similarly, special prism glasses can help improve vision for those patients who are so kyphotic that they cannot look ahead while walking. There are many AS patient support groups in various countries that provide useful pamphlets and information about the disease and its management, as well as advice about life and health insurance, jobs, working environment, wide-view mirrors, and other useful items (1).

In extreme cases where the disease has progressed to a severe stage, surgery is helpful. Total hip replacement yields very good results and prevents partial or total disability from severe hip disease. Vertebral wedge osteotomy may be needed for correction of severe kyphosis in some patients, although it carries a relatively high risk of paraplegia.

The ankylosed osteoporotic spine in AS is unduly susceptible to fracture even after a relatively minor trauma, including events that may not be remembered or recalled by the patient. The fracture line is usually transverse, and the cervical spine is the most common site, usually at C5–C6 or C6–C7 level. The fracture may not be readily visible on roentgenography, and a bone scan or magnetic resonance imaging can be helpful in its detection. The possibility of spinal fracture should be excluded in any patient with advanced AS who complains of neck or back pain after even a mild trauma. The fracture may result in spondylodiscitis (or discovertebral destruction) and pseudoarthrosis.

The reported incidence of spondylodiscitis in AS is 5% to 6%, and the site of lesion is most commonly at T11–L1. Spondylodiscitis, however, can occur spontaneously in many AS patients in the absence of any trauma. It is asymptomatic in about one-half of the patients and usually pursues a benign clinical course. Some patients may require a degree of bed rest and localized immobilization rather than exercise so as to allow fibrous and bony ankylosis to occur. This is probably one of the few indications where some simple form of brace may be needed.

Muhammad Asim Khan, MD

1. Khan MA (ed): Ankylosing spondylitis and related spondyloarthropathies. Spine: State of the Art Reviews. Philadelphia, Hanley & Belfus, Inc., 1990, pp 497–688
2. Khan MA: Ankylosing spondylitis. In: Rheumatology, 1st ed., Edited by Klippel JH, Dieppe P. London, Mosby, 1994
3. Resnick D, Niwayama G: Ankylosing spondylitis. In: Diagnosis of Bone and Joint Disorders. Edited by Resnick D, Niwayama G. Philadelphia, W. B. Saunders, 1981, pp 1040–1102
4. Khan MA, Kushner I: Diagnosis of ankylosing spondylitis. In: Progress in Clinical Rheumatology, vol. 1. Edited by Cohen AS. Orlando, Grune and Stratton, 1984, pp 145–178
5. Khan MA, van der Linden SM: Ankylosing spondylitis and associated diseases. Rheum Dis Clin N Am 16:551–579, 1990
6. Zeidler H, Mau W, Khan MA: Undifferentiated spondyloarthropathies. Rheum Dis Clin N Am 18:187–202, 1992
7. Burgos-Vargas R, Petty RE: Juvenile ankylosing spondylitis. Rheum Dis Clin N Am 18:123–142, 1992
8. Rosenbaum JT: Acute anterior uveitis and spondyloarthropathies. Rheum Dis Clin N Am 18:143–152, 1992
9. Bergfeldt L, Edhag O, Vedin L, et al: Ankylosing spondylitis: an important cause of severe disturbances of the cardiac conduction system. Prevalence among 223 pacemaker-treated men. Am J Med 73:187–191, 1982
10. Carette S, Graham DC, Little HA, et al: The natural disease course of ankylosing spondylitis. Arthritis Rheum 26:186–190, 1983
11. Boushea DK, Sundstrom WR: The pleuropulmonary manifestations of ankylosing spondylitis. Semin Arthritis Rheum 18:277–281, 1989
12. Suarez-Almazor ME, Russell AS: Anterior atlantoaxial subluxation in patients with spondyloarthropathies: association with peripheral disease. J Rheumatol 15:973–975, 1988
13. Tussous MW, Skerhut HE, Story JL, et al: Cauda equina syndrome of long-standing ankylosing spondylitis: case report and review of the literature. J Neurosurg 73:441–447, 1990
14. Lance NJ, Curran JJ: Amyloidosis in a case of ankylosing spondylitis with a review of the literature. J Rheumatol 18:100–103, 1991
15. Chang C-P, Schumacher HR: Light and electron microscopic observations on the synovitis of ankylosing spondylitis. Semin Arthritis Rheum 22:54–65, 1992
16. Khan MA, Khan MK: Diagnostic value of HLA–B27 testing in ankylosing spondylitis and Reiter's syndrome. Ann Intern Med 96:70–76, 1982
17. Sparling MJ, Bartleson JD, McLeod RA, et al: Magnetic resonance imaging of arachnoid diverticula associated with cauda equina syndrome in ankylosing spondylitis. J Rheumatol 16:1335–1337, 1989
18. Ahlström H, Feltelius N, Nyman R, et al: Magnetic resonance imaging of sacroiliac joint inflammation. Arthritis Rheum 33:1763–1769, 1990
19. Wilkinson M, Bywaters EGL: Clinical features of ankylosing spondylitis; as seen in a follow-up of 222 hospital referred cases. Ann Rheum Dis 17:209–228, 1958
20. Dougados M, van der Linden S, Juhlin R, et al: The European Spondylarthropathy Study Group preliminary criteria for the classification of spondylarthropathy. Arthritis Rheum 34:1218–1227, 1991
21. Guillemin F, Briancon S, Pourel J, et al: Long-term disability and prolonged sick leave as outcome measurements in ankylosing spondylitis. Arthritis Rheum 33:1001–1006, 1990

C. Reiter's Syndrome

In 1916, Hans Reiter described the case of a cavalry officer who developed arthritis, nongonococcal urethritis, and conjunctivitis following a bout of bloody diarrhea. This clinical triad was recognized as a syndrome by Bauer and Engleman in 1942. In 1973 a genetic predisposition to Reiter's syndrome was established. Eighty percent of patients were positive for the histocompatibility antigen HLA–B27 compared to 6% of the Caucasian population. Using the presence of this HLA antigen, Arnett and colleagues were able to classify 13 patients into a category of *incomplete Reiter's syndrome*. These patients demonstrated asymmetric oligoarthritis of the lower extremities but no conjunctivitis or urethritis. The clinical course of incomplete Reiter's syndrome was identical to the full syndrome; these patients evidently represented subsets of the same disease.

It has become clear that Reiter's syndrome develops in a genetically susceptible host following an infection by bacteria such as *Chlamydia trachomatis* in the genitourinary tract or by *Salmonella, Shigella, Yersinia,* or *Campylobacter* in the gastrointestinal tract. Fragments of *Yersinia*, *Salmonella*, and *Chlamydia* have been identified in the synovial tissues of patients with Reiter's syndrome, but intact organisms have not been cultured.

Reiter's syndrome is considered to be only one clinical manifestation of reactive arthritis, which may occasionally be accompanied by a variety of extraarticular symptoms such as uveitis, bowel inflammation, and carditis. These may occur in the classic triad of Reiter's syndrome or in a more limited spectrum; sometimes even as an isolated event, such as isolated uveitis or carditis. Currently, there is no official definition for the term *Reiter's syndrome*, and many alternative designations such as sexually acquired reactive arthritis (SARA); BASE syndrome (B27, arthritis, sacroiliitis, and extra-articular inflammation); and the ESSG (European Spondyloarthropathy Study Group) classification criteria have been proposed. Indeed the need for such a term as Reiter's syndrome may soon be relegated to history as the pathogenesis becomes better understood. It is still widely used in the literature, however, to describe the full-blown manifestations of some cases of reactive arthritis (see Chapter 20F).

EPIDEMIOLOGY

The incidence of Reiter's syndrome has not been well documented because of the variable nature of its presentation. In Rochester, Minnesota, the incidence has been estimated at 3.5/100,000 in males under the age of 50 (1). During epidemics of enteric infections with *Shigella* and *Salmonella* 1% to 4% of unselected populations subsequently develop arthritis. Reiter's syndrome has been reported worldwide, but it is rare in blacks. Patients of African descent are frequently HLA–B27 negative, although they may have an antigen that cross-reacts with HLA–B27 such as HLA–B7, Bw22, or B42 (2). Furthermore, the HLA–B27 subtype, B*2703, found in black Africans is so far not associated with the spondylarthropathies. Reiter's syndrome is rarely seen in children; most reported cases are postenteric rather than postvenereal. Traditionally it has been claimed that Reiter's syndrome is 20 times more frequent in men than women. With the recognition that the initiating infectious episode might be silent cystitis or cervicitis, the male-to-female ratio is more likely 5:1. Postdysenteric reactive arthritis shows an equal sex distribution (3).

CLINICAL FEATURES

Musculoskeletal

Arthritis typically appears within one to three weeks of the inciting urethritis or diarrhea. Constitutional symptoms are usually mild and fever, if present, is low grade. However, an occasional patient may have high fever, weight loss, and severe malaise. Joint stiffness, myalgia, and low back pain are prominent early symptoms. The back discomfort radiates into the buttocks and thighs and is made worse by bed-rest and inactivity.

Typically only a few joints are involved in an asymmetric pattern: the knees, ankles, feet, and wrists are most commonly affected. Many joints are only moderately swollen but tender, stiff, and restricted in range of motion. The knee can become markedly swollen early in the course followed by popliteal cyst dissection and rupture.

The distinctive arthropathy of Reiter's syndrome includes a local enthesopathy. The principal target of inflammation is located at the tendinous insertion into bone rather than or in addition to the synovium. In the fingers and toes this gives the appearance of a uniformly swollen *sausage digit*; this contrasts with rheumatoid arthritis where the inflammation is confined to the synovium and the phalangeal shafts are normal. The presence of a sausage digit is of diagnostic value since this suggests Reiter's syndrome or psoriatic arthritis.

In the ankle, the enthesopathic process causes chronic hindfoot swelling and pain. The Achilles tendon and plantar fascia are inflamed at the site of insertion into the calcaneus as are the ligaments around the ankle and subtalar joints. Reiter's syndrome should always be suspected in a young man who presents with subacute arthritis of the knees, chronic hindfoot pain, metatarsalgia, and tenderness in the low back over the sacroiliac joints. The spine is prominently affected in those patients with severe, chronic, or recurrent disease. A few patients with long-standing Reiter's syndrome may develop axial disease indistinguishable from ankylosing spondylitis. Childhood Reiter's syndrome typically presents as severe heel pain and plantar fasciitis (4).

Urogenital Tract

Reiter's syndrome followed nongonoccocal urethritis in 3% of patients attending a venereal disease clinic in London. Men experience increased frequency of and burning during urination. Examination of the penis reveals meatal erythema and edema, and a clear mucoid discharge can be expressed. Pyuria is best detected in a first-void urine. Prostatitis is common and has been reported in up to 80% of patients. Hemorrhagic cystitis may develop and may clear spontaneously. Silent cystitis or cervicitis without urethritis may be the only urogenital involvement in women; salpingitis and vulvovaginitis have also been reported. Urogenital symptoms do not necessarily indicate infection at that site. Patients who develop postdysenteric Reiter's syndrome may experience a sterile urethritis within one to two weeks of the initial bout of diarrhea. It is therefore difficult at times to determine whether the arthritis is postdysenteric or postvenereal.

Mucous Membrane and Skin

Two characteristic sites of lesions, on the penis and on the skin, are diagnostic of Reiter's syndrome. Small shallow painless ulcers of the glans penis and urethral meatus, termed *balanitis circinata*, have been described in 25% of post-*Chlamydia* and post-*Shigella* Reiter's syndrome. In uncircumcised patients, the lesions are moist, and they are asymptomatic unless secondarily infected. On the circumcised penis, the lesions harden to a crust that may scar and cause pain.

Keratoderma blenorrhagica is a hyperkeratotic skin lesion that is seen in 12% to 14% of patients. It begins as clear vesicles on erythematous bases and progresses to macules, papules, and then to small keratotic nodules. The lesions are frequently found on the soles of the feet, but may involve the toes, scrotum, palms, penis, trunk, and scalp. They cannot be distinguished either clinically or microscopically from pustular psoriasis, and their presence or course does not predict or correlate with the course of the disease. Keratotic material also accumulates under the nail and lifts it from the nail-bed.

Superficial oral ulcers are an early and transient feature of the disease. They begin as vesicles and progress to small, shallow, sometimes confluent ulcers. Because they are often painless, they may go unnoticed by the patient.

Eye

In 40% of patients there is unilateral or bilateral apparently noninfectious conjunctivitis. This most often occurs early in the disease and is usually mild as well as transient. A more significant involvement is uveitis that is acute and unilateral; however, subsequent attacks may also affect the other eye. Reiter's syndrome was the most frequently diagnosed systemic disease (17 cases) in a survey of 236 patients reviewed at a uveitis clinic (5). The inflammation is anterior (iritis) and tends to spare the choroid and retina. Hypopyon, keratitis, corneal ulceration, posterior uveitis, optic neuritis, and intraocular hemorrhage are rare complications.

Gastrointestinal Tract

The precipitating episode of diarrhea is often mild and transient, but occasionally it may be bloody and prolonged. Enteric infections by *Shigella dysenteriae* or *flexneri*, *Salmonella enteritidis* or *typhimurium*, *Yersinia enterocolitica* or *pseudotuberculosis*, and *Campylobacter jejuni*, (6) may give rise to Reiter's syndrome. The arthritis usually appears after a one to three week period following the onset of infectious symptoms.

Heart and Other

In 10% of patients with severe and longstanding disease, aortic regurgitation develops as a result of inflammation and scarring of the aortic wall and valvular cusps. Conduction defects sometimes occur early, the most common being a prolonged P–R interval, but second and third degree atrio–ventricular blocks have also been reported.

Unusual complications include IgA glomerulonephritis, renal amyloidosis, cranial and peripheral neuropathies, thrombophlebitis, purpura, and livedo reticularis.

Reiter's Syndrome and Human Immunodeficiency Virus

Reiter's syndrome was the first rheumatic disease to be recognized in association with human immunodeficiency virus (HIV) infection. Symptoms of arthritis may precede any overt signs of HIV disease. Treatment of Reiter's syndrome with agents such as methotrexate and azathioprine may further suppress the immune response and provoke a full expression of the acquired immunodeficiency syndrome (7) (see Chapter 44).

RADIOLOGIC FINDINGS

Sacroiliitis occurs in 10% of patients with early disease. Its presence can confirm the diagnosis of Reiter's syndrome in a patient with a suggestive asymmetric oligoarthritis. Eventually up to 70% of patients with chronic Reiter's syndrome show either unilateral (early) or bilateral (late) sacroiliac abnormalities (8). Asymmetric paravertebral comma-shaped ossification is a distinctive finding in Reiter's syndrome and psoriatic arthritis, typically involving the lower three thoracic and upper three lumbar vertebrae. Squaring of vertebrae is uncommon. Atlantoaxial subluxation is rare, but five cases have recently been reported.

Soft tissue swelling is prominent around affected joints, but bone density is surprisingly well-preserved even in chronic disease. Joint space narrowing is often restricted to the small joints of the hands and feet where erosions with indistinct margins and fluffy periostitis can be seen. Linear periostitis occurs along metacarpal, metatarsal, and phalangeal shafts, and exuberant periosteal spurs with indistinct margins can be seen along the sites of tendinous insertion into bone such as the calcaneus, ischial tuberosity, and trochanter.

LABORATORY FINDINGS

The first group of laboratory tests to be considered are those that attempt to document the presence of a specific bacterial infection. Since chronic antimicrobial therapy is possibly beneficial in *Chlamydia*-induced Reiter's syndrome (8), it is now important to look for *Chlamydia* in every case of Reiter's syndrome. *Chlamydia trachomatis* is an obligate intracellular parasite that cannot be grown on artificial media. Culture techniques are unreliable. It is better to submit urethral swabs and cervical cytobrushings for either direct fluorescent antibody and enzyme-immunoassay tests or preferably DNA-probe for chlamydial ribosomal RNA. Stool cultures are useful for confirming the diagnosis of infection by an appropriate triggering microbe even when bowel symptoms are unapparent or mild, and these can support the diagnosis of reactive arthritis in an otherwise undefined case (9).

The second group of laboratory tests reflects the presence of inflammation. A moderate neutrophilic leukocytosis, elevated erythrocyte sedimentation rate, and C-reactive protein are common during the acute illness. These slowly return to normal as the disease subsides. Chronic cases show a mild normocytic anemia. Antinuclear antibody and rheumatoid factor are negative, and C3 and C4 levels, being acute phase reactants, are raised. Synovial fluid may be mildly to severely inflammatory and may include large macrophages with vacuoles that contain nuclear debris and whole leukocytes. These are sometimes called Reiter's cells, but they are not specific for Reiter's syndrome. Synovial biopsies show nonspecific inflammatory changes although often with more neutrophil infiltration than in rheumatoid

arthritis (6). Recent reports of success in identifying infectious antigens or RNA in synovium and synovial fluid suggest that immunohistochemistry, polymerase chain reaction, or molecular hybridization of these specimens may become more useful (10).

HLA–B27 typing is occasionally helpful when characteristic extraarticular features are absent. There is increasing evidence that the possession of the HLA–B27 antigen correlates with axial disease, carditis (11), and uveitis.

COURSE AND PROGNOSIS

The natural history of Reiter's syndrome is highly variable and probably related to the particular infective organism and host factors, including the presence or absence of HLA–B27. Most patients experience hectic symptomatic episodes of arthritis lasting several weeks to six months (6). A few patients have only a single self-limiting period of arthritis, but 15% to 50% have recurrent bouts. Recent evidence suggests that recurrent arthritis may be caused by unapparent chlamydial infection of the synovium (12). The presence of heel pain has been reported to correlate with a poorer prognosis (13). A few patients (3%) may develop axial disease indistinguishable from ankylosing spondylitis. About 20% develop chronic peripheral or axial arthritis and may become unemployed or be forced to change their occupations (14). The presence of HLA–B27 correlates with persistent low back pain and sacroiliitis but not with residual symptoms in peripheral joints (15).

TREATMENT

Nonsteroidal antiinflammatory drugs (NSAIDs) are the primary agents for treating joint symptoms. Indomethacin at 100 mg/day divided into four doses and taken with food is often effective, but the dosage may have to be incrementally raised to 200 mg/day. At this dose side effects such as headaches, lightheadedness, and abdominal distress are common. Bed rest is sometimes helpful, but prolonged splinting of joints should be avoided because of the tendency toward fibrous ankylosis and muscle atrophy. When the most severe symptoms subside, range of motion and isometric strengthening exercises are prescribed. Residual pain and tenderness in the plantar fascia or retrocalcaneal bursa should be treated with local corticosteroid injections so that the ankle can be mobilized early to avoid heel cord shortening and fibrous ankylosis. Care must be taken to avoid direct injection into the Achilles tendon, which may cause tendon rupture. Intraarticular injection of depot corticosteroids can provide temporary relief for swollen knees and other joints. Topical corticosteroids and keratolytic agents are useful for keratoderma blenorrhagica. Oral lesions resolve spontaneously and require no treatment.

Other NSAIDs are often effective. Phenylbutazone works in an occasional patient who is refractory to other NSAIDs. It is a valuable drug in treating the HIV-positive patient. With any NSAID, at least a month's treatment at maximum dosage is usually required before its effectiveness can be evaluated. When NSAIDs fail to control the arthritis, sulfasalazine at 2,000 mg/day may be added. Sulfasalazine has been reported to be effective in open studies (16), and several large cooperative trials are now in progress. The reason for its efficacy is not yet clear.

Because microbial antigens have been demonstrated to persist in the synovial membrane and fluid of patients with reactive arthritis, the question of whether long-term antimicrobial therapy could improve outcome has been raised. Previous uncontrolled and short-term antibiotic trials have been inconclusive. A recent double-blind, placebo-controlled study (17) of three months duration evaluating treatment with a lysine conjugate of tetracycline showed that patients with *Chlamydia*-triggered reactive arthritis recovered more quickly, whereas those with post-*Yersinia* and post-*Campylobacter* arthritis failed to show any improvement. These results have been confirmed. Another study based on the Inuit population showed that early treatment of chlamydial infections before arthritic symptoms may lower the incidence of arthritis. These findings indicate the importance of searching for chlamydial infection in all cases of reactive arthritis. The next logical step would be to study the effect of long-term treatment of postdysenteric cases of reactive arthritis with an effective antibiotic such as trimethoprim/sulfa or a quinolone.

Aggressive and unremitting Reiter's syndrome may benefit from immunosuppressive drugs such as methotrexate (18) or azathioprine (19). Patients should undergo HIV antibody testing before such therapy or the use of systemic corticosteroids. Sulfasalazine can be safely used in HIV-positive patients (20), and etretinate has been suggested to be beneficial (21). Skin lesions may respond to zidovudine (22).

Peng Thim Fan, MD
David T. Y. Yu, MD

1. Michet CJ, Machado EBV, Ballard DJ, et al: Epidemiology of Reiter's syndrome in Rochester, Minnesota: 1950–1980. Arthritis Rheum 31:428–431, 1988
2. Arnett FC, Hochberg MC, Bias WB: Cross-reactive HLA antigens in B27-negative Reiter's syndrome and sacroiliitis. Johns Hopkins Med J 141:193–197, 1977
3. Lahesmanaa-Rantala R and Toivanen A: Clinical spectrum of reactive arthritis. Reactive Arthritis. Edited by Toivanen A, Toivanen P. Boca Raton, Florida, CRC Press, 1988, pp 1–13
4. Gerster J-C, Piccinin P: Enthesopathy of the heels in juvenile onset seronegative B–27 positive spondyloarthropathy. J Rheumatol 12:310–314, 1985
5. Rosenbaum JT: Characterization of uveitis associated with spondyloarthritis. J Rheumatol 16:792–796, 1989
6. Schumacher HR Jr, Magge S, Cherian PV: Light and electron microscopic studies on the synovial membrane in Reiter's syndrome. Immunocytochemical identification of chlamydial antigen in patients with early disease. Arthritis Rheum 31:937–946, 1988
7. Winchester R, Bernstein DH, Fischer HD, et al: The co-occurrence of Reiter's syndrome and acquired immunodeficiency. Ann Intern Med 106:19–26, 1987
8. Ahlstrom H, Feltelius N, Nyman R, et al: Magnetic resonance imaging of sacroiliac joint inflammation. Arthritis Rheum 33:1763–1769, 1990

9. Valtonen VV, Lerisalo M, Pentikainen PJ, et al: Triggering infections in reactive arthritis. Ann Rheum Dis 44:399, 1985
10. Rahman MU, Cheema MA, Schumacher HR, et al: Molecular evidence for the presence of chlamydia in the synovium of patients with Reiter's syndrome. Arthritis Rheum 35:521–529, 1992
11. Bergfeldt L, Edhag O, Rajs J: HLA–B27-associated heart disease: clinopathologic study of three cases. Am J Med 77:961–967, 1984
12. Rahman MU, Schumacher HR, Hudson AP: Recurrent arthritis in Reiter's syndrome: a function of inapparent chlamydial infection of the synovium? Sem Arthritis Rheum 21:259–266, 1992
13. Fox R, Calin A, Gerber RC, et al: The chronicity of symptoms and disability in Reiter's syndrome: an analysis of 131 consecutive patients. Ann Intern Med 91:190–193, 1979
14. Arnett FC: Seronegative spondylarthropathies. Bull Rheum Dis 37:1–12, 1987
15. Leirisalo-Repo M, Suoranta H: Ten-year follow-up study of patients with *Yersinia* arthritis. Arthritis Rheum 31:533–537, 1988
16. Trnavsky K, Peliskova Z, Vacha J: Sulphasalazine in the treatment of reactive arthritis. Scan J Rheumatol Suppl 67:76–79, 1988
17. Lauhio A, Leirisalo-Repo M, Lahdevirta J, et al: Double-blind, placebo-controlled study of three-month treatment with lymecycline in reactive arthritis, with special reference to *Chlamydia* arthritis. Arthritis Rheum 34:6–14, 1991
18. Lally EV, Ho G, Jr.: A review of methotrexate therapy in Reiter's syndrome. Sem Arthritis Rheum 15:139–144, 1985
19. Calin A: A placebo controlled cross-over study of azathioprine in Reiter's syndrome. Ann Rheum Dis 45:653–655, 1986
20. Youssef PP, Bertouch JV, Jones PD: Successful treatment of human immunodeficiency virus-associated Reiter's syndrome with sulfasalazine. Arthritis Rheum 35:723–724, 1992
21. Louthrenoo W: Successful treatment of severe Reiter's syndrome associated with human immunodeficiency virus infection with etretinate: report of two cases. J Rheumatol 20:1243–1246, 1993
22. Keat A, Rowe I: Reiter's syndrome and associated arthritides. Rheum Dis Clin North Am 17:25–42, 1991

D. Psoriatic Arthritis

Epidemiologic studies have generally but not uniformly confirmed an increased prevalence of inflammatory arthritis in association with psoriasis. While the ideal population-based study remains to be performed, the concept of psoriatic arthritis as a distinct disease has been accepted.

ETIOLOGY AND PATHOGENESIS

A complex interplay of immune, genetic, and environmental factors appear to influence disease expression. Immune perturbations in some patients have included elevated serum IgG and IgA, IgG rheumatoid factor, and the presence of immune complexes. Early family studies suggested an increased prevalence of psoriatic arthritis in the families of patients with the disease (1).

Studies of the major histocompatibility complex (MHC) in patients with psoriasis and psoriatic arthritis utilizing traditional micro-lymphocytotoxicity have been hampered by small sample size, ethnic diversity, and the likelihood of multiple genetic influences. Psoriasis is associated with B13, B17, B37, and most importantly CW6. Subsets of psoriatic arthritis patients have an increased prevalence of B27, B38, B39, CW1, CW2, DRW4 and DRW7. B27 correlates with spinal disease (2).

Environmental factors, including infectious agents and physical trauma, are also likely important. The clinical similarity of reactive arthritis and psoriatic arthritis suggests careful attention to bacteria and other infectious agents. Early Scandinavian studies first drew attention to streptococci in the pathogenesis of psoriasis. More recently, investigators (3) have shown that in psoriasis vulgaris patients, peripheral blood lymphocytes have enhanced mitogenic responses to sonicated group A streptococci compared to normal controls.

An immunohistologic study (4) suggested cross-reactivity between Group A, C, and G streptococcal cell surface antigen M protein and skin component keratin. The authors proposed that molecular mimicry between streptococcal and epidermal components could allow T cell clones directed against streptococci to initiate the psoriatic process in susceptible individuals.

Class II molecules have been shown on psoriatic keratinocytes in patients with psoriatic arthritis. Gram-positive bacteria concentrate in psoriatic plaques. Individuals with psoriatic arthritis produce antibodies against these bacteria to a greater degree than individuals with psoriasis alone or normal individuals (5,6).

The precise influence of human immunodeficiency virus (HIV) on the psoriatic process is not fully understood. Progressive and severe arthritis has been described (7), but whether the prevalence of skin and joint disease is increased remains controversial (2). One study described 9 of 18 HIV-associated psoriasis patients with arthritis, but distinguishing psoriatic arthritis from Reiter's syndrome in these patients was difficult (8).

The concurrence of HIV and psoriatic arthritis suggests that CD_4 helper cells are not critical to disease expression and seems to support the notion that the secondary infections could play a role in the clinical expression of skin and joint disease. Joint trauma and overuse could summon infectious agent-stimulated immunocompetent cells like macrophages (Langerhan's cells) to the injured or abused joint, tendon, ligament, or bursa inciting local inflammation.

CLINICAL FEATURES

Joint Disease

The pattern of joint involvement varies widely. About 95% of patients with psoriatic arthritis have peripheral joint involvement. The majority of these have more than five involved joints. Others have a pauciarticular asymmetric arthritis or exclusive distal interphalangial involvement (9, Fig. 20D–1). Another 5% have exclusive spinal involvement. About 20% to 40% have spinal involvement with one of the forms of peripheral joint

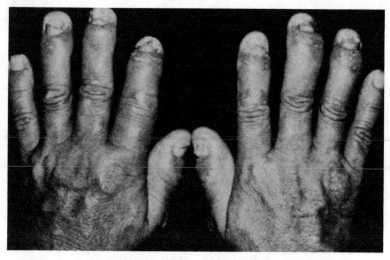

Fig. 20D–1. Swelling and deformity of distal interphalangeal joints are present together with typical psoriatic involvement of the skin and nails. Nail changes associated with psoriasis may include discoloration, fragmentation, pitting, and lifting up of the distal portion of the nail (onycholysis). Several digits, including the left thumb and index finger, are diffusely swollen, suggesting a sausagelike appearance (from Perlman SG, Barth WF: Comprehensive Therapy 5:60–66, 1979).

disease (9,10). Rare patients may have a *bamboo spine* typical of ankylosing spondylitis.

Stiffness in the spine or in peripheral joints after inactivity that lasts at least 30 minutes in the morning is an important clue to the presence of psoriatic arthritis. Inflammation is not limited to joints and spine, but also occurs at the periosteum, along tendons, and at the areas of insertion points into bone (enthesopathy). These sites of inflammation appear to be factors in the development of *sausage digits*, which are typical of psoriatic arthritis and Reiter's syndrome.

Dermatologic and Other Features

Although arthritis can antedate detectable rash, the definite diagnosis of psoriatic arthritis cannot be made without evidence of skin or nail changes typical of psoriasis. One may need to search areas such as the scalp, umbilical, and perianal area for small lesions. Psoriatic skin lesions are macular or papular with characteristic scales. Bleeding often occurs at sites of scale removal. The papulosquamous eruption is generally clearly delineated from surrounding normal skin. Lesions take numerous shapes, but are most often round and located over extensor surfaces. Nail involvement may be an early diagnostic clue, although nail findings are not specific to psoriasis. Some pitting and transverse or longitudinal ridging may be normal variants. Oil droplet discoloration, subungal hyperkeratosis, and onycholysis more strongly suggest psoriasis. Interestingly, 80% of those with psoriasis who have arthritis, but only 20% without joint disease, express nail abnormalities.

Systemic involvement is largely limited to eye inflammation, which occurs in 30% of patients. Findings include conjunctivitis, iritis, episcleritis, and keratoconjunctivitis sicca (11). Aortic insufficiency has also been reported. An associated myopathy has been suggested.

Gender distribution is about equal. Psoriasis and psoriatic arthritis are rare in children under age 13. Usual age of onset is 30 to 50 years, with skin disease usually preceding joint disease by months or even years.

LABORATORY AND RADIOLOGIC FINDINGS

Laboratory abnormalities are mild and nonspecific. Slight elevation of erythrocyte sedimentation rate and mild normocytic normochromic anemia of chronic disease are occasionally seen. Hyperuricemia has occurred, particularly with severe psoriasis.

Synovial fluid findings are also nonspecific. Mildly inflammatory cell counts ranging from 2–15,000 cells/mm³ with predominance of neutrophils and reduced viscosity are the usual findings. Occasional massive effusions can have leukocyte counts in the 100,000/mm³ range.

The psoriatic synovium has many similarities to the synovium in rheumatoid arthritis (RA) with lymphocyte and plasma cell infiltrate. Microvascular changes are seen with light and electron

microscopy (12). A propensity toward synovial fibrosis has been consistently observed.

Radiographic features include distal interphalangeal erosive disease that can evolve into terminal whittling of the more proximal bone at the interphalangeal joints and *pencil-in-cup* appearance. In severe cases osteolysis with complete joint destruction or joint ankylosis can occur (13). Spinal involvement includes sacroiliitis that is unilateral or asymmetric in the early stages but can progress to bilateral fusion. The distribution of involvement in the axial skeleton is less predictable than in ankylosing spondylitis. Isolated, sometimes unusually large and irregular, marginal or non-marginal syndesmophytes may be seen at any level of the spine (10). Atlantoaxial, lateral, and subaxial subluxations of the cervical spine have been described (14). Enthesopathy may lead to radiographic evidence of periostitis.

Generally, psoriatic arthritis has a favorable prognosis in comparison to RA. A five year follow-up study (15) of 126 treated psoriatic arthritis patients showed slowing of the rate of progression of joint damage assessed radiographically. The proportion of patients with at least five damaged joints doubled from 19% to 41% over the five years. About 7% of these patients were rheumatoid factor positive at presentation, but patients with rheumatoid nodules were excluded.

TREATMENT

Basic management utilizing nonsteroidal antiinflammatory drugs, exercise, physical therapy, and education is similar to treatment of RA. Patients should be instructed to try to obtain a full range of motion of all joints daily, but not to overuse and abuse inflamed joints. Constitutional symptoms such as fatigue are less common than in RA but should be respected with periods of rest.

Suppression of the skin disease may be important in helping to control the arthritis. Sunlight, topical petroleum products, and corticosteroids are useful, but patients with recalcitrant skin disease should be referred to a dermatologist.

Articular, bursal, and tendon involvement can be temporarily suppressed by injectable long-acting corticosteroids. Frequently prolonged remission is observed. Care should be observed not to inject into the tendon or tendon's insertion, which could possibly weaken the structure. Careful preparation of the skin should be carried out if either injection or surgery is to be conducted through psoriatic plaques. Oral corticosteroids are generally not recommended.

Psoriatic arthritis patients with polyarticular progressive disease should be considered for second-line therapy. A blinded prospective trial of oral gold with NSAID versus NSAID and placebo in psoriatic arthritis showed modest benefit that did not reach statistical significance (16). Injectable gold is likely more effective (17).

Methotrexate has been recognized as an effective treatment of psoriatic arthritis for 35 years. Weekly administration of methotrexate in three divided doses at 12-hr intervals has been widely used. Administration over 36 hrs is thought to inhibit the cell cycle in the proliferative epidermis. Both skin and joints are likely to improve. Precautions and side effects are similar to those observed in RA. Liver biopsy should be considered after 1.5 to 2.2 g total dose.

Methoxypsoralen and long wave ultraviolet A light (PUVA) has been shown to be helpful for peripheral, but not for axial, psoriatic arthritis (18).

Antimalarials have been reportedly effective (15), but some individuals have experienced marked exacerbation of the skin disease following treatment. Sulfasalazine has recently been reported to be efficacious (19) and is currently under study in a multicenter Veterans Administration trial.

Dietary manipulation with polyunsaturated ethyl ester lipids (20) and oral administration of 1, 25-dihydroxyvitamin D_3 (calcitriol) (21) appeared of potential value in pilot studies. Antibiotics deserve future study (22).

Hip and knee joint prostheses have been used successfully. One surgical study in the hand showed post-operative stiffness was a greater problem in psoriatic arthritis than in RA (23). This could reflect a post-traumatic exacerbation of the arthritis.

Frank B. Vasey, MD

1. Moll JMH, Wright V: Familial occurrence of psoriatic arthritis. Ann Rheum Dis 32:181–201, 1973
2. Arnett FC, Reveille JD, Davic M: AIDS and Rheumatic Disease. Rheumatic Disease Clinics of NA 17:1;58–78, 1991
3. Baker BS, Powles AU, Malkoni AK, et al: Altered cell mediated immunity to group A haemolytic streptococcal antigens in chronic plaque psoriasis. Br J Dermatol 125:30–42, 1991
4. McFadden J, Valdimorsson H, Fry L: Cross reactivity between streptococcal M surface antigen and human skin. Brit J Dermatol 125:443–447, 1991
5. Vasey FB, Dietz CB, Fenske NA, et al: Possible involvement of group A streptococci in the pathogenesis of psoriatic arthritis (PsA). J Rheumatol 9:5:556–560, 1982
6. Rahman MU, Ahmed S, Schumacher HR, et al: High levels of antipeptidegly-can antibodies in psoriatic and other seronegative arthritides. J Rheumatol 17:621–2, 1990
7. Espinoza LR, Berman A, Vasey FB, et al: Psoriatic arthritis and acquired immunodeficiency syndrome. Arthritis Rheum 31:1034–40, 1988
8. Reveille JD, Conant MA, Davic M: Human immunodeficiency virus-associated psoriasis, psoriatic arthritis and Reiter's syndrome: a disease continuum? Arthritis Rheum 33:1574–78, 1990
9. Gladman DD, Shuckett R, Russell ML, et al: Psoriatic arthritis (PsA): an analysis of 220 patients. Q J Med 62:127–141, 1987
10. Lambert JR, Wright V: Psoriatic spondylitis: a clinical and radiological description of the spine in psoriatic arthritis. Q J Med 184:411–425, 1979
11. Lambert JR, Wright V: Eye inflammation in psoriatic arthritis. Ann Rheum Dis 35:354–356, 1976
12. Espinoza LR, Vasey FB, Espinoza CG, et al: Vascular changes in psoriatic synovium: a light and electron microscopy study. Arthritis Rheum 25:677–684, 1982
13. Martel W, Stuck KJ, Dworin AM, et al: Erosive osteoarthritis and psoriatic arthritis: radiologic comparison in the hand, wrist and foot. Am J Roentgenol 127:579–584, 1976
14. Yeadon C, Dumas JM, Karsh J: Lateral subluxation of the cervical spine in psoriatic arthritis: a proposed mechanism. Arthritis Rheum 26:109–112, 1983
15. Gladman DD, Stafford-Brady F, Chi-Hsing C: Longitudinal study of clinical and radiological progression in psoriatic arthritis. J Rheumatol 17:809–12, 1990
16. Palif J, Hill J, Capell HA, et al: A multicenter double blind comparison of auronofin, intramuscular gold thiomalate and placebo in patients with psoriatic arthritis. Br J Rheumatol 29:280–283, 1990
17. Dorwart BB, Gall EP, Schumacher HR, et al: Crysotherapy in psoriatic arthritis: efficacy and toxicity compared to rheumatoid arthritis. Arthritis Rheum 21:513–515, 1978
18. Kammer GM, Soter NA, Gibson DJ, et al: Psoriatic arthritis: a clinical immunologic and HLA study of 100 patients. Semin Arthritis Rheum 9:75–97, 1979
19. For M, Kitas GD, Waterhouse L, et al: Sulphasalazine in psoriatic arthritis: a double-blind placebo-controlled study. Br J Rheumatol 29:46–49, 1990
20. Lassus A, Dahlgren AL, Halpern MJ, et al: Effects of dietary supplementation with polyunsaturated ethyl ester lipids (angiosan) in patients with psoriasis and psoriatic arthritis. J Int Med Res 18:68–73, 1990
21. Huckins D, Felson DT, Holick M: Treatment of psoriatic arthritis with oral 1,25-dihydroxy vitamin D_3: a pilot study. Arthritis Rheum 33:1723–1727, 1990
22. Rosenberg EW, Noah PW, Zanolli MD, et al: Use of rifampin with penicillin and erythromycin in the treatment of psoriasis. J Am Acad Dermatol 14:761–4, 1986
23. Belsky MR, Feldon P, Millender LH, et al: Hand involvement in psoriatic arthritis. J Hand Surg 7:203–207, 1982

E. Enteropathic Arthritis

Inflammatory rheumatic disease is generally considered an enteropathic arthritis if the gastrointestinal tract is directly involved in the pathogenesis. A wide spectrum of other inflammatory rheumatic diseases may be accompanied by gastrointestinal manifestations or intestinal complications, but not all of these diseases can be classified as enteropathic arthritides. Rheumatic diseases, with intestinal manifestations not directly related to the cause of the arthritis, include the vasculitic syndromes that may have abdominal symptoms as part of their course. There may be gastrointestinal hemorrhage, protein-losing enteropathy and sometimes perforation, initiated by vasculitic inflammation of the abdominal arteries.

Systemic sclerosis may be complicated by a motility dysfunction of the entire gastrointestinal tract leading to malabsorption and constipation. In amyloidosis, familial Mediterranean fever, and collagenous colitis, the arthritis and intestinal disease may occur synchronously, without any known direct causative relationship. In 29 patients with collagenous colitis, monarticular reactive arthritis was detected in 2 patients (7%) (1), and coexisting autoimmune diseases were detected in 5 patients. Collagenous colitis therefore seems to be related indirectly to the spectrum of autoimmune diseases. Behcet's disease may have prominent gastrointestinal involvement.

The greater part of the enteropathic arthritides in which there is a direct causative relationship between the intestines and joint disease, belongs among the spondylarthropathies (2): arthritis associated with inflammatory bowel diseases (ulcerative colitis and Crohn's disease), the reactive arthritides triggered by enterogenic bacteriae, some of the undifferentiated spondylarthropathies, and Whipple's disease. Other forms of enteropathic arthrit-ides include the arthritides following intestinal bypass surgery, and arthritis associated with coeliac disease.

IDIOPATHIC INFLAMMATORY BOWEL DISEASES

The locomotor disorders observed in ulcerative colitis and Crohn's disease share many features and will be discussed together.

Intestinal Symptoms

Crohn's disease is characterized by the classic triad of abdominal pain, weight loss, and often diarrhea. Disease onset may be insidious and progression subclinical. Abdominal pain is frequent but not severe. Weight loss in the range of 10% to 20% of body weight is common. Low-grade fever and general debility are common complaints. At a later stage fistulae and abscesses may appear.

In ulcerative colitis, diarrhea and intestinal blood loss are the most common abdominal manifestations. Diarrhea is almost always present, while fever and weight loss are less common. In ulcerative colitis the mucosa is diffusely and continuously involved. The lesions, including superficial ulcerations, edema, friability, and microabscesses, are confined to the colonic mucosa. In Crohn's disease the lesions may occur in the entire gastrointestinal tract, although the terminal ileum and colon are predominantly involved. The lesions are usually ulcerative but their distribution is patchy. They can occur superficially as in ulcerative colitis, but frequently are transmural and granulomatous. Apthoid ulceration, pseudopyloric metaplasia, and sarcoid-like granulomas are virtually pathognomonic findings. Sometimes it is difficult to distinguish between ulcerative colitis and Crohn's disease. In the presence of confined colonic involvement, the histologic appearance may be comparable.

Peripheral Arthritis

Peripheral arthritis occurs in 17% to 20% of patients, with a higher prevalence in Crohn's disease (3). In a recent study (4), however, articular involvement was described in 49 of 79 (62%) consecutive patients with active ulcerative colitis. The arthritis is pauciarticular, mostly asymmetric, and frequently transient and migratory. Large and small joints, predominantly of the lower limbs, are involved. The arthritis usually is nondestructive and many episodes subside within six weeks. Recurrences are common. Sausage-like fingers and toes may occur. Enthesopathies, especially inflammation of the Achilles tendon or insertion of the plantar fascia, are known manifestations, and may also involve the knee or other sites. Clubbing and, rarely, periostitis may occur in Crohn's disease. The peripheral arthritis may become chronic in some cases. Destructive joint lesions of small joints and hips have been described (5).

In most cases intestinal symptoms antedate or coincide with the joint manifestations, but the articular symptoms may precede the intestinal symptoms by years (5). There is evidence that in some cases of spondylarthropathies, Crohn's disease could remain subclinical, joint and tendon inflammation being the only clinical manifestation (6). In ulcerative colitis, there is a more distinct temporal relationship between attacks of arthritis and flares of bowel disease. Surgical removal of the diseased part of the colon can induce remission of the peripheral arthritis. In Crohn's disease, colonic involvement increases the susceptibility to peripheral arthritis, but surgical removal has little effect on the joint disease (7).

Raised serum indicators of inflammation (especially C-reactive protein), thrombocytosis, and hypochromic anemia are common findings. The synovial fluid analysis findings are nonspecific and consistent with inflammatory arthritis, showing a cell count ranging from 1,500 to 50,000 cells/mm^3. Cultures are negative. Synovial biopsies have been limited, but granulomas have been reported in some patients with Crohn's disease (8).

There is substantial evidence favoring a genetic basis for both ulcerative colitis and Crohn's disease. They are believed to be genetically linked, since both occur within the same families (9). No significant association with HLA antigens has been demonstrated, and the frequency of HLA–B27 is within the normal range in patients with peripheral arthritis alone.

Axial Involvement

Axial involvement is identical in both diseases. The true prevalence of sacroiliitis is difficult to estimate since the onset is frequently insidious. Prevalence rates of 10% to 20% for sacroiliitis and 7% to 12% for spondylitis (10) have been described although the actual figures are probably higher. Recently, ankylosing spondylitis (20 patients) and unclassifiable spondylarthritis (14 patients) were found in 34 of 79 patients (43%) with ulcerative colitis (4). Men are three times more likely to develop these diseases than women.

The clinical picture may be indistinguishable from uncomplicated ankylosing spondylitis (AS). The patient complains of an inflammatory low back pain, thoracic or cervical pain, buttock pain, or chest pain. Limitation of motion in the lumbar or cervical region and reduced chest expansion are characteristic clinical signs. Peripheral arthritis may be associated. The onset of axial involvement does not parallel that of bowel disease and frequently precedes it (3). The course is also totally independent of the course of the intestinal disease. Bowel surgery does not alter the course of any associated sacroiliitis or spondylitis.

Radiologically, the axial involvement is often indistinguishable from uncomplicated AS. The frequency of asymmetric sacroiliitis may be higher than in idiopathic AS.

Sacroiliitis and spondylitis are, to a lesser degree than in uncomplicated AS, associated with HLA–B27. The prevalence of

HLA–B27 ranges between 50% and 60%, although it is lower when only sacroiliitis is present. Ankylosing spondylitis patients not carrying the HLA–B27 antigen are at a higher risk of developing inflammatory bowel disease then HLA–B27 positive AS patients. The frequency of HLA-BW62 is significantly increased in spondylarthritic patients with Crohn's disease-like lesions on bowel biopsy (11). The HLA B27–B44 phenotype may place patients at a high risk of developing the common manifestations of Crohn's disease and AS (12). It has been postulated that the peripheral arthritis is a manifestation of inflammatory bowel disease, while the axial involvement is an associated disorder (10).

Extraintestinal and Extraarticular Features

A variety of cutaneous, mucosal, serosal, and ocular manifestations may occur in inflammatory bowel disease. Skin lesions are most frequently associated and occur in 10% to 25% of patients. *Erythema nodosum* parallels the activity of bowel disease, tends to occur in patients with active peripheral arthritis, and is probably a disease-related manifestation (10). *Pyoderma gangrenosum* is a more severe but less common extraarticular manifestation, not related to the bowel and joint disease, and is probably an associated disorder. Leg ulcers and thrombophlebitis also may be associated.

Ocular manifestations, predominantly anterior uveitis, frequently accompany inflammatory bowel disease (3% to 11%). Uveitis is often acute in onset, unilateral, and transient, but recurrences are common (13). It generally spares the choroid and retina; however, a chronic course with lesions in the posterior part of the eye has been described. Granulomatous uveitis is rare but may be present in Crohn's disease. Acute anterior uveitis is more closely related to the axial involvement and to HLA–B27. Conjunctivitis and episcleritis have also been described.

Pericarditis is an uncommon complication, but secondary amyloidosis with involvement of major organs can be seen in Crohn's disease.

Therapy

The pharmacologic and physical treatment of the peripheral arthritis and spondylitis is the same in inflammatory bowel disease as in AS. Nonsteroidal antiinflammatory drugs (NSAIDs) are the first choice, although they may cause an exacerbation of the intestinal symptoms in ulcerative colitis. Intraarticular corticosteroid injections may be beneficial in monarticular chronic forms. Sulfasalazine, which was successfully used to treat the colonic inflammation in both diseases, has been found effective in the peripheral manifestations of the spondylarthropathies (14), especially if intestinal inflammation is present, and may help the peripheral arthritis of inflammatory bowel disease. Oral corticosteroids may reduce synovitis, but are ineffective for the axial symptoms. They should be used systemically only if they are necessary to control bowel disease.

Intestinal surgery is infrequently indicated in the treatment of inflammatory bowel disease and can only influence the peripheral arthritis in ulcerative colitis.

UNDIFFERENTIATED SPONDYLARTHROPATHIES

A large number of patients with clinical, laboratory, radiologic, and genetic features of the spondylarthropathies cannot be classified into one of the known clinical entities. They are referred to as having *undifferentiated spondylarthropathies*. Some of them could be included within the enteropathic arthritides, since ileocolonoscopic studies have disclosed the presence of ileocolonic inflammation in about 65% of spondylarthropathic patients even without clinical intestinal symptoms (15). Repeat ileocolonoscopy demonstrated a strong relationship between the persistence of intestinal inflammation and joint inflammation (16). This supports the hypothesis that the bowel triggers the joint disease in many spondylarthritic patients.

The intestinal lesions either resemble acute bacterial enteritis and can be classified as *acute* (Fig. 20E–1), or they resemble idiopathic inflammatory bowel disease and are then termed

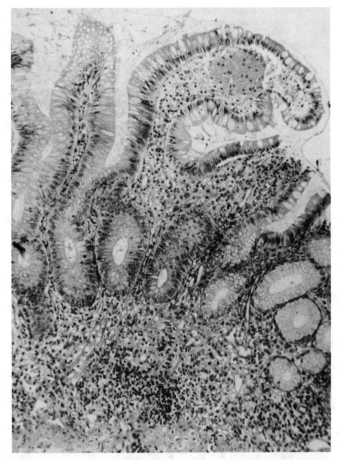

Fig. 20E–1. Acute ileitis: The villi are swollen and blunted. The epithelium is hyperplastic. The lamina propria is infiltrated by plasma cells, lymphocytes and polymorphonuclear cells (HE × 160).

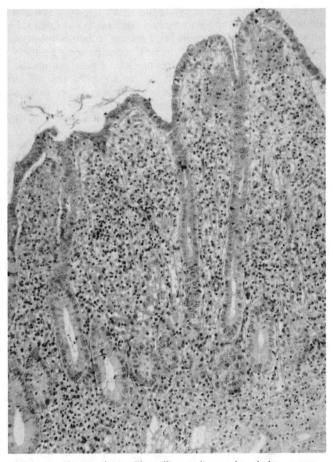

Fig. 20E–2. Chronic ileitis: The villi are distorted and the crypts are irregular. Some are covered with metaplastic cells. The lamina propria contains basal lymphoid follicles and is diffusely infiltrated by mononuclear cells (HE × 160).

chronic (17; Fig. 20E–2). A comparison of different features of both forms of bowel inflammation revealed that the clinical, laboratory, and radiologic manifestations observed in patients with chronic lesions resemble features of inflammatory bowel disease and AS, while patients with acute lesions have features similar to those seen in enterogenic reactive arthritis (18).

The clinical picture, extraarticular manifestations, and treatment are the same as in other forms of spondylarthropathies related to either inflammatory bowel disease or enterogenic reactive arthritis.

WHIPPLE'S DISEASE

Whipple's disease is a multisystem disorder characterized in its fully expressed form by steatorrhea, severe weight loss, fever, arthritis, serositis, lymphadenopathy, leukocytosis, and often thrombocytosis. The main intestinal symptoms are diarrhea with steatorrhea and weight loss.

Whipple's disease occurs most often in men (90%), and the joint symptoms may antedate the intestinal complaints by more than five years. Arthritis flares are not related temporally to exacerbations of intestinal symptoms. Arthralgia is a common finding. The arthritis is polyarticular, symmetrical, and usually transient, but may become chronic. Synovial effusions contain between 4,000 and 100,000 cells/mm³, consisting mainly of polymorphonuclear cells. Radiologic lesions are rare. The incidence of sacroiliitis and spondylitis is controversial, as well as the relationship with HLA–B27. A variety of ophthalmologic and neurologic syndromes may occur, including anterior and posterior uveitis, vitritis, ocular palsies, and progressive encephalopathy.

Whipple's disease is probably a form of enterogenic arthritis, caused by an infection of the intestine. Characteristic periodic acid shiff (PAS) staining deposits are found in the macrophages of the small intestine and in the mesenteric nodes. These cells also contain rod-shaped free bacilli best seen by electron microscopy (19). These bacilliform bodies are considered to be the etiologic agent, because they disappear when the patients are successfully treated with antibiotics. Some synovial morphologic studies suggest that the joint can also be directly invaded by the causative organism. Recently, a unique 1321-base bacterial 16 SrRNA sequence was amplified from duodenal tissue of five patients with Whipple's disease, but not from duodenal tissue of 10 patients without the disorder (20). Phylogenetic analysis showed the bacterium to be a gram-positive actinomycete which is being designated *Tropheryma whippelii*. The polymerase chain reaction for this sequence now provides a specific test for the disease.

A correct diagnosis is important, since the condition responds very well to appropriate antibiotic therapy, usually tetracycline 1 g/day, which has to be continued for more than one year. However, functional abnormalities of the macrophages may persist after successful treatment, indicating a possible immunogenetic predisposition of the affected individual.

INTESTINAL BYPASS ARTHRITIS

Intestinal bypass surgery (jejunocolostomy or jejunoileostomy), which had been a popular treatment for morbid obesity, may give rise to an arthritis–dermatitis syndrome, sometimes associated with renal, hepatic, and hematologic disorders.

Polyarthritis develops in 20% to 80% of cases (21). Symptoms appear 2 to 30 months following surgery. The arthritis is polyarticular, symmetric, and migratory, affecting both upper and lower limb joints. Chronic involvement occurs in one-fourth of the patients. The duration of the arthritis is unpredictable, and there is no relationship between the joint symptoms and abnormal bowel movements. Radiographic deformities or erosions are not seen. Sacroiliac and spine involvement, although uncommon, have been described. In 66% to 80% of the patients a variety of dermatologic abnormalities are present. Erythema nodosum, maculae progressing to papules and vesiculopustules, urticaria, and nodular dermatitis have been described. Other associated features are Raynaud's phenomenon, paresthesia, pericarditis, pleuritis, glomerulonephritis, retinal vasculitis, and superficial thrombophlebitis.

The pathogenesis involves bacterial overgrowth and mucosal alterations in the blind loop. The disease seems to be immuno-mediated: cryoprecipitates and other circulating complexes containing immunoglobulins, complement, bacterial antibodies, and antigens are found in the serum (21,22). Bacterial overgrowth in the blind loop could be responsible for a substantial increase of antigenic stimulation.

Nonsteroidal antiinflammatory drugs are usually sufficient to control the arthritis. Oral antibiotics, such as tetracycline, clindamycin, or metronidazole, given intermittently or continuously, can reduce the symptoms through a reduction of bacterial overgrowth. Only surgical reanastomosis of the bypassed segment of the intestine gives complete resolution of all symptoms and may be necessary in refractory cases.

COELIAC DISEASE

Coeliac disease (gluten-sensitivity enteropathy) is known to be associated with abnormal intestinal permeability. Dermatitis herpetiformis and autoimmune disorders have been associated with the disease.

Patients may have diarrhea (usually steatorrhea) as the main feature. Constitutional disturbances such as lassitude, weight loss and malaise, and varied symptoms such as neuropathy and osteomalacia may occur. Bowel symptoms are absent in 50% of the patients. The pattern of arthritis varies widely, but is mainly polyarticular and symmetric, predominantly involving the large joints, hips, knees, and shoulders. Joint destruction is rarely seen. A higher frequency of HLA–B8, DR3 has been described.

There is often a striking response of the joint manifestations to a gluten-free diet (23). Interestingly, rechallenge may not cause a relapse of the arthritis.

H. Mielants, MD
E.M. Veys, MD

1. Roubenoff R, Ratain J, Giardiello I, et al: Collagenous colitis, enteropathic arthritis, and autoimmune diseases: results of a patient survey. J Rheumatol 16: 1229–1232, 1989
2. Wright V: Seronegative polyarthritis: a unified concept. Arthritis Rheum 21: 618–633, 1978
3. Gravallese EM, Kantrowitz FG: Arthritic manifestations of inflammatory bowel disease. Am J Gastroenterol 83:703–709, 1988
4. Scarpa R, Del Puente A, D'Arienzo A, et al: The arthritis of ulcerative colitis: clinical and genetic aspects. J Rheumatol 19:373–377, 1992
5. Haslock I: Arthritis and Crohn's disease. Ann Rheum Dis 32:479–486, 1973
6. Mielants H, Veys EM: The gut in the spondyloarthropathies. J Rheumatol 17:7–10, 1990
7. Isdale A, Wright V: Seronegative arthritis and the bowel. Ballière's Clinical Rheumatology. The gut and rheumatic diseases 3:285–301, 1989
8. Al-Hadidi S, Khath G, Chatwal P, et al: Granulomatous arthritis in Crohn's disease. Arthritis Rheum 27:1061–1062, 1984
9. Kirsner JB: Genetic aspects of inflammatory bowel disease. Clin Gastroenterol 2:557–562, 1973
10. Schorr-Resnick B, Brandt LJ: Selected rheumatologic and dermatologic manifestations of inflammatory bowel disease. Am J Gastroenterol 83:216–223, 1988
11. Mielants H, Veys EM, Joos R, et al: HLA-antigens in seronegative spondyloarthropathies, reactive arthritis and arthritis in ankylosing spondylitis: relation to gut inflammation. J Rheumatol 14:466–471, 1987
12. Purrmann J, Zeidler H, Bertrams J, et al: HLA antigens in ankylosing spondylitis associated with Crohn's disease: increased frequency of the HLA phenotype B27, B44. J Rheumatol 15:1658–1661, 1988
13. Rosenbaum T: Characterization of uveitis associated with spondyloarthritis. J Rheumatol 16:792–796, 1989
14. Nissila M, Lethinen K, Leirisalo-Repo M, et al: Sulphasalazine in the treatment of ankylosing spondylitis. Arthritis Rheum 31:1111–1116, 1988
15. Mielants H, Veys EM, Cuvelier C, et al: Ileocolonoscopic findings in seronegative spondyloarthropathies. Br J Rheumatol 27(suppl II):95–105, 1988
16. Mielants H, Veys EM, Joos R, et al: Repeat ileocolonoscopy in reactive arthritis. J Rheumatol 14:456–458, 1987
17. Cuvelier C, Barbatis C, Mielants H, et al: The histopathology of intestinal inflammation related to reactive arthritis. Gut 28:394–402, 1987
18. Mielants H, Veys EM, Goemaere S, et al: Gut inflammation in the spondyloarthropathies: clinical, radiologic, biologic and genetic features in relation to the type of histology: a prospective study. J Rheumatol 18:1542–1551, 1991
19. Fleming JL, Wiesner RH, Shorter RC: Whipple's disease: clinical, biochemical and histopathologic features and assessment of treatment in 29 patients. Mayo Clin Proc 63:539–552, 1988
20. Relman DA, Schmidt TM, MacDermott RP, et al: Identification of the uncultured bacillus of Whipple's disease. N Eng J Med 327:293–301, 1992
21. Wands JR, La Mont TJ, Mann E, et al: Arthritis associated with intestinal bypass procedure for morbid obesity: complement activation and characterization of circulatory cryoproteins. N Engl J Med 294:121–124, 1976
22. Clegg DO, Zone JJ, Samuelson CD, et al: Circulating immune complexes containing secretory IgA in jejuno-ileal bypass disease. Ann Rheum Dis 44:239–244, 1985
23. Chakravarty K, Scott DGI: Oligoarthritis—a presenting feature of occult coeliac disease. Brit J Rheum 31:349–350, 1992

F. Reactive Arthritis After Infectious Enteritis

Reactive arthritis (ReA) refers to a sterile synovitis with clinical or microbiologic evidence of an antecedent extraarticular infection. In most common usage of the term reactive arthritis, the antecedent infection is primarily gastrointestinal or genitourinary. A confounding feature in reactive arthritis is that the primary site of inflammation or portal of entry of the pathogen may not be apparent on examination. Studies with ileocolonoscopy have identified lesions in the small bowel reminiscent of Crohn's disease occurring even in the absence of gastrointestinal symptoms (1). This suggests that clinical clues to the nature and site of the antecedent infection may be few. An unexplained oligoarthritis in a young patient should occasion a comprehensive search for the inciting event, employing all of the historical, physical, serologic, and microbiologic clues available.

PATHOGENESIS

The gastrointestinal pathogens implicated in reactive arthritis are predominantly *Yersinia*, *Salmonella*, *Shigella* and *Campylobacter* (2). In the sexually transmitted category, *Chlamydia* has the best substantiated causal relationship to reactive arthritis.

These arthritogenic agents are all intracellular pathogens, having the capability of surviving, or even thriving, in the intracellular milieu of an infected cell. The sequelae of these infections in susceptible patients may be limited to the joints as in reactive arthritis, or may involve characteristic extraarticular sites of inflammation as well, as in Reiter's syndrome.

The pathogenic steps between gastrointestinal or genitourinary infection may proceed by several routes (3). Deposition of circulating immune complexes resulting in synovitis can be seen in the intestinal bypass syndrome. Circulating immune complexes can be detected after *Yersinia* infection, whether complicated by reactive arthritis or not (4). This remains a conjectural mechanism for the induction of synovitis. Some gastrointestinal pathogens such as *Clostridium difficile* may produce an arthritogenic toxin, but this has yet to be demonstrated definitively for the organisms usually associated with reactive arthritis. Molecular mimicry, which refers to an autoimmune reaction that results from cross-reactivity of microbial and host antigens, is also a possible mechanism. This theory has drawn support from sequence homology between HLA–B27, an enzyme of *K. pneumoniae* (5), and a plasmid from an arthritogenic *S. flexneri* (6).

Studies using monoclonal antibodies have also demonstrated cross-reactivity of B27 and certain microbial antigens (7,8). Such antibodies may be demonstrable in patients' sera (9).

The mechanism with the most supportive evidence at present is in situ antigen deposition and local retention of phlogistic bacterial components. Monoclonal antibody staining of synovial fluid mononuclear cells has demonstrated bacterial lipopolysaccharide in patients with post-*Yersinia* reactive arthritis (10–12) and post-*Salmonella* reactive arthritis (13). Indirect evidence of local antigen deposition is provided by profiles of synovial fluid T cell proliferation against candidate bacterial antigens. These studies indicate higher proliferation indices in synovial fluid compared with peripheral blood, and may reveal the nature of the provocative microbe by distinctive proliferation patterns (14). Despite these findings, it has not been possible to demonstrate intact organisms either by culture methodology or by polymerase chain reaction.

CLINICAL FEATURES

Reactive arthritis is typically characterized by an asymmetric oligoarthritis, predominantly of the lower extremities. Knees, ankles, and metatarsophalangeal joints are most commonly affected, but upper extremity involvement is also seen (15). Enthesopathy can be expressed as Achilles tendinitis or plantar fasciitis, and heel pain is suggestive for the spondylarthropathies because of this feature. Back pain is not uncommon although radiographic sacroiliitis is seen in the acute phase in only 28% (16). The extraarticular manifestations often provide important diagnostic clues in the setting of the arthritis, but if these occur temporally removed from the joint disease, a diagnostic puzzle may ensue with the patient seeing an ophthalmologist or urologist before a rheumatologist. Urethritis can be manifested by urethral discharge and dysuria in men, whereas cervicitis in women is generally asymptomatic. Conjunctivitis may be mildly or markedly symptomatic with a local burning sensation. Uveitis is generally associated with pain, photophobia, and sometimes loss of visual acuity. Mucocutaneous involvement may entail circinate balanitis, keratoderma blenorrhagica, and oral mucosal ulcers that may be painless or painful. Some cases thus have features that can be considered "Reiter's syndrome."

There are no diagnostic laboratory tests for evaluating a patient with suspected reactive arthritis. The erythrocyte sedimentation rate is generally elevated but is nonspecific. Chronic inflammation may be accompanied by the anemia of chronic disease. Serum immunoglobulins are generally normal, except in the case of post-dysenteric reactive arthritis, in which an elevation of serum IgA levels is commonly seen. Identification of possible pathogens that may have triggered the disease requires a thorough culture of stool, urethra, and synovial fluid or tissue on appropriate media. Anti-*Chlamydia* antibodies are sufficiently common in the general population to be of limited diagnostic value, whereas elevated anti-*Yersinia* antibodies are more strongly supportive of a recent infection. HLA–B27 occurs in 7% of the normal Caucasian North American population. Conversely, 15% to 25% of reactive arthritis patients may be negative for HLA–B27, with cross-reacting group antigens accounting for most of these patients. Thus, in an individual patient HLA–B27 falls short of a diagnostic test; however, in a patient with suggestive clinical features (in which the pre-test probability is higher), HLA–B27 status may help the clinician categorize the disease process.

The natural history of reactive arthritis varies in the literature and may be influenced by a survivor bias in which self-limited cases are often lost to follow-up. Recurrent attacks have been described over long periods in up to 40% of patients (17). In the study of Leirisalo et al (16), a more severe course in the acute phase as well as the occurrence of sacroiliitis was associated with HLA–B27. Axial radiographic changes occurred in 50% of B27-positive individuals compared with 16% of B27 negative individuals. The development of sacroiliac changes did not correlate with the number of attacks. Long-term disability of significant degree was reported in 25% of cases at a follow-up period of 5.6 years in the study by Fox et al (18).

The differential diagnosis for reactive arthritis and Reiter's syndrome spans a range of rheumatic diseases. The most important exclusion is septic arthritis. Appropriate cultures of synovial fluid and potential portals of entry should be included in the initial evaluation. The most common diagnosis to exclude is gonococcal arthritis. Both Reiter's syndrome and disseminated gonococcal infection can involve tenosynovitis, urethritis, conjunctivitis, and dermatitis. Colitic arthropathy reflecting underlying Crohn's disease or ulcerative colitis can present a picture of post-diarrheal arthritis. Endoscopy and radiographic gastrointestinal studies may be needed to exclude this possibility.

TREATMENT

As noted with Reiter's syndrome there is recent evidence to suggest that tetracycline therapy might shorten the course of post-*Chlamydia* reactive arthritis but this does not seem to be true in other reactive arthritis patients (19). The value of antibiotics is not established for disease triggered by intestinal pathogens.

Generally the newer nonsteroidal antiinflammatory drugs (NSAIDs) are superior to aspirin in controlling the synovitis of reactive arthritis. Diclofenac or indomethacin are generally well tolerated by the young patient population that constitutes the majority in this disease, but dyspepsia and gastritis can be a problem with higher dose regimens. Control of synovitis may necessitate sustained, high-dose NSAID therapy. Sulfasalazine may be useful adjunct if the clinical response to NSAIDs is not adequate (20). Whether sulfasalzine functions primarily as an antibiotic or an anti-inflammatory agent is unresolved. Intraarticular corticosteroid injections can be of benefit, particularly in monarthritis or oligoarthritis. Oral steroids are rarely indicated for joint disease; the synovitis of reactive arthritis may be more steroid-resistant than is rheumatoid arthritis (RA).

For patients with a chronic course unresponsive to these measures, management is more difficult. Methotrexate (10–15 mg/week) is well tolerated, with similar precautions as would apply to the RA patient (21). Mucositis that develops after treatment with methotrexate may result from drug toxicity or from the underlying disease. Uveitis should be managed jointly by a rheumatologist and an ophthalmologist. Generally local steroid drops will suffice, but oral corticosteroids may be required in severe cases.

Patient education plays an important part of the management of reactive arthritis. A discussion about sexually transmitted pathogens as potential contributors to reactive arthritis is appropriate even if the current illness followed enteritis. For the patient who has had previous postdysenteric reactive arthritis and is planning travel to an area of endemic intestinal pathogens, there is currently no proven role for prophylactic antibiotic therapy, and one can only exercise the logical travel precautions regarding local food and water consumption.

Robert D. Inman, MD

1. Mielants H, Veys EM, Goethals K, van der Straeten C, et al: Destructive hip lesions in seronegative spondyloarthropathies: relation to gut inflammation. J Rheumatol 17:335–340, 1990
2. Keat AC: Reiter's syndrome and reactive arthritis in perspective. N Engl J Med 309:1606–1615, 1983
3. Inman RD: Arthritis and enteritis: an interface of protean manifestations. J Rheumatol 14:406–410, 1987
4. Laheshaa-Rantala R, Granfors K, Kekomaki R, et al: Circulating *Yersinia*-specific immune complexes after acute yersiniosis: a follow-up study of patients with and without reactive arthritis. Ann Rheum Dis 46:121–126, 1987
5. Schwimmbeck PL, Yu DTY, Oldstone MBA: Autoantibodies to HLA–B27 in the sera of HLA–B27 patients with ankylosing spondylitis and Reiter's syndrome. J Exp Med 166:173–181, 1987
6. Stieglitz H, Fosmire S, Lipsky P: Identification of a 2-Md plasmid from *Shigella flexneri* associated with reactive arthritis. Arthritis Rheum 33:937–946, 1989
7. Raybourne RB, Bunning VK, Williams KM: Reaction of anti-HLA-B monoclonal antibodies with envelope proteins of *Shigella* species. J Immunol 140:3489–3495, 1988
8. Youg Z, et al: A monoclonal anti-HLA-B27 antibody which is reactive with a linear sequence of the HLA-B27 protein is useful for the study of molecular mimicry. Clin Exp Rheumatol 7:513–519, 1989
9. Tsuchiya N, Husby G, Williams RC, Stieglitz H, Lipsky PE, Inman RD:

Autoantibodies to the HLA-B27 sequence cross-react with the hypothetical peptide from the arthritis-associated Shigella plasmid. J Clin Invest 86:1193–1203, 1990

10. Granfors K, Jalkanen S, von Essen R, et al: *Yersinia* antigens in synovial fluid cells from patients with reactive arthritis. N Eng J Med 320:216–221, 1989

11. Hammer M, Zeidler H, Klimsa S, et al: *Yersinia enterocolitica* in the synovial membrane of patients with *Yersinia*-induced arthritis. Arthritis Rheum 33:1795–1800, 1990

12. Merilahti-Palo R, Soderstrom KO, Lahesmaa-Rantala R, et al: Bacterial antigens in synovial biopsy specimens in *Yersinia*-triggered reactive arthritis. Ann Rheum Dis 50:87–90, 1991

13. Granfors K, Jalkanen S, Lindberg AA, et al: *Salmonella* lipopolysaccharide in synovial cells from patients with reactive arthritis. Lancet 2:685–688, 1990

14. Gaston JSH, Life PF, Granfors K, et al: Synovial T lymphocyte recognition of organisms that trigger reactive arthritis. Clin Exp Immunol 76:348–353, 1989

15. Inman RD, Johnston MEA, Hodge M, et al: Post-dysenteric reactive arthritis: a clinical and immunogenetic study following an outbreak of salmonellosis. Arthritis Rheum 31:1377–1383, 1988

16. Leirisalo M, Skylv G, Kousa M, et al: Follow-up study on patients with Reiter's disease and reactive arthritis, with special reference to HLA–B27. Arthritis Rheum 25:249–259, 1982

17. Hawkes JG: Clinical and diagnostic features of Reiter's disease: a follow-up study of 39 patients. New Zeal Med J. 78:347–357, 1973

18. Fox R, Calin A, Gerber RC, et al: The chronicity and symptoms and disability in Reiter's syndrome: an analysis of 131 consecutive patients. Ann Intern Med 91:190–198, 1979

19. Lauhio A, Leirisalo-Repo M, Lahdevirta J, et al: Double-blind placebo-controlled study of three-month treatment with lymecycline in reactive arthritis, with special reference to *Chlamydia trachomatis*. Arthritis Rheum 34:6–14, 1991

20. Mielants H, Veys E: HLA–B27 related arthritis and bowel inflammation. I. Sulfasalzine in HLA–B27 related reactive arthritis. J Rheumatol 12:287–293, 1985

21. Lally EV, Ho G: A review of methotrexate in Reiter's syndrome. Semin Arthritis Rheum 15:139–145, 1985

21. RHEUMATIC FEVER

Rheumatic fever is an acute inflammatory condition that follows a Group A beta-hemolytic streptococcal infection and involves joints, heart, skin, central nervous system, and subcutaneous tissue. The most relevant clinical manifestations are polyarthritis, carditis, subcutaneous nodules, Sydenham's chorea, and erythema marginatum.

EPIDEMIOLOGY

The incidence of rheumatic fever has declined steadily in the last decades, leading to the near disappearance of the disease in developed countries. In the poorer areas of the world, incidence has been substantially reduced, although in some of them its frequency is still high (1,2).

The steep descent in mortality due to the disease began before the introduction of antibiotics, and was attributed to general improvement in health conditions, less crowding, and better access to medical care. Additional elements could be related to changes in host susceptibility and modifications in the virulence of streptococci (3). With the advent of penicillin and clear treatment guidelines for streptococcal pharyngitis, the number of cases diminished even further (4).

Recently, several outbreaks have occurred in the United States (3,5). The cause for this resurgence is not clear, but the reappearance of heavily encapsulated, highly virulent rheumatogenic streptococcal strains may be important. Also, the decrease in the general awareness of the disease and the relaxation of some epidemiologic control measures, particularly related to prophylaxis in large groups, may have contributed (3).

PATHOGENESIS

The link between streptococci and acute rheumatic fever has been clearly established both clinically and epidemiologically (3,6,7). The incidence of an acute rheumatic episode after a streptococcal pharyngitis is in the range of 0.5% to 3%. Although the pharyngeal infection may be clinically inapparent, it can be evidenced by culture or increasing antibody titers to diverse streptococcal antigens in 95% of patients. Furthermore, appropriate treatment clearly prevents the disease as well as its recurrences (6,7). Interestingly, skin or other streptococcal infections usually do not cause the disease.

Certain strains of streptococci are more frequently associated with outbreaks of acute rheumatic fever, suggesting that they are more "rheumatogenic" than others. Particularly M serotypes 1, 3, 5, 6, 14, 18, 19, and 24 have been repeatedly isolated from different epidemics. Some of these organisms form mucoid colonies on culture, characteristic of encapsulated organisms with increased virulence. Such increased virulence is probably due to their greater resistance to (or possibly decreased breakdown following) phagocytosis (3,6,7). Other factors in the pathogenesis are related to the streptococcal M protein structure, which shares certain epitopes with heart myosin and sarcolemmal membrane proteins (3). This molecular mimicry has also been described in patients with chorea, in whom antibodies against subthalamic and caudate neurons correlating with disease activity have been found (8).

Recent data suggest that molecular mimicry may be enhanced by the active participation of T cells, since M protein may act as a superantigen stimulating subsets of T cells with specificity for self antigens (9). CD4[+] helper T cells predominate in the infiltrate of heart valves removed during cardiac surgery (10). Circulating immune complexes may also play a role in pathogenesis. During an acute episode, 90% of patients have circulating immune complexes, and a decrease in their titers was associated with disease remission (11). Anticardiolipin antibodies have also been found circulating in acute rheumatic fever, although their influence in the acute episode and its potential sequelae is still unclear (12).

A genetic predisposition has been postulated, based on an increase in family incidence, and on the fact that affected individuals have a much higher rate of recurrence after a streptococcal pharyngitis (6,7). This predisposition to develop an immune response leading to an episode of rheumatic fever has been the focus of a number of studies. No significant association with class I HLA antigens has been found, but an increase in HLA type II antigens DR2 and DR4 was established in black and Caucasian patients, respectively (13). Additionally, monoclonal antibody D8/17, directed against B cell alloantigens independent from the HLA system, identified 90% of patients versus 14% of healthy controls (14). These studies could lead to better identification of susceptible individuals to whom efforts in prevention of streptococcal infections can be particularly directed.

CLINICAL ASPECTS

Rheumatic fever may develop at any age, but it is infrequent in early infancy and after age 30. Peak incidence is between 5 and 20 years of age, although in some countries a shift into older age groups may be a trend (6,7,15).

Acute *polyarthritis* is the most frequent initial symptom, occurring in 85% to 95% of patients. Usually it is migratory, affecting joints one after another while subsiding in those previously involved, although occasionally it can be additive. In most of the patients, large joints such as knees, ankles, elbows, and shoulders are affected. In a minority, arthritis of the small joints of hands and feet as well as neck and lumbar pain has been described (15). The symptoms are usually severe, develop acutely, sometimes in hours or overnight, with prominent periarticular inflammation. Myalgias, prostration, and fever are frequently associated. The entire episode lasts two to four weeks and is very responsive to salicylates and probably to other nonsteroidal antiinflammatory agents. In adults, it may have longer duration and be more resistant to treatment, sometimes acquiring additive features that suggest a different entity.

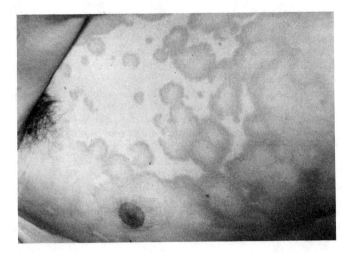

Fig. 21–1. Erythema marginatum in rheumatic fever. This circinate eruption extends centrifugally, sometimes leaving residual hyperpigmentation. Individual lesions usually appear as open or closed rings with sharp outer edges, but macular rings with pale centers also occur. Fusion of adjacent rings produces a polycyclic configuration (from the Revised Clinical Slide Collection).

A chronic articular noninflammatory sequel of rheumatic fever is *Jaccoud's arthropathy*, described particularly in patients who have had several acute episodes (16) (Fig. 21–1). The same changes may be seen in the feet although less frequently. Erosions are almost never seen on roentgenogram, and the articular space is unaffected. Occasionally a "hook" lesion may be observed on the ulnar aspect of the metacarpal heads. Treatment is usually not required for Jaccoud's arthropathy. It should be noted however, that these deformities are not specific for rheumatic fever and have been reported in other arthritides such as systemic lupus erythematosus (7).

Cardiac involvement, the most ominous clinical manifestation of rheumatic fever, is described in 30% to 90% of patients following an acute episode. It is virtually always associated with a murmur and may lead to severe valvular damage. Carditis, however, may be clinically silent in its initial stages in up to 50% of patients who already have established valvular disease when first seen (7). The main features include tachycardia disproportionate to the degree of fever and persistent during sleep, valvular lesions, cardiomegaly, heart failure, pericarditis, extrasystoles, and conduction disturbances such as first degree atrioventricular block (6,7,17).

The appearance or change in character of established organic murmurs are also characteristic of acute carditis, and although valvular sequelae tend to be more frequent in children than in adults, they can be seen in 15% to 25% of all patients. Mitral insufficiency is its most common acute manifestation, followed by a mid-diastolic mitral flow murmur. Occasionally a minimal aortic regurgitation is also found.

In patients with prior valvular damage, the diagnosis may be difficult, and only strict observation as to the emergence of new murmurs or recent onset of cardiac failure may help (6,7). Detection of carditis has been simplified with the use of new diagnostic methods such as bidimensional Doppler echocardiography (6,7,17).

Pericarditis, clinically evidenced as faint and transient friction rubs, may be a feature of acute carditis, although it rarely presents as the sole finding. It is confirmed by echocardiography. Cardiomegaly and cardiac failure, in the absence of severe chronic valvular disease, can also appear. Electrocardiographic changes, such as prolongation of the P–R interval, and extrasystoles, are common and should not be used as evidence of carditis in the absence of cardiomegaly or significant murmurs (6,7).

Established mitral regurgitation, aortic insufficiency, or mitral stenosis are the most important chronic consequences of acute rheumatic fever. Their frequency is higher in patients who have more than one episode of the disease, so that 50% to 100% have valvular damage after two or more recurrences (7,15). A minority of patients following an acute bout present with an unremmiting course leading to multiple valvular disease and cardiac failure (6,7).

Sydenham's chorea is usually a late neurologic event of an acute rheumatic episode, appearing weeks or months after a streptococcal infection when other symptoms have abated. Its frequency has declined in recent years affecting 5% to 10% of all patients, although in one recent series that number reached 30% (5,7,17). It may be an isolated symptom or associated with valvular damage, which is noticed later in the course of the disease. Clinically, it has a gradual onset with emotional lability, followed by the development of abrupt, short, nonrhythmical involuntary movements, incoordination, weakness, and purposeless grimacing. There is also inability to maintain a fixed posture, with tendency to pronate the hands. These findings may be unilateral and tend to disappear during sleep (6,7,18).

Subcutaneous nodules are observed in 3% to 5% of cases, mostly in children who also have carditis and are usually asymptomatic. They locate on extensor surfaces of elbows and forearms and occasionally in other areas such as the scalp. Nodules may persist up to 4 weeks (6,7).

Erythema marginatum is a nonpruritic evanescent rash of the trunk and extremities that spares the face. It is characteristic of the acute episode, is seen in 3% to 15% of cases, and is also particularly associated with carditis. It has an irregular reddish pink peripheral rim that extends outward with a blanching interior. In rare instances, it is observed late, after other signs are disappearing (6,7,17).

Fever up to 39°C commonly accompanies acute polyarthritis, and rarely carditis. It subsides spontaneously after two or three weeks, and remits promptly with aspirin (7). Other less common symptoms that may lead to diagnostic confusion in the early phases of the disease include acute abdominal pain, pneumonitis, epistaxis, glomerulitis, and hepatitis (7,17).

LABORATORY FINDINGS

Laboratory tests in acute rheumatic fever are useful to evaluate the inflammatory nature of the disease and adequately document a streptococcal infection. The erythrocyte sedimentation rate and C-reactive protein are increased in all patients during the acute stage. These correlate with clinical activity except when chorea is the only presenting symptom. They normalize as the disease remits. The sedimentation rate may be affected by anemia or cardiac failure, which does not occur with C-reactive protein. Leukocytosis can also be found (6,7,17).

Proof of streptococcal infection, which is asymptomatic in a high proportion of patients, is a very important feature in the correct diagnosis of the disease. Demonstration of streptococcal pharyngitis can be achieved with conventional throat swab cultures or rapid detection tests. Although rapid detection tests are highly specific, their variable sensitivity makes them less reliable (3,17,19). However, since these methods are positive in only 20% of patients during the acute episode, the confirmation of an antecedent streptococcal infection relies mainly on antibody testing. Antistreptolysin O (ASO) is positive in 80% to 85% of patients, particularly if changes between acute and convalescent determinations are sought. Titers over 1/200 are more acceptable evidence of recent infection, since levels below these can be seen in populations where streptococcal infections are highly prevalent. In endemic areas, the appropriate diagnostic titers should be defined locally. Antideoxyribonuclease B, unfortunately not universally available, is the test of choice to be done together with ASO, thus increasing the sensitivity to 95% (17,19).

Other antibodies to streptococcal antigens, such as antihyaluronidase, antistreptokinase, and antidiphosphopyridine dinucleotidase, may also be carried out. A commercially available latex agglutination test designed to study all these antibodies simultaneously in one reaction is currently not recommended (7,17,19).

Diverse ancillary laboratory studies may be helpful in the differential diagnosis of the disease. Synovial fluid analysis shows a sterile inflammatory reaction, usually with less than 20,000 cells/mm³ (mainly polymorphonuclear) without crystals. Synovial biopsy can show mild inflammatory changes, with minimal hyperplasia of lining cells (15). Subcutaneous nodule histopathology reveals mainly edema, fibrinoid necrosis, and mononuclear infiltrate (7). Determinations of serum complement, immunoglobulin levels, or antinuclear antibodies do not assist in the diagnosis. Although immune complexes are elevated during the acute phase, they do not have current clinical application (11).

Documentation of carditis can be enhanced with two-dimensional echo doppler studies. However, CPK–MB isoenzymes, nuclear magnetic resonance of the heart, or endomyocardial biopsies have not contributed significantly so far.

DIAGNOSIS, COURSE, AND CLINICAL CONSEQUENCES

The diagnosis of acute rheumatic fever is based on clinical features, plus evidence of an antecedent streptococcal infection. None of the symptoms by themselves, except for chorea, are sufficiently characteristic or pathognomonic of the disease. The Jones criteria, introduced in 1944 and subsequently revised, brilliantly combined both clinical and laboratory aspects in the guidance for accurate diagnosis of rheumatic fever (20) (see Appendix 5).

The presence of two major criteria and one minor, or one major and two minor, in addition to evidence of prior streptococcal infection are highly suggestive of the disease (20). The separation between major and minor criteria is based principally on the importance of the symptoms. These criteria were introduced more as a diagnostic guide than a rigid rule. They continue to be extremely helpful in conceptually unifying the disease.

Some exceptions to these criteria have been pointed out. When chorea is the only major criteria present, the level of anti-streptococcal antibodies in serum may be normal due to the long time elapsed from the infection to the beginning of the symptoms. Other eventual difficulties in the application of these criteria may arise from the interpretation of certain clinical situations. Because arthritis is the most frequent presenting symptom during the acute stage, a possible pitfall in the application of the Jones criteria is adequate differentiation from arthralgias. In some patients, particularly children, the articular pains may be described as severe, but no clear evidence of inflammation can be observed. In this situation, particularly if the titers of anti-streptococcal antibodies are increased, it may be appropriate to consider arthralgia as suggestive of active disease, and follow the patient closely. Similarly, in cases with prior carditis and established valvular damage, recurrences can be difficult to define. Changing murmurs or echocardiographic evidence of heart failure are strong arguments in favor of an acute episode, if a streptococcal infection is proven.

Of the Jones major criteria, the most important prognostic event is carditis, which usually develops in the first two weeks. When it does not manifest during the first episode, it rarely appears during a recurrence. In patients who already have chronic valvular sequelae, however, a recurrence usually worsens existing damage. Mitral insufficiency is the most frequent expression of valvular damage during an acute episode, and can be reversed in a majority of patients if adequate prophylaxis is maintained (6,7). Although aortic regurgitation may start during the acute attack, it may be clinically insignificant and detected later in the course of the disease. Another late feature is the combination of severe mitral and aortic regurgitation, which is highly suggestive of chronic rheumatic sequelae (7).

Mitral stenosis also requires months or years to become established, although it may follow an episode of isolated chorea or constitute the initial finding in previously asymptomatic patients. Recurrences commonly appear in the first five years after the acute attack, declining thereafter. They tend to be more frequent in patients who developed carditis in the first episode or who have valvular sequelae (6,7).

Subcutaneous nodules and erythema marginatum are generally of limited assistance in the diagnosis. They are relatively infrequent and usually appear in severe acute episodes that also have carditis.

The course followed by a patient after a first attack of rheumatic fever is highly variable and unpredictable (6,7). Ninety percent of the episodes last less than three months, and only a minority persist longer in the form of unremittent rheumatic carditis or prolonged chorea.

The differential diagnosis of acute rheumatic fever has been expanding. Particularly when polyarthritis is the main presenting problem, other possibilities need to be considered, including reactive arthritis, ankylosing spondylitis, gonococcal arthritis, subacute bacterial endocarditis, Lyme disease, viral infections, acute leukemia, Still's disease, and serum sickness (6,7). When carditis is the outstanding feature, additional diagnostic options include congenital lesions, mitral valve prolapse, infection with *Yersinia enterocolitica*, viral myocarditis, Lyme disease, and systemic lupus erythematosus with valvular disease (7). In all these situations, evidence of a prior streptococcal infection is a significant argument in favor of acute rheumatic fever, particularly if there is a curve with rising titer of antibodies. However, the possibility of a coincidental streptococcal infection with another disease must be considered.

TREATMENT

Treatment of the acute episode of rheumatic fever is directed to the eradication of the streptococcus and suppression of the acute inflammatory response. Once this is accomplished, prevention of recurrences is the major objective.

After the diagnosis is firmly established, eradication of infection is achieved by a single dose of intramuscular benzathine penicillin (600,000 units in children or 1,200,000 in adults). An alternative is oral phenoxymethyl penicillin (250,000 units 4 times daily for 10 days) if appropriate compliance is assured. Erythromycin is a choice in those allergic to penicillin. Sulfa derivatives do not eradicate the streptococcus from the pharynx and are not recommended (6,7,17,19).

Bed rest is advised during the acute stage. In patients without carditis, it may be limited to two or three weeks, with gradual resumption of normal activities. When carditis is present, bed rest should be prolonged to at least four weeks, and if cardiac failure or cardiomegaly are apparent, it should be extended to eight weeks or until complications subside (7,17).

Treatment of acute arthritis is based on the use of salicylates, although other nonsteroidal antiinflamatory drugs may be equally helpful. Evident improvement is usual when salicylates are given in doses ranging from 80–100 mg/kg/day, divided in three or four doses and maintained for a minimum of three or four weeks. If treatment is abandoned too soon, articular symptoms may recur.

Corticosteroids can be used in the presence of carditis. Although there is the impression that they may shorten the acute phase of the disease, they have no proven influence on the development of valvular sequelae. Dosages equivalent to 40–60 mg/day of prednisone are used for two to three weeks, followed by a gradual withdrawal (7,17). Aspirin and prednisone can be used together, particularly if articular symptoms reappear when prednisone is tapered.

Secondary prophylaxis, a major breakthrough in the control of the disease, is extremely important. It should be carefully planned, once the acute stage has been adequately controlled, to avoid recurrences or further cardiac damage by repeated infections. Prophylaxis is achieved with monthly Benzathine penicillin (1,200,000 units by intramuscular injection). In highly endemic areas or in patients with severe cardiac sequelae, it has been suggested that prophylaxis should be repeated every three weeks (17,19). Oral phenoxymethyl penicillin (250,000 units daily) can also be used in compliant patients.

Depending on the weight of the patient, sulfadiazine (500–1,000 mg/day orally), is the treatment of choice in individuals allergic to penicillin. Duration of secondary prophylaxis is a crucial question. Although there is no absolute consensus, some guidelines are firmly established and should be followed.

It is well known that the risk of a new episode of rheumatic fever is higher within the first five years following an acute attack, and all patients should have prophylaxis at least during this period of time or until they reach 18 years of age (7,17,19). In those patients who have had carditis, but without residual valvular damage, prophylaxis may be prolonged particularly if they live in poor or crowded areas and are at high risk of repeated streptococcal infections. When chronic valvular sequelae are present, prophylaxis is indefinite or until the chances of recurrence are definitely reduced. Prophylaxis is also indicated in patients with chorea, in whom the same principles can be applied. In addition, it should be maintained after cardiac surgery. Secondary prophylaxis requires special follow-up, and attention has to be given to patients at high risk to maximize adherence.

Leonardo Guzman, MD

1. Gordis L: The virtual dissapearance of acute rheumatic fever in the United States: Lessons in the rise and fall of the disease. Circulation 72:1155, 1985
2. World Health Organization: Community control of rheumatic heart disease in developing countries: a major health problem. WHO chronicle 34:336–345, 1980
3. Bisno AL: Group A streptococcal infections and acute rheumatic fever. N Engl J Med 325:783–793, 1991
4. Maselli BF, Chute CG, Walker AM, et al: Penicillin and the marked decrease in morbidity and mortality from rheumatic fever in the United States. N Engl J Med 318:280–286, 1988
5. Veasey LG, Wiedmeir SE, Orsmond GS, et al: Resurgence of acute rheumatic fever in the intermountain area of the USA. N Engl J Med 316:421–427, 1987
6. Stollerman GH: Rheumatic Fever. Harrison's principles of internal medicine, 12th Ed. Edited by Wilson JD. New York, McGraw Hill, 1991, pp 933–938
7. Taranta A, Markowitz M: Rheumatic Fever, 2nd Ed. Dordrecht, Kluwer Academic, 1989
8. Ayoub EM, Kaplan E: Host parasite interaction in the pathogenesis of rheumatic fever. J Rheumatol (suppl 30)18:6–13, 1991
9. Tomai M, Kotb M, Majumdar G, et al: Superantigenicity of M protein. J Exp Med 172:359–362, 1990
10. Raizada V, Williams RC, Chopra P, et al: Tissue distribution of lymphocytes in rheumatic heart valves as defined by monoclonal anti T cell antibodies. Am J Med 74:90–96, 1983
11. Yoshinoya S, Pope RM: Detection of immune complexes in acute rheumatic fever and their relationship to HLA B–5. J Clin Invest 65:136–145, 1980
12. Figueroa F, Berrios X, Gutierrez M, et al: Anticardiolipin antibodies in acute rheumatic fever. J Rheumatol 19:1175–1180, 1992
13. Ayoub EM, Barrett DJ, Maclaren NK, et al: Association of class II human histocompatibility leukocyte antigens with rheumatic fever. J Clin Invest 77:2019–1026, 1986
14. Gibofsky A, Khanna A, Suh E, et al: The genetics of rheumatic fever: relationship to streptococcal infection and autoimmune disease. J Rheumatol (Suppl 30) 18:1–5, 1991
15. Guzman L, Reginato AJ, Wohlk N: La fiebre reumatica del adulto. Rev Esp Reumatol 18:288–293, 1991
16. Bywaters EGL: The relation between the heart and joint disease including rheumatoid heart disease and chronic post rheumatic arthritis (type Jaccoud). Br Heart J 12:101–131, 1950
17. Rheumatic fever and rheumatic heart disease. Report of a World Health Organization study group. WHO Tech Rep Ser 764:1–58, 1988
18. Aron AM, Freeman JM, Carter S: The natural history of Sydenham's chorea. Review of the literature and long term evaluation with emphasis on cardiac sequelae. Am J Med 38:83–95, 1965
19. Dajani AS, Bisno AL, Chung KJ, et al: Prevention of rheumatic fever: A statement for health professionals by the committee on rheumatic fever, endocarditis and Kawasaki diseases of the Council on Cardiovascular Disease in the young. The American Heart Association. Circulation 78:1082–1086, 1988
20. Stollerman GH, Markowitz M, Taranta A, et al: Jones criteria (revised) for guidance in the diagnosis of rheumatic fever. Circulation 32:664–668, 1965

22. PEDIATRIC RHEUMATIC DISEASES
A. *Nonarticular Rheumatism, Juvenile Rheumatoid Arthritis, Juvenile Spondylarthropathies*

The rheumatic diseases of childhood are not rare and now include at least 120 illnesses associated with arthritis or related musculoskeletal syndromes (1,2). Although classification, diagnosis, and treatment of the pediatric and adult rheumatic diseases are generally similar, important differences exist. Differences include the central role of the parent in all aspects of care and the major influences of a child's growth and development on therapeutic interventions, compliance, and prognosis.

A major change in pediatric rheumatology during the past decade has been the recognition that soft tissue or *nonarticular* rheumatism now constitutes almost 40% of new cases, including problems such as limb pains, benign hypermobility syndrome, fibrositis and reflex sympathetic dystrophy (RSD). The pediatric spondylarthropathies are more frequently recognized, and the postinfectious (reactive) forms of arthritis, vasculitis syndromes, and Lyme disease, are now widely diagnosed. These entities need to be excluded before a differential diagnosis shifts to juvenile rheumatoid arthritis (JRA). Systemic lupus erythematosus (SLE), dermatomyositis, scleroderma, Kawasaki disease, and other less common conditions are still important problems. Metabolic, endocrine, neuropathic, and bone and cartilage disorders are only rarely causes of arthritis in childhood. A broad spectrum of miscellaneous conditions, however, should be considered whenever there is an atypical presentation of childhood extremity pains or arthritis; for example, neoplasia often masquerades as a pediatric rheumatic disease. Joint infections of bacterial or viral origin, inherited conditions, congenital anomalies, musculoskeletal trauma, and osteonecrosis must also be excluded.

NONARTICULAR RHEUMATISM

Limb pains (growing pains) are the most common soft tissue rheumatic syndrome in childhood. These pains often occur in the late afternoon or at night, usually in the muscles and other soft tissues of the calves, shins, and thighs. They are intermittent, self-limited, and often follow high levels of athletic or play activities. They are not associated with systemic symptoms or with physical or laboratory evidence of inflammation. The prevalence of limb pains may be as high as 13% in boys and 18% in girls. They most commonly develop in the child who falls asleep uneventfully, awakes with major lower limb complaints, and yet often looks totally well by the following morning. While moist heat, extremity massage, and acetaminophen or ibuprofen may appear beneficial to some concerned parents, education about the benign nature and excellent prognosis for limb pains often leads to prompt improvement. There is no evidence that these pains are related to physical growth, and restriction of physical activity is unnecessary.

The benign hypermobility joint syndrome is another important cause of periarticular complaints. Joint pains in these children are often related to increased or unusual physical activity. Hypermobility of joints occurs in 12% of normal children (3), has a definite familial tendency, and may be associated with an increased frequency of ankle and wrist sprains, shoulder or elbow dislocations, subluxation of the patellae, and scoliosis. Arthralgias are most frequent at the knees (40%), fingers and hands (40%), and hips (20%). Patients are often slender, are more often girls (11:4), and may have episodic joint effusions, but do not have an underlying connective tissue disorder such as the Ehlers–Danlos or Marfan syndromes. Diagnostic maneuvers suggestive of the hypermobility syndrome include: passive apposition of the thumb to the palmar side of the forearm, hyperextension of the fingers parallel to the forearm, knee or elbow active hyperextension $\geq 10°$, and placing the palms on the floor with the knees fully extended. Management requires education, guidance about choice of sports or physical activities, and assurance that many patients improve as they get older. Children wishing to continue sports often benefit from prophylactic ibuprofen one hour before and again one hour after their activity.

A psychosomatic etiology for musculoskeletal pain may be found in up to 11% of new pediatric rheumatology clinic referrals, particularly among adolescent females (4). Back pain, multiple pain sites, incongruent affect, highly stressed or abnormal family milieu, and identifiable pain role models are common findings. The closely related reflex neurovascular (sympathetic) dystrophy syndrome, with associated autonomic dysfunction, often appears to be a stress-related disorder and commonly exhibits features of parental enmeshment.

The primary fibromyalgia (fibrositis) syndrome, characterized by fatigue, nonrestorative sleep, and numerous tender points, is increasingly common in adolescents. Up to 28% of adult patients diagnosed with fibromyalgia may have their onset of symptoms during childhood (5). Although the causes are unknown, poor sleep, high ambient noise, significant family dysfunction, and endogenous depression are often seen in children with fibromyalgia. There is no evidence of associated histopathologic or serologic changes (see Chapter 41, Fibrositis-fibromyalgia syndrome). One study of 33 children with primary fibromyalgia, diagnosed over a three-year period, emphasized the association of generalized aches and pains, stiffness, waking up tired, chronic headaches, and irritable bowel syndrome (5). Management of all pediatric musculoskeletal pain syndromes should focus on identification and relief of psychological and lifestyle causes of stress and anxiety, altering sleep behaviors, education, and improved physical conditioning. Currently, prognosis and outcome are not well understood.

JUVENILE RHEUMATOID ARTHRITIS

Juvenile rheumatoid arthritis is characterized by chronic synovial inflammation of unknown cause. It affects an estimated 65,000 to 70,000 children in the United States (6). The disease may develop at any age during childhood, and girls are more often affected than boys; however, sex and age ratios differ in the various subgroups of JRA. Diagnosis of definite JRA requires at least six consecutive weeks of objective synovitis, and assignment to onset subtype should occur only after six months of active disease. Adherence to these important criteria, along with a careful history and physical evaluation, will generally lead to a correct diagnosis.

Alternative nomenclature to JRA remains controversial, with *juvenile chronic arthritis* used by some European investigators, while other American researchers prefer *juvenile arthritis*. These latter terms both can encompass the childhood spondylarthropathies and related conditions, and thus neither descriptor achieves a desirable level of specificity (7). The current American College of Rheumatology (ACR) classification of syndromes considered to be juvenile rheumatoid arthritis, as outlined in Appendix 6, includes three onset subtypes: pauciarticular, polyarticular, and systemic. Whether these subtypes are distinctive diseases resulting from different causes or varying responses to common factors is unknown.

No laboratory test is diagnostic for JRA, although the presence of rheumatoid factors (RF), antinuclear antibodies (ANA), and certain HLA antigens may assist in classifying patients (8). Baseline joint roentgenograms are important to allow assessment of later bone growth or damage, but they are not diagnostic except when revealing late, characteristic articular damage (1,2). No clear evidence of a genetic predisposition for juvenile forms of arthritis exists, except in the case of pauciarticular disease in older children and familial spondylarthropathies, which may be associated with HLA–B27 (2,6,8).

Subtypes of JRA

Systemic onset. About 10% of children with JRA have a systemic onset. The ratio of boys to girls is approximately equal, and it can begin at any age during childhood. Spiking quotidian or diquotidian fevers, often associated with an evanescent, salmon-pink centripetal rash, may occur at any time during the day, but most often during the late afternoon or early evening. Diffuse lymphadenopathy, hepatosplenomegaly, and pericardial or pleural effusions are common. Fatigue, muscle atrophy, and weight loss are occasionally severe. Leukocytosis and anemia may occur, but ANAs and RFs are generally absent.

Systemic manifestations are usually self-limited and rarely life-

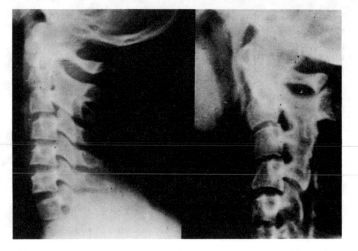

Fig. 22A–1. Lateral projections of the cervical spine in juvenile rheumatoid arthritis. **L**, Narrowing of interspace C2-C3 with obliteration of the apophyseal articulation. **R**, Extensive fusion of the posterior articulations of C2, C3, and C4. The normal cervical lordosis is lost, and some degree of kyphosis is seen at this level. There is a decrease in the anteroposterior diameter of the fifth and sixth vertebrae on the right, usually the result of disease early in life (from the Revised Clinical Slide Collection on the Rheumatic Diseases).

threatening, although severe pericarditis, myocarditis, or anemia demand prompt intervention. Musculoskeletal findings early in the disease may consist only of recurrent arthralgias, myalgias, or transient arthritis, which are maximal with fever spikes. About one-half of these children will have more than one systemic attack. These can range from days to months in duration, recur after an interval of many years, and are usually unexpected.

In most children with systemic onset JRA, chronic polyarthritis develops within weeks to months after disease onset, but sometimes it does not occur until years later. About 50% of patients ultimately have severe, chronic arthritis, which continues after systemic manifestations have subsided (2,8). Alternatively, affected children may have recurrent systemic manifestations of unknown frequency after they have reached adulthood, and chronic arthritis may continue (see Chapter 23).

Polyarticular onset. Arthritis in five or more joints occurs in approximately 40% of children with JRA, and often presents insidiously with malaise, weight loss, low-grade fever, mild organomegaly, adenopathy, anemia, and growth retardation. Cervical spine involvement, most often at the C2–C3 apophyseal joints, is frequent but can also be found in systemic onset disease (Fig. 22A–1). Polyarticular JRA may begin at any age during childhood, with girls being affected more often than boys (3:1). Three-fourths of patients have symmetric joint involvement.

Rheumatoid factors are detected by latex or sheep cell agglutination in only 15% to 20% of children with polyarthritis, most of whom are at least eight years old when the disease begins (8). Antinuclear antibodies are detected in 40% to 60% of patients with polyarticular JRA, regardless of whether they are RF positive or negative. Children who are consistently RF-positive have more erosions, rheumatoid nodules, and vasculitis. They also have a worse prognosis than those who are RF-negative. Destructive, disabling arthritis occurs in as many as 50% of JRA patients with RF, but in perhaps only 10% to 15% of RF-negative patients. Indeed, RF-positive JRA closely resembles classic adult onset rheumatoid arthritis.

Some investigators propose separation of polyarticular onset JRA into RF negative and positive groups, with only the latter continuing to be called juvenile rheumatoid arthritis. Additional "hidden" IgM and IgG rheumatoid factors can be detected by various immunosorbent techniques in 40% to 60% of children who are seronegative by classic agglutination methods. The clinical significance of these hidden rheumatoid factors awaits further definition (9).

Systemic and polyarticular JRA can cause growth retardation and delay of secondary sexual characteristics in up to one-third of patients. Localized effects of inflammation on epiphyseal growth can result in bony overgrowth or undergrowth of long tubular bones, around affected joints, and at the mandible (micrognathia) due to temporomandibular joint arthritis. Overall, many of these children will be below the third percentile for height. These growth disturbances are made worse by treatment with corticosteroids.

Pauciarticular onset. This subtype occurs in up to 50% of children with juvenile rheumatoid arthritis. Such patients have arthritis affecting four or fewer joints within the first six months of disease, and about one-half have only one joint involved, most commonly the knee. Several subgroups of pauciarticular JRA have been suggested. One subgroup is characterized by early childhood onset (generally before age six) and female preponderance. These patients often have ANA, but are RF-negative (10). In some combination, the knees, ankles, wrists, or elbows are most frequently affected. The hips are usually spared, and sacroiliitis is not seen. Although synovitis may be chronic, the prognosis for joint function is most often good. Systemic features do not occur.

Inflammation of the anterior uveal tract (iridocyclitis) develops in 10% to 50% of children with pauciarticular JRA (11). Generally, iridocyclitis begins concurrently with or occasionally precedes joint complaints, but it may develop as long as 5 to 10 years later. Iridocyclitis is often chronic and insidious, with great potential for ocular damage including band keratopathy, posterior synechiae, and secondary cataracts (30%); glaucoma (20%); and visual loss or even blindness. Since these children rarely have or complain of photophobia, red eyes, or visual changes, early detection can occur only with regular slitlamp examinations by an ophthalmologist.

Another subgroup of pauciarticular childhood arthritis manifests strong male preponderance and older age at onset. More than one-half of these patients have HLA–B27, but rheumatoid factors and ANA are absent (1,8). Family histories may be positive for chronic back pain, enteritis, colitis, or psoriasis. The arthritis is asymmetric, affects predominantly lower extremity joints, and early hip involvement is common. Enthesopathy is often present. Sacroiliitis may be present at onset and can be either silent or symptomatic. Attacks of acute self-limited iridocyclitis may occur. Many of these children with pauciarticular, self-limited arthritis may represent early or incomplete expression of spondylarthropathy.

Treatment

Early diagnosis and comprehensive therapy of JRA are important to minimize deformity and maximize normal growth and development. Although JRA is often chronic, the prognosis for most children is good. At least 75% of patients eventually enter long periods of disease quiescence or remission, with little or no residual disability (12). Many parents and children are alarmed by the diagnosis; thus, effective treatment begins with detailed education of the patient, parents, and the child's community. Attention to counseling needs are important, and schools should also be actively involved.

The immediate therapeutic goals for JRA are relief of symptoms, maintenance of joint range of motion and muscle strength in patients seen early in their illness, and rehabilitation of those seen later in the disease. Physical, emotional and pharmacologic aspects of therapy are all important. Several unique aspects of pain perception in young people, however, should be recognized.

Many children with objective arthritis complain little of joint pain, particularly if they are younger than 10 years old, have long-standing disease, or are experiencing adolescent denial. Rather, they limit or modify any motion that would result in pain; thus, pediatric complaints of severe joint discomfort or pain at rest are distinctly unusual (13). Morning gelling and stiffness after periods of immobility, such as sitting in the classroom, are common in children. Diagnosis and follow-up assessment of treatment responses in the pediatric arthritides require careful, age-appropriate functional assessment, evaluation of ambulation, and parental description of subtle changes in play activities. The lack of verbally accurate descriptions of pain, discomfort, or dysfunction in young children is a significant impediment to optimal care.

Parents, physicians, and patients may develop a false sense of security related to a lack of complaints.

Although aspirin remains the single most effective, and least expensive, antiinflammatory medication for JRA, public acceptance in the U.S. has been severely compromised by its association with the occurrence of Reye's syndrome. Aspirin should be started at a dosage of 75–90 mg/kg/day. Marked systemic or polyarticular involvement may require incremental increases to a level of 100–120 mg/kg/day if good results are not obtained at lower dosages. Serum salicylate levels should be monitored to achieve a range of 18–25 mg/dl. Levels above 30 mg/dl do not increase therapeutic benefit but do increase side effects (1,2). Giving aspirin with snacks, meals, or antacids helps minimize gastrointestinal irritation. Some children may be more tolerant of swallowing an enteric-coated tablet, and liquid choline salicylate may be useful for young children who are unable or unwilling to swallow tablets.

Elevated serum transaminase levels are intermittently found in some children taking aspirin and are more common as the dose increases. Enzyme values, decreased appetite, and vague abdominal discomfort return to normal when the aspirin is briefly stopped and then resumed at a 20% lower dose.

Reye's syndrome, including persistent vomiting and alterations in behavior or mentation, occurs more frequently in children who are treated with aspirin for fever accompanying viral infections such as chickenpox or influenza. Serum transaminase levels are elevated due to fatty metamorphosis of the liver. Both the overall use of aspirin and the frequency of Reye's syndrome appear to be decreasing. Children with JRA undergoing long-term treatment with high doses of salicylate have not been shown to have any increased frequency of clinical Reye's syndrome. However, aspirin should be briefly discontinued following exposure to, or infection with, varicella, influenza, or unknown viruses. This does not adversely affect the course of JRA.

Many children with JRA are now treated with other nonsteroidal antiinflammatory drugs (NSAIDs). Ibuprofen, tolmetin, naproxen, and fenoprofen have been approved for use in patients under 14 years of age. For patients over 14, any of the NSAIDs can be employed. Indomethacin may be useful as a night-time adjunct to reduce morning stiffness, for pericarditis, or for persistent enthesopathy. Because exacerbations often occur after brief remissions, aspirin and other NSAIDs should be continued for 12 to 18 months after all clinical manifestations of disease have disappeared.

If JRA is incompletely responsive to aspirin or other NSAIDs after several months, intramuscular gold therapy may be added. Gold is as effective in the treatment of children as it is in adults (14). It is given at a dosage of 1 mg/kg each week, up to a maximum of the adult dosage of 50 mg weekly. Therapy should be monitored by blood counts, urinalyses, and physical examinations. Gold is often continued for several years. Oral weekly pulse methotrexate, 10 mg/M^2, is now often substituted if gold is ineffective, or may be started before gold (15). Cumulative data from 183 children in five studies showed 15% had mild and reversible side effects; however, 60% to 90% demonstrated significant benefit (16). Methotrexate should be considered early for the treatment of severe, long-standing, corticosteroid-dependent, or rapidly progressive JRA.

Hydroxychloroquine and D-penicillamine have been used in JRA with results less favorable than those seen in adults. Use is generally only adjunctive, or for methotrexate or gold treatment failures (17).

Systemic corticosteroids are contraindicated in the treatment of JRA, except for patients with severe polyarthritis or systemic disease that have incompletely responded to methotrexate or an adequate trial of gold. Oral corticosteroid therapy should begin with an alternate day regimen, and must include good parent and patient education about growth suppression and other toxicities. Very rarely, advancement to daily dosages will be required if improvement is inadequate. Another approach for the severely ill child, particularly early in the disease while awaiting the benefits of methotrexate or gold, is to give two to three daily doses (1 gm/M^2; 1 gm maximum) of methylprednisolone pulse therapy. There is no indication for systemic corticosteroids in pauciarticular or mild polyarticular JRA. Disabling pain or flexion contracture in one or a few joints may occasionally be treated by intraarticular corticosteroid injections (18).

Management of iridocyclitis depends on early detection, always in cooperation with an ophthalmologist. Topical corticosteroids, dilating agents, and close follow-up will often control ocular inflammation. If not, systemic corticosteroids may be required. Immunosuppressive agents such as chlorambucil or cyclophosphamide can be successfully used in severe, unremittent iritis due to JRA, but these remain strictly experimental approaches, requiring experienced supervision (11). There is suggestive evidence that NSAIDs, gold, and methotrexate may delay onset, or at least ameliorate, the severity of iridocyclitis in JRA.

Muscle weakness and atrophy, decreased endurance, and contractures are features of JRA that contribute significantly to disability. Exercises to maximize muscle strength, joint ranges of motion, and function are extremely valuable. Evaluations by physical and occupational therapists are important. Treatment plans should reflect the child's level of maturity; be performed daily; and be adopted by child, parents, and school as part of their normal activities of daily living. Written guidelines are available from the Arthritis Foundation and from the National Arthritis Information Clearinghouse.

Morning baths are excellent to relieve stiffness, but are difficult for busy families. An auxillary electric blanket plugged into a timer, set to activate one hour before the child arises, is an effective alternative. Emphasis on good posture should start at diagnosis. Wrist contractures may be reduced by the use of resting splints, a soft cervical collar may retard neck flexion deformities, and daily adoption of the prone position for extended periods may reduce hip flexion contractures. Serial casting, splinting, or soft tissue releases, particularly of the knees, ankles, and fingers, may be required to reduce unyielding contractures. Such interventions must always be combined with active physical therapy. Bed rest is contraindicated, and children with JRA should be encouraged to be physically active, as tolerated.

Synovectomy does not benefit the course of JRA, but may be helpful for pain reduction in rare instances. Total joint replacements may greatly improve function in long-standing disease, but must await full bone growth near affected joints. Early closure of epiphyses, although complicated by reduced total bone size, may permit surgery by the early to mid teenage years.

Children with JRA should be strongly encouraged to be self-sufficient and responsible to an age-appropriate extent, should attend regular schools, and lead as normal lives as possible. Adaptive devices may be helpful in achieving independence in some cases. Vocational and psychological counseling are often beneficial for teenagers, even in the absence of significant disabilities. The goal of all treatment for JRA is to optimize health status and functional outcomes (19).

JUVENILE SPONDYLARTHROPATHIES

Ankylosing spondylitis, Reiter's syndrome, psoriatic arthritis, and the spondylarthropathies associated with regional enteritis and ulcerative colitis, often present diagnostic difficulty in children (2,20–22). Enthesopathy may be present historically or on examination. Early arthritis can simulate pauciarticular JRA. There usually is no clinical or roentgenographic evidence of sacroiliac or spine involvement for months to years after onset. The spondylarthropathies occur more often in boys than in girls, frequently manifest as asymmetric lower extremity or large joint arthritis, and commonly occur in children who have a positive family history. Other features include involvement of the first metatarsophalangeal joint and an inflammatory enthesopathy that occurs particularly at the insertions of the plantar fascia, Achilles tendons, and infrapatellar ligaments. Palpation and percussion of the heels, sacroiliac joints, and costochondral junctions are important techniques in children, as is a detailed search for early eczema or psoriaform lesions.

HLA–B27 typing may be of some diagnostic and prognostic aid in children, because of incomplete spondylopathic disease expression, less accurate histories, infrequent clinical back symptoms, and often sparse family histories from young parents. Roentgenograms of the sacroiliac joints and back are rarely abnormal at disease onset in children, and only 20% become abnormal even after five years of illness.

Juvenile ankylosing spondylitis (JAS) may comprise 10% of children with arthritis, but the absence of uniform diagnostic criteria for JAS remains a major problem (2). Ninety percent of children with JAS have HLA–B27 (1,2,8), with a 7:1 ratio of boys to girls. Disease onset is from late childhood to adolescence. Peripheral arthritis characteristically develops before back involvement in JAS, and joints of the lower extremities, especially hips, are most commonly affected. About 25% of children will exhibit polyarticular arthritis. Only one-fourth of children with JAS have axial or sacroiliac symptoms at onset. Roentgenograms are of little help in diagnosis of early disease due to the normally widened, irregular, and poorly defined sacroiliac margins in children. Evidence of enthesopathy should always be sought in children with arthritis, and its presence should prompt careful examination of the back and sacroiliac joints, a Schöber test, and good follow up (20). Acute iritis, pulmonary disease, and aortic valve insufficiency may develop in JAS, as they do in adults. Good prognostic and outcome information is not yet available.

Reiter's syndrome (RS) in children most frequently develops as a reactive arthritis following *Shigella*, *Salmonella*, or *Yersinia* associated diarrhea (80%) (21). Children with RS as young as 18 months have been reported. This disorder is probably significantly under-recognized in children, because conjunctivitis, minimal pyuria, dysuria, diarrhea, and brief extremity complaints are common pediatric problems. Onset can be acute, febrile, and polyarticular, with protean features mimicking systemic onset JRA. In some children, weight loss and enthesitis are dramatic. Mucocutaneous manifestations of RS are less common in children than adults, and the ratio of boys to girls is only about 4:1. Erythrocyte sedimentation rates are often very high, and 90% of children with RS are HLA–B27 positive. The potential for long-term disability from Reiter's syndrome is also important.

Psoriatic arthritis occurs in 10% to 15% of children with all forms of chronic arthritis. Diagnostic skin changes may lag behind joint disease by up to 15 years. Nail pitting, ridging, or onycholysis, and atypical rash behind the ears, at the scalp line, umbilicus, or extensor surfaces may provide early clues (22). A positive family history of psoriasis occurs in 40% of cases, girls exceed boys by 2:1, and one-half have a pauciarticular onset arthritis. Involvement of the toes, a single small joint such as a distal interphalangeal or dactylitis are suggestive of the diagnosis. Intermittent, usually pauciarticular arthritis is also a common complication of pediatric regional enteritis and ulcerative colitis. The cumulative prevalence of joint involvement is 10%.

Management of childhood spondylarthropathies includes education; physical treatment modalities; and attention to school, growth and development, and remaining as active as possible. Pharmacotherapy may begin with aspirin or ibuprofen, but tolmetin sodium or indomethacin are often added or substituted relatively quickly in difficult cases, and may be followed by either sulfasalazine or oral weekly methotrexate. Severe inflammatory bowel disease or aggressive iridocyclitis may require systemic corticosteroids as adjunctive treatment.

Bernhard H. Singsen, MD, MPH

1. Jacobs JC: Pediatric Rheumatology for the Practitioner. New York, Springer-Verlag, 1982, pp 1–556

2. Cassidy JT, Petty RE: Textbook of Pediatric Rheumatology, 2nd ed. New York, Churchill Liningstone, 1990, pp 1–607

3. Gedalia A, Person DA, Brewer EJ, et al: Hypermobility of the joints in juvenile episodic arthritis/arthralgia. J Pediatr 107:873–876, 1985

4. Sherry DD, McGuire T, Mellins E, et al: Psychosomatic musculoskeletal pain in childhood: clinical and psychological analyses of 100 children. Pediatrics 88: 1093–1099, 1991

5. Yunus MG, Masi AT: Juvenile primary fibromyalgia syndrome: a clinical study of 33 patients and matched normal controls. Arthritis Rheum 28:138–145, 1985

6. Singsen BH: Epidemiology of the rheumatic diseases of childhood. Rheum Dis Clin North Am 16:581–599, 1990

7. Hanson V: From Still's disease and JRA to JCPA, JCA, and JA: medical progress or biased ascertainment? J Rheumatol 9:819–820, 1982

8. Lang BA, Shore A: A review of current concepts on the pathegenesis of juvenile rheumatoid arthritis. J Rheumatol (suppl 21) 17:1–15, 1990

9. Moore TK, Osborn TG, Weiss RD, et al: Autoantibodies in juvenile arthritis. Semin Arthritis Rheum 13:329–336, 1986

10. Melin-Aldana H, Giannini EH, Glass DN: Immunogenetics of early onset pauciarticular juvenile rheumatoid arthritis. J Rheumatol (suppl 26) 17:2–15, 1990

11. Hemady RK, Baer JC, Foster CS: Immunosuppressive drugs in the management of progressive, corticosteroid-resistant uveitis associated with juvenile rheumatoid arthritis. Internat Ophthalmol Clin 32:241–252, 1992

12. Hanson V, Kornreich H, Bernstein, et al: Prognosis of juvenile rheumatoid arthritis. Arthritis Rheum 20(suppl):279–284, 1977

13. Beales JG, Keen JH, Holt PJL: The child's perception of the disease and the experience of pain in juvenile chronic arthritis. J Rheumatol 10:61–65, 1983

14. Brewer EJ, Jr., Giannini EH, Barkely E: Gold therapy in the management of juvenile rheumatoid arthritis. Arthritis Rheum 23:404–411, 1980

15. Wallace CA, Bleyer WA, Sherry DD, et al: Toxicity and serum levels of methotrexate in children with juvenile rheumatoid arthritis. Arthritis Rheum 32:667–681, 1989

16. Rose CD, Singsen BH, Eichenfield AH, et al: Safety and efficacy of methotrexate therapy in juvenile rheumatoid arthritis. J Pediatr 117:653–659, 1990

17. Grondin C, Malleson P, Petty RE: Slow-acting anti-rheumatic drugs in chronic arthritis of childhood. Semin Arth Rheum 18:38–47, 1988

18. Allen RC, Gross KR, Laxer RM, et al: Intraarticular triamcinolone hexacetonide in the management of chronic arthritis in children. Arthritis Rheum 29:997–1001, 1986

19. Singsen BH: Health status (arthritis impact) in children with chronic rheumatic diseases: current measurement issues and an approach to instrument design. Arthritis Care and Res 4:87–101, 1991

20. Burgos-Vargas R, Petty RE: Juvenile ankylosing spondylitis. Rheum Dis Clin North Am 18:123–142, 1992

21. Rosenberg AM, Petty RE: Reiter's disease in children. Am J Dis Child 133:394–398, 1979

22. Shore A, Ansell BM: Juvenile psoriatic arthritis—an analysis of 60 cases. J Pediatr 100:529–535, 1982

B. Kawasaki Disease

Kawasaki disease, or acute infantile febrile mucocutaneous lymph node syndrome, is an acute febrile disease occurring predominantly in infants and children under five years of age (1,2). The male-to-female ratio is 1.3 to 1.5:1. The most serious clinical manifestation is the development of coronary artery aneurysms. Some of the aneurysms produce stenotic or occlusive lesions that may cause myocardial infarction or sudden death. Autopsy findings reveal coronary artery aneurysms with thrombosis in most of the fatal cases. The fatality rate in Japan is 0.1% to 0.3%.

CLINICAL FEATURES

In general, abrupt high fever without prodromal symptoms characterizes the onset of this disease. Usually, remittent or continuous fever ranging from 38°C to 40°C lasts for one to two weeks, with the mean peak fever reached between 39.0°C and 39.9°C. The longer the fever continues, the higher the possibility of coronary artery aneurysms.

Within two to five days after disease onset, conjunctival injection, redness of the lips and oral mucous membranes, and a polymorphous exanthem on the trunk, extremities or both occur. The skin lesions are not accompanied by vesicles or crusting. There is redness of the palms and soles and indurative edema of the hands (Fig. 22B–1) and feet. Occasionally, cervical adenopathy occurs. Symptoms may appear simultaneously or one after another at intervals. When the fever subsides, symptoms usually disappear.

From 10 to 15 days after the onset of the illness, desquamation of the skin occurs, beginning at the tip of the fingers and spreading over the palm up to the wrist. About two months after the

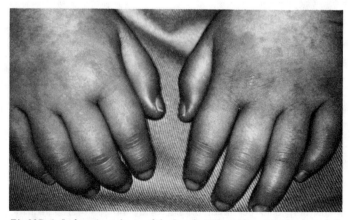

Fig 22B–1. *Indurative edema of the hands with erythema is characteristic of Kawasaki disease.*

Table 22B–1. Diagnostic criteria for Kawasaki disease

At least five of the following requirements must be fulfilled:
1. Fever persisting five days or more
2. Peripheral extremities:
   Initial stage: Reddening of palms and soles, indurative edema
   Convalescent stage: Membranous desquamation from fingertips
3. Polymorphous exanthema
4. Bilateral conjunctival congestion
5. Lips and oral cavity: Reddening of lips, strawberry tongue, diffuse injection of oral and pharyngeal mucosa
6. Acute nonpurulent cervical lymphadenopathy

onset, transverse furrows frequently appear in the nails of the fingers and toes.

Mild pancarditis frequently occurs in the acute stage. Auscultation may reveal a gallop rhythm and distant heart sounds. Two-dimensional echocardiography demonstrates coronary aneurysms or dilatation in approximately 40% of all patients during the period of one to four weeks from disease onset (3,4). Thirty days after onset, however, the rate decreases to approximately 20% of all patients, and by 60 days after onset the rate is reduced to approximately 10%. At one year after onset, only 3% to 5% of patients continue to show coronary aneurysms.

Recent coronary angiographic studies have revealed that large aneurysms with a diameter of more than 8 mm do not show regression, and the possibility of developing stenosis or occlusion in such patients is very high (5). The prognosis is favorable for patients with aneurysms of less than 8 mm in diameter.

Other features that may occur include diarrhea, abdominal pain, gall bladder hydrops, paralytic ileus, arthralgia or arthritis, aseptic meningitis, facial palsy, hemiplegia, and encephalopathy.

The diagnostic criteria for Kawasaki disease (2) are listed in Table 22B–1. At least five items should be present for the clinical diagnosis. Patients with four of the principal symptoms, however, may be diagnosed as having Kawasaki disease when coronary aneurysm is recognized by two-dimensional echocardiography or coronary angiography.

LABORATORY FINDINGS

During the acute phase of the illness, laboratory findings reveal leukocytosis with a left shift in the differential, thrombocytosis, increased erythrocyte sedimentation rate, and an elevated C-reactive protein. Serum transaminase levels are often elevated. Urinalysis may reveal proteinuria and increased leukocytes in the urine sediment.

An electrocardiogram may show different degrees of PQ and QT interval prolongation, low voltage, ST and T wave changes, and arrhythmias.

EPIDEMIOLOGY AND ETIOLOGY

Kawasaki disease occurs internationally (5–8) and in all races, but is especially common among Japanese children. By the end of 1990, 105,627 cases had been reported in Japan. Between 1979 and 1986, there were three major epidemics of the disease. Each of the epidemics lasted approximately six months.

In the United States and Korea, outbreaks have been reported in several cities at two- to four-year intervals. There have been reports of Kawasaki disease from almost every country in the world.

Several etiologic hypotheses have been proposed, including infection with *Rickettsia*, mite antigen, *Propionibacterium acnes* and retrovirus (9,10). None of these reports has been confirmed.

Some researchers now think that a microorganism acts as a trigger to disturb the immune system and thus gives rise to immunoregulatory abnormalities that cause the features of the disease (11). Marked activation of T cells and monocyte/macrophages can be demonstrated, including an expansion of a cell population that expresses the T-cell receptor variable regions V beta 2+ and V beta 8.1+ (12). Recent findings suggest that the cytokine interleukin–1 mediates an increased expression of activation antigens on endothelial cells (13).

TREATMENT

For the acute phase of Kawasaki disease, high-dose intravenous gammaglobulin treatment with aspirin is indicated. The recommended dose of gammaglobulin is 400 mg/kg/day for four or five days (14). Recently, infusion therapy with a single dose of gammaglobulin (2gm/kg/8–10 hours) has been reported to be effective (15). The dose of aspirin is 30 to 100 mg/kg/day (16).

Kawasaki disease patients should be admitted to the hospital and closely monitored for coronary artery changes using two-dimensional echocardiography. For patients with coronary aneurysms that persist, low-dose aspirin, 3–5 mg/kg/day, should be administered until the aneurysms disappear.

Patients with large aneurysms or myocardial infarction should be monitored with selective coronary angiography as well as two-dimensional echocardiography. In rare instances, coronary bypass surgery should be considered (17).

Tomisaku Kawasaki, MD

1. Kawasaki T: Clinical features of Kawasaki syndrome. Acta Paediatr Jpn 25:79–90, 1983
2. Diagnostic Guidelines for Kawasaki Disease, 4th rev ed, September 1984, prepared by The Japan Kawasaki Disease Research Committee, c/o Department of Pediatrics, Japanese Red Cross Medical Center, Tokyo, Japan
3. Kato H, Koike S, Yamamoto M, et al: Coronary aneurysms in infants and young children with acute febrile mucocutaneous lymph node syndrome. J Pediatr 86:892–898, 1975
4. Nakano H, Ueda K, Saito A, et al: Repeated quantitative angiograms in coronary arterial aneurysm in Kawasaki disease. Am J Cardiol 56:846–851, 1985
5. Kato H, Ichinose E, Kawasaki T: Myocardial infarction in Kawasaki disease: clinical analysis in 195 cases. J Pediatr 108:923–927, 1986
6. Yanagawa H, Nakamura Y, Kawasaki T, et al: Nationwide epidemic of Kawasaki disease in Japan during winter of 1985–1986. Lancet ii:1138–1139, 1986
7. Melish ME, Hicks RM, Larson EJ: Mucocutaneous lymph node syndrome in the United States. Am J Dis Child 103:599–607, 1976
8. Lee DB: Epidemiologic survey of Kawasaki syndrome in Korea (1976–1984). J Catholic Med College 38:13–19, 1985
9. Shulman ST, Rowley AH: Does Kawasaki disease have a retroviral aetiology? Lancet ii:545–546, 1986
10. Burns JC, Geha RS, Schneeberger, et al: Polymerase activity in lymphocyte culture supernatants from patients with Kawasaki disease. Nature 323:814–816, 1986
11. Leung DYM, Collins T, Lapierre LA, et al: Immunoglobulin M antibodies present in the acute phase of Kawasaki syndrome lyse cultured vascular endothelial cells stimulated by gamma interferon. J Clin Invest 77:1428–1435, 1986
12. Abe J, Kotzin BL, Jujo K, et al: Selective expansion of T cells expressing T–cell receptor variable regions V beta 2 and V beta 8 in Kawasaki disease. Proc Natl Acad Sci 89:4066–4070, 1992
13. Leung DY, Cotran R, Kurt-Jones E, et al: Endothelial cell activation and high interleukin–1 secretion in the pathogenesis of acute Kawasaki disease. Lancet 2:1298–1302, 1989
14. Furusho K, Kamiya T, Nakano H, et al: High-dose intravenous gammaglobulin for Kawasaki disease. Lancet ii:1055–1058, 1984
15. Newburger JW, Takahashi M, Beiser AS, et al: A single intravenous infusion of gammaglobulin as compared with four infusions in the treatment of acute Kawasaki syndrome. N Engl J Med 324:1633–1639, 1991
16. Kato H, Koike S, Yokoyama T: Kawasaki disease: effect of treatment on coronary artery involvement. Pediatrics 63:175–179, 1979
17. Kitamura S, Kawachi K, Oyama C, et al: Severe Kawasaki heart disease treated with an internal mammary artery graft in pediatric patients. J Thorac Cardiovasc Surg 89:860–866, 1985

C. Other Pediatric Rheumatic Diseases

The spectrum of other pediatric rheumatologic diseases includes inflammatory systemic connective tissue diseases along with infectious diseases, malignancies, mechanical problems such as orthopedic conditions, genetic abnormalities, and psychological dysfunction. Overall, pediatric connective tissue diseases are less common than their adult counterparts. The recently published experience of a pediatric rheumatology clinic serving a population of 290,000 in Canada gives an idea of how commonly the different diagnoses are made in a referral setting (1). Of 875 children seen with musculoskeletal complaints, a definite diagnosis was made in 58%. Thirty-eight percent of the total (335 children) had a classic inflammatory arthropathy, the most common being juvenile rheumatoid arthritis (JRA) and spondylarthropathy, which together accounted for 30% of the total. Seven percent (62 children) had other connective tissue diseases. In order of decreasing frequency these were vasculitis, systemic lupus erythematosus (SLE), dermatomyositis, and scleroderma (Tables 22C–1). Other causes of musculoskeletal symptoms are shown in Table 22C–2.

VASCULOPATHIES

Vasculitis can be both a primary childhood disease and a feature of other syndromes such as dermatomyositis and SLE. The classification of the primary vasculitis syndromes includes leukocytoclastic vasculitis (Henöch–Schönlein purpura, anaphy-

lactoid purpura, hypersensitivity vasculitis); polyarteritis nodosa, both cutaneous and generalized; Kawasaki disease (covered in Chapter 22B); and granulomatous diseases including Wegener's granulomatosis (2). Recently, antiphospholipid vasculopathy has been recognized in childhood.

Henöch–Schönlein Purpura

One of the most common forms of vasculitis in childhood is Henöch–Schönlein purpura, a syndrome consisting of rash, arthritis, abdominal pain, and renal dysfunction. The signs and symptoms persist for several days to weeks. Henöch–Schönlein purpura usually occurs in previously healthy 5 to 15 year-old children, with a prior history of upper respiratory infection and no previous drug exposure. The characteristic cutaneous lesions consist of palpable purpura located most commonly on the buttocks and lower extremities and accentuated in areas of pressure such as around the waist or sock line (Fig. 22C–1). The lesions come in crops with recurrences occurring in up to one-half of the children. The rash progresses from red to purple to brown. Regional subcutaneous edema of the extremities, scalp, eyes, or scrotum can occur early in the disease. Approximately 80% of cases will have arthritis or arthralgias of the large joints; small joints may also be affected. There are no long-term arthritic deformities. Gastrointestinal manifestations, which usually present with cramping umbilical pain, occur in 20% to 40% of

Table 22C–1. *Inflammatory rheumatic disease diagnoses in 337 children**

Disease or condition	Patients with Diagnosis
Juvenile rheumatoid arthritis	
Pauciarticular	97
Polyarticular	42
Systemic	17
Total	156
Spondylarthropathies	
Seronegative enthesopathy arthropathy syndrome (excluding patients with diagnoses of another spondyloarthropathy)	54
Reactive arthritis	22
Arthritis associated with inflammatory bowel desease	8
Ankylosing spondylitis	7
Reiter's syndrome	6
Psoriatic arthritis	5
Acne arthropathy	1
Behcet's disease	1
Total	104
Connective tissue or collagen vascular disease	
Henoch-Schönlein purpura	20
Kawasaki's disease	13
Systemic lupus erythematosus	10
Localized or linear scleroderma	7
Dermatomyositis	5
Raynaud's disease	4
Neonatal lupus	1
Polyarteritis	1
Wegener's granulomatosis	1
Total	62
Other rheumatic diseases	
Acute rheumatic fever	7
Arthropathy associated with cystic fibrosis	4
Reflex sympathetic dystrophy	1
Sarcoidosis	1
Total	13

*From reference 1, with permission.

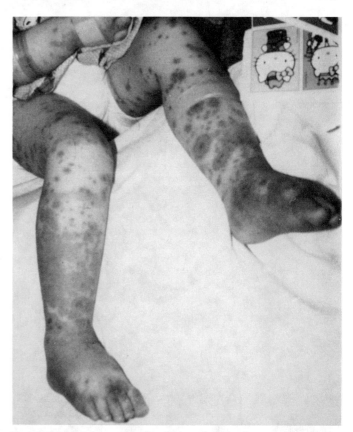

Fig. 22C–1. *Five-year old girl with Henöch–Schönlein purpura showing coalescing purpura over the extremities and swelling in both feet.*

cases and are usually present within a week of onset of the rash. Complications of gastrointestinal involvement include bleeding, intussusception, infarction, and perforation. Approximately 50% of children will develop nephritis ranging from microscopic hematuria and proteinuria to nephrotic syndrome and renal failure. Five to ten percent of children with this syndrome develop serious renal disease; usually this occurs within one to three months of onset. Most cases run their course within four weeks. Recurrences can occur up to two years later, are more common in older children, and often are associated with an upper respiratory infection.

No laboratory test is specific for Henöch–Schölein purpura. The platelet count is normal, which differentiates this syndrome from thrombocytopenic purpura. The white blood count is usually elevated, and a normochromic anemia is common. Serum IgA and IgM are elevated in one-half of the children and antinuclear antibodies and rheumatoid factors are not found. A skin biopsy may help in the diagnosis by showing a leukocytoclastic vasculitis with deposition of IgA and C_3 in the vessel wall.

Prognosis is good, with only 5% of patients progressing to renal failure. Treatment should consist of supportive care with maintenance of hydration and nutrition. Corticosteroids are usually not required unless there is serious gastrointestinal disease. The treatment of the renal disease is controversial, with most studies concluding that steroids alone are unhelpful.

Polyarteritis Nodosa and Other Vasculopathies

Polyarteritis nodosa or vasculitis of the small- and medium-sized vessels has been reported throughout childhood. Infantile polyarteritis nodosa or polyarteritis nodosa before the age of one are now considered to be under the category of Kawasaki disease. Most children with polyarteritis nodosa are between 9 and 11 years of age and do not meet the criteria for Kawasaki disease. The clinical manifestations are similar to adult polyarteritis nodosa (see Chapter 17).

Wegener's granulomatosis is uncommon in childhood with about 30 cases reported in the literature (3). The clinical findings are similar to those found in adults. Other vasculopathies such as antiphospholipid syndrome, Takayasu's arteritis and Behcet's syndrome also occur rarely in children. Antiphospholipid syndrome may present as chorea or lower extremity thrombosis (4). Takayasu's arteritis is rare in childhood and presents with hypertension and abnormal pulses. The abdominal aorta is the most frequent large vessel involved. Behcet's syndrome (Chapter 29) is also uncommon in childhood (5). Two very rare types of vasculopathy seen primarily in childhood are Moya Moya and Mucha–Habermann disease. Moya Moya is a description of an angiographic finding showing multiple stenoses of vessels around the circle of Willis with telangiectatic collateral vessels giving the appearance of a "puff of smoke" (6) (Fig. 22C–2). Children typically present with a stroke. Mucha–Habermann disease is a

Table 22C–2. *Other musculoskeletal disease diagnoses in 538 children*

Nonrheumatic Condition	Patients with Diagnosis
Mechanical (patella-femoral knee pain, Scheuermann's disease, benign hypermobility, enthesitis)	79
Infection (osteomyelitis, discitis, septic arthritis, postviral myositis or arthritis)	33
Neoplastic	
malignant	11
benign (osteoid osteoma, leukemia, neuroblastoma)	4
Other diseases (growing pains, serum sickness, ITP)	70
Conditions not yet diagnosed (arthralgia, back pain, arthritis)	272
Diagnoses of connective tissue diseases suspected not firmly established	23
Referrals to rule out a diagnosis (neonatal lupus, JRA as cause of uveitis)	45

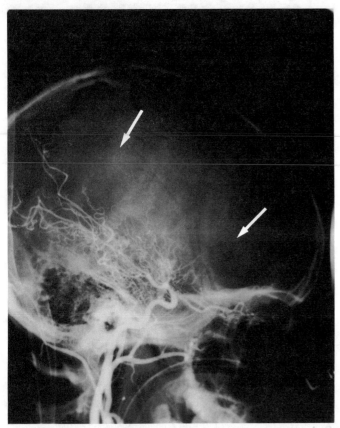

Fig. 22C–2. *Arteriogram demonstrating "puff of smoke" vascular abnormality seen in Moya Moya disease.*

cutaneous perivasculitis. The skin lesions resemble chicken pox lesions that become atrophic and scarred. The lesions can occur in association with fever and large joint arthritis (7).

SYSTEMIC LUPUS ERYTHEMATOSUS

Systemic lupus erythematosus is rare under the age of five years. The incidence increases with age until adulthood. The female to male ratio in children is 4.3:1. The incidence is about 0.6/100,000. Previously it was believed that pediatric SLE had a worse prognosis than adult SLE, but recent studies have shown children do as well as adults.

The presenting signs and symptoms of SLE in childhood are similar to those in adults (Chapter 11), although systemic features such as fever (76%), lymphadenopathy (40%), and nephritis (87%) are slightly more common in childhood onset than adult onset SLE (8). Almost all children have some form of renal disease ranging from minimal or mesangial glomerulonephritis, to focal proliferative glomerulonephritis, to diffuse proliferative glomerulonephritis. Membranous glomerulonephritis can also occur. Central nervous system involvement and cognitive disturbance may be subtle. Pulmonary symptoms can be found in 19% to 36% of cases with pleuritic chest pain being one of the most common symptoms. Arthritis and arthralgia are frequent but rarely cause residual problems except for osteonecrosis, which tends to be more frequent in pediatric cases. Destructive arthritis is rare except in children whose disease begins with a JRA-like illness (9).

The prognosis for children with SLE has improved over the last 30 years with 10-year survival at 80% in the 1980s versus 20% in the 1960s. A large study of children with SLE and renal disease showed that proteinuria, hematuria, hypertension, and biopsy-proven diffuse proliferative glomerulonephritis are all significant predictors of renal failure (10). The most common causes of death are infection and renal failure. Growing attention is being paid to an increased incidence of atherosclerosis in young adults who have had SLE since childhood. Accelerated atherosclerosis in this population may be due to coronary vasculitis or the effects of corticosteroids on lipid profiles.

Given the increase in survival of children with SLE, physicians need to focus more attention on the morbidity of the disease and complications of therapy. In a recent study of the morbidity of childhood SLE, approximately 84% of cases had a noninfectious or drug-related complication such as cataracts, osteopenia, diabetes, impotence, Cushingoid facies, short stature, osteonecrosis, or neuropsychological dysfunction. Eighty-eight percent of patients had chronic organ dysfunction at a five-year follow-up (11).

The current approach to treatment of the child with SLE at high risk for renal failure is still controversial. The use of pulse cyclophosphamide has been shown to be safe and efficacious in studies with children after one year of follow-up (12). Only one long-term study involving a small group of children has been reported. Over one-half of the children had worsening of their renal disease either during therapy or shortly after discontinuing intravenous cyclophosphamide. Because most children who develop SLE do so during adolescence, physicians need to be knowledgeable about adolescent stages of physical and psychological development and the effect of chronic disease on the adolescent and family. Issues of appearance, compliance, independence, career maturity, and pregnancy become central in treating adolescents with chronic illnesses.

Drug-induced lupus syndromes occur in children exposed to anticonvulsants such as diphenylhydantoin, methylphenylhydantoin, and other drugs including trimethadione, hydralazine, sulfonamide, sulfasalazine, and chlorpromazine.

Neonatal SLE

Children born to mothers with clinical SLE or more commonly, mothers who are asymptomatic but carry Sjogren's antibody Ro (SS–A) and La (SS–B), or both may develop certain manifestations of SLE in the neonatal period (13). This neonatal disease may be mediated by the transplacental passage of the SS–A and SS–B antibodies. Affected infants can develop transient abnormalities such as thrombocytopenia, neutropenia, hepatosplenomegaly, and cutaneous lesions including erythema annulare and discoid lupus lesions. The most serious complications of neonatal SLE involve permanent cardiac sequelae including congenital heart block, myocarditis, endocardial fibroelastosis, and other cardiac defects. The transient features regress in several weeks to months consistent with the normal half-life of maternal IgG in infants. Treatment of the transient autoimmune abnormalities is rarely necessary. However, treatment of the cardiac complications often requires a pacemaker.

JUVENILE DERMATOMYOSITIS

Juvenile dermatomyositis is an idiopathic inflammatory disease of the skin and muscle, often characterized by vasculitis in skin, muscle, and the gastrointestinal tract. The histologic presence of vasculitis, the onset of calcinosis and lack of association with malignancy in childhood are features distinctive of childhood dermatomyositis. Diagnosis requires presence of the typical rash, plus three of the following four criteria: 1) elevated muscle derived enzymes; 2) symmetric proximal muscle weakness; 3) evidence of vasculitis or chronic inflammation on muscle biopsy; and 4) an electromyogram confirming inflammatory myopathy. Polymyositis is much less common in children than adults. Juvenile dermatomyositis occurs most commonly between the ages of 5 and 14 and is more common in girls. The etiology is unknown but both genetics and infectious agents are felt to be important. There is serologic evidence in some studies that coxsackieviruses B and A-9 are causative agents, and echo virus has been implicated as the cause of a dermatomyositis-like illness in children with agammaglobulinemia.

In the majority of cases, children with juvenile dermatomyositis present with proximal muscle weakness that causes difficulty running, climbing stairs, or getting up from the floor. Unlike bacterial myositis, muscle pain is not a frequent complaint. Up to 20% of children with juvenile dermatomyositis have arthritis. Contractures are also seen, especially in children with a subacute onset. The characteristic rash may include a heliotrope discolor-

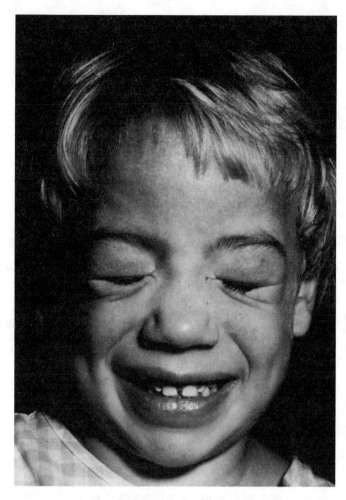

Fig. 22C–3. *The face of this child with dermatomyositis demonstrates heliotrope discoloration of the upper eyelids, periorbital edema, malar rash, and dry shiny erythematous involvement of the upper forehead. The facial rash of this disease can resemble that seen in SLE. The rash is frequently photosensitive and may be associated with mild alopecia (from the Revised Clinical Slide Collection on the Rheumatic Diseases).*

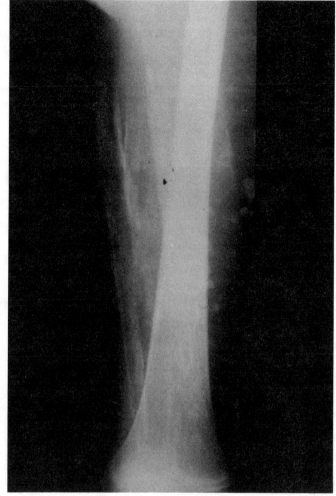

Fig. 22C–4. *Soft tissue calcification is seen in this radiograph of a child with juvenile dermatomyositis.*

ation of eye lids (Fig. 22C–3), telangiectasias, erythema of sun-exposed area of the upper torso or extensor surfaces of the extremities, and erythematous, scaling papules of the knuckles or proximal interphalangeal joints. These rashes can occur before or after the onset of myositis, or even in the absence of myositis. Ectopic calcification in the skin and muscles occurs in up to 50% of children but causes significant functional disability in only a small number (Fig. 22C–4). The diffuse vasculitis can result in telangiectasias of the nail beds and upper eye lids, and ulcerations of the digits, around the eyes, and in the skin folds of the axilla and groin. Gastrointestinal involvement can lead to poor absorption of medications, ulceration, and perforation. Myocarditis is common in up to 50% of children having abnormal electrocardiograms. Restrictive pulmonary findings on pulmonary function tests are sometimes found even when there are no symptoms.

Laboratory findings include elevated muscle enzymes as in adults, increased levels of factor VIII related antigens, and positive antinuclear antibody in up to 70% of patients. Antibodies to Jo–1 and PM–1 antigens are not found.

The differential diagnosis of juvenile dermatomyositis includes myositis secondary to other connective tissue diseases such as JRA, SLE, mixed connective tissue disease, and scleroderma; myositis secondary to bacterial or viral infection; drugs; trauma; and overuse of muscles. Neuromuscular diseases and myopathies, such as muscular dystrophy, and endocrine abnormalities such as hypothyroidism can cause elevated muscle enzymes and may mimic juvenile dermatomyositis.

The prognosis is good with less than 7% mortality. Various clinical courses have been described: monocyclic lasting approximately two years (80% of cases), chronic polycyclic, and chronic continuous. Those patients with the chronic form of the disease tend to have calcinosis and functional disability in adulthood. Standard treatment consists of prednisone, 2 mg/kg/day at onset, with a slow taper over two years once muscle enzyme elevations have normalized. To prevent or improve contractures, physical therapy is instituted once the muscles are less inflamed. In refractory cases methotrexate has been advocated, but controlled trials evaluating the efficacy of methotrexate in juvenile dermatomyositis are lacking (14).

OVERLAP SYNDROMES

Children with overlap syndromes or undifferentiated connective tissue disease, similar to their adult counterparts (Chapter 16) have more than one defined connective tissue disease (SLE, scleroderma, dermatomyositis), either at the same time or over time or incomplete syndromes. Children with overlap syndromes are rare, and only a few small series have been described (15). When compared to adult series, children with overlap syndromes appear to have an increased incidence of renal involvement, thrombocytopenia, pericarditis, Sjogren's syndrome, and skin rash. Treatment is based on the organ system involved and the degree of disease activity. The overall course appears less severe if the disease does not transform into one of the major connective tissue diseases such as juvenile dermatomyositis, SLE or systemic sclerosis.

SYSTEMIC SCLEROSIS

Systemic sclerosis (scleroderma) is rare in children (16). Less than 3% of all cases occur before age 16, and less than 1.5% develop before age 10. This disease in childhood differs from the

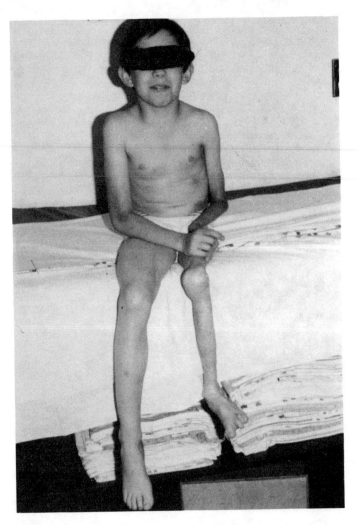

Fig. 22C–5. Boy with linear scleroderma effecting the upper and lower extremities resulting in growth abnormalities.

adult disease in that localized forms are more common than either limited or diffuse sclerosis. In children the skin, muscles, tendons, joints, and bones are affected often resulting in severe growth abnormalities. This pattern may reflect a predilection for structures with high collagen turnover in the developing child. Localized sclerosis includes a spectrum of skin lesions from morphea through linear type lesions. Morphea lesions can start with erythema and evolve into patches of firm, white, fibrotic skin. They may be single, multiple, or may coalesce. Linear type lesions have skin changes distributed along a dermatome pattern and can be self-limiting lasting three to four years. Linear scleroderma can involve atrophy of not only skin but also the underlying soft tissues, muscle, periosteum, and bone leading to extensive atrophy of a limb or marked growth defects (Fig. 22C–5). One linear localized lesion called coup de sabre involves the forehead and scalp and extends down over the face. Growth defects with or without joint contractures may be the presenting feature. Children with localized disease can be difficult to diagnose. They may appear to have juvenile arthritis but present with tendon nodules, stiffness, and limited motion and contractures of the joints with little evidence for synovitis. Prognosis of localized sclerosis except for the growth abnormalities is excellent; progression of localized scleroderma to diffuse systemic sclerosis in childhood is very rare.

Diffuse skin involvement with and without visceral involvement can occur in the pediatric age group. Approximately 50% of those with diffuse skin involvement will have visceral involvement. Children with internal organ involvement can be asymptomatic and detailed investigation should be performed. The generalized form of systemic sclerosis in childhood with Raynaud's phenomenon, skin, musculoskeletal, gastrointestinal, pulmonary, cardiac, and renal involvement is similar to that in adults

and treatment is also similar. For children, orthopedic, plastic, or facio-maxillary surgery may be required for severe growth defects.

Other sclerosis-like syndromes have been described in childhood. Eosinophilic fasciitis is similar to that seen in adults. Children with insulin-dependent diabetes can develop sclerosis-like skin changes of the hands associated with joint contractures. Most of these children have had long-standing diabetes and are over 12 years of age. Sclerotic skin changes are also seen in 90% of children with graft-versus-host reaction after bone marrow transplant.

REFLEX SYMPATHETIC DYSTROPHY

Reflex sympathetic dystrophy (RSD) is a pain amplification syndrome commonly seen in adolescents. It is associated with diffuse swelling, tenderness, and autonomic dysfunction (coolness, sweating, and mottling of the skin). The adolescent often refuses to move the affected extremity due to pain. Occasionally children with RSD appear to have "la belle indifference" when the affected limb is moved (17). Radiographs can demonstrate osteopenia if the RSD has been present for six to eight weeks. Technetium bone scans can show both an increase (early phase) and a decrease (late phase) in uptake of the affected limb. Treatment is most effective if the pain is controlled. Psychiatric treatment is used if necessary, and range of motion and use of the affected limb is restored through physical therapy.

MISCELLANEOUS CONDITIONS

Arthritis is a common finding in childhood. Many of the causes are discussed in other chapters, such as the arthritis associated with immunodeficiency (Chapter 44), arthritis associated with heritable disorders of connective tissue (Chapter 42), the syndromes associated with bone and joint dysplasias (Chapter 46), and hematologic diseases (Chapter 35). Several other conditions unique to children that are not covered elsewhere are mentioned below.

Transient or Toxic Synovitis of the Hip

This is one of the most common causes of hip pain in children between the ages of 3 and 10. This condition is often preceded by an upper respiratory tract infection and occurs most commonly in boys. Unilateral pain in the hip, thigh, or knee comes on either suddenly or gradually and can last for an average of six days. Low grade fever is often present. On physical examination there is a significant loss of internal rotation and abduction of the hip; laboratory studies usually show a normal white blood count (WBC) and erythrocyte sedimentation rate (ESR). If there is a high fever with an elevated WBC and ESR, a septic hip must be ruled out. Treatment of toxic synovitis of the hip consists of traction, bedrest, analgesics, and anti-inflammatories as needed. Long-term sequelae include Legg–Calvé–Perthes disease in approximately 1.5%, coxa magna, and osteoarthritis (18).

Granuloma Annulare/Benign Rheumatoid Nodule

Granuloma annulare is an asymptomatic subcutaneous nodular lesion that often develops over bony prominences and spontaneously regresses (19). Histologically this resembles a classic rheumatoid nodule. It is rare that a child with granuloma annulare or benign rheumatoid nodules will later develop arthritis. All routine laboratory tests are normal. Resolution of the lesions tends to occur months to years later.

Discitis

Discitis is a self-limited inflammation in the disc space (20). There is considerable debate as to whether or not it is secondary to an infectious process. Discitis occurs throughout childhood, but peak age of onset is between 1 and 3 years. Most often it presents in a young patient who has a low-grade fever and refuses to walk or sit. Older patients describe back pain and stiffness.

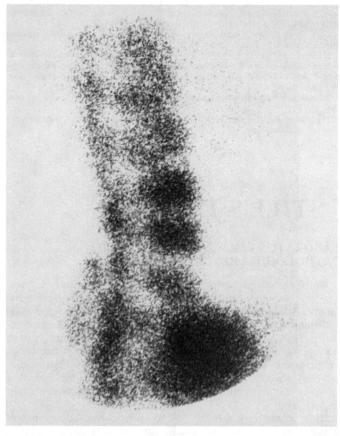

Fig. 22C–6. *Technetium bone scan demonstrating increased uptake in the lower lumbar vertebrae in four-year old boy with discitis.*

The lower lumbar vertebrae are most commonly affected. Palpation of the spine often reveals localized tenderness. A technetium bone scan is usually diagnostic (Fig. 22C–6). Treatment is supportive, including the use of back braces. Antibiotics are often started until blood cultures are negative.

Chronic Recurrent Multifocal Osteomyelitis

This condition is characterized by acute or insidious onset of multifocal areas of bone pain and bone lesions resembling osteomyelitis. Low-grade fevers are often present, and the course is one of recurrences and remissions. Biopsy material from the lesions are negative for any bacteria or fungus and show chronic inflammatory cells, necrosis, and new bone formation. Antibiotics are not helpful, but nonsteroidal antiinflammatory drugs may improve the painful episodes. In conjunction with the bone lesions, cutaneous complications (pustulosis palmaris et plantaris and psoriasis), oligoarthritis, and sacroiliitis have been described (21).

Infantile Cortical Hyperostosis

This is a rare disease presenting in an infant usually under four months of age. The symptoms and signs include fever, swelling, tenderness, and erythema of affected areas. Asymmetric enlargement of the mandible, shoulder, or large bones are most commonly affected. Radiographs show marked cortical thickening with irregular bone shape. The etiology is unknown, and it is usually self-limited lasting weeks to months (22).

Neuroblastoma

The differential diagnosis of fever and arthritis in a child includes malignancy. In children, leukemia (Chapter 35) and neuroblastoma are the most common. Neuroblastoma, a tumor of the sympathetic nervous system, is the most common tumor to produce skeletal metastases in childhood. Bone scintigraphy may be used to determine the location of the bone lesions.

Chronic Infantile Neurologic, Cutaneous, and Articular Syndrome

This syndrome is present from birth in a majority of the 30 cases reported. Distinctive features include systemic signs and symptoms, skin rash, joint inflammation, and central nervous system involvement. Most of the children are born prematurely and have a low birth weight. The course is one of recurring episodes of fever, lymphadenopathy, splenomegaly, arthritis, and rash. The rash appears at birth or shortly thereafter and consists of migratory, nonpuritic urticaria that is not vasculitic on biopsy. Joint involvement consists of swelling and warmth that is most pronounced during the febrile episodes. Non-axial joints are affected, with the knee being the most common. Over time there is overgrowth of the epiphyses resulting in contractures. The synovium and synovial fluid are normal or only mildly inflammatory. Central nervous system involvement is characterized by decreased mental capacity and chronic meningeal inflammation with headaches and seizures that worsen with age. There are visual abnormalities including optic atrophy, uveitis, and keratitis, as well as progressive deafness. The radiographic findings of the long bones are distinctive, showing flared, irregular, cupped metaphyses with enlarged, irregular and fragmented epiphyses. These abnormalities lead to growth retardation. The children have enlarged heads with frontal bossing and a saddle back nose along with clubbing of the fingers and toes. Laboratory studies show evidence of systemic inflammation with anemia, leukocytosis, thrombocytosis, and increased ESR. There is often early death or severe disability. The etiology is unknown and although the findings suggest a neonatal or intrauterine infection, none has been found (23).

Kashin–Beck and Mseleni Disease

An endemic symmetric, progressive, polyarthritic bony dysplasia has been described in children in Russia, northern China, and Korea called Kashin–Beck disease. The initial symptom of joint pain occurs in the school-age child and results in early osteoarthritis, dwarfing, and bone dysplasia (24). Another bone dysplasia resulting in irregular shape of the epiphysis and mild stunting of growth in the hips, knees, and ankles is found in the Mseleni area of northern Zululand giving it the name of Mselenic disease. Both bony dysplastic diseases are felt to be secondary to a nutritional deficiency or toxin in the food such as fungal infected grain (25).

Patience White, MD

1. Rosenberg AM: Analysis of a pediatric rheumatology clinic population. J Rheumatol 17:827–830, 1990
2. Dillon MJ: Vasculitis syndromes, Pediatric Rheumatology Update. Edited by Woo P, White P, Ansell B. New York, Oxford University Press, 1990, pp 227–242
3. Hall SL, Miller LC, Duggan E: Wegener's granulomatosis in pediatric patients. J Pediatric 106:739–744, 1985
4. Vlachogyiannopoulos PG, Dimov G, Siamopoulou-Mavridov A. Chorea as a manifestation of the anti-phospholipid syndrome in childhood. Clin Exp Rheum 9:303–305, 1991
5. Lang BA, Laxer RM, Thorner P, et al: Pediatric onset of Behcet's syndrome with myositis: Care report and literature review illustrating unusual features. Arthritis Rheum 33:418–428, 1990
6. Carlson CB, Harvey FH, Loop J: Progressive alternating hemiplegia in early childhood with basal artery stenosis and telangiectasia (Moya Moya syndrome). Neurology 23:734–744, 1973
7. Ellsworth JE, Cassidy JT, Ragsdale CG, et al: Mucha–Habermann disease in children: The association with rheumatic diseases. J Rheumatol 9:319–324, 1982
8. Hirsch R, White P: Systemic lupus erythematosus in children. Current Pediatrics 1:85–88, 1991
9. Ragsdale CG, Petty RE, Cassidy JT, et al: Clinical progression of apparent juvenile rheumatoid arthritis to systemic lupus erythematosus. J Rheumatol 7:50–55, 1980
10. Curdy DK, Lehman TJA, Bernstein B, et al: Lupus nephritis: Prognostic factors in children. Pediatrics 89:240–246, 1992
11. Lacks S, White P: Morbidity associated with childhood systemic lupus erythematosus. J Rheumatol 17:941–945, 1990
12. Lehman TJA, Sherry DD, Wagner-Weiner L, et al: Intermittent intravenous cyclophosphamide therapy for lupus nephritis. J Pediatr 114:1055–1060, 1989
13. Buyon JR, Winchester R: Congenital complete heart block. Arthritis Rheum 33:609–614, 1990
14. Miller LC, Sisson BA, Tucker LB, et al: Methotrexate treatment of childhood dermatomyositis. Arthritis Rheum 35:1143–1149, 1992

15. Allen RC, St-Cyr C, Maddison PH, et al: Overlap connective tissue syndromes. Arch Dis Child 61:284–288, 1986
16. Black C: Juvenile scleroderma, Paediatric Rheumatology Update. Edited by Woo P, White PH, Ansell B. New York, Oxford University Press, 1990, pp 194–208
17. Sherry DD, Weisman R: Psychologic aspect of childhood reflex neurovascular dystrophy. Pediatrics 81:572–578, 1988
18. Wingstrand H: Transient synovitis of the hip in the child. Aeta Orthrop Scand 57(Suppl):219, 1986
19. Trohan AP, Pachman LM, Esterly NB: Granuloma annulare. Arthritis Rheum 30:117–118, 1987
20. Crawford AH, Kucharzyle DW, Ruder R, et al: Discitis in children. Clin Orthop 206:70–79, 1991
21. Laxer RM, King S, Manson D, et al: Chronic recurrent multifocal osteomyelitis (CRMO)—a review of seven cases. Arthritis Rheum 30:S80, 1987
22. Caffey J: Infantile cortical hyperostosis: A review of the clinical and radiographic features. Proc R Soc Med 50:347, 1957
23. Prieur AM and Lovell D: The chronic, infantile, neurological, cutaneous, and articular syndrome (CINCA Europe, IOMID USA), Paediatric Rheumatology Update. Edited by Woo P, White PH, Ansell B. New York, Oxford University Press, 1990, pp 147–160
24. Sokoloff L: Kashin–Beck disease. Rheum Dis Clin North Am 13:101–104, 1987
25. Lockisentro G, Fellingham SA, Wittman W, et al: Mseleni joint disease: the pilot study. S Afr Med J 47:2283–2293, 1973

23. ADULT ONSET STILL'S DISEASE

Adult onset Still's disease is a form of polyarthritis associated with systemic manifestations identical to those described in children with systemic onset juvenile rheumatoid arthritis or Still's disease (1). Adult onset Still's disease has been increasingly recognized since Bywaters' description in 1971 (1). Adult onset Still's disease usually affects young adults, although the disease may be observed rarely in individuals older than 70 years of age. Both sexes are affected equally.

CLINICAL PRESENTATION

Common clinical features include sudden onset of high spiking fever, sore throat, and an evanescent erythematous salmon-colored rash (2–12) (Table 23–1). Fever and rash are often the only initial manifestations. The rash is maculopapular and mainly involves the trunk and extremities. Very often the rash is only seen during temperature spikes. In most patients it is nonpruritic and nonscarring, but occasionally itching can be prominent and residual skin hyperpigmentation is seen.

The musculoskeletal manifestations are important features and consist of myalgias and arthralgias, and oligoarticular or polyarticular arthritis. Arthritis usually affects the proximal interphalangeal (PIP) joints, metacarpophalangeal (MCP) joints, wrists, knees, hips, and shoulders. Synovitis is usually mild and can be transient, although some patients develop severe disability and progressive destruction of hip joints (7,11). Peripheral lymph node enlargement may be seen. Less often, patients present with splenomegaly, hepatomegaly, abdominal pain, pleuritis, pericarditis, and pneumonitis. Renal and central nervous system manifestations may develop, but are uncommon. A few patients with peripheral neuropathy have been reported. Although visceral involvement usually is not associated with organ failure, occasionally severe hepatic insufficiency, acute respiratory failure, congestive heart failure, cardiac tamponade, pericardial constriction, intravascular coagulation, severe anemia, and necrotizing lymphadenopathy may occur (7,12,13).

Table 23–1. *Clinical manifestations in 283 patients with adult onset Still's disease (adapted from references 9 and 12, with permission)*

Manifestation	Percent of Patients
Arthralgias	100
Fever > 39°C	97
Arthritis	94
Rash	87
Sore throat	64
Lymphadenopathy	63
Splenomegaly	52
Hepatomegaly	43
Pleuritis	31
Pericarditis	29
Abdominal pain	21
Nervous system involvement	7
Renal involvement	5
Eye involvement	4
Subcutaneous nodules	1

LABORATORY, RADIOGRAPHIC, AND PATHOLOGIC FEATURES

Nonspecific abnormalities are evident in laboratory studies. The erythrocyte sedimentation rate is elevated, often above 100 mm/hr. Peripheral neutrophilic leukocytosis, usually over 15,000 cells/mm^3 has been reported in most patients. A leukemoid reaction also may be seen as well as persistent and progressive normocytic, normochromic anemia in the absence of hemolysis or gastrointestinal bleeding. Elevation of serum hepatocellular enzymes can be seen with active disease alone and as a result of administration of nonsteroidal antiinflammatory drugs (NSAIDs).

High serum ferritin levels, up to 10 times the upper limit of normal, are often seen and usually correlate with disease activity (10,14). The ferritin level may be useful to support the clinical diagnosis and to monitor the effects of therapy (10). Characteristically, antinuclear antibodies and rheumatoid factor tests are negative, although in some series a few patients with low positive titers have been reported (8,10). Antistreptolysin O titers may be elevated as well, but on serial testing the titers remain constant. Associations with leukocyte histocompatibility antigens have been reported for the loci of HLA–B8, Bw35, B44, DR4, DR5, and DR7. These studies are not helpful in supporting a clinical diagnosis or in predicting the outcome of visceral or articular manifestations or drug side effects (12). A few patients have been described with rising titers of antibodies against mumps, rubella viruses, and *Yersinia enterocolitica*, although no viruses or bacteria have been isolated from inflamed articular tissues (15).

Periarticular demineralization can be the only radiographic finding. Bone erosions and subluxation are uncommon. There is a peculiar tendency for fusion of the carpometacarpal and intercarpal joints that is considered characteristic of the disease (Fig. 23–1). Involvement of the upper cervical apophyseal joints, tarsal and temporomandibular joints, and terminal phalangeal joints can be seen in up to 50% of the patients who have been followed for more than 10 years (11).

Examination of synovial fluid reveals a high leukocyte count and predominance of polymorphonuclear cells (7). The synovium shows signs of mild, chronic, nonspecific synovitis with moderate synovial cell proliferation, variable degree of vascular engorgement, and scattered or diffuse infiltrates with lymphocytes and plasma cells. The histopathologic findings in skin and visceral lesions are nonspecific (7,12).

DIAGNOSIS

The diagnosis of Still's disease is a clinical one. Differential diagnosis includes other conditions associated with high fever, sore throat, rash, and arthritis (16). These conditions include infections such as bacterial endocarditis, meningococcemia, gonococcemia, rubella, hepatitis B, parvovirus B19, secondary syphilis, Lyme disease, and toxic shock syndrome. Other conditions to include in the differential diagnosis are reactive arthritis, rheumatic fever, Reiter's syndrome, serum sickness, drug allergy, erythema multiforme, systemic lupus erythematosus,

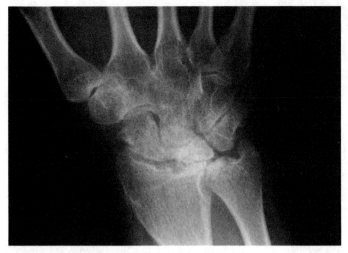

Fig. 23-1. *Radiograph illustrating ankylosis of the second and third carpometacarpal and intercarpal joints in a patient with adult onset Still's disease. Note also radioulnar erosion and radiocarpal disease.*

systemic vasculitis (including Kawasaki disease), as well as myeloproliferative or lymphoproliferative disorders (leukemia, angioblastic lymphadenopathy, and lymphoma).

Several reports have proposed diagnostic criteria to assist in the clinical diagnosis of individual cases and serve as classification criteria for clinical studies (7,8,10). However, none of these criteria has been validated. A combination of a high, spiking fever, arthritis persisting for at least six weeks, an evanescent maculopapular rash, and leukocytosis with neutrophilia or one of the other minor manifestations (Table 23-1) indicates a high probability or "definite" diagnosis of adult onset Still's disease. A probable diagnosis may be considered in the presence of fever, arthritis, rash, or neutrophilic leukocytosis, and any of the minor manifestations such as serositis, sore throat, hepatic or other organ involvement, splenomegaly, or lymphadenopathy. A recurrent or more chronic course of fever, arthritis, and rash, recognized after long-term observation and associated with articular radiologic manifestations similar to those seen in childhood Still's disease may provide the most firm diagnosis and could be considered as classic adult onset Still's disease. Important diseases to be excluded are infectious, neoplastic, and connective tissue disorders (16).

TREATMENT

Management of patients with adult onset Still's disease is based on the use of NSAIDs, corticosteroids, and second-line agents including cytotoxic drugs (7-9). Efficacy of any of these drugs has been difficult to evaluate because of the remittent disease course, variable treatment indications, different doses, and lack of controls. In about 20% of the reported patients, the systemic manifestations and arthritis are controlled with the administration of high-dose salicylate or aspirin (3.2-4.5 g/day) or the administration of other NSAIDs.

In patients with life-threatening complications or abnormal serum liver enzymes, one should consider the early use of corticosteroids. Liver failure, with or without disseminated intravascular coagulation, has been described in a small number of patients with adult onset Still's disease taking high doses of aspirin or other NSAIDs (7,12,16). Serum liver enzymes, complete blood count, blood urea nitrogen (BUN), and creatinine must be monitored weekly at the beginning of NSAID therapy. Patients who fail to improve or develop toxicities from NSAIDs generally respond to prednisone or a similar corticosteroid. Prednisone doses of 1-2 mg/kg/day are adequate for most patients. In a few patients, lower doses ranging from 5-20 mg may be effective. In those patients requiring prolonged high-dose corticosteroid therapy to control the high fever and other systemic manifestations or in whom the arthritis progresses relentlessly, slow-acting drugs including gold, hydroxychloroquine, and penicillamine; and immunosuppressive agents such as cyclophosphamide, azathioprine, and low-dose methotrexate have been used (7-9,17,18). With each of these agents there is adequate immediate response in some patients, but no information about long-term effects and side effects of such medications in adult onset Still's disease is available (19,20).

Prognosis is usually good. A few patients, however, develop progressive, severe joint damage requiring hip or knee replacement. Rarely, patients have died as a result of septicemia, tuberculosis, or peritonitis during corticosteroid therapy; or intravascular coagulation, liver failure, or sudden unexplained death while receiving NSAIDs (7-9,11,12,19).

Antonio Reginato, MD

1. Bywaters EGL: Still's disease in the adult. Ann Rheum Dis 30:121-133, 1971
2. Bujak JS, Aptekar RG, Decker JL, et al: Juvenile rheumatoid arthritis presenting in the adult as fever of unknown origin. Medicine 52:431-444, 1973
3. Medsger TA, Christy WC: Carpal arthritis with ankylosis in late onset Still's disease. Arthritis Rheum 19:232-242, 1976
4. Elkon KB, Bywaters EGL, Inman RQ, et al: Adult onset Still's disease: long-term follow-up and immunologic studies. Ann Rheum Dis 39:187-188, 1980
5. Larson EB: Adult Still's disease: evolution of a clinical syndrome and diagnosis, treatment, and follow-up of 17 patients. Medicine 63:82-91, 1984
6. Wouters JMGW, Reekers P, Van de Putte LBA: Adult-onset Still's disease: disease course and HLA associations. Arthritis Rheum 29:415-418, 1986
7. Reginato AJ, Schumacher HR, Baker DJ, et al: Adult onset Still's disease: experience with 23 patients and literature review with emphasis on organ failure. Semin Arthritis Rheum 17:39-57, 1987
8. Cush JJ, Medsger TA Jr., Christy WC, et al: Adult-onset Still's disease: clinical course and outcome. Arthritis Rheum 30:186-194, 1987
9. Ohta A, Yamaguchi M, Kaneoka H, et al: Adult onset Still's disease: review of 228 cases from the literature. J Rheumatol 14:1139-1146, 1987
10. Ohta A, Yamaguchi M, Tsunematsu T et al: Adult onset Still's disease: a multicenter survey of Japanese patients. J Rheumatol 17:1058-1063, 1990
11. Cabane J, Agnes M, Ziza JM, et al: Comparison of long-term evolution of adult onset and juvenile onset Still's disease, both followed-up for more than 10 years. Ann Rheum Dis 49:283-285, 1990
12. Pouchot J, Sampalis JS, Beudet F, et al: Adult Still's disease: manifestations, disease course, and outcome in 62 patients. Medicine 70:118-136, 1991
13. Ohta A, Masumoto Y, Ohta T, el al: Still's disease associated with necrotizing lymphadenitis (Kikuchi's disease): report of 3 cases. J Rheumatol 15:981-983, 1988
14. Blasa Criado A, Niguel-Mendieta E: Serum ferritin can be useful in adult onset Still's disease. J Rheumatol 16:412-413, 1989
15. Luder AS, Naphtali V, Porat EB, et al: Still's disease associated with adenovirus infection and defect in adenovirus directed natural killing. Ann Rheum Dis 48:781-786, 1989
16. Reginato AJ, Falasca GF: Fever in the patient with rheumatic diseases. Critical Care of the Patient with Immunologic Diseases. Edited by Mandel B., In press
17. Burgeois P, Palazzo E, Belmatoug N, et al: Low dose methotrexate in adult Still's disease: second line treatment or steroid sparing? Arthritis Rheum 32: S63, 1989
18. Kraus A, Alarcon-Segovia D: Fever in adult onset Still's disease: response to methotrexate. J Rheumatol 18:918-920, 1991
19. Juvenile and adult systemic-onset Still's disease. Editorial. Lancet 376:92, 1990
20. Lipton JH, Messner HA: Chronic myeloid leukemia in a woman with Still's disease treated with 198Au synoviorthesis. J Rheumatol 18:734-735, 1991

24. OSTEOARTHRITIS
A. Epidemiology, Pathology, and Pathogenesis

Osteoarthritis (OA), the most common joint disease, is characterized by progressive loss of articular cartilage, appositional new bone formation in the subchondral trabeculae, and formation of new cartilage and new bone at the joint margins (osteophytes). Evidence of cartilage repair is present until the disease becomes far advanced. Low grade synovitis is often seen and is considered to be secondary to the changes in the hard tissues within the joint. Clinical features can include pain in the involved joint, which is typically worse with activity and relieved by rest; stiffness after periods of immobility (gelling); enlargement of the joint; instability; limitation of motion; and functional impairment. Periarticular muscle atrophy is common and the associated weakness may contribute to disability.

Depending on the absence or presence of an identifiable local or systemic etiologic factor, osteoarthritis has been classified into idiopathic (primary) and secondary forms. Criteria for classification of OA of the knee, hip, and hand have been developed recently by the American College of Rheumatology (formerly American Rheumatism Association) (Appendix 8). They permit classification of the disease on the basis of various combinations of clinical, radiographic, and laboratory parameters. For each of the above sites the criteria provide approximately 90% sensitivity and 90% specificity. The classification criteria are not intended for use as *diagnostic* criteria; rather, they facilitate standardized reporting of cases for research purposes and permit consistency in communication.

ECONOMIC IMPACT

The economic impact of OA is enormous. To demonstrate the relative impact of the two diseases, Kramer et al (1) applied accepted prevalence estimates for OA and rheumatoid arthritis (RA) to health care utilization and disability data from the 1976 National Health Interview Survey (NHIS). The greater severity of RA, compared to OA, was apparent in higher per capita estimates of annual physician visits, days of restricted activity and work loss, and hospitalization rates. However, when disease prevalence figures were applied to estimates of health care utilization and disability, the greater prevalence of OA suggested an aggregate economic impact some 30-fold greater than that of RA. For example, there were 68 million work loss days per year for OA versus 2 million for RA. Furthermore, more recent analyses of 1984–1986 NHIS data (2) indicate that the proportion of the total direct medical costs of musculoskeletal diseases attributable to OA may be increasing as hospitalization rates and length of stay for patients with RA have decreased.

Analysis of costs incurred by ambulatory patients with RA and with OA showed that, on average, patients spent $147 for arthritis medications, aids, and devices, and $207 for outpatient visits (in 1979 dollars). In addition to these direct dollar costs, they averaged nearly seven days of restricted activity per month. Among working patients, 2.5 work days per month were lost due to arthritis; 30% reported that they were unemployed or retired because of poor health. Notably, costs for patients with OA were as high as those for RA, with the exception of higher outpatient charges for RA (3). Furthermore, an analysis performed a decade ago indicates that the morbidity of OA resulted in nearly 4 million hospitalizations annually (1). Due to the sharp increase in total joint arthroplasty since that time, this figure will now be much higher.

EPIDEMIOLOGY

Prevalence, Age, Sex. Radiographic evidence of OA can be found at some site in the majority of people older than 65 years of age. More than 80% of those over the age of 75 are affected. Osteoarthritis is a major cause of disability, and knee OA is more likely to result in disability than osteoarthritis of any other joint.

Estimates of the true prevalence of OA are imprecise because of the difficulties associated with diagnosis; estimates of its incidence are unavailable because of the lack of longitudinal data and difficulties associated with defining disease onset.

The prevalence of OA at all joint sites increases progressively with age, which is the most powerful risk factor for the disease. For example, the National Health and Nutrition Examination Survey (NHANES) found that the prevalence of knee OA increased from <0.1% in people 25–34 years old to 10% to 20% in those 65–74 years old. Women were about twice as likely as men to be affected, and black women were twice as likely as white women to have knee OA (4). Others have found an even higher prevalence of knee OA. In the Framingham study the prevalence was 30% between age 65–74 years (5), and virtually every study that has examined people more than 75 years old has found a prevalence greater than 30% in this subset of the population, with more disease among women than men. Osteoarthritis of the hip is somewhat less common than knee OA and does not exhibit this female preponderance, suggesting a difference in disease etiology at these two sites.

Racial differences exist for both the prevalence of OA and the pattern of joint involvement. For example, in Hong Kong, the Chinese have a lower prevalence of hip OA than Caucasians; similarly, in South African blacks, East Indians and native Americans, hip OA is much less common than in Caucasians (6). Whether these differences are genetic or due to differences in joint usage related to lifestyle or occupation is not known.

It is important to note that fewer than one-half of all those with radiographically identifiable OA have symptoms. Therefore, risk factors for pain and disability must be differentiated from those related to the pathologic changes (the radiograph is a surrogate for joint pathology). In any given joint, OA may result from a combination of local etiologic factors, such as trauma, and generalized osteoarthritis, which may be due to a genetic predisposition (7), chondrocalcinosis, generalized hypermobility (8), or other factors. For example, patients with a tendency to primary OA, as manifest by Heberden's nodes, are more likely than those without nodal OA to develop secondary OA of the knee after meniscectomy (9).

Obesity. Increased body mass has been associated with an increased prevalence of knee OA in both cross-sectional and longitudinal studies. Most convincing in this regard are the Framingham data (10), which showed that being overweight as a young adult—long before any symptoms of osteoarthritis had developed—strongly predicted the appearance of knee OA in the subsequent 36-year period of follow-up. For those in the highest quintile for body mass index at the baseline examination, the relative risk for developing knee OA during this period was 1.5 for men and 2.1 for women. For severe OA, the relative risk rose to 1.9 for men and 3.2 for women, suggesting that obesity plays an even larger role in the etiology of the most serious cases. In a strain of guinea pigs that develops spontaneous knee OA, diet restriction resulting in a 28% decrease in body weight led to a 40% reduction in the severity of OA (11). Obese human subjects who have not yet developed OA can significantly reduce their risk; weight loss of only 5 kg was associated with a 50% reduction in the odds of developing symptomatic knee OA (12). Notably, OA of the hip does not demonstrate this striking association with obesity.

Bone Density. Related to the association between obesity and knee OA is the apparent inverse relationship between OA and osteoporosis, although the question of whether this relationship is, in fact, real is not settled (13). It has been suggested that the less dense subchondral bone in osteoporosis absorbs load better than normal bone, so that less stress is transferred to the overlying articular cartilage. Evidence to support this general hypothesis includes the finding of a higher than expected prevalence of OA in subjects with osteopetrosis (14) and in those with greater than average bone mineral density (bone mass). Obesity, which is common in OA patients, may be a common denominator, since it is associated with a greater than normal bone mass at virtually all skeletal sites (15).

Trauma and Repetitive Stress. Both major trauma and repetitive use have been implicated as causes of OA. Studies of humans and of animal models convincingly demonstrate that a loss of anterior cruciate ligament integrity or damage to the meniscus (or meniscectomy) can lead to knee OA (15). Although damage to the articular cartilage may occur at the time of injury, even normal articular cartilage will degenerate when the joint is unstable.

When major trauma is excluded, there are no convincing data to support an association between specific sports and arthritis, although this may be due to the lack of good long-term studies and the difficulties associated with retrospective assessment of activities. Thus, repetitive use of the type associated with athletics—even long-term running (17)—does not appear to cause the joint degeneration associated with repetitive occupational use, such as that seen in jackhammer operators, cotton mill workers, shipyard workers, coal miners and others (18). While selection bias, such as early discontinuation of the athletic activity by those with damaged joints, may account for the discrepancy, it also may be due to the intensity and duration of the activity. Most occupational use involves repeated exposure over many hours of the day, whereas even serious athletes expose their joints to injury at a much lower frequency.

Genetic Factors. The mother of a woman with distal interphalangeal joint OA (Heberden's nodes) is twice as likely to exhibit the same changes—and the proband's sister three times as likely—as the mother and sister of a non-affected woman. The mechanism appears to involve autosomal dominant transmission in women and recessive inheritance in men. The prevalence of Heberden's nodes is 10 times greater in women than in men.

The discovery of a point mutation in the cDNA cloning for type II collagen in several generations of a family with chondrodysplasia and polyarticular secondary OA provides a clear example of the disease developing in association of a generalized genetic defect in the matrix of articular cartilage (19,20). Local stresses related to joint use and the degree of deformity due to the chondrodysplasia presumably influenced the appearance of OA in some joints, but not others, in affected members of the kindred. The prevalence of genetic abnormalities in collagen or other matrix macromolecules in subjects with what appears presently to be idiopathic OA remains to be determined.

PATHOLOGY

The pathology of OA reflects both damage to the joint and reaction to that damage. The most striking gross changes are usually seen in the load-bearing areas of articular cartilage. Although contemporary descriptions emphasize the progressive loss of articular cartilage that occurs in this disease, in the earlier stages the cartilage is *thicker* than normal (21). An increase in water content, reflecting damage to the collagen network of the tissue, leads to swelling of the cartilage and is associated with an increase in the net rate of synthesis of proteoglycans, the molecules that contribute elasticity to the tissue and endow it with its ability to resist compression. The increase in proteoglycan synthesis, which represents a repair effort by the chondrocytes, may result in an increase in the total proteoglycan concentration of the tissue. This process may be reflected by an increase in staining of the tissue with toluidine blue or Safranin-O in histochemical studies. Thus, the earlier stages of OA—which may last years or decades in humans—are characterized by hypertrophic repair of the articular cartilage (21,22).

With disease progression, however, the joint surface thins and the proteoglycan concentration diminishes, leading to softening of the cartilage. The integrity of the surface is lost and vertical clefts develop (*fibrillation*) (Fig. 24–1). With joint motion the fibrillated cartilage is lost, exposing underlying bone. Areas of fibrocartilaginous repair may appear, but these are inferior to pristine hyaline articular cartilage in their ability to withstand mechanical stress. The chondrocytes replicate, forming clusters

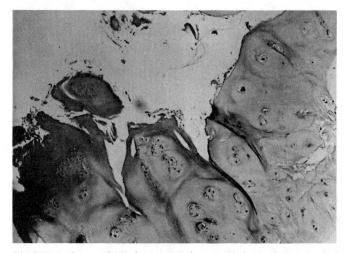

Fig. 24A–1. Osteoarthritic human cartilage: pathologic changes include surface fibrillation, vertical fissure formation, and clusters (clones) of proliferating cells; cartilage components are being released into the synovial cavity.

called *clones*. Later, however, the remaining cartilage becomes hypocellular.

While loss of articular cartilage represents the pathologic hallmark of OA, remodelling and hypertrophy of bone are also major features. Appositional bone growth occurs in the subchondral region, leading to the sclerosis that may be seen radiographically. The abraded bone in the floor of the ulcerated cartilage may take on the gross appearance of ivory. Microfractures of subchondral trabeculae may be seen. Bone cysts, reflecting localized osteonecrosis, form beneath the surface and weaken the osseous support for the overlying cartilage. Growth of cartilage and bone at the joint margins leads to osteophytes, or *spurs*, which alter the contour of the joint and may restrict movement. Radiographic evidence of osteophytes, in the absence of other bony changes such as subchondral cysts or sclerosis, may be a manifestation of aging, and not of osteoarthritis (23).

Soft tissue changes include a patchy chronic synovitis (24) and thickening of the joint capsule, which may further restrict movement. Periarticular muscle wasting is common. These changes may play a major role in symptoms and disability.

PATHOGENESIS

Although the most obvious changes in the osteoarthritic joint occur in the cartilage, OA should not be viewed simply as a disease of cartilage. It does not represent the failure of a single tissue, but of an *organ*—the diarthrodial joint. Just as congestive heart failure may be due to primary disease of the myocardium, pericardium, or endocardium, the primary abnormality in OA may reside in the articular cartilage, synovium, subchondral bone, ligaments, or neuromuscular apparatus. Nonetheless, given the marked changes that occur in the OA cartilage, it is essential to appreciate the importance of this tissue in normal joint physiology. Joint cartilage plays two essential roles: first, it provides a remarkably smooth bearing surface, permitting virtually frictionless movement of one bone over the other within the joint; second, it spreads and transmits load, preventing concentration of stress within the joint.

Essentially, OA develops in two settings: when the biomaterial properties of the articular cartilage and underlying subchondral and bone are normal, but excessive loads on the joint cause the tissues to fail; or when the applied load is reasonable but the biomaterial properties of the cartilage or bone are inferior.

Although articular cartilage is highly resistant to wear under conditions of repeated oscillation, repetitive impact loading leads to joint failure (25). This accounts for the high prevalence of OA in specific joints related to vocational or avocational overload. In general, the earliest progressive degenerative changes occur at those sites within the joint that are subject to the greatest compressive loads. It has been suggested that more than 80% of all cases of idiopathic osteoarthritis of the hip reflect subtle developmental defects, such as acetabular dysplasia or slipped femoral epiphysis, which increase joint congruity and concentrate loads.

Even if the stresses within the joint are normal, conditions that reduce the ability of the articular cartilage or subchondral bone to deform may lead to OA. For example, in ochronosis the accumulation of homogentisic acid polymers leads to stiffening of the cartilage; in osteopetrosis stiffening of the subchondral trabeculae, rather than of the cartilage, occurs. In both conditions severe, generalized OA is common (26). Osteoarthritis in familial chondrodysplasia due to a mutation in the cDNA coding for type II collagen, mentioned above, illustrates development of the disorder in association with a generalized defect in the articular cartilage matrix.

MECHANISMS PROTECTING THE JOINT FROM STRESS

The major load on articular cartilage results from the contraction of muscles that stabilize or move the joint (27). In normal walking, three to four times the weight of the body is transmitted through the knee joint; during a deep knee bend the patellofemoral joint is subjected to a load of up to 10 times body weight. Adaptive mechanisms must protect the joint from these physiologic loads. Although articular cartilage is an excellent shock absorber in terms of its bulk properties, at most sites it is only 1–2 mm thick, making it too thin to serve as the sole shock-absorbing structure in joints. The additional protective mechanisms that are needed are provided by both subchondral bone and periarticular muscles.

Passive protection. In the normal unloaded state the opposing surfaces of joints are incongruent. Under load, deformation occurs (28), maximizing the contact area and minimizing the stress (force per unit area). Deformation of the cartilage provides the self-pressurized hydrostatic weeping lubrication needed for effortless motion. However, with increasing load, cartilage deformation alone is insufficient; deformation of the underlying bone must also occur. Under high loads, this is more important than deformation of cartilage in reducing stress.

The highly elastic cancellous subchondral bone, although 10 times stiffer than cartilage, is much softer than cortical bone and serves as a major shock absorber. By providing it with a pliable bed that absorbs energy, cancellous bone protects the overlying cartilage (28).

Recent work has indicated that some 30% of the stiffness of normal subchondral bone is due to hydraulic factors, rather than to the intrinsic material properties of the trabeculae themselves (29). As a result of appositional bone growth in the subchondral trabeculae, intraosseous blood flow is altered in OA, resulting in venous engorgement and medullary hypertension (30,31) which may increase the hydraulic stiffness of the bone. In OA, furthermore, the subchondral plate thickens (32), limiting transmission of compressive stresses from the cartilage to the underlying trabecular network and intertrabecular hydraulic system and providing a mechanical basis for articular cartilage damage. If the load is excessive, the subchondral trabeculae will fracture. These microfractures then heal with callus formation and remodeling. Since the remodeled trabeculae may be stiffer than normal, however, a significant increase in the number of microfractures in subchondral bone may be detrimental to normal joint function (33). Under such circumstances the bone cannot deform normally with load, the increase in congruity of joint surfaces that occurs with loading is diminished, stresses are concentrated at contact sites on the articular cartilage, and the cartilage fails.

Active protection. Active shock-absorbing mechanisms involve the use of muscles and joint motion in *negative work*. While muscle contraction can move a joint, muscles can also act as large rubber bands. When a slightly stretched muscle is subjected to greater stretch as a result of joint motion, it can absorb a large amount of energy. Most of the muscle activity generated during ambulation is not used to propel the body forward but to absorb energy to decelerate the body.

When we negotiate a jump off a ledge or table top we normally land on our toes, come down on our heels, and straighten our flexed knees and hips. During this smooth action, our muscles absorb energy. As we dorsiflex our ankles we stretch our gastrocnemius–soleus complex; as we straighten our knees we stretch our quadriceps; as we straighten our hips we stretch our hamstrings. The amount of energy absorbed by this mechanism is enormous. Indeed, the energy produced by normal walking is great enough to tear all the ligaments of the knee. That this does not occur routinely attests to the importance of active energy absorption.

Small unexpected loads for which we are unprepared are much more damaging to joints than large ones that have been anticipated. Consider what happens when we come down stairs, misjudge a step and abruptly slip a couple of steps: because our muscles are not prepared to accommodate the load we feel a sharp jolt. To prepare the neuromuscular apparatus to handle an impact load requires approximately 75 msec. Thus, falls of very brief duration do not afford sufficient time to bring protective muscular reflexes into play. Under such conditions, the load is transmitted to the cartilage and bone. In contrast, during a fall from a greater height, sufficient time is available for activation of the appropriate reflexes, the energy of impact is absorbed by the lengthening of the muscles surrounding the joint and movement of the joint, and the articular cartilage is thereby protected. Both muscle atrophy, which may occur in association with OA, and an increase in the latent period of the reflex, which may occur with peripheral neuropathy due to aging or other causes, will reduce the effectiveness of this shock-absorbing mechanism.

After a femoral nerve block, the load rate in normal individuals who have no force transient profile during gait increases more than two-fold to approximately 150 times body weight/second (34). This suggests that a force transient can be caused by failure to decelerate the lower extremity prior to heel strike. In normal individuals, minor incoordination in muscle recruitment, resulting in failure to decelerate the leg, may generate rapidly applied impulsive forces as high as 65 times body weight/second at heel strike. Whether this micro-incoordination of neuromuscular control is a risk factor for OA remains to be established, but the possibility is intriguing.

CARTILAGE LOSS IN OSTEOARTHRITIS

As indicated above, cartilage loss is central to OA. The cartilage is slowly degraded, with a progressive decrease in the content of proteoglycans. Since the rates of synthesis of proteoglycans, collagen, hyaluronan, and DNA all are increased in OA, catabolic activity of the tissue is extraordinarily high. Although wear may be a factor in cartilage loss, it is believed that lysosomal proteases (cathepsins) and neutral metalloproteinases, such as stromelysin, collagenase, and gelatinase, account for much of the loss of cartilage in this disease.

The concentration of collagenase in the cartilage increases with advancing severity of the disease and presumably accounts for the destruction of matrix collagen. Despite an increase in hyaluronan synthesis (35), a reduction in cartilage hyaluronan content develops (36), indicating accelerated degradation of the backbone of the proteoglycan aggregate. A specific hyaluronidase has not been isolated from cartilage, but several lysosomal enzymes can cleave hyaluronic acid and chondroitin-6 sulfate.

The slowly progressive loss of cartilage is associated with a loss of aggrecan (37), resulting in a loss of compressive stiffness and elasticity and an increase in hydraulic permeability. The water content of the cartilage is increased and a change occurs in the arrangement and size of the collagen fibers within the matrix. The biochemical data are consistent with a defect in the collagen network of the cartilage, perhaps due to disruption of the "glue" that binds adjacent collagen fibers together in the matrix (38). This is perhaps the earliest matrix change to occur in OA, and it appears to be irreversible. The aggregation defect may be due to an alteration in the hyaluronan-binding region of the proteoglycan monomer, a quantitative deficiency in hyaluronan, or a deficiency in link protein, and is of considerable importance since the proteoglycans are less constrained than normal within the collagen network. Sites of cleavage have been noted in link protein from osteoarthritic cartilage, but are no different from those in link from normal adult cartilage.

While the cells in normal adult articular cartilage do not divide, in osteoarthritic cartilage the chondrocytes undergo active cell division. The new cells are very active metabolically and produce increased quantities of collagen, proteoglycan, and hyaluronan. However, the new products do not aggregate well and are not adequately stabilized in the extracellular matrix, so that the mechanical properties of the matrix are inferior to those of normal cartilage. As indicated above, prior to the loss of cartilage mass and proteoglycan depletion, the marked repair activity of the chondrocytes may lead to an increase in proteoglycan concentration, associated with thickening of the cartilage (20). Evidence that this phenomenon of hypertrophic repair is common in the earlier stages of OA in both humans and experimental animals is provided by a variety of data from both humans and experimental models (39–42). It is obviously inaccurate to call OA degenerative joint disease.

Many investigators consider that interleukin–1 (IL–1) drives the progression of cartilage breakdown in OA. This cytokine is produced by mononuclear cells, including synovial lining cells, and synthesized by chondrocytes. It stimulates the synthesis and secretion of latent collagenase, latent stromelysin, latent gelatinase, and tissue plasminogen activator (43). Intraarticular injection of IL–1 leads rapidly to loss of proteoglycans from articular cartilage of normal rabbits (44). A similar effect is seen after incubation of normal cartilage from young animals with IL–1 in vitro. The number of IL-1 receptors on chondrocytes in osteoarthritic cartilage is greater than that on normal chondrocytes (45), perhaps accounting for the greater sensitivity of the former to IL-1 and suggesting an explanation for the increased levels of matrix metalloproteinases in the diseased cartilage. These observations must be viewed with some caution, however, since IL–1 has little effect on proteoglycan release from adult canine, porcine, or human articular cartilage (46). Although it can be argued that the effects of IL–1 may be focal, rather than diffuse, data suggest that all chondrocytes in the OA joint exhibit enhanced biosynthetic activity.

Whether their synthesis and release is stimulated by IL–1 or by other factors such as altered mechanical stresses, the neutral metalloproteinases, cathepsins, and plasmin, which can activate the latent forms of the neutral metalloproteinases, all appear to be involved in failure of the cartilage in OA. Plasminogen, the substrate for plasmin, may be synthesized by the chondrocytes or may enter the cartilage by diffusion from the synovial fluid. Tissue inhibitor of matrix metalloproteinases (TIMP) and plasminogen activator inhibitor, both of which are synthesized by the chondrocyte, limit the degradative activity of the neutral metalloproteinases and plasminogen activator, respectively. A stoichiometric imbalance appears to exist in osteoarthritic cartilage between levels of active enzyme, which may be several-fold higher than those in normal cartilage, and the level of TIMP, which may be only modestly increased (47).

Growth factors drive repair processes that, in some cases may heal the cartilage lesion or at least stabilize the process (48). These growth factors modulate catabolic as well as anabolic pathways of chondrocyte metabolism. Not only do they increase proteoglycan synthesis but, by down-regulating chondrocyte receptors for IL–1, they decrease proteoglycan degradation. Thus, these homeostatic mechanisms may maintain the joint in a reasonable functional state for years. The repair tissue, however, often does not hold up as well under mechanical stresses as normal hyaline cartilage. Eventually, at least in some cases, the rate of proteoglycan synthesis falls off, the cells are no longer able to maintain the matrix, and end-stage OA develops, with full-thickness loss of cartilage.

Kenneth D. Brandt, MD
Charles W. Slemenda, DrPH

1. Kramer JS, Yelin EH, Epstein WV: Social and economic impacts of four musculoskeletal conditions: a study using national community-based data. J Rheumatol 26:901–907, 1983
2. Yelin EH, Felts WR: A summary of the impact of musculoskeletal conditions in the United States. Arthritis Rheum 33:750–755, 1990
3. Liang MH, Larson M, Thompson M, et al: Costs and outcomes in rheumatoid arthritis and osteoarthritis. Arthritis Rheum 27:522–529, 1984
4. Davis MA, Ettinger WH, Neuhaus JM, et al: Knee osteoarthritis and physical functioning: evidence from the NHANES I epidemiologic followup study. J Rheumatol 18:591–598, 1991
5. Felson DT, Naimark A, Anderson J, et al: The prevalence of knee osteoarthritis in the elderly: the Framingham osteoarthritis study. Arthritis Rheum 30:914–918, 1987
6. Peyron JG, Altman RD: The epidemiology of osteoarthritis. Osteoarthritis. Diagnosis and Medical/Surgical Management, 2nd ed. Edited by: Moskowitz RW, Howell DS, Goldberg M, Mankin HJ. Philadelphia, Penn. WB Saunders Company. 1992, pp 15–17
7. Kellgren JH, Lawrence JS, Bier F: Genetic factors in generalized osteoarthrosis. Ann Rheum Dis 22:237–255, 1963
8. Bird HA, Tribe CR, Bacon PA: Joint hypermobility leading to osteoarthrosis and chondrocalcinosis. Ann Rheum Dis 37:203–211, 1978
9. Doherty M, Watt I, Dieppe P: Influence of primary generalized osteoarthritis on development of secondary osteoarthritis. Lancet 11:8–11, 1983
10. Felson DT, Anderson JJ, Naimark A, et al: Obesity and knee osteoarthritis: the Framingham study. Ann Int Med 109:18–24, 1988
11. Bendele AM, Hulman JF: Effects of body weight restriction on the development and progression of spontaneous osteoarthritis in guinea pigs. Arthritis Rheum 34:1180–1184, 1991
12. Felson DT, Zhang Y, Anthony JM, Naimark A, Anderson JJ: Weight loss reduces the risk for symptomatic knee osteoarthritis in women. Ann Intern Med 117:535–539, 1992
13. Knight SM, Ring EFJ, Bhalla AK: Bone mineral density and osteoarthritis. Ann Rheum Dis 51:1025–1026, 1992
14. Cameron HV, Dewar FP: Degenerative osteoarthritis associated with osteopetrosis. Clin Orthop Rel Res 127:148–149, 1977
15. Slemenda CW, Hui SL, Williams CJ, et al: Bone mass and anthropometric measurements in adult females. Bone and Mineral 11:101–109, 1990
16. Brandt KD, Myers SL, Burr D, et al: Osteoarthritic changes in canine articular cartilage, subchondral bone, and synovium fifty-four months after transection of the anterior cruciate ligament. Arthritis Rheum 34:1560–1570, 1991
17. Panush RS, Schmidt C, Caldwell JR, et al: Is running associated with degenerative joint disease? JAMA 255:1152–1154, 1986
18. Lindberg H, Montgomery F: Heavy labor and the occurrence of gonarthrosis. Clin Orthop 214:235–236, 1987
19. Knowlton RG, Katzenstein PL, Moskowitz RW, et al: Genetic linkage of a polymorphism in the type II pro-collagen gene (COL2A) to primary osteoarthritis associated with mild chondrodysplasia. N Engl J Med 322:526–530, 1990
20. Vikkula M, Palotie A, Ritvaniemi P: Early-onset osteoarthritis linked to the type II procollagen gene. Arthritis Rheum 36:401–409, 1993
21. Adams ME, Brandt KD: Hypertrophic repair of canine articular cartilage in osteoarthritis after anterior cruciate ligament transection. J Rheum 18:428–435, 1991
22. Braunstein EM, Brandt KD and Albrecht M: MRI demonstration of hypertrophic articular cartilage repair in osteoarthritis. Skeletal Radiol 19:335–339, 1990
23. Hernborg J, Nilsson BE: The relationship between osteophytes in the knee joints, osteoarthritis and aging. Acta Orthop Scand 44:69–74, 1973
24. Myers SL, Brandt KD, Ehlich JW, et al: Synovial inflammation in patients with early osteoarthritis of the knee. J Rheum 17:1662–1669, 1990
25. Radin EL, Paul IL: The response of joints to impact loading. I. In vitro wear. Arthritis Rheum 14:356–362, 1971
26. Schumacher JR Jr: Secondary osteoarthritis. Osteoarthritis—Diagnosis and Management, 2nd edition. Edited by Moskowitz RW, Howell DS, Goldberg VM, Mankin HJ. WB Saunders Co. Philadelphia, Penn., 1992, pp 367–398
27. Reilly DT, Mertens M: Experimental analysis of the quadriceps muscle force and patello-femoral joint reaction force for various activities. Acta Orthop Scand 43:126–137, 1972
28. Radin EL, Paul IL: Does cartilage compliance reduce skeletal impact loads? The relative force attenuating properties of articular cartilage, synovial fluid, periarticular soft-tissues and bone. Arthritis Rheum 13:139–144, 1970
29. Ochoa JA, Heck DA, Brandt KD, Hillberry BM: The effect of intertrabecular fluid on femoral head mechanics. J Rheumatol 18:580–584, 1991
30. Hulth A: Circulatory disturbances in osteoarthritis of the hip. A venographic study. Acta Orthop Scand 8:81–91, 1958
31. Arnoldi CC, Linderholm H, Mussbichler H: Venous engorgement and intraosseous hypertension in osteoarthritis. J Bone Joint Surg 54B:409–421, 1972
32. Dedrick KD, Goldstein SA, Brandt KD, O'Connor BL, Goulet RW, Albrecht M: A longitudinal study of subchondral plate and trabecular bone in cruciate-deficient dogs with osteoarthritis followed for up to 54 months. Arthritis Rheum In press.
33. Radin EL, Parker HG, Pugh JW, et al: Response of joints to impact loading. III. Relationship between trabecular microfractures and cartilage degeneration. J Biomech 6:51–57, 1973
34. Radin EL, Yang KH, Riegger C, et al: Relationship between lower limb dynamics and knee joint pain. J Orthop Res 9:398–405, 1991
35. Ryu J, Treadwell BV, Mankin HJ: Biochemical and metabolic abnormalities in normal and osteoarthritic human articular cartilage. Arthritis Rheum 27:49–57, 1984
36. Sweet MBE, Thonar E-J, Immelman AR, et al: Biochemical changes in6 progressive osteoarthritis. Ann Rheum Dis 36:387–398, 1977
37. Mankin HJ, Dorfman H, Lippiello L, et al: Biochemical and metabolic abnormalities in articular cartilage from osteoarthritic human hips. II. Correlation of morphology with biochemical and metabolic data. J Bone Joint Surg 53A:523–537, 1971
38. Smith GN Jr, Brandt KD: Hypothesis: Can type IX collagen "glue" together intersecting type II fibers in articular cartilage matrix? A proposed mechanism. J Rheum 19:14–17, 1992

39. Bywaters EGL: The metabolism of joint tissues. J Pathol Bacteriol 44:247–268, 1937

40. Châteauvert JMD, Grynpas MD, Kessler MJ, et al: Spontaneous osteoarthritis in rhesus macaques. II. Characterization of disease and morphometric studies. J Rheumatol 17:73–83, 1990

41. Vignon E, Arlot M, Hartmann D, Moyen B, Ville G: Hypertrophic repair of articular cartilage in experimental osteoarthritis. Ann Rheum Dis 142:82–88, 1983

42. McDevitt CA, Muir H, Pond MJ: Canine articular cartilage in natural and experimentally induced osteoarthritis. Biochem Soc Trans 1:287–289, 1973

43. Dodge GR, Poole AR: Immunohistochemical detection and immunochemical analysis of type II collagen degradation in human normal, rheumatoid, and osteoarthritic articular cartilages and in explants of bovine articular cartilage cultured with interleukin–1. J Clin Invest 83:647–661, 1989

44. Pettipher ER, Higgs GA, Henderson B: Interleukin–1 induces leukocyte infiltration and cartilage proteoglycan degradation in the synovial joint. Proc Natl Acad Sci USA 83:8749–8753, 1986

45. Martel-Pelletier J, McCollum R, DiBattista J, Faure M-p, Chin JA, Fournier S, Sarfati M, Pelletier J-P: The interleukin-1 receptor in normal and osteoarthritic human chondrocytes. Arthritis Rheum 35:530–540, 1992

46. Nietfeld JJ, Wilbrink B, Den Otter W, et al: The effect of human IL–1 on proteoglycan metabolism in human and porcine cartilage explants. J Rheumatol 17:818–826, 1990

47. Dean DD, Martel-Pelletier J, Pelletier J-P, et al: Evidence for metalloproteinase and metalloproteinase inhibitor (TIMP) imbalance in human osteoarthritic cartilage. J Clin Invest 84:678–685, 1989

48. Morales TI: Cartilage proteoglycan homeostasis: Role of growth factors. Cartilage Changes in Osteoarthritis. Edited by Brandt KD. Indiana University School of Medicine, Indianapolis, Ind., 1990, pp 17–21

B. Clinical Features and Treatment

SIGNS AND SYMPTOMS

Signs and symptoms of osteoarthritis (OA) are usually local, but if they are more generalized, a systemic form of connective tissue disease is suggested. Clinical symptoms usually show positive correlation with radiologic abnormalities. In a given patient, however, the lack of correlation between joint symptoms and pathologic findings may be striking.

Pain early in the disease course occurs after joint use and is relieved by rest. Later, pain occurs with minimal motion or even at rest. At this stage of the disease night pain is common. Cartilage has no nerve supply and is insensitive to pain. Pain arises from other intraarticular and periarticular structures.

Acute inflammatory flares may be precipitated by trauma or, in some patients, by crystal-induced synovitis in response to crystals of calcium pyrophosphate or apatite. Joint stiffness is relatively short-lived and localized. Local tenderness may be elicited, especially if synovitis is present.

Pain on passive motion and *crepitus*, a feeling of crackling as the joint is moved, are prominent findings. Joint enlargement results from synovitis, increased amounts of synovial fluid, or proliferative changes in cartilage and bone.

Hand. *Heberden's nodes* are spurs formed at the dorsolateral and medial aspects of the distal interphalangeal joints. Flexor and lateral deviations of the distal phalanx are common. Similar changes at the proximal interphalangeal joints are called *Bouchard's nodes*.

In most patients, Heberden's nodes develop slowly over months or years. In other patients, onset is rapid and associated with moderately severe inflammatory changes. Gelatinous cysts resembling ganglia may precede the appearance of the node itself. Involvement of the first carpometacarpal joints leads to tenderness at the base of the first metacarpal bone and a squared appearance of the hand. Common involvement of the trapezioscaphoid joint has been emphasized (1).

Knee. Osteoarthritis of the knee is characterized by localized tenderness over various components of the joint and pain on passive or active motion. Crepitus can often be detected, and muscle atrophy is seen secondary to disuse. Disproportionate losses of cartilage localized to the medial or lateral compartments of the knee lead to secondary genu varus or valgus.

Chondromalacia patellae, seen most often in young adults, is associated with softening and erosion of patellar articular cartilage. Pain, localized around the patella, is aggravated by activity such as walking hills or stairs. Chondromalacia patellae likely represents a final common pathway of conditions affecting the knee, such as meniscal tears, hypermobility, or abnormal patellar positions, which lead to altered joint biomechanics and eventual degenerative change.

Hip. Osteoarthritic changes in the hip lead to an insidious onset of pain, often followed by a limp. Pain is usually localized to the groin or along the inner aspect of the thigh, although patients often complain of pain in the buttocks, sciatic region, or the knee due to pain referral along contiguous nerves. Physical examination shows loss of hip motion, initially most marked on internal rotation or extension.

Foot. Osteoarthritis of the first metatarsophalangeal joint is aggravated by tight shoes. Irregularities in joint contour can be palpated. Tenderness is common, particularly when the overlying bursa at the medial aspect of the joint is secondarily inflamed.

Spine. Osteoarthritis of the spine results from involvement of the intervertebral discs, vertebral bodies, or posterior apophyseal articulations. Involvement of the lumbar spine is seen most commonly at the L3–L4 area. Associated symptoms include local pain and stiffness, and radicular pain due to compression of contiguous nerve roots. Cauda equina syndrome with sphincter dysfunction may result. Large anterior osteophytes in the cervical spine give rise at times to dysphagia or respiratory tract symptoms. Compression of nerve roots or the cord itself leads to variable neurologic deficits.

Spinal stenosis, commonly seen in the lumbar spine, results from degenerative spurs, disc herniation, ligamentous hypertrophy, and spondylolisthesis. Pain in the legs may be constant or intermittent, and is often worsened by exercise, simulating intermittent claudication.

Other Joints. Osteoarthritis may occur in joints generally considered protected from development of OA, including elbows (2), shoulders, and interphalangeal joints of toes (3); consider occupational factors or metabolic diseases when unusual joints are involved.

Variant Forms

Certain so-called variant forms of primary OA have been defined. Patients with *primary generalized osteoarthritis* reveal involvement of the distal and proximal interphalangeal joints of the hands, the first carpometacarpal joint, knees, hips, and metatarsophalangeal joints. Radiologic changes often exceed clinical findings. These cases may represent a more severe form of ordinary OA, differing only in the number and severity of joints involved.

Erosive inflammatory osteoarthritis involves primarily the distal or proximal interphalangeal joints of the hands (4). Painful inflammatory episodes are associated with eventual development of joint deformity and ankylosis. After a variable period of years of intermittent acute flares, the joints often become asymptomatic. Bony erosions are prominent on roentgenograms. A relationship to Sjogren's syndrome has been described (5).

Diffuse idiopathic skeletal hyperostosis is characterized by flowing ossification along the anterolateral aspect of the vertebral bodies (6). Disc narrowing does not appear to be a part of the process, so that this disease is more a source of confusion with OA than a variant (see Chapter 47).

Secondary osteoarthritis produces clinical findings and radiologic changes similar to those of the primary form of the disease. Some underlying causes are listed in Table 24B–1.

LABORATORY AND RADIOLOGIC FINDINGS

Laboratory evaluations other than radiologic studies are helpful primarily in excluding other joint diseases. The erythrocyte sedimentation rate is normal in most patients but may be elevated

Table 24B–1. *Underlying causes of secondary osteoarthritis*

Heritable metabolic disorders
  Alkaptonuria
  Wilson's disease
  Hemochromatosis
  Morquio's disease
Multiple epiphyseal dysplasia
Slipped capital femoral epiphysis
Congenital dislocation of the hips
Neuropathic arthropathy (Charcot joints)
Hemophilic arthropathy
Acromegalic arthropathy
Paget's disease of bone (osteitis deformans)
Rheumatoid arthritis
Gout
Septic and tuberculous arthritis

slightly in patients with erosive inflammatory or generalized forms of the disease. Synovial fluid study reveals minimal abnormalities. Viscosity is good, and the cell count is slightly increased over normal but virtually always less than $1,000/mm^3$. Calcium pyrophosphate dihydrate or apatite crystals are seen in many osteoarthritic joint effusions. Scintigraphic abnormalities defined by pertechnetate joint scanning may precede the development of roentgenographic signs and clinical manifestations, but such studies are of limited clinical utility. Studies of serum and synovial markers of joint tissue components revealed increased serum keratan sulphate concentrations in patients with OA (7), and elevations of synovial fluid proteoglycan epitopes related to acute knee injury (8). However, the use of such markers for diagnostic and prognostic purposes remains investigational at this time (9).

Studies comparing roentgenograms with pathologic changes defined by arthroscopy confirmed that plain roentgenograms were frequently insensitive in defining mild to moderate articular cartilage degeneration (10). At the time of significant cartilage loss, roentgenographic findings frequently suggested absent or minimal disease. Conversely, standing anteroposterior knee radiographs often suggested joint space narrowing in the presence of normal tibiofemoral articular cartilage. Characteristic progressive changes include joint space narrowing, subchondral bony sclerosis (eburnation), marginal osteophyte formation, and cyst formation (Fig. 24B–1). Ankylosis is uncommon except in patients with the erosive inflammatory form of the disease. Osteoporosis is not a component of degenerative change. Newer imaging modalities including computed tomography, magnetic

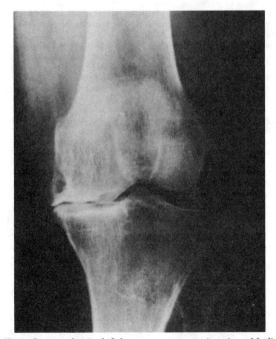

Fig. 24B–1. *Osteoarthritis, left knee, anteroposterior view. Medial compartment changes are characterized by structural cartilage loss with joint space narrowing and subchondral bony sclerosis.*

resonance imaging, and ultrasonographic techniques are helpful in the differential diagnosis of non-osteoarthritic lesions such as internal joint derangements, but provide little additional information in routine study of OA joints.

DIFFERENTIAL DIAGNOSIS

Since OA is a ubiquitous disease and may present in various forms, a number of diagnostic considerations should be entertained, depending on the specific joint involvement. Changes in patients with inflammatory OA of the hands, for example, may suggest a diagnosis of seronegative rheumatoid arthritis. Psoriatic arthritis or Reiter's syndrome, which frequently involve distal interphalangeal joints, may also lead to diagnostic confusion. Osteoarthritis of the hip may be simulated by avascular necrosis or pigmented villonodular synovitis, and OA of the knee may be simulated by mechanical internal joint derangements, chronic infections, or osteochondritis, among others.

Although the diagnosis of OA is usually straightforward, atypical presentations lead to diagnostic difficulties. Such atypical presentations include the occurrence of OA in a joint infrequently involved, such as the elbow; the presence of OA associated with a significant degree of inflammation such as in erosive inflammatory arthritis of the hands; or OA associated with crystal deposition disease such as pyrophosphate or apatite. Neurologic abnormalities due to spinal OA are at times mistaken for those seen in primary neurologic disorders.

TREATMENT

The selection of a specific therapeutic program must be individualized. Many patients require only reassurance that they have no generalized crippling form of rheumatoid disease.

Physical Therapy

Protection of joints from overuse is important, especially if weight-bearing joints are involved. Forces on the lower extremity are increased three- to four-fold when weight is shifted to each leg in walking. Appliances such as canes, when indicated, are beneficial for joint protection.

Weight reduction should be advised, especially in patients with marked obesity. Physical therapy relieves pain and associated muscle spasm and maintains and regains joint range of motion. Simple measures such as hot applications or warm tub baths may alleviate pain. Evidence suggests that exercise such as running is not deleterious to normal joints when the criterion used is loss of roentgenographic space (11). Such activities should be individualized in the presence of OA of weight-bearing joints. Frequently, modified programs such as race-walking or stationary bicycle use without high stress loads may be tolerated.

Drug Therapy

Analgesic agents such as acetominophen, administered on a regular basis, are frequently effective in OA pain management (12). Other analgesic agents such as propoxyphene hydrochloride may be used temporarily as needed. Narcotic preparations, required only occasionally for acute flares, should be very limited in use. Although aspirin, particularly in the enteric-coated form, is tolerated by many patients, the newer nonsteroidal antiinflammatory drugs (NSAIDs) (see Chapter 55) are generally associated with decreased toxicity and increased compliance. These agents share a number of side effects including rash, gastrointestinal upset, peptic ulceration, occasional vague psychic reactions, and tinnitus. Nonacetylated salicylates such as salsalate and choline magnesium trisalicylate as well as acetaminophen may be associated with fewer gastrointestinal reactions.

Oral or parenteral therapy with adrenal corticosteroids is not indicated in the treatment of OA. Intraarticular injections of corticosteroids, however, may be beneficial when used judiciously in the management of acute joint flares. Injections should be infrequent, especially if given in weight-bearing joints. Joint deterioration may be accelerated due to masking of pain with subsequent joint overuse or to a direct deleterious effect of these drugs on cartilage. Pericapsular and ligamentous injections in areas of tenderness around involved joints can provide relief with less hazard.

Surgery

Orthopedic surgical procedures of use in treating OA include arthroplasty, osteotomy, fusion, and partial or total prosthetic replacement. Angulation osteotomy is particularly helpful for correcting joint malalignment when significant varus of valgus deformities of the knee are present in unicompartmental disease. Pain may be relieved by bringing healthy articular cartilages into position.

Hip and knee replacement procedures produce striking symptomatic relief and improved range of motion in patients with disabling OA. Potential benefits of prosthetic replacements must be weighed against associated complications, including infection, phlebitis, pulmonary emboli, nerve injury, and eventual failure of the prosthesis itself by loosening or fracture. The use of porous surface implants to allow bone ingrowth for biologic fixation may lessen prosthesis failures related to loosening.

Advances in arthroscopic technique have led to increased surgical management earlier in the disease course. The joint can be irrigated and debrided to remove loose bodies and to smooth out irregular joint surfaces. Also, superficial degenerated areas of cartilage can be treated by abrasion chondroplasty, in which remaining cartilage is removed down to bleeding bone, with the expectation that the denuded surface will be covered by regenerated functional cartilage. Abrasion procedures may represent a valid adjunct to joint debridement for OA, but more information is required to substantiate their effectiveness and to determine which lesions are most suitable for successful treatment. Joint irrigation alone to remove cartilage fragments and debris present in synovial fluid may provide temporary relief of OA symptoms in some patients (13). This procedure, too, needs further study and validation.

Management of Specific Joints

Hands. Hot soaks, paraffin wax applications, and avoidance of aggravating repetitive trauma may be helpful in OA of the hands. Analgesics and NSAIDs are useful. Local steroid injections into or around involved joints are particularly beneficial when only one or two joints are symptomatic. Osteoarthritis of the first carpometacarpal joint responds temporarily to judicious use of intraarticular steroids. Splinting may be helpful. Joint arthroplasty or arthrodesis may be necessary if these conservative measures fail.

Hip. Osteoarthritis of the hip requires heat, rest from weight bearing, and appropriate range-of-motion exercises. Analgesic and antiinflammatory drugs are helpful. Stress is reduced by the use of crutches, canes, or a walker. Hip replacement procedures are generally recommended for advanced disease.

Knee. Patients with OA of the knee similarly benefit from physical therapy for range of motion and quadriceps strengthening, avoidance of joint over-use, and analgesic/antiinflammatory medication. Use of a cane in the hand opposite the affected knee is often beneficial. Local steroid injections may be considered for acute flares, but more than occasional use should be avoided. Total prosthetic replacements of the knee provide relief of pain and improved ambulation.

Spine. Acute cervical spine symptoms benefit from the use of a collar and traction, particularly when nerve root pain is prominent. Patients with acute or subacute symptoms involving the lumbar spine should use a lumbosacral corset for abdominal support. A firm mattress is helpful.

Experimental Agents

Approaches to the specific management of OA, by which the disease process might be prevented, retarded, or reversed, are based on a search for agents that inhibit cartilage degradation, stimulate cartilage repair, or both. Several agents have been shown capable of stabilizing cartilage in vitro, or interrupting the disease process in experimental models. Examples include growth peptides that stimulate cartilage metabolic synthetic activities (14); tamoxifen, which inhibits estrogen responses (15); low-dose steroids, which may inhibit proteoglycan destruction by proteases (16); a glycosaminoglycan-peptide complex with effects that may be related to growth stimulating peptides or inhibition of cytokines (17); and a polysulphated glycosaminoglycan that inhibits proteolytic enzymes (18). All have been shown capable of experimental amelioration of OA changes in various model systems. These investigations provide promise that clinically useful agents can be developed for a more direct therapeutic approach in the management of OA.

Roland W. Moskowitz, MD
Victor M. Goldberg, MD

1. Patterson AC: Osteoarthritis of the trapezioscaphoid joint. Arthritis Rheum 18:375–379, 1975
2. Doherty M, Preston B: Primary osteoarthritis of the elbow. Ann Rheum Dis 48:743–747, 1989
3. McKendry RJR: Nodal osteoarthritis of the toes. Arthritis Rheum 16:126–134, 1986
4. Ehrlich GE: Inflammatory osteoarthritis. I. The clinical syndromes. J Chron Dis 25:317–328, 1972
5. Shuckett R, Russell ML, Gladman DF: Atypical erosive osteoarthritis and Sjogren's syndrome. Ann Rheum Dis 45:281–288, 1986
6. Resnick O, Shapiro RF, Weisner KB, et al: Diffuse idiopathic skeletal hyperostosis (ankylosing hyperostosis of Forestier and Rotes–Querol). Semin Arthritis Rheum 7:153–187, 1978
7. Mehraban F, Finegan CK, Moskowitz RW: Serum keratan sulphate: quantitative and qualitative comparisons in inflammatory versus non-inflammatory arthritides. Arthritis Rheum 34:383–392, 1991
8. Lohmander LS, Dahlberg L, Ryd L, Heinegard D: Increased levels of proteoglycan fragments in the knee joint after injury. Arthritis Rheum 32:1434–1442, 1989
9. Brandt KD: A pessimistic view of serologic markers for diagnosis and management of osteoarthritis. Biochemical, immunologic, and clinical pathologic barriers. J Rheumatol 16(Suppl 18):39–42, 1989
10. Brandt KD, Fife RS, Braunstein EM, et al: Radiographic grading of the severity of knee osteoarthritis: relation of the Kellgren and Lawrence grade to a grade based on joint space narrowing, and correlation with arthroscopic evidence of articular cartilage degeneration. Arthritis Rheum 34:1381–1386, 1991
11. Lane NE, Bloch D, Jones A, et al: Running and osteoarthritis: a controlled study. Long distance running, bone density, and osteoarthritis. JAMA 255:1147–1151, 1986
12. Bradley JD, Brandt KD, Katz BP, et al: Comparison of an anti-inflammatory dose of ibuprofen, an analgesic dose of ibuprofen, and acetaminophen in the treatment of patients with osteoarthritis of the knee. N Engl J Med 325:87–91, 1991
13. Chang RW, Falconer J, Stulberg SD, et al: A randomized, controlled trial of arthroscopic surgery versus closed-needle joint lavage for patients with osteoarthritis of the knee. Arthritis Rheum 36:289–296, 1993
14. Denko CW, Boja B, Moskowitz RW: Growth promoting peptides in osteoarthritis: insulin, insulin-like growth factor–1, growth hormone. J Rheumatol 17:1217–1221, 1990
15. Rosner IA, Boja BA, Goldberg VM, et al: Tamoxifen therapy in experimental osteoarthritis. Curr Ther Res 34:409–414, 1983
16. Colombo C, Butler M, Hickman L, et al: A new model of osteoarthritis in rabbits. II. Evaluation of anti-osteoarthritic effects of selected antirheumatic drugs administered systematically. Arthritis Rheum 26:1132–1139, 1983
17. Moskowitz RW, Reese JH, Young RG, et al: The effects of Rumalon, a glycosaminoglycan peptide-complex (GP-C), on experimentally-induced osteoarthritis. J Rheumatol 18:205–209, 1991
18. Carreno MR, Muniz OE, Howell DF: The effect of glycosaminoglycan polysulfuric acid ester on articular cartilage in experimental osteoarthritis: effects on morphologic variables of disease severity. J Rheumatol 13:490–497, 1986

25. NEUROPATHIC ARTHROPATHY

Neuropathic arthropathy, commonly called *Charcot joint*, is a severe destructive arthropathy that is a consequence of impaired joint sensation. Charcot (1868) first described this arthropathy in a patient with tabes dorsalis and emphasized the role of the "trophic nerve center" controlling bone and joint nutrition. Many neurologic diseases, including both upper and lower motor neuron disorders, have been reported in association with neuropathic arthropathy (Table 25–1).

PATHOGENESIS

The pathogenesis of neuropathic arthropathy is not clearly understood. Two theories have been proposed. The neurovascular theory postulates that alterations of the sympathetic nervous system lead to increased blood flow to bone, causing active bone hyperemia and bone resorption (1). The neurotraumatic theory speculates that joint damage is primarily caused by repetitive injury to the insensitive joint. In all likelihood, both mechanisms may play a role at different phases of the disease process. The neurovascular changes occur initially. Later, when a joint insensitive to pain is repetitively injured, the neurotraumatic process contributes to progressive joint destruction and repair (2).

CLINICAL MANIFESTATIONS

Neuropathic arthropathy can present in two forms depending on the pathogenesis. Acute neuropathic arthropathy, the atrophic or resorptive form, presents rapidly in a period of a few weeks. The affected joint is swollen, warm, and erythematous indicating hyperemia. The joint may be painful. This form typically involves a nonweight-bearing joint (3) and is often undiagnosed or mistaken as severe infection or an aggressive bone tumor.

Chronic neuropathic arthropathy, the hypertrophic form, is more commonly recognized. It usually develops over a longer period of time and involves weight-bearing joints. Initially the joint involvement may closely mimic osteoarthritis, but later the joint is swollen and enlarged with joint effusion and/or hypertrophic osteophytes. Neurologic changes, including loss of deep pain sensation and loss of deep tendon reflexes, are usually evident, although they may not be readily detectable early (4).

Progression of the disease varies widely. Many patients have a sudden collapse of the joint because of intraarticular or juxtaarticular fractures, whereas others progress more slowly. Spontaneous fractures, dislocation, and infection are common complications. These can lead to further progressive joint destruction.

Diabetes mellitus, tabes dorsalis, and syringomyelia are the three most common causes of neuropathic arthropathy. Diabetic neuroarthropathy occurs in approximately 0.15% of diabetic patients (5). The forefoot and midfoot are most commonly involved (see Chapter 38), followed by ankle, knee, spine and the upper extremity joints. In patients with tabes dorsalis, lower extremity joints are most commonly involved (6). Polyarticular involve-

Table 25–1. *Conditions associated with neuropathic arthropathy*

Diabetes mellitus
Tabes dorsalis
Syringomyelia
Spinal cord or peripheral nerve injury
Leprosy
Amyloidosis
Multiple sclerosis
Myelomeningocele
Congenital insensitivity to pain
Tumor invading nerve
Familial dysautonomia
  (Riley–Day syndrome)
Familial interstitial hypertrophic polyneuropathy
  (Dejerine–Sottas disease)
Hereditary sensory radicular neuropathy
Peroneal muscular atrophy (Charcot–Marie–Tooth Disease)

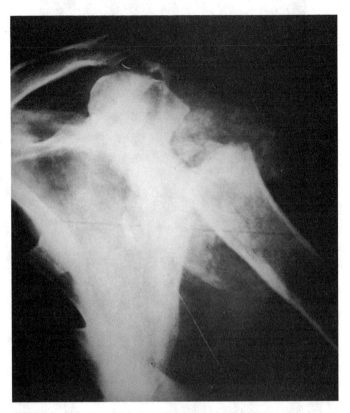

Fig. 25–1. Anteroposterior view of a shoulder of a patient with syringomyelia showing the classic atrophic form of neuropathic arthropathy. There is total resorption of the humeral head. The remaining edge is sharp and normally mineralized. Soft tissue swelling and bone debris are present.

ment can occur. Approximately one-third of patients with syringomyelia have neuropathic arthropathy predominantly in the upper extremity joints and the cervical spine (7).

RADIOLOGIC FINDINGS

In acute neuropathic arthropathy, soft tissue swelling around the joint is usually present. Extensive bone resorption occurs without evidence of bone repair. The transitional zone between the resorbed bone and the remaining bone is sharp. Bone around the resorbed area is normally mineralized (8). Poorly marginated fuzzy bone contours (as occur in septic arthritis) are not evident unless joint infection is superimposed. Bone debris can be seen around the resorbed area (Fig. 25–1).

Early radiographic changes of the hypertrophic form of neuropathic arthropathy may mimic osteoarthritis (OA). In the late stage, severe osteoarthritic changes with massive periarticular new bone formation, large osteophytes, bony fragments accompanying bony dislocation, and subluxation are present resulting in the appearance of a severely disrupted joint (Fig. 25–2). Pathologic fractures of unusual location and orientation are frequently seen. Intraarticular bony fusion is an uncommon finding. A mixed pattern of radiographic findings can present in the same joint. The combination of bone resorption and bone eburnation with osteophytosis and fragmentation are commonly seen, especially in the weight bearing joint.

SYNOVIAL FLUID AND PATHOLOGIC FINDINGS

Noninflammatory fluids and serosanguinous or hemorrhagic effusions are frequently described in neuropathic arthropathy, but a case with severe inflammatory effusion mimicking septic arthritis has been reported (9). Bone and cartilage fragments as well as calcium pyrophosphate dihydrate (CPPD) crystals can

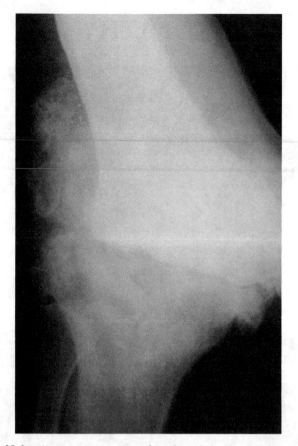

Fig. 25–2. *Anteroposterior view of a tabetic knee showing the classic hypertrophic changes; joint subluxation, osteophytosis and fragmentations and bone debris are present.*

fibrous tissue and mononuclear cells. Multiple fragments of bone and cartilage embedded in the deep layer of synovium are characteristic findings that can be seen even in the early stage of the disease (11). Similar findings can occasionally be seen in severe OA.

The articular ends of the joint are devoid of cartilage. The subchondral bone appears eburnated, shiny, and may be deformed or distorted (4). The underlying bone is replaced by numerous vascular channels. The remaining bone trabeculae are surrounded by dilated vessels and bone is actively resorbed by osteoclasts (2).

MANAGEMENT

Conditions that cause neurologic disorders should be corrected promptly if possible to prevent progression of the neurologic deficit. Immobilization of the affected joint or reduction of weight bearing are recommended. An orthosis should be fitted properly to prevent abnormal stress that can aggravate joint destruction. Arthrodesis has a high failure rate due to non-union, pin fracture, or infection. However, successful knee arthrodesis has been reported and usually requires adequate bone resection, debridement, and firm internal fixation (12). Total joint replacement is generally contraindicated due to rapid loosening and subluxation of the prosthesis. Amputation should be considered in an advanced, destructive case or a case complicated with infection.

Worawit Louthrenoo, MD

1. Delano PJ: The pathogenesis of Charcot's joint. Am J Roentgenol 56:189–200, 1946
2. Brower AC, Allman RM: Pathogenesis of the neurotrophic joint: neurotraumatic vs. neurovascular. Radiology 139:349–354, 1981
3. Norman A, Robbins H, Milgram JE: The acute neuropathic arthropathy—a rapid, severely disorganizing form of arthritis. Radiology 90:1159–1164, 1968
4. Katz I, Rabinowitz JG, Dziadiw R: Early changes in Charcot's joints. Am J Roentgenol 86:965–974, 1961
5. Sinha S, Munichoodappa CS, Kazak GP: Neuro-arthropathy (Charcot's joints) in diabetes mellitus. (Clinical study of 101 cases.) Medicine 51:191–210, 1972
6. Jaffe HL: Metabolic, Degenerative and Inflammatory Diseases of Bone and Joint. Philadelphia, Lea & Febiger, 1972, pp 847–874
7. Skall-Jensen J: Osteoarthropathy in syringomyelia. Analysis of seven cases. Acta Radiol 38:382–388, 1952
8. Brower AC: The acute neuropathic joint. Arthritis Rheum 31:1571–1573, 1988
9. Louthrenoo W, Ostrov BE, Park YS, et al: Pseudoseptic arthritis: an unusual presentation of neuropathic arthropathy. Case report with studies on synovial membrane and synovial fluid. Ann Rheum Dis 50:717–721, 1991
10. Bennett RM, Mall JC, McCarty DJ: Pseudogout in acute neuropathic arthropathy. A clue to pathogenesis? Ann Rheum Dis 33:563–567, 1974
11. Horwitz T: Bone and cartilage debris in the synovial membrane. Its significance in the early diagnosis of neuro-arthropathy. J Bone Joint Surg 30A:579–588, 1948
12. Drennan DB, Fahey JJ, Maylahn RJ: Important factors in achieving arthrodesis of the Charcot knee. J Bone Joint Surg 53A:1180–1193, 1971

also be identified in synovial fluids (10). Severe joint destruction reminiscent of neuropathic arthritis can also be seen in some patients with CPPD or apatite crystals in joint fluid but no neurologic problems.

Synovial changes in neuropathic arthropathy are more dramatic than those in OA. In the acute stage, the synovium is edematous, congested, and infiltrated with polymorphonuclear cells (8,9). In the more chronic stage, the joint capsule is thickened with fibrous tissue. Synovial tissue in the form of pannus grows and invades cartilage. The synovium is replaced with

26. INFECTIOUS ARTHRITIS
A. Bacterial Agents

Acute bacterial infection in a joint typically produces pain, tenderness, and loss of function. The patient may or may not have additional symptoms that suggest an infection, such as fever. The availability of effective antibiotics against most infecting organisms should have made septic arthritis an unimportant clinical entity or historic curiosity. However, septic arthritis continues to be a serious cause of morbidity, mortality, joint damage, and functional disability. Establishment of infection in articular tissues initiates host defense mechanisms that may erradicate the infection but may also damage articular tissues. Increased numbers of individuals with chronic medical illnesses, advanced age, immunosuppression, and prosthetic joints have changed the anticipated clinical presentations that provoke diagnostic consideration of joint infection. Delayed diagnosis in these vulnerable patients reduces the likelihood of a successful treatment outcome. Understanding of pathogenic mechanisms important in septic arthritis provides the basis for interpreting clinical findings, making therapeutic decisions, and directing research studies to improve therapeutic outcome.

PATHOGENIC MECHANISMS IN ARTICULAR INFECTION

Bacteria reach joints in several ways: 1) as a result of trauma, surgery, or arthrocentesis; 2) by contiguous extension from an adjacent focus of osteomyelitis, a soft tissues abscess, an infected prosthesis, or wound infection; and 3) through the blood stream from a remote focus of infection such as cellulitis, respiratory, urinary, or gastrointestinal tract infections. Following direct injection of organisms into the joint cavity, bacteria rapidly multiply in the liquid culture medium of the synovial fluid, are phagocytosed by the synovial lining cells, and are either killed or form abscesses within the synovial membrane. If organisms reach the synovium via the blood stream, they multiply in enlarging subsynovial abscesses until they break into the articular cavity and extend throughout the joint.

Staphylococcus aureus strains from human osteomyelitis and septic arthritis and from a strain that produced joint infection in mice have been shown to bind bone sialoprotein, or type I collagen. This suggests the ability of bacteria to localize in a joint may be related to the interaction of *S. aureus* with the extracellular matrix components (1). Bacterial products such as endotoxin (lipopolysaccharide) from gram negative organisms, cell wall fragments from gram positive organisms, and immune complexes stimulate synovial cells to release tumor necrosis factor (TNF) alpha and interleukin 1 (IL-1) beta, which trigger the infiltration of articular tissues by polymorphonuclear leukocytes (PMNs) and their activation. Bacteria are phagocytosed by vacuolated synovial lining cells and PMNs. The phagocytic cells have bactericidal systems that are more or less successful in killing the bacteria depending on the virulence factors of the infecting organism. Bacterial components form antigen–antibody complexes that activate the classic pathway of complement. Bacterial toxins activate the alternative complement pathway producing the pro-inflammatory split products C3a and C5a. The PMNs are both the primary cellular host defense system and a potential source of irreversible joint damage and destruction. The phagocytic killing of bacteria also results in PMN autolysis with release of lysozomal enzymes into the joint, leading to synovial, ligament, and cartilage damage. The PMNs stimulate arachidonic acid metabolism, release collagenase, and release proteolytic enzymes and more IL-1 to amplify the inflammatory response (2).

Bacteria also induce changes in articular cartilage by mechanisms independent of the inflammatory response reactions as described above. Multiplying bacteria adhere to the articular cartilage surface by binding of the bacterial cell wall glycocalyx to collagen fibrils in the articular cartilage. The collagen fibrils become fragmented permitting invasion of the articular cartilage by bacteria (3). Bacterial products have direct effects on chondrocytes causing inhibition of proteoglycan synthesis and an increase in protease activity. Chondrocyte stimulation by *S. aureus* conditioned culture medium, IL-1, and bacterial polysaccharides results in induction of RNA expression and protein synthesis with increased protease activity. The increased protease activity may be due to increased production of proteases, inactivation of protease inhibitors, or by production of an activator of latent proteases. The chondrocyte proteases persist in the cartilage and continue proteolytic degradation of cartilage with release of collagen and proteoglycan from the matrix, even after the infection is eradicated by antibiotics (4). Bacterial toxins also activate the coagulation system causing intravascular thrombosis of the subsynovial vessels and fibrin deposition on the surface of the synovium and articular cartilage. The layer of fibrin provides an acellular gelatinous nidus for bacterial replication. Subsynovial microvascular obstruction causes ischemia and necrosis, thus permitting further abscess formation (5). Activation of the coagulation system and fibrin deposits activate the fibrinolytic mechanism with formation of plasmin, which destroys the protein core and polysaccharides in cartilage matrix.

After the initial acute, necrotic synovitis, the synovial membrane proliferates (pannus) and erodes articular cartilage and subchondral bone. A chronic synovitis may persist. It has been theorized that cartilage is altered by infection to become antigenic and, together with the adjuvant effects of bacterial components, causes a persistent, immune-mediated, "sterile" synovitis. Persistence of endotoxin or lipopolysaccharide from gram-negative organisms can also stimulate chronic synovitis.

CO-MORBIDITY FACTORS AND THE CLINICAL PRESENTATIONS OF SEPTIC ARTHRITIS

Most articular infections involve a single joint, but 20% are polyarticular. Joints commonly involved include the knee (50%), hip (13%), shoulder (9%), wrist (8%), ankle (8%), elbow (7%), and the small joints of the hand or foot (5%) (6). Many patients are febrile although shaking chills occur in only 20%. The absence of fulminant or severe symptoms tends to decrease consideration of infection and delay diagnosis. Co-morbidity factors modify the risk and frequency of septic arthritis in various groups of patients. The clinical picture is also shaped by these co-morbidity factors, because their distinctive features should prompt earlier recognition and diagnosis of joint infection. Co-morbidity factors important in septic arthritis include age extremes (children and the elderly), co-existant systemic diseases, prosthetic joints, arthrocentesis, and intravenous drug use. Systemic diseases most often associated with septic arthritis include chronic liver disease, diabetes mellitus, malignancy, sickle cell anemia, rheumatoid arthritis (RA), and systemic lupus erythematosus (SLE). Immunosuppressive therapy also increases the risk of joint infection. In chronic liver disease, bacteremias may be prolonged because collateral vessels can permit shunting of organisms past the reticuloendothelial system of the liver. The appearance of joint pain in one of these illnesses should prompt a search for infectious arthritis. Specific organisms causing septic arthritis also carry companion features that should prompt consideration of bacteremia with metastatic suppurative arthritis (6).

Septic Arthritis in Children

Joint infection in children is monarticular in 93% of cases, and one-half of the cases occur in children less than 2 years of age. Septic arthritis in an infant may present with limited spontaneous movement of a limb (pseudoparalysis), irritability, and low grade or no fever. Joints infected tend to involve the large joints of the lower extremities, such as the knee (39%), hip (26%), and ankle (13%). Potential sources of infection in children include otitis media, umbilical catheters, central lines, femoral venipunctures, meningitis, and adjacent osteomyelitis. In the neonate, septic arthritis often occurs with osteomyelitis because metaphyseal vessels communicate with epiphyseal vessels and because the metaphysis of the proximal femur, proximal humerus, proximal radius, and distal lateral tibia are intracapsular. Causative organisms in acute septic arthritis in children depend on the age of the child and the setting in which the infection was acquired. *Neisseria gonorrhoeae* causes less than 10% of septic arthritis, but it is the most common cause of polyarticular septic arthritis in children. Gram stain of the synovial fluid is positive in one-third and culture positive in two-thirds of all septic arthritis in children. Blood cultures are positive in one-third to one-half of the cases and may be the only method to identify the causative organism. In one-third of the septic arthritis cases the causative organism is not identified (7,8).

Radiographs of infected joints may show joint space widening and soft tissue swelling but no changes of osteomyelitis until the infection is present more than 7 to 14 days. Radioisotope scanning with [99m]Technetium is only 77% accurate because vasospasm, abscess formation, or vascular thrombosis may offset the increased uptake. [67]Gallium has an accuracy of 91%, but the radiation dose is higher.

Definitive antibiotic selection should be adjusted when culture results and susceptibility testing are available. Parenteral antibiotics should be continued until there has been significant clinical improvement. Oral antibiotics should then be administered in doses several times the usual dose. Infection in the hip requires urgent surgical decompression to prevent osteonecrosis in the femoral head. Other joints usually respond satisfactorily to repeated needle drainage of synovial pus. Residual abnormality is seen in 25% of infected joints.

Septic Arthritis in the Elderly

In adults with septic arthritis, approximately 40% are over age 60. However, the actual incidence of septic arthritis in the elderly is quite low (9). In this older age group, 75% of the infections occur in joints with prior arthritis, and 75% involve the hip or knee. The majority have significant co-morbidity from diabetes (24%), malignancy (19%), renal failure (14%), other diseases such as rheumatoid arthritis, SLE, chronic lung disease, or alcoholism (14%). Steroid use is seen in up to one-third of these cases. The diagnosis of joint infection is usually not considered on admission because the paucity of signs fails to suggest sepsis. Only 10% of elderly patients are febrile, and only one-third have marked leukocytosis, but the erythrocyte sedimentation rate (ESR) is usually significantly elevated. Joint culture, blood culture, or both yield positive results in most cases. An extraarticular source of infection is evident in approximately 75% of the cases (urinary tract infection, pneumonia, osteomyelitis); infection is due to direct innoculation in approximately 25% of patients (trauma or wound infections). Mortality ranges from 30% to only 5% in a rural elderly population with gram-negative joint infections. Nevertheless, permanent joint damage is substantial. Thirty percent of infected joints progress to osteomyelitis, and 50% of the survivors have a poor functional outcome (9,10).

Joint Infection in Rheumatoid Arthritis

Rheumatoid arthritis patients have an increased incidence of joint infections (0.3% to 3.0%), with a higher mortality and a poor functional outcome in most survivors. Articular infection in RA is seen more in older men with an average disease duration of 20 years. Patients frequently have another serious medical illness and are commonly on prednisone (11). Infection is polyarticular in nearly one-half of the patients. Periarticular features such as infected adjacent bursae, spontaneous drainage, and sinus tract formation may be the presenting manifestation. Fever and leukocytosis are not prominant features, but the ESR is usually elevated and declines with adequate therapy. Duration of symptoms prior to diagnosis is often prolonged because of minimal symptoms or attribution of symptoms to the underlying arthritis. One-third have positive blood cultures; extraarticular sources of infection are commonly found in the skin, lung, or urinary tract. Approximately 2% of the joint infections occur after an intraarticular injection of corticosteroid.

Recurrent infection in the same joint occurs in up to one-third of patients, and there is a three-fold higher mortality for those with polyarticular infection. Analysis of outcome data relative to initial surgical drainage indicates a good outcome in 66% versus only 44% good outcome with medical therapy. Approximately 25% of the medically treated RA patients eventually need surgery. The infected rheumatoid joint needs more aggressive treatment to preserve joint function, to prevent recurrence, and to lower mortality (11,12).

Joint Infection in IV Drug Users

Intravenous drug abuse (IVDA) is increasingly associated with infection of joints. In a recent report, 37% of septic arthritis cases occurred in IVDA and many of these patients were HIV positive (13). Joint infection in IVDA occurs predominantly in the joints and bones of the axial skeleton but also in the peripheral joints. Most infections are due to S. aureus (45%) which is often methicillin resistant, Streptococci (9%) or gram-negative organisms such as Enterobacter, Pseudomonas aeruginosa (40%) and Serratia marcesens (5%). Gram-negative joint infections tend to be more indolent and difficult to diagnose than the more fulminant staphylococcal joint infections. Outbreaks of acute systemic candidiasis in addicts using contaminated brown heroin diluted with lemon juice produce a clinical syndrome of ocular, cutaneous, and costochondral junction or sternoclavicular joint infection. An elevated ESR and leukocytosis are present in more than 60% of the cases but radiographs are abnormal in only 30%. 99^m-Technetium bone scans are usually abnormal and especially helpful in the evaluation of the axial skeleton joints. Increasing numbers of IVDAs are becoming HIV positive, (up to 30% depending on geographical area) thus increasing a population at risk for joint infection and AIDS-associated arthritis [see Chapter 44]. Both acute joint infection with common bacteria and more indolent infections with mycobacteria, fungi and unusual opportunistic organisms occur in HIV-infected patients and must be considered in the differential diagnosis.

Joint Infections After Bites

Joint infections after animal bites are usually due to S. aureus or organisms of the oral flora common to the specific animal.

Pasteurella multocida causes one-half of the infections following cat or dog bites producing marked erythema, pain, and swelling in the small joints of the hand within 24 hours of the bite. P. multocida is sensitive to penicillin, but joint infections should also be surgically debrided. Other infections following dog and cat bites include Pseudomonas species, Moraxella, and Haemophilus species. Rat bites cause infection with Streptobacillus moniliformis or Spirillum minus, producing fever, rash, and joint pain with regional adenopathy. Penicillin is effective.

Joint infections following human bites are often indolent requiring a week to become manifest and are due to gram-negative bacillus Eikenella corrodens, S. aureus, group B streptococci, or oral anaerobes such as a fusobacterium, peptostreptococci, and bacteroides species. Human bites should be treated with penicillin or ampicillin for three to five days.

Joint Infection following Intraarticular Injections

The risk of joint infection following intraarticular corticosteroid injection is well-recognized but is probably less than 0.01%. Early acute septic arthritis, within one week after arthrocentesis, occurs from direct bacterial inoculation during the arthrocentesis or from bacterial contamination of the injection tract. The acute infection is usually associated with suggestive clinical signs of fever, abrupt increase in pain, and swelling of the joint. Septic arthritis developing one week to three months after intraarticular glucocorticoid injection probably occurs after bacteremia from a remote site of infection. Long-lasting immunosuppressive effects of the crystalline corticosteroids or the antecedent joint disease may provide a locus of impaired resistance during episodes of bacteremia. The late infection is often not suspected because of the delay after the injection. Systemic symptoms may be absent and local joint symptoms may not be severe or may be disregarded, especially in patients with underlying arthritis or those on immunosuppressive drugs (14).

Infections in Prosthetic Joints

Approximately 200,000 prosthetic joint arthroplasties are performed yearly in the United States. Infection is the most devastating complication of prosthetic joint surgery, because it leads to prosthesis loosening, failure, and sepsis. The rate of early prosthetic joint infections (<12 months) is 2% or less and the annual rate of late infection (>12 months) is 0.60% (15). The estimated cost of an infected prosthesis is $50,000, requires up to five hospital admissions for treatment and carries a mortality of up to 20%. With 1,000 to 2,000 early prosthesis infections per year and an increasing number of late infections in an expanding population of at risk patients with prostheses, the costs are at least $10 million annually (15,16). There is a substantially increased risk of prosthetic joint infection in patients with RA (2- to 5-fold increase); in joints with prior surgery and revision arthroplasties (2- to 8-fold increase); and in joints with prior infection. Infection risk is also increased if there is a concurrent infection at a distant site, if the patient is being treated with corticosteroid therapy, and if the operation time for the surgery is prolonged (15). The presence of infection anywhere in the body is a contraindication to elective prosthesis implantation. Joint replacement should be delayed until infection is eradicated.

Two-thirds of prosthetic joint infections occur within one year of surgery and are due to intra-operative innoculations of bacteria into the joint or post-operative bacteremias. Early post-operative bacteremias are due to skin infections, pneumonia, and dental or urinary tract infections that may seed the newly implanted prosthesis. In prosthetic infections occurring within one year of surgery there is usually a history of a post-operative wound infection that appeared to resolve, satisfactory post-operative recovery for many months, and the development of persistent joint pain at rest and on weight bearing. Patients may become acutely ill with a fulminant, septic joint, and shock, especially with early S. aureus infection. However, patients may not be febrile and have minimal local joint signs of infection especially with the low virulence S. epidermidis infections. Many patients have persistent leukocytosis and almost all have elevated ESR.

Early infection rates have been reduced to less than 2% by the administration of peri-operative antibiotics so that bactericidal levels of antibiotics are present in the tissues during surgery; the use of clean air systems for operating rooms; and improved surgical technique or experience. Post-operative prophylactic antibiotics should be brief to avoid promotion of antibiotic resistant infections. Prompt treatment of wound infections, decompression of hematomas, vigorous treatment of post-operative pneumonias and urinary tract infections, and early removal of intravenous and urinary catheters decrease the risk of early post-operative bacteremias. Organisms causing early prosthetic infections are *S. aureus* (50%), mixed infections (30%), gram negatives (10%) and anaerobes (5%). The use of antibiotic impregnated cement remains controversial because of concerns regarding prolonged toxicity and efficacy (17).

One-third of prosthetic joint infections occur one year or more after surgery. Extraarticular sites of infection such as pneumonia, urinary tract infections, instrumentation, skin infections, and dental procedures produce intermittant bacteremias. The patient usually has an uneventful surgery and more than one year of satisfactory functional recovery before the onset of pain in the prosthetic joint. Interestingly, approximately 25% reported injury from a fall within two weeks of pain onset, and approximately 20% have prior revisions. The diagnostic dilemma is differentiation of septic from aseptic loosening of the prosthesis. Infected patients usually do not have fever or leukocytosis, but most have an elevated ESR. Most patients require removal of the prosthesis; reimplantation is often complicated by reinfection (38%). Organisms isolated from late infected prostheses are 75% gram positive and 25% gram negative organisms with staphylococci, streptococci, *E. coli*, and anaerobes accounting for 86% of all infections (15).

The current recommendations (16) to prevent infection of joint prostheses are: 1) search for and eradicate any foci of infection in dental, genitourinary, gastrointestinal, or cutaneous sites before the joint surgery; 2) discontinue corticosteroids and immunosuppressive drugs or reduce to the lowest possible dose prior to surgery; 3) administer pre-operative antibiotics so that bactericidal tissue levels are attained at the time of surgery; 4) treat any infection after joint surgery at once; and 5) use prophylactic antibiotics for procedures likely to produce bacteremia in patients with high risk for prosthetic infections.

Treatment of joint prosthesis infections is arduous and prolonged. For the infected, non-loose prosthesis, surgical arthrotomy with meticulous debridement of all abscesses and devitalized tissues, catheter placement for suction drainage, and prolonged antibiotics are recommended. If the prosthesis is loose, a one- or two-stage revision (debridement, removal of prosthesis and all cement, followed by implantation of a new prosthesis) using antibiotic impregnated cement is preferred. There is a high rate of reinfection (38%) in new implants whether replaced immediately or after two to three months of antibiotic therapy. If the infection cannot be eradicated or the patient's medical condition precludes revision surgery, excision arthroplasty is required. If insufficient bone stock remains after debridement, removal of an infected prosthesis, and arthrodesis will provide a better functional limb than excision arthroplasty.

FEATURES OF SPECIFIC ORGANISMS CAUSING SEPTIC ARTHRITIS

Gram-positive organisms cause 65% to 85% of nongonococcal bacterial arthritis, gram negative bacilli cause 10% to 15%, and less than 5% are caused by mixed aerobic and anaerobic infections. More indolent infections with mycobacteria and fungi cause less than 5% of joint infections. The frequency distribution of individual organisms causing nongonococcal septic arthritis varies in different clinical situations. Therapeutic decisions must be made before or without causative organism identification. Initial therapy selection is based on the synovial fluid gram stain (revealing in 50% to 60%) and the most likely causative organism given the clinical setting. Ongoing therapy is later modified according to SF culture results, specific antibiotic sensitivity testing results, and whether clinical response indicates improvement.

Gram negative bacilli cause approximately 10% of all joint infections and tend to be seen in the very young, elderly patients, those with severe trauma or serious underlying medical illnesses (renal failure or transplantation, prosthetic joints, SLE, RA, diabetes, malignancy) and in IV drug users. The source of infection is commonly identified in the urinary tract or skin. Mortality rates have decreased from approximately 20% before 1980 to 5% after 1980. Poor joint outcome has decreased from 70% to 33%. Improved outcome is probably due to more effective antibiotics and improved control of underlying medical illnesses. Outcomes should be good in nearly 100% if the patient can be managed medically and in 55% if surgical drainage is required for control of the infection (10). *N. gonorrhoeae* joint infection is discussed separately because clinical presentation and therapeutic response are distinctive.

POLYMICROBIAL AND ANAEROBIC INFECTIONS

Up to 10% of joint infections are polymicrobial and are seen following penetrating trauma or recent surgery. Anaerobic joint infections are uncommon (1%), often caused by multiple organisms, and occur following trauma or penetrating injury to the limbs, in prosthetic joints, in the compromised host, or following gastrointestinal surgery for malignancy. The most common anaerobes in post-operative or trauma-induced joint infection are Peptococcus and Peptostreptococcus species. *B. fragilis* is the major pathogen found in anaerobic infections in patients with debilitating medical illnesses. Other anaerobic organisms include Fusobacterium species, anaerobic diphtheroids or corynebacteria, and clostridium species. Most cases of anaerobic joint infection are monarticular, involving the hip and knee in 80%. Foul smelling synovial fluid and air within the joint or surrounding soft tissue on radiograph should suggest anaerobic infection. One-half of the anaerobic infections are mixed. Infection of the hip may occur by direct extension of a retroperitoneal or pelvic abscess often in the setting of malignancy or chemotherapy (10). Extraarticular sites of anaerobic infection include the abdomen, genital tract, periodontal abscesses, sinusitis, and decubiti.

DISSEMINATED GONOCOCCAL INFECTIONS

N. gonorrhoeae, (GC) a gram-negative intracellular and extracellular diplococcus, produces septic arthritis in the small joints of the hands, wrists, elbows, knees, and ankles and rarely the axial skeletal joints. There are one to three million cases of GC per year in the US. Approximately 1% of these cases develop bacteremia and arthritis (disseminated gonococcal infection or DGI). Disseminated gonococcal infection is generally discussed as a separate entity from other forms of suppurative bacterial arthritis, because it is the most common form of acute bacterial arthritis and has a distinctive clinical picture and excellent response to appropriate therapy (18). Gonococcal strains with pili on their surface adhere to mucosal surfaces and can resist phagocytosis by PMNs. Understanding of the pathogenesis of DGI is based on experimental animal studies in which nonviable bacteria and GC lipopolysaccharide produced arthritis in rabbits. The early phase of DGI is likely an immune complex disease that resolves spontaneously. Affected individuals presumably have foci of infection within mucosal surfaces that can intermittantly cause bacteremia and the clinical manifestations of DGI. In some cases the bacteremia is sufficient to establish a synovial infection and cause true septic arthritis. *N. gonorrhoeae* may also cause gonococcal osteomyelitis with a subacute pattern of pain or swelling without fever or rash, often in the small joints of the hand or foot.

A frequent presentation of gonococcal arthritis (or DGI) is in a sexually active individual with a five to seven day history of fever, shaking chills, multiple skin lesions (petechiae, papules, pustules, hemorrhagic bullae, or necrotic lesions), fleeting migratory polyarthralgias, and tenosynovitis in the fingers, wrists, toes, and ankles that typically evolves into a persistent mono or oligoarthritis. Skin lesions occur in up to 50%, starting as an erythematous macule that progresses to a papule, then pustule

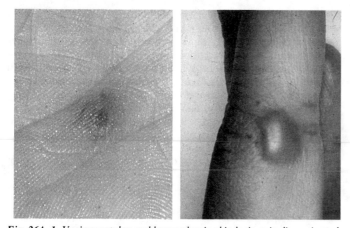

Fig. 26A–1. Vesicopustular and hemorrhagic skin lesions in disseminated gonococcal infection. Left, a pustule with a necrotic center surrounded by inflammation. Right, large hemorrhagic blister (bulla) with fluid that may be positive for the inciting organism (from the Revised Clinical Slide Collection on the Rheumatic Diseases).

with necrosis or ulceration on the trunk and extremities including palms and soles. The oral mucosa is spared. Lesions of different ages are usually present at the same time (Fig. 26A–1). Affected individuals may not have symptoms of genitourinary tract infection: 80% of men and women with DGI have asymptomatic local GC infection, urethritis (up to 50% asymptomatic), cervicitis (majority asymptomatic), proctitis (90% asymptomatic) or pharyngitiis (most asymptomatic). Women are often menstruating or pregnant. Additional risk factors for DGI infection include inherited deficiencies of the late complement components (C5, C6, C7, C8).

Isolation of the organism can be difficult, because it is very sensitive to drying. Blood cultures are often positive during the first week, but cultures from joints with early tenosynovitis are often negative. Cultures of synovial fluid from joints with frank purulent arthritis are usually positive, and fluid from skin lesions may be positive. The operational rule for diagnosis is to culture all orifices and plate at the bedside on chocolate agar or Thayer Martin medium (synovial fluid, blood, cervix, urethra, rectum, pharynx, and skin lesion fluid). Proof of infection by culture of the organism requires 24 hrs, but treatment must be initiated according to diagnosis based on the characteristic clinical features described above. Antibiotics should be administered to eradicate all foci of infection and prevent further recurrences of bacteremia. Treatment for DGI in the early febrile tenosynovitis phase or the later frank arthritis is the same. The strains that cause DGI are those which have pili on their surface and are generally sensitive to penicillin. Strains that carry a plasmid for production of Beta-lactamase (penicillinase) are resistant to penicillin but sensitive to spectinomycin. The strains of penicillinase-producing N. gonorrhoeae are predominant in the Far East and West Africa and are rapidly increasing in the United States and Europe especially in prostitutes and the urban poor. Current treatment recommendations are initial ceftriaxone 1 g/day for 7 days; if found to be sensitive, penicillin 10–20 million units/day or ampicillin 4 g/day for 7 days (19). Daily needle aspiration of synovial fluid should be performed as long as it continues to accumulate. Gonococcal infections usually do not require surgical debridement and drainage and most often do not produce permanent joint damage.

A similar arthritis–dermatitis syndrome may be produced by N. meningitidis, which may be increasing in frequency in urban areas. N. meningitidis, a gram negative diplococcus, may produce septic arthritis in the setting of a relatively mild upper respiratory tract infection or severe clinical illness with shock and meningoencephalitis. Petechial lesions on mucous surfaces, trunk, and lower extremities should suggest this as a diagnostic possibility.

DIAGNOSTIC APPROACH TO SEPTIC ARTHRITIS

Clinical suspicion and an extraarticular focus of infection should prompt a search for septic arthritis. A positive gram stain and culture of the synovial fluid are the fundamental criteria for the diagnosis of bacterial arthritis, but are revealing in only one-half to three-fourths of patients. Delay in diagnosis occurs when the anticipated clinical picture is altered. Fever may be absent or only low grade in 50% of the cases. Blood tests usually have nonspecific abnormalities. Peripheral white blood cell counts are elevated in approximately one-half of cases, but the ESR and C reactive protein are usually elevated. Blood cultures are positive in approximately 50% of the cases and may be the only method to identify the causative organism.

Synovial fluid analysis is the most important test in acute septic arthritis. The white blood cell count (WBC) is intensely inflammatory ($>50,000/mm^3$) in 50% to 70% of the cases and moderately inflammatory ($2,000–50,000/mm^3$) in the remainder. The percentage of PMNs is usually greater than 85%. The synovial fluid WBC may be low within the first 72 hours, but will be higher if repeated 12 to 48 hours later. Synovial fluid glucose is often less than 25% of the serum glucose, but may also be low in other forms of arthritis such as RA. Lactic acid is usually elevated because of increased glucose utilization and anaerobic conversion to lactic acid. Levels of lactic acid usually correlate with a fall in synovial fluid pH, but may be normal in gram-negative infections or if antibiotics have been administered. Urate and calcium pyrophosphate crystals may be seen in infected synovial fluids presumably because of "leaching" out from intraarticular deposits during infection. The finding of crystals should not dissuade one from the diagnosis of joint sepsis.

Gram stain of synovial fluid will reveal organisms in 50% to 70% of infected joints and will distinguish gram-positive from gram-negative organisms but not staphylococci from streptococci. Fluid should be cultured aerobically and anaerobically. If gonococcal infection is likely, chocolate agar or medium should be plated as soon as the specimen is obtained to avoid drying. The use of blood culture bottles for synovial fluid may improve the frequency of bacteria isolation. The operational rule should be to culture all orifices, body fluids, and foci of infection.

Early in acute bacterial arthritis the only radiographic abnormality evident is soft tissue swelling and signs of synovial effusions. A plain radiograph should be obtained at the time of diagnosis to search for a contiguous focus of osteomyelitis and to provide a baseline to monitor adequacy of treatment. After 10 to 14 days of bacterial infection, destructive changes of joint space narrowing (reflecting cartilage destruction) and erosions or foci of subchondral osteomyelitis become evident (Fig. 26A–2). Gas formation within the joints suggests infection with E. coli or anaerobes.

99mTechnetium methylene diphosphonate bone scans demonstrate increased uptake with increased blood flow in the septic synovial membrane and at metabolically active bone (Fig. 26A–3). 67Gallium citrate or 111indium labeled WBC scans may demonstrate enhanced activity in septic joints. Gallium tends to concentrate at sites of increased protein concentration and leukocytes whereas technetium uptake results from increased

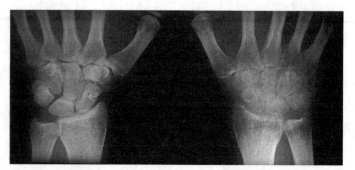

Fig. 26A–2. Staphylococcus arthritis in wrists. The carpus and adjacent bones reveal soft tissue swelling and localized osteopenia. There is narrowing of multiple joints and irregularity of adjacent bony margins.

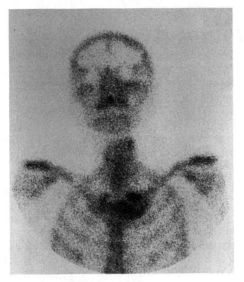

Fig. 26A-3. *Technetium radioisotope scan of septic sternoclavicular joint shows increased uptake in medial clavicle and first rib.*

blood flow. Fluroscopy can be very helpful during aspiration of the axial joints. Bone scans normally may show increased uptake for one year after prosthesis insertion. After one year, increased uptake occurs with septic or aseptic loosening of the prosthesis. Gallium has a low sensitivity for prosthesis infection and the utility of indium-WBC scans has not been established.

THERAPEUTIC APPROACH TO SEPTIC ARTHRITIS

Initial antibiotic selection for bacterial arthritis is directed by the clinical setting, including age, antecedent history, extraarticular foci of infection, and co-morbidity factors together with synovial fluid gram stain findings. The initial antibiotic regimen should be modified when culture results identify the causative organism (usually available in 1–2 days) and adjusted when sensitivities of the causative organism are known (usually by day 3 or 4). Parenteral administration should generally be continued for two weeks then followed by oral antibiotics for 1–2 weeks given at 2–3 times the usual dose. Duration of antibiotic therapy must be determined by the clinical response (20). Infections due to streptococci and haemophilus can be eradicated usually in two weeks. Staphylococcal infections require longer treatment especially in those with prior arthritis. Parenteral antibiotics produce synovial fluid antibiotic concentrations required to eradicate bacteria, therefore intraarticular injection of antibiotics is unnecessary. Synovial fluid bactericidal levels should be measured if infection is not responding promptly.

Acute nongonococcal septic arthritis cannot be treated successfully by antibiotics alone. The joint must be aspirated adequately to drain intraarticular pus. Adequate drainage is accomplished by daily needle aspiration, lavage of peripheral joints, or arthroscopic lavage and debridement of the axial and larger peripheral joints (21). Surgical arthrotomy is required for drainage and debridement of septic hips, septic joints with co-existent osteomyelitis, and joint infections that are not controlled within 5 to 7 days by needle or arthroscopic drainage. Arthroscopy permits disruption of abscesses, removal of necrotic synovium, lysis of intraarticular adhesions, and irrigation under visualization. Outcome of needle drainage was shown to be comparable to arthrotomy or arthroscopy as initial treatment in accessible joints (21). In children, arthroscopy has been shown to be as good as

arthrotomy but allows for earlier recovery and avoids the need for repeated aspirations. Evidence is accumulating that treatment of infected rheumatoid joints should include early, aggressive surgical debridement and drainage (11,12).

Pain in an infected joint causes the patient to hold the joint in flexion, which can lead to contractures. It has been standard therapy to splint infected joints to reduce pain; however, recent studies advocate continuous passive motion and active range of motion with muscle strengthening exercises when the effusion is reduced (18).

The clinical outcome for septic arthritis is dependent on several factors. The duration of symptoms prior to appropriate treatment is important. Only one out of four patients have complete recovery if treated after more than a week of symptoms, but one-half have good recovery if treated in less than eight days. Other factors are the number of infected joints, the age of the patient, the degree of immunocompetence of the host, the normalcy of the joint architecture prior to the infection, sensitivity of the infecting organism to minimally toxic antibiotics, duration of positive synovial fluid cultures, extent of surgical debridement or drainage required to control infection, treatability of the extraarticular site of infection, and the age of the patient. Outcome is generally poor if synovial fluid cultures are positive for greater than six days after antibiotics have been started, if infection is polyarticular especially in patients with RA, and if infection is caused by a gram negative bacillus (11,22).

Maren L. Mahowald, MD

1. Bremel T, Lange S, Yacoub A, et al: Experimental staphylococcus aureus arthritis in mice. Infect Immun 59:2615–2623, 1991

2. Saez–Lorens X, Jafari HS, Olsen KD, et al: Induction of suppurative arthritis in rabbits by Haemophilus endotoxin, tumor necrosis factor–alpha, and interleukin–1 beta. J Infect Dis 163:1267–1272, 1991

3. Alderson M, Speers D, Emslie K, et al: Acute hematogenous osteomyelitis and septic arthritis—Single Disease. J Bone Joint Surg 68:268–271, 1986

4. Williams RI, Smith R, Schurman D: Septic arthritis: Staphylococcal induction of chondrocyte proteolytic activity. Arthritis Rheum 33:533–541, 1990

5. Mahowald ML: Animal modes of infectious arthritis. Clin Rheum Dis 12:403–421, 1986

6. Goldenberg DL. The evaluation of patients with nongonococcal bacterial arthritis, Infections in the Rheumatic Diseases. Edited by Espinoza L, Goldenberg D, Arnett F, Alarcon G. Orlando; Grune & Stratton, 1988, pp 3–20

7. Morrissy RT: Bone and joint infection in the neonate. Pediatr Ann 18:33–44, 1989

8. Fink CW, Nelson JD: Septic arthritis and osteomyelitis in children. Clin Rheum Dis 12:423–435, 1986

9. Vincent GM, Amirault JD: Septic arthritis in the elderly. Clin Orthop 251:241–245, 1990

10. Newman ED, Davis DE, Harrington TM: Septic arthritis due to gram negative bacilli: Older patients with good outcome. J Rheum 15:659–662, 1988

11. Gardner GC, Weisman NH: Pyarthrosis in patients with rheumatoid arthritis: a report of 13 cases and a review of the literature from the past 40 years. Am J Med 88:503–511, 1990

12. Goldenberg DL: Infectious arthritis complicating rheumatoid arthritis and other chronic rheumatic disorders. Arthritis Rheum 32:496–502, 1989

13. Brancos MA, Peris P, Miro JM, et al: Septic arthritis in heroin addicts. Semin Arth Rheum 21:81–87, 1991

14. Ostensson A, Geborek P: Septic arthritis as a non-surgical complication in rheumatoid arthritis: Relation to disease severity and therapy. Brit J Rheumatol 30:35–38, 1991

15. Maderazo EG, Judson S, Pasternak H: Late infections of total joint prostheses: a review and recommendations for prevention. Clin Orthop 229:131–142, 1988

16. Blackburn WD, Alarcon GS: Prosthetic joint infections: a role for prophylaxis. Arthritis Rheum 34:110–117, 1991

17. Maguire JH: Advances in the control of perioperative sepsis in total joint replacement. Rheum Dis Clin N Am 14:519–535, 1988

18. Goldenberg DL, Reed JI: Bacterial arthritis. N Engl J Med 312:764–771, 1985

19. Center for Disease Control. 1989 sexually transmitted diseases treatment guidelines. MMWR 38:1–43, 1990

20. Smith J: Infectious Arthritis. Infec Dis Clin N Amer 4(3):523–538, 1990

21. Broy SB, Schmid FR: A comparison of medical drainage (needle aspiration) and surgical drainage (arthrotomy or arthroscopy) in the initial treatment of infected joints. Clin Rheum Dis 12:501–522, 1986

22. Meijers K, Dijkmans B, Hermans J, et al: Non-gonococcal infectious arthritis: A retrospective study. J Infect 14:13–20, 1987

B. Viral and Less Common Agents

The occurrence of acute inflammatory arthritis in some viral infections has long been recognized. The development of chronic arthralgia or arthritis following an acute infection in some patients has spurred the search for virally induced alterations in the immune system or persistent viral infection. The number of patients in the rheumatologic population with post-viral arthralgia or arthritis may be significant, but diagnosis of acute infection is rarely confirmed by acute phase serology or viral isolation, because patients often present late in their course. As improvements in biotechnology provide simpler and more sensitive tests for viral diagnosis, and options for specific antiviral treatment become available, it may become necessary to consider specific viruses in the differential diagnosis of arthritis.

PARVOVIRUS B19

Infection with human parvovirus, designated B19, may be responsible for as many as 12% of patients presenting with recent onset polyarthralgia or polyarthritis (1). The B19 parvovirus is common and widespread, causing the common childhood exanthem *erythema infectiosum*, or fifth disease, characterized by red cheeks that look as if they had been slapped and a lacy or blotchy rash of the torso and extremities. Approximately 10% of children with fifth disease have arthralgias, and 5% have arthritis, usually short lived. Up to 60% of adults have serologic evidence of past infection. However, up to 78% of infected symptomatic adults develop joint symptoms. Outbreaks of erythema infectiosum occur in late winter and spring, but summer and fall outbreaks have also been observed. Sporadic cases may occur throughout the year (2).

Whereas the B19 infection is usually mild or even asymptomatic in children, adults tend to have a more severe, flu-like illness. Adults usually lack the facial rash. The reticular rash on the torso or extremities may be subtle or absent. Arthralgia is more prominent than frank arthritis. The distribution of involved joints is rheumatoid-like with prominent symmetric involvement of metacarpophalangeal, proximal interphalangeal, knee, wrist, and ankle joints. Patients usually experience sudden onset followed in two weeks by improvement. Joint symptoms in infected adults are usually self-limited, but a minority of adults may have symptoms for up to five years, the longest follow-up to date. The course in those with chronic symptoms includes intermittent flares. Only one-third are symptom-free between flares (1). Morning stiffness is prominent. About one-half of the patients meet diagnostic criteria for rheumatoid arthritis (see Appendix 1). Rheumatoid factor is usually absent in parvovirus B19 arthropathy, but transiently low to moderate titer rheumatoid factor as well as anti-DNA and anti-lymphocyte antibodies may be found in some patients acutely (3). Joint erosions and rheumatoid nodules have not been reported. Specific serologic diagnosis is possible. However, there is a brief opportunity to make the diagnosis based on the presence of anti-B19 IgM antibodies, which may be elevated for only two months following an acute infection. Joint symptoms occur one to three weeks following initial infection; anti-B19 IgM antibodies are usually present at the time of onset of rash or joint symptoms. The high prevalence of anti-B19 IgG antibodies in the adult population limits its diagnostic usefulness. Appropriate treatment includes nonsteroidal antiinflammatory agents. Parvovirus B19 has also been shown to cause most cases of transient aplastic crisis in patients with chronic hemolytic anemias, some cases of hydrops fetalis with fetal loss, and chronic bone marrow suppression in immunocompromised patients (4).

HEPATITIS VIRUSES

Hepatitis B virus infection may cause an immune complex mediated arthritis. Significant viremia occurs early in infection. Soluble immune complexes with circulating anti-hepatitis B surface antigen are formed as anti-hepatitis B surface antigen antibodies are produced. Arthritis onset is sudden and often severe. Joint involvement is usually symmetric and migratory or additive, but simultaneous involvement of several joints at onset may occur. The joints of the hand and knee are most often affected, but wrists, ankles, elbows, shoulders, and other large joints may be involved as well. Arthritis and urticaria may precede jaundice by days to weeks and may persist several weeks after jaundice. While arthritis is usually limited to the pre-icteric prodrome, those patients who develop chronic active hepatitis or chronic hepatitis B viremia may have recurrent arthralgias or arthritis. Polyarteritis nodosa and mixed essential cryoglobulinemia are two entities frequently associated with chronic hepatitis B viremia (5). Hepatitis A infection is rarely associated with arthralgia and rash during acute infection, or with cryoglobulinemia in chronic infection (6). Hepatitis C virus has recently been associated with cryoglobulinemia.

RUBELLA VIRUS

Rubella virus is the sole member of the genus rubivirus in the Togaviridae family of RNA viruses. Rubella infection leads to a high incidence of joint complaints in adults, especially in women. Joint symptoms may occur one week before or after onset of the characteristic rash. Joint involvement is usually symmetric and may be migratory, resolving after a few days to two weeks. Arthralgias are more common than frank arthritis. Stiffness is prominent. The proximal interphalangeal and metacarpophalangeal joints of the hands, knees, wrists, ankles, and elbows are most frequently involved. Periarthritis, tenosynovitis, and carpal tunnel syndrome are known complications. In some patients, symptoms may persist for several months or years (7).

Live attenuated vaccines have been employed in rubella vaccination. A high frequency of post-vaccination arthralgia, myalgia, arthritis, and paraesthesias have been associated with some vaccine preparations. The HPV77/DK12 strain is the most arthritogenic of the vaccine strains that have been available in the United States. The pattern of joint involvement is similar to natural infection. Arthritis usually occurs two weeks after innoculation and lasts less than a week, although symptoms may persist in some patients for more than a year. The currently used vaccine (RA 27/3) may cause post-vaccination joint symptoms in 15% or more of recipients (8).

In children, two syndromes of rheumatologic interest may occur. In the *arm syndrome*, a brachial radiculoneuritis causes arm and hand pain and dysesthesias that are worse at night. The *catcher's crouch* syndrome is a lumbar radiculoneuropathy characterized by popliteal fossa pain on arising in the morning. Those affected assume a catcher's crouch position. The pain gradually decreases through the day. Episodes may recur for up to one year, but there is no permanent damage (8,9). Both syndromes occur one to two months after vaccination. The initial episode may last up to two months, but recurrences are usually shorter in duration.

HUMAN IMMUNODEFICIENCY VIRUS

Several musculoskeletal syndromes have been described in human immunodeficiency virus (HIV) infected patients (10). Whether these are attributable to HIV infection itself or to co-infection with other agents remains controversial. The caprine arthritis encephalitis virus, a goat retrovirus, causes an inflammatory destructive arthritis and lends support to the notion that HIV infection alone may have musculoskeletal manifestations. This is covered in more detail in Chapter 44.

ALPHAVIRUSES

The alphavirus genus of the Togaviridae family includes a number of arthritogenic viruses responsible for major epidemics of febrile polyarthritis in Africa, Australia, Europe, and Latin

America. All are mosquito-borne, the specific species depending on the virus and the locale. The known viral pathogens in this genus include Chikungunya fever virus, O'nyong-nyong virus, Ross River virus, Sindbis virus, Mayaro virus, and Barmah Forest virus (11,12).

Chikungunya fever virus (Chikungunya means "that which bends up") causes abrupt onset of fever, myalgia, and sudden severe pain in one or more joints. Symptoms occur 3 to 12 days after a bite by infected *Aedes* species mosquitos. Maculopapular skin eruption occurs two to five days after onset. Petechiae may occur. Acute disease resolves within 10 days, but joint pain and swelling may last weeks to months.

O'nyong-nyong ("joint breaker") virus is characterized by sudden onset headache, retroorbital pain, chills, and severe symmetric polyarthralgia. A majority of patients develop a morbilliform rash by day 4 of their illness. Postcervical adenitis is often prominent. Residual joint pain often persists. The virus is transmitted by *Anopheles* mosquitos.

Ross River virus is responsible for epidemics of acute febrile polyarthritis in the islands of the South Pacific and in Australia, where it is endemic. Outbreaks occur most frequently in the late summer and fall. The first symptom is usually sudden onset joint pain. Wrists, ankles, metacarpophalangeals, interphalangeals, and knees are most commonly affected. Most patients develop a macular or maculopapular rash, although vesicular, papular, or petechial lesions may also be seen. In a few patients with Chikungunya fever virus or Ross River virus infection, arthritis may persist for years.

Barmah Forest virus is an alphavirus originally isolated from mosquitos in Australia and recently shown to cause febrile polyarthritis (12).

OTHER VIRUSES

Apart from specific viral infections noted above, in which arthralgia and arthritis are typically prominent features, there are a host of commonly encountered viral syndromes in which joint involvement is occasionally seen. Children with varicella have been reported to rarely develop brief monarticular or pauciarticular arthritis, which is thought to be viral in origin. This must be differentiated from the occasional bacterial arthritis due to contiguous bacterial spread from an infected vesicle. Adults who develop mumps occasionally develop small or large joint synovitis lasting up to several weeks. Arthritis may precede or follow parotitis by up to four weeks.

Infection with adenovirus and coxsackieviruses A9, B2, B3, B4, and B6 have been associated with recurrent episodes of polyarthritis, pleuritis, myalgia, rash, pharyngitis, myocarditis, and leukocytosis. Epstein–Barr virus-associated mononucleosis is frequently accompanied by polyarthralgia, but frank arthritis is rare. Polyarthritis, fever, and myalgias due to echovirus infection have been reported in only a few cases. Arthritis associated with herpes simplex virus or cytomegalovirus infections is likewise rare. Vaccinia virus has been associated with post-vaccination knee arthritis in only two reported cases.

LESS COMMON NON-VIRAL AGENTS

Syphilis

Syphilis is a rare cause of arthritis but should not be overlooked; the incidence of syphilis is increasing. *Saber shins* are a classic manifestation of congenital syphilis. In older children, painless effusions, especially of the knees (Clutton's joints), may occur (13).

In acquired primary syphilis, transient bone pain may be prominent. The tibia, humerus, and cranium are most frequently involved, but roentgenograms are normal. In secondary syphilis, pain and tenderness with overlying soft tissue swelling may be seen in superficial bones such as anterior tibia, sternum, ribs, and frontal calvarium. Symptoms and signs are variable, but are characteristically worse at night. Proliferative periostitis is the most common radiographic change and may cause marked cor-

tical thickening. The tibia, sternum, ribs, and calvarium are most significantly involved, but changes may also be seen in the femur, fibula, clavicle, hands, and feet. Periostitis in the adult, involving clavicles or tibiae, is frequently syphilitic. Destructive bony lesions suggest syphilitic osteomyelitis or osteitis, but these are less common than periostitis. Areas of lysis may be seen in the skull, although any bone may be affected. Skull involvement may present as headache with localized swellings. In the long bones, lytic foci, periostitis, and epiphyseal separation may be seen. Syphilitic arthritis, especially of the sternoclavicular joints, may complicate the picture (13,14).

Tertiary syphilis may be complicated by gummatous osseous lesions. Pathologically, the lesion resembles a tubercle with necrosis of adjacent bone. Lytic and sclerotic areas of bone may reach large size and be associated with pathologic fracture. Periostitis adjacent to gummatous lesions is frequent. Nongummatous osseous lesions consisting of periostitis, osteitis, or osteomyelitis may occur in conjunction with or in the absence of gummatous bony lesions.

Charcot joints, characteristically of the knees, result from loss of proprioception due to tabes dorsalis in tertiary syphilis. Hip, ankle, shoulder, elbow, spine, and other joints may also be affected. The frequency of direct syphilitic involvement of the joint is low. Penicillin remains the mainstay of syphilis treatment.

Tuberculous Arthritis

Tuberculous arthritis should be considered in the differential diagnosis of monarticular and pauciarticular arthritis at any age. The arthritis is frequently insidious in onset. It tends to lack some of the usual signs of active inflammation, especially erythema and heat (15,16). *Pott's disease*, tuberculous involvement of the spine, classically involves the thoracolumbar junction. Anterior destruction of vertebral bodies and discs eventually leads to angulation of the spine and kyphosis (gibbus deformity) (13,15) (Fig. 26B–1). While constitutional signs of tuberculosis (fever,

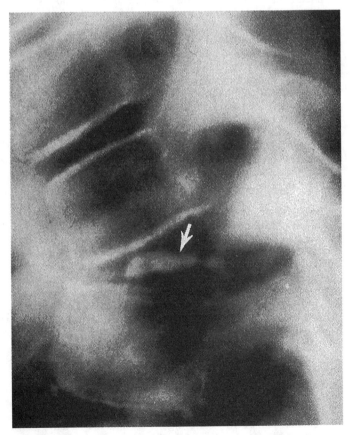

Fig. 26B–1. Tuberculous spondylitis (Pott's disease), showing destruction of the infected vertebrae (arrow) with angulation of the spine resulting in kyphosis (gibbous deformity). The adjacent vertebrae appear normal (from reference 13, with permission).

malaise, or weight loss) may be present, active pulmonary tuberculosis is rare. A history of past infection may be absent. A positive skin test for tuberculosis is helpful, although a negative test in the presence of anergy does not rule out the diagnosis. Diagnosis is based on finding acid-fast bacilli in synovial fluid, or more readily in caseating granulomas in biopsied synovium. Synovial fluid or tissue cultures are positive 90% of the time. Tuberculosis and its complications should be considered in patients with acquired immune deficiency syndrome (AIDS) or a history of immigration from an endemic area. Atypical mycobacterial infections also occur and should particularly be considered in the setting of immune compromise, especially AIDS. Long-term therapy with multiple anti-tuberculous drugs is required for eradication of infection.

Leprosy

Leprosy may be acquired in the United States in Texas or Louisiana. Additional patients may come from endemic areas abroad, such as Mexico. *Lepromatous leprosy* may cause polyarthralgia or polyarthritis. *Erythema nodosa leprosum* is an associated finding and consists of nodose lesions of the legs, arms, trunk, or all three. Malaise and fever may occur. *Swollen hands syndrome* is another presentation of leprosy with acid-fast bacilli found through the subcutaneous tissues. Thickening of peripheral nerves and typical skin changes suggest the diagnosis, which is made by identifying *Mycobacterium leprae* in aspirates of skin lesions, synovium, periarticular tissues or in scrapings of the nasal septum (17,18). Multiple drug treatment regimens are required; nifampin, dapsone, and clofazimine are first-line drugs.

Brucella Arthritis

Brucellosis (Mediterranean fever, Malta fever, undulant fever) is caused by one of four species of gram-negative coccobacilli: *B. abortus* (cattle), *B. suis* (hogs), *B. melitensis* (goats), and in a few cases, *B. canis* (dog). Human infection is acquired through abraded skin or via ingestion of infected tissue or milk. Veterinarians and slaughterhouse workers are at special risk. In areas of the world where ingestion of fresh milk or cheese is common, brucellosis is not limited to those in an occupation at risk (19).

The acute form of the disease is associated with bacteremia. Fever, which may be high, is accompanied by diaphoresis, polyarthralgias, myalgias, headache, and general malaise. Fever is less prominent in the subacute form occurring more than eight weeks but less than one year after infection. Constitutional symptoms of diaphoresis and weight loss may be undulant, hence the term *undulant fever*. Hepatosplenomegaly is common. Leukopenia may be noted in acute and subacute forms of brucellosis. Ocular and urologic damage may occur. Patients with chronic disease have frequent arthralgias and often low grade fever. Uveal tract lesions, hepatic dysfunction, and anemia are common.

Peripheral arthritis is the most common articular manifestation of brucellosis. The majority of cases are monarticular and involve the large, weight-bearing joints of the lower extremity, such as the knee, hip, or ankle. Rarely, the arthritis may have a symmetric rheumatoid-like distribution. Sacroiliitis is most commonly seen in the chronic form. The articular surfaces of the sacroiliac joint are usually blurred on roentgenograms, but erosions are infrequent. Spondylitis occurs in about one-tenth of patients and is most common in the lumbar spine. The characteristic changes are erosions at the anterosuperior margin of the vertebral body with disc narrowing. Unlike Pott's disease (tuberculous spondylitis), brucella spondylitis is characterized by early repair with sclerosis and formation of "parrot-beak" osteophytes. The concurrence of erosion and osteoblastic repair suggest the diagnosis of brucella spondylitis (13) (Fig. 26B–2). Brucella osteomyelitis is rare. Tendonitis, bursitis, and epicondylitis have been reported in brucellosis. Failure to isolate organisms in some instances suggests that peripheral arthritis may be reactive in some cases.

Diagnosis of brucellosis is based on a positive culture, or rising or high titer brucella serology. A definitive diagnosis is difficult. Culture of bone marrow may be helpful. About 50% of synovial

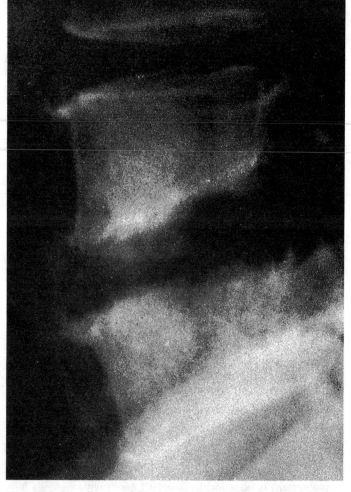

Fig. 26B–2. Brucellar spondylitis showing irregular erosions of adjacent vertebral surfaces and osteoblastic repair characterized by anterior osteophytes and early sclerosis. The anterior osteophytes may become prominent giving a "parrot-beak" appearance (from reference 13, with permission).

fluid cultures are positive in peripheral arthritis. Special medium is required for optimal culture results. Synovial biopsy typically shows cellular infiltrates and granuloma formation.

Treatment of acute and subacute forms of brucellosis is difficult and relies on oral tetracyclines given for one month initially, but five months may be required in difficult cases. Some authors suggest adding rifampin to decrease the incidence of relapse.

Fungal Arthritis

Fungal arthritis usually presents as an indolent monarthritis, much like tuberculous arthritis. Coccidioidomycosis occurs in the southwestern United States. It may present with erythema nodosum, periarthritis, and bihilar lymphadenopathy. This triad is also seen in sarcoidosis (where it is known as Lofgren's syndrome); therefore, the two entities must be differentiated. In coccidioidomycosis, the triad is a hypersensitivity reaction to primary infection and resolves spontaneously within weeks. Persistent arthritis is uncommon, resulting from hematogenous spread or extension from contiguous osteomyelitis. The most commonly involved joints are knees, wrist and hand, ankle, elbow, and foot, in order of decreasing frequency. Arthritis progression is slow and indolent. Diagnosis is by synovial biopsy and culture (15).

Blastomycosis occurs as a primary pulmonary infection in the central and southern United States. Hematogenous spread to skin and bone may occur. Monarthritis is uncommon, but may occur in a middle-aged man typically involving the knee, ankle, or elbow. Constitutional signs and symptoms may accompany pulmonary and skin disease. The organism may be isolated from sputum, skin, and synovial fluid (15,20).

Sporotrichosis typically occurs in agricultural or mine workers, or gardeners following minor skin trauma. Indolent arthritis occurs rarely, involving the knee, hand, wrist or ankle, in order of decreasing frequency. More than one joint is involved in about 50% of the patients. Alcoholism or myeloproliferative disease predisposes to infection. Diagnosis is by synovial histology and culture (15,21).

Candida arthritis is rare. It is usually seen in the setting of immune compromise. Some infections may be indolent. The knee is typically involved, with polyarticular involvement occurring in 40% of infections. Osteomyelitis may occur in up to 65% of patients. Mortality is high (15).

Treatment of fungal arthritis is limited to amphotericin B, ketoconazole, or fluconazole. Surgery is reserved for debridement of involved bone or synovium in those patients with coccidioidomycosis or sporotrichosis, who fail to respond to antifungal agents alone.

Mycoplasma Arthritis

Mycoplasma pneumoniae infection is often associated with nonspecific arthralgias and myalgias. In some patients a migratory polyarthritis of medium-sized joints such as the shoulder, elbows, knees, and ankles may occur three to eight days after onset of initial illness and may last two months. In a few patients, symptoms may last up to one year (22).

Stanley J. Naides, MD

1. White DG, Woolf AD, Mortimer PP, et al: Human parvovirus arthropathy. Lancet 1:419–421, 1985
2. Naides SJ: Erythema infectiosum (fifth disease) occurrence in Iowa. Amer J Public Health 78:1230–1231, 1988
3. Solonika CA, Anderson MJ, Laskin CA: Anti-DNA and antilymphocyte antibodies during acute infection with human parvovirus B19. J Rheumatol 16:777–781, 1989
4. Naides SJ, Scharosch LL, Foto F, et al: Rheumatologic manifestations of human parvovirus B19 infection in adults. Initial two-year clinical experience. Arthritis Rheum 33:1297–1309, 1990

5. Inman RD: Rheumatic manifestations of hepatitis B virus infection. Sem Arth Rheum 11:406–420, 1982
6. Inman RD, Hodge M, Johnston ME, et al: Arthritis, vasculitis, and cryoglobulinemia associated with relapsing hepatitis A virus infection. Ann Int Med 105:700–703, 1986
7. Smith CA, Petty RE, Tingle AJ: Rubella virus and arthritis. Rheum D Clin N Amer 13:265–274, 1987
8. Adverse Effects of Pertussis and Rubella Vaccines. A Report of the Committee to Review the Adverse Consequences of Pertussis and Rubella Vaccines. Edited by Howson CP, Howe CJ, Fineberg HV. Washington, D.C., National Academy Press, 1991, pp 187–205
9. Schaffner W, Fleet WF, Kilroy AW, et al: Polyneuropathy following rubella immunization: A follow-up study and review of the problem. Amer J Dis Child 127:684–688, 1974
10. Winchester R, (ed): AIDS and Rheumatic Disease. Rheum Dis Clin N Am, volume 17:1, W. B. Saunders Company, Philadelphia, 1991
11. Peters CJ, Dalrymple JM: Alphaviruses. Virology, 2nd ed. Edited by Fields BN, Knipe DM, Chanock RM, et al. New York, NY, Raven Press, 1990, pp 713–761
12. Nash P, Harrington T: Acute Barmah Forest polyarthritis. Aust N Zealand J Med 21:737–738, 1991
13. Resnick D, Niwayama G: Osteomyelitis, septic arthritis, and soft tissue infection: The organisms. Diagnosis of Bone and Joint Disorders, 2nd ed. Edited by Resnick D, Niwayama G. Philadelphia, Penn., W. B. Saunders Company, 1988, pp 2647–2754
14. Reginato AJ, Schumacher HR, Jimenez S, et al: Synovitis in secondary syphilis: Clinical, light and electron microscopic studies. Arthritis Rheum 22:170–176, 1979
15. Hoffman GS, Sentochnik DE: Mycobacterial and fungal infections. Textbook of Rheumatology, 3rd ed.. Edited by Kelly WN, Harris ED, Ruddy S, et al. Philadelphia, Penn., W. B. Saunders Company, 1989, pp 1589–1601
16. Evanchick CC, Davis DE, Harrington TM: Tuberculosis of peripheral joints: An often missed diagnosis. J Rheum 13:187–189, 1986
17. Albert DA, Weisman MH, Kaplan R: Rheumatic manifestations of leprosy (Hansen's disease). Medicine 59:442–448, 1980
18. Chavez-Legaspi M, Gomez-Lopez A, De La Torre CG: Study of rheumatic manifestations and serologic abnormalities in patients with lepromatous leprosy. J Rheum 12:738–741, 1985
19. Gotuzzo E, Carrillo C: Brucella arthritis. Infections in the Rheumatic Diseases. Edited by Espinoza L, Grune and Stratton, Inc. New York, NY 1988, pp 31–41
20. Bayer AS, Scott VJ, Guze LB: Fungal, arthritis. IV. Blastomycotic arthritis. Sem Arth Rheum 9:145–151, 1979
21. Bayer AS, Scott VJ, Guze LB: Fungal arthritis. III. Sporotrichal arthritis. Sem Arth Rheum 9:66–74, 1979
22. Hernandez LA, Urquhart GED, Dick WC: Mycoplasma pneumoniae infection and arthritis in man. Brit Med J 2:14–16, 1977

27. LYME DISEASE

Lyme disease is a complex multisystem illness caused by the tick-borne spirochete *Borrelia burgdorferi* (1). The illness, which closely mimics several other rheumatic diseases, usually occurs in stages, with remissions, exacerbations, and different clinical manifestations at each stage. It is important to make the correct diagnosis since Lyme borreliosis is usually curable by appropriate antibiotic therapy.

Borrelia burgdorferi, the causative agent of Lyme disease, is a fastidious, microaerophilic bacterium that grows best at 33°C in Barbour–Stoenner–Kelly medium (2). Except for erythema migrans skin lesions, culture of the spirochete from patient specimens has been difficult. *B. burgdorferi* has recently been divided into three different species: group 1 is called *B. burgdorferi*; group 2 is named *B. garinii*; and group 3 is still called by the number, VS461 (3). To date, American isolates have been group 1, whereas European isolates have included all three groups. These differences probably account for the clinical variations in the disease in different geographic regions.

The Lyme disease spirochete is transmitted primarily by certain ixodid ticks that are a part of the *Ixodes ricinus* complex. *Ixodes dammini* (now reported to be the same species as *I. scapularis*) is the principal vector in the northeastern and midwestern United States and *I. pacificus* is the vector in the west. Although the illness has been recognized in 47 states, most cases have occurred along the northeastern coast from Massachusetts to Maryland, in the midwest in Wisconsin and Minnesota, and on the west coast in northern California and Oregon (4). Lyme borreliosis is widely disseminated throughout Europe— from France to Scandinavia to Russia—where *I. ricinus* is the vector. Cases have also been noted in China, Japan, and Australia.

CLINICAL FEATURES

After an incubation period of 3 to 32 days, erythema migrans occurs at the site of the tick bite in about 80% of patients (5). The lesion usually begins as a red macule or papule that expands slowly to form a large annular lesion, often with a bright red outer border and partial central clearing. Because of the small size of ixodid ticks, most patients do not remember the preceding tick bite. The center of the lesion sometimes becomes intensely erythematous and indurated, vesicular, or necrotic. In other instances, the expanding lesion remains an even, intense red; several red rings are found within the outside one; or the central area turns blue before it clears. Although the lesion can be located anywhere, the thigh, groin, and axilla are particularly common sites. The lesion is warm to touch, but is not often painful.

In some patients, the Lyme disease spirochete remains localized to this skin lesion and regional lymph nodes, and is sometimes accompanied by minor constitutional symptoms. In most patients, the organism spreads hematogenously to many different sites. Within days after the onset of erythema migrans, these patients often develop secondary annular skin lesions, which are similar in appearance to the initial lesion (Fig. 27–1). Skin involvement is frequently accompanied by severe headache, mild

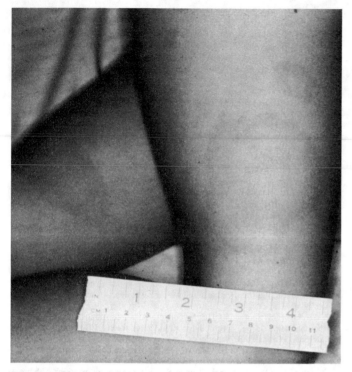

Fig. 27-1. *Thigh of child shows erythema chronicum migrans, the initial skin lesion of Lyme disease. Secondary annular skin lesions are apparent on the other leg (from Steere et al. Ann Intern Med 86:685-698, 1977).*

neck stiffness, fever, chills, myalgias, arthralgias, and profound malaise and fatigue. Less common manifestations include generalized lymphadenopathy or splenomegaly, hepatitis, sore throat, nonproductive cough, testicular swelling, conjunctivitis, iritis, or panophthalmitis. Except for fatigue and lethargy, which are often constant, the early signs and symptoms of Lyme disease are typically intermittent and changing. Even in untreated patients, the early symptoms usually improve or disappear within several weeks.

Neurologic Abnormalities

Symptoms suggestive of meningeal irritation may occur at the beginning of Lyme disease when erythema migrans is present, but are usually not associated with a spinal fluid pleocytosis or objective neurologic deficit at that time. After several weeks, about 15% of untreated patients develop frank neurologic abnormalities, including meningitis, subtle encephalitic signs, cranial neuritis (including bilateral facial palsy), motor and sensory radiculoneuritis, plexitis, mononeuritis multiplex, or myelitis, alone or in various combinations (6). Cerebrospinal fluid typically shows a lymphocytic pleocytosis, often with elevated protein. Even in untreated patients, these manifestations usually improve or disappear within weeks or months.

Months to years later, usually following long periods of latent infection, chronic neurologic manifestations may develop (7). The most common form of chronic central nervous system involvement is a subtle encephalopathy affecting memory, mood, or sleep. These patients often have evidence of memory impairment on neuropsychological tests and abnormal cerebrospinal fluid analyses with elevated protein or intrathecal antibody production to the spirochete. Most of these patients also have an axonal polyneuropathy manifested by either distal paresthesias or spinal or radicular pain. Electromyography generally shows extensive abnormalities of proximal and distal nerve segments. Leukoencephalitis, a rare manifestation of Lyme disease, is a severe neurologic picture that may include spastic paraparesses, upper motor-neuron bladder dysfunction, and lesions in the periventricular white matter.

Cardiac Involvement

Within several weeks after the onset of illness, about 8% of untreated patients develop cardiac involvement. The most com-

mon abnormality is fluctuating degrees of atrioventricular block (first degree, Wenckebach, or complete heart block) (8). Some patients have more diffuse cardiac involvement including electrocardiographic changes of acute myopericarditis, radionuclide evidence of left ventricular dysfunction, or rarely, cardiomegaly or pancarditis. The duration of cardiac involvement is usually only weeks, but severe involvement may be fatal. One case of chronic cardiomyopathy caused by *B. burgdorferi* has been reported (9).

Arthritis and Other Musculoskeletal Symptoms

If musculoskeletal symptoms occur early in the illness, the typical pattern is one of migratory pain in joints, tendons, bursae, muscle, or bone. The pain is usually without joint swelling, and lasts hours or several days in one or two locations at a time (5). Months later, about 60% of untreated patients in the United States develop frank arthritis (10). The typical pattern is brief, intermittent attacks of monarticular or oligoarticular arthritis in a few large joints, especially knees. Although the pattern varies, episodes of arthritis often become longer during the second or third years of illness, lasting months rather than weeks. In about 10% of these patients, chronic arthritis—defined as one year or more of continual joint inflammation—begins during this period. Chronic Lyme arthritis, which usually affects only one or both knees, may lead to erosion of cartilage and bone. Even among patients with chronic arthritis, objective joint swelling for longer than five or six years is rare, although brief episodes of joint pain may still occur after the period of frank arthritis (11). A few patients have been reported with osteomyelitis, panniculitis, or myositis.

Acrodermatitis

Acrodermatitis chronica atrophicans, a late skin manifestation of Lyme borreliosis, usually begins with an ill-defined area of erythema, edema, and induration, most commonly at an acral site (12). Gradually, the erythema fades and is replaced by atrophic skin. The final picture evolves over months to years, producing a wrinkled area of skin resembling cigarette paper. The disorder has been observed mainly in elderly women. Below the skin lesions, patients may have subluxation of small joints of the hand, periostitis, or erosion of cartilage and bone.

Congenital Infection

Two provocative case reports have suggested that *B. burgdorferi* may cause congenital infection. However, subsequent prospective studies have failed to identify a single case of maternal-fetal transmission of the Lyme disease spirochete (13). If congenital infection occurs in Lyme disease, it is rare.

PATHOGENESIS

After injection into the skin, *B. burgdorferi* may migrate outward producing erythema migrans and may spread hematogenously to other organs. The spirochete has been cultured from blood, skin, cerebrospinal fluid, and joint fluid, and has been seen in skin, myocardial, retinal, and synovial lesions. These findings and the usual response of all stages of the disease to antibiotic therapy suggest that the organism invades and persists in affected tissues throughout the illness.

Initially the immune response seems to be suppressed. For a period of weeks after the first several weeks of infection, there is often evidence of B cell hyperactivity with elevated total and specific serum IgM levels, cryoprecipitates, circulating immune complexes, and sometimes rheumatoid factor, antinuclear antibodies, or anticardiolipin antibodies in low titer. Over a period of months to years, the specific cellular and humoral immune responses develop to an increasing array of spirochetal antigens (14,15). As the specific immune response develops, the disease often seems to localize to a few joints that become markedly inflamed. At that time, antigen-reactive mononuclear cells are concentrated in joint fluid (15).

Chronic Lyme arthritis is associated with an increased frequency of HLA–DR4 and secondarily, HLA–DR2 alleles (16). Similar to rheumatoid arthritis and to the other forms of chronic inflammatory arthritis, synovium in Lyme disease shows villous hypertrophy, synovial cell hyperplasia, prominent microvasculature, fibrin deposition, lympho-plasmacellular infiltration, and sometimes, pseudolymphoid follicles (17). In several patients, spirochetes have been seen in and around blood vessels using immunohistologic techniques, but the number of organisms seems to be exceedingly small (17). Joint fluid white cell counts range from 500–110,000 cells/mm^3 (average: 25,000 cells/mm^3), most of which, in patients with high white cell counts, are polymorphonuclear leukocytes.

LABORATORY FINDINGS

Serologic testing is currently the only practical laboratory aid in diagnosis. After the first several weeks of infection, most patients have a positive antibody test to B. burgdorferi, determined by ELISA (14). As with any serologic test, antibody testing in Lyme disease is subject to false-negative and, more often, false-positive results. Western blotting is often helpful in sorting out false-positive results in patients who have indeterminant responses by ELISA (14). Early antibody responses are often directed against the 21 kDa outer-surface protein C(OspC), the 41 kDa flagellar protein, and the 58 kDa heat shock protein of the spirochete. Later, responses often develop to spirochetal polypeptides at 18, 21, 28, 30, 39, 41, 45, 58, 66, and 93 kDa. At least 5 of these 10 most frequent bands are required for a positive IgG blot. However, serologic testing for this disorder is not standardized and different laboratories may get different results. In addition, patients with past infection often remain seropositive, and a small percentage of patients have asymptomatic infection. If these patients develop another illness, the positive serologic test for Lyme disease may cause diagnostic confusion. In about 5% of patients who receive antibiotic therapy during the first several weeks of infection, the spirochete may still survive in protected niches and cause subtle joint or neurologic symptoms. In these patients, the humoral immune response may be aborted, but a cellular immune response to the spirochete can usually be demonstrated by T cell proliferative assay (18).

TREATMENT

The various manifestations of Lyme disease can usually be treated successfully with oral antibiotic therapy, except for objective neurologic abnormalities, which seem to require intravenous therapy (1). For early Lyme disease, doxycycline, 100 mg/twice daily, or amoxicillin, 500 mg/four times daily, are effective therapy (19), but doxycycline should not be given to children or pregnant women. Cefuroxime, 500 mg/twice daily, seems to be an effective alternative in patients with penicillin allergy (20). Erythromycin, 250 mg/four times daily, is less effective clinically, but is another alternative in patients with allergies to other medications. In children under age 12, amoxicillin is effective in divided dosages of 50 mg/kg/day; in cases of penicillin allergy, erythromycin (30 mg/kg/day) can be given. For patients with infection localized to the skin, 10 days of therapy is generally sufficient. For patients with disseminated infection, a longer course of 20 to 30 days may be needed. Approximately 15% of patients with early infection experience a Jarisch–Herxheimer-like reaction during the first 24 hours of therapy.

In patients with objective neurologic abnormalities, parenteral antibiotic therapy is usually necessary except perhaps for patients with facial palsy alone (1). Intravenous ceftriaxone, 2 g/day for 30 days is most commonly used for this purpose (21), but intravenous penicillin G, 20 million units/day in divided doses, may also be effective. In patients with high-degree atrioventricular block or a PR interval of greater than 0.3 seconds, intravenous antibiotic therapy and cardiac monitoring are recommended. In patients with complete heart block or congestive heart failure, corticosteroids may be of benefit if there is no improvement on antimicrobial therapy alone within 24 hours.

For patients with arthritis, oral regimens given for 30 days are generally successful, but the response may be slow. Patients with chronic arthritis, primarily those with the HLA–DR4 allele and antibody reactivity to outer-surface protein A (OspA) and OspB of B. burgdorferi, may not respond to either oral or intravenous antibiotic therapy (22). Intraarticular steroids and nonsteroidal antiinflammatory agents may be tried in these patients. If there is no response within 6 to 12 months, arthroscopic synovectomy may be helpful (23).

VACCINE DEVELOPMENT

Although reinfection may occur in patients treated early in the course of Lyme disease, this has not been observed in patients with late disease. Thus, it would appear that protective immunity can be achieved eventually with the natural infection, but the necessary components of the protective response are not yet known. In an experimental animal model of Lyme disease, mice vaccinated with recombinant OspA have been shown to be protected from infection with B. burgdorferi, both by antibody-mediated killing of the spirochete within the host and by destruction of the organism within the tick prior to disease transmission (24,25). However, the efficacy and safety of OspA immunization have not yet been demonstrated in human subjects.

Allen C. Steere, MD

1. Steere AC: Lyme disease. N Engl J Med 321:586–596, 1989
2. Barbour AG, Hayes SF: Biology of Borrelia species. Microbiol Rev 50:381–400, 1986
3. Baranton G, Postic D, Saint Girons I, et al: Delineation of Borrelia burgdorferi sensu stricto, Borrelia garinii sp. nov., and group VS461 associated with Lyme borreliosis. Int J Syst Bacteriol 42:378–383, 1992
4. Centers for Disease Control: Lyme disease—United States 1991–1992. MMWR 42:345–350, 1993
5. Steere AC, Bartenhagen NH, Craft JE, et al: The early clinical manifestations of Lyme disease. Ann Intern Med 99:76–82, 1983
6. Pachner AR, Steere AC: The triad of neurologic manifestations of Lyme disease: meningitis, cranial neuritis, and radiculoneuritis. Neurology 35:47–53, 1985
7. Logigian EL, Kaplan RF, Steere AC: Chronic neurologic manifestations of Lyme disease. N Engl J Med 323:1438–1444, 1990
8. Steere AC, Batsford WP, Weinberg M, et al: Lyme carditis: cardiac abnormalities of Lyme disease. Ann Intern Med 93:8–16, 1980
9. Stanek G, Klein J, Bittner R, et al: Isolation of Borrelia burgdorferi from the myocardium of a patient with longstanding cardiomyopathy. N Engl J Med 322:249–252, 1990
10. Steere AC, Schoen RT, Taylor E: The clinical evolution of Lyme arthritis. Ann Intern Med 107:725–731, 1987
11. Szer IS, Taylor E, Steere AC: The long-term course of children with Lyme arthritis. N Engl J Med 325:159–163, 1991
12. Asbrink E, Hovmark A: Early and late cutaneous manifestations of Ixodes-borne Borreliosis. Ann NY Acad Sci 539:4–15, 1988
13. Williams CL, Benach JL, Curran AS, et al: Lyme disease during pregnancy: a cord blood serosurvey. Ann NY Acad Sci 539:504–506, 1988
14. Dressler F, Whalen J, Reinhardt B, et al: Western blotting in the serodiagnosis of Lyme disease. J Infect Dis 167:392–400, 1993
15. Yoshinari NH, Reinhardt BN, Steere AC: T cell responses to polypeptide fractions of Borrelia burgdorferi in patients with Lyme arthritis. Arthritis Rheum 34:707–713, 1991
16. Steere AC, Dwyer E, Winchester R: Association of chronic Lyme arthritis with HLA–DR4 and HLA–DR2 alleles. N Engl J Med 323:1438–1444, 1990
17. Steere AC, Duray PH, Butcher EC: Spirochetal antigens and lymphoid cell surface markers in Lyme synovitis: comparison with rheumatoid synovium and tonsillar lymphoid tissue. Arthritis Rheum 31:487–495, 1988
18. Dressler F, Yoshinari NH, Steere AC: The T cell proliferative assay in the diagnosis of Lyme disease. Ann Intern Med 115:533–539, 1991
19. Massarotti EM, Luger SW, Rahn DW, et al: The treatment of early Lyme disease. Am J Med 92:396–403, 1992
20. Nadelman RB, Luger SW, Frank E, et al: Comparison of cefuroxime acetil and doxycycline in the treatment of early Lyme disease. Ann Intern Med 117:273–280, 1992
21. Dattwyler RJ, Halperin JJ, Volkman DJ, et al: Treatment of late Lyme borreliosis—randomized comparison of ceftriaxone and penicillin. Lancet 1:1191–1194, 1988
22. Kalish RA, Leong JM, Steere AC: Association of treatment-resistant chronic Lyme arthritis with HLA–DR4 and antibody reactivity to OspA and OspB of Borrelia burgdorferi. Infect Immun 61:2774–2779, 1993
23. Schoen RT, Aversa JM, Rahn DW, et al: Treatment of refractory chronic Lyme arthritis with arthroscopic synovectomy. Arthritis Rheum 34:1056–1060, 1991
24. Fikrig E, Barthold SW, Kantor FS, et al: Long-term protection of mice from Lyme disease by vaccination with OspA. Infect Immun 60:773–777, 1992
25. Fikrig E, Telford SR, Barthold SW, et al: Elimination of Borrelia burgdorferi in ticks feeding on OspA-immunized mice. Proc Natl Acad Sci USA 89:5418–5421, 1992

28. SARCOIDOSIS

Sarcoidosis is a systemic, chronic, granulomatous disease of unknown etiology, chiefly striking individuals 20 to 40 years of age (1–3). Although sarcoidosis most notably involves the lungs, it can affect nearly any organ system and thereby mimic other rheumatic diseases capable of causing fever, arthritis, uveitis, myositis, and rash.

PATHOGENESIS

While the cause of sarcoidosis is unknown, the host immune response clearly plays a central role in pathogenesis (4–6). Sarcoidosis is characterized by disseminated noncaseating granulomas. The sarcoid granuloma contains a central follicle of tightly packed epithelioid cells and multinucleated giant cells surrounded by lymphocytes, macrophages, monocytes, and fibroblasts. In the lung, the initial inflammation is an alveolitis composed chiefly of activated $CD4^+$ (helper) T cells whose cytokines recruit other cells to help form the granulomas (4). These alveolar T cells also preferentially express specific antigen receptors, which suggests that they are responding to a specific stimulus such as an organism or self-antigen (7). Granulomas are widely distributed in sarcoidosis, being found in the lung (86% of patients), lymph nodes (86%), liver (86%), spleen (63%), heart (20%), kidney (19%), bone marrow (17%), and pancreas (6%) (1,8). Granulomas mediate disease by compressing tissues, secreting cytokines that provoke constitutional symptoms, recruiting inflammatory cells whose products injure local tissues, and elaborating growth factors that cause fibrosis (3,5,10). In addition, activated monocytes in granulomas convert 25 hydroxyvitamin D to 1,25 dihydroxyvitamin D, which can increase intestinal absorption of calcium and cause hypercalcemia (9).

The peripheral blood reveals the dichotomy of features of depressed cellular immunity and enhanced humoral immunity (8). Depressed cellular immunity is evidenced by lymphopenia, a low helper/suppressor T cell ratio (0.8/1 in sarcoid patients versus 1.8/1 in normals), and cutaneous anergy. In contrast, the activated humoral immunity is manifested by polyclonal gammopathy and autoantibody production. Approximately 20% to 30% of patients have rheumatoid factor or antinuclear antibodies.

CLINICAL FEATURES

Sarcoidosis occurs most often in American blacks and northern European Caucasians. The prevalence of American blacks (40/100,000) is eight times higher than that of American Caucasians (3,6). Women are slightly more frequently affected than men.

Patients with sarcoidosis commonly present with one of four problems, which are: pulmonary symptoms (40% to 45%), constitutional symptoms (25%), extrathoracic inflammation (25%), including rheumatic manifestations or asymptomatic hilar adenopathy on chest roentgenogram (5% to 10%) (3,8).

Pulmonary Involvement. Respiratory symptoms are the most common presenting complaints, and include dry cough, dyspnea, and nonspecific chest pain. Hemoptysis, rare at initial presentation, may be recurrent, massive, and even fatal in those who develop mycetomas in pulmonary cysts (3).

Regardless of initial symptoms, over 90% of patients with sarcoidosis have an abnormal chest roentgenogram. Four types are recognized (3). Type 0 is normal and occurs in fewer than 10% of patients. Type 1 is most common (43%) and shows enlargement of hilar, mediastinal, and often right paratracheal lymph nodes. Type II, found in 24%, exhibits the adenopathy found in Type I, plus pulmonary infiltrates. Type II is most common in patients presenting with symptomatic respiratory disease. Type III occurs in 13% and demonstrates infiltrates without adenopathy. Pleural effusions are rare in sarcoidosis.

This classification has prognostic significance. Approximately 80% of patients with Type I chest films will remit within two years (3). In contrast, only 30% to 50% of patients with Type II and fewer than 20% of patients with Type III will remit.

Constitutional Symptoms. Fever, weight loss, fatigue, and malaise are the presenting symptoms in 25% of patients. Fever is frequently associated with hepatic granulomas.

Rheumatic Manifestations. Arthritis occurs in 10% to 15% of patients (11–15). Two patterns of joint disease are recognized, classified by whether the arthritis occurs early (within the first six months after onset of sarcoidosis) or late in the course. The first form, in which arthritis is part of the initial presentation, is most frequent. The arthritis often begins in one or both ankles and may occasionally spread in additive fashion to involve the knees and other joints. The axial skeleton is spared. Monarthritis in this early phase is unusual. Periarticular swelling is more common than frank joint effusion. When joint effusions are found they are usually non-inflammatory. Tenosynovitis and heel pain can also occur. The pain is often periarticular and more severe than the few objective signs of inflammation would suggest. Erythema nodosum is strikingly associated with early arthritis, occurring in 66% of patients. The syndrome of acute arthritis, erythema nodosum, and bilateral hilar adenopathy (Lofgren's syndrome) has an excellent prognosis with a 90% remission rate. Radiographs of sarcoidosis patients with acute arthritis almost never show bony or cartilaginous changes. The duration of acute arthritis averages several weeks but may be as short as several days and as long as three months. Few patients have multiple attacks of arthritis.

The second form of arthritis begins six months or more after the onset of sarcoidosis (11). Late joint disease is generally less dramatically symptomatic and less widespread. The knees are the most commonly involved joints, followed by the ankles and proximal interphalangeal joints. The average number of joints involved is two to three; monarthritis can occur. Synovial effusions are noninflammatory or moderately inflammatory, as evidenced by synovial fluid white blood cell counts of $250-6,200/cc^3$ with 56% to 100% mononuclear cells (15). Synovial histology is often less inflammatory than in rheumatoid arthritis, but occasionally reveals granulomas. In contrast to early arthritis, late disease is associated with chronic, cutaneous sarcoidosis and not with erythema nodosum. Late arthritis can be either transient or chronic. The chronic form often manifests itself by *dactylitis*, a sausage-like swelling of a digit frequently with overlying cutaneous sarcoidosis. Despite considerable deformity, activities of daily living are not greatly impaired and pain is not intense. Radiographic changes are infrequent, but destructive and cystic changes can occur and are most often noted in the middle and distal phalanges of the hand (Fig. 28–1). Cystic lytic lesions in the middle portion of the phalanx are typical. Less obvious but also characteristic are sclerosis or diffuse trabecular changes giving a honeycomb appearance. Patients with dactylitis most frequently demonstrate these radiographic findings, but some patients have findings without arthritis.

There are several other rheumatic manifestations of sarcoidosis (Table 28–1). Sarcoidosis of the larynx, nasal turbinates, and nasal cartilage can resemble Wegener's granulomatosis. Eye disease eventually develops in 22% of patients with sarcoidosis. Uveitis, a feature of several rheumatic diseases, is the most common ocular manifestation (16). Patients may also develop lachrymal gland enlargement, conjunctival nodules, parotid enlargement and keratoconjunctivitis (similar to that seen in Sjogren's syndrome), and proptosis (similar to that seen in Wegener's granulomatosis). Clinically evident sarcoidosis of the skeletal muscles resembles polymyositis, with slowly progressive proximal weakness, an elevated creatinine phosphokinase, and a myopathic pattern on electromyography. Muscle involvement can be asymptomatic. Muscle biopsy may reveal granulomatous myositis (17). Mononeuritis multiplex, facial nerve palsy, and parotid gland enlargement are signs common to sarcoidosis and

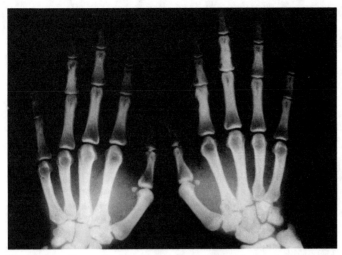

Fig. 28–1. Radiograph of the hands of a patient with chronic sarcoidosis showing multiple punched out bony lesions and swelling of the tissues around the joints.

other rheumatic diseases (see Table 28–1). Sarcoidosis can cause hyperuricemia. Patients with sarcoidosis sometimes develop arthritis from other causes: septic arthritis, especially fungal, should be considered when a patient on chronic corticosteroids develops a monarthritis.

Other Extrathoracic Manifestations. Peripheral lymphadenopathy is one of the most common manifestations of sarcoidosis, seen in 75% of patients. Typical patients have non-tender nodes ranging in size from 1–5 cm, involving at least the cervical and also often the axillary, epitrochlear, and inguinal regions (1–3). Skin involvement occurs in one-third of patients and serves as a marker for prognosis (3). Erythema nodosum occurs early and is associated with an excellent prognosis. Papules, nodules, plaques, and scaling lesions, which can disfigure, are associated with chronic sarcoidosis. Most patients (86%) have hepatic granulomas, but only 20% have hepatomegaly or elevated liver enzymes, especially the alkaline phosphatase. Jaundice, intrahepatic cholestasis, postnecrotic cirrhosis, and portal hypertension without cirrhosis have been reported. Neurosarcoidosis occurs in 5% of patients. It is rarely the sole presenting sign of sarcoidosis (3,18). Central nervous system manifestations include basilar meningitis, hydrocephalus, intracranial mass lesions, seizures, and neuroendocrine disorders, such as hypopituitarism and diabetes insipidus. Heart involvement leads to tachyarrhythmias, cardiomyopathy, or sudden death. Cor pulmonale complicates severe pulmonary disease. Renal manifestations of sarcoidosis include membranous glomerulonephritis, nephrocalcinosis, renal calculi, and renal insufficiency, with or without hypercalcemia (2). In the absence of massive hemoptysis, anemia is not a prominent feature of sarcoidosis. Leukopenia (WBC < 4,000/cc^3) occurs in 28% of patients, mild eosinophilia (>5% eosinophils) in 34%, and hypercalcemia in 19%. Although the serum angiotensin converting enzyme (ACE) level is elevated in 60% of patients with sarcoidosis, it is also increased in many other disorders (3,8).

DIAGNOSIS AND MANAGEMENT

No single finding or laboratory test establishes the diagnosis of sarcoidosis. Therefore, the diagnosis depends on a compatible clinical picture, histologic evidence of noncaseating granulomas, and exclusion of other possible causes. A tissue diagnosis is not necessary for asymptomatic patients with a classic chest radiograph, since such patients are exceedingly unlikely to have any other disorder. In symptomatic patients, one must exclude other causes, especially infections or lymphoma.

Most patients with sarcoidosis do well. Many, especially those with a Type I chest radiograph, remit spontaneously. However, 25% of patients develop pulmonary disability, and 10% of patients die from progressive sarcoidosis. Treatment depends on the specific manifestations. Asymptomatic hilar adenopathy requires no therapy. Many patients with early or late sarcoid arthritis respond to nonsteroidal antiinflammatory drugs, including salicylates (8,11,15). Colchicine can be effective especially for acute sarcoidosis arthropathy. Mucocutaneous sarcoidosis often improves with chloroquine (3). Corticosteroids are indicated for severe lung disease, liver disease, hypercalcemia, cardiac inflammation, posterior uveitis, neurosarcoidosis, and severe sarcoidosis elsewhere (3). The initial prednisone dose is 40 mg/day; divided daily doses are more effectively control fever. The dose is tapered, 5 mg every two weeks, to 15 mg/day. The dose is then held steady for four to eight months to make certain that the improvement has plateaued, and then, if possible, tapered off completely (19). Efficacy of immunosuppressive drugs is not established. Assessing treatment response depends chiefly on careful clinical examination, supplemented by changes in key laboratory tests like the chest radiograph and pulmonary function tests. The newer techniques of bronchoalveolar lavage, serum ACE levels, and gallium lung scanning have helped research into pathogenesis but not yet altered patient management (3).

David B. Hellmann, MD

1. Longscope WT, Freiman DG: A study of sarcoidosis: based on a combined investigation of 160 cases including 30 autopsies from the Johns Hopkins Hospital and Massachusetts General Hospital. Medicine 31:1–132, 1952
2. Mayock RL, Bertrand P, Morrison CE, et al: Manifestations of sarcoidosis: analysis of 145 patients, with a review of nine series selected from the literature. Am J Med 35:67–89, 1963
3. Bascom RA, Johns CJ: The natural history and management of sarcoidosis. Advances in Internal Medicine, Vol. 31. Edited by Stollerman GH, Harrington WJ, et al. Chicago, Yearbook Medical Publishers, Inc., 1986, pp 213–241
4. Keogh BA, Hunninghake GW, Line BR, et al: The alveolitis of pulmonary sarcoidosis: evaluation of natural history and alveolitis-dependent changes in lung function. Am Rev Respir Dis 128:256–265, 1983
5. Crystal RG, Roberts WC, Hunninghake GW, et al: Pulmonary sarcoidosis: a disease characterized and perpetuated by activated lung T-lymphocytes. Ann Intern Med 94:73–94, 1981
6. Thomas PD, Hunninghake GW: Current concepts of the pathogenesis of sarcoidosis. Am Rev Respir Dis 135:747–760, 1987
7. Tamura N, Moller DR, Balbi B, et al: Preferential usage of the T-cell antigen receptor β-chain constant region Cβ1 element by lung T-lymphocytes of patients with pulmonary sarcoidosis. Am Rev Respir Dis 143:635–639, 1991
8. Stobo JD, Hellmann DB: Sarcoidosis. In: Rheumatology and Immunology, 2nd ed. Edited by Cohen AS, Bennet JD. Orlando, Grune and Stratton, pp 301–309, 1986
9. Mason RS, Frankel T, Chan Y, et al: Vitamin D conversion by sarcoid lymph node homogenate. Ann Intern Med 100:59–61, 1984
10. McFadden RG, Vickers KE, Fraher LJ: Lymphocyte chemokinetic factors derived from human tonsils: modulation by 1,25-dihydroxyvitamin D (calcitriol). Am J Respir Cell Mol Biol 4:42–49, 1991
11. Gumpel JM, Johns CJ, Shulman LE: The joint disease of sarcoidosis. Ann Rheum Dis 26:194–205, 1967
12. Spilberg I, Siltzbach LE, McEwen C: The arthritis of sarcoidosis. Arthritis Rheum 12:126–137, 1969

Table 28–1. Rheumatic manifestations of sarcoidosis

Manifestation	Frequency in Sarcoidosis (% of Patients)	Differential Diagnosis
Arthritis	15	Rheumatoid arthritis, rheumatic fever, SLE, gonococcal arthritis, gout, spondyloarthropathies
Parotid gland enlargement	5	Sjogren's syndrome
Upper airway disease, (sinusitis, laryngeal inflammation, saddle nose deformity)	3	Wegener's granulomatosis
Uveitis	19	
Anterior	18	Spondyloarthropathies
Posterior	7	Behcet's
Keratoconjunctivitis	5	Sjogren's
Proptosis	1	Wegener's granulomatosis
Myositis	4	Polymyositis
Mononeuritis multiplex	1	Systemic vasculitis
Facial nerve palsy	2	Lyme disease

13. Kaplan H: Sarcoid arthritis: a review. Arch Intern Med 112:924–935, 1963
14. Shaw RA, Holt PA, Stevens MB: Heel pain in sarcoidosis. Ann Intern Med 15:675–677, 1988
15. Palmer DG, Schumacher HR: Synovitis with non-specific histological changes in synovium in chronic sarcoidosis. Ann Rheum Dis 43:778–782, 1984
16. Jabs DA, Johns CJ: Ocular involvement in chronic sarcoidosis. Am J Ophthalmol 102:297–301, 1986

17. Wolfe SM, Pinals RS, Aelion JA, et al: Myopathy in sarcoidosis: clinical and pathologic study of four cases and review of the literature. Semin Arthritis Rheum 16:300–306, 1987
18. Chapelon C, Ziza JM, Piette JC, et al: Neurosarcoidosis: signs, course and treatment of 35 confirmed cases. Medicine 69:261–276, 1990
19. Johns CJ, Zachary JB, Ball WC Jr: A ten-year study of corticosteroid treatment of pulmonary sarcoidosis. Johns Hopkins Med J 134:271–283, 1974

29. BEHCET'S SYNDROME

Originally described as a triad of recurrent aphthous oral and genital ulcerations with uveitis, Behcet's disease is now known as a multisystem illness. Other targeted organs can include skin, joints, veins, arteries, gastrointestinal tract, meninges, and brain. The disease is both more common and more aggressive in the Eastern Mediterranean and Far East than in North America.

DIAGNOSTIC CRITERIA

A set of diagnostic criteria has been developed (1) (Table 29–1). Recurrent oral ulceration is mandatory for diagnosis. A notable aspect of this set of criteria is the heavy reliance on mucocutaneous lesions. Some features such as cerebral vasculitis and arterial aneurysms could not be included as diagnostic criteria due to their rarity in the studied patients.

Since few North American patients have cutaneous pathergy, it seems reasonable to substitute any one of the following features: aseptic meningitis, cerebral vasculitis, recurrent phlebitis, arteritis with aneurysm, or discrete bowel ulceration. Incomplete forms of the syndrome probably exist; for instance, some recurrent aphthous stomatitis and aphthous vulvitis in young women.

CLINICAL FEATURES

The oral lesions are the first to appear and the last to leave. In untreated patients activity often waxes and wanes over 20 years with eventual subsidence (see Table 29–2).

Multiple painful oral aphthous ulcers, seen in all patients, range in size from a few mm to 2 cm, are rounded, and appear in crops anywhere on the mucous membrane of the mouth and pharynx. The ulcers heal in one to three weeks, usually without scarring. Patients have oral lesions 50% to 100% of the time.

Genital ulcerations, resembling the oral ulcerations, are likely to occur on the labia minora, cervix, penis, and scrotum (Fig. 29–1). Genital recurrences are less common than oral, perhaps occurring three to four times per year.

Hypopyon, an extreme form of anterior uveitis is now uncommon in North American patients possibly due to antiinflammatory treatment. There is usually an interval of several years between the onset of mucosal ulcers and eye disease. Typically, eye disease manifests as painless blurring of vision in one or both eyes due to some combination of anterior and posterior uveitis and retinal vasculitis. An ophthalmologic examination, with slit lamp biomicroscopy and fundoscopy, reveals cellular infiltrates or retinal infarctions. Eastern patients may become blind within five years of onset, but ocular disease appears to be milder in North American patients.

Cutaneous lesions are pleomorphic and seldom distinctive. Papules, pustules (especially perianal), nodose lesions, and folliculitis are seen. The pathergy reaction is an erythematous or pustular response, at least 0.5 cm in diameter, developing 24 to 48 hours after the forearm skin is pricked with a sterile disposable 25-gauge needle (2). This test is positive in most patients reported from the Middle and Far East, but is less common in patients from North America. The criteria for this phenomenon are variously described and need standardization.

About one-half of all patients will experience, during exacerbations, mild synovitis in large or small joints. The arthritis is seldom erosive. Synovial fluid cell counts are in the inflammatory range, often with a predominance of polymorphonuclear leukocytes (PMN). Synovial biopsies can show predominantly PMN or mononuclear infiltrates (3). A sacroiliitis is sometimes seen, but only in HLA–B27 positive patients.

Central nervous system inflammation can present as meningitis with headache, fever, and stiff neck associated with cerebrospinal fluid (CSF) pleocytosis (4). In the acute stage, polymorphonuclear cells appear in the CSF, but after a few days lymphocytes predominate. When vasculitis occurs in the brain, CSF pleocytosis accompanies it. Focal neurologic deficits with corticospinal tract lesions may present as hemiparesis or quadriparesis, at times with cerebellar ataxia or pseudobulbar palsy. Magnetic resonance imaging (MRI) in acute phases reveals areas of increased signal in the periventricular white matter, brain stem, and cerebellum. Neurologic deficits may be irreversible. Cerebral angiography sometimes reveals evidence of vasculitis in medium-sized arteries. Dural vein thrombosis can cause persistent headache and elevated CSF pressure. The venous occlusions can be proved by digital subtraction angiography or MRI.

Deep vein phlebitis affecting the leg veins can ascend to the inferior vena cava (5). Other veno-occlusive syndromes include superior vena caval occlusion and Budd–Chiari syndrome as well as superficial phlebitis. Pulmonary embolism is rare. Vasculitic arterial aneurysms may cause lesions in an extremity or in the abdomen and, even when resected, can recur at the anastomosis. Such aneurysms can affect the aorta or its branches as well as the pulmonary arterial circulation (6). A virtually pathognomonic presentation is pulmonary artery-bronchus fistula presenting as life-threatening hemoptysis. Recognition of this lesion, as with other vasculitic aneurysms, can be life saving. Prompt pulmonary arteriography pinpoints the leaking aneurysm(s), thus permitting selective resection of the diseased lung segment. The blood vessels of patients with prominent venous or arterial disease are

Table 29–1. Diagnostic criteria for Behcet's disease*

Oral ulcerations	Recurrent aphthous ≥ 3 attacks/year
PLUS ANY *TWO* OF:	
Genital ulcerations	Recurrent aphthous
Eye inflammation	Uveitis anterior posterior
	Vitreous cells on slit lamp
	Retinal vasculitis
Skin lesions	Erythema nodosum
	Pseudo-folliculitis
	Papulo-pustular
	Acneiform nodules
Pathergy test	2 mm erythema 24–48 hours after #25 needle pricked to depth of 5 mm

* For inclusion, each criterion must be confirmed by a physician.

Table 29–2. Approximate frequency of systemic features

	Percentage
Aphthous stomatitis	100
Genital ulcerations	70–90
Uveitis	60–80
Synovitis	50
Cutaneous lesions	60
Central nervous system	10–30
Major vessel occlusion/aneurysm	10–37

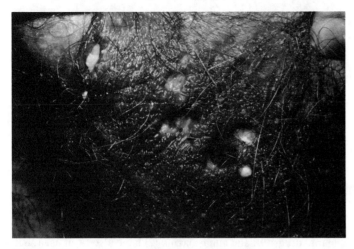

Fig. 29–1. Scrotal ulcers in a patient with Behcet's syndrome.

cytes generate supernatants with greater neutrophil-potentiating activity than controls (13). This has been a rationale for the use of colchicine. Japanese investigators are examining a possible abnormal immune response to streptococcal antigens. Another candidate antigen is herpes simplex virus I (14). Upregulation of $\gamma\delta$ receptors on CD8 T lymphocytes suggests exposure to a microbial antigen (15).

TREATMENT

Corticosteroids have a palliative effect and are useful if applied early as topical applications, such as triamcinolone in gel, to mucosal ulcers. Dapsone and colchicine are sometimes helpful. Thalidomide may reduce mucosal lesions but is virtually unavailable. There is controversy over whether recurrent phlebitis in Behcet's disease can be prevented by anticoagulation. It appears that warfarin may be ineffective in severe cases. Heparin can be used pending the time required for immunosuppressive regimens to work. Most treatments have not been evaluated in controlled trials, although trials of alpha-interferon (IFN-α) are underway.

For posterior uveitis, retinal vasculitis, or cerebral vasculitis, corticosteroid alone are inadequate. Chlorambucil, 0.1 mg/kg/day, is often effective in suppressing these serious phases. Tapering of the dose is allowed, and most patients can expect to be on chlorambucil for up to 2.5 years (16). Relapses require retreatment. Azathioprine appears to be less effective (17). Cyclosporine in doses of 10 mg/kg/day may also suppress ocular and oral manifestations (18).

J. Desmond O'Duffy, MD

unusually susceptible to trauma. Phlebitis can occur at intravenous sites and aneurysms at arterial puncture sites.

Mucosal ulcerations can be found anywhere in the gastrointestinal tract but favor the terminal ileum, cecum, and ascending colon (7). Clinically they may present as abdominal pain, bleeding, or perforation. Endoscopically these discrete ulcerations must be distinguished from granulomatous colitis. This is facilitated if adequate histology is available, such as after local resection.

Nephritis is rare, but secondary amyloidosis has been reported. Hepatitis and pulmonary involvement are also rare.

Differential diagnosis can be complex and includes other more common diseases such as Crohn's disease, cicatrical pemphigoid, lichen planus, herpes simplex and somatization disorders that can all have ulcerating lesions.

PATHOLOGY AND IMMUNOPATHOGENESIS

The cause of Behcet's disease is unknown. The early pathology of oral ulcers reveals emigration of lymphocytes and plasma cells from dermal blood vessels (8). Liquification-degeneration at the dermoepidermal junction leads to necrosis and slough (that is, an aphthous ulcer). Histology of the genital ulceration is equally nonspecific, but vasculitis is sometimes seen. Enucleated eyes have revealed venous and arterial occlusions. Lesions resembling erythema nodosum may contain either round cell or neutrophilic infiltrates in the dermis. Frank necrotizing vasculitis in skin is rare, but leukocytoclastic vasculitis in palpable purpura can be seen. Cerebral lesions in the active stage show perivascular infiltrates, but late lesions reveal gliosis and demyelination (9).

The CSF in active central nervous system disease contains an elevated cell count, typically lymphocytic with elevated IgA, IgG, and IgM index (10). Arterial aneurysms result from a panarteritis. Little is known about the pathogenesis of the venous occlusions; presumably they are vasculitis with superimposed thrombosis (11).

Acute phase reactants are sometimes elevated in active disease. Circulating immune complexes are elevated in about 50% of the patients. HLA–B51, a split of HLA–B5, is more common in patients, especially among those from Japan and the Eastern Mediterranean. Studies of cellular and humoral immunity are usually normal, but in preactive phases patients have a reduced number and function of T4 lymphocytes (12). Patients' lympho-

1. International Study Group for Behcet's Disease: Criteria for diagnosis of Behcet's disease. Lancet 335:1078–1080, 1990

2. Friedman-Birnbaum R, Bergman R, Aizen E: Sensitivity and specificity of pathergy test results in Israeli patients with Behcet's disease. Cutis 45:261–264, 1990

3. Abdou NI, Schumacher HR, Colman RW: Behcet's disease: possible role of secretory component deficiency, synovial inclusions, and fibrinolytic abnormality in the various manifestations of the disease. J Lab Clin Med 91:409–422, 1978

4. O'Duffy JD, Goldstein NP: Neurologic involvement in seven patients with Behcet's disease. Am J Med 6:170–178, 1976

5. Wechsler B, Piette JC, Conard J, et al: Deep venous thrombosis in Behcet's disease: 106 localizations in a series of 177 patients. La Presse Medicale 16(14)661–664, 1987

6. Lie JT: Cardiac and pulmonary manifestations of Behcet's syndrome. Path Res Pract 183:347–352, 1988

7. Lee RG: The colitis of Behcet's syndrome. Am J Surg Pathol 10:888–893, 1986

8. Lehner T: Pathology of recurrent oral ulceration and oral ulceration in Behcet's syndrome: light, electron, and fluorescence microscopy. J Pathol 97:481–494, 1969

9. McMenemey WH, Lawrence BJ: Encephalomyelopathy in Behcet's disease: report of necropsy findings in two cases. Lancet 2:353–358, 1957

10. Hirohata S, Takeuchi A, Miyamoto T: Association of cerebrospinal fluid IgM index with central nervous system involvement in Behcet's disease. Arthritis Rheum 29(6):793–796, 1986

11. O'Duffy JD: Vasculitis in Behcet's disease. Rheum Clinic of North America 16(2):423–431, 1990

12. Sakane T, Kotani H, Takada S, Tsunematsu T: Functional aberration of T cell subsets in patients with Behcet's disease. Arth Rheum 25(11):1343–1351, 1982

13. Niwa Y, Mizushima Y: Neutrophil-potentiating factors released from stimulated lymphocytes: special reference to the increase in neutrophil-potentiating factors from streptococcus-stimulated lymphocytes of patients with Behcet's disease. Clin Exp Immunol 79:353–360, 1990

14. Young C, Lehner T, Barnes CG: CD4 and CD8 cell responses to herpex simplex virus in Behcet's disease. Clin Exp Immunol 73:6–10, 1988

15. Fortune F, Walker J, Lehner T: The expression of $\gamma\delta$ T cell receptor and the prevalence of primed, activated, and IgA-bound T cells in Behcet's disease. Clin Exp Immunol 82:326–332, 1990

16. Matteson EL, O'Duffy JD: Treatment of Behcet's disease with chlorambucil. Behcet's Disease: Basic and Clinical Aspects, Edited by O'Duffy JD. New York, Marcel Dekker, Inc., 1991, pp 575–580

17. Yazici H, Pazarli H, Barnes CG, et al: A controlled trial of azathioprine in Behcet's syndrome. New Eng J Med 322(5):281–285, 1990

18. Masuda K, Urayama A, Kogure M, et al: Double-masked trial of cyclosporine versus colchicine and long-term open study of cyclosporine in Behcet's disease. Lancet 1(8647):1093–1095, May 1989

30. PERIODIC SYNDROMES

Several clinical syndromes are characterized by intermittent inflammatory synovitis, with complete resolution during the intervals between attacks. Residual joint damage occurs only rarely. Little is known about their underlying causes or pathogenesis. Familial Mediterranean fever (FMF) is a genetic disorder. The clinical picture usually includes extraarticular manifestations. Intermittent hydrarthrosis and palindromic rheumatism are limited to the joints and paraarticular tissues. Other syndromes, which may sometimes include intermittent joint swelling, are discussed elsewhere in the *Primer*. Among these are systemic lupus erythematosus (SLE), inflammatory bowel disease, crystal-induced synovitis, Behcet's syndrome, Lyme disease, HIV infection, and joint swelling in angioedema and other allergic or inflammatory cutaneous disorders.

PALINDROMIC RHEUMATISM

In 1944, Hench and Rosenberg introduced the term *palindromic rheumatism* to describe a recurring acute arthritis and periarthritis with symptom-free intervals of days to months between attacks (1). Men and women are equally affected, with onset usually between the third and sixth decades (2). Occasionally, the initial attack may occur in childhood, and several cases in the same family have been reported.

Each attack begins suddenly in one or two joints, often in the late afternoon or evening, with pain that may be intense, reaching a peak within a few hours. Swelling, warmth, and redness over or near the affected joint are noted shortly after the onset of pain. In typical cases minor attacks may not be accompanied by swelling and redness, but since the diagnosis is based on clinical findings, it should not be made until definite local signs of inflammation have been observed. These signs usually disappear in one to three days, but may remain for as long as a week. The episodes occur irregularly and attacks in individual joints may overlap. Any appendicular joint may be affected, but the knees, wrists, and shoulders are most commonly involved; attacks are experienced occasionally in the vertebral column and temporomandibular joints. Periarticular attacks are marked by painful swelling of the fingerpads, heels, and other soft tissues. Poorly circumscribed subcutaneous nodules may also be present transiently. Constitutional symptoms are uncommon, but some patients have low-grade fever during attacks.

Examination of the synovium and joint fluid reveals a nonspecific, subacute, inflammatory reaction with no crystals (3). Microvascular injury is prominent in synovial biopsies. Elevations of the erythrocyte sedimentation rate (ESR) and various acute-phase reactants may occur during an attack, but these values are generally normal between attacks. Serum and synovial fluid complement levels are not depressed (4,5). Except for soft tissue swelling at the time of the attack, no specific radiologic findings are present.

The extended clinical course is variable. Less than 10% of patients experience a spontaneous remission, but many continue to have attacks without developing persistent synovitis or permanent joint damage. In 30% to 40% of patients the disorder evolves into typical rheumatoid arthritis (RA) (2-4,6). These patients often have rheumatoid factor during the palindromic phase, but conversion from seronegativity to seropositivity may also occur during the evolution of the disease (4). The presence of typical persistent rheumatoid nodules also has been reported during the palindromic phase before chronic synovitis develops (7).

As palindromic rheumatism evolves into RA, the individual attacks may become more frequent but less severe. More joints are involved simultaneously, and morning stiffness becomes prominent. Rarely, palindromic rheumatism represents an early phase of SLE or some other connective tissue disease (2,3,6). Except for its relationship to RA, there is little or no insight into the etiology of palindromic rheumatism or the pathogenesis of the acute attacks.

The treatment of individual attacks of palindromic rheumatism is difficult to evaluate because of their brief duration, but antiinflammatory drugs do not appear to have a significant impact. Attempts to prevent attacks by regular administration of antiinflammatory drugs, including low-dose corticosteroids, are seldom successful. Prophylactic colchicine has been advocated (8), but experience with this approach is limited. The most consistently successful therapy has been with injectable gold salts (6). Chrysotherapy may be initiated during the palindromic phase if attacks are sufficiently severe, frequent, and disabling. The mode of gold administration is similar to its use in RA. Long-term results cannot be evaluated in the absence of a controlled trial, but about one-half of the patients respond. Penicillamine, antimalarial drugs (9), and sulfasalazine (2) have also been used, but experience is limited.

INTERMITTENT HYDRARTHROSIS

The term *intermittent hydrarthrosis* has been used to describe recurrent effusions of unknown cause that occur with equal frequency in both sexes starting in the third to fifth decade (10). In contrast with palindromic rheumatism, the attacks come at regular intervals, usually with involvement of one knee or occasionally another large joint. Both knees are usually affected, but seldom simultaneously. Fluid accumulates over 12–24 hours, accompanied by minimal discomfort or signs of inflammation. The effusion resolves within an additional two to four days. Between attacks the joints appear entirely normal.

Laboratory studies, including the ESR, are normal, even during attacks. Joint fluid may be normal or may show a slight increase in leukocytes. There are no roentgenographic abnormalities except for the demonstration of an effusion. Pathologic changes of mild inflammation in the synovium have been reported, but clinical evolution into RA is rare. No treatment has been shown to abort or prevent attacks, and no recent studies have addressed cases such as these.

FAMILIAL MEDITERRANEAN FEVER

Familial Mediterranean fever is an autosomal recessive hereditary disease of unknown etiology encountered in ethnic groups of east Mediterranean origin and expressed somewhat more frequently in men (11–14). The onset is usually during childhood with recurrent attacks of systemic illness occurring at irregular intervals. Each attack is accompanied by fever and one or more inflammatory manifestations, including (in order of frequency) peritonitis, arthritis, pleuritis, and an erysipelas-like rash (15). Spontaneous resolution of each episode occurs within a few days. Before the diagnosis of FMF is made, peritonitis may lead to unnecessary surgery for an acute abdominal emergency.

Joint involvement is more likely to be expressed as arthralgia, but there may be frank synovitis with acute painful effusions in large joints, such as the knee, ankle, hip, or elbow. When oligoarthritis occurs, the pattern is usually asymmetric. Pain is usually disproportionate to swelling and, although there may be some warmth, erythema is rare. Severe attacks of arthritis often persist longer than other manifestations of FMF, sometimes for two or three weeks. Chronic synovitis may result in periarticular osteopenia and, rarely, in residual joint damage.

Laboratory abnormalities include elevated ESR and joint fluid leukocyte counts during attacks. Synovial biopsy shows nonspecific inflammation.

Amyloidosis, a frequent late complication of FMF (16), usually presents with proteinuria and progressive renal failure (see Chapter 36).

Neutrophil activation plays an important role in the pathogenesis of FMF. Deficiency of a partially characterized inhibitor of the complement-derived chemotactic anaphylotoxin C5a has been demonstrated in synovial and peritoneal fluids in FMF. This may lead to diminished inhibition of neutrophil chemotaxis, thereby enhancing the inflammatory response (17,18). The gene that encodes the inhibitor protein has not been cloned, but it appears to be located on the short arm of chromosome 16 in an Israeli population (19).

Treatment during attacks of FMF is aimed at symptomatic relief. Corticosteroids are ineffective. Prophylactic colchicine (1.2–1.8mg/day) has been demonstrated to reduce the frequency of attacks (20) and may delay the progression of amyloidosis (21).

Robert S. Pinals, MD

1. Hench PS, Rosenberg EF: Palindromic rheumatism: a "new", oft recurring disease of joints (arthritis, periarthritis, para-arthritis) apparently producing no articular residues: report of 34 cases; its relation to "angioneural arthrosis," "allergic rheumatism," and rheumatoid arthritis. Arch Intern Med 73:292–321, 1944
2. Guerne PA, Weisman MH: Palindromic rheumatism: part of or apart from the spectrum of rheumatoid arthritis. Am J Med 93:451–460, 1992
3. Schumacher HR: Palindromic onset of rheumatoid arthritis: clinical, synovial fluid, and biopsy studies. Arthritis Rheum 25:361–369, 1982
4. Williams MH, Sheldon PJHS, Torrigiani G, et al: Palindromic rheumatism: clinical and immunological studies. Ann Rheum Dis 30:375–380, 1971
5. Wajed MA, Brown DL, Currey HLF: Palindromic rheumatism: clinical and serum complement study. Ann Rheum Dis 36:56–61, 1977
6. Mattingly S: Palindromic rheumatism. Ann Rheum Dis 25:307–317, 1966
7. Schreiber S, Schumacher HR, Cherian PV: Palindromic rheumatism with rheumatoid nodules: a case report with ultrastructural studies. Ann Rheum Dis 45:78–81, 1986
8. Schwartzberg M: Prophylactic colchicine therapy in palindromic rheumatism. J Rheumatol 9:341–342, 1982
9. Youssef W, Yan A, Russell AS: Palindromic rheumatism: a response to chloroquine. J Rheumatol 18:35–37, 1991
10. Weiner AB, Ghormley RK: Periodic benign synovitis: idiopathic hydrarthrosis. J Bone Joint Surg 38A:1034–1055, 1956
11. Sohar E, Gafni J, Pras M, et al: Familial Mediterranean fever: a survey of 470 cases and review of the literature. Am J Med 43:227–253, 1967
12. Heller H, Gafni J, Michaeli D, et al: The arthritis of familial Mediterranean fever (FMF). Arthritis Rheum 9:1–17, 1966
13. Danar DA, Kwanth, Stern RS, et al: Familial Mediterranean fever, Am J Med 82:829–832, 1987
14. Gedalia A, Adara A, Gorodischer R: Familial Mediterranean fever in children. J Rheumatol 19 (Suppl 35):1–9, 1992
15. Majeed HA, Quabazard A, Hijazi Z, et al: The cutaneous manifestations in children with familial Mediterranean fever (recurrent hereditary polyserositis): a six-year study. Q J Med 75:607–616, 1990
16. Knecht A, DeBeer FC, Pras M: Serum amyloidosis: protein in familial Mediterranean fever. Ann Intern Med 102:71–72, 1985
17. Matzner Y, Przezinski A: C5a-inhibitor deficiency in peritoneal fluids from patients with familial Mediterranean fever. N Engl J Med 311:287–290, 1984
18. Matzner Y, Ayesh SK, Hochner-Celniker, D, et al: Proposed mechanism of the inflammatory attacks in familial Mediterranean fever. Arch Int Med 150:1289–1291, 1990
19. Pras E, Aksentijevich I, Gruberg L, et al: Mapping of a gene causing familial Mediterranean fever to the short arm of chromosome 16. N Engl J Med 326:1509–1513, 1992
20. Dinarello CA, Wolff SM, Goldfinger SE, et al: Colchicine therapy for familial Mediterranean fever: a double-blind trial. N Engl J Med 291:934–937, 1974
21. Zemer D, Pras M, Sohar E, et al: Colchicine in the prevention and treatment of the amyloidosis of familial Mediterranean fever. New Engl J Med 314:1001–1005, 1986

31. GOUT
A. Epidemiology, Pathology, and Pathogenesis

Gout, is a disease in which tissue deposition of crystals of monosodium urate occurs from supersaturated extracellular fluids and results in one or more clinical manifestations. These include: 1) recurrent attacks of severe acute or chronic articular and periarticular inflammation, also termed *gouty arthritis*; 2) accumulation of articular, osseous, soft tissue, and cartilaginous crystalline deposits, called *tophi*; 3) renal impairment, also referred to as *gouty nephropathy*; and 4) uric acid calculi in the urinary tract (1). Hyperuricemia, defined as serum urate concentration more than two standard deviations (SD) above the mean established in the individual laboratory for the sex of the patient (generally above 7.0 mg/dL in males or above 6.0 mg/dL in females), reflects the metabolic derangement in extracellular fluids that predisposes to the clinical events. Although hyperuricemia is a pathogenetic common denominator through which diverse etiologic factors give rise to the clinical syndrome, this chemical aberration is most often insufficient for the expression of gout. Therefore, asymptomatic hyperuricemia in the absence of gout is not a disease state.

EPIDEMIOLOGY OF GOUT AND HYPERURICEMIA

The prevalence of gout has increased over the last few decades in the United States and in a number of other countries with a high standard of living. Gout is predominantly a disease of adult men, with a peak incidence in the fifth decade. In 1986, the prevalence of self-reported gout in the United States was estimated at 13.6/1,000 men, and 6.4/1,000 women (2). Thus, gout is the most common cause of inflammatory arthritis in men over age 30, and is probably the second most common form of inflammatory arthritis in the United States. In addition, gout frequently results in significant short-term disability, occupational limitations, and utilization of medical services, making the disease a significant public health problem.

Gout rarely occurs in men before adolescence or in women before menopause. Serum urate concentrations rise from normal childhood mean values of 3.5–4.0 mg/dL to adult levels during puberty in young men. In contrast, urate levels remain rather constant in women until menopause. The discrepancy in serum urate levels between the sexes during the reproductive years appears to stem from the action of estrogens, which promote renal excretion of uric acid (1). Serum urate levels in women rise after cessation of menses.

Hyperuricemia is demonstrable in at least 5% of asymptomatic Americans on at least one occasion during adulthood. One study reported hyperuricemia in 13.2% of hospitalized adult men. Despite the prevalence, evidence suggests that fewer than one in five hyperuricemic individuals will at any point develop clinically apparent urate crystal deposition. The relatively infrequent occurrence of gout in this population is likely to be accounted for, at least in part, by relatively mild increases in urate levels in the majority of hyperuricemic individuals (serum urate less than 9.0 mg/dL) and by transient hyperuricemia, particularly likely to occur in response to dietary alterations or to ingestion of a variety of drugs.

Duration and magnitude of hyperuricemia are directly related to the likelihood of subsequent development of gouty arthritis or uric acid urolithiasis (1,3). Nevertheless, recent data on the long-term effects of hyperuricemia and gout indicate that, in the absence of uric acid overproduction, hyperuricemia (at least up to 13 mg/dL in men and 10 mg/dL in women) is tolerated with little apparent jeopardy to renal function (3).

PATHOGENESIS OF HYPERURICEMIA

Uric acid is the normal end product of the catabolism of purines (1,4). Gout in humans arises from the species-wide lack of the enzyme uricase. Uricase oxidizes uric acid, which is only sparingly soluble in body fluids, to the highly soluble compound allantoin. The lack of uricase subjects humans to the risk of tissue deposition of crystalline forms of uric acid. This jeopardy is compounded by a complex array of renal mechanisms of uric acid handling that promote a net retention of more than 90% of the serum urate filtered at the glomerulus. Uric acid clearance suffi-

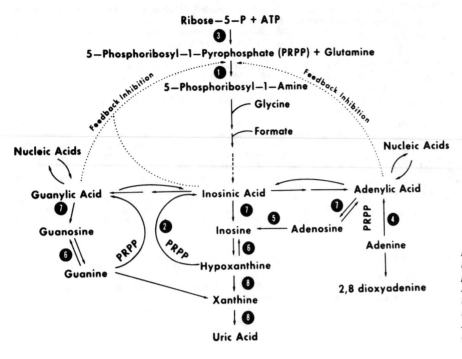

Fig. 31A–1. Schematic outline of purine metabolism: 1) amidophosphoribosyltransferase; 2) hypoxanthine–guanine phosphoribosyltransferase; 3) PRPP synthetase; 4) adenine phosphoribosyltransferase; 5) adenosine deaminase; 6) purine nucleoside phosphorylase; 7) 5'-nucleotidase; 8) xanthine oxidase (adapted from Seegmiller, Rosenbloom, and Kelley: Science 155:1682–1684, 1967).

cient to balance production is usually achieved in humans at plasma concentrations below the limit of solubility of monosodium urate in plasma (about 7 mg/dL at 37°C). Nevertheless, the margin of safety is relatively narrow, as indicated by the normal adult mean (±SD) serum urate concentrations (5.1 ± 1.0 mg/dL in men, and 4.0 ± 1.0 mg/dL in women).

Many genetic and environmental influences prompt the chain of events governing uric acid formation, transport, and disposal. Any one of a combination of derangements in these processes can lead to hyperuricemia and gout. Among environmental factors modifying serum urate concentration are weight, diet, lifestyle, social class, and hemoglobin level. An example of the interplay of genetic and environmental factors in determining hyperuricemia is provided by the higher mean serum urate level encountered in Filipinos living in the United States in comparison with individuals of identical racial stock living in the Phillipines. The limited ability of members of this population group to excrete uric acid provides an inherited basis for this tendency toward hyperuricemia, which is manifested when a diet with a relatively high purine content, such as the usual American diet, is ingested. The familial occurrence of gout, known for nearly 2,000 years, is reported by about 20% of affected patients, and hyperuricemia has been demonstrated in one-fourth of first-degree relatives of gout patients (1).

Purine metabolism and biochemistry

In humans, uric acid is derived both from the ingestion of foods containing purines and from the endogenous synthesis of purine nucleotides, which are building blocks in the synthesis of nucleic acids. The synthesis of purine nucleotides involves alternative biochemical pathways that are closely regulated (Fig. 31A–1). In the pathway of purine synthesis de novo, a purine ring is synthesized from small molecule precursors of uric acid, sequentially added to a ribose-phosphate backbone donated by 5-phosphoribosyl 1-pyrophosphate (PRPP). The first reaction committed to the pathway, catalyzed by the enzyme amidophosphoribosyltransferase (reaction 1, Fig. 31A–1), is the major site of the regulation of the pathway (1,4) by means of an antagonistic interaction between inhibition by purine nucleotide products and activation by PRPP, a substrate usually present in limited concentrations in the cell. Additional sites of control of purine nucleotide production have been identified at the level of the PRPP synthesis (reaction 3) and at the distal branch point governing

distribution of newly formed nucleotides into adenylate and guanylate derivatives (1,4).

The alternative pathway of purine nucleotide synthesis involves two enzymes, adenine phosphoribosyltransferase (reaction 4) and hypoxanthine–guanine phosphoribosyltransferase (HGPRT, reaction 2), which catalyze reactions between PRPP and the respective purine base substrates in the single-step synthesis of purine nucleotides. Among the factors governing the relationship between rates of purine base salvage and purine synthesis de novo are the availability of PRPP and the concentrations of the nucleotide products common to both pathways (1,4).

The catabolic steps that generate uric acid from nucleic acids and free purine nucleotides involve degradation through purine nucleoside intermediates to hypoxanthine and xanthine. The latter are ultimately oxidized to uric acid in sequential reactions catalyzed by the enzyme xanthine oxidase (reactions labeled 8).

Urate circulates in the plasma mainly in unbound form. The major route of uric acid disposal is renal excretion, which accounts for about two-thirds of the loss of this compound from the body under steady state conditions. Bacterial oxidation of urate secreted into the gut is the major mechanism of extrarenal urate disposal.

The total miscible urate pool averages about 1,200 mg (range 800–1,600 mg) in normal men and is about one-half this value in normal women. Since uric acid synthesis averages about 750 mg/day in men, an estimated two-thirds of the urate pool is turned over daily (1,4). Urinary uric acid excretion averages about 425 ± 80 mg/day in normal adult men receiving a purine-free diet and is the major adjustable mechanism for maintaining urate hemeostasis. The capacity of extrarenal uric acid disposal to compensate for abrupt changes in urate pool size is greatly limited in comparison with that of the kidney, which is capable of considerable increases in urinary uric acid excretion in response to increased filtered urate load. Chronic hyperuricemia and gout are invariably characterized by substantial expansion of the total uric acid pool and urate supersaturation of the extracellular space.

The above considerations suggest a number of potential mechanisms for excessive uric acid accumulation and thus hyperuricemia. In fact, only increased uric acid production and diminished uric acid excretion by the kidney, operating alone or in combination, have been demonstrated to contribute substantially to the hyperuricemia of patients with gout. This finding permits a

Table 31A–1. *Classification of hyperuricemia*

Uric acid overproduction
Primary hyperuricemia
  Idiopathic
  HGPRT deficiency (partial and complete)
  PRPP synthetase superactivity
Secondary hyperuricemia
  Excessive dietary purine intake
  Increased nucleotide turnover
    (e.g. myeloproliferative and lymphoproliferative disorders, hemolytic diseases, psoriasis)
  Accelerated ATP degradation
    glycogen storage diseases (types I, III, V, VII)
    fructose ingestion, hereditary fructose intolerance
    hypoxemia and tissue underperfusion
    severe muscle exertion
    ethanol abuse
Uric acid underexcretion
Primary hyperuricemia
  Idiopathic
Secondary hyperuricemia
  Diminished renal function
  Inhibition of tubular urate secretion
    competitive anions (e.g. keto- and lactic acidosis)
  Enhanced tubular urate reabsorption
    dehydration, diuretics
  Mechanism incompletely defined
    hypertension
    hyperparathyroidism
    certain drugs (e.g. cyclosporine, pyrazinamide, ethambutol, low dose salicylates)
    lead nephropathy

convenient subclassification of patients according to the respective mechanism responsible for hyperuricemia; that is, overproduction or underexcretion of uric acid or both mechanisms (Table 31A–1).

CAUSES AND CLASSIFICATION OF HYPERURICEMIA

Patients with hyperuricemia can be classified in a variety of ways with one useful method shown in Table 31A–1. In this scheme, *primary hyperuricemia* refers to those circumstances in which elevated serum urate levels or manifestations of urate deposition appear to be consequences of inherently disordered uric acid metabolism not associated with another acquired disorder and in which the gout syndrome is a prominent feature of the clinical picture. In contrast, *secondary hyperuricemia* refers to circumstances in which gout is a minor clinical feature secondary to any of a number of genetic or acquired processes. Classification of the type indicated here is useful in directing diagnostic attention, guiding rational therapy, and identifying patient populations in which deranged mechanisms of purine nucleotide synthesis or aberrations of renal uric acid handling can be studied with greater efficiency.

Uric Acid Overproduction

Perhaps 10% of patients with hyperuricemia or gout excrete excessive quantities of uric acid in a 24-hour urine collection (more than 1,000 mg excreted while on a normal diet) (1). Isotopic labeling studies almost invariably demonstrate increased rates of uric acid synthesis (overproduction) in such individuals. Overproduction of uric acid occurs with some frequency in a variety of acquired and genetic disorders characterized by excessive rates of cell and, therefore, nucleic acid turnover, such as myeloproliferative and lymphoproliferative diseases, hemolytic anemias and anemias associated with ineffective erythropoiesis, and psoriasis. These disorders constitute examples of secondary hyperuricemia and gout with uric acid overproduction.

In another group (probably not more than one-tenth of all patients with uric acid overproduction) manifestations of urate

deposition reflect primary, identifiable inherited derangements in mechanisms regulating purine nucleotide synthesis de novo. Specifically, in both partial deficiency of HGPRT and milder forms of superactivity of PRPP synthetase, early adult-onset gout and a high incidence of uric acid urinary tract stones constitute the usual clinical phenotype (1,5,6). Severe HGPRT deficiency is associated with spasticity, choreoathetosis, mental retardation, and compulsive self-mutilation (Lesch–Nyhan syndrome) (5). In some individuals, regulatory defects in PRPP synthetase are accompanied by sensorineural deafness and neurodevelopment defects (6). Intracellular accumulation of PRPP is a result of diminished utilization of this regulatory substrate in purine base salvage. This drives purine synthesis de novo at an increased rate in HGPRT deficiency. In the case of variant forms of PRPP synthetase with excessive activity, increased PRPP availability for purine synthesis results from increased rates of PRPP generation (7). Thus, aberrations of both of these enzymes result in increased uric acid synthesis by increasing PRPP availability and altering the balance of control of purine synthesis toward increased production. Both of these enzymes are produced from X-linked genes, and thus hemizygous men are affected. In addition, postmenopausal gout and urinary tract stones can occur as the phenotype of carrier women. Importantly, hyperuricemia detected in prepubertal boys always suggests that one of these enzymatic defects could be the cause.

Last, an increase in the net intracellular degradation of the adenine nucleotide, ATP, has been proposed as a common thread linking hyperuricemia in several conditions (Table 31A–1) (8–11). In particular, the accelerated degradation of ATP to AMP via the conversion of acetate to acetyl CoA in the metabolism of ethanol appears to be a critical mechanism in causing overproduction of uric acid and hyperuricemia associated with alcohol ingestion (9). In this regard, a history of heavy alcohol consumption is recognized in many individuals with gout (9,12).

Uric Acid Underexcretion

The great majority of patients with primary hyperuricemia or gout (up to 90%) show a relative deficit in the renal excretion of uric acid. Excretion of normal amounts of uric acid is accomplished in these individuals only when serum urate concentrations are inappropriately high. Uric acid clearance in these gouty underexcreters is decreased compared with normal individuals whose serum urate levels are rendered comparable via feedings of purine-rich diets (1,4).

Virtually all plasma urate is filtered at the glomerulus, with greater than 95% of the filtered load undergoing proximal tubular (presecretory) reabsorption (1,4). Subsequent proximal tubular secretion contributes the major share of excreted uric acid, and postsecretory tubular reabsorption is an additional important mechanism of renal uric acid handling. A number of kindreds with relatively early onset gout and a reduced fractional excretion of urate have been described (13,14); however, there is no evidence that most primary uric acid underexcreters with gout constitute a population with a single genetic or acquired renal defect. A diminished tubular secretory rate may contribute to hyperuricemia in some of these patients, and the possibilities of increased tubular reabsorption or diminished uric acid filtration in other patients with renal urate retention have not been dismissed. It is also uncertain whether the proposed tubular abnormalities reflect primary defects in transport mechanisms or are the result of interfering metabolites that impair tubular processes, such as those that accumulate in the course of other genetic and acquired metabolic disorders. A precedent for the latter possibility is the contribution of lactic acid-induced diminished renal urate secretion to the hyperuricemia of type 1 glycogen storage disease.

Pharmacologic agents that alter renal tubular function, either as a major action or as an unintended side effect, are also contributors to the occurrence of gout with uric acid underexcretion. Among the offending agents are diuretics (15,16), cyclosporine (17,18), and low dose salicylates (1,4). Low doses, below 2 g/day of salicylates, suppress tubular secretion and induce hyperuricemia, whereas high doses also suppress reabsorption and can result in hyperuricosuria. Until very recently, approximately 25% of the American population over age 65 was taking prescribed thiazide diuretics; this appears to account for increases in the number of elderly women presenting with gout (15,16). Alcohol use also decreases urate excretion. The metabolism of ethanol gives rise to an increase in the concentration of blood lactate. Like a number of other organic acids, lactic acid blocks the renal excretion of uric acid, presumably through inhibition of tubular secretion. If the blood lactate levels rise and then remain above 20–25 mg/dL for a sufficient time, uric acid output by the kidneys is sharply reduced. Cryptic forms of acquired renal impairment can also be manifested initially by gouty arthritis, as demonstrated by the high incidence of this disorder among chronically lead-intoxicated users of unbonded whiskey in the southeastern United States (19). Finally, patients with gout, as a group, have a relatively high incidence of other diseases that predispose to renal insufficiency such as hypertension and diabetes mellitus (1).

PATHOGENESIS OF URATE CRYSTAL DEPOSITION

In most instances, urate crystallizes as a monosodium salt in oversaturated joint tissues (4). As mentioned above, only a minority of individuals with sustained hyperuricemia develop tophi and gouty arthropathy. The reasons for this are poorly understood at present. The decreased solubility of sodium urate at the lower temperatures of peripheral structures such as the toes and ears may help explain why urate crystals deposit in these areas (1,4,20). However, the predilection for marked urate crystal deposition in the first metatarsophalangeal joint may also relate to repetitive minor trauma at this articulation. The observations that hemiplegia appears to have a sparing effect on the development of tophi and acute gout on the paretic side, and that tophi and acute gout occur in interphalangeal joints at the location of Heberden's nodes (20,21), suggests the potential importance of connective-tissue structure and turnover in urate crystal deposition.

Urate tophi have been found in synovial membrane at the time of the first gouty attack (reviewed in 20). Urate crystals found in joint fluid at the time of the acute attack may derive from rupture of preformed, arthroscopically detectable synovial deposits or may have precipitated de novo, as exemplified in certain instances by the recognition of urate spherulites (22). Declines in serum urate levels caused by antihyperuricemic drugs may promote the release of urate crystals from tophi via a decrease in the size of crystals, with consequent loosening of packed crystals and the formation of gaps at the periphery of urate crystal deposits.

In some individuals with gout, urate crystals can be found in asymptomatic metatarsophalangeal and knee joints that have never been involved in an acute attack of gout. Furthermore, patients with asymptomatic hyperuricemia may have urate crystals in metatarsophalangeal joint fluid. These findings confirm that gout can exist in an asymptomatic state.

PATHOLOGY OF GOUT

The histopathology of the tophi (Fig. 31A–2) shows a chronic foreign body granuloma surrounding a core of monosodium urate crystals. The inflammatory reaction around the crystals consists mostly of mononuclear cells and giant cells. A fibrous capsule is usually prominent. Crystals within the tophi are needle-shaped and are often arranged radially in small clusters. Crystals can be dissolved by water-based fixatives, so caution must be exercised in handling these specimens when obtained for diagnosis. The DeGolantha stain can be used to stain urates black; crystals can also be identified by compensated polarized light in frozen or alcohol-fixed specimens. Other potentially important components in tophi include lipids, glycosaminoglycans, and proteins (20).

In parenchymal renal disease of gout, the kidneys are usually small and equally affected. The cortical area is reduced in width and scars can been seen through the capsule. Many of these changes can be related to associated hypertension and infection (1). Even before the availability of effective urate-depleting

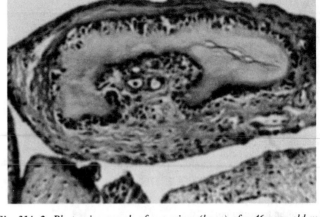

Fig. 31A–2. Photomicrograph of synovium (knee) of a 46-year-old man who sustained repeated attacks of gouty arthritis for 15 years. Note large tophaceous deposit in the synovial villus with surrounding histiocytic reaction. Crystals are dissolved from tophi unless tissue is processed with absolute alcohol.

drugs, renal parenchymal urate deposits were only occasionally present.

Histologic examination of kidneys from patients with gouty nephropathy may reveal that urate crystals are located primarily in the medullary interstitium, papillae, and pyramids. Like other tophi, they may be surrounded by a chronic inflammatory reaction with foreign body giant cells. Nephrosclerosis and other evidence of hypertensive disease are also common. The pelvis may contain uric acid stones.

PATHOGENESIS OF GOUTY INFLAMMATION

Gout was the first disease in which crystals were identified in joint effusions and subsequently incriminated in the pathogenesis of the arthritis. Intraarticular injection of urate crystals was shown to induce gout-like attacks even in normal individuals. However, the finding of crystals in synovial fluids of asymptomatic joints (20) illustrates that factors other than simply the presence of crystals may be important in the modulation of the inflammatory reaction.

Urate crystals appear to be directly able to initiate and sustain intense attacks of acute inflammation because of their capacity to stimulate the release of several inflammatory mediators, such as C5a, bradykinin, and kallikrein, via proteolysis of serum proteins and via the generation and secretion of many mediators from phagocytes, synovial lining cells and other cells; for example cyclooxygenase and lipoxygenase metabolites of arachidonic acid, lysosomal proteases, interleukin-1 (IL-1), tumor necrosis factor alpha (TNF), IL-6, and IL-8 (20,23,24). Neutrophil influx is promoted both by chemotactic factors, and by endothelial activation by IL-1 and TNF. The ingress of neutrophils is the most important event for the development of acute urate crystal-induced synovitis (20). Intraarticular neutrophils can be activated both by direct contact with crystals and by exposure to the rich soup of soluble mediators. These events support prolonged ingress of neutrophils, which is likely vital for perpetuation of acute gouty inflammation because of the limited functional lifespan (days) of normal neutrophils. The systemic release from the gouty joint into the venous circulation of IL-1, TNF, IL-6, and IL-8 appears responsible for systemic manifestations, such as fever, leukocytosis, and hepatic acute phase protein response (1).

The acute gouty attack may be self-limited by certain changes in not only the physical properties of intraarticular urate crystals, which include their size, shape, and possibly most important the proteins and other materials bound to the crystals (26,27) but also in the balance between pro- and anti-inflammatory soluble factors (release of IL-1 inhibitors and transforming growth factor beta) (20,25). However, the precise mechanisms that spontaneously limit acute gouty inflammation remain to be defined.

Robert Terkeltaub, MD

1. Levinson D, Becker MA: Clinical gout and pathogenesis of hyperuricemia. Arthritis and Allied Conditions, 12th ed. Edited by McCarty DJ and Koopman WJ. Philadelphia, Lea & Febiger, 1993, pp 1773–1805

2. Lawrence RC, Hochberg MC, Kelsey JL, et al: Estimates of the prevalence of selected arthritic and musculoskeletal diseases in the United States. J Rheumatol 16:427–441, 1989

3. Campion EW, Glynn RJ, DeLabry LO: Asymptomatic hyperuricemia. Risks and consequences in the normative aging study. Am J Med 82:421–426, 1987

4. Palella TD, Kelley WN: Purine and deoxypurine metabolism. Textbook of Rheumatology. Edited by Kelley WN et al. Philadelphia, W.B. Saunders, pp 337–352, 1989

5. Wilson JM, Stout JT, Palella TD, et al: A molecular survey of hypoxanthine-guanine phosphoribosyltransferase deficiency in man. J Clin Invest 77:188–195, 1986

6. Becker MA, Puig JG, Matoes FA, et al: Inherited superactivity of phosphoribosylpyrophosphate synthetase: association of uric acid overproduction and sensorineural deafness. Am J Med 85:383–390, 1988

7. Becker MA, Losman MJ, Wilson J, et al: Superactivity of human phosphoribosylpyrophosphate synthetase due to altered regulation by nucleotide inhibitors and inorganic phosphate. Biochim Biophys Acta 882:168–176, 1986

8. Fox IH, Palella TD, and Kelley WN: Hyperuricemia: a marker for cell energy crisis. N Engl J Med 317:111, 1987

9. Faller J, Fox I: Ethanol induced hyperuricemia, evidence for increased urate production by activation of adenine nucleotide turnover. N Engl J Med 307:1598–1602, 1982

10. Mineo I, Kono N, Hara N, et al: Myogenic Hyperuricemia. A common pathophysiologic freature of glycogenosis types III V, and VII. N Engl J Med 317:75–80, 1987

11. Seegmiller JE, Dixon RM, Kemp GJ, et al: Fructose-induced aberration of metabolism in familial gout identified by ^{31}P magnetic resonance spectroscopy. Proc Natl Acad Sci 87:8326–8330, 1990

12. Birchall MA, Henderson HP: Alcohol and response to treatment of gout. Brit Med J 296:1641–1642, 1988

13. Calabrese G, Simmonds HA, Cameron JS, et al: Precocious familial gout with reduced fractional urate clearance and normal purine enzymes. Q J Med, New Series 75, 277:441–450, 1990

14. Editorial. Precocious familial gout. Lancet. ii:412, 1990

15. Macfarlane DG, Dieppe PA. Diuretic-induced gout in elderly women. Brit J Rheum 24:155–157, 1985

16. Langford HG, Blaufox MD, Borhani NO, et al: Is thiazide-produced uric acid elevation harmful? Arch Intern Med 147:645–649, 1987

17. Lin H, Rocher LL, McQuillan MA, et al: Cyclosporine-induced hyperuricemia and gout. N Engl J Med 321:287–292, 1989

18. Kahl LE, Thompson ME, Bartley P, et al: Gout in the heart transplant recipient: physiologic puzzle and therapeutic challenge. Am J Med 87:289–294, 1989

19. Reynolds PP, Knapp MJ, Baraf HSB: Moonshine and lead: relationship to the pathogenesis of hyperuricemia in gout. Arthritis Rheum 26:1057–1064, 1983

20. Terkeltaub R: Pathogenesis and treatment of crystal-induced inflammation. Arthritis and Allied Conditions, 12th ed. Edited by McCarty DJ and Koopman, W. Philadelphia, Lea and Febiger, 1993, pp 1819–1833

21. Simkin PA, Campbell PM, Larson EB: Gout in Heberden's nodes. Arthritis Rheum 26:94–97, 1983

22. Fiechtner JJ, Simkin PA: Urate spherulites in gouty synovia. JAMA 245:1533–1536, 1981

23. di Giovine FS, Malawista SE, Thornton E, et al: Urate crystals stimulate production of tumor necrosis factor alpha from human blood monocytes and synovial cells. Cytokine mRNA and protein kinetics, and cellular distribution. J Clin Invest 87:1375–1381, 1991

24. Terkeltaub R, Zachariae C, Santoro D, et al: Monocyte-derived neutrophil chemotactic factor/IL–8 is a potential mediator of crystal-induced inflammation. Arthritis Rheum 34:894–903, 1991

25. Terkeltaub R. Editorial: What stops a gouty attack? J Rheumatol 19:8–10 1992.

26. Ortiz-Bravo E, Sieck M, Schumacher HR: Changes in the proteins coating monosodium urate crystals during active and subsiding inflammation. Arthritis Rheum, 1993 (in press)

27. Rosen MS, Baker D, Schumacher HR: Products of polymorphonuclear cell injury inhibit IgG enhancement of monosodium urate-induced superoxide production. Arthritis Rheumatism 29:1480–1484, 1986

B. Clinical and Laboratory Features

STAGES OF GOUTY ARTHRITIS

Four phases can be identified in the evolution of gout: asymptomatic hyperuricemia, acute gouty arthritis, intercritical gout, and chronic tophaceous gout.

Asymptomatic Hyperuricemia

Asymptomatic hyperuricemia, as noted above, is not strictly gout as by no means all patients with hyperuricemia will develop gout. It seems very likely, however, that in many patients there is an asymptomatic deposition of urate crystals in connective tissues that occurs before the first episode of acute gouty arthritis. This would be true of asymptomatic gout.

Acute Gouty Arthritis

The acute arthritis of gout is the most common early clinical manifestation. Indeed, the clinical picture is often typical enough to strongly suggest the diagnosis. The metatarsophalangeal (MTP) joint of the first toe is involved most often, and is affected at some time in 75% of patients. The ankle, tarsal area, and the knee are also commonly involved. A wrist or finger joint is less often involved during the early attacks. The first episode of acute gouty arthritis frequently begins fairly abruptly in a single joint, often during the night, so that the patient awakes with dramatic unexplained joint pain and swelling.

Affected joints are usually warm, red, and tender. The diffuse periarticular erythema that often accompanies the attacks (Fig. 31B–1) can be confused with cellulitis or thrombophlebitis. In 1683 Thomas Sydenham, himself a victim of the disease, described the attacks as follows:

The victim goes to bed and sleeps in good health. About two o'clock in the morning he is awakened by a severe pain in the great toe; more rarely in the heel, ankle, or instep. The pain is like that of a dislocation, and yet the parts feel as if cold water were poured over them. Then follow chills and shivers, and a little fever. The pain, which was at first moderate, becomes more intense. With its intensity, the chills and shivers increase. After a time this comes to its height, accommodating itself to the bones and ligaments of the tarsus and metatarsus. Now it is a violent stretching and tearing of the ligaments—now it is a gnawing pain, and now a pressure and tightening. So exquisite and lively meanwhile is the feeling of the part affected that it cannot bear the weight of the bedclothes nor the jar of a person walking in the room. The night is passed in torture, sleeplessness, turning of the part affected and perpetual change of posture.

Early attacks tend to subside spontaneously over 3–10 days even without treatment. Desquamation of the skin overlying the affected joint may occur when the inflammation subsides. Patients are often completely symptom free after an acute attack. Subsequent episodes may occur more frequently, involve more joints, and persist longer. Polyarticular gout occasionally occurs in patients having their first attack. Usually, patients with more than one joint inflamed are those with more prolonged disease and suboptimal management (1). Some mild arthralgias between attacks may be caused by gout, but other causes should also be sought for such symptoms. Acute attacks may be triggered by a specific event recognizable by patients or their physicians, such as trauma, alcohol, drugs, surgical stress, or acute medical illness.

Swings in the level of serum urate may precede episodes of gouty arthritis. This often occurs early in the course of treatment with uricosuric drugs or allopurinol or after the administration of various drugs that affect renal handling of uric acid, such as diuretics.

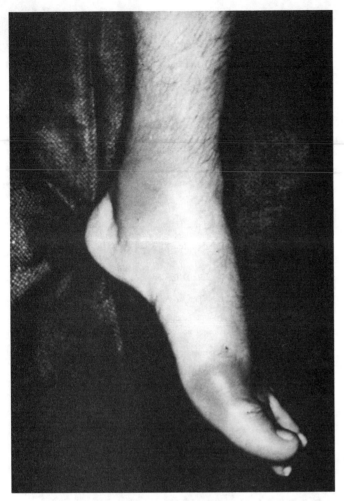

Fig. 31B–1. Acute gouty arthritis at the first metatarsophalangeal joint and ankle joint.

Intercritical Gout

The intervals between attacks constitute the intercritical stage of gout. In the beginning, the intercritical periods are usually without symptoms or abnormal physical findings. Even during an asymptomatic period, monosodium urate crystals can often be aspirated from previously involved joints or from joints that have never been overtly affected (2). Monosodium urate crystals have been found in up to 97% of synovial fluids from asymptomatic joints previously inflamed and in 22% from knees that have never been inflamed in patients with untreated gout (3). Some crystals from these asymptomatic joints lie within synovial cell or mononuclear leukocyte vacuoles, raising questions as to the role of such low grade inflammation in indolent joint damage or as to what prevents the evolution of clinically detectable inflammation. Since crystal deposition persists between attacks, a definitive diagnosis can still be made even during this asymptomatic period.

Chronic Tophaceous Gout

Clinically evident subcutaneous monosodium urate crystal-containing tophi occur in only fairly advanced gout, although microtophi appear to be present in the synovial membrane even at an early stage (2). Tophi are generally first noted some time after onset, on the average of about 10 years after the first episode of arthritis. Tophi occur most often in the synovium, subchondral bone, olecranon bursa, infrapatellar and Achilles tendons, subcutaneous tissue on the extensor surface of the forearms, overlying joints, and still (but less often than previously) on the helix of the ear. Tophi are especially common in previously damaged joints like Heberden's nodes in post-meno-

pausal women (4). They are less often seen in the aortic walls, tricuspid and mitral valves, nasal cartilage, eyelids, cornea, and sclerae. Even in advanced cases, tophi have never been reported in the central nervous system, because the concentration of uric acid in spinal fluid is very low, ranging from 0.25–1.0 mg/dL in normal and gouty patients (5).

Tophi are easily confused with rheumatoid nodules unless aspirated or biopsied for diagnosis. About 50% of inadequately treated patients may eventually develop overt tophaceous deposits, but this may require many years. Their presence is generally but not invariably associated with more frequent and severe inflammatory episodes.

Deforming arthritis can develop as a result of the erosion of cartilage and subchondral bone caused by crystal deposition and the chronic inflammatory reaction. Tophaceous formation in tendon sheaths of the hand and wrist may cause trigger fingers or carpal tunnel syndrome. Chronic gouty arthritis can mimic rheumatoid arthritis, although it tends to be less symmetric than typical rheumatoid disease, and it can involve any joint. Tophaceous material, which is white and chalky, can be aspirated from superficial tophi and occasionally extrudes spontaneously through the overlying skin. It can be recovered for polarized light examination to confirm the presence of crystals and cultured to exclude infection.

RENAL DISEASE

Renal parenchymal compromise and renal stones may occur in patients with gout. Proteinuria and mild hypertension have been reported in 20% to 40% of patients, but both are usually benign in idiopathic gout. More severe forms of renal disease with nephrosclerosis or other decline in renal function are usually associated with aging, more severe hypertension, renal calculi, pyelonephritis, lead nephropathy, and inherited enzyme deficiency (6). As noted above, some renal disease is a cause of hyperuricemia. This accounts for some early age of onset gout and some gout in unusual situations like in women with SLE (7).

The risk of urolithiasis is clearly increased in patients with gout. Fessel found that the risk of urolithiasis was 1 stone in 852 normouricemic patients/yr, 1 in 295 patients/yr in persons with asymptomatic hyperuricemia, and 1 in 114 patients/yr in established gout (8). The frequency of stone formation parallels the increase in serum uric acid, acidity of the urine, and urinary uric acid concentration. The prevalence of urolithiasis increased from 11% in patients with urinary uric acid excretion of 300 mg/day to 50% in patients with values over 1,100 mg/day. Uric acid stones are usually radiolucent, small, and round, but they sometimes contain calcium salts and are radiopaque. Yu and Gutman (9) also found that the incidence of calcium stones was increased in patients with gout.

Striking increases in serum urate levels, as high as 40–60 mg/dL, may occur in patients with leukemia or lymphoma as a result of the rapid breakdown of the cellular nucleic acids after aggressive treatment with corticosteroids, irradiation, or alkylating agents. The precipitation of uric acid in the renal tubules of these patients may lead to urinary obstruction with prolonged oliguria. This hazard can be prevented or reversed by administering allopurinol.

COMPLICATIONS AND ASSOCIATED DISEASES

The development of hyperuricemia in arterial hypertension appears to be related to an abnormality in uric acid transport by the renal tubules. Diabetes mellitus, cardiac and cerebral atherosclerosis, and hypertriglyceridemia (10) also occur more frequently among patients with gout. The precise explanation for these associations is not known, although a common connection with obesity has been suggested.

The connection of gout with gluttony and the belief that the attacks of articular inflammation follow intemperance and venery

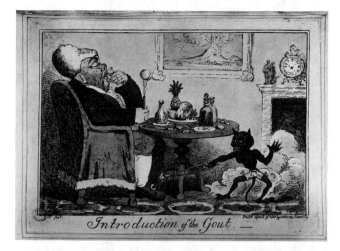

Fig. 31B–2. Introduction of the Gout. *Copper-plate engraving by George Cruikshank, published by SW Fores, London, 1818. Note the decanter of wine on the table of the pinguid/gastronome and the illustration of a volcanic (gouty) eruption in the picture on the dining room wall (reproduced by permission of the Trustees of the British Museum).*

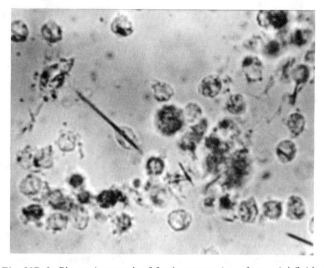

Fig. 31B–3. *Photomicrograph of fresh preparation of synovial fluid obtained from the inflamed knee of a 45-year-old man with acute gouty arthritis. Note numerous small and large needle-shaped crystals of monosodium urate monohydrate that have been engulfed by neutrophilic leukocytes.*

date to ancient times and serve as the basis for the extensive use of the gouty foot as a symbol of overindulgence in satirical works throughout the centuries (Fig. 31B–2). The association of primary gout with overeating and alcoholism is well documented. Approximately one-half of gouty individuals weigh 15% or more than their ideal weights, and 75% or more exhibit hypertriglyceridemia, the frequency of which appears to be correlated with obesity (11). The observation that uric acid synthesis is accelerated when the diet is fortified with protein, and reports of the occasional correction of hyperuricemia in obese individuals by severe weight reduction suggest that chronically excessive food intake may be important in persistent elevation of serum urate levels. In general, however, adherence to a strict low-purine diet results in only a modest reduction in the concentration of serum urate, usually no more than 2 mg/dL (12).

Avascular necrosis of bone, involving particularly the head of the femur, may occur with increased frequency in gouty individuals (13). In some instances, this association is related to chronic alcoholism.

ROENTGENOGRAPHIC FINDINGS

Roentgenograms are not usually of any positive diagnostic value during the initial attack, but they do show soft tissue swelling surrounding the affected joint. Roentgenograms can be useful to help exclude septic changes, chondrocalcinosis, or calcific periarthritis that can clinically resemble acute gouty arthritis. The articular tophi of later chronic gout tend to produce irregular asymmetric soft tissue swelling. Calcifications of the tophi can occur.

The bony erosions that can also occur in chronic disease are round or oval in shape and surrounded with a sclerotic margin (14). These erosions may be intraarticular or periarticular; a thin overhanging edge of displaced bone may seen. Joint spaces are preserved until late in the course of the disease.

LABORATORY FINDINGS

The demonstration of monosodium urate crystals is now generally considered to be mandatory for establishing the diagnosis of gout as an explanation to acute arthritis, because serum urate levels can be misleading. Even during asymptomatic periods, monosodium urate crystals can be recovered from many joints (2). Only a single drop of fluid is necessary for the detection of tell-tale crystals, and even the small amount of synovial fluid obtainable from the first MTP joint suffices in many cases.

The crystals, which are either intra- or extracellular and are typically rod- or needle-shaped ($3-20\mu$), are usually visible with a light microscope (Fig. 31B–3). A polarizing microscope produces

a more definitive picture of the crystals, however, which are birefringent and bright yellow, parallel to the axis of slow vibration marked on the polarizing microscope compensator (negative elongation).

Synovial fluid leukocytes are elevated from 20,000–100,000 cells/mm³ in acute gouty arthritis and contain predominantly neutrophils. Effusions appear cloudy as a result of the high concentrations of cells and crystals. Occasionally masses of crystals produce a thick, pasty white joint fluid. Since infection can coexist with urate crystals, joint fluid cultures should also be obtained if the diagnosis is in question.

The value of serum uric acid levels in the diagnosis of the acute attack is limited. Serum uric acid levels can be normal at the time of acute gouty arthritis. Some normal levels are explained by high (uricosuric) doses of aspirin or recent institution of a uricosuric agent. Whatever the reasons, a normal serum uric acid level does not exclude the diagnosis of acute gout. In almost all patients, serum uric acid levels will be elevated at some time. Serum urate measurements are important in following treatment. Some patients have elevated serum uric acid due to drugs or other causes and do not have gout.

A 24-hour urine uric acid measurement is valuable in assessing the risk of renal stones, in elucidating underlying factors in the gout, and in determining the type of treatment. Urinary excretion of uric acid greater than 750–1000 mg/day on a regular diet suggests one of the diseases that causes overproduction of uric acid. Diuretics, aspirin, alcohol consumption, contrast radiology, or phenylbutazone can affect uric acid excretion for several days and should be avoided before measurements. Colchicine and indomethacin do not interfere with urate excretion. Laboratory tests are also useful for ruling out other diseases associated with gout, such as renal insufficiency, hyperlipidemia, and diabetes.

Guillermo A. Tate, MD
H. Ralph Schumacher, Jr, MD

1. Lawry GV, Fan PT, Bluestone R: Polyarticular versus monoarticular gout: a prospective, comparative analysis of clinical features. Medicine 67:335–343, 1988

2. Agudelo CA, Weinberger A, Schumacher HR, et al: Definite diagnosis of gouty arthritis by identification of urate crystals in asymptomatic metatarsophalangeal joints. Arthritis Rheum 22:559–560, 1979

3. Pascual E: Persistence of monosodium urate crystals and low-grade inflammation in the synovial fluid of patients with untreated gout. Arthritis Rheum 34: 141–145, 1991

4. Lally EV, Ho G, Kaplan SR: The clinical spectrum of gouty arthritis in women: Arch. Int Med 146:2221–2225, 1986

5. Wyngaarden JB: Uric Acid. Encyclopedia of Medicine, Surgery, Specialities, Edited by Piersol GM, Philadelphia, Davis, 1955, pp 341

6. Yu T-F, Berger L, Dorph DT, et al: Renal function in gout. V. Factors influencing the renal hemodynamics. Am J Med 67:766–771, 1979

7. Veerapen K, Schumacher HR, Van Lindhoudt D, et al: Tophaceous gout in young patients with systemic lupus erythematosus. J Rheum 20:721–724, 1993

8. Fessel WJ: Renal outcomes in gout and hyperuricemia. Am J Med 67:74–82, 1979

9. Yu T-F: Uric acid nephrolitiasis in gout: predisposing factors. Ann Intern Med 67:1133–1148, 1967

10. Allard C, Goulet C: Serum Uric acid, not a discriminator of coronary heart disease in man and women. Can Med Assoc J 109:986–988, 1973

11. Yu T-F, Dorph DJ, Smith H: Hyperlipidemia in primary gout. Semin in Arth Rheum 7:97–113, 1977

12. Rodnan GP: The pathogenesis in aldermanic gout (abstract). Arth Rheum 23:137, 1980

13. Mielants H, Veys EM, DeBussere A, et al: Avascular necrosis and its relationship with lipid and purine metabolism. J Rheumatol 2:430–436, 1975

14. Watt I, Middlemiss H: The radiology of gout. Clin Radiol 26:27–36, 1975

C. Treatment

In each stage of gout that may require therapy—acute, intercritical, or tophaceous—there is effective medical management, which in most situations should be successful and without excessive complications. After the diagnosis of gout, the treatment goals should be to provide rapid and safe relief of the pain of acute arthritis, to prevent further attacks, and to prevent destructive arthropathy and the formation of tophi or kidney stones.

Coexistent illness may directly influence the safety and efficacy of drugs used in gout; particular attention must be paid to abnormalities of the gastrointestinal, renal, hepatobiliary, and hematopoietic systems. Toxicity and effectiveness of drugs used are influenced by renal function; therefore, pretreatment knowledge of serum creatinine is mandatory. Furthermore, the inappropriate use of colchicine may be prevented by a pretreatment white blood count and differential as well as liver function studies.

An informed patient is a great help in the ideal management of gout. The physician should instill awareness of the early signs of gout and the importance of early treatment as a major determinant of therapeutic success. The patient should also understand the treatment goals and the distinguishing characteristics of the drugs used to attain them.

ACUTE GOUT

Colchicine

Its venerable history does not exempt colchicine from controversy. Current rheumatology texts and editorials have questioned its continued role in the treatment of acute gout because of its toxicity.

To date there has been only one placebo controlled trial of colchicine in the treatment of acute gout (1). Of 43 patients randomized to receive either colchicine or placebo, two-thirds of those receiving colchicine exhibited a 50% decrease in baseline scores of clinical severity and pain within 48 hours, as did one-third of those treated with placebo. This study is faulted by the long delay (mean 38 hours) between the onset of symptoms and the initiation of treatment. In all other studies, data has been accumulated by review rather than by prospective experimentation. Colchicine does seem to be less effective when used after the first several days of an episode.

Gutman and Yu reported that pain subsided within 48 hours in 80% of 536 gouty attacks treated with colchicine (2). Others have reported similar success with colchicine in nonselected gout patients. It has been suggested that the prompt response of arthritis to colchicine is diagnostic of gout, with more than 90% of attacks reported to respond to colchicine when it is given within the first few hours of symptoms. Other crystal induced arthropathies may also respond to colchicine, however (3).

Though usually effective, the oral administration of colchicine may cause gastrointestinal toxicity in up to 80% of patients (2). Nausea, vomiting, diarrhea, and cramping abdominal pain may be severe, leading to hypovolemia, electrolyte disarray, and metabolic alkalosis. The gradual use of small repeated doses is intended only to minimize gastrointestinal toxicity; gradual dosing affords no therapeutic advantage.

Avoidance of gastrointestinal toxicity is one of the advantages of intravenous colchicine administration, which is also of use in the postoperative patient in whom oral intake is restricted. The speed with which intravenous colchicine may act is also advantageous. Some patients may experience improvement within 30 minutes when therapy is initiated soon after the onset of joint pain. With proper use, the only anticipated side effects of intravenous colchicine are thrombophlebitis, if the drug is not diluted properly, and skin sloughing if it is extravasated.

The improper use of colchicine, particularly the intravenous form, has led to serious toxicity and fatality (4). Excessive dosage may produce bone marrow suppression, renal failure, disseminated intravascular coagulation, hypocalcemia, cardiopulmonary failure, seizures, and death. The report of two deaths at one teaching hospital represented 2% of the patients treated with intravenous colchicine during a four-year period (5). In these patients, colchicine-induced granulocytopenia was profound and a major contributor to fulminant illness. Advanced age, renal insufficiency, and the concurrent use of both oral and intravenous preparations was common to both patients. Similar observations have been made regarding other reported cases of colchicine toxicity or fatality. The average dose associated with fatality has been 16 mg, but doses as low as 7 mg given over three days have been fatal, while doses as high as 40–60 mg have been survived (6).

Severe toxicity and fatality have also been reported with oral administration of excessive doses. In prophylactic use, oral colchicine has been associated with a neuromuscular syndrome. Colchicine-induced myopathy resembles polymyositis with proximal muscle weakness, elevated creatine kinase levels, and abnormalities on electromyography. The myopathy may resolve spontaneously over several weeks, but more subtle polyneuropathy caused by colchicine resolves more slowly (6).

All reported cases of death, severe toxicity, or neuromuscular disease involved unusually high doses of colchicine, renal insufficiency, advanced age, or the use of both oral and intravenous preparations during a short period of time (4). The mechanism of action and elimination kinetics of colchicine offer insight into its toxicity. Colchicine inhibits the polymerization of microtubules by binding their protein subunits and preventing their aggregation. Membrane dependent functions such as chemotaxis and phagocytosis may, therefore, be disrupted. Other unknown mechanisms are almost certainly present since trimethylcolchicinic acid, a congener of colchicine that does not bind to microtubular structures, is also effective in the treatment of gout (7). Reflecting microtubular binding in cells such as polymorphonuclear leukocytes, plasma levels decay rapidly as colchicine is concentrated intracellularly. Only 10% of an intravenous dose is excreted during the first 24 hours; with sensitive assays, colchicine can be detected in granulocytes and in urine 10 days after administration. Thus, an important determinant of toxicity is the cumulative dose over 7–10 days relative to renal function (4). Colchicine undergoes entero–hepatic circulation, and liver disease or extrahepatic biliary obstruction may potentiate its toxic effects.

Wallace and Singer have provided cogent recommendations for the intravenous use of colchicine (8) including the following: 1) a single intravenous dose should not exceed 3 mg, and the total cumulative dose for an attack should not exceed 4 mg in a 24-hour period; 2) patients should receive no more colchicine by any route for seven days after a full intravenous dose; 3) the dosage should be reduced and perhaps halved in the presence of renal or hepatic disease and in the older patient even with apparently normal renal function; and 4) absolute contraindications to intravenous colchicine include combined renal and hepatic disease, glomerular filtration rate (GFR) less than 10 ml/min, and extrahepatic biliary obstruction.

Relative contraindications include significant intercurrent infection, preexisting bone marrow suppression, and immediate prior use of oral colchicine. Colchicine for intravenous use should be diluted in 20 ml of normal saline and administered over 10–20 minutes through a secured intravenous line to avoid thrombophlebitis or extravasation. In none of the reported cases of extreme toxicity were these requirements fulfilled. Their application should greatly increase the safety of intravenous colchicine administration.

Similar constraints apply to the use of oral colchicine, whether for acute gout or its prophylaxis. In patients with estimated GFR less than 50–60 ml/min, doses should be halved (8). In general, it is better not to mix oral and intravenous colchicine during any attack or in a 7–10 day time period; therefore, colchicine is administered as 0.5 mg tablets taken hourly until one of three endpoints is reached: 1) significant improvement of pain and inflammation; 2) gastrointestinal toxicity, or 3) a maximum total dose of 8 mg, assuming normal renal and hepatic function. Patients should be provided with advice on symptomatic measures to treat gastrointestinal toxicity in addition to discontinuing the drug.

Nonsteroidal Antiinflammatory Drugs

Although no placebo controlled trials have been reported, nonsteroidal antiinflammatory drugs (NSAIDs) are probably used more often than colchicine for acute gout. Many agents are reportedly effective; however, the comparative efficacy and toxicity of NSAIDs have not been studied adequately. In general, NSAIDs are started in their recommended maximal doses at the first sign of an attack. The dose is lowered within a day or two and continued until the arthritis has resolved. When used in this way, the response rate of NSAIDs approaches that of oral colchicine. NSAIDs may be more effective than colchicine in the well-established attack.

Although less toxic than colchicine, NSAIDs may cause significant side effects. Most common are dyspepsia and gastrointestinal side effects: gastritis, peptic ulceration, and gastrointestinal bleeding. Nonsteroidal antiinflammatory drugs should be avoided in patients with active or recent peptic ulcer disease and in patients requiring anticoagulation (see Chapter 55).

Caution should be used in prescribing NSAIDs in patients with renal insufficiency or conditions associated with impaired renal blood flow such as congestive heart failure because NSAIDs may exacerbate renal insufficiency or induce hyporeninemic hypoaldosteronism through their inhibition of intrarenal prostaglandin formation. They may worsen hypertension, induce sodium retention, and cause edema. Rarely, they may cause interstitial nephritis or papillary necrosis. Aspirin-associated bronchospasm or urticaria are relative contraindications to NSAID use. Among NSAIDs, many physicians prefer indomethacin for acute gout.

Corticosteroids and Adrenocorticotrophic Hormone

Corticosteroids and adrenocorticotrophic hormone (ACTH) have traditionally been used when colchicine and NSAIDs were contraindicated or ineffective. As used in gout, corticosteroids and ACTH have minimal toxicity. There are reports of relapse or early recurrence complicating their use; however, a recent study of corticosteroids in acute gout noted relapse infrequently (9). Response time was comparable to that of NSAIDs. A single unblinded trial compared ACTH with indomethacin in monarticular gout and reported similar efficacy (10).

For acute gout, 20–40 mg doses of prednisone or its equivalent are administered daily for three to four days and then gradually tapered over one to two weeks. If oral administration is problematic, the hospitalized patient can be treated with equivalent doses of intravenous methylprednisolone. Adrenocorticotrophic hormone is given as an intramuscular injection of 40–80 IU;

some have recommended following the initial dose with 40 IU every 6–12 hours for several days if necessary.

Aspiration and intraarticular depot steroid injection with 10–40 mg of triamcinolone and 2–10 mg dexamethasone is a useful alternative in the patient who has gout in one or two large joints. Full drainage of the joint alone may be helpful. If septic arthritis is suspected after aspiration, injection should be deferred until synovial fluid has been cultured, as 38 cases of concurrent septic and gouty arthritis have been reported (11). Joint aspiration and injection may be a nontoxic therapeutic option in the elderly patient with renal insufficiency, peptic ulcer disease, or other intercurrent illness. It is also an appropriate option for recalcitrant gout.

Most often, gout will respond to corticosteroids or ACTH when NSAIDs and colchicine have failed. In some situations, however, optimal treatment may not be possible because of delay in therapy or intercurrent illness. When delayed relief of pain is anticipated, administration of narcotics is appropriate as with any other similarly painful condition.

PROPHYLACTIC TREATMENT OF INTERCRITICAL GOUT

The decision to employ prophylactic therapy in individual patients depends on issues such as toxicity, cost, compliance, and patient tolerance of acute attacks. Unless there is an overriding indication, prophylactic therapy ought not be considered until the patient has established a pattern of frequency. Twenty-five percent of persons whose first attack occurred during the 12-year period of the Heart Disease Epidemiology Study had only the single attack (7). The patient may be better served by education regarding recognition of the incipient flare, the use of colchicine or NSAIDs to abort or mitigate the attack, and recognition of the signs of developing tophaceous gout which is not prevented by colchicine. Education should make clear the potential for dangerous toxicity if the drug is used in any way other than as prescribed.

In some patients, behavioral modification may significantly reduce the frequency of gouty attacks (7). Weight reduction may yield beneficial reduction in serum urate, and dietary purine restriction may be an adjunct to therapy, though urate reduction is usually modest. As it may both increase production and impair excretion of uric acid, alcohol should be avoided. Furthermore, dehydration and repetitive trauma, as encountered in certain exercises or occupations, may be avoidable causes of gouty attacks. Thus, modification of diet and lifestyle may reduce the frequency of acute attacks and may render daily drug therapy unnecessary. Also, diuretics and other drugs known to contribute to hyperuricemia can be eliminated if possible.

When gouty attacks are frequent or when urate-lowering therapy is being initiated, daily oral colchicine may be given to reduce their frequency. A single double-blind, placebo-controlled study supports the prophylactic efficacy of one 0.5 mg colchicine tablet twice daily (12). Gutman and Yu (2) reported that in 208 patients prophylactic therapy rendered 74% free of attacks and moderated attack severity in 20%. For optimal effectiveness, 65% required 1 mg/day and 25% required 0.5 mg/day. The smallest daily dose providing acceptable control of attacks should be used to minimize the risk of toxicity.

The protracted use of small daily doses of colchicine appears to be relatively safe (6). When used chronically for familial Mediterranean fever, few serious problems have been reported with doses of 1.0–1.5 mg/day, although diarrhea occurred commonly and steatorrhea was observed rarely. Although there have been rare reports of colchicine-associated azoospermia, the literature does not document any clear effect on fertility. Thirty-four patients who received colchicine for gout prophylaxis reportedly fathered apparently normal children. In women with familial Mediterranean fever, miscarriage and infertility rates have not apparently changed with the advent of colchicine therapy.

HYPERURICEMIA AND URATE LOWERING AGENTS

Hyperuricemia alone is not a disease state and is seldom a reason for treatment. However, over a period of years moderate hyperuricemia may lead to gouty arthritis, tophus formation, and less commonly, nephrolithiasis. Although there is little long-term risk of tophus formation in the patient with a plasma urate level of 7–8 mg/dl, there is increasing risk with higher levels such that 50% of nonselected gout patients develop tophi by examination or radiography if left untreated (13).

The treatment of hyperuricemia in patients with recurrent or chronic gout implies a long-term commitment to daily therapy and behavioral change. Foods with high purine content, such as visceral meats, sardines, shellfish, turkey, salmon, trout, beans, peas, asparagus, and spinach, should be restricted, particularly in patients on uricosuric drugs and in those patients who cannot tolerate urate-lowering treatment. When possible, the concurrent use of drugs with hyperuricemic effects (such as pyrazinamide, ethambutol, thiazide or loop diuretics) and low dose salicylates should be avoided.

The goal of treatment is consistent maintenance of serum urate less than 6 mg/dl at 37°C, which should allow solubilization of crystalline urate. Lower levels are often needed for resorption of cutaneous or osseous tophi and reduction of attack frequency. For example, some argue that as the ambient temperature of skin and extremities is closer to 30°C, serum urate levels less than 5 mg/dl may be needed to allow dissolution of urate deposits. One recent study examined radiographic changes occurring over 10 years of urate-lowering therapy (14). Achieving normouricemia did not appear to translate into radiographic improvement of intraosseous tophi as often as expected, and the authors expressed concern that deeper reduction of serum urate may be necessary even when symptom control is good.

Uricosuric drugs or xanthine oxidase inhibitors are selected according to patient need. Because only 10% of patients are overexcretors of uric acid (11), uricosuric therapy is rarely inappropriate on these grounds. Both allopurinol and uricosuric drugs are available in generic form with roughly comparable prices for average effective doses. Although occurring with similar frequency, uricosuric drug toxicity tends to be far less severe than that seen with xanthine oxidase inhibitors. Once-daily allopurinol dosing is convenient, but differences in toxic potential suggest the use of uricosuric agents in the absence of contraindications.

Probenecid is the uricosuric used most often. As with all urate-lowering drugs, therapy should be started during a stable attack-free period, as initiation during an acute flare can lead to prolongation of the flare. Probenecid is started at 0.5 g/day and advanced slowly to not more than 1 g twice daily or until the targeted urate level is reached. To avoid acute attacks, prophylactic colchicine may be needed for as long as the first six months of therapy or until tophi are gone. For therapy to succeed, the patient should meet the following requirements: 1) glomerular filtration rate should exceed 50–60 ml/min; 2) the patient must drink at least 2 liters of fluids daily and maintain good urine flow even at night, 3) there should be no history of nephrolithiasis or excessive urine acidity; and 4) the patient must be able to avoid all salicylate ingestion as even low doses can inhibit the drug's effect. With advancing age, GFR falls, and few patients over 60–65 years of age can adequately respond to most uricosuric drugs.

The most common side effects of probenecid therapy are rash or gastrointestinal upset. The adverse effect of most concern, however, is urate nephrolithiasis. Occurring at times despite patient efforts to maintain high urine volume, the formation of stones indicates that uricosuric therapy may be inappropriate, and allopurinol is preferred in such patients. If a uricosuric is absolutely necessary, urinary alkylinization to pH 6.0–6.5 may be effective in increasing urate solubility; potassium citrate in doses of 30–80 meq/day may help prevent urate nephrolithiasis. Such complex and inconvenient multi-drug regimens are rarely indicated.

Sulfinpyrazone, as a potent uricosuric, can also promote urate nephrolithiasis and should be used with similar precautions. Sulfinpyrazone has a mild antiplatelet effect and, like probenecid,

is inhibited by aspirin. Gastrointestinal side effects are seen in approximately 5% of patients (11). A congener of phenylbutazone, sulfinpyrazone may be ulcerogenic, and in rare cases, bone marrow suppression may occur. The drug is slowly advanced from 100 mg to approximately 800 mg daily in divided doses until the desired level of serum urate is reached. Available in Europe, benzbromarone is a more potent uricosuric, which may be effective even in the face of moderate renal insufficiency or salicylate use.

In clinical practice the xanthine oxidase inhibitor allopurinol is often required. Allopurinol should be reserved for patients in whom there is urate overproduction, nephrolithiasis, or other contraindications to uricosuric therapy. It is the preferred drug in renal insufficiency, but its toxicity occurs most frequently when the GFR is reduced. Typically, a dose of 300 mg/day can be started as initial therapy; however, beginning doses of 100 mg or less are appropriate in the elderly, in those with frequent attacks, or in patients with GRF less than 50 ml/min (11).

In addition to dyspepsia, headache, and diarrhea, a pruritic papular rash occurs in 3% to 10% of those receiving allopurinol. In perhaps 10% of these, the syndrome of allopurinol hypersensitivity may occur with a mortality of 20% to 30% (11). Characteristic toxic features may include fever, urticaria, leukocytosis, eosinophilia, interstitial nephritis, acute renal failure, granulomatous hepatitis, and toxic epidermal necrolysis.

In situations where the need to reduce hyperuricemia is great, allopurinol hypersensitivity may be overcome through cautious desensitization. In an oral regimen, slow daily escalation of dose from 8 mcg to 300 mg over 30 days may be successful. In one such case, however, symptoms of hypersensitivity recurred after several weeks of well-tolerated therapy at full dosage (15). A rapid intravenous regimen for desensitization has been used successfully in a patient who failed oral desensitization (16). After a 0.1 mcg intradermal skin test, intravenous allopurinol was infused in 5 increments from 0.1 mcg to 500 mcg at 15 minute intervals. Doses were then advanced at 30 minute intervals from 1.0 mg to 50 mg in 5 further increments. One hour later, 100 mg was given intravenously, and the following morning, 300 mg was given orally. Thereafter, daily 300 mg doses of allopurinol were tolerated without incident. Oxypurinol, the active metabolite of allopurinol, can also be used cautiously as this will be tolerated by some patients sensitive to allopurinol.

Several drug interactions involving urate-lowering agents should be noted. For unknown reasons, the concomitant administration of allopurinol and ampicillin is associated with increased frequency of rash. Probenecid inhibits the excretion of the penicillins as well as of indomethacin, dapsone, and acetazolamide. Probenecid may also affect the metabolism of rifampin and heparin. If probenecid is used to enhance preformed urate excretion in the tophaceous patient on allopurinol, dosage adjustment is necessary as allopurinol may increase the half-life of probenecid, while probenecid accelerates the excretion of allopurinol. Thus, higher allopurinol doses may be needed and probenecid may be effective in relatively low doses.

It is reasonable to question whether the initiation of urate-lowering therapy implies the need for lifelong treatment. Gast (17) reported his experience with 10 patients of whom five had experienced no recurrence 33 months after the discontinuation of urate-lowering therapy. The other five patients had recurrent attacks first occurring at 15.8 months on average. Such data suggests that discontinuing urate-lowering therapy may be well-tolerated at least for short periods after years of normouricemia and presumed depletion of total body urate.

GOUT IN THE TRANSPLANT HOST

New technologies often give rise to new therapeutic challenges. Such is the case in recipients of organ transplants in whom gout is relatively common. Although a variety of factors in these patients may raise serum urate, cyclosporine A appears to be the most significant. Treatment of the acute attack and reduction of hyperuricemia may both be difficult in the transplant host. Without regard to the organ transplanted, renal function is often impaired in these patients. Like NSAIDs, cyclosporine may interfere with renal prostaglandin formation, thus decreasing renal blood flow; their concomitant use may have an additive effect on renal function (18). Colchicine use may be hazardous in the patient on azathioprine whose granulocyte count is decreased. Corticosteroids and ACTH may be ineffective, as most transplant patients are on chronic corticosteroid therapy at the time of their attack. In the patient with marginal renal function or white blood cell count, the safest alternative to colchicine and NSAIDs may be articular injection. Synovial fluid culture should be performed routinely in such patients.

The management of hyperuricemia may be similarly complex. The patient with GFR below 50 ml/min will not respond to uricosurics. Tophi may be present, dictating the use of allopurinol even in the patient with an adequate GFR. Yet, allopurinol causes potentiation of the action of azathioprine, which as a purine analogue is metabolized by xanthine oxidase. The use of allopurinol requires a 50% to 75% reduction of azathioprine dose (18). Even with frequent monitoring of white cell count, the therapeutic margin between leukopenia and inadequate immunosuppression is dangerously narrow.

Parks W. Pratt, MD
Gene V. Ball, MD

1. Allen MJ, Reid C, Gordon TP, et al: Does colchicine work? Results of the first controlled study in gout. Aust NZ J Med 17:301–304, 1987
2. Gutman AB: Treatment of primary gout: the present status. Arthritis Rheum 8:911–20, 1965
3. Wallace SL, Bernstein D, Diamond H: Diagnostic value of the colchicine therapeutic trial. JAMA 199:525–528, 1967
4. Moreland LM, Ball GV: Colchicine and gout. Arthritis Rheum 34:782–786, 1991
5. Roberts WN, Liang MH, Stein SH: Colchicine in acute gout: reassessment of risks and benefits. JAMA 257:1920–1922, 1987
6. Putterman C, Ben–Chetrit E, Caraco Y, et al: Colchicine intoxication: clinical pharmacology, risk factors, features, and management. Semin Arthritis Rheum 21:143–155, 1991
7. Wallace SL: Colchicine and new antiinflammatory drugs for the treatment of acute gout. Arthritis Rheum 18(suppl):847–851, 1975
8. Wallace SL, Singer JZ: Review: systemic toxicity associated with the intravenous administration of colchicine-guidelines for use. J Rheumatol 15:495–499, 1988
9. Groff GD, Franch WA, Raddaty DA: Systemic steroid therapy for acute gout: a clinical trial and review of the literature. Semin Arthritis Rheum 19:329–336, 1990
10. Axelrod D, Preston S: Comparison of parenteral adreno-corticotropic hormone with oral indomethacin in the treatment of acute gout. Arthritis Rheum 31:803–805, 1988
11. Wallace SL, Singer JZ: Therapy in gout. Rheum Dis Clin North Am 14:441–457, 1988
12. Paulus HE, Schlosstein LH, Godfrey RC, et al: Prophylactic colchicine therapy of intercritical gout. A placebo-controlled study of probenecid-treated patients. Arthritis Rheum 17:609–614, 1987
13. Yu TF: Pathogenesis and medical management of chronic gouty arthritis. Clin Orthop Rel Res 71:40–45, 1970
14. McCarthy GM, Barthelemy CR, Veium JA, et al: Influence of antihyperuricemic therapy and the clinical and radiographic progression of gout. Arthritis Rheum 34:1489–1494, 1991
15. Unsworth J, Blake DR: Desensitization to allopurinol: a cautionary tale. Ann Rheum Dis 46:646, 1987
16. Halz–LeBlanc BAE, Reynolds WJ, MacFadden DK: Allopurinol hypersensitivity in a patient with chronic tophaceous gout: success of intravenous desensitization after failure of oral desensitization. Arthritis Rheum 34:1329–1331, 1991
17. Gast LF: Withdrawal of longterm antihyperuricemic therapy in tophaceous gout. Clin Rheumatol 6:70–73, 1987
18. West C, Carpenter BJ, Hakala TR: The incidence of gout in renal transplant incipients. Am J Kidney Dis 10:369–372, 1987

32. CALCIUM PYROPHOSPHATE DIHYDRATE CRYSTAL DEPOSITION DISEASE

Specific identification of calcium pyrophosphate dihydrate (CPPD) crystals ($Ca_2P_2O_7 \cdot 2H_2O$) in synovial fluid (1) permits differentiation of this crystal deposition disease from other inflammatory and degenerative arthritides. The preferred name for the disease thus incorporates its only specific feature. The term *chondrocalcinosis* (2) is often used to describe the radiologic appearance of calcified joint cartilage. However, CPPD crystals are deposited in tendons, ligaments, articular capsules, and synovium as well as in cartilage. Moreover, cartilaginous calcification can consist of orthophosphates such as dicalcium phosphate dihydrate ($CaHPO_4 \cdot 2H_2O$), octacalcium phosphate, hydroxyapatite ($Ca_5OH(PO_4)_3 \cdot H_2O$) (3), and in uremic patients, calcium oxalate (4).

Pathologic surveys indicate that about 4% of the adult population have articular CPPD crystal deposits at the time of death at or near age 72 years. Radiologic surveys also show a steadily increasing prevalence with age, so that nearly 50% of individuals have evidence of chondrocalcinosis by the ninth decade of life (1). The incidence of clinically symptomatic disease is about one-half that of classic gout. The male-to-female ratio is about 1.4:1, but other series show a predominance in women.

ETIOLOGIC CLASSIFICATION

Arthritis associated with CPPD crystal deposition can be classified as hereditary, sporadic (idiopathic), or associated with various metabolic diseases or trauma (Table 32–1). Most patients with familial disease show an autosomal dominant pattern of inheritance and have not had any of the putative associated metabolic diseases. A thorough study of patients with sporadic disease would probably result in their reclassification as either hereditary or metabolic disease-associated. Because of the high prevalence of CPPD crystal deposition, the condition has often been reported as associated with other conditions. Based on the frequency of such reports and the relative rarity of some of these

Table 32–1. *Classification of CPPD crystal deposition disease (1)*

I. Hereditary
   Slovakian (Hungarian gene), Chilean (Spanish gene), Japanese, Dutch, Swedish, French, Swiss-German, Mexican-American, French-Canadian
II. Sporadic (idiopathic) increases with age
III. Associated with metabolic disease:
   Hyperparathyroidism, familial hypocalciuric hypercalcamia, hemochromatosis, hemosiderosis, hypothyroidism, gout, hypomagnesemia, hypophosphatasia, amyloidosis
IV. Associated with joint trauma or surgery

possible "associated" conditions, the most likely true associations are listed in Table 32–1, although none have been proven to be associated by rigorously controlled studies. The association with aging is best documented. In series of patients with hyperparathyroidism or hemochromatosis, those showing CPPD deposition are significantly older (1).

The routine study of a patient newly diagnosed with CPPD crystal deposition should include evaluation of serum calcium, magnesium, phosphorus, alkaline phosphatase, ferritin, iron and iron-binding capacity, glucose, thyroid-stimulating hormone, and uric acid. Further studies should be obtained if abnormal values are found.

CLINICAL FEATURES

"Pseudogout" is only one of a number of clinical patterns shown by symptomatic patients. The occurrence of both joint inflammation and joint degeneration may occur independently or overlap, thus simulating many other rheumatic diseases and leading to diagnostic confusion. A patient may show one disease pattern early, usually inflammatory, and later manifest another pattern, usually degenerative.

Acute pseudogout is marked by inflammation in one or more joints lasting for several days or more. These self-limited attacks can be as abrupt in onset and as severe as true acute gout, although the average attack is less painful. Subpainful "petite" attacks occur, as with gout. The knee is the site of almost one-half of all attacks, although involvement of nearly all other synovial joints, including the first metatarsophalangeal joint, has been noted. Provocation of acute attacks by surgery is common in both gout and pseudogout (8.3% of 168 gout patients vs. 9.4% of 106 patients with pseudogout) (5). Severe illness, such as stroke or myocardial infarction, provoked acute attacks in 20.3% of 167 subjects with gout and in 24% of 104 patients with pseudogout. About 25% of patients show this pattern, with men predominating. Patients are usually asymptomatic between acute attacks.

About 5% of patients show multiple joint involvement, usually symmetric, with low-grade inflammation lasting for weeks or months. Morning stiffness, fatigue, synovial thickening, flexion contractures, and elevated erythrocyte sedimentation rate often lead to a misdiagnosis of rheumatoid arthritis (RA). As in true gout, about 10% of patients with CPPD deposits have positive tests for IgM rheumatoid factor (5). The negative association of RA with urate gout does not appear to hold for CPPD deposition; about 1% of our patients with such crystals have fully expressed typical RA.

Nearly one-half of all patients have progressive degeneration of numerous joints. The knee joints are most commonly affected, followed by the wrists, metacarpophalangeal joints, hips, shoulders, elbows, and ankles. Although there is some overlap with the patterns of joint involvement in primary osteoarthritis (for example, hip and knee), the pattern of joint degeneration associated with CPPD crystal deposits is distinctive. Distal interphalangeal and proximal interphalangeal joint involvement, manifested by Heberden's and Bouchard's nodes, and first carpometacarpal joint involvement are no more common than would be expected by chance alone in an elderly population. Symmetric involvement is the rule, although degeneration may be more advanced on one side, especially where severe trauma or fracture has occurred. Flexion contractures of the affected joints and deformities of the knees are common. Valgus knee deformities are especially suggestive of underlying CPPD crystal deposits (1). Patients with chronic symptoms of this "pseudo-osteoarthritis" pattern may have superimposed episodes of joint inflammation.

A severe destructive arthropathy has been associated with CPPD crystal deposition. Neurologic examination in most cases is entirely within normal limits. Three consecutive cases of mild tabes dorsalis were reported, however, with Charcot arthropathy involving the knees and polyarticular CPPD crystal deposition, leading to the speculation that tabetic neurotrophic joints develop in that 5% of the population with underlying CPPD crystal deposition (1).

Some patients, especially those with familial disease, have shown straightening and stiffening of the spine, simulating ankylosing spondylitis (1). True bony ankylosis of joints has been reported. Other patients have been thought to have rheumatic fever because of short-lived acute attacks of migratory arthritis in numerous joints. Still others with mild attacks have been thought to have psychogenic joint complaints. Injury can trigger acute pseudogout, which may be ascribed to the traumatic event. When a bloody joint effusion is obtained, CPPD crystal deposition should be included in the differential diagnosis.

Most joints with radiologically evident CPPD calcification are not symptomatic, even in patients with symptoms in other joints. Many patients with CPPD crystal deposits have no joint symptoms.

RADIOLOGIC FEATURES

The typical appearance of punctate and linear densities in articular hyaline or fibrocartilaginous tissues is diagnostically helpful. The most characteristic sites of crystal deposition are illustrated in Fig. 32–1. When the deposits are typical and unequivocal, the radiographic appearance is nearly specific, but

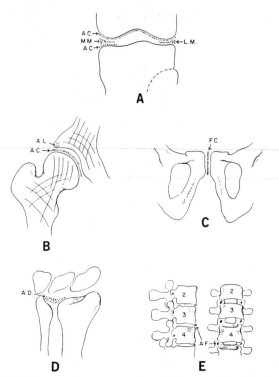

Fig. 32–1. Diagrammatic representation of characteristic sites of CPPD crystal deposition. A, A.C. = articular cartilage; L.M. and M.M. = lateral and medial meniscus in knee joint shown in anteroposterior projection. B, A.L. = acetabular labrum in anteroposterior projection of hip joint. C, F.C. = fibrocartilaginous symphysis pubis in anteroposterior projection of pelvis. D, A.D. = articular disc of the wrist in anteroposterior projection. E, A.F. = anulus fibrosus of intervertebral discs in anteroposterior and lateral views. (Reproduced courtesy of the Bulletin on the Rheumatic Diseases)

interpretation of atypical or faint deposits is often difficult. Fine detail roentgenograms of thin parts, such as hands, and focal-spot magnification views of thick parts, such as knees, may be helpful.

Calcific deposits may also occur in articular capsule, ligaments, and tendons. Synovial deposits have been so massive as to be mistaken for chondromatosis (1). Although the earliest calcific deposits occur in radiographically normal cartilage, degenerative changes often supervene with the passage of time (6). A patient can be screened for CPPD crystal deposits with four well-exposed roentgenograms: an anteroposterior (AP) view of both knees, an AP view of the pelvis for hips and symphysis pubis, and a posteroanterior view of the hands. If these views show no evidence of crystal deposits, it is most unlikely that further study will prove fruitful.

Crystals may or may not be seen in fluid from joints radiographically negative for calcification, especially those showing extensive joint space narrowing. Changes in MCP joints, such as squaring of the bone ends, subchondral cysts, and hooklike osteophytes, described as characteristic features of the arthritis associated with hemochromatosis, are also found in patients with CPPD crystal deposition alone. A controlled study showed that these changes occur more frequently in patients with CPPD crystal deposits and hemochromatosis than in those with only crystal deposits (1). Another controlled study of the radiographic appearance of joint degeneration associated with CPPD crystal deposits disclosed certain differences from typical osteoarthritis, in addition to the difference in the pattern of affected joints already cited (1). One of these differences is isolated patellofemoral joint space narrowing or isolated wrist joint degeneration. Such differences may provide helpful clinical clues and are incorporated into the diagnostic criteria given in Table 32–2.

PATHOGENESIS OF INFLAMMATION

Acute pseudogout is thought to represent a dose-related inflammatory host response to CPPD crystals shed from cartilaginous tissues contiguous with the synovial cavity (1). Phagocyto-

Table 32–2. *Revised diagnostic criteria for CPPD crystal deposition disease*

Criteria

I. Demonstration of CPPD crystals (obtained by biopsy, necropsy, or aspirated synovial fluid) by definitive means (e.g., characteristic "fingerprint" by x-ray diffraction powder pattern or by chemical analysis)

II. (a) Identification of monoclinic and/or triclinic crystals showing none or a weakly positive birefringence by compensated polarized light microscopy

   (b) Presence of typical calcifications in roentgenograms

III. (a) Acute arthritis, especially of knees or other large joints, with or without concomitant hyperuricemia

   (b) Chronic arthritis, especially of knees, hips, wrists, carpus, elbow, shoulder, and metacarpophalangeal joints, especially if accompanied by acute exacerbations. The chronic arthritis shows the following features helpful in differentiating it from osteoarthritis:

     1. Uncommon site—e.g., wrist, MCP, elbow, shoulder

     2. Appearance of lesion radiologically—e.g., radiocarpal or patellofemoral joint space narrowing, especially if isolated (patella "wrapped around" the femur)

     3. Subchondral cyst formation

     4. Severity of degeneration—progressive, with subchondral bony collapse (microfractures), and fragmentation, with formation of intraarticular radiodense bodies

     5. Osteophyte formation—variable and inconstant

     6. Tendon calcifications, especially Achilles, triceps, obturators

Categories

A. Definite—Criteria I or II(a) plus (b) must be fulfilled

B. Probable—Criteria II(a) or II(b) must be fulfilled

C. Possible—Criteria III(a) or III(b) should alert the clinician to the possibility of underlying CPPD deposition

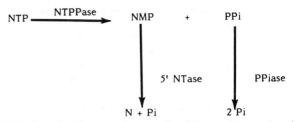

Fig. 32–3. *Postulated enzymatic cascade of inorganic pyrophosphate (PPi) production from nucleoside triphosphate (NTP). Elevated NTP pyrophosphohydrolase and 5' nucleotidase activities and decreased inorganic pyrophosphate activity in chondrocalcinosic cartilages all favor PPi accumulation. 5'NTase = 5'nucleotidase; PPiase = inorganic pyrophosphatase; Pi = inorganic phosphate; N = nucleotide; NMP = nucleoside monophosphate. (Reproduced courtesy of Lea & Febiger)*

sis of crystals by neutrophilic phagocytes (Fig. 32–2) results in release of lysosomal enzymes and cell-derived chemotactic factors. Membranolysis by CPPD crystals is much less striking than that induced by sodium urate crystals, and binding of IgG by these latter crystals is several orders of magnitude greater (1). Details of the interaction between crystals and neutrophilic leukocytes have been reviewed recently (7).

Colchicine in therapeutic concentrations is remarkably effective in blocking the release of chemotactic factor from neutrophils in vitro induced by CPPD or other crystals. Colchicine given intravenously is also effective in the treatment of pseudogout (1). The effectiveness of oral colchicine is less predictable in pseudogout than in gout, but both the number and duration of acute attacks were significantly reduced by colchicine (1.2 mg/day) in a randomized double-blinded multicenter study (1).

PATHOGENESIS OF CRYSTAL DEPOSITION

Plasma levels and urinary excretion of inorganic pyrophosphate (PPi) are not altered in patients with CPPD crystal deposition. Synovial fluid PPi is elevated in most joints afflicted with

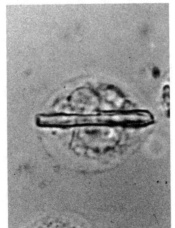

Fig. 32–2. *Neutrophilic leukocyte in fresh preparation of synovial fluid from an 84-year-old woman with acute inflammation of the knee (pseudogout). Note rod-shaped crystal of calcium pyrophosphate dihydrate.*

CPPD crystal deposition, but similar elevations are found in joint fluids from patients with osteoarthritis or other forms of joint disease. Synovial fluid PPi levels correlate with the degree of osteoarthritis as graded radiologically, irrespective of the clinical diagnosis, and a kinetic study of joint fluid PPi turnover showed a similar relationship. Joint fluid PPi levels were consistently lower during an acute attack than they were later when the inflammation had subsided, probably due to more rapid equilibration with plasma due to increased synovial blood flow during the acute inflammation (1).

Articular chondrocytes are the most likely source of the excess synovial fluid PPi, because cartilage slices in organ culture have been shown to liberate PPi into the surrounding medium. Such release occurred from both adult and immature hyaline and fibrocartilage from several species of animals, including humans.

More PPi was produced when adenosine triphosphate (ATP) was added to extracts of cartilages containing CPPD crystals than was produced by osteoarthritic or normal cartilages (1). It was postulated that ATP was enzymatically hydrolyzed to adenosine monophosphate and PPi by a nucleoside triphosphate pyrophosphohydrolase (Fig. 32–3), an ectoenzyme with broad substrate reactivity (8). Nucleoside triphosphate pyrophosphohydrolase activity was higher in the synovial fluid of patients with CPPD deposition and osteoarthritis than in fluid of patients with RA or gout (9) and correlated directly with the concentration of PPi. In addition to elevated nucleoside triphosphate pyrophosphohydrolase activity in detergent extracts of cartilages with CPPD deposition, higher levels of 5' nucleotidase activity and lower levels of alkaline phosphatase and inorganic pyrophosphatase activity were found as compared with osteoarthritic or normal cartilage (10). These aberrations would favor the accumulation of PPi in the ectoenzyme system shown in Fig. 32–3. ATP, a substrate for ectonucleoside triphosphate pyrophosphohydrolase, has been identified in both plasma and synovial fluid and is higher in fluids from joints containing CPPD crystals (11).

Intracellular PPi levels were twice those of control subjects in the cells of affected members of a French kindred with familial CPPD deposition (12). A generalized metabolic abnormality phenotypically expressed only in chondrocytes was postulated. Inorganic pyrophosphate levels in skin fibroblasts from patients with both sporadic and familial CPPD crystal deposition were significantly elevated compared with those from normal persons or subjects with osteoarthritis. Activity of ectonucleoside triphosphate pyrophosphohydrolase was elevated in fibroblasts from sporadic, but not familial, CPPD crystal deposition (13). Enzyme activity correlated with intracellular inorganic pyrophosphate concentration (13). It is likely that there are at least two ectonucleoside triphosphate pyrophospho-hydrolases, one on the chondrocyte membrane and the other localized to matrix vesicles derived from chondrocytes (14). Safranin O staining of the chondrocytes surrounding developing but not mature CPPD crystal deposits occurs in both the hereditary and sporadic forms of the disease. Such cells were present in deposits in hyaline or fibrocartilage and in lesions developing in focal areas of chondroid metaplasia in tendons, ligaments, and synovium (15). The matrix of cartilages and synovial membranes that harbor CPPD crystal deposits is also abnormal (16). Alterations in the collagen, proteoglycans, and other matrix components may also contribute to localization of crystals.

It is likely that CPPD crystal deposition may represent a final common pathway of various antecedent metabolic aberrations just as the sodium urate crystal represents a final common pathway of the various mechanisms leading to hyperuricemia.

CRYSTAL CLEARANCE FROM JOINTS

Radiolabeled synthetic CPPD crystals injected into human and rabbit joints were removed in inverse proportion to crystal size over a period of several weeks (rabbits) to several months (humans) (17). Endocytosis and intracellular dissolution by fixed synovial macrophagelike cells were the mechanisms of crystal clearance. Manipulation of extracellular variables affecting CPPD crystal solubility had no effect on clearance rate constants (18), while alteration of the intracellular environment (iron loading of synovial cells) had a pronounced effect (19). Joint fluid crystal concentrations probably represent the net effect of shedding from cartilage and synovial endocytosis and dissolution.

TREATMENT

Unlike gout, there is no way to remove CPPD crystals from joints. Treatment of the putative associated diseases such as hyperparathyroidism, hemochromatosis, or myxedema does not result in resorption of CPPD crystal deposits. In fact, thyroid hormone replacement for the latter condition is reported to result in emergence of symptomatic disease (20). Acute attacks in large joints can be treated by thorough aspiration alone or combined with injection of microcrystalline corticosteroid esters. Nonsteroidal antiinflammatory drugs are often very useful. The predictable effects of colchicine given intravenously and its successful use in prevention of attacks were discussed in the section on pathogenesis of inflammation. Whether crystal removal would prevent or slow the devolutionary degenerative cartilaginous and bony changes in an important but unanswered question.

Daniel J. McCarty, MD

1. Ryan LM, McCarty DJ: Calcium pyrophosphate crystal deposition disease: pseudogout, articular chondrocalcinosis. Arthritis and Allied Conditions: A Textbook of Rheumatology, 12th ed. Edited by DJ McCarty and WJ Koopman. Philadelphia, Penn., Lea & Febiger, 1993, pp 1835–1855

2. Zitnan D, Sitaj S: Articular chondrocalcinosis. Ann Rheum Dis 22:142, 1963
3. McCarty DJ, Lehr JR, Halverson PB: Crystal populations in human synovial fluid: identification of apatite, octacalcium phosphate, and tricalcium phosphate. Arthritis Rheum 26:1220–1224, 1983
4. Hoffman GS, Schumacher HR, Paul H: Calcium oxalate microcrystalline-associated arthritis in end stage renal disease. Ann Intern Med 97:36–42, 1982
5. Wallace SL, Robinson H, Masi AT: Preliminary criteria for the classification of the acute arthritis of primary gout. Arthritis Rheum 20:895, 1977
6. Zitnan D, Sitaj S: Natural course of articular chondrocalcinosis. Arthritis Rheum (suppl) 19:363–390, 1976
7. Terkeltaub RA: Pathogenesis and treatment of crystal-induced inflammation. Arthritis and Allied Conditions: A Textbook of Rheumatology, 12th ed. Edited by DJ McCarty and WJ Koopman, Philadelphia, Penn., Lea & Febiger, 1993, pp 1819–1833
8. Ryan LM, Wortmann RL, Karas B, et al: Cartilage nucleoside triphosphate (NTP) pyrophosphohydrolase. I. identification as an ecto-enzyme. Arthritis Rheum 27:404–409, 1984
9. Rachow JW, Ryan LM: Adenosine triphosphate pyrophosphohydrolase and pyrophosphatase activities in human synovial fluids. Clin Res 31:806A, 1983
10. Tenenbaum J, Muniz O, Pita JC, et al: Comparison of phosphohydrolase activities from articular cartilage in calcium pyrophosphate deposition disease and primary osteoarthritis. Arthritis Rheum 24:492–500, 1981
11. Ryan LM, Rachow JW, McCarty DJ: Synovial fluid ATP: a potential substrate for the production of inorganic pyrophosphate. J Rheumatol 18:716–720, 1991
12. Lust G, Faure G, Netter P, et al: Evidence of a generalized metabolic defect in patients with hereditary chondrocalcinosis: increased inorganic pyrophosphate in cultured fibroblasts and lymphoblast. Arthritis Rheum 24:1517–1521, 1981
13. Ryan LM, Wortmann RL, Karas B, et al: Pyrophosphohydrolase activity and inorganic pyrophosphate content of cultured human skin bibroblasts: elevated levels in some patients with calcium pyrophosphate dihydrate deposition disease. J Clin Invest 77:1689, 1986
14. Masuda I, Hamada J, Derfus B, et al: A unique nucleoside triphosphate pyrophosphohydrolase. Arthritis Rheum (in press)
15. Ishikawa K: Chondrocytes that accumulate proteoglycans and inorganic pyrophosphate in the pathogenesis of chondrocalcinosis. Arthritis Rheum 28:118–119, 1985
16. Beutler A, Rothfuss S, Clayburne G, et al: Calcium pyrophosphate dihydrate crystal deposition in synovium. Relationship to collagen fibers and chondrometaplasia. Arthritis Rheum 36:704–715, 1993
17. McCarty DJ, Palmer DW, Halverson PB: Clearance of calcium pyrophosphate dihydrate crystals in vivo I. Studies using 169Yb labeled triclinic crystals. Arthritis Rheum 22:718–727, 1979
18. McCarty DJ, Palmer DW, James C: Clearance of calcium pyrophosphate dihydrate crystals in vivo II. Studies using triclinic crystals doubly labeled with 45Ca and 85Sr. Arthritis Rheum 22:1122–1131, 1979
19. McCarty DJ, Palmer DW, Garancis JC: Clearance of calcium pyrophosphate dihydrate in vivo III. Effects of synovial hemosiderosis. Arthritis Rheum 24:706–710, 1981
20. Dorwart BB, Schumacher HR: Joint effusions chondrocalcinosis and other rheumatic manifestations in hypothyroidism: clinicopathologic study. Am J Med 59:780–789, 1975

33. APATITES AND MISCELLANEOUS CRYSTALS

PRINCIPLES AND PATHOGENESIS

A wide variety of particles other than monosodium urate monohydrate (MSUM, the gout crystal) and calcium pyrophosphate dihydrate (CPPD) can sometimes be found in joint tissues and fluids (Table 33–1). Of those listed, the basic calcium phosphates, particularly carbonated apatites (hydroxyapatite, $Ca_{10}(PO_4)_6.OH$, with CO_3 partially substituting for OH groups) are encountered most frequently. Deposits of any of these particles may be associated with arthritis or with periarticular syndromes.

The relationship between deposition of these crystals and the rheumatic diseases is complex. Crystal formation may be the result of joint damage, rather than its cause. An example of this phenomenon in a different tissue is the calcification of an old tuberculous focus in the lung. Similar "secondary" calcification can occur in articular tissues. However, the crystals can also cause disease; either through biologic or biomechanical pathways. For example, if a shower of particles is released from a deposit, they can induce an acute inflammatory reaction in the tissue, as in acute calcific periarthritis. In view of the potential complexity of these interactions, it is important not to equate the identification of a particle with a disease.

Mixtures of apatites and other types of crystal can also occur,

there being a particularly strong relationship between CPPD deposits in joints, and the presence of apatite. This adds to the confusion of nomenclature in the literature (1).

Crystal Identification

Compensated polarized light microscopy is the standard technique used to find MSUM and CPPD crystals in synovial fluids or tissue samples. Crystals of cholesterol and calcium oxalate also grow to form particles of sufficient size and characteristic morphology to be identifiable with this technique. Various lipids, proteins and other particles can also be seen as birefringent particles in a polarized light microscope, without it being possible to make a clear identification. In contrast, basic calcium phosphate crystals cannot usually be seen by any form of light microscopy. Individual apatite crystals are usually rod or needle shaped and they vary in length from 50–500 nm. However, they tend to clump into rounded aggregates that can sometimes be seen as small shiny, coin-like objects of around 1–5 μm diameter in the light microscope.

Special stains have been used in an attempt to screen synovial fluids and other samples for the presence of clumps calcium containing crystals. The one used most is Alizarin red S, a calcium stain (2). Clumps of apatite tend to stain up with a "halo"

Table 33–1. *Some crystals and other particles identified in joint tissues and synovial fluids**

Monosodium urate monohydrate crystals
Spherulites of urates

Calcium pyrophosphate dihydrate crystals

Basic calcium phosphates: Apatites
                               Tricalcium phosphate
                               Octacalcium phosphate

Dicalcium phosphate dihydrate (Brushite)

Calcium magnesium phosphate (Whitlokite)

Calcium carbonates (Calcite and Aragonite)

Calcium oxalates (monohydrate and dihydrate)

Lipids: Cholesterol crystals
       "Liquid lipid crystals"
       Lipid spherulites

Protein crystals such as cryoglobulins, hematoidin crystals, and
    Charcot–Leyden crystals

Steroid crystals

Plant thorns, sea urchin spines, and other extrinsic particles

Metal, plastic, and cement fragments from implants

Cartilage fragments

* Combinations or mixtures of two or more types of particle in the same joint are seen more commonly than would be expected by chance

of the Alizarin red around the crystal aggregate, and a pale center, giving a fairly characteristic "onion skin" appearance (Fig. 33–1). However, both false-positive and false-negative results can occur with this technique, and it is not crystal specific. Definite identification requires the use of more sophisticated techniques.

The electron microscope will provide more magnification, and hence visualization of smaller particles, including individual hydroxyapatite crystals. In addition, a variety of analytical tools can be used in conjunction with electron microscopy, including elemental analysis and electron diffraction (3).

If larger quantities of the material are available, x-ray powder diffraction and infra-red spectroscopy can also be used to analyze mineral deposits. Both techniques can deal with relatively small quantities, and identify the different components of a mixed crystal deposit. Infra-red spectroscopy is a particularly helpful technique if equipped with modern Fourier transform facilities, as it provides a very quick, accurate analysis of the chemical bonds in a sample (4).

Recently, a variety of other new techniques have been de-scribed. These include methods for the extraction and quantification of particles from synovial fluids and tissues by using protease digestion and hypochlorite cleaning of samples (5), and single crystal identification by Raman spectroscopy (6). However, use of these specialized techniques, often only available in reference laboratories, is rarely warranted. At present, the identification of large amounts of apatite particles in joints can help support diagnoses of calcific periarthritis or apatite-associated dialysis arthropathy, but in most other situations will rarely affect clinical decisions—either diagnostic or therapeutic—so the major application of the technology is for research purposes only.

Etiology and Pathogenesis

Crystal formation requires a sufficient concentration of the solutes (supersaturation), nucleation of the crystals, and subsequent growth. Each step is dependent on different factors. Body fluids are normally close to or at the point of supersaturation with respect to a variety of salts, such as calcium carbonates; changes in local or systemic metabolism can easily create conditions for the formation of a variety of other salts.

Connective tissues contain natural inhibitors of crystal formation, which may be lost in disease or with aging. Thus the formation of crystals in and around joints might be due to local or general metabolic disturbances raising solute concentration, to local loss of inhibitors of nucleation and growth, or to the presence or unmasking of nucleating surfaces (such as collagen fibrils) or growth promoters. In most cases, apatite formation appears to depend more on local tissue damage than on any local or general metabolic disturbance, whereas the contrary is true in the case of oxalate crystal formation. Crystals of lipids and proteins probably form when some local conditions favor massive release of their constituents into a tissue space.

Crystal-induced tissue damage can result from a variety of pathways; most depend on the shedding of some of the particles into a free tissue space from preformed deposits in cartilage or other structures. Nearly all biologic crystals are capable of inducing an acute inflammatory response. This depends on the surface charge and "atomic roughness" of the crystal surface, which in turn controls their ability to interact with proteins and cell membranes (7). Apatite crystals can also be phagocytosed by synovial lining cells and macrophages, resulting in the production of proteases, cytokines, and growth factors, as well as the classic mediators of inflammation (8). As a result, it is possible that these crystals induce chronic inflammation, tissue damage, and cellular hypertrophy in and around the joints, as well as acute inflammation. Finally, it is possible that the particles also induce mechanical disruption of the tissues. The presence of a deposit of hard, inflexible crystal aggregates in cartilage or other soft tissues is likely to alter the tissue's ability to respond to mechanical loading. Furthermore, if the crystals are shed into the surrounding spaces, mechanical abrasion of the surface of cartilage or other structures may occur (9).

DISEASE ASSOCIATIONS

Apatite

Apatite deposition is encountered in three main circumstances in rheumatology: in the subcutaneous tissues in association with connective tissue diseases, in periarticular tissues, especially around the shoulder, and within osteoarthritic and other pathological joints.

Subcutaneous Tissues. Many of the connective tissue diseases can lead to the formation of apatite in the subcutaneous tissues in the hand and elsewhere. Raynaud's phenomenon is usually prominent, and poor tissue vascularity, low temperatures, as well as damage to collagen and other elements of the subcutaneous connective tissues, may be important in pathogenesis. Limited cutaneous scleroderma or the "CREST" syndrome of scleroderma (calcinosis, Raynaud's, esophageal disease, sclerodactyly and telangectasia) is the most common cause, and in some cases the calcification is extensive and the main feature of the disorder

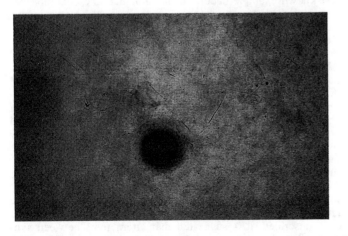

Fig. 33–1. *Alizarin red-S stain of a clump of apatite crystals in synovial fluid, showing the characteristic "halo" appearance.*

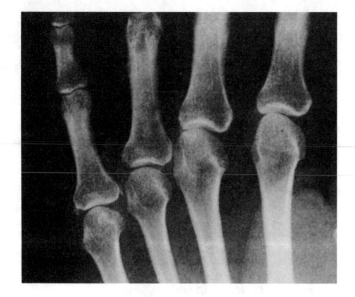

Fig. 33–2. *Small periarticular and capsular calcifications at metacarpophalangeal joints in a patient with apatite crystal deposition disease and recurrent acute arthritis and periarthritis (courtesy of Dr HR Schumacher, Jr).*

(Fig. 33–2). The deposits slowly grow and dissolve in different parts of the hand; they may set up minor local inflammatory responses. They can rupture through the skin, discharging chalky lumps, and can become secondarily infected. In addition, their bulk alone can interfere with hand function.

Periarticular Tissues. The formation of apatite in periarticular tissues around the shoulder is relatively common, being seen in up to 5% of shoulder radiographs in adults. Other sites that can be involved include the hip, knee, and other joints. In the majority of cases the deposits form in tendons; the supraspinatus is most often involved (10).

The causes of this phenomenon are not clear. Occasional cases are familial, and in renal disease the same sites tend to be involved as in idiopathic calcific periarthritis, arguing that some systemic predisposition may be involved. However, local factors are probably more important. Poorly vascularized areas of the tendon and damaged tendons are susceptible, suggesting that connective tissue changes favoring surface nucleation of apatite are important; cell-driven calcification has also been postulated. Chondrometaplasia in tendons may also favor calcification (11).

The majority of the deposits probably remain asymptomatic. In a minority, crystal shedding leads to the release of a shower of crystals into surrounding tissue spaces, such as the subacromial bursa. This can result in a dramatic, intense inflammatory reaction, with severe pain and disability. In any severe, acute shoulder syndrome, this diagnosis should be suspected. Attacks may follow trauma, but are usually spontaneous; the onset is abrupt, and there is usually marked tenderness and complete inability to move the shoulder. Serial radiographs will show that the normal appearance of an inert deposit, with well defined edges, changes to a fluffy, indistinct appearance at the start of an attack (12). As the attack progresses, the calcific density will become hazy and may disappear completely, usually reforming some months or years later. This presumably reflects the shedding of crystals and reformation of the apatite deposit. The clinical course is usually one of slow spontaneous resolution of the symptoms with complete recovery, although severe inflammation can persist for many days or weeks. Chronic tendinitis or a capsulitis of the shoulder can follow an attack.

Treatment with nonsteroidal antiinflammatory drugs and rest is usually sufficient. Aspiration can be attempted, and in some cases a thick, toothpaste-like material may be obtained, with relief of symptoms. Local steroids can relieve symptoms, but may not be beneficial in the long-term, as there is some evidence that they can promote further calcification, in addition to the risk of causing more damage to the tendons. In severe or prolonged cases surgical removal of the deposit is indicated.

Acute calcific tendinitis or bursitis (acute apatite periarthritis) can occur almost anywhere in the body. It is occasionally multifocal, and familial cases have been reported. Patients with a history of one attack are prone to recurrences. It can affect patients of any age, although most attacks occur in young adults. The contribution of calcification to chronic tendon and bursal problems around the shoulder and elsewhere is unclear. In one survey, it was estimated that 7% of shoulder syndromes could be explained in this way (13), but it is difficult to know to what extent the deposits are the cause or the effect of the problem.

Joints. Intraarticular apatite has been associated with three different types of clinical presentation: acute synovitis, osteoarthritis, and rapidly progressive joint destruction in the elderly.

Acute synovitis is occasionally caused by apatite. Cases have been described, some arising from the rupture of periarticular deposits into a neighboring joint, but the phenomenon is uncommon (14). It is important to remember that acute arthritis due to other diseases, including sepsis, may result in the presence of apatite in the synovial fluid, perhaps due to "strip-mining" release of crystals from preformed deposits in the cartilage.

Osteoarthritis (OA) is frequently associated with apatite crystal deposition. Crystal aggregates have been described in the cartilage, both superficially and around the chondrocytes, as well as in the synovium (15). About 50% of OA synovial fluids will have aggregates that stain positively with Alizarin Red S, and analytical electron microscopy will reveal individual apatite crystals in many cases (16,17). It is unclear how much of this material is released from preformed calcific deposits in the cartilage or synovium, and how much is released from the underlying bone as a secondary phenomenon. It appears that there may be several forms of crystal that can form in the cartilage in OA (18,19). The role of apatite deposition in the pathogenesis of OA is also disputed (20). In view of the ability of the crystals to cause inflammation and tissue damage, some researchers believe that it may have an important role. Most consider it to be largely a secondary, relatively unimportant factor. The known association between synovial fluid apatite and more severe radiographic changes (21), and the presence of more cartilage fragments and CPPD crystals in the synovial fluid, does not resolve this argument, and there are no other clear differences between OA patients with or without evidence of crystal deposition. In practice, there is little value in searching for apatite in OA, because its presence should have little influence on clinical decision making.

Destructive arthropathies tend to be associated with the release of cartilage and bone fragments into the synovial fluid. Sometimes CPPD deposition is associated with destructive arthritis, and mixtures of apatite and CPPD crystals are commonly seen in such cases. In addition, a variety of special forms of destructive arthritis of the elderly have been described, in which apatite crystals are found in abundance, usually without CPPD, and in which the apatite may be of pathogenic significance. The best known example occurs in the shoulder; the condition has been described by many authors in many countries, and is known by many names, including "senile haemorrhagic arthritis" (France where it was first described), "apatite associated destructive arthritis" (UK) and "Milwaukee shoulder" (USA) (22,23). The condition almost exclusively affects elderly women, and is characterized by shoulder pain and disability, large cool effusions, destruction of the rotator cuff and radiographic evidence of damage to both sides of the glenohumeral joint without a bony response of the sort seen in OA. It should not be confused with "cuff-tear arthropathy" a common condition of the elderly in which there is upward migration of the humeral head but no destruction of the glenohumeral joint, or with OA (with or without CPPD) of the shoulder. The synovial fluid of "Milwaukee shoulder" patients is frequently blood-stained, contains numerous apatite aggregates but few cells, and according to some authors, high levels of proteases (24). In view of the experimental work described, it is suggested that interactions between synovial cells and apatite crystals lead to the release of cytokines and proteases, which then induce the massive destruction of soft tissues and bone seen in the condition. The alternative view is that the apatite is being shed as a result of the destruction.

This form of shoulder disease is sometimes accompanied by similar forms of rapidly destructive, atrophic joint disease at other sites, including the knee, and less commonly the hip, joints of the hindfoot, or other sites. It has also been suggested that other rapidly destructive forms of OA, such as analgesic hip, are analogous conditions (25). No satisfactory form of treatment has been described, although the natural history of the condition appears to be a tendency to partial resolution. Symptoms may subside somewhat, the effusion resolves, and the radiographic changes stabilize. The patient may be left with a severely destroyed "flail" shoulder. Joint replacement can relieve pain in refractory cases.

Miscellaneous Crystals

Calcium oxalate crystals can be deposited in bone and articular tissues in both primary and secondary hyperoxaluria (26). Primary hyperoxaluria is a rare syndrome associated with premature death and widespread organ involvement. The secondary form is associated with chronic renal failure, especially in patients on hemodialysis and those given ascorbic acid supplements (ascorbic acid metabolizes to oxalate). The crystals can be deposited in joints and tendon sheaths as well as bones and other periarticular tissues, causing arthritis and tenosynovitis. The condition has a predilection for the hands.

Lipids can also form crystals in articular tissues. Cholesterol crystals form relatively large pleotropic plates, easily identified by polarized light microscopy. They are rare, and most often seen in chronic cysts or effusions of rheumatoid patients; their presence has not been shown to be of any definite clinical significance (27). Various other forms of lipid spherules can also be found in synovial fluids, particularly following joint trauma; they may give rise to the striking "Maltese Cross" appearance. Their significance is also unclear, although when found in profusion, may contribute to synovitis (28).

Numerous other particles are occasionally found in joint tissues and fluids (Table 33–1), including extrinsic agents that have penetrated the skin, such as plant thorns, fragments of cartilage or of prosthetic joint materials, and crystals of proteins. Caution must be used in the interpretation of particles seen in joint fluids, because contaminants and inexperience can lead to false positives in identification, and it is difficult to ascribe any pathologic significance to their presence. Cartilage particles, steroid crystals, and contaminants from syringes, glassware, or dust can all produce birefringent material in specimens.

Paul Dieppe, MD

1. Simkin P: The taxonomy of gout. JAMA 260:1258, 1988
2. Paul H, Reginato AJ, Schumacher HR: Alizarin red S staining as a screening test to detect calcium compounds in synovial fluid. Arthritis Rheum 26:191–200, 1983
3. Dieppe PA, Calvert P: Crystals and joint disease. London, Chapman and Hall, 1983
4. McCarthy DS, Lehr JR, Halverson PB: Crystal populations in human synovial fluid. Identification of apatite, octacalcium phosphate and bicalcium phosphate. Arthritis Rheum 26:1220–1224, 1983
5. Swan AJ, Heywood BR, Dieppe PA: Extraction of calcium containing crystals from synovial fluids and articular cartilage. J Rheumatol 19:1763–1773, 1992
6. McGill N, Dieppe PA, Bowden M, Gardiner DJ, Hall M: Identification of pathological mineral deposits by Raman microscopy. Lancet 337:77–78, 1991
7. Mandel NS: The structural basis of crystal-induced membranolysis. Arthritis Rheum 19:439–445, 1976
8. Terkeltaub RA, Gunsberg MH: The inflammatory reaction to crystals. Rheum Dis Clin North Am 14:353–364, 1988
9. Clift SE, Dieppe PA, Harris B, Hayes A: The functional response of articular cartilage containing crystals. Biomaterials 10:329–333, 1989
10. Faure G, Dalcusi G: Calcific tendonitis: a review. Ann Rheum Dis 42(suppl): 49–53, 1983
11. Uhthoff HK, Sarkor K, Maynard JA: Calcifying tendinitis. A new concept of its pathogenesis. Clin Orthop 118:164–168, 1976
12. McCarthy DJ, Gatter RA: Recurrent acute inflammation associated with local apatite deposition. Arthritis Rheum 9:804–819, 1966
13. Bosworth BM: Calcium deposits in the shoulder and subacromial bursitis. A survey of 12,222 shoulders. JAMA 116:2477–2482, 1941
14. Fam AG, Rubenstein J: Hydroxyapatite pseudopodagra. Arthritis Rheum 32:741–747, 1989
15. Dieppe PA, Crocker P, Corke C, et al: Synovial fluid crystals Q J Med 1979
16. Gibilisco PA, Schumacher HR, Hollander JL, Soper KA: Synovial fluid crystals in osteoarthritis. Arthritis Rheum 28:511–515, 1985
17. Carroll GJ, Stuart RA, Armstrong JA: Hydroxyapatite crystals are a frequent finding in osteoarthritic synovial fluid, but are not related to increased concentrations of keratan sulphate or interleukin. J Rheumatol 18:861–866, 1991
18. Halverson PB, McCarthy DJ: Identification of hydroxyapatite crystals in synovial fluid. Arthritis Rheum 22:389–395, 1979
19. Ali SY, Rees JA, Scotford CA: Micro crystal deposition in cartilage and in osteoarthritis. Base and Mineral 17:115–118, 1993
20. Dieppe PA, Watt I: Crystal deposition in osteoarthritis: an opportunistic event? Clin Rheum Dis 11:367–392, 1985
21. Halverson PB, McCarthy DJ: Patterns of radiographic abnormalities associated with calcium phosphate and calcium pyrophosphate dehydrate crystal deposition in the knee. Ann Rheum Dis 45:603–605, 1986
22. Camnion GV, McCrae F, Alwan W, Watt I, Bradfield J, Dieppe PA: Idiopathic destructive arthritis of the shoulder. Semin Arthritis Rheum 17:232–245, 1988
23. Halverson PB, McCarthy DJ: Clinical aspects of basic calcium phosphate deposition. Rheum Dis Clin North Am 14:427–440, 1988
24. Halverson PB: Arthropathies associated with basic calcium phosphate crystals. Scanning Microscopy 6:791–797, 1992
25. Doherty M, Holt M, MacMillan P, Watt I, Dieppe PA: A reappraisal of analgesic hip. Ann Rheum Dis 45:272–276, 1986
26. Hoffman G, Schumacher FR, Paul H, et al: Calcium oxalate micro crystalline associated arthritis in end stage venal disease. Ann Intern Med 97:36–42, 1982
27. Reginato AJ: Lipid microspherule-associated acute monoarticular arthritis. Arthritis Rheum 26:1166, 1986
28. Reginato AJ, Schumacher HR, Allan DA, et al: Acute monoarthritis associated with liquid lipid crystals. Ann Rheum Dis 44:537–543, 1985

34. STORAGE AND DEPOSITION DISEASES

This chapter covers a number of osteoarthropathies associated with either systemic deposition of normal material such as metal ions or storage of abnormal material such as some specific lipids (1). Hemochromatosis and Wilson's disease are characterized by cellular deposition of the normal metal ions: iron and copper, respectively. In the case of Gaucher's, Fabry's, and Farber's disease, cellular storage of abnormal lipids is characteristic. In hemochromatosis, rheumatic complaints may provide the first clue to the presence of an underlying systemic disorder, whereas with alkaptonuria, Gaucher's disease, and multicentric reticulohistiocytosis, arthritis evolves as a predominant feature.

HEMOCHROMATOSIS

Idiopathic hemochromatosis is a common hereditary disorder characterized by excessive body iron stores and the deposition of hemosiderin causing tissue damage and organ dysfunction (2). Arthropathy was recognized as a feature of idiopathic hemochro-

matosis in 1964, and since then it has become a well known clinical manifestation of the condition (3).

The disorder rarely appears before age 40 unless there is a family history, and men are affected 10 times more frequently than women, who appear to be protected by menstruation. Increased intestinal iron absorption and visceral deposition can lead to hepatic cirrhosis, cardiomyopathy, diabetes mellitus, pituitary dysfunction (including hypogonadism), sicca syndrome, and skin pigmentation (mostly due to melanin). Although arthropathy was traditionally not regarded as a classic feature of hemochromatosis, it is a common early feature and a potentially disabling complication.

Idiopathic hemochromatosis is an autosomal recessive disorder with the gene located near the HLA–A locus on chromosome six (4). Although HLA–A3 and –B7 appear to be common antigens, homozygous and heterozygous patterns are consistent only within individual pedigrees without crossover. Within given pedigrees, homozygous and heterozygous genotypes correlate with major or minor iron loads, respectively. The expression of hemochromatosis with arthritis is most common in homozygotes who show the heaviest iron overload (5).

Although serum iron studies may rarely be normal in hemochromatosis, a marked elevation of serum ferritin is characteristic. The diagnosis is best suggested by screening for the detection of an increase in serum iron concentration with at least 60% saturation of serum iron-binding transferrin. Diagnosis may then be confirmed by liver biopsy showing hemosiderin in parenchymal cells. Biopsy can also show any degree of fibrosis, cirrhosis, or even hepatoma. Screening the relatives of hemochromatosis probands with ferritin and transferrin saturation is important, because early phlebotomy therapy can reduce body iron stores before tissue damage occurs. Although HLA typing is useful in predicting the risk of hemochromatosis in apparently healthy relatives, it gives no indication of body iron stores. Prolonged excessive iron ingestion, such as in the South African Bantu, and repeated blood transfusion in chronic hypoproliferative anemia and thalassemia may also result in iron deposition. Without tissue damage this iron overload is known as *hemosiderosis*; with tissue damage it is called *secondary hemochromatosis*. Iron deposition predominantly in macrophages as occurs in hemosiderosis is associated with less tissue damage and end-organ dysfunction than in idiopathic hemochromatosis.

The arthropathy of hemochromatosis is characterized by chronic arthritis of the peripheral joints and spine. One–half of the cases show chondrocalcinosis, and these patients may have attacks of pseudogout. Arthritis develops in more than one–half of patients showing classic features of hemochromatosis and may be the only presenting feature.

Clinically, the presenting feature in about 50% of the cases is chronic progressive arthritis affecting predominantly the second and third metacarpophalangeal (MCP) and proximal interphalangeal (PIP) joints, thus resembling rheumatoid arthritis (RA) in joint distribution (Fig. 34–1). The dominant hand may be solely or more severely affected. Along with the wrists, these joints are mildly tender, often indurated with limited motion, and without true morning stiffness. Larger joints, including the shoulders, hips, and knees, may also be affected. Hemochromatotic arthritis of larger joints may, at times, be rapidly progressive.

The detection of an osteoarthritis-like disease involving MCP and wrist joints, particularly in men during the fourth and fifth decades of life, should alert the clinician to the possibility of underlying hemochromatosis. Arthropathy may be seen in individuals as young as age 26, and may sometimes develop after phlebotomy therapy is started.

Radiologically, the irregular joint narrowing and sclerotic cyst formation at the MCP joints are indicative of an osteoarthritis-like process. Although the distal interphalangeal (DIP) joints may be affected, the carpometacarpal joint changes of generalized osteoarthritis (OA) are not a feature. Somewhat similar MCP changes can occur in calcium pyrophosphate dihydrate (CPPD) deposition without hemochromatosis and in manual laborers. Hip joint involvement has been striking in most series. The radiologic changes resemble OA except that in hemochromatosis there may be less osteophytosis.

Chondrocalcinosis is characteristic of the arthropathy and a radiographic feature at some time in about 50% of patients (5). The hyaline cartilage of the shoulder, wrists, hip, and knees, and the fibrocartilage of the triangular ligament of the wrists and symphysis pubis may be affected. The finding of chondrocalcinosis should always suggest the possibility of hemochromatosis. Some degree of diffuse osteoporosis may be present, presumably due to hypogonadism, but a direct effect of iron on bone is also possible.

Yersinia septic arthritis or septicemia is an unusual complication that may occur in patients with hemochromatosis because of a microbial requirement for an iron-rich environment (6).

The synovial fluid in hemochromatosis has good viscosity, with leukocyte counts often below 1,000/mm³. During acute episodes of pseudogout, synovial fluid leukocytosis with calcium pyrophosphate crystals can be found. Except for such episodes, the erythrocyte sedimentation rate is usually normal. With chronic liver disease rheumatoid factor tests may be positive.

Needle biopsy of the liver provides the most definitive evidence of iron overload in hemochromatosis. In idiopathic hemochromatosis, iron deposits affect parenchymal hepatic cells, whereas reticuloendothelial cells are most affected in secondary forms. Synovial biopsy in hemochromatosis shows iron deposition in the type B (synthetic) lining cells of synovium, whereas in RA, traumatic hemarthrosis, hemophilia, and villonodular synovitis, deposits may tend to form more prominently in the deeper layers or in the phagocytic type A lining cells. Hemosiderin deposits may also be found in the chondrocytes. The amount of iron excreted in the urine after administration of the iron-chelating agent deferoxamine correlates with the presence of parenchymal hepatic iron in hemochromatosis. Magnetic resonance imaging can help suggest increased hepatic iron stores and may have some value for early detection of iron overload or rapid evaluation of treatment.

The pathogenesis of the arthritis is not fully established. Osteoarthritis-like joint changes do not necessarily develop in relation to synovial iron. Iron in chondrocytes may be important. The relationship of chondrocalcinosis to iron overload is also intriguing. The low frequency of chondrocalcinosis in patients with hemophilia and RA weighs against synovial hemosiderin as a cause of chondrocalcinosis. It is speculated that ionic iron might inhibit pyrophosphatase activity and lead to a local concentration of calcium pyrophosphate in the joint. The pathologic evidence of deposition of calcium crystals in cartilage appears to be even more common than evidenced on radiographs.

When hemochromatosis is diagnosed, it is imperative to obtain biochemical screening of at least first-degree relatives of the patient for medical preventive reasons. Aggressive phlebotomy therapy can prevent or reverse much organ damage. Weekly phlebotomies are generally needed until iron is depleted and mild anemia is present. Phlebotomy may not prevent the progression of arthritis in hemochromatosis, but in some cases arthritis may improve after this therapy (3). Iron-chelating therapy with deferoxamine is effective but impractical, because it is expensive and must be administered intravenously. However, new oral iron chelators are being tested and may prove valuable.

Arthritis symptoms may be controlled by nonsteroidal antiinflammatory drugs (NSAIDs), but agents requiring hepatic metabolism should probably be avoided. Prosthetic hip, knee, and shoulder arthroplasties can be performed when required. Only procedures employing total joint replacement prostheses should be utilized since the cartilage on both sides of the joint is affected.

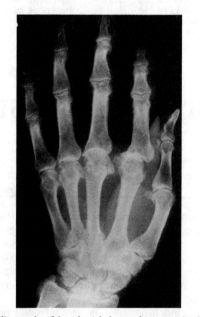

Fig. 34–1. Radiograph of hand with hemochromatosis. Note the joint space narrowing, cystic subchondral lesions, joint space irregularity, mild subluxation, bony sclerosis, and small osteophytes in the metacarpophalangeal joints. Chondrocalcinosis is in the ulnar carpal joint, and soft tissue has calcified around the interphalangeal joint of the thumb (illustration provided by Dr HR Schumacher, Jr).

ALKAPTONURIA (OCHRONOSIS)

Alkaptonuria (ochronosis), a rare, inherited disorder transmitted by a recessive gene, results from a complete deficiency of the enzyme homogentisic acid oxidase (7). This deletion causes accumulation of homogentisic acid, a normal intermediate in the metabolism of phenylalanine and tyrosine, which is excreted in the urine. Alkalinization and oxidation of this acid causes the urine to turn black. Some homogentisic acid is retained in the body and deposited as a pigmented polymer in the cartilage and, to a lesser degree, in skin and sclerae. The darkening of these tissues by this pigment is designated *ochronosis*. Because ochronotic pigment is preferentially deposited in cartilage, a degenerative arthropathy is an inevitable late complication of alkaptonuria.

The pigment, which is found in the deeper layers of the articular cartilage, is bound to collagen fibers, causing this tissue to lose its normal resiliency and become brittle and fibrillated. The erosion of this abnormal cartilage leads to a denudation of subchondral bone and the penetration of tiny shards of pigmented cartilage into the bone, synovium, and release into the joint cavity (8). These pigmented cartilage fragments likely become a nidus for the formation of osteochondral bodies.

A progressive degenerative arthropathy develops, with symptoms usually beginning in the fourth decade of life. The features of the arthropathy include arthritis of the spine (ochronotic spondylosis) and arthritis of the larger peripheral joints, with chondrocalcinosis, formation of osteochondral bodies, and synovial effusions (ochronotic peripheral arthropathy).

Initially, the spinal column is affected with pigment found in the annulus fibrosus and nucleus pulposus of the intervertebral discs (Fig. 34–2). Later the knees, shoulders, and hips deteriorate. In contrast to the picture in primary OA, the small peripheral joints are spared. In adults, the first sign of spondylosis may be an acute disc syndrome. Eventually, it clinically resembles ankylosing spondylitis, with progressive lumbar rigidity and loss of stature.

Stiffness and loss of joint mobility are the predominant complaints at peripheral joints, with pain less prominent. Knee effusions, crepitus, and flexion contractures are common, but other signs of articular inflammation are ordinarily absent. Fragments of darkly pigmented cartilage can occasionally be found floating in the joint fluid. Osteochondral bodies, which form in response to the deposition of cartilaginous fragments in the synovium, are often palpable in and around the knee joint and may reach several centimeters in diameter.

Nonarticular features of ochronosis include bluish discoloration and calcification of the ear pinnae, triangular pigmentation of the sclera, and pigmentation over the nose, axillae, and groin. Prostatic calculi are common in men, and cardiac murmurs may develop from valvular pigment deposits.

Among the earliest features visible on roentgenograms are multiple vacuum discs of the spine. Eventually, the entire spine shows ossification of the discs and/or narrowing and collapse of discs with later fusion. Chondrocalcinosis may affect the symphysis pubis, costal cartilage, and ear helix. In contrast to ankylosing spondylitis, the sacroiliac and apophyseal joints are not affected. Rarely, both conditions may coexist (9). The roentgenographic appearance of the peripheral joints, resembles that in primary OA with loss of cartilage space, marginal osteophytes, and eburnation of the subchondral bone. Unlike primary OA, however, degeneration of the shoulders and hips is more severe, and osteochondral joint bodies are seen.

The diagnosis of alkaptonuria is suspected when the patient gives a history of passing dark urine or when fresh urine turns black on standing or on alkalinization. Some individuals do not have this typical history, however, and the diagnosis is made only after the detection of a false-positive urine test for glucose or the onset of arthritis. Moreover, if knee arthroscopy is performed, dark pigmented cartilage and synovium may be seen. A specific enzymatic method permits quantitation of homogentisic acid in urine and blood.

Synovial fluid is usually clear, yellow, and viscous and does not darken with alkalinization. At times the fluid may be speckled with many particles of debris resembling ground pepper (Fig. 34–3). Leukocyte counts of a few hundred cells are predominantly mononuclear. Occasionally, the cytoplasm of mononuclear and polymorphonuclear cells contains dark inclusions of phagocytosed ochronotic pigment. Centrifugation and microscopic examination of synovial fluid sediment may show fragments of pigmented cartilage. Effusions may contain CPPD crystals and yet show no inflammation. Pigmented cartilage fragments are embedded in synovium and are often surrounded by giant cells (7,8) (Fig. 34–3).

No effective treatment is available for the underlying metabolic disorder, although in the future, replacement of the missing enzyme is a conceivable therapy. Large amounts of ascorbic acid might show deposition of ochronotic pigment, but long-term effects of this therapy are unknown. Surgical removal of osteo-

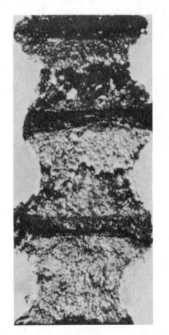

Fig. 34–2. Part of a lumbar vertebral column of 49-year-old woman with alkaptonuria who died of renal failure (ochronotic nephrosis). Blackened intervertebral discs are thin and focally calcified. This patient had incapacitating pain since age 36, with progressive limitation of back motion. Microscopic examination of the discs, which splintered easily, revealed nonrefractile granular pigment (illustration provided by Dr J Cooper and reproduced with permission of Cooper J, Moran TJ: Studies on ochronosis. I. Report of case with death from ochronotic nephrosis. Arch Pathol 61:46–53, 1957).

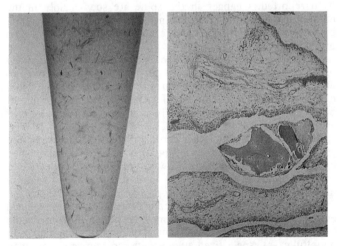

Fig. 34–3. Ochronosis: synovial fluid and synovium (gross and microscopic). On the left, the synovial fluid reveals numerous dark particles and shards having the appearance of ground pepper. On the right, a low power microscopic view of the synovium shows fragments of darkly pigmented cartilage (H&E) (from J Rheumatol 1:45–53, 1974).

chondral loose bodies from the knee joint is warranted when these interfere with motion. In a number of patients, prosthetic joint replacement has been successful (10).

WILSON'S DISEASE

Wilson's disease (hepatolenticular degeneration) is a rare metabolic disorder in which deposition of copper leads to dysfunction of the liver, brain, and kidneys. It is inherited as an autosomal recessive trait, and patients aged 6 to 40 years are affected.

The fundamental defect underlying these abnormalities is unknown. Total body copper is increased with accumulation of copper occurring in the liver, leading to cirrhosis; in the cornea, causing characteristic Kayser–Fleischer rings; in the basal ganglia, leading to lenticular degeneration and movement disorders; and in the kidneys, causing renal tubular damage. An arthropathy may develop in as many as 50% of affected adults. Arthritis is rare in children. Patients usually develop hepatic or neurologic symptoms in childhood or adolescence. Liver disease is the most common presentation between 8–16 years of age with symptoms of jaundice, nausea, vomiting, and malaise. Acute hepatic failure may rarely develop. Neurologic symptoms are rare before age 12. Dysarthria and decreased coordination of voluntary movements are the most common complaints. Other presenting symptoms include acute hemolytic anemia, arthralgias, renal stones, and renal tubular acidosis.

The arthropathy is characterized by mild premature OA of the wrists, MCP joints, knees, or spine. Occasionally, joint hypermobility also may be found. Ossified bodies of the wrists may be associated with subchondral cysts. Chondromalacia patellae, osteochondritis dissecans, or chondrocalcinosis of the knee may be associated with mild knee effusions. The arthropathy tends to be mild in patients treated early in life with copper chelation therapy, but it may be more severe in patients with untreated disease of longer duration. A few patients have had acute or subacute polyarthritis resembling RA. These cases are possibly a result of the penicillamine therapy used for the disease.

Synovial biopsies show hyperplasia of synovial lining cells with mild inflammation. Calcium pyrophosphate deposition has been described and copper is detectable by elemental analysis of joint cartilage. Limited data are available concerning morphologic changes in joints. Microvilli formation, intimal cell hyperplasia, chronic inflammatory infiltrates, and vascular changes have been reported in synovium. Joint fluids may have low leukocyte counts.

Radiologic features may include subchondral cysts, joint space narrowing, sclerosis, marked osteophyte formation, and multiple calcified loose bodies, especially at the wrist. Unlike hemochromatosis, involvement of the hip and MCP joints is uncommon. Periostitis at the femoral trochanters and other tendinous insertions, periarticular calcifications, and chondrocalcinosis have been reported. Changes in the spine are seen mainly in the midthoracic to lumbar areas and include squaring of the vertebral bodies, intervertebral joint space narrowing, osteophytes, and osteochondritis.

Skeletal manifestations of Wilson's disease include generalized osteoporosis in as many as 50% of patients, usually asymptomatic, unless spontaneous fractures occur. Osteomalacia, Milkman pseudofractures, and renal rickets have been reported. Some cases are from areas where nutritional deficiencies may also affect skeletal abnormalities.

Although Kayser–Fleischer corneal rings, if found, are pathognomonic of Wilson's disease, the diagnosis is best established by laboratory investigations. Low serum copper and decreased serum ceruloplasmin levels occur in most cases, and in symptomatic patients urinary copper excretion is increased. Biliary excretion of copper is also markedly decreased. Microchemical evidence of copper deposition may be obtained from needle biopsy of the liver, but histochemical methods are unreliable. In doubtful cases, specialized studies with radioactive copper may be necessary.

The pathogenesis of the arthropathy is unclear. Its presence does not correlate with neurologic, hepatic, or renal disease. Although chondrocalcinosis has been observed in patients with Wilson's disease, most light and transmission electron microscopic studies have not detected crystals in synovial fluids or in cartilage and synovial biopsies. Copper has been found in the articular cartilage by elemental analysis of a few patients with Wilson's disease and could theoretically cause tissue damage mediated by oxygen-derived free radicals (11).

Although the arthropathy is generally milder than that seen in hemochromatosis, its causes may similarly involve metal-induced injury deposition of CPPD and the development of chronic arthritis.

Copper chelation with penicillamine along with dietary copper restriction is the treatment of choice. Whether penicillamine can control the arthropathy is uncertain, but contemporary series suggest that nowadays the arthropathy is milder because of earlier diagnosis and more intensive chelation therapy. Side effects from penicillamine reported in patients with Wilson's disease rarely include acute polyarthritis, polymyositis, or a lupus-like syndrome. Otherwise, symptomatic measures suffice to control arthritis symptoms.

GAUCHER'S DISEASE

Gaucher's disease is a lysosomal glycolipid storage disease in which glucocerebroside accumulates in the reticuloendothelial cells of the spleen, liver, and bone marrow. It is an autosomal recessive disorder caused by subnormal activity of the hydrolytic enzyme glucocerebrosidase. Although the gene for Gaucher's disease is located on chromosome 1 in the q21 region, real understanding of its transmission came with the cloning and sequencing of both complementary DNA (cDNA) and the gene (12).

Fortunately, the most severe forms of Gaucher's disease are extremely rare, whereas milder forms are encountered frequently, particularly in the Jewish population. Its clinical subdivisions are as follows: Type 1, the most common form is the adult or chronic type that accounts for more than 99% of cases. It is a common familial disorder in Ashkenazi Jews, while other types occur in all ethnic groups. It is defined by the lack of neurologic involvement, and affected adults present with accumulation of glucocerebroside in the reticuloendothelial system causing organomegaly, hypersplenism, conjunctival pingueculae, skin pigmentation, and osteoarticular disease. It has the best prognosis. Type 2, the infantile form, is a fulminating disorder with severe brain involvement and death within the first 18 months of life. Type 3, the intermediate or juvenile form, begins in early childhood and shows many features of the chronic form, with or without central nervous system dysfunction. All the cells of the body are deficient in glucocerebroside activity in Gaucher's disease, but it is the glycolipid-engorged macrophages that account for all the non-neurologic features of the disease.

Skeletal involvement is characteristic of type 1 and to a lesser extent type 3, but not type 2 disease. Musculoskeletal involvement is rarely the first symptom. Patients usually present with lymphadenopathy, hepatosplenomegaly, or signs and symptoms of hypersplenism. Nevertheless, rheumatic complaints may appear early in the course of Gaucher's disease. Pain in the hip, knee, or shoulder is caused by disease of adjacent bone. In young individuals, the most common complaint is chronic aching around the hip or proximal tibia. This may last a few days, but is usually recurrent. Another complaint is excruciating pain (bone crisis) involving the femur and tibia with tenderness, swelling, and erythema. Monarticular hip or knee degeneration is typical, and unexplained migratory polyarthritis sometimes occurs. Bony pain tends to lessen with age.

Other skeletal features include pathologic long bone fractures, vertebral compression, and osteonecrosis of the femoral or humeral heads or proximal tibia. The osteonecrosis can develop slowly, or rapidly with bone crisis. These crisis usually affect only one bone area at a time and since acute-phase reactants and bone scans are usually positive, the clinical picture of acute osteomyelitis is mimicked (pseudoosteomyelitis). Surgical drainage in these cases should be avoided as it commonly leads to infection and chronic osteomyelitis.

Some patients with type 1 disease have few or no features of the disease. In these cases, the condition may be discovered only when bone marrow is examined for some other reason, or if mild thrombocytopenia is investigated.

Asymptomatic radiologic areas of rarefaction, patchy sclerosis, and cortical thickening are common. Involvement of the femur is thought to be a barometer of bone symptoms. Widening of the distal femur with the radiologic appearance of an Erlenmeyer flask is a frequent finding, but flaring of the bones can occur in the tibia and humerus as well. Magnetic resonance imaging also may be valuable in distinguishing the different types of bony changes and monitoring progression (13). The pathogenesis of cortical collapse and the contribution of the histiocytic Gaucher cells is not clearly understood. Arthroplasty and complete joint replacement is often necessary, but loosening of prostheses occurs more often than in other disorders. Bleeding can be an operative problem.

When bone pain or other articular symptoms appear, the serum acid phosphatase and the angiotension-converting enzymes are usually elevated. The most reliable method however, for diagnosing Gaucher's disease is the determination of leukocyte β-glucosidase. In the past, the diagnosis has been confirmed by examination of bone marrow aspirate for the Gaucher cell, a large lipid storage histiocyte. This cell should be differentiated from globoid cells of another lysosomal storage disorder, Krabbe's disease (galactocerebrosidosis). Bone biopsy is not recommended because of the risk of secondary infection. Needle biopsy of the liver for assay of glucocerebroside may be performed, but washed leukocytes and extracts of cultured skin fibroblasts are easily obtained for glucocerebrosidase testing. These assays may also be used to detect heterozygous carriers. Amniocentesis has been used for the prenatal detection of diseased fetuses. When the diagnosis is established, genetic counselling for family members or prospective parents is recommended. Although enzyme assays are useful for genetic screening, DNA analysis using the polymerase chain reaction are much more precise (14). Interestingly, the incidence of monoclonal gammopathy, multiple myeloma, and chronic lymphocytic leukemia have been reported to be increased in adult Gaucher's disease.

Until recently, therapy of Gaucher's disease was mostly symptomatic, based on control of pain and infection. In adults, splenectomy may control hypersplenism, but then bone disease may accelerate. Partial splenectomy has been recommended as protection against post-splenectomy infection and for its hepatic and bone sparing effect.

With the commercial availability of replacement enzyme, the modified glucocerebroside (alglucerase), effective treatment of Gaucher's disease has become a reality. Periodic intravenous infusions of the enzyme over many months result in regression of the features of Gaucher's disease (12). The treatment appears safe without significant side effects; however, it is not recommended for patients with minimal disease. Although lower doses than originally described can be effective, a drawback of this treatment is still its high cost (15). With the development of a recombinant-enzyme preparation, however, it should become available to a wider range of patients at reasonable cost. Bone marrow transplantation and gene transfer therapy using viral vectors are other experimental approaches not yet practical because of their greater risks compared to enzyme replacement.

FABRY'S DISEASE

Fabry's disease is a lysosomal lipid storage disease in which glycosphingolipids accumulate widely in nerves, viscera, skin, and osteoarticular tissues (16).

It is a sex-linked inherited disease caused by a deficiency of the enzyme, α–galactosidase A. The gene responsible for expression of this enzyme has been localized to the middle of the long arm of the X chromosome. Linkage studies have identified cDNA markers to provide a simple method of diagnosing the disease in carriers or affected fetuses by amniocentesis (16).

As a slowly progressive disorder predominately affecting men, clinical features are widespread and nonspecific so that diagnosis is often missed or delayed. In childhood the deposition is particularly marked in and around blood vessels, giving rise to the characteristic rash of dark blue or red angiokeratomas or angiectases around the buttocks, thighs, and lower abdomen. When diffuse, it is referred to as *angiokeratoma corporis diffusum* and is almost always associated with hypohydrosis.

The kidneys are the main target organ, and proteinuria gradually develops in childhood or adolescence with abnormal urinary sediments including birefringent lipid crystals (Maltese crosses). Progressive renal disease leads to renal failure. Cardiovascular and cerebrovascular deposition of the sphingolipid parallels the renal disease, with vascular insufficiencies or sudden death. Ocular changes are severe. A characteristic corneal opacity seen by slit lamp examination occurs early and can be helpful in diagnosis even in heterozygous women.

The rheumatologist may become involved because of the gradual development of polyarthritis with degenerative changes and flexion contractures of the fingers, particularly of the DIP joints. Foam cells have been described in the synovial vessels and connective tissues. Radiographs may show infarct-like opacities of bone and osteoporosis of the spine. Osteonecrosis of the hip and talus have been described. Eighty percent of children or young adults undergo painful crises of burning paresthesias of the hands and feet and later of whole extremities. These attacks are associated with fever and elevations of the erythrocyte sedimentation rate.

Understanding the inheritance pattern means that genetic counseling should be offered to affected families. Measurement of α-galactosidase to α-galactosidase activity ratios in leukocytes and fibroblasts provides reasonable discrimination between carriers and non-carriers. Identification of DNA is reserved for people showing equivocal results.

Treatment is not satisfactory. Anti-platelet medication may suppress vascular damage. Burning paresthesias may benefit from phenytoin or carbamazepine. Without dialysis or transplantation, most affected men succumb to renal failure before age 50. Understanding of the basic molecular defect enhances the prospect for, as in the case of Gaucher's disease, direct enzyme replacement and eventual gene transfer therapy.

FARBER'S DISEASE

Farber's disease is a lysosomal lipid storage disease in which a glycolipid ceramide accumulates widely in many tissues including the skin and musculoskeletal system (17).

It is an autosomal recessive disorder caused by a deficiency of the enzyme acid ceramidase. Affected children show disease manifestations by the age of four months and die before the age of four years.

A hoarse cry from thickened vocal cords or swollen painful joints may be the first feature. The appearance of tender, subcutaneous nodules follows, and the early occurrence of nodules correlates with shortened survival. All the extremities may be swollen and tender, but this gives way to more localized joint swelling with nodules around the fingers, wrists, elbows, and knees. Joint contractures develop later especially affecting the fingers and wrists. The gastrointestinal, cardiovascular, and nervous systems gradually become involved with death from respiratory disease.

Diagnosis can be confirmed by demonstrating a deficiency of acid ceramidase both in leukocytes and fibroblasts.

LIPOCHROME HISTIOCYTOSIS

Lipochrome histiocytosis is an extremely rare lysosomal storage disease associated with pulmonary infiltrates, splenomegaly, hypergammaglobulinemia, polyarthritis, and increased susceptibility to infection (18). The disorder is familial and histiocytes show lipochrome pigment granulation. Peripheral blood leukocytes exhibit impaired activity.

MULTICENTRIC RETICULOHISTIOCYTOSIS

Multicentric reticulohistiocytosis is a rare dermatoarthritis of unknown cause, characterized by the cellular accumulation of histocytes and multinucleated giant cells in skin and joints (19).

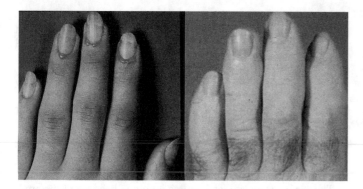

Fig. 34–4. The fingers of a 16-year-old girl on the left reveal multiple, reddish-brown, tender papulonodules that are periungual in distribution. On the right is a hand of another patient with multiple nodules in the fingers. These nodules are firm, can fluctuate in size, and may disappear spontaneously (from the Revised Clinical Slide Collection).

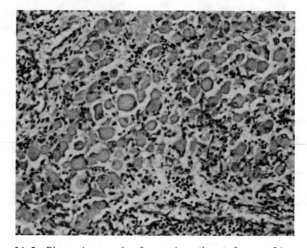

Fig. 34–5. Photomicrograph of synovium (knee) from a 54-year-old woman with multicentric reticulohistiocytosis shows numerous histiocytes and multinucleated giant cells that contain large amounts of periodic acid-Schiff (PAS)-positive material (from Arthritis and Allied Conditions).

The most common presentation is a painful destructive polyarthritis resembling RA. The joint manifestations may precede the appearance of skin lesions in most patients, but the appearance and location of the skin nodules are not entirely characteristic of RA (Fig. 34–4). Although a self-limited form may be seen in childhood, adult multicentric reticulohistiocytosis predominantly affects middle-aged women. The onset is insidious and is characterized by polyarthritis, skin nodules, and in many cases xanthelasma. Small papules and bead-like clusters around the nailfolds are characteristic, with nodulation of the skin of the face and hands. Skin nodules are yellowish, purple, or brown in color and are of varying size, occurring over the hands (Fig. 34–4), elbows, face and ears. Oral, nasal, and pharyngeal mucosa involvement is seen in one-fourth of patients, sometimes with ulceration. Various visceral sites may also be affected.

Symmetric polyarthritis resembles RA when PIP joints are affected, and psoriatic arthritis when involvement of DIP joints predominates. Tenosynovial involvement may also occur. Remission of polyarthritis may be seen after many years of progressive disease.

Early radiographs show "punched out" bony lesions resembling gouty tophi followed by severe joint destruction. Spinal involvement with erosions and subluxations including atlantoaxial damage may occur.

No specific laboratory abnormality has yet been demonstrated, and the diagnosis is established by examination of biopsies of affected tissues. Both the skin and synovium (Fig. 34–5) are infiltrated by large, multinucleated giant cells. The cytoplasm has a ground-glass appearance and stains positively for lipids and glycoproteins with periodic acid-Schiff stain (PAS positive). Definitive analysis of the contents of these cells has not been made, but glycolipids, triglycerides, cholesterol, and phosphate esters appear to be present. These histiocytes also elaborate cytokines that contribute to synovial cell proliferation. Other inflammatory cells, particularly lymphocytes, are also present. Synovial fluid leukocyte counts range from 220–79,000 cells/mm^3, with mononuclear cells predominating. Scanning the synovial fluid Wright-stained smear or wet preparation is important, as can be a synovial biopsy, since giant cells or large, bizarre macrophages may point to the diagnosis (19).

There is no known cause or familial association, and the pathogenesis is unknown. Mycobacteria have been suggested as a possible cause. Rheumatoid factor is not present. Some patients develop positive reactions to tuberculin (PPD positive). There are case descriptions with associated Sjogren's syndrome and polymyositis. Multicentric reticulohistiocytosis has also been implicated with a variety of malignancies (20). Death due to the

disease itself has not been reported, but patients may be left with severe joint disability.

There is no specific treatment; however, corticosteroids or topical nitrogen mustard may improve the skin lesions and cyclophosphamide may control both skin and joint disease (21). Spontaneous remission of skin and arthritis, however, are not uncommon, especially in childhood.

Duncan A. Gordon, MD

1. Rooney PJ: Hyperlipidemias, lipid storage disorders, metal storage disorders and ochronsis. Curr Opin Rheumatol 3:166–71, 1991
2. Nichols GM, Bacon BR: Hereditary hemochromatosis: pathogenesis and clinical features of a common disease. Am J Gastroenterol 84:851–862, 1989
3. Schumacher HR, Straua PC, Krikker MA, et al: The arthropathy of hemochromatosis. Recent studies. Ann NY Acad Sci 526:224–233, 1988
4. Edwards CQ, Skolnick MH, Kushner JP: Hereditary hemochromatosis. contributions of genetic analysis. Prog Hematol 12:43–71, 1981
5. Mathews JL, Williams HJ: Arthritis in hereditary hemochromatosis. Arthritis Rheum 30:1137–1141, 1987
6. Adams PC, Gregor J: Hemochromatosis and yersinosis. Can J Gastroenterol 4:160–162, 1990
7. Schumacher HR, Holdsmith DE: Ochronotic arthropathy. I. clinicopathologic studies. Semin Arthritis Rheum 6:207–246, 1977
8. Gaines JJ, Tom GD, KhanKhanian N: The ultrastructural and light microscopic study of the synovium in ochronotic arthropathy. Hum Pathol 18:1160–1164, 1987
9. Gemignini G, Olivieri I, Semeria R, et al: Coexistence of ochronosis and ankylosing spondylitis. J Rheumatol 17:1707–1709, 1990
10. Kottinen YT, Hoikka AV, Landtman M, et al: Ochronosis; a report and a case and a review of the literature. Clin Exp Rheumatol 7:435–444, 1989
11. Menerey KA, Eider W, Brewer GJ, et al: The arthropathy of Wilson's disease: clinical and pathologic features. J Rheumatol 15:331–337, 1988
12. Beutler E: Gaucher's disease—current concepts. Engl J Med 325:1354–1360, 1991
13. Cremin BJ, Davey H, Goldblatt J: Skeletal complications of type 1 Gaucher's disease. The magnetic resonance features. Clin Radiol 41:244–247, 1990
14. Mistry PK, Smith SJ, Ali M, et al: Genetic diagnosis of Gaucher's disease. Lancet 339:889–892, 1992
15. Figueroa ML, Rosenbloom BE, Kay AC, et al: A less costly regimen of alglucerase to treat Gaucher's disease. N Engl J Med 327:1632–1636, 1992
16. Anon: Anderson–Fabry Disease (editorial) Lancet 336:24–25, 1990
17. Chanoki M, Ishii M, Fukaik, et al: Farber's lipogranulomatosis in siblings: light and electron microscopic studies. Br J Dermatol 121:779–785, 1989
18. Rodey GE, Park BH, Ford DK, et al: Defective bacteriocidal activity of peripheral blood leukocytes in lipochrome histiocytosis. Am J Med 49:322–327, 1970
19. Krey PR, Comerford FR, Cohen AS: Multicentric reticulohistiocytosis: fine structural analysis of the synoviam and synovial fluid cells. Arthritis Rheum 17:615–633, 1974
20. Kenik JG, Fok F, Hueter CJ, et al: Multicentric reticulohistiocytosis in a patient with malignant melanoma; a response to cyclophosphomide and a unique cutaneous feature. Arthritis Rheum 33:1047–1051, 1990
21. Pandhi RK, Vaswani N, Ramam M, et al: Multicentric reticulohistiocytosis response to dexamethosone pulse therapy. Arch Dermatol 126:251–252, 1990

35. ARTHROPATHIES ASSOCIATED WITH HEMATOLOGIC DISEASES AND MALIGNANT DISORDERS

HEMOPHILIC ARTHROPATHY

The hemophilias are sex-linked disorders with historic significance. They occur in 1 of every 10,000 males. Because one-third are due to new mutations, the diagnosis may not be suspected at birth. The basic problem is a deficiency of key factors of the intrinsic clotting system. In classic hemophilia (hemophilia A), factor VIII or antihemophilic globulin is absent or present in small amounts, and in Christmas disease (hemophilia B), factor IX or plasma thromboplastin is lacking. Von Willebrand's disease and factor V deficiency, autosomal clotting disorders, have abnormalities similar to the hemophilias, yet hemarthroses are rare.

Approximately 85% of hemophilic patients have hemophilia A. The lower the amounts of factor VIII, the more severe are the bleeding diatheses and clinical symptoms. For example, patients with less than 2% of normal factor may have spontaneous bleeding into internal organs at birth or in infancy, those with levels below 10% often have significant problems in childhood, while individuals with levels over 20% may have milder episodes of hemorrhage occurring only after severe trauma or surgery (1).

Intraarticular hemorrhage is a common problem and most often involves large joints, particularly the knees, ankles, and elbows. The joint becomes warm, swollen, and very tender. Due to an increase in volume and intraarticular pressure, the patient keeps the joint in flexion. With recurrent bleeding, the joint remains swollen and flexion deformities develop. Contractures of elbows and knees may result, and in young children involvement of the ankle can lead to equinus deformity. Hemorrhage into muscles, causing hematomas and pseudotumors, may lead to palsies that in turn contribute to flexion deformities and instability of joints.

The exact mechanism of joint damage in hemophilia is not completely understood. Because of the absence of prothrombin and fibrinogen in normal fluid and the absence of tissue thromboplastin in the synovium, blood in the joint remains liquid. In hemophilia where intrinsic clotting is abnormal, bleeding apparently continues until stopped by intraarticular pressure. Reabsorption of the plasma follows, and there is activation of platelets and gradual phagocytosis of red cells by synovial lining cells and macrophages. With recurrent episodes of bleeding, the synovium becomes hyperplastic and hypertrophic, and encroaches on the cartilage. Hemosiderin is found in lining cells, in the sublining areas, and even within chondrocytes. Whether hemosiderin or iron itself is toxic to chondrocytes is not known, but the end result is cartilage breakdown. Intraosseous hemorrhage may contribute to cartilage loss by removing its support. The hypertrophic synovium forms a pannus, which is fibrous with few lymphocytes (Fig. 35–1). Evidence of immunologic processes, such as immunoglobulin deposition and complement activation, is lacking. Some patients have circulating immune complexes and decreased total complement, but these do not correlate with clinical or pathologic findings. Activated macrophages in the advancing synovium, the presence of plasminogen activator, collagenases, and prostaglandins all mediate cartilage destruction (1,2).

As can be expected, radiologic changes include osteopenia, joint space narrowing, and subchondral cyst formation. Radiographic findings characteristic of hemophilia include epiphyseal irregularities in young children, widening of the femoral intercondylar notch (Fig. 35–2), squaring of the inferior patella, and enlargement of the proximal radius in the elbow. Since it can outline cartilaginous changes and better define the hypertrophied synovium, magnetic resonance imaging has been shown to be helpful, especially prior to synovectomy (3).

The treatment for an acute bleeding episode in hemophilia is

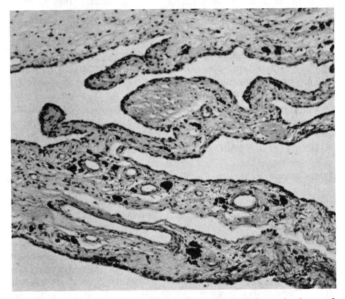

Fig. 35–1. *Photomicrograph of synovium obtained from the knee of a 76-year-old man with classic hemophilia (factor VIII deficiency) who had repeated episodes of hemarthrosis and developed severe osteoarthritis. Note heavy deposits of iron-containing pigment (hemosiderin) in lining cells and deeper portions of the synovium (from Arthritis and Allied Conditions).*

the immediate infusion of factor VIII, the dose depending on the patient's weight and known deficit. The joint has to be placed at rest with as much extension as is comfortable. Ice applications, analgesics, and nonsteroidal antiinflammatory drugs (NSAIDs) may be helpful. Intraarticular corticosteroids have been used to help stop bleeding but are not advocated by all.

Arthrocentesis is mandatory when infection is suspected, but it should be done until sufficient factor replacement has been given. Synovial fluid findings in hemophilia have shown a low leukocyte count and a predominance of monocytes (75%). Glucose and

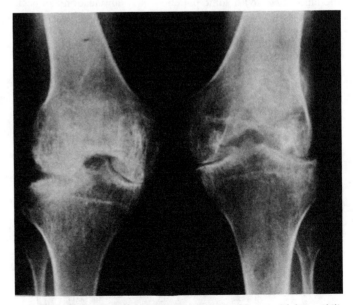

Fig. 35–2. *Radiograph of the knees of a 23-year-old man with hemophilia and repeated hemarthroses. Note loss of articular cartilage, bony overgrowth, and widening of the left intercondylar notch.*

lactic acid are usually normal. While septic arthritis in hemophilia has been rare, the incidence has increased because many patients have become infected with the human immunodeficiency virus.

At this time more hemophiliac patients die of acquired immunodeficiency syndrome (AIDS) than of any other cause. Fortunately, tests to control contamination of plasma-derived factor preparations are now in place; monoclonal production of human recombinant DNA–derived factor VIII may obviate this problem (4).

Home therapy with hemophilic factor, which began in the late 1960s, has had a beneficial effect on the mortality and, to some extent, on the morbidity of patients. The problems of arthropathies are still paramount, however. Physiotherapy to maintain joint motion and strengthen muscles is extremely important. Arthroscopic synovectomies before cartilage destruction, and joint replacement afterward, have had good outcomes. Until recombinant factor VIII preparations are more easily available and until gene therapy is perfected, monitoring patients for spontaneous and traumatic hemarthroses will remain the mainstay of therapy.

SICKLE CELL DISEASE

Osteoarticular symptoms in the hemoglobinopathies can be due to involvement of bone and joints secondary to ischemic events or to the actively proliferating bone marrow (5). One in five patients with sickle cell crisis may have acute bone or periarticular pain. Fewer patients have a true arthropathy with tenderness, swelling, and effusion of a large joint. The synovial fluid is usually noninflammatory with a predominance of mononuclear cells. Most attacks subside spontaneously with hydration, rest, and analgesia, but they may last up to two weeks. Ankle arthritis associated with leg ulcers may occur and then disappear when the skin ulcers heal. Muscle necrosis has been described in a few patients during crises.

In about one-third of infants with sickle cell disease, there is a well-known presentation of acute, diffuse swelling and tenderness of fingers or toes, the so-called hand–foot syndrome, or *sickle cell dactylitis* (Fig. 35–3). This is usually the first manifestation of sickle cell disease, or more rarely sickle cell–hemoglobin C disease (S–C) or S-thalassemia, and is presumably due to infarction or tissue anoxia. Periostitis of metacarpals and metatarsals may be seen in roentgenograms 10–14 days after the acute episode. Unless complicated by infection, the swelling subsides in a matter of weeks (6).

The most serious ischemic episodes of homozygous sickle cell disease lead to osteonecrosis, including infarctions of diaphyseal bone (Fig. 35–4). Osteonecrosis is also seen in sickle–thalassemia and S–C disease. The overall incidence of ischemic necrosis of the hip is 10%. With some patients, this complication can occur as early as age 5. Unfortunately, the results of total hip replacement in sickle cell disease are poor. In one multicenter study the majority continued to have pain and limitation of motion, and in one series, 5 of 27 patients needed a revision of the prosthesis within four and one-half years (7).

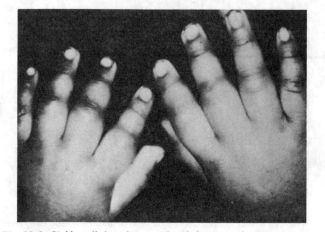

Fig. 35–3. Sickle cell dactylitis or "hand–foot" syndrome.

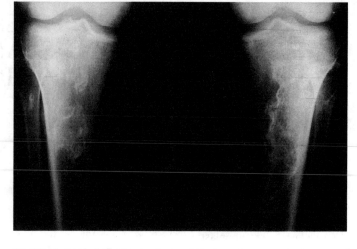

Fig. 35–4. Sickle cell anemia: knees. This posteroanterior projection of both knees demonstrates moderate osteopenia and coarse sparse trabeculae. The medullary cavity is widened throughout with atrophy of the cortices. Small bone infarcts are seen in the femoral shafts. The joints are intact (from Revised Clinical Slide Collection on the Rheumatic Diseases).

Children with sickle cell disease are clearly prone to infections, particularly with salmonella. Defective opsonization of bacteria, an ineffective spleen, impaired phagocytosis, and the probable spread of organisms from hypoxic intestine to areas of necrotic bone, may all play a role. Salmonella osteomyelitis is increased at all stages of the disease; in one series the incidence was 71% (8). Acute presentations of osteomyelitis must be differentiated from ischemic necrosis, which is said to be 50 times more common than infection. Combined technetium and gallium scintigraphs usually show increased uptake in osteomyelitis, while scans of infarcted bone can show decreased perfusion.

There are numerous radiologic alterations in the hemoglobinopathies due to hyperactive bone marrow, including widening of medullary cavities, thinning of cortices, coarsening and irregularity of trabeculae, and cupping of vertebrae. Sclerosis of terminal phalanges has also been described (8).

Gouty arthritis is a rare complication of sickle cell disease. Children are usually normouricemic despite increased erythropoiesis and urate overproduction. Forty percent of adults, however, become hyperuricemic with impaired renal tubular function, probably due to sickle cell disease itself. Few adult patients, however, have been documented with urate crystals in synovial fluid during an acute attack of arthritis.

The mortality and morbidity of sickle cell anemia is variable. Recently, it has been shown that in patients over the age of 20, the death rate correlates with the number of painful crises. Although sickle cell disease can be diagnosed prenatally and bone marrow transplantation is feasible, the side effects of the latter procedure are still unacceptable to most parents (9). Treatments that aim at increasing fetal hemoglobin may improve outcomes.

THALASSEMIA

Osteoporosis, pathologic fractures, and epiphyseal deformities can occur in β-thalassemia. There is also a form of chronic arthritis involving the ankles, and less commonly the knees, that has been described in young adults. Pain, tenderness, and mild swelling occur from weight bearing, producing microfractures in areas of active hematopoiesis and osteopenia. The synovium shows hyperplasia with deposition of hemosiderin, but no synovitis or evidence of inflammation in synovial fluid is observed. Because of many transfusions, a secondary form of hemochromatosis may develop. Osteonecrosis of the hip, common in sickle cell anemia, is rare in thalassemia (6).

MYELOMATOSIS

Two-thirds of patients with multiple myeloma present with bone pain, primarily of the back or chest wall. The pain is usually exacerbated by movement and is gradual in onset. Fractures may cause acute pain, however, and sudden disability can occur from hip or compression fractures of the spine. Classically, roentgenograms of bone show well-circumscribed, lytic lesions in the vertebrae, ribs, sternum, skull, pelvis, or proximal long bones. These areas result from malignant plasma cell proliferation with secretion of multiple cytokines, which stimulate bone resorption and hypercalcemia. Patients show a monoclonal gammaglobin spike or excessive light chain excretion in the urine, and eventually develop disseminated disease. A very small percentage of patients show generalized osteoporosis only.

Since most patients have an onset of symptoms in the seventh decade, differentiation from senile osteoporosis may be difficult. Technetium bone scans are usually negative except in areas of fracture or concomitant osteoarthritis. Gallium citrate scans, on the other hand, may be positive in areas of marked myelomatous activity. Computed tomography and magnetic resonance imaging have been more successful in delineating vertebral lesions, especially spinal cord compression. Osteosclerotic myeloma is rare and is characterized by an indolent disease course, smaller monoclonal spikes on serum protein electrophoresis, and a high association with peripheral neuropathy. Patients with plasma cell dyscrasia, polyneuropathy, organomegaly, endocrinopathy, monoclonal spikes, and scleroderma-like skin changes have been described, the so-called POEMS syndrome (10). Both autologous and allogeneic bone marrow transplantations have been carried out in multiple myeloma patients. The results are promising, but large, formal clinical trials are needed.

Almost all forms of myelomatosis, especially light chain disease and IgA myeloma, may be complicated by amyloid deposition (see Chapter 36). Carpal tunnel syndrome due to the amyloid deposits deep to the flexor retinaculum is common. Patients may present with a symmetric polyarthritis, particularly of the hands, wrists, shoulders, and knees. Synovial fluid analysis reveals low leukocyte counts with predominantly mononuclear cells. Rarely, patients may have counts up to 10,000 cells/mm³ with a greater percentage of polymorphonuclear leukocytes. Because both small and large joints are symmetrically involved and amyloid-containing skin nodules are often present, the clinical picture may be very similar to rheumatoid arthritis. Biopsy of the synovium or capsule and examination of the synovial fluid sediment may show Congo red staining material even in the absence of other clinical features of amyloidosis and negative rectal biopsies (11).

WALDENSTROM'S MACROGLOBULINEMIA

Waldenstrom's macroglobulinemia, which is characterized by excessive monoclonal IgM synthesis by plasma cells or their B cell precursors, presents a variable picture with anemia, lymphadenopathy, hepatosplenomegaly, bleeding tendencies, hyperviscosity, and cryoglobulin-related symptoms. Although the bone marrow shows benign plasmacytoid lymphocytes, some patients gradually develop multiple myeloma or malignant lymphoma (6). Joint abnormalities as described in multiple myeloma are extremely rare, but destructive bone lesions have been found. An occasional patient with amyloidosis has been described, usually of the primary or AL type.

CANCER AND ARTHRITIS

Malignancies have been associated with a number of connective tissue diseases, particularly with dermatomyositis, Sjogren's syndrome, systemic lupus erythematosus (SLE), systemic sclerosis (scleroderma), and following immunosuppressive therapy. These, along with hypertrophic osteoarthropathy, a distinct symptom complex associated with solid tumors, are described elsewhere in the *Primer*. Primary malignant tumors of the joint, such as synovial sarcomas, are very rare and are discussed in Chapter 37. The following sections deal primarily with malignancies that give rise to diffuse musculoskeletal symptoms, either directly via metastatic invasion of bone and joints as most often occurs with lung and breast carcinoma or indirectly as paraneoplastic syndromes and with the hematologic malignancies.

Carcinoma Polyarthritis

Carcinoma polyarthritis is considered to be a paraneoplastic process in which presumed factors from the tumor cause an arthritis. Since the joint symptoms may be present before the cancer is suspected, the patient may be mistakenly diagnosed and managed as having rheumatoid disease. Most patients have a high erythrocyte sedimentation rate, negative serology, and, when reported, a mildly inflammatory synovial fluid. The clinical picture may be especially confusing in some cases since rheumatoid factor is positive in up to 20% of patients and even antinuclear antibodies may be positive with malignancy. There are few distinctive features in this form of arthritis, but the onset late in life and sparing of wrists and small joints should raise suspicion. In women, 80% with polyarthritis have had breast carcinoma. The most convincing confirmation is the disappearance of the arthritis when the tumor is resected and reappearance of arthritis when the carcinoma recurs. Unfortunately, most patients die without experiencing a remission.

A number of unusual associations have been reported with specific cancers (12) such as palmar fasciitis and ovarian carcinoma, polyarthritis with pancreatic cancer (13), and even with a malignant histiocytoma of the heart (14). In the latter, the fluid aspirated from the knee had 500 WBC/mm³ and 30% granulocytes and 70% mononuclear cells. The synovial fluid taken from the patient with pancreatic cancer was yellow-green and creamy, with many fat globules and necrotic cells (13).

Leukemia

Musculoskeletal symptoms are clearly associated with the leukemias, most commonly in children with acute or chronic lymphocytic leukemia. The incidence of joint involvement in adults with leukemia has been reported as 13.5%. Symptoms vary from bone pain and arthralgias to arthritis. Most patients develop an asymmetric, additive, or migratory polyarthritis, but at least one-third may show bilateral involvement of small and large joints mimicking rheumatoid arthritis. Knees, ankles, and shoulders are most commonly affected. Involvement of joints may be due to leukemic infiltration of the synovium, periosteal elevation of the intra- and paraarticular bone, hemorrhage into the joint, or rarely, crystal-induced inflammation. In a number of patients, however, no definite cause can be determined. In spite of the presence of circulating immune complexes, synovial fluid does not show a marked reduction of complement nor are there vascular abnormalities as described in hypertrophic osteoarthropathy. Synovial fluid leukocyte counts range from 50–45,000 cells/mm³. Usually, polymorphonuclear cells predominate. A few fluids show blast cells, and some synovial membranes reveal infiltration of leukemic cells, although others are unremarkable or show mild inflammation.

A significant recent advance has been the use of monoclonal antibodies to type leukemic cells in the synovium or in synovial fluid. In one study (15), synovial fluid mononuclear cells reacted with antibodies to a common lymphoblastic antigen, and leukemic infiltration of the synovium was later documented at autopsy. Both gout and pseudogout have occurred in association with lymphocytic and myelocytic leukemia; however, calcium pyrophosphate dihydrate arthritis, described in several elderly patients, may have been coincidental.

Arthritis may antedate the diagnosis of leukemia by weeks to months, or it can occur simultaneously with abnormal hematologic findings. The arthritis may also occur during an exacerbation of chronic leukemia. In one report of six children, three had a positive antinuclear antibody test that clouded the initial evaluation. Treatment with NSAIDs or cytotoxic drugs may alleviate the joint symptoms but not necessarily the hematologic abnormalities. When the leukemia is adequately treated, however, the arthritis responds readily.

Lymphoma

Although bone involvement in lymphoma constitutes 10% of all extranodal lymphomas, joint symptoms, which are confused with specific forms of arthritis, are only occasionally reported. Indeed, only 10 patients have been described with joint manifestations of lymphoma. Some of these have had contiguous involvement of bone, but four have had the malignancy apparently arising from the synovium. In those with monarticular arthritis, synovial fluid findings have shown from 1,000–10,500 leukocytes/mm³ with normal or atypical lymphocytes or mononuclear cells. Immunocytologic techniques to characterize these cells have not been carried out in most patients.

In the largest series of lymphomas occurring in bone, 4 of 14 patients had polyarthralgias ranging from four months to several years in duration. At the time of diagnosis, all had advanced disseminated disease, and a rheumatologic diagnosis had not been made on these young patients. Three men died within two years, while a 22 year-old woman was doing well two and a half years after radiation and chemotherapy (16).

Two patients with cutaneous T cell lymphomas (mycosis fungoides) had polyarthritis resembling rheumatoid arthritis. One patient with a positive rheumatoid factor and antinuclear antibodies was treated with anti-CD4 monoclonal antibodies, which improved the skin disease and arthritis, but did not cause a remission. The second patient improved with radiation (17,18).

ANGIOIMMUNOBLASTIC LYMPHADENOPATHY

The recently described disorder of angioimmunoblastic lymphadenopathy is characterized by lymphadenopathy, hepatosplenomegaly, and constitutional symptoms. Fever, weight loss, urticarial or maculopapular rash, pleuritis, pericarditis, hemolytic anemia, and hypergammaglobulinemia are classic features (19). Arthritis may be present in a number of patients, and SLE, adult onset Still's disease, Sjogren's syndrome, and cryoglobulinemia have been mistakenly diagnosed. A symmetric inflammatory polyarthritis is often present with joint fluid leukocytes up to 20,000 cells/mm³. Two patients had 70% and 88% synovial fluid neutrophils, but one patient had 93% mononuclear cells, identified primarily as T helper/inducer cells by monoclonal antibody studies (20).

Lymph node biopsy shows a distinctive picture with infiltration of T lymphocytes, plasma cells, histiocytes, eosinophils, and immunoblasts and destruction of nodal architecture. Marked proliferation or "arborization" of venules is characteristic. The T cells take on cell markers of peripheral T-cell lymphomas when malignancy develops.

Angioimmunoblastic lymphadenopathy appears to be an exaggerated B cell response to a T cell defect following exposure to drugs, viruses, or other unknown antigen(s). Clinical manifestations can appear like infections with the HIV virus. A small number of patients have had Sjogren's syndrome, a few had rheumatoid arthritis, and one patient had SLE with antinuclear and anti-DNA antibodies.

About one-third of patients progress to malignant lymphoma, one-fourth have a hectic course with corticosteroid and cytotoxic therapy and the remainder appear to have self-limiting disease. Early diagnosis and early aggressive therapy is usually indicated.

Phoebe R. Krey, MD

1. Madhok R, York J, Sturrock RD: Haemophilic arthritis. Ann Rheum Dis 50:588–591, 1991
2. Madhok R, Bennett D, Sturrock RD, et al: Mechanisms of joint damage in an experimental model of hemophilic arthritis. Arthritis Rheum 31:1148–1155, 1988
3. Yulish BS, Lieberman JM, Strandjord SE, et al: Hemophilic arthropathy: assessment with MR imaging. Radiology 164:759–762, 1987
4. Schwartz RS, Abildgaard CF, Aledort LM, et al: Human recombinant DNA-derived antihemophilic factor (factor VIII) in the treatment of hemophilia A. N Engl J Med 323:1800–1805, 1990
5. Sturrock RD: Hematologic disorders with rheumatic manifestations. Curr Opin Rheumatol 1:551–553, 1989
6. Isenberg DA, Schoenfeld Y: The rheumatologic complications of hematologic disorders. Semin Arthritis Rheum 12:348–358, 1983
7. Milner PF, Kraus AP, Sebes JI, et al: Sickle cell disease as a cause of osteonecrosis of the femoral head. N Engl J Med 325:1476–1481, 1991
8. Bennett OM, Namnyak SS: Bone and joint manifestations of sickle cell anemia. J Bone Joint Surg 72:494–499, 1990
9. Platt OS, Thorington BD, Brambilla DJ, et al: Pain in sickle cell disease. N Eng J Med 325:11–16, 1991
10. Fam AG, Rubinstein JD, Cowan DH: POEMS syndrome. Arthritis Rheum 29:233–241, 1986
11. Lakhanpal S, Li CY, Gertz MA, et al: Synovial fluid analysis for diagnosis of amyloid arthropathy. Arthritis Rheum 30:419–423, 1987
12. Schwarzer AC, Schrieber L: Rheumatic manifestations of neoplasia. Curr Opin Rheumatol 3:145–154, 1991
13. van Klaveren RJ, de Mulder PHM, Boerbooms AMT, et al: Pancreatic carcinoma with polyarthritis, fat necrosis, and high serum lipase and trypsin activity. Gut 31:953–955, 1990
14. Berkelbach van der Sprenkel JW, Timmermans AJM, Elbers HRJ, et al: Polyarthritis as the presenting symptom of a malignant, fibrous histiocytoma of the heart. Arthritis Rheum 28:944–947, 1985
15. Fam AG, Voorneveld C, Robinson JB, et al: Synovial fluid immunocytology in the diagnosis of leukemic synovitis. J Rheumatol 18:293–296, 1991
16. Reimer RR, Chabner BA, Young RC, et al: Lymphoma presenting in bone: results of histopathology, staging and therapy. Ann Intern Med 87:50–55, 1977
17. Berger RG, Knox SJ, Levy R, et al: Mycosis fungoides arthropathy. Ann Intern Med 114:571–572, 1991
18. Seleznick MJ, Aguilar JL, Rayhack J, et al: Polyarthritis associated with cutaneous T cell lymphoma. J Rheumatol 16:1379–1382, 1989
19. Steinberg AD, Seldin MF, Jaffee ES, et al: NIH Conference: angioimmunoblastic lymphadenopathy with dysproteinemia. Ann Intern Med 108:575–584, 1988
20. McHugh NJ, Campbell GJ, Landreth JJ, et al: Polyarthritis and angioimmunoblastic lymphadenopathy. Ann Rheum Dis 46:555–558, 1987

36. THE AMYLOIDOSES

For more than a century, pathologists have described organs infiltrated with a homogeneous eosinophilic material that bound the organic dye Congo Red. Virchow's designation of all such deposits as *amyloid* (starch-like) has been retained, despite increasing recognition of its inaccuracy. Over the last 20 years, the notion that there is a single amyloid substance appearing during the course of a number of diseases has been replaced by a body of data showing that there are many amyloidoses, each representing a different protein, specific for each disease. Resulting organ compromise is related to the location, quantity, and rate of deposition.

The main reason for the assignment of these disorders to the realm of the rheumatologist is the association of long-standing inflammatory joint disease with amyloid deposition in the kidneys, liver, and spleen. Clinical amyloid arthropathy is seen infrequently, but does occur in the amyloid associated with immunoglobulin L-chain deposition (AL), the amyloid formed by β_2 microglobulin in patients with chronic renal failure, and in rare patients with transthyretin (TTR) associated familial disease.

All the amyloids share certain basic characteristics (Table 36–1). Fifteen discrete fibril precursors have been identified in hu-

Table 36–1. Criteria for definition of amyloid

1. Homogeneous, hyaline, eosinophilic material on H&E stain
2. Crystal violet metachromasia
3. Stains with alkaline Congo Red
4. Apple green positive birefringence with polarized light after Congo Red staining
5. Fibrillar structure on electron microscopy
6. Salt extraction yields P-component from all forms of amyloid
7. Tissue extraction with distilled water or low ionic strength buffers yields opalescent solution of fibrils 70–90 A diameter which precipitate in 0.0075–0.01 M NaCl
8. Fibril is unique for each form of amyloid

man diseases during the last two decades (Table 36–2). Several more conditions have been noted in which amyloid material has been found in tissues, but the nature of the protein(s) is not yet known. At least two additional molecules, apolipoprotein AII and insulin, have been seen only in deposits in animals with amyloid (1).

It is uncertain what makes a protein amyloidogenic. All have

Table 36–2. *Chemical classification of the human amyloidoses*

Amyloid Protein	Precursor Protein	Clinical Syndrome
AL	Immunoglobulin L-chain	Primary amyloid; multiple myeloma
AH	Immunoglobulin H-chain	Primary amyloid; multiple myeloma
AA	apo-SAA	Inflammation associated familial Mediterranean fever; Muckle-Wells
ATTR	Transthyretin (TTR)	Familial amyloidotic polyneuropathy; senile systemic amyloidosis; isolated vitreous amyloid
AGEL	Gelsolin	Familial amyloidotic polyneuropathy-Finnish lattice corneal dys.
AApoAI	Apolipoprotein A1	Familial amyloidotic polyneuropathy Van Allen
Aβ_2M	Beta$_2$ microglobulin	Dialysis-associated amyloidosis
Aβ	Beta-protein precursor	Alzheimers; Down's Syndrome; HCHWA* (Dutch)
ACys	Cystatin C	HCHWA* (Iceland)
ACal	Calcitonin	Medullary carcinoma of the thyroid
AIAPP	Islet amyloid polypeptide	Insulinoma; type II diabetes mellitus
AANF	Atrial natriuretic factor	Isolated atrial amyloid
AScr	Scrapie (prion) protein	Creutzfeldt-Jakob; Gerstmann-Straussler-Scheinker syndrome
AFIBα	Fibrinogen α chain	Hereditary non-neuropathic
ALYS	Lysozyme	Ostertag; hereditary, non-neuropathic

*HCHWA: Hereditary cerebral hemorrhage with amyloidosis

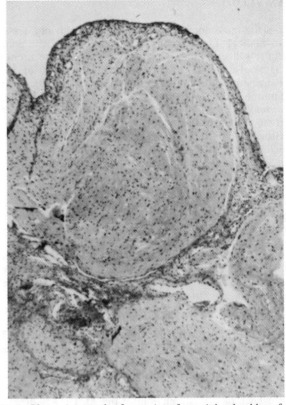

Fig. 36–1. *Photomicrograph of synovium from right shoulder of a 56-year-old woman with myelomatosis who dislocated her right humerus following a fall. At the time of open reduction of this dislocation, large deposits of amyloid were found in the glenoid fossa. Note large mass of amyloid covered by a thin rim of synovium. The material in this nodule stained metachromatically with crystal violet (from Arthritis and Allied Conditions).*

substantial beta pleated sheet structure, but that in itself is insufficient (2). There appear to be certain size constraints, with all fibril subunits ranging from 3,500 to 30,000. A variety of pathogenetic modes are involved. Increased local or systemic production of a precursor as a result of a prolonged normal stimulus to the synthesizing cell, or monoclonal proliferation of a cell producing the amyloidogenic protein, may be responsible. There may be decreased excretion of the precursor, as in the amyloid of chronic renal failure. Structural abnormalities of a normal protein secondary to a germline mutation may also predispose to fibril formation. Finally there may be a defect in an undefined process responsible for the normal degradation and disposition of either single proteins or a group of proteins that have amyloidogenic properties when present at levels only slightly higher than normal.

The diagnosis of any form of amyloid is made by the demonstration of material that is homogeneous in conventional histology, binds Congo Red with a characteristic birefringence when viewed under polarized light, binds metachromatic dyes, such as thioflavine T or crystal violet, and is fibrillar in its ultrastructural appearance (Fig. 36–1). Biopsies of clinically affected organs have a high yield, but sampling of more accessible tissues may also have a good return with lower risk (Table 36–3).

Each form of amyloid is defined by the nature of the fibril protein. It is now possible to stain pathologic specimens with antibodies specific for many of the precursors, thereby establishing the nature of the deposits and the character of the responsible disease (3). An antiserum to a second protein, common to all deposits (the P-component), can be used in addition to Congo Red staining, to confirm the nature of the tissue material as an amyloid (4). The P-component is derived from a serum precursor (serum amyloid P-component), which behaves as an acute phase reactant in the mouse, but not in humans (5). It shares structural features with C-reactive protein and has been grouped with the latter and several other proteins as members of the pentraxin family. The role of the P-component in the pathogenesis of amy-

loid deposition is unclear; however, recent studies have shown that intravenously injected purified P-component will bind to deposited fibrils in tissues. Based on this observation, radiolabeled P-component has been used as a reagent for gamma scanning to determine the presence and extent of deposits in both experimental animals and patients with clinical disease (6). Although the technique requires an increased level of sensitivity, particularly for assaying peripheral nerve and brain, and a more discriminating way of analyzing cardiac deposition because of the heart's large intracavitary blood pool, it should prove valuable, particularly in assessing responses to treatment.

Table 36–3. *Diagnosis of some of the amyloidoses by biopsy*

Tissue	Positive	AL	AA	FA	Uncl
Gingiva	19/26				
	11/19	7/10	4/9		
	6/32				
Marrow		39/80			
Rectal	47/62	5/5	19/27	14/18	9/12
			*6/115		
			*2/47		
		24/31			
Subcut. fat			*2/47		
	28/32	18/19	4/6	6/7	
	9/12	2/3	7/9		
	70/83	46/52	12/18	12/13	
		20/28			
Renal	21/24				
		29/30			
Hepatic	13/27				

*RA patients only
FA: Familial Amyloid
These data compiled from studies published since late 1940's.

AL AMYLOID

While the most common clinical form of amyloid deposition seen in medical practice in the U.S. is the beta protein plaque of Alzheimer's disease, that most likely to come to the attention of rheumatologists is AL disease, either in the form of primary amyloidosis or in the course of multiple myeloma (7). The usual presentation is renal with proteinuria, renal failure, or both. The former may be massive in the context of a full-blown nephrotic syndrome, or relatively mild. True nephropathic proteinuria must be distinguished from the excretion of large amounts of free monoclonal light chains, sometimes described in light chain myeloma. The latter is usually associated with renal disease, such as myeloma kidney, with the dominant urine protein being the monoclonal light chain responsible for the formation of the characteristic tubular casts. In amyloid nephropathy the monoclonal component is usually minor in the glomerular leakage pattern of proteinuria. The amount of urinary protein may diminish with the onset of renal insufficiency. Occasionally renal tubular disorders precede renal failure. Both concentration and acidification defects have been described. Hypertension can occur and the kidneys may be small, enlarged or normal in size. Enlargement usually occurs early in the disease. As in all forms of proteinuric nephropathy, intravenous urography should be carried out with care.

The second most common presentation of AL disease is restrictive cardiomyopathy. Echocardiography has made detection relatively straightforward, showing noncompliant hemodynamics, thickening of the interventricular septum and valve leaflets, and the presence of "sparkling" of the ventricular echoes (8). The presence of cardiac amyloid of the AL (or any other) type can be definitively established by endomyocardial biopsy. The biopsy sample is stained with the appropriate immunohistochemical reagents to identify monoclonal light chain deposition. Coronary deposition of AL and AA amyloid have been noted but myocardial deposits of AA are rare. Both digoxin and nifedipine toxicity have been reported in patients with cardiac amyloid deposition (9,10). Evidence suggests that the two drugs are bound to the fibrils, and their effective concentrations are disproportionately increased in the myocardial deposits.

A dominant neuropathic presentation of AL is seen in about 20% of patients (7). Symptoms are sensorimotor with the first manifestation frequently carpal tunnel syndrome; but lower extremity involvement is also seen. Biopsy of an involved nerve or the sural nerve usually reveals amyloid deposition.

Periarticular amyloid deposition has been reported in AL disease, presenting as a pseudoarthritis (11). However, joint effusions may also be present with amyloid fibrils found in fluid obtained by arthrocentesis. A soft tissue *shoulder pad sign* may be the major physical finding in the patient (Fig. 36–2).

A potentially fatal complication of AL disease is an acquired deficiency of clotting factor X (12). In vivo studies carried out in a patient with such a defect suggested that the factor was bound to the fibrils in the deposits. However, analyses of amyloid deposits from another patient failed to identify factor X associated with the fibrils, nor could in vitro binding to fibrils be demonstrated. Thus, while factor binding to fibrils seems likely, its definitive demonstration has not yet been achieved.

Fibrils from the deposits of 60 patients with AL have been obtained by the distilled water extraction procedure in sufficient quantity to establish the subunit size, light chain class and subclass, and in many cases partial or full amino acid sequence (13). Lambda light chains are the precursor more than twice as often as kappa. Fibrils belonging to all light chain v-region subclasses have been identified. In comparison with all human light chains that have been sequenced, serum and urine light chains and fibrils from patients with AL disease have statistically significant increases in the proportion of proteins belonging to the v_λ VI and v_κ I subclasses. Most deposits contain light chain fragments beginning with a normal amino terminus. Fewer than 10% contain only intact light chains. About one-quarter contain both intact chains and one or more fragments, while 10% contain fragments 12 kDa or smaller. The last suggests why 10% to 15% of AL tissue deposits may not stain with commercially available

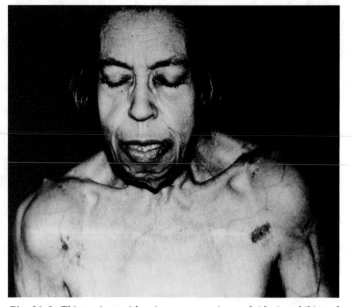

Fig. 36–2. *This patient with primary systemic amyloidosis exhibits advanced macroglossia, resulting in inability to close her mouth. Purpura is present around eyelids, lips, and anterior thorax. Solid firm masses of amyloid have caused prominence of both shoulders, known as the shoulder pad sign (from the Revised Clinical Slide Collection on the Rheumatic Diseases).*

antisera specific for light chain constant region determinants. These data are most consistent with some form of proteolysis playing a major role in the pathogenesis of the disease. Biosynthetic data from two laboratories suggest a possible role for the synthesis of abnormal chains in addition to the production of free monoclonal light chains of the same class as the deposited protein in all patients, including the 10% to 20% who show no monoclonal light chains in the serum or urine. In 80%–90% of patients serum and urine immunoelectrophoresis will reveal the Ig precursor.

Two randomized trials of melphalan and prednisone in regimens similar to those used in the treatment of multiple myeloma have not shown statistically significant increases in survival of treated patients, but both trials suffered from design flaws. Nonetheless, it appeared that approximately 20% of patients treated had some benefit (14). Preliminary data from two current randomized, prospective, double-blind trials also indicate that the combination is moderately effective. No additional therapeutic effect was noted when colchicine was added to the regimen (15).

β_2 MICROGLOBULIN AMYLOID

The second form of amyloid deposition associated with a significant articular presentation is the deposition of β_2 microglobulin in patients with chronic renal disease (16). (see also Chapter 40). Originally all the reported patients presenting with the syndrome of joint pain, carpal tunnel syndrome, and osteonecrosis had been on dialysis, usually for a mean period of seven years. More recently the condition has been reported after shorter periods of renal support. At least one case has been identified in which the patient had not been dialyzed. In each case, the deposited protein was found to be β_2 microglobulin, the 12,500 d polypeptide component of class I proteins of the major histocompatibility complex. Studies of fibrils extracted from the deposits reveal that the subunit is the intact polypeptide, of normal amino acid sequence, either as monomer or dimers.

AA AMYLOID

The third rheumatologically associated form of amyloid deposition is found in patients with rheumatoid arthritis RA and familial Mediterranean fever, consisting of the AA (Amyloid A) protein (17,18). The AA protein was discovered as an amyloid fibril that was found to have a serum precursor, serum amyloid A (SAA). The latter has a polypeptide weight of 12,500 d, but circulates as an apoprotein of HDL in a molecular complex of about 250 kDa. It behaves as an acute phase reactant in man and in all species in which it has been studied. It is synthesized primarily in the liver, in response to elevated levels of the cytokine IL–6, which in turn responds to IL–1 and tumor necrosis factor (TNF). The fibril subunit has a normal sequence with a molecular size of 7,500 d, although a range of various size polypeptides has been found in various preparations. It has been suggested that humans are polymorphic in their ability to degrade SAA to small peptides and that when the production of SAA is increased in inflammatory disease, some individuals are incapable of completely digesting the increased substrate load. Digestion is incomplete, and the 7,500 d intermediate product is fibrillogenic. While reasonable, the hypothesis has not been rigorously tested.

Clinically, older autopsy studies of patients with RA indicated that as many as 25% had significant tissue amyloid deposits; severity of the deposition correlated with the extent and duration of disease. More recent analyses of sequential patients by rectal biopsy or subcutaneous fat aspiration have shown that about 5% have detectable deposits with perhaps one-third of these displaying clinical disease, usually renal or hepatic deposition. In much of the world, AA deposition is common in the course of chronic infectious diseases such as leprosy, tuberculosis, and osteomyelitis. The frequency in the course of noninfectious inflammatory diseases such as juvenile rheumatoid arthritis is also much higher in Europe (10%) and the United Kingdom than it is in the U.S. (1%).

Investigations of the genetic predisposition to AA deposition have been encouraged by the discovery that the amyloid found in some well-defined groups of patients with the apparently autosomal recessive disorder familial Mediterranean fever was the AA protein (19). Virtually all Sephardic Jews and many Turks who display the clinical features of the disease (episodes of fever, arthralgias, and abdominal or pleuritic inflammation), develop renal amyloidosis, usually by the end of the second decade of life. Ashkenazi Jews, Armenians, and other groups display the episodic disease, but do not develop amyloid; therefore, two discrete events may be involved. In the first, presumably controlled by a gene or genes inherited in an autosomal recessive manner, there is a low threshold for triggering an inflammatory response. In non-Ashkenazi Jews, linkage has been established between the disease and a marker on chromosome 16 (20). The second, perhaps related to an inability to process the SAA produced in the course of the inflammation, is associated with renal amyloid deposition.

Fortunately, it has now been established that daily colchicine administration can abort both the acute episodes and the development of amyloid in susceptible individuals (21).

OTHER TYPES

Five different sites of amyloid deposition have been associated with aging, apparently without other predisposing disease (1). The fibril precursors have been identified in four of these: the beta protein of Alzheimer's disease (brain); islet associated polypeptide (pancreas), perhaps associated with type II diabetes mellitus; atrial natriuretic factor, the fibril of isolated atrial amyloid; and transthyretin, the fibril precursor of senile systemic (cardiac) amyloid. The precursor of human aortic amyloid has not yet been identified. Interestingly, mutant forms of both the beta protein and transthyretin have been associated with more severe, autosomal dominant forms of amyloid deposition in tissue sites similar to those seen in late onset conditions (22). While beta protein deposition has only been found to be significant in the brain, the mutant TTRs produce severe sensorimotor and autonomic neuropathy, vitreopathy, and nephropathy along with the cardiomyopathy. Some patients with the latter come to the attention of rheumatologists when they present with Charcot joints.

Additional rare, familial, autosomal dominant forms of amyloidosis have been associated with the deposition of mutant forms of several other proteins including gelsolin (Finnish familial amyloidotic polyneuropathy and lattice corneal dystrophy), cystatin C (Icelandic kindreds with hereditary cerebral hemorrhage with amyloidosis), apolipoprotein Al (Van Allen form of familial amyloidotic polyneuropathy), lysozyme (Ostertag hereditary, non-neuropathic amyloidosis), and the alpha chain of fibrinogen (22–24).

Many of the proteins contain within their structures a sequence of amino acids that have the capacity in vitro to associate either with the same or another sequence in adjacent molecules to form fibrils that are no longer soluble under physiologic conditions. It is likely that these stretches of sequence are constrained by the internal environments of the molecules in which they are embedded. If these constraints are lessened or removed (by mutation, proteolytic nicking, or incorporation of an oligosaccharide) or made less relevant by a local increase in concentration, a process of nucleation can occur that results in fibril formation. It is possible that most or all tissues have a complement of proteases capable of disposing of small amounts of such structures. When the capacity is exceeded by an increased substrate load, or is reduced by other physiologic or pathologic processes, the fibrils accumulate with resultant organ compromise. Only by understanding these phenomena will rational approaches to the therapy of these conditions be possible.

Joel Buxbaum, MD

1. Amyloid and Amyloidosis 1990. Edited by Natvig, JB, Forre O, Husby G, et al. Dordrecht, Kluwer Academic Publ. 1991.
2. Glenner, GG. Amyloid deposits and amyloidosis. The β-fibrilloses, N Engl J Med 302:1283–1292, 1980
3. Gallo GR, Feiner HD, Chuba JV, et al: Characterization of tissue amyloid by immunofluorescence microscopy. Clin Immunol Immunpathol 39:479–490, 1986
4. Gallo GR, Picken M, Frangione B, et al: Nonamyloidotic monoclonal immunoglobulin deposits lack amyloid P-component. Mod Pathol 1:453–456, 1988
5. Hind CRK: Amyloidosis and Amyloid P-component. New York, NY, Wiley, 1989
6. Hawkins PN, Cavender JP, Pepys MB: Evaluation of systemic amyloidosis by scinigraphy with ^{125}I labeled serum amyloid P-component. N Engl J Med 323:508–513, 1990
7. Kyle RA, Greipp PR: Amyloidosis (AL) clinical and laboratory features in 229 cases. Mayo Clin Proc 58:665–683, 1983
8. Cueto–Garcia L, Tajik J, Kyle RA, et al: Serial echocardiographic observations in patients with primary systemic amyloidosis: an introduction to the concept of early (asymptomatic) amyloid infiltration of the heart. Mayo Clin Proc 59:589–597, 1984
9. Rubinow A, Skinner M, Cohen AS: Digoxin sensitivity in amyloid cardiomyopathy. Circulation 63:1285–1288, 1981
10. Gertz MA, Falk RH, Skinner M, et al: Worsening of congestive heart failure in amyloid heart disease treated by calcium channel blocking agents. Am J Cardiol 55:1645, 1985
11. Wiernik PH, Amyloid joint disease. Medicine 51:465–479, 1972
12. Greipp Pr, Kyle RA, Bowie EJW: Factor X deficiency in amyloidosis: a critical review. Am J Hematol 11:443–450, 1981
13. Buxbaum JN: Mechanisms of disease: monoclonal immunoglobulin deposition. Hematol/Oncol Clinics of N Am 6:323, 1992.
14. Gertz MA, Kyle RA, Greipp PR: Response rates and survival in primary systemic amyloidosis. Blood 77:257–262, 1991
15. Proceedings VIIth International Symposium on Amyloidosis, Kingston, Ontario, July 11–15, 1993
16. Gejyo F, Yamada T, Odani S, et al: A new form of amyloid protein associated with chronic hemodialysis was identified as Beta 2 Microglobulin. Bioch Biophys Res Commun 129:701–706, 1985
17. Sletten K, Husby G: The complete amino acid sequence of nonimmunoglobulin amyloid fibril AS in rheumatoid arthritis. Eur J Biochem 41:117–125, 1974
18. Levin M, Franklin EC, Frangione B, et al: The amino acid sequence of a major non-immunoglobulin component of some amyloid fibrils. J Clin Invest 51:2773–2776, 1972
19. Heller H, Sohar L, Sherf L: Familial Mediterranean fever. Arch Intern Med 102:50–71, 1958
20. Pras E, Aksentijevich I, Gruberg L, et al: Mapping of a gene causing Familial Mediterranean Fever to the short arm of chromosome 16. N Engl J Med 326:1509, 1992.
21. Zemer D, Revach M, Pras M, et al: A controlled trial of colchicine in preventing attacks of familial Mediterranean fever. N Engl J Med 291:932–934, 1974
22. Jacobson DR, Buxbaum JN: Genetic aspects of amyloidosis. Adv Hum Genet 20:69–123, 1991
23. Benson MD, Liepnieks J, Uemichi T, et al: Hereditary renal amyloidosis associated with a mutant fibrinogen alpha chain. Nature genetics 3:252, 1993.
24. Pepys MB, Hawkins PN, Booth DR, et al: Human lysozyme gene mutations cause hereditary systemic amyloidosis. Nature 362:553, 1993.

37. NEOPLASMS OF THE JOINTS

Primary true neoplasms of joints, tendon sheaths, and bursae are rare (1,2). The majority arise from the synovium and are benign. A number of non-neoplastic, traumatic, or inflammatory lesions can produce tumor-like swellings in or around the joints and be confused with true joint neoplasms (Table 37–1).

BENIGN NEOPLASMS AND TUMORAL CONDITIONS

Pigmented Villonodular Synovitis

Pigmented villonodular synovitis is an uncommon benign disease, of unknown etiology, characterized by circumscribed or diffuse nodular thickening of the synovial lining of joints, tendon sheaths, or bursae with the production of locally invasive, tumor-like growths (1–7). The lesion consists of masses of matted, reddish-brown, synovial villous projections, intermingled with sessile and pedunculated nodular excrescences. Areas of hemorrhage and brown hemosiderin deposits are commonly present. The lesion may encroach on the articular cartilage and burrow into the subchondral bone, producing surface erosions and thin-walled cysts.

Histologic examination shows marked proliferation of synovial lining cells and the formation of numerous villi, fronds, and lobulated masses that fuse together to form nodules. There is a dense heterogeneous, subsynovial, cellular infiltrate, which consists predominantly of large, polyhedral or round, mononuclear cells, and a variable number of lipid-laden macrophages (foam or xanthoma cells), hemosiderin-laden macrophages, scattered multinucleated giant cells, fibroblasts, and lymphocytes (Fig. 37–1). Cleftlike spaces are occasionally present. Large mononuclear cells are the most characteristic finding. Electron microscopic studies have demonstrated two populations of these cells: macrophagelike cells (type-A synovial lining cells), and fibroblastlike cells (type-B lining cells), suggesting derivation of the lesion from the synovium. The condition is considered by many to be a true, slowly progressive, locally invasive but nonmalignant, nonmetastasizing neoplasm of synovial tissue (2).

Three forms of the disease have been identified: 1) a diffuse lesion involving much of the synovium of a joint, tendon sheath, or bursa (*diffuse pigmented villonodular synovitis*); 2) a solitary, intraarticular nodular lesion (*localized nodular synovitis*); and 3) an isolated, discrete lesion involving the tendon sheath (*localized nodular tenosynovitis*, or *giant cell tumor of tendon sheath*) (1–5). The histologic appearance is essentially identical in all three.

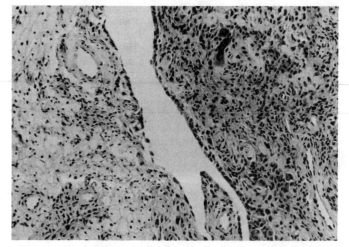

Fig. 37–1. *Diffuse pigmented villonodular synovitis: histopathologic section showing polyhedral histiocytes, scattered multinucleated giant cells, foam cells, lymphocytes, and hemosiderin deposits (magnification ×250).*

Diffuse pigmented villonodular synovitis. Diffuse pigmented villonodular synovitis usually involves the knee (80%), but may occasionally involve the hip, ankle, other joints, tendon sheaths, or bursae. Multiple lesions are extremely rare. It occurs most frequently in young adults; the sex incidence is equal. Insidious pain, limitation of movement, and monarticular joint swelling are the most common presenting complaints. The involved joint is swollen and tender, and exhibits limited movement, synovial thickening, and sometimes palpable synovial masses. Recurrent serosanguinous, dark brown, or xanthochromic joint effusions, in the absence of a history of trauma, are a useful diagnostic clue. Recently, lipid microspherules and lipid-laden foam cells have been demonstrated in some synovial fluids (8).

The most common radiographic finding is soft tissue swelling with thickening and lobulation of the synovium. Calcification does not occur, but increased density of the synovium secondary to hemosiderin deposition may be observed. Bony changes are found in long-standing cases and consist of pressure erosions of articular surfaces, clusters of thin-walled subchondral cysts, and joint space narrowing (3,5,6). Arthrography, sonography, computed tomography (CT), and magnetic resonance imaging (MRI) improve the diagnostic accuracy particularly in the early stages of the disease (5,6,9). Magnetic resonance imaging is particularly useful in defining the entire synovial lesion and the extent of bone erosions (5,6,9). The diagnosis is best made by arthroscopy, which reveals the shaggy, proliferative, brown-stained synovium, and allows a definitive tissue biopsy under direct vision.

Total synovectomy, with meticulous excision of the entire synovium, is the treatment of choice (2,3,5,6). However, the recurrence rate is high (20% to 40%), presumably due to incomplete removal of the lesion. Recurrent lesions can be treated by arthroscopic resection, intraarticular yttrium-90 radiation synovectomy (10), or by radiotherapy. Reconstructive surgery, including total hip or knee arthroplasty, is indicated for those with extensive joint destruction (6).

Localized nodular synovitis. Localized pigmented villonodular synovitis, affecting only one area of the synovium, occurs less frequently than the diffuse form (1–3,5,6). It usually presents as a solitary, sessile or pedunculated, lobulated nodule in either the medial or lateral compartment of the knee joint.

Intermittent pain, swelling, and episodes of "locking" and "giving way" of the knee are the principal complaints. A mass is sometimes palpable in the medial or lateral compartment, and the condition is often mistaken for a meniscal tear or a parameniscal cyst. Synovial effusions are less sanguinous than those in the diffuse form. Arthroscopy combined with synovial biopsy offers

Table 37–1. *Types of tumors of joints, tendon sheaths, and bursae*

Benign
  Neoplasms and tumoral conditions
    Pigmented villonodular synovitis
    Synovial chondromatosis (osteochondromatosis)
    Other benign tumors: lipoma including lipoma arborescens, chondroma, hemangioma, fibroma
  Tumor-like lesions
    Synovial cysts, parameniscal cyst, posttraumatic intraarticular synovial hematoma, intraarticular ossicles, ganglion, bursitis, nodules, tumoral calcinosis.
Malignant
  Primary
    Synovial sarcoma (malignant synovioma): biphasic, monophasic, and poorly differentiated
    Clear cell sarcoma
    Epithelioid sarcoma
    Synovial chondrosarcoma
  Secondary
    Metastatic carcinomatous arthropathy
    Contiguous spread of malignant bone tumors
    Joint invasion by leukemia, lymphoma, myeloma

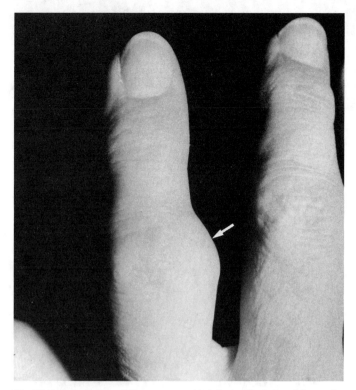

Fig. 37–2. *Localized nodular tenosynovitis (giant cell tumor of the tendon sheath) of the index finger (arrow).*

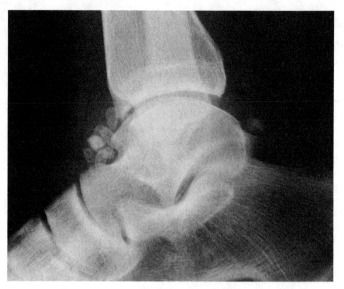

Fig. 37–3. *Synovial osteochondromatosis of the ankle: lateral radiograph, showing multiple calcified bodies of various sizes with good preservation of the articular cartilage.*

the best means of diagnosis. Surgical excision of the lesion is generally curative.

Localized nodular tenosynovitis. Localized nodular tenosynovitis, also called giant cell tumor of the tendon sheath or fibroxanthoma of the tendon sheath, is the most common form of pigmented villonodular synovitis (1–3,5–7). The lesion occurs most frequently in the tendon sheaths of the hand but occasionally involves the foot. It is the second most frequent soft tissue mass of the hand after ganglia. A *ganglion* is a thin-walled, sac filled with a viscous fluid, often in continuity with a joint or tendon sheath. The dorsum of the wrist is the most common site.

Localized nodular tenosynovitis occurs most frequently in young and middle-aged women. It presents as a discrete, multi-lobulated, nodular, slowly-growing mass affixed to a tendon sheath, most often the flexor sheath of the index or middle fingers (Fig. 37–2). Radiographs show a soft tissue swelling and sometimes an underlying bony pressure erosion. It may occur more often than expected by chance in patients with rheumatoid arthritis (RA) (3). Surgical excision is the treatment of choice.

Synovial Chondromatosis (Osteochondromatosis)

Synovial chondromatosis is a rare benign disorder of unknown etiology, characterized by the formation of multiple foci of metaplastic hyaline cartilage in the synovial membrane of joints, tendon sheaths, or bursae (Fig. 37–3) (1,2,11,12). Microscopic and ultrastructural studies indicate that the cartilaginous nodules develop as a result of metaplastic transformation of subsynovial fibroblasts to chondrocytes. The term *synovial osteochondromatosis* is used when endochondral ossification occurs within the cartilaginous masses. As the cartilaginous nodules grow, they form multiple sessile or pedunculated masses within the thickened synovial membrane. The nodules often undergo calcification or ossification, and many become detached from the synovium into the joint cavity forming loose bodies. Three overlapping phases of the disease have been described: 1) an early active phase with cartilage metaplasia in the subsynovial tissue but no loose bodies, 2) an intermediate phase with active intrasynovial disease and loose bodies, and 3) a late phase with multiple loose bodies but no intrasynovial disease.

The knee is the most frequently involved joint but the hip, elbow, shoulder, ankle, or other joints may be affected. Multiple joint involvement, and extraarticular synovial chondromatosis affecting a bursal lining or tenosynovial sheath, are rare. The disease occurs in young and middle-aged adults, and is twice as common in men as in women. It typically presents as a chronic, slowly progressive, monarticular arthropathy in an otherwise healthy individual. Symptoms include intermittent pain, stiffness, swelling, and episodes of "locking" and giving way. Limitation of movement, synovial thickening, crepitus, palpable loose bodies, and sometimes a small effusion are the main findings.

The radiographic finding of multiple stippled calcifications within the confines of the joint capsule is highly diagnostic of synovial osteochondromatosis. However, milder forms of the disease can be confused with osteoarthritis (OA) associated with loose bodies (secondary synovial osteochondromatosis), and with synovial calcification secondary to chronic calcium pyrophosphate crystal deposition disease. Both CT and MRI examinations are helpful in defining the nature of the lesions and their intraarticular origin. In doubtful cases, the diagnosis can be confirmed by arthroscopic examination and synovial biopsy under direct vision. Arthroscopy is particularly useful in assessing the extent of the disease (localized vs generalized), and the condition of the articular cartilage (12).

Although synovial chondromatosis may be self-limiting and undergo spontaneous regression, mechanical derangement from the pedunculated cartilaginous masses and loose bodies can damage the joint and cause secondary osteoarthritic changes. Removal of all loose bodies and surgical synovectomy with complète excision of the abnormal synovium are, therefore, recommended (11). Partial surgical or arthroscopic synovectomy and removal of loose bodies are indicated in those with localized disease (11,12). Removal of loose bodies alone is sometimes adequate in late phases of the disease. The recurrence rate is generally low, and the lesion rarely undergoes malignant transformation into synovial chondrosarcoma (1,2).

Other Benign Tumors

Other benign joint tumors include lipoma, chondroma, hemangioma, and fibroma (1). True intraarticular *lipoma* is extremely rare. It presents as a lobulated fatty mass, most frequently located in the infrapatellar fat pad of the knee. *Lipoma arborescens* (or diffuse articular lipomatosis) is a more common diffuse lesion, characterized by numerous villous and polypoid fatty synovial projections and appears most often in the suprapatellar region of the knee (1,13). It occurs either as a primary lesion, or more commonly, in association with OA or traumatic lesions of the knee. Gradual knee swelling with pain, intermittent clear effusions, and restriction of movements are the main presenting symptoms. The diagnosis can be confirmed by arthroscopy. Treatment consists of surgical or arthroscopic synovectomy and correction of any underlying mechanical knee problem.

Intracapsular solitary chondroma is a rare, benign, circumscribed neoplasm of hyaline cartilage that may demonstrate partial calcification. It presents as an intracapsular or intraarticular mass usually located in the infrapatellar region of the knee (1).

Synovial hemangioma is a rare condition that occurs most often in the knee joint (1). Two forms are recognized: a circumscribed, true hemangioma and a diffuse hemangiomatous form involving part of or all of the entire synovial membrane and adjacent tissues and bone. The diagnosis is suspected in children and young adults presenting with recurrent, otherwise unexplained episodes of knee hemarthrosis. The lesion can be demonstrated by arteriography, radionuclide angiography, CT, arthrography or arthroscopy. Surgical excision, whenever possible, is the treatment of choice.

MALIGNANT TUMORS

Primary Malignant Tumors

Primary malignant neoplasms of the joints and periarticular tissues are rare (1,2,14–17). Synovial sarcoma is the principal lesion, which primarily occurs in the paraarticular regions, usually in close association with tendon sheaths, bursae, or joint capsules. Clear cell sarcoma of tendons and aponeuroses (16), and epithelioid sarcoma (17) are two other malignant tumors with an origin in the paraarticular and periarticular fascial and tendinous tissues of the extremities.

Synovial sarcoma. Synovial sarcoma or malignant synovioma, is a highly malignant fibroblastic neoplasm of adolescents and young adults (1,2,14,15). It often originates within the fascial planes of the thigh or leg, in the vicinity of the knee or foot, but it may occur in the foot, hand, back or at other nonarticular sites such as abdominal wall. The tumor seldom originates within the joint; articular involvement nearly always results from extension of a nearby primary tumor.

Histologic examination shows a characteristic *biphasic* (bimorphic) cellular pattern with large, polyhedral, cuboidal, mucincontaining epithelial-like cells lining clefts, tubules and irregular gland-like spaces, or arranged in cords or nests, and spindle-shaped stromal cells resembling fibroblasts (Fig. 37–4). In other tumors, one of these two cell populations may predominate, giving rise to a *monophasic* (monomorphic) synovial sarcoma, most commonly of the spindle cell type and less frequently of the epithelial cell pseudoglandular type. A rare third type of poorly differentiated synovial sarcoma carries a worse prognosis. Focal areas of hemorrhage, necrosis, cystic degeneration and calcification are commonly present in the tumor, and foci of calcification occur in about 30% of lesions.

Although there are similarities between synovial sarcoma and normal synovium, a synovial origin has never been proven (2,14,15). Ultrastructural and immunohistochemical studies of synovial sarcoma have shown a number of dissimilarities from normal synovium: 1) presence of a distinct basal lamina between epithelial and stromal cells, 2) specialized cell junctions including desmosomes and maculae adherentes, and 3) positive stains for proteins of cytoskeletal components (cytokeratins in the epithelial-like cells and vimentin in stromal spindle-shaped cells), and less frequently for epithelial membrane antigen and carcinoembryonic antigen. Current evidence suggests that synovial sarcoma is derived from primitive mesenchymal cells capable of differentiating into epithelial and fibroblast spindle-shaped cells (2,14,15).

The usual clinical presentation of synovial sarcoma is a slowly growing, deep-seated, mass adjacent to the knee or foot. Pain and tenderness occur in about 50% of patients. The most common radiographic finding is a paraarticular, lobulated, soft tissue swelling. Speckled calcification occurs in 30% of lesions and

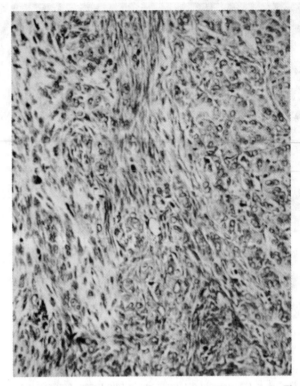

Fig. 37–4. *Photomicrograph of synovial sarcoma (synovioma). There is an inextricable admixture of two types of malignant cells: one is present in clumps and cords of polyhedral and ovoid cells that are epithelioid in appearance; the other consists of fibroblastlike elements with large fusiform nuclei.*

produces a characteristic radiographic appearance (Fig. 37–5). Erosion of the underlying bone is observed in about 20% of patients. Arteriography, CT, and MRI are useful in defining the anatomic location of the mass and its relation to adjacent soft tissue prior to surgical planning (18).

A treatment approach utilizing radical surgery, radiotherapy, and combination chemotherapy has improved the overall prognosis of synovial sarcoma. However, the recurrence rate is high,

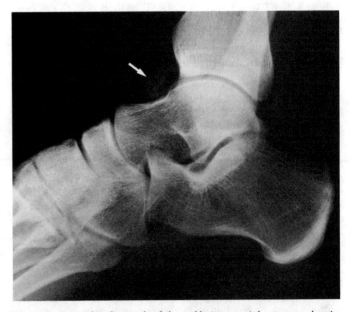

Fig. 37–5. *Lateral radiograph of the ankle in synovial sarcoma showing a cluster of fine speckled calcifications anterior to the joint (**arrow**) (courtesy of Dr J Rubenstein).*

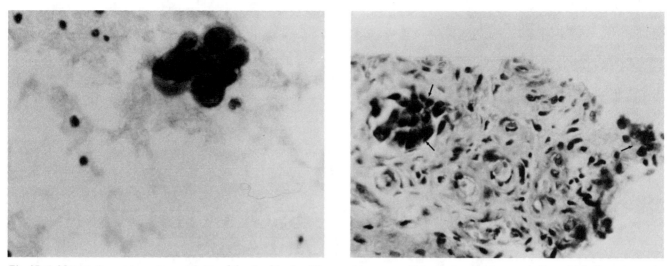

Fig. 37–6. *Metastatic carcinomatous arthritis of the shoulder in a 77-year-old woman with lung adenocarcinoma: A. Synovial fluid cytology, showing clumps of neoplastic cells with pleomorphic, eccentric, hyperchromatic, multiple nuclei; large irregular nucleoli; and distinct cell membranes (Papanicolaou stain). B. Synovial membrane of the right shoulder showing nests of carcinomatous metastases (magnification ×400).*

nosis of synovial sarcoma. However, the recurrence rate is high, with distant metastases to the lungs, regional lymph nodes, bones, and other sites. The five-year survival rate is about 55%; at 10-years survival is about 40% (1,2). Favorable clinical and histologic variables include young age, small tumors (under 5 cm in diameter), a highly grandular biphasic sarcoma with a low mitotic count (<15 per 10 high power field) and presence of calcification within the tumor (2,19).

Clear cell sarcoma. Clear cell sarcoma is a rare malignant tumor of tendons, fascial aponeuroses, and ligaments (1,2,16,20). Its exact cell of origin is not known. The tumor is more common in young adults and is characterized by a slowly growing mass that is usually painless. It is most commonly located in the foot, particularly near the Achilles tendon or plantar aponeurosis. It consists of nests and clusters of fusiform and polygonal cells with clear cytoplasm, pale vesicular nuclei, and prominent nucleoli. Use of MRI may help to define the infiltrative margins of the lesion and its peritendinous or periaponeurotic location (18).

Several lines of evidence suggest that clear cell sarcoma represents a soft tissue malignant melanoma of neuroectodermal origin (1,2,16,20). Melanin can be demonstrated in the tumor by histochemical staining, and ultrastructural studies have confirmed the presence of premelanosomes. Immunoperoxidase stains for the neuroectodermal marker, S-100 protein, and for HMB–45, a melanoma-specific monoclonal antibody, are usually positive (16). Chromosomal abnormalities, similar to those associated with malignant melanoma, have also been noted (20). These observations indicate that the tumor probably originates from melanogenic cells that have migrated during embryonic life from the neural crest into the vicinity of tendons and fasciae.

The prognosis is poor. The lesion is highly malignant with marked propensity for local recurrence and distant metastases.

Epithelioid sarcoma. Epithelioid sarcoma is a rare, malignant, soft tissue neoplasm of tendinous and fascial structures (1,2,17). It consists of irregular nodular masses made up of two types of cells: numerous large polygonal epithelioid cells and a few spindle-shaped cells. This biphasic cellular pattern and the findings from ultrastructural, enzyme, and immunohistochemical studies suggest that the lesion may be a variant of synovial sarcoma. Epithelioid sarcoma often presents as a rapidly growing, nodular lesion along tendon sheaths or fascial planes, usually in the upper extremity (hand, wrist or forearm). Central necrosis of tumor nodules and ulceration of the overlying skin are common.

The clinical course is one of recurrent tumor and ultimately distant metastases. The five-year survival rate is about 70% (17).

Synovial chondrosarcoma. Primary synovial chondrosarcoma is extremely rare. Most cases are either malignant transformation of a preexistent synovial chondromatosis or direct spread from a primary metaphyseal bone chondrosarcoma.

Secondary Malignant Tumors

Secondary involvement of joints occurs as a complication of contiguous spread of primary bone sarcomas, carcinomatous metastases, or invasion by leukemia, lymphoma, or myeloma.

Metastatic carcinomatous arthropathy. Arthritis is rarely caused by metastatic carcinomatous deposits in and around joints. This often occurs as a late complication of the primary tumor, usually carcinoma of the lung. Joint involvement is typically monarticular, affecting principally the knee but occasionally the hip, ankle, or other joints including even the digits. Joint effusions are commonly hemorrhagic and reaccumulate rapidly after aspiration. Tumor cells can be demonstrated in the synovial fluid (Fig. 37–6A). Radiographs may reveal juxtaarticular osteolytic lesions. Arthroscopic or percutaneous needle synovial biopsy may reveal carcinomatous invasion of the synovium (Fig. 37–6B) (see also Chapter 35).

Involvement of joints by primary bone tumors. Primary metaphyseal malignant bone tumors, including osteosarcoma, chondrosarcoma, and fibrosarcoma, can directly invade adjacent joints by direct extension beneath the joint capsule, along intraarticular ligaments, or less frequently, across the articular cartilage.

Subperiosteal osteoid osteomas. Juxtaarticular osteoid osteomas are sometimes associated with a mild "reactive" synovitis of the neighboring joint, with articular pain often worse at night and relieved by aspirin, stiffness, and swelling mimicking monarthritis (21).

Adel G. Fam, MD

1. Schajowicz F: Tumors and Tumor-like Lesions of Bone and Joints. New York, NY, Springer-Verlag, 1981, pp 519–567
2. Enzinger FM, Weiss SW: Soft Tissue Tumors, 2nd ed. St. Louis, Mo CV Mosby, 1988, pp 638–688, 861–881
3. Myers BW, Masi AT, Feigenbaum SL: Pigmented villonodular synovitis and tenosynovitis: a clinical epidemiologic study of 166 cases and literature review. Medicine 59:223–238, 1980
4. Schumacher HR, Lotke P, Athreya B, et al: Pigmented villonodular synovitis: light and electron microscopic studies. Semin Arthritis Rheum 12:32–43, 1982
5. Goldman AB, DiCarlo EF: Pigmented villonodular synovitis. Diagnosis and differential diagnosis. Radiol Clin N Am 26(6):1327–1347, 1988
6. Schwartz HS, Unni KK, Pritchard DJ: Pigmented villonodular synovitis. A retrospective review of affected large joints. Clin Orthop 247:243–255, 1989
7. Moore JR, Weiland AJ, Curtis RM: Localized nodular tenosynovitis: experience with 115 cases. J Hand Surg 9A:412–417, 1984
8. Ugai K, Kurosaka M, Hirohata K: Lipid microspherules in synovial fluid of patients with pigmented villonodular synovitis. Arthritis Rheum 31:1442–1446, 1988
9. Weisz GM, Gal A, Kitchener PN: Magnetic resonance imaging in the diagnosis of aggressive villonodular synovitis. Clin Orthop 236:303–306, 1988
10. Gumpel JM, Shawe DJ: Diffuse pigmented villonodular synovitis: non-surgical management. Ann Rheum Dis 50:531–533, 1991
11. Maurice H, Crone M, Watt I: Synovial chondromatosis. J Bone Joint Surg 70-B:807–811, 1988
12. Coolican MR, Dandy DJ: Arthroscopic management of synovial chondroma-

10. Gumpel JM, Shawe DJ: Diffuse pigmented villonodular synovitis: non-surgical management. Ann Rheum Dis 50:531–533, 1991

11. Maurice H, Crone M, Watt I: Synovial chondromatosis. J Bone Joint Surg 70-B:807–811, 1988

12. Coolican MR, Dandy DJ: Arthroscopic management of synovial chondromatosis of the knee. Findings and results in 18 cases. J Bone Joint Surg 71-B:498–500, 1989

13. Hallel T, Lew S, Bansal M: Villous lipomatous proliferation of the synovial membrane (lipoma arborescens). J Bone Joint Surg 70(A):264–270, 1988

14. Ghadially FN: Is synovial sarcoma a carcinosarcoma of connective tissue? Ultrastruct Pathol 11:147–151, 1987

15. Ordónez NG, Mahfouz SM, Mackay B: Synovial sarcoma: an immunohistochemical and ultrastructural study. Hum Pathol 21:733–749, 1990

16. Mechtersheimer G, Tilgen W, Klar E, et al: Clear cell sarcoma of tendons and aponeuroses: case presentation with special reference to immunohistochemical findings. Hum Pathol 20:914–917, 1989

17. Bos GD, Pritchard DJ, Reiman HM, et al: Epithelioid sarcoma. An analysis of fifty-one cases. J Bone Joint Surg 70-A:862–870, 1988

18. Wetzel LH, Levine E: Soft-tissue tumors of the foot: value of MR imaging for specific diagnosis. AJR 155:1025–1030, 1990

19. Cagle LA, Mirra JM, Storm FK, et al: Histologic features relating to prognosis in synovial sarcoma. Cancer 59:1810–1814, 1987

20. Bridge JA, Sreekantaiah C, Neff JR, et al: Cytogenetic findings in clear cell sarcoma of tendons and aponeuroses. Malignant melanoma of soft parts. Cancer Genet Cytogenet 52:101–106, 1991

21. Brabants K, Geens S, Van Damme B: Subperiosteal juxtaarticular osteoid osteoma. J Bone Joint Surg 68B:320–324, 1986

38. ARTHROPATHIES ASSOCIATED WITH ENDOCRINE DISEASES

Musculoskeletal complaints may be the first clue in the detection of certain endocrine diseases and are often curable by treatment of the underlying disorder (1). The presence of carpal tunnel syndrome, fibromyalgia, joint hyperlaxity, crystal deposition disease, capsulitis of the shoulder (periarthritis), proximal myopathy, or osteopenia should raise the diagnostic possibility of a causative or contributory endocrinopathy.

HYPERPARATHYROIDISM

Hyperparathyroidism causes osteitis fibrosa cystica, subperiosteal bone resorption, generalized muscular aching and stiffness, joint laxity, osteoarthritis, erosive arthritis of the hands, back pain, vertebral fractures mimicking senile osteoporosis, and spontaneous tendon avulsion and rupture. Hyperparathyroid neuropathy is associated with proximal lower extremity weakness and atrophy, muscle aching after use, intact deep tendon reflexes, and normal creatine kinase levels. Even asymptomatic patients with elevated serum and parathyroid hormone (PTH) levels have been found to have paresthesias, muscle cramps, and stocking glove loss of pain and vibratory sensation (2). In hyperparathyroidism resulting from renal failure, ischemic skin necrosis and vascular and periarticular calcifications (due to apatite crystal deposition) are also seen. In dialysis patients with extreme levels of serum PTH, destructive erosive spondylarthropathy has been halted with parathyroidectomy (3).

Thirty-five percent of hyperparathyroid patients have chondrocalcinosis (4). Acute postoperative arthritis may be due to gout or pseudogout; both can coexist with hyperparathyroidism (refer to Chapters 31–32).

HYPOPARATHYROIDISM

With *hypoparathyroidism*, a disease similar to ankylosing spondylitis with normal sacroiliac joints has been reported (5). The patient may have hypocalcemic muscular cramps, subcutaneous calcification (nodules), and carpopedal spasm with tingling. Vitamin D and calcium replacement alleviate the neuromuscular complaints. *Pseudohypoparathyroidism* (hypocalcemia resistant to parathormone) is associated with shortened metacarpals and metatarsals.

HYPERTHYROIDISM

Hyperthyroid patients may complain of muscle weakness, bone pain caused by osteopenia, or shoulder periarthritis. The muscular weakness can result from thyrotoxic myopathy, periodic paralysis, or myasthenia gravis. Shoulder-hand syndrome can complicate the adhesive capsulitis (6). Restoration to the euthyroid state improves or halts many of these abnormalities. Diffusely swollen hands and feet associated with periostitis (thyroid acropachy) also occur in Graves' disease. This acropachy is generally unaffected by treatment of the thyrotoxicosis. Roent-

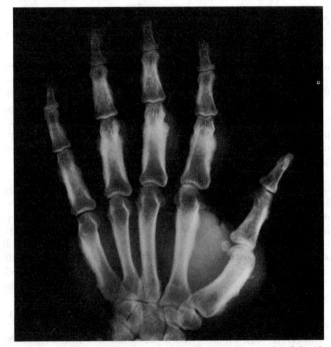

Fig. 38–1. *Thyroid acropachy showing an extreme example of the characteristic periosteal reaction in the hand.*

genograms often show periosteal reaction at the shafts of involved digits (Fig. 38–1). Propylthiouracil treatment of hyperthyroidism has resulted in vasculitis (7) and systemic lupus erythematosus.

Musculoskeletal symptoms may occur with Hashimoto's thyroiditis. Thyroiditis occurs with increased frequency in rheumatoid arthritis (RA) and possibly with eosinophilic fasciitis, mixed connective tissue disease, and systemic sclerosis (8).

HYPOTHYROIDISM

Primary *hypothyroidism* may be heralded by myalgias and other fibromyalgia-like complaints. Peripheral joints in myxedema can be affected by symmetric joint swelling mimicking RA (9). Joint fluid in hypothyroidism, unlike RA, is usually highly viscous and has low white cell counts of less than 1,000 cells/mm^3. Calcium pyrophosphate dihydrate (CPPD) crystal deposition disease (pseudogout) can coexist in many myxedematous patients. Crystals may be found in synovial fluids without any evidence of joint inflammation until thyroid replacement is begun; acute pseudogout may develop after replacement. Some series of patients with mild hypothyroidism have shown no increased incidence of CPPD deposition, but a recent meta-analysis did show the association. Muscle weakness may be associated with very high levels of creatine kinase activity, causing confusion with polymyositis. The presence of otherwise unexplained carpal tunnel syndrome should also suggest the possibility of hypothyroidism. Thyroid replacement results in striking resolution of most of these rheumatic complaints. Untreated hypothyroidism may predispose patients to clofibrate-induced myopathy (10). Hyperuricemia can result from decreased renal urate clearance.

ADRENAL DISORDERS

Cortisol excess (*Cushing's syndrome*), whether idiopathic or from treatment with glucocorticoids, may cause severe osteoporosis with compression fractures of spine and ribs, osteonecrosis (especially of the femoral head), and proximal muscle wasting. Creatine kinase levels are normal in steroid myopathy. Septic arthritis occurs more frequently with cortisol excess.

In *adrenal insufficiency*, severe muscle cramps and muscle contractures of the legs are reversible with steroid replacement (11). Pseudorheumatism (diffuse muscle, joint, and bony aching, as well as noninflammatory joint effusions) occurs when exogenous corticosteroids are withdrawn. Adrenal insufficiency appears to occur with increased frequency in the antiphospholipid syndrome (12).

Pheochromocytoma has presented with rhabdomyolysis and myoglobinuric renal failure, possibly due to catecholamine-mediated vasoconstriction and skeletal muscle ischemia (13).

PITUITARY DISORDERS

Acromegalic arthropathy results from the action of excessive growth hormone on cartilage, bone, and periarticular soft tissue. Early cartilage hypertrophy causes the joint space to appear widened on roentgenogram. This cartilage is friable, ulcerates at weight-bearing surfaces, and undergoes subsequent premature osteoarthritic narrowing. The cartilage and connective tissue overgrowth is manifested clinically by hypermobility of the spine, wrists, ankles, and knees. Carpal tunnel compression is also common. Roentgenograms of fingers show characteristic broad distal tufts and narrowed waists of the digits. Early diagnosis is now possible by serum human growth hormone levels and computerized tomography scan of the sella turcica. Prompt treatment may lead to dramatic resolution of some polyarthritis and spinal pain (14).

Men with prolactin-secreting pituitary tumors and *hypogonadism* have low bone mass. This can be reversed with testosterone replacement and bromocriptine, transphenoidal surgery, or radiation of the tumor (15).

In congenital vasopressin-resistant diabetes insipidus, serum urate concentration may be elevated as high as 15 mg/dl as a result of decreased renal clearance of urate.

DIABETES MELLITUS

Diabetes mellitus may be associated with several rheumatic problems (16). *Charcot joints* occur as a complication of neuropathy, predominantly in the tarsometatarsal area (Fig. 38–2). These may not be completely painless and can be confused with osteomyelitis, to which diabetics are also susceptible. Periarthritis of the shoulder, carpal tunnel syndrome, and flexor tendinitis in the palms also occur, as well as a peculiar form of digital sclerosis resembling scleroderma of the hands. Unlike scleroderma (skin thickening caused by increased synthesis of collagen), diabetic finger sclerosis reflects decreased removal of skin collagen and possibly increased tissue hydration (17). Increases

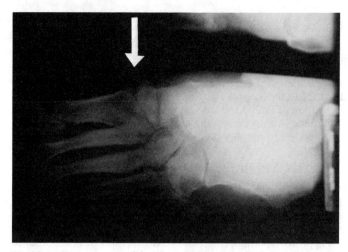

Fig. 38–2. *Tarsometatarsal destruction (arrow) in a diabetic neuropathic foot.*

in lysyloxidase-dependent cross links of collagen also appear to be involved (18). Adult and juvenile diabetics also experience painless contractures of the proximal interphalangeal and distal interphalangeal joints. Recognition of such joint contractures is important, because microvascular complications, such as nephropathy and retinopathy, probably parallel the presence of these contractures. A diffuse scleroderma-like induration of the back and trunk that has been termed *scleredema* also occurs in diabetics.

Bonnie B. Dorwart, MD

1. Bland JH, Frymoyer JW, Newberg AH, et al: Rheumatic syndromes in endocrine disease. Semin Arthritis Rheum 9:23–65, 1979
2. Turken SA, Cafferty M, Silverberg SJ, et al: Neuromuscular involvement in mild, asymptomatic primary hyperparathyroidism. Am J Med 87:553–557, 1989
3. McCarthy JT, Dahlberg PJ, Krieghauser JS, et al: Erosive spondyloarthropathy in long-term dialysis patients: relationship to severe hyperparathyroidism. Mayo Clin Proc 63:446–452, 1988
4. Pritchard MH, Jessop JD: Chondrocalcinosis in primary hyperparathyroidism. Ann Rheum Dis 36:146–151, 1977
5. Chaykin LB, Frame B, Sigler JW: Spondylitis: a clue to hypoparathyroidism. Ann Intern Med 70:995–1000, 1969
6. Wohlgethan JR: Frozen shoulder in hyperthyroidism. Arthritis Rheum 30:936–939, 1987
7. Houston BD, Crouch ME, Brick JE, et al: Apparent vasculitis associated with propylthiouracil use. Arthritis Rheum 30:936–939, 1979
8. Gordon MB, Klein I, Dekker A, et al: Thyroid disease in progressive systemic sclerosis: increased frequency of glandular fibrosis and hypothyroidism. Ann Intern Med 95:431–435, 1981
9. Dorwart BB, Schumacher HR: Joint effusions, chondrocalcinosis, and other rheumatic manifestations in hypothyroidism. Am J Med 59:780–790, 1975
10. Hattori N, Shimatsu A, Murabe H, et al: Clofibrate-induced myopathy in a patient with primary hypothyroidism. Jpn J Med 29:545–547, 1990
11. Shapiro MS, Trebich C, Shilo L, et al: Myalgias and muscle contractures as the presenting signs of Addison's disease. Postgrad Med J 64:222–223, 1988
12. Asherson RA, Hughes RA: Hypoadrenalism, Addison's disease and antiphospholipid antibodies. J Rheumatol 18:1–3, 1991
13. Shemin D, Cohn PS, Zipin SB: Pheochromocytoma presenting as rhabdomyolysis and acute myoglobinuric renal failure. Arch Intern Med 150:2384–2385, 1990
14. Lacks S, Jacobs RP: Acromegalic arthropathy: a reversible rheumatic disease. J Rheumatol 13:634–636, 1986
15. Greenspan SL, Oppenheim DS, Klibanski A: Importance of gonadal steroids to bone mass in men with hyperprolactinemic hypogonadism. Ann Intern Med 110:526–531, 1989
16. Gray RB, Gottlieb NL: Rheumatic disorders associated with diabetes mellitus: literature review. Semin Arthritis Rheum 6:19–34, 1976
17. Seibold JR, Uitto J, Dorwart BB, Prockop DJ: Collagen synthesis and collagenase activity in dermal fibroblasts from patients with diabetes and digital sclerosis. J Lab Clin Med 105:664–667, 1985
18. Buckingham B, Reiser KM: Relationships between the content of lysyloxidase dependent cross-links in skin collagen, nonenzymatic glycosylation and long term complications in type I diabetes. J Clin Invest 86:1046–1054, 1990

39. HYPERLIPOPROTEINEMIA AND ARTHRITIS

Diseases of the joints and tendons are underrecognized features of certain of the heritable disorders of lipoprotein metabolism. Musculoskeletal signs and symptoms, sometimes the first indication of lipid disorders, may alert the clinician to the underlying illness, thus facilitating more rapid diagnosis, dietary modification, and drug therapy.

TYPE II HYPERLIPOPROTEINEMIA

Several studies have described rheumatic syndromes associated with type II hyperlipoproteinemia. Articular disease is strikingly common in individuals afflicted with this disorder. Migratory polyarthritis occurs in 50% of young patients homozygous for type II hyperlipoproteinemia. Arthritis has been reported to occur principally in large peripheral joints, including the knees and ankles, but it may also occur in small joints of the lower and upper extremities. The joints are severely inflamed, red, hot, and swollen. Joint disease may be polyarticular and symmetric or oligoarticular. Episodes tend to be self-limited, lasting several days to two weeks. In some patients, the illness resembles rheumatic fever because of evanescent arthritis, increased erythrocyte sedimentation rate (ESR), increased antistreptolysin O titers, and the coincidence of atherosclerotic aortic valvular disease with aortic insufficiency. The valvular disease is a direct result of the hyperlipoproteinemia, and the elevated ESR is a result of high density lipoproteins, which accelerate red cell sedimentation (1–3).

In patients heterozygous for type II hyperlipoproteinemia, monarticular involvement of the knee or first metatarsophalangeal joint of the great toe is seen. Migratory polyarthritis involving up to six joints has been reported in some patients. Involved joints include the knee, proximal interphangeal joints, wrist, elbow, shoulder, and hip. In some patients, this polyarthritis is actually an inflammatory periarthritis or polytendinitis. In fact, recurrent Achilles tendinitis is a common problem in such patients. Synovial fluids from affected joints have had low white blood cell counts and have not generally contained crystals. Positively birefringent incompletely explained crystals were reported from a retrocalcaneal bursa adjacent to a xanthoma (4). These articular, tendinous, and periarticular findings have been reported in children, adolescents, and adults (5–7).

TYPE IV HYPERLIPOPROTEINEMIA

An arthropathy resembling that seen in type II hyperlipoproteinemia occurs in patients with type IV hyperlipoproteinemia (8–10). It should be noted that some individuals reported with the type IV variant actually may have had familial combined hyperlipidemia. Individuals within a single family with the combined variant may exhibit any one of three separate phenotypes, including types IIA, IIB, and type IV hyperlipoproteinemia, and may spontaneously convert from one lipoprotein phenotype to another. The patients with type IV hyperlipoproteinemia may have an asymmetric arthritis involving both small and large joints, including the proximal interphalangeal joints and the metacarpophalangeal joints in the hands, wrists, shoulders, knuckles, knees, tarsal, and metatarsophalangeal joints. In some patients the inflammatory disease is mild and persistent, while others experience episodic and recurrent disease. Morning stiffness of moderate duration is characteristic of the illness. Paraarticular hyperesthesia has been described by some patients. In a recent controlled study, oligoarthritis has been reported to occur with increased frequency in patients with mixed hyperlipidemia (11).

Synovial fluid is relatively noninflammatory and contains no crystals. In some patients with type IV disease, roentgenograms show prominent paraarticular bone cysts (Fig. 39–1). One such cyst contained material that was grossly yellow and mucinous and showed only fibrous tissue and fat cells on microscopic examination. There were no granulomas, cholesterol deposits, or

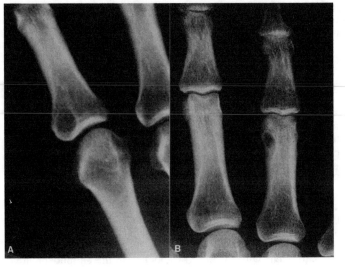

Fig. 39–1. *Paraarticular bone cysts are seen in the hands of two patients (panels A and B) with type IV hyperlipoproteinemia.*

lipid-laden histiocytes. Synovial biopsy in one patient revealed moderate hyperplasia of the synovial villi, prominent stromal vessels, and a moderate mononuclear infiltrate. In this patient an effort was made to ascertain the relationship between serum triglyceride levels and the degree of inflammation. Synovial biopsies performed after several days on a diet high in carbohydrates and calories showed a marked increase in synovial lipids and synovial inflammatory infiltrate. Four other patients experienced decreased articular inflammation after reduction or normalization of serum lipid levels. A relationship between tissue levels of arachidonic acid substrate and joint inflammation in these patients is possible.

OTHER HYPERLIPOPROTEINEMIAS

Reports of other skeletal lesions associated with hyperlipoproteinemia have been published. One patient with type V hyperlipoproteinemia had cystic lesions in both proximal femurs that contained yellow tissue, revealing foamy histiocytes and a granulomatous reaction around cholesterol clefts on microscopic examination (12).

Other investigators have noted joint changes resulting from infiltration of foam cells in subchondral bone in secondary hyperlipoproteinemia, such as that seen in patients with biliary cirrhosis. Secondary hyperlipoproteinemia associated with the nephrotic syndrome, pancreatitis, alcoholism, hypothyroidism, and diabetes mellitus may be seen. Whether this leads to musculoskeletal complaints in such cases is not known.

XANTHOMAS IN HYPERLIPOPROTEINEMIAS

Patients with type II hyperlipoproteinemia exhibit tendinous, tuberous, and periosteal xanthomas as well as xanthelasma, corneal ulcers, and early, rapidly progressive atherosclerosis. Tendinous xanthomas are located in Achilles and patellar tendons and in the extensor tendons of the hands and feet (13). Tendon xanthomas have also been found in the plantar fascia and in periosteum overlying the lower tibia and the peroneal tendons. These xanthomas reside within the tendon fibers rather than on the tendon sheath, and they cannot be separated from the tendon on movement. They contain large lipid-filled histiocytes within the collagenous connective tissue and are composed primarily of cholesterol and phospholipid. Tuberous xanthomas are soft subcutaneous masses occurring over extensor surfaces, especially on the elbows, knees, and hands, as well as on the buttocks. Individuals homozygous for type II hyperlipoproteinemia develop extensive xanthomas in childhood, whereas those who are heterozygous develop tendinous xanthomas after age 30 and lack tuberous xanthomas.

Tendinous and tuberous xanthomas also occur in type III and type IV hyperlipoproteinemia (1). A distinctive clinical feature of the type III disorder is lipid deposition, or plane xanthomas, in the palms of the hands. Types I, IV, and V hyperlipoproteinemia are characterized by eruptive xanthomas over the knees, buttocks, shoulders, and back.

Cerebrotendinous xanthomatosis is a rare, familial, and apparently autosomal recessive disorder characterized by progressive cerebellar ataxia, dementia, spinal cord paresis, subnormal intelligence, tendon xanthomas, and cataracts (14). Cholestanol, or dihydrocholesterol, accumulates in the nervous tissue, tendons, and other tissues. The underlying defect has not been identified, and no specific treatment is available. Tendon xanthomas appear as early as the second decade, but they are usually first noted in the third or fourth decade. The Achilles tendons are the most common sites, but xanthomas may also occur in the triceps tendons, at the tibial tuberosities, and in the extensor tendons of the hands. Tuberous xanthomas and xanthelasma may occur also.

Tendon xanthomas also constitute a feature of β-sitosterolemia, another rare familial lipid storage disease marked by the accumulation of plant sterols in the blood and tissues (15). These individuals have an increased intestinal absorption of dietary β-sitosterol, but the underlying metabolic defect has not yet been defined. The patient's serum cholesterol level may be normal or moderately elevated. Inheritance is autosomal recessive. Tendon xanthomas, indistinguishable histologically from those found in hyperlipoproteinemia, appear during childhood, initially in the extensor tendons of the hands and later in the patellar, plantar and Achilles tendons.

Tendinous, tuberous, and eruptive xanthomas have also been observed in patients with type II or type IV hyperlipoproteinemia associated with the development of multiple myeloma, as well as in some patients with myelomatosis without definite hyperlipoproteinemia (16). Myeloma protein may interfere with lipid transport by at least two mechanisms. One involves heparin–paraprotein interaction and results in heparin resistance and impaired uptake of the remnant of glyceride-rich lipoproteins. The other involves the formation of complexes among myeloma protein, lipoprotein, and cholesterol.

Robert B. Buckingham, MD

1. Frederickson DS, Levy RI, Lees RS: Fat transport in lipoproteins: an integrated approach to mechanisms and disorders. N Engl J Med 276:34–44, 1967
2. Khachadurian AK: Migratory polyarthritis in familial hypercholesterolemia (type II hyperlipoproteinemia). Arthritis Rheum 11:385–393, 1968
3. Rimon D, Cohen L: Hypercholesterolemic (type II hyperlipoproteinemic) arthritis. J Rheumatol 16:703–705, 1989
4. Schumacher HR, Michaels R: Recurrent tendinitis and Achilles tendon nodule with positively birefringent crystals in a patient with hyperlipoproteinemia. J Rheum 16:1387–1389, 1989
5. Glueck CJ, Levy RI, Fredrickson DS: Acute tendinitis and arthritis: presenting symptom of familial type II hyperlipoproteinemia. JAMA 206:2895–2897, 1968
6. Rooney PJ, Third J, Madkour MM, et al: Transient polyarthritis associated with familial hyperbetalipoproteinemia. Q J Med 187:249–259, 1978
7. Mathon G, Gagne C, Brun D, et al: Articular manifestations of familial hypercholesterolemia. Ann Rheum Dis 44:599–602, 1985
8. Buckingham RB, Bole GG, Bassett DR: Polyarthritis associated with type IV hyperlipoproteinemia. Arch Intern Med 135:286–290, 1975
9. Goldman JA, Glueck CJ, Abrams NR, et al: Musculoskeletal disorders associated with type IV hyperlipoproteinemia. Lancet 2:449–452, 1972
10. Menkes CJ, Laoussadi S, Auvert L, et al: Oligo-arthritis associated with type IV hyperlipoproteinemia. Presse Medicale 16:1414–1418, 1987
11. Klemp P, Halland AM, Majoos FL, et al: Musculoskeletal manifestations in hyperlipidaemia: a controlled study. Ann Rheum Dis 52:44–48, 1993
12. Siegelmann SS, Schlossberg I, Becker NH, et al: Hyperlipoproteinemia with skeletal lesions. Clin Orthop 87:228–232, 1972
13. Fahey JJ, Stark HH, Donovan WF, et al: Xanthoma of the Achilles tendon. J Bone Joint Surg 55A:(1) 1197–1211, 1973
14. Truswell AS, Pfister PJ: Cerebrotendinous xanthomatosis. Br Med J 1:353–354, 1972
15. Shulman RS, Bhattacharyya AK, Connor WE, et al: Beta-sitosterolemia and xanthomatosis. N Engl J Med 294:482–483, 1976
16. Neufeld ARH, Morton HS, Halpenny GW: Myelomatosis with xanthomatosis multiforme. Can Med Assoc J 91:374–380, 1964

40. MUSCULOSKELETAL PROBLEMS IN DIALYSIS PATIENTS

Patients treated with prolonged hemodialysis are now surviving longer and are increasingly developing musculoskeletal problems. Renal osteodystrophy, crystal deposition and β_2 microglobulin amyloidosis are presently recognized as the major etiologic factors.

RENAL OSTEODYSTROPHY

Secondary Hyperparathyroidism

Hyperparathyroid bone disease remains the most frequent form of renal osteodystrophy. Primary factors of uremic hyperparathyroidism are hyperphosphatemia, deficient generation of 1,25-dihydroxyvitamin D by the kidney, low calcium intake and absorption, and insensitivity of the parathyroid gland to the suppressive effects of calcium on parathyroid hormone (PTH) secretion (1). Preventive treatments include the use of high dialysate calcium concentration and control of phosphatemia by dietary phosphorus restriction, and prescription, as phosphorus binders, of calcium acetate, or carbonate with meals. Further enrichment of diet with calcium supplements between meals, and vitamin D derivatives may also be necessary. The use of aluminum containing phosphate binders is now drastically restricted because of the risk of aluminum intoxication.

Secondary hyperparathyroidism is usually asymptomatic but may be the source of bone pain or polyarthralgia. Serum alkaline phosphatase activity, osteocalcin, and immunoreactive 1-84 PTH concentrations are increased (2). Serum phosphate levels are usually elevated, whereas the level of serum calcium is variable. The most characteristic radiologic feature is subperiostal resorption of bone, which is seen most clearly on the radial border of the middle phalanges. Bone resorption may also lead to acroosteolysis of the phalangeal tufts, to widening of the acromioclavicular and sacroiliac joints or of the pubic symphisis, and to small articular erosions. The frequency of these erosions increases with dialysis duration (3), but erosions do not correlate with symptoms (4) and are not always related to hyperparathyroidism. More advanced hyperparathyroidism may be responsible for painful erosions at the sites of tendon attachment, which bear a high risk of tendon rupture. The skull may be affected and exhibit a "pepperpot" appearance. Osteosclerosis of the spine may be observed, with vertebral bodies showing a "rugger jersey" appearance, due to resorption of bone from their central portion. Brown tumors are rare and must be differentiated from amyloid cysts. Extraskeletal calcifications can develop, particularly in the eye, periarticular tissues, small blood vessels, or skin, leading to pruritus.

Secondary hyperparathyroidism can be treated by 1-alphahydroxylated vitamin D derivatives, provided that calcium and phosphorus serum levels can be controlled, and that no extensive soft tissue or vascular calcifications develop. Pulse intravenous administration of these sterols seems particularly effective, due to direct negative effect on PTH secretion obtained by high concentrations (1). When hyperparathyroidism is too advanced or resists medical management, subtotal parathyroidectomy is indicated.

Aluminum-Induced Bone Disease

Aluminum-induced bone disease follows intoxication from high aluminum content in the dialysate solution or prolonged ingestion of aluminum-containing phosphate binders. Control of the solution and avoidance of phosphate binders that contain aluminum have led to a dramatic decrease of its frequency. Affected patients typically experience bone pain, proximal muscle weakness, and pathologic fractures, particularly of the first ribs (5,6). Serum calcium level is normal or elevated, especially if the patient receives vitamin D. Serum alkaline phosphatase activity and intact parathormone concentration are normal or low. Aluminum serum levels are elevated either spontaneously or after deferoxamine mesylate infusion (7). Bone histology demonstrates heavy staining for aluminum, decreased cellular activity, and either increased or normal osteoid, respectively characterizing the two histologic forms of the disease: osteomalacia and adynamic bone disease. Elimination of the source of intoxication and treatment with deferoxamine mesylate can cure this disabling osteopathy.

Adynamic Bone Disease

Adynamic bone histology recently has been described in dialysis patients, in the absence of aluminum intoxication (8). This condition seems to be related to overtreatment of hyperparathyroidism and could favor the development of osteoporosis in the long run; however, it has not been proved to be responsible for clinical symptoms thus far.

MUSCULAR INVOLVEMENT

Muscular cramps are common during the hemodialysis procedure and are thought to be due to extracellular volume contraction (9). A proximal myopathy may affect dialysis patients. It is usually due to aluminum intoxication or abnormal vitamin D metabolism and very rarely to excessive phosphorus binding, leading to hypophosphatemia. Severe secondary hyperparathyroidism may be responsible for arterial calcification and muscular infarction.

DISORDERS OF MICROCRYSTALLINE ORIGIN

Periarticular calcifications are common and are related to hyperphosphatemia and high serum calcium × phosphorus product, secondary hyperparathyroidism, and long-term survival with hemodialysis. Such calcifications are composed of calcium phosphate (mainly apatite) crystals. They are usually asymptomatic, but apatite can induce acute articular, or more frequently, periarticular inflammatory episodes. Despite careful search for crystals and infectious agents, some acute joint and bursal effusions remain unexplained. Occasionally, calcium deposits grow into pseudotumoral masses. Apatite deposition in dialysis patients has been held responsible for some joint erosions (10) and has also been demonstrated in intervertebral discs of patients with destructive arthropathy of the spine (11).

Calcium oxalate crystal deposition can occur at various sites, including bone, synovium, and cartilage and is one cause of synovial calcification or chondrocalcinosis in dialysis patients. This state has been primarily observed in patients with diets supplemented by vitamin C, a precursor of oxalate (12,13). Gout and calcium pyrophosphate crystal deposition disease are rare despite the frequency of hyperuricemia and of gout before dialysis (4) and the presence of secondary hyperparathyroidism.

BONE AND JOINT INFECTIONS

Bone and joint infections are well-documented complications of hemodialysis and require urgent management with appropriate antibiotics. Immune defenses of patients treated with hemodialysis are impaired, and the arteriovenous fistula is a potential source of hematogenous spread. Intra- or periarticular steroid injections are also an important source of infection and should be avoided in these patients. Unusual infections can include listeriosis associated with secondary iron overload after transfusions.

DIALYSIS ARTHROPATHY AND β_2 MICROGLOBULIN AMYLOID

The deposition of β_2 microglobulin amyloid in articular and periarticular tissues of dialysis patients has been well documented in the last decade (14). Carpal tunnel syndrome is a prominent feature of the disease, although edema, uremic nephropathy, and crystal deposition may also have roles in some carpal tunnel syndromes. A chronic amyloid arthropathy is also frequently observed and includes chronic arthralgias (particularly of the shoulders), chronic joint swelling, finger tendon tenosynovitis, large subchondral bone erosions that affect predominantly the hip and the wrist, and destructive arthropathies. Shoulder pain may be related to amyloid thickening of the rotator cuff tendons or subacromial bursa, which can lead to a chronic impingement syndrome (15). Recurrent hemarthrosis may also occur and is associated with blood anticoagulation during the dialysis procedure. Some patients may even develop a pseudorheumatoid arthropathy, with grossly symmetric amyloid infiltration and morning stiffness of short duration. The diagnosis can be established by examination of synovial fluid (16) as well as by biopsy. Systemic deposits are rare but may be responsible for intestinal hemorrhage or cardiac dysfunction (14). Lack of β_2 microglobulin catabolism by the deficient kidney and unsatisfactory elimination of the molecule through dialysis membranes are important in the pathogenesis of the disorder. β_2 microglobulin amyloid deposits have been observed even before the start of dialysis therapy (17), but the frequency of dialysis arthropathy increases with the length of patient survival. Up to 65% of individuals who have received 10 or more years of maintenance hemodialysis may be affected (18). The use of more permeable membranes may delay the onset of the disease, but has been thus far unable to totally prevent its development.

Thomas Bardin, MD

1. Delmez JA, Slatopolsky E: Recent advances in the pathogenesis and therapy of uremic secondary hyperparathyroidism. J Clin Endocrinol Metab 72:735–739, 1991

2. Cohen Solal ME, Sebert JL, Boudailliez B, et al: Comparison of intact, midregion and carboxy terminal assays of parathyroid hormone for the diagnosis of bone disease in hemodialysis patients. J Clin Endocrinol Metab 73:516–524, 1991

3. Rubin LA, Fam AG, Rubinstein, et al: Erosive azotemic osteoarthropathy. Arthritis Rheum 27:1086–1094, 1984

4. Chou CT, Wasserstein A, Schumacher HR, et al: Musculoskeletal manifestations in hemodialysis patients. J Rheumatol 12:1149–1153, 1985

5. Parkinson IS, Ward MK, Keer DNS: Dialysis encephalopathy, bone disease and anaemia: the aluminum intoxication syndrome during regular haemodialysis. J Clin Pathol 34:1285–1294, 1981

6. Kriegshauser JS, Swee RG, McCarty JT, et al: Aluminum toxicity in patients undergoing dialysis: radiological findings and prediction of bone biopsy results. Radiology 164:399–403, 1987

7. Milliner DS, Nebecker HG, Ott SM, et al: Use of the deferoxamine infusion test in the diagnosis of aluminum related osteodystrophy. Ann Intern Med 101:775–780, 1984

8. Morinière P, Cohen-Solal MH, Belbriks S, et al: Disappearance of aluminic bone disease in a long term asymptomatic dialysis population restricting Al(OH)3 intake: emergence of an idiopathic adynamic bone disease not related to aluminum. Nephron 53:93–101, 1989

9. Milutinovitch J, Graefe V, Follete WC, et al: Effect of hypertonic glucose on the muscular cramps of hemodialysis. Ann Intern Med 90:926–928, 1979

10. Schumacher HR, Miller JL, Ludivico C: Erosive arthritis associated with apatite crystal deposition. Arthritis Rheum 24:31–37, 1981

11. Kuntz D, Naveau B, Bardin T, et al: Destructive spondylarthropathy in hemodialyzed patients: a new syndrome. Arthritis Rheum, 27:369–375, 1984

12. Hoffman GS, Schumacher HR, Paul H, et al: Calcium oxalate microcrystalline-associated arthritis in end stage renal disease. Ann Intern Med 97:36–42, 1982

13. Reginato AJ, Kurnik B: Calcium oxalate and other crystals associated wtih kidney diseases and arthritis. Sem Arthritis Rheum 18:198–224, 1989

14. Gejyo F, Brancaccio D, Bardin T: Dialysis amyloidosis. Milan, Witchig, 1989, Vol. 1

15. Okutsu I, Ninomiya Y, Takatori Y, et al: Endoscopic management of shoulder pain in long-term haemodialysis patients. Nephrol Dial Transplant 6:117–119, 1991

16. Muñoz–Gomez J, Gomez-Pérez R, Solé–Arques M, et al: Synovial fluid examination for the diagnosis of synovial amyloidosis in patients with chronic renal failure undergoing haemodialysis. Ann Rheum Dis 46:324–326, 1987

17. Zingraff J, Noel LH, Bardin T, et al: Beta-2 microglobulin amyloidosis as a complication of chronic renal failure (letter). N Engl J Med 323:1070–1071, 1990

18. Bardin T, Zingraff J, Kuntz D, et al: Dialysis related amyloidosis. Nephrol Dial Transpl 1:151–154, 1986

41. THE FIBROMYALGIA SYNDROME

The fibromylagia syndrome (FMS) is commonly misunderstood and remains a source of some controversy among physicians and of confusion to patients. The most important clinical features of patients felt to have this syndrome are diffuse achiness, stiffness, and fatigue, coupled with an examination that demonstrates multiple tender points in specific areas. Although the pathophysiology has yet to be elucidated, FMS does not appear to be an inflammatory process, so the term *fibrositis* has been abandoned. Patients may have no underlying disease or may have concomitant entities as diverse as rheumatoid arthritis (RA), osteoarthritis (OA), Lyme disease, or sleep apnea. In the absence of an underlying condition, FMS is characterized by a strong female predominance (>75% in most series) with a peak incidence in the 20 to 60 year old age group (1). Fibromyalgia has been observed in up to 15% of patients from rheumatology practices and 5.7% from general medical practices (1).

CLINICAL FEATURES

Patients with FMS most frequently complain of a generalized achiness. The achiness tends to be concentrated in axial locations, such as the neck and lower back, and is often accompanied by diffuse stiffness, which is worse in the morning, occasionally mimicking that seen with RA. The upper part of the trapezius muscles are commonly involved. These symptoms, although chronic, can vary in intensity from day to day. They are commonly exacerbated by environmental stimuli, such as vigorous physical exercise, inactivity, poor sleep, emotional stress, and adverse weather conditions. Painful flares of an underlying condition, such as a peripheral arthritis or lower back problem, may also aggravate FMS. Pain has been found to be similar in magnitude to that experienced in RA (2). One study demonstrated that 30% of FMS patients changed their type of employment and 17% stopped work due to this syndrome (1).

Other problems encountered in association with symptoms of FMS include irritable bowel syndrome, tension headaches, paresthesias, and the sensation of swollen hands. Irritable bowel syndrome has been documented in up to 50% of cases (1). The headaches frequently begin with neck discomfort. Despite the common complaint of paresthesias in the upper extremities, nerve conduction studies are for the most part within normal limits. Objective examination of the hands usually fails to reveal any swelling.

Fatigue, which is often prominent, may be due to dysfunctional sleep (3). Patients frequently experience nonrestorative or nonrefreshing sleep. A majority of patients will admit to a sleep problem on questioning, although some may actually deny poor sleep. The same patients who deny poor sleep may admit to light sleep, multiple awakenings at night, or fatigue that begins 30 minutes to several hours after arising rather than immediately on awakening. These complaints can be difficult to interpret as they are not uncommon in the general population.

Criteria for the diagnosis of FMS were established by a multicenter trial sponsored by the American College of Rheumatology (ACR) (4, Appendix 7). The proposed criteria consist of widespread pain in combination with tenderness of at least 11 of 18 specific tender point sites (Fig. 41–1). These criteria were developed after testing multiple variables in a population of known FMS patients against matched rheumatology patient controls. While the criteria were sensitive enough to distinguish between these two groups, there was no difference noted among patients who had FMS with or without an associated rheumatic disease. Thus, it was suggested to abandon the terms *primary* and *secondary* FMS. The criteria are important in defining patients on research protocols. Until the pathophysiology of this entity is clarified, clinicians need to consider the possibility that patients with typical complaints but fewer tender points may still have similar processes affecting them as in those with classic FMS.

On physical examination of the FMS patient, regardless of other findings from underlying illnesses, tenderness to palpation

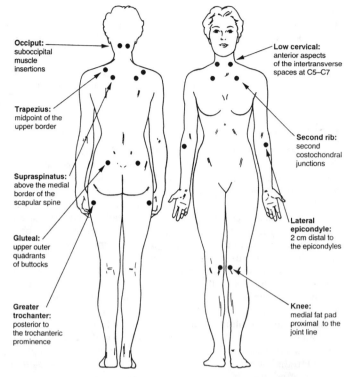

Fig. 41–1. *Location of specific tender points in fibromyalgia*

is noted over characteristic locations using a moderate amount of pressure. There is clearly a subjective component to a tender point examination. Some physicians may not press hard enough, while others press too hard, or the patient may be obese or wearing protective clothing during the examination leading to an altered interpretation. An instrument called a *dolorimeter*, which distributes pressure equally over a discrete point, has therefore been used to more objectively study these patients. The pressure required to produce pain in a given area can be recorded. Various authors have emphasized the importance of having non-tender control points, such as the mid-forehead or anterior thigh, in establishing a diagnosis of FMS; however, these are not included in the ACR criteria. These control sites may be useful in distinguishing FMS from a conversion reaction, which has been referred to as *psychogenic rheumatism*, in which there may literally be tenderness everywhere (5). However, there is some evidence that FMS patients may have a lowered threshold for pain on palpation and so-called control points are occasionally tender.

There is a conspicuous lack of laboratory and radiographic abnormalities attributable to FMS. It is reasonable to obtain screening blood chemistries, a complete blood count, and erythrocyte sedimentation rate (ESR). These tests should be normal unless there is another underlying disorder. In the proper context, antinuclear antibody, rheumatoid factor, creatine kinase, magnesium, Lyme titer, or thyroid function tests may be obtained. Radiographs limited to very symptomatic areas may be useful in selected patients. A sleep study may be appropriate in patients with a history suggestive of particular types of sleep disturbances. For example, the complaint of daytime sleepiness or loud snoring and long respiratory pauses noted by a spouse is suggestive of sleep apnea and may warrant a sleep study.

Since FMS can be found in association with a wide variety of conditions, the concomitant diagnosis of FMS may be obscured by an underlying entity such as RA. Upper torso pain in the setting of RA, for example, may be erroneously assumed to be due to cervical arthritis. Likewise, in new patients presenting with symptoms suggesting FMS, a search should be made for an underlying condition.

Table 41–1. *Differential features of FMS and myofascial pain syndrome*

Feature	FMS	Myofascial Pain
Pain	Diffuse	Local
Fatigue	Common	Uncommon
AM stiffness	Common	Uncommon
Tender points	Diffuse	Local
Treatment	Exercise	Local measures
	Sleep medication	
Prognosis	Tends to be chronic	Resolves with treatment though may recur

Table 41–2. *Conditions associated with sleep disturbance and FMS*

Symptoms	Diagnoses to Consider
Headaches, rhinitis	Sinusitis
Nocturia	Diabetes mellitus, diuretic use, interstitial cystitis
Dry mouth	Sjögren's syndrome Anticholinergic medication
Snoring, daytime sleepiness	Sleep apnea
Kicking at night	Nocturnal myoclonus
Morning facial pain	Bruxism, TMJ disorder
Joint pain, swelling	Rheumatologic condition

DIFFERENTIAL DIAGNOSIS

The differential diagnosis of FMS includes other conditions that present as nonarticular musculoskeletal pain or stiffness with limited physical findings. Some of these include localized nonarticular musculoskeletal pain (which has been termed *myofascial pain*), polymyalgia rheumatica, axial arthritis, hypothyroidism, electrolyte imbalance, osteomalacia, metabolic myopathies, eosinophilia–myalgia syndrome, early collagen disease, psychogenic rheumatism, and chronic fatigue syndrome (CFS). *Myofascial pain* is a term used for a localized, unilateral muscular pain that has an equal sex distribution and is not associated with generalized achiness, stiffness, or fatigue (Table 41–1). This condition often responds to local therapy such as stretching, heat, local anesthetic, or corticosteroid injections. Also, it is important to identify and eliminate pain aggravating activities.

In an elderly individual presenting with shoulder and hip girdle pain and an elevated ESR, polymyalgia rheumatica should be considered. Patients with psychogenic rheumatism may have a strange affect with bizarre exaggerated complaints.

Chronic fatigue syndrome is defined as disabling fatigue of at least six months duration, usually accompanied by symptoms suggestive of a viral infection (6). Although fatigue predominates, patients frequently complain of generalized achiness and have tender points similar to FMS patients (6). The overlap of symptoms between CFS patients and FMS patients with no apparent underlying disease (previously called primary FMS) is striking. In one study, 50% of patients with FMS described a viral-like component to their condition, including recurrent pharyngitis, adenopathy, and low grade fevers (7). Evidence for an Epstein–Barr virus infection is not increased in FMS patients as opposed to controls; however, it has been known for a long time that patients who develop infectious mononucleosis can develop persistent fatigue and achiness. Recently, it appears that other infectious agents have also been associated with these symptoms. These agents include the Lyme spirochete (8), human immunodeficiency virus (9), and parvovirus B19 (10). Since the viral-like symptoms and fatigue predominate in CFS, patients tend to see internists and infectious disease specialists, while FMS patients with prominent aching and stiffness seek out rheumatologists.

Entities associated with FMS may include almost any chronic condition that produces pain. The mechanism of this association may be related to a sleep disturbance. Groups of patients with RA and degenerative arthritis both have fragmented sleep with multiple arousals to lighter sleep stages and actual awakenings due to nocturnal motion, presumably secondary to pain. One sleep study found that a group of patients with RA had an average of 3.4 awakenings and 43.2 arousals (abrupt change to a lighter stage of sleep) per hour (11). Despite feeling fatigued during the day, most of these patients were almost completely unaware of the frequency of these nocturnal events. This illustrates the lack of precision in obtaining a sleep history.

Primary sleep disturbances such as sleep apnea and nocturnal myoclonus have also been associated with FMS (3). The common link among these conditions appears to be fragmented sleep. In sleep apnea, sleep disruption is caused by either obstruction of the upper airways or decreased respiratory signalling from the central nervous system. Nocturnal myoclonus, on the other hand, is manifested by involuntary leg motion during sleep. Arousals and awakenings in both sleep apnea and nocturnal myoclonus occur in a manner analogous to that seen with arthri-

tis. Fibromyalgia associated with these conditions tends to dissipate when the underlying problem is treated, with subsequent improvement of sleep. Table 41–2 lists some conditions associated with a sleep disturbance and FMS.

PATHOPHYSIOLOGY AND ETIOLOGY

The etiology of FMS is unknown. To fully understand the pathophysiology, it is necessary to explain the characteristic tender points and the fatigue. Biopsies of tender points from FMS patients have revealed no clear-cut histologic abnormalities when compared with controls (12). Some data suggest decreased blood flow and diminished high energy phosphate metabolism in these areas (13). There is evidence from some but not all authors that FMS patients may have a generalized lower pain threshold (14).

A subset of patients may have various immunologic abnormalities such as dermal–epidermal immune complex deposition that suggests an autoimmune link (14). Another subset may have mild endocrinologic dysfunction such as an abnormal hypophyseal–adrenal axis, manifested by an abnormal dexamethasone suppression test (16). The existence of other biochemical abnormalities, such as low brain endorphin or increased substance P levels, have received little support. There are some data, however, that blood serotonin may be decreased (16). This is of interest because serotonin is an important neurotransmitter in brain centers involved with pain, sleep, and mood.

Due to the lack of objective findings in the presence of complaints, patients are often considered to have a non-organic root to their illness. The association of tension headaches, irritable bowel syndrome, and stress-exacerbated symptoms further corroborate for the physician that the patient may have a psychiatric problem. Although there appears to be an increased incidence of prior depression in FMS patients (and depression in their families), the majority of patients do not have a primary major depression at the time of diagnosis (17). The chronic pain component in FMS may make the interpretation of psychological tests imprecise. Not uncommonly, FMS patients develop a reactive depression to this chronic, poorly understood, and disabling condition. Although nocturnal antidepressants have been used effectively in this syndrome, the doses employed to improve the quality of sleep are generally nontherapeutic for major depression.

There are several pieces of information as noted above that suggest a link between FMS and a sleep disturbance. Moldofsky, using healthy young controls, was able to reproduce the signs and symptoms of FMS by disrupting non-rapid eye movement (non-REM) stage 3–4 sleep with an auditory stimulus (3). This stage of sleep is characterized by high amplitude, low frequency delta waves on EEG recordings and has been termed *delta wave sleep*. Control subjects deprived of REM sleep, the stage associated with dreaming, did not manifest these symptoms. Delta wave sleep, which is the deepest stage of sleep, is more highly preserved in evolution than REM sleep and may therefore have an important restorative function. It had been noted in sleeping FMS patients that the low frequency EEG waves of stage 3–4 sleep were interrupted by high frequency alpha waves. This was termed *alpha wave intrusion*. Controlled, blinded studies are needed to determine the importance of this finding. It has already been observed that FMS patients whose symptoms improve following therapy may continue to manifest alpha wave intrusion on the sleep EEG.

TREATMENT

The initial therapeutic approach should include patient education and reassurance. The patient should be informed that FMS is not a psychiatric disturbance and furthermore, symptoms seen in FMS are not uncommon in the general population. It should be made clear that FMS is not deforming or life threatening.

Although FMS is frequently a chronic problem, effective treatments are available. Blinded, randomized placebo-controlled studies of amitriptyline (3), cyclobenzaprine (18), and alprazolam (19) given at bedtime, have all been demonstrated to be effective in treating FMS. These medications are usually helpful in achieving a more restorative sleep; however, the dosage and timing are important. Drowsiness and anticholinergic side effects can undermine positive actions. Tricyclic antidepressants with less anticholinergic side effects appear to be better tolerated, and long-term compliance may be superior. Treatment should be initiated at the lowest available dose of whatever medication is chosen. The dosage can be increased until restorative sleep is achieved or adverse effects are encountered. Medication may be more effective if taken one to two hours before bedtime. Hypnotic agents such as flurazepam, temazepam, and triazolam appear to be less useful in general, since FMS patients usually do not have a problem initiating sleep. There is a good chance that if the sleep improves, the pain may dissipate over time.

Antiinflammatory medications such as nonsteroidal antiinflammatory drugs (NSAIDs) and corticosteroids have not been effective as single agents. However, in one study ibuprofen enhanced the efficacy of alprazolam (19). Certainly, any coexistant disease should be treated appropriately. The addition of an NSAID to treat an underlying tendinitis or degenerative arthritis, for example, may also be beneficial for associated FMS. In general, narcotics should be avoided.

Other forms of therapy have included psychological counseling, biofeedback, acupuncture, occasional tender point injections with local anesthetics or corticosteroids, ultrasound treatments, massage, and exercise. Aerobic exercise appears to be more beneficial than simple stretching (20). Heat, in the form of whirlpools or ultrasound, coupled with electrical stimulation may be of temporary benefit. Daily exercise programs, although often helpful, may exacerbate the condition if administered prematurely and incorrectly. It is important to be sensitive to the pace at which the patient advances the exercise program. A good rule is to begin exercise at a low energy level, concentrating mostly on stretching, and then progress gradually to more strenuous aerobic exercises.

It is important to identify and treat patients with an underlying depression. In these instances, it is preferable to prescribe a tricyclic antidepressant at night rather than a benzodiazepine.

Psychiatric consultation should be sought if the situation is unclear; however, this is unnecessary in the majority of patients.

The literature that has addressed the prognosis of patients with FMS has emphasized the chronic nature of this entity in most patients (21). Patients who are younger and those with less severe presentations tend to have a better outcome. Even patients who respond to therapy may continue to complain of a lower level of persistent but tolerable pain.

Bruce Freundlich, MD
Lawrence Leventhal, MD

1. Wolfe F: Fibromyalgia: the clinical syndrome. Rheum Dis Clin NA 15:1–17, 1989
2. Leavitt F, Katz RS, Golden HE, et al: Comparison of pain properties in fibromyalgia patients and rheumatoid arthritis patients. Arthritis Rheum 29:775–781, 1986
3. Moldofsky H: Sleep and fibrositis syndrome. Rheum Dis Clin NA. 15:90–103, 1989
4. Wolfe F, Smythe HA, Yunus MB, et al: The American College of Rheumatology 1990 criteria for the classification of fibromyalgia. Report of the multicenter criteria committee. Arthritis Rheum 33:160–172, 1990
5. Yunus M, Masi AT, Calabro JJ, et al: Primary fibromyalgia (fibrositis): clinical study of 50 patients with matched normal controls. Semin Arthritis Rheum 11:151–170, 1981
6. Shafran SD: The chronic fatigue syndrome. Am J Med 90:730–739, 1991
7. Buchwald D, Goldenberg DL, Sullivan JL, et al: The "chronic, active Epstein–Barr virus infection" syndrome and primary fibromyalgia. Arthritis Rheum 30:1132–1136, 1987
8. Sigal LH: Summary of the first 100 patients seen at a Lyme Disease Referral Center. Amer J Med 88:577–581, 1990
9. Buskila D, Gladman DD, Langevitz P, et al: Fibromyalgia in human immunodeficiency virus infection. J Rheumatol 17:1202–1206, 1990
10. Leventhal LJ, Naides SJ, Freundlich B: Fibromyalgia and parvovirus infection. Arthritis Rheum 34:1319–1342, 1991
11. Mahowald MW, Mahowald ML, Bundlie SR, et al: Sleep fragmentation in rheumatoid arthritis. Arthritis Rheum 32:974–983, 1989
12. Yunus MB, Kalyan–Raman UP: Muscle biopsy findings in primary fibromyalgia and other forms of nonarticular rheumatism. Rheum Dis Clin NA 15:115–133, 1989
13. Bennett RM: Muscle physiology and cold reactivity in the fibromyalgia syndrome. Rheum Dis Clin NA 15:135–147, 1989
14. Simms RW, Goldenberg DL, Felson DT, et al: Tenderness in 75 anatomic sites: distinguishing fibromyalgia patients from controls. Arthritis Rheum 31:182–187, 1988
15. Caro XJ: Is there an immunologic component to the fibrositis syndrome? Rheum Dis Clin NA 115:169–185, 1989
16. Russell IJ: Neurohormonal aspects of fibromyalgia syndrome. Rheum Dis Clin NA 15:149–167, 1989
17. Goldenberg DL: Psychiatric and psychologic aspects of fibromyalgia syndrome. Rheum Dis Clin NA. 15:105–113, 1989
18. Bennett RM, Gatter RA, Campbell SM, et al: A comparison of cyclobenzaprine and placebo in the management of fibrositis. A double-blind controlled study. Arthritis Rheum 31:1535–1542, 1988
19. Russell IJ, Fletcher EM, Michalek JE, et al: Treatment of primary fibrositis/fibromyalgia syndrome with ibuprofen and alprazolam. A double-blind, placebo-controlled study. Arthritis Rheum 35:552–560, 1991
20. McCain GA, Bell DA, Mai FM, et al: A controlled study of the effects of a supervised cardiovascular fitness training program on the manifestations of primary fibromyalgia. Arthritis Rheum 31:1135–1141, 1988
21. Felson DT, Goldenberg DL: The natural history of fibromyalgia. Arthritis Rheum 29:1522–1526, 1986

42. HERITABLE DISORDERS OF CONNECTIVE TISSUE

The molecular composition and organization of connective tissue (see Chapters 2 and 3) are extraordinarily complex, and much remains unknown about the genes—their number, structure, chromosomal location, and regulation—that control synthesis, organization, and metabolism of this tissue. Thus far, the genes that specify more than 50 proteins involved in connective tissue metabolism have been mapped (1). Mutations in the genes for these proteins cause a variety of disorders. Another dozen disorders for which the basic defect is not yet known have also been localized to specific chromosome regions (1). Mutation is the hallmark of this group of conditions; each of the heritable disorders of connective tissue obeys Mendel's laws, and each is caused by an aberration in one component of connective tissue.

The phenotypic characterization of these disorders, crude as it

may be, still outstrips biochemical or genetic understanding. Over 200 conditions are called heritable disorders of connective tissue. The more common and familiar ones have prevalences of 1:10,000 to 1:50,000; many are less prevalent. Recently, families have been described in which much more frequent disorders, such as osteoarthritis (2), osteoporosis (3), and aortic aneurysms (4), are due to mutations in various collagens. An exciting area for the future is to determine the extent to which genetic variation underlies common rheumatic diseases.

The subclassification of these disorders is unsatisfactory, and must ultimately be based on pathobiology. Several phenotypic groupings are traditionally employed (5–7). These are: 1) disorders of fibrous elements, such as osteogenesis imperfecta, Ehlers–Danlos syndromes, pseudoxanthoma elasticum, and Marfan syndrome; 2) disorders of proteoglycan metabolism, including the mucopolysaccharidoses; 3) osteochondrodysplasias and dysostoses, such as achondroplasia, the spondyloepiphyseal dysplasias, and the metaphyseal dysplasias; and 4) inborn errors of metabolism that secondarily affect connective tissue, such as homocystinuria and alkaptonuria (see Chapter 34).

MARFAN SYNDROME

Patients with Marfan syndrome have abnormalities in multiple organs and tissues, especially the skeletal, ocular, cardiovascular, pulmonary, and central nervous systems (8). Diagnosis remains based solely on clinical features and the autosomal dominant inheritance pattern. The basic defect in all cases studied thus far is in fibrillin (9), the principal constituent of extracellular microfibrils (10). These 10–14 nm structures are ubiquitous, and form the substructure for deposition of elastin during formation of elastic fibers. Thus, fibrillin is a functionally important molecule in organs containing elastic fibers, such as arteries, ligaments, and lung parenchyma. In other tissues, such as the zonular fibers of the eye, at the epidermal–dermal junction, and in the perichondrium, microfibrils are not associated with elastin. Defective fibrillin neatly explains the pleiotropic manifestations of Marfan syndrome. The current challenges are to understand the molecular and cellular pathogenesis of each manifestation in Marfan syndrome, and the range of expression of fibrillin mutations, including disorders that are distinct from this syndrome.

Skeletal manifestations include excessive stature; abnormal body proportions, with a long arm span and an abnormally low ratio of the upper segment to the lower segment (dolichostenomelia) (11); elongated digits (arachnodactyly); anterior thoracic deformity (pectus excavatum, carinatum, or an asymmetric combination) (12); abnormal vertebral column curvature (loss of thoracic kyphos, resulting in a "straight back," and scoliosis); hyperextensibility or, less often, congenital contractures of appendicular joints; protrusio acetabulae (13); and pes planus, with a long, narrow foot. Most patients have myopia, and about one-half have subluxation of the lenses (ectopia lentis). The ascending aorta, beginning in the sinuses of Valsalva, gradually dilates in association with fragmentation of the medial elastic fibers; aortic regurgitation and dissection result and are the main causes of death. Mitral valve prolapse occurs in 80% and leads to severe mitral regurgitation in about 10%, usually in childhood. Hernias are frequent, and apical bullae lead to pneumothorax in 5% (14). Striae distensae over the pectoral, deltoid and lumbar areas are a helpful diagnostic sign. Dural ectasia, producing erosion of lower lumbar and sacral vertebrae, is usually an incidental finding on computed tomography (CT) or magnetic resonance imaging (MRI), but may lead to pelvic meningoceles or radicular problems (15).

Management is both palliative and preventive. The size of the ascending aorta should be followed by echocardiography, β-adrenergic blockade is used to reduce stress on the aortic wall, and composite graft replacement is undertaken when the aortic diameter is greater than twice expected (16). Scoliosis should be aggressively managed in the child and adolescent with bracing; when curvature exceeds 40°, surgical stabilization should be considered. Hormonal advancement of pubarche can modulate excessive stature and reduce the time when vertebral curvature can worsen. Most patients do not dislocate joints. Patients may be disposed to develop degenerative arthropathy in middle-age.

HOMOCYSTINURIA

Homocystinuria usually refers to an inborn error in the metabolism of methionine due to deficient activity of the enzyme cystathionine β-synthase (17). Clinical features are superficially similar to those of Marfan syndrome and include ectopia lentis, tall stature, dolichostenomelia, arachnodactyly, and anterior chest and spinal deformity. Generalized osteoporosis, "tight" joints, arterial and venous thrombosis, malar flush, mental retardation, and autosomal recessive inheritance are features of homocystinuria not found in Marfan syndrome, whereas aortic aneurysm and mitral prolapse are not features of homocystinuria. Back pain

and vertebral collapse due to osteoporosis occur in some patients. Most have no specific arthropathy.

The pathogeneses of the three cardinal manifestations—mental retardation, connective tissue disorder and thrombosis—are not understood. One hypothesis holds that sulfhydryl groups of homocysteine and methionine interfere with collagen cross-linking. If true, this is a form of thiolism such as occurs from prolonged administration of penicillamine, a compound structurally similar to homocysteine. Fibrillin is rich in cysteine, and intra- and inter-chain disulfide bonds are crucial to the formation and function of microfibrils. Some of the phenotypic resemblance of homocystinuria to Marfan syndrome may be due to disruption of microfibrils by the reactive sulfhydral moiety of homocysteine.

About one-half of patients respond biochemically and clinically to large doses of vitamin B_6 (usually more than 50 mg pyridoxine/day). Adequate levels of folate and vitamin B_{12} are required for therapeutic and biochemical response. Preexisting mental retardation and ectopia lentis are not reversed by pyridoxine treatment in patients who show biochemical correction, emphasizing the need for early diagnosis and therapy (18). This is now feasible since many states include testing for elevated blood methionine as part of newborn screening. Unfortunately, some pyridoxine-responders may escape detection in the typical screening protocols. In pyridoxine-nonresponders, a low methionine diet and oral betaine therapy (to stimulate remethylation of homocysteine to methionine) are the usual treatments; this approach is successful if the diet and vitamin are tolerated.

STICKLER SYNDROME

The Stickler syndrome is a relatively common, autosomal dominant condition with severe progressive myopia, vitreal degeneration, retinal detachment, progressive sensorineural hearing loss, cleft palate, mandibular hypoplasia, hyper- and hypomobility of joints, variable epiphyseal dysplasia, and variable disability resulting from joint pain, dislocation, or degeneration (19). This condition, also called progressive arthroophthalmopathy, is under-diagnosed, due to patients often not having the full syndrome and to the clinician's failure to obtain a detailed family history that might suggest a hereditary condition. The diagnosis should be strongly considered in 1) any infant with congenitally enlarged (swollen) wrists, knees or ankles, particularly when associated with the Robin anomalad (hypognathia, cleft palate, and glossoptosis); 2) any young adult with degenerative hip disease; and 3) anyone suspected of Marfan syndrome who has hearing loss, degenerative arthritis, or retinal detachment. In some families, the Stickler syndrome is linked to the $\alpha 1(II)$ procollagen locus on chromosome 12 (20). The identification of mutations in type II collagen, the structural macromolecule of both cartilage and the vitreous, is proceeding.

EHLERS–DANLOS SYNDROMES

The Ehlers–Danlos syndromes (EDS) are a group of disorders whose wide phenotypic variability is largely due to extensive genetic heterogeneity (1,5,21,22). The cardinal features relate to the joints and skin: hyperextensibility of skin (Fig. 42–1), easy bruisability, increased joint mobility, and abnormal tissue fragility. Internal manifestations tend to occur only in specific types of EDS. Nine types are now accepted on the basis of phenotypic and inheritance characteristics (Table 42–1). Within individual types, however, biochemical studies have demonstrated considerable heterogeneity. Extensive phenotypic and biochemical characterization fails the clinician as often as it helps; about one-half of all patients who have at least one "cardinal" feature defy categorization.

Ehlers–Danlos type I (gravis form) and *type II* (mitis form) have generalized hyperextensibility of joints and skin, bruisability and fragility of the skin with gaping wounds from minor trauma, and poor retention of sutures. Congenital dislocation of the hips in the newborn, habitual dislocation of joints in later life, joint effusions, clubfoot, and spondylolisthesis are all consequences of this loose-jointedness. Hemarthroses and "hemarthritic disability" have been described and are analogous to the

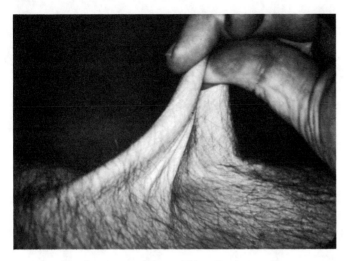

Fig. 42–1. Skin hyperextensibility in Ehlers–Danlos syndrome.

bruisability of the skin in this syndrome. Scoliosis is sometimes severe. Both of these types are inherited as autosomal dominant traits and show wide variability; hence, their differentiation is subjective. The biochemical defects have not been characterized in either type. Management of both EDS I and II stresses prevention of trauma and great care in treating wounds.

Ehlers–Danlos type III (benign hypermobility form) has less marked skin involvement than the previous two types. Joint hyperextensibility ranges from extreme to moderate. Many people with mild joint laxity without joint instability are often labeled as having type III, particularly if relatives show a similar manifestation. In some cases, such labeling does more harm than good, unless it is made quite clear that little disability is likely.

Ehlers–Danlos type IV (arterial form) is by far the most serious type because of a propensity for spontaneous rupture of arteries and bowel (21,23). The unifying pathogenetic theme is abnormal production of type III collagen. Skin involvement is variable, with thin, nearly translucent skin present in some, and mildly hyperextensible skin the only feature in others. Joint laxity is also variable, but is generally limited to the digits. Inheritance is usually autosomal dominant, and many cases are sporadic occurrences in their pedigree, suggesting they are heterozygous for a new mutation.

Ehlers–Danlos type VI (ocular–scoliotic form) is characterized by fragility of the ocular globe, marked joint and skin hyperextensibility, a propensity to severe scoliosis, and autosomal recessive inheritance. Collagen in skin contains little hydroxylysine because of deficiency of the enzyme that hydroxylates selected lysyl residues in the nascent collagen chains. Vitamin C is a necessary cofactor of lysyl hydroxylase and pharmacologic doses may be beneficial (24).

Ehlers–Danlos type VII (arthrochalasis multiplex congenita) is typified by profound loose-jointedness, congenital dislocations, moderately short stature, and variable skin involvement. The underlying defect is an inability to cleave the N-propeptide from type I procollagen, which is necessary for conversion to mature collagen (1).

JOINT INSTABILITY SYNDROMES

The cardinal manifestation of familial joint instability, which once was classified as an Ehlers–Danlos type (5), is instability of numerous appendicular joints, with recurrent dislocation the usual presenting complaint (25). Joint hyperextensibility is variable but usually mild, and skin involvement is uncommon. This syndrome is not rare and often is associated with considerable disability. Autosomal dominant inheritance with marked variability within a family is the rule, emphasizing the need for a comprehensive family history, including examination of close relatives if possible. The biochemical defect is unknown.

The *Larsen syndrome* is characterized by congenital dislocations; a characteristic facies of prominent forehead, depressed nasal bridge, and widely spaced eyes; joint dislocations; and skeletal dysplasia (5,26). Dislocation occurs at the knees (characteristically anterior displacement of the tibia on the femur), hips, and elbows. The metacarpals are short with cylindrical fingers that lack the usual tapering. Cleft palate, hydrocephalus, abnormalities of spinal segmentation, and moderate-to-severe short stature have occurred in some. Several instances of multiple affected siblings with normal parents are known, suggesting autosomal recessive inheritance, but parent–child involvement also occurs, consistent with dominant inheritance. Thus, two clinically indistinguishable forms of the Larsen syndrome may exist.

OSTEOGENESIS IMPERFECTA SYNDROME

Several phenotypically distinct osteogenesis imperfecta syndromes exist (1,5,21). These disorders share osseous, ocular, dental, aural, and cardiovascular involvement. The classification enjoying current application is based on inheritance pattern and clinical criteria (Table 42–2) (5).

Type I osteogenesis imperfecta is the most common form. It is autosomal dominant and is associated with considerable intrafamilial variability. One patient might be markedly short of stature,

Table 42–1. *Ehlers-Danlos syndromes*

Type	Inheritance	Skeletal Features	Other Features	Basic Defect
I	AD	marked joint hypermobility	skin hyperextensibility & fragility	?
II	AD	less severe than type I		?
III	AD	marked joint mobility	mild skin hyperextensibility	?
IV	AD, AR	hypermobile digits	thin skin; bowel & areterial rupture	↓ procollagen III
V	X-L	similar to type II		?
VI	AR	marked joint hypermobility	rupture of ocular globe	↓ lysyl hydroxylase
VII	AD, AR	marked joint hypermobility & dislocations, short stature	minimal skin changes	↓ type I procollagen N-peptide cleavage
VIII	AD	variable joint hypermobility	peridontitis	?; some with ↓ type III collagen
X	AD	mild joint hypermobility	mild skin changes; mitral valve prolapse	? ↓ serum fibronectin

According to revised terminology (5), the condition once termed EDS Type IX (or X-linked cutis laxa) has been reclassified as a disorder of copper metabolism. The condition once termed EDS Type XI has been reclassified as a disorder of joint instability. According to convention, EDS Types IX and XI will now be vacant. AD = autosomal dominant; AR = autosomal recessive; X-L = x-linked.

Table 42-2. *Osteogenesis imperfecta syndromes*

Type	Inheritance	Skeletal Features	Sclerae	Other Features
IA	AD	variable bony fragility & short stature, Wormian bones	blue	opalescent teeth, hearing loss
IB	AD	variable bony fragility & short stature, Wormian bones	blue	normal teeth, hearing loss
II	AD	*in utero* fractures, little calvarial calcium	blue	pulmonary hypertension, neonatal death usual
III	most sporadic	variable fragility, deformity, scoliosis, joint laxity	variable	some with opalescent teeth
IVA	AD	variable bony fragility & short stature, Wormian bones	normal	opalescent teeth, hearing loss
IVB	AD	variable bony fragility & short stature, Wormian bones	normal	normal teeth, hearing loss

with frequent fractures and much disability, while an affected relative leads an unencumbered, vigorous life. Defects in the genes for both α1(I) and α2(I) procollagen can cause this syndrome (27).

Type II osteogenesis imperfecta encompasses the classic congenital variants, nearly all of which are lethal in infancy, if not in utero. Most cases arise as the result of a new mutation (the phenotype thus being dominant, if the patient could live and reproduce), in either α1(I) or α2(I) procollagen. Rare patients have affected siblings and normal parents; in some of these cases, a parent has been shown to have the mutation at low level in the gonads, resulting in the potential for multiple affected offspring (27).

Type III osteogenesis imperfecta comprises severe skeletal deformity, kyphoscoliosis, short stature, and variable fractures. It usually occurs sporadically, suggesting new mutations or autosomal recessive inheritance.

Type IV osteogenesis imperfecta is phenotypically and genetically similar to type I, only rarer and not associated with blue sclerae.

The natural histories of the skeletal involvement among these types bear similarities. Brittle bones are a unifying theme; sometimes fractures occur in utero, particularly in type II, and permit radiographic antenatal diagnosis. In such cases, the limbs are likely to be short and bent at birth and multiple rib fractures give a characteristic "beaded" appearance on radiographs. Other patients with types I or IV have few fractures or may escape them entirely, although the presence of blue sclerae, opalescent teeth, or deafness indicates the presence of the mutant gene. Brittleness and deformability result from a defect in the collagenous matrix of bone. The skeletal aspect of osteogenesis imperfecta is, therefore, a hereditary form of osteoporosis. *Codfish vertebrae* (scalloping of the superior and inferior vertebral bodies by pressure from the expansile intervertebral disc) or flat vertebrae are observed, particularly in older patients in whom senile or postmenopausal changes exaggerate the change, or young patients who are immobilized after fractures or orthopedic surgery.

The frequency of fractures usually decreases at puberty for patients with types I, III, and IV. Pseudoarthrosis occurs because of failure of union of fractures. Hypertrophic callus occurs frequently in patients with osteogenesis imperfecta and may be difficult to distinguish from osteosarcoma. Debate continues as to whether the risk of true osteosarcoma is increased in any form of osteogenesis imperfecta; the risk is not great, but worthy of consideration whenever skeletal pain occurs in the absence of fracture, particularly in an older patient. Joint laxity is sometimes striking in type I. Dislocation of joints can result from deformity secondary to repeated fractures, lax ligaments, or rupture of tendons.

The differential diagnosis of osteogenesis imperfecta includes idiopathic juvenile osteoporosis, Cheney syndrome (osteoporosis, multiple Wormian bones, acroosteolysis), pycnodysostosis (dwarfism, brittle bones, absent mandibular ramus, persistent cranial fontanelles, acroosteolysis), and hypophosphatasia. Recently, osteoporosis in one family was found to be due to a mutation in type I collagen (3). This finding emphasizes that identifying mutations in a particular gene does not necessarily facilitate clinical diagnosis. Furthermore, patients with common

problems that are not thought to be syndromic may harbor defects in one or another of the components of the extracellular matrix.

OSTEOCHONDRODYSPLASIAS

The largest and most diverse group of disorders affecting the bony skeleton are the osteochondrodysplasias (6,28). The osseous skeleton, which is the largest specialized connective tissue, participates in many of the generalized heritable disorders of connective tissue discussed earlier. In addition, the skeleton is subject to a large number of gene-determined derangements, with primary effects apparently limited to bone and cartilage, as exemplified by multiple epiphyseal dysplasia.

The types of osteochondrodysplasias are legion. Each is unusual, and most physicians, even specialists such as orthopedists, radiologists, and rheumatologists, encounter them rarely. Little is known of etiopathogenesis and, until recently, little was known even of their natural history or histopathology. No definite therapy is available for most. Diagnostic criteria and nomenclature have been chaotic until international committees established some order (6), but the older literature can be misleading because the diagnoses do not conform to current practice.

Most of the skeletal dysplasias fall into the category of disproportionate dwarfism (commonly called *dwarfs*) or proportionate dwarfism (commonly but inappropriately called *midgets*). Many people with proportionate short stature do not have a defect in the extracellular matrix, but rather have deficiency of growth hormone. Disproportionate dwarfs tend further to fall into short-limb or short-trunk groups, of which achondroplasia and the Morquio syndrome are, respectively, prototypes.

Achondroplasia

Achondroplasia is the most common and easily diagnosed osteochondrodysplasia causing short stature (29). Manifestations include rhizomelic, short-limbed dwarfism; macrocephaly with prominent forehead and midfacial hypoplasia; thoracolumbar kyphosis in infancy that may persist; lumbosacral lordosis that develops during childhood; bowed legs with elongated fibulae; flexion contractures of the elbows; knee joint instability; trident hand; delayed development of motor skills; and average intelligence (30,31). Compression of the spinal cord may occur at any level, most often at the foramen magnum, posing a life-threatening risk in infancy, or in the lower thoracolumbosacral region at any age, producing upper motor neuron, lower motor neuron, cauda equina, or mixed deficits (32). The radiologic features are large skull with midface hypoplasia and restricted foramen magnum; lack of normal increase in interpedicular distance from upper to lower lumbar vertebrae; square iliac wings with a short, narrow sciatic notch; rhizomelic shortening of limbs; and short, thick tubular bones. Cranial CT or MRI shows large ventricles, usually without any clinical sign of increased intracranial pressure. The head circumference should be followed carefully in pediatric patients, and neurologic and CT evaluations should be obtained if the circumference begins to deviate from the percentile range for that patient on growth charts specifically constructed for achondroplasia. Laminectomy and suboccipital resection are effective methods of relieving neurologic problems (33).

Multiple Epiphyseal Dysplasia

The child with multiple epiphyseal dysplasia comes to medical attention because of short stature or changes in the heads of the femora, similar to those in Legg–Calve–Perthes disease (see Chapter 46), leading to abnormality of gait (7,28). In the third and fourth decades, the patient develops osteoarthritis of the hips and, to a lesser extent, of other joints. The vertebral bodies may be involved, most noticeable as mild platyspondyly, although not as severe as in the spondyloepiphyseal dysplasias (30). Precocious osteoarthritis of the hips coupled with short stature should raise the suspicion of multiple epiphyseal dysplasia. The diagnosis is corroborated by the finding of sloping at the distal end of the tibia. This condition is a mendelian dominant disorder of wide clinical variability. Some families with multiple epiphyseal dysplasia show especially striking changes in the hands, with short fingers and painless deformity at the proximal interphalangeal joints. The cause of this disorder is unknown.

Spondyloepiphyseal Dysplasias

The spondyloepiphyseal dysplasias are a heterogeneous group of conditions sharing radiologic abnormalities of epiphyseal ossification and platyspondyly, and little else. The Stickler syndrome is near the mild end of the clinical spectrum. Two more severe and less common phenotypes, spondyloepiphyseal dysplasia congenita and tarda, are differentiated by age of onset, radiography, and inheritance pattern (6,7,30). In the former, the newborn is dwarfed with a short barrel chest, mild rhizomelic limb shortening, and relatively normal hands (34). Additional features include a cleft palate, myopia, retinal detachment, subluxation of C_1–C_2, and marked retardation of epiphyseal ossification. In later life, patients are often severely short-statured, develop hearing loss, and have mobility problems resulting from hip and knee deformities. Most cases are sporadic and likely represent new mutations with an autosomal dominant condition. Defects in type II collagen have been demonstrated in some cases (35). A mutation in the $\alpha 1(II)$ procollagen gene has also been found in a family with "juvenile osteoarthritis," (2) suggesting that this diagnosis represents the mildest form of spondyloepiphyseal dysplasia yet described.

The tarda form is often not recognized until early adolescence. By that time, the child being evaluated for mild short stature will have the characteristic radiographic changes, especially in the lumbar vertebrae, of flattened bodies with dense, humped centra (30). The sternum often protrudes, and later severe osteoarthropathy of the hips and knees produces disability. The common spondyloepiphyseal dysplasia tarda is X-linked, and males have much more severe arthritic complications.

Mucopolysaccharidoses

The mucopolysaccharidoses are the result of inborn errors of mucopolysaccharide metabolism. While phenotypically diverse, the individual disorders share mucopolysacchariduria and deposition of mucopolysaccharides in various tissues (36). Numerous distinct types of mucopolysaccharidoses can be distinguished on the basis of combined phenotypic, genetic, and biochemical analysis (Table 42–3). Relative short stature is the rule in all forms of mucopolysaccharidosis, and can be profound in types IH (Hurler syndrome), II (Hunter syndrome), IV (Morquio syndrome, the prototypic "short trunk" form of dwarfism), and VI (Maroteaux–Lamy syndrome). Radiologically, the skeletal dysplasia is quite similar in character in all but type IV, differing among the others largely in severity (30). Although the term *dysostosis multiplex* has been used, it is not specific for the mucopolysaccharidoses, because similar changes occur in a variety of storage disorders.

Table 42–3. The mucopolysaccharidoses

Type	Eponym	Clinical Findings	Enzyme Deficiency
MPS I H	Hurler	clouding of cornea, grave manifestations, death usually before age 10	α-L-iduronidase
MPS I S	Scheie	stiff joints, cloudy corneae aortic valve disease, normal intelligence	α-L-iduronidase
MPS I H/S	Hurler-Scheie	intermediate phenotype	α-L-iduronidase
MPS II, severe	Hunter, severe	no corneal clouding, grave manifestations, death before 15 years	iduronate sulfatase
MPS II, mild	Hunter, mild	survival to 30s to 60s, fair-to-normal intelligence; obstruction of airways, sleep apnea	iduronate sulfatase
MPS IIIA	Sanfilippo A	mild coarse facies & short stature, severe mental retardation	heparan N-sulfatase
MPS IIIB	Sanfilippo B	same as IIIA	N-acetyl-α-D-glucosaminidase
MPS IIIC	Sanfilippo C	same as IIIA	acetyl-CoA:α-glucosaminide N-acetyltransferase
MPS IIID	Sanfilippo D	same as IIIA	N-acetylglucosamine-6-sulfate sulfatase
MPS IVA	Morquio A	severe, distinctive bone changes, cloudy cornea, aortic regurgitation, thin enamel	galactosamine-6-sulfate sulfatase
MPS IVB	Morquio B	mild bone changes, cloudy corneae hypoplastic odontoid, normal enamel	β-galactosidase
MPS VI, severe	Maroteaux-Lamy classic severe	severe osseous and corneal changes, valvular heart disease, striking WBC inclusions, normal intellect, survival to 20s or beyond	arylsulfatase B (N-acetylgalactosamine 4-sulfatase)
MPS VI, milder forms	Maroteaux-Lamy	mild-moderately severe changes	arylsulfatase B (N-acetylgalactosamine 4-sulfatase)
MPS VII	Sly	hepatosplenomegaly, dysostosis multiplex, mental retardation, WBC inclusions	β-glucuronidase

The chief radiologic features include a thick calvaria; an enlarged, J-shaped sella turcica; a short and wide mandible; biconvex vertebral bodies; hypoplasia of the odontoid; broad ribs; short and thick clavicles; coxa valga; metacarpals with widened diaphyses and pointed proximal ends; and short phalanges.

Survival to adulthood without severe retardation occurs with types IS (Scheie syndrome), II mild, IV, and VI. In these forms, progressive arthropathy and transverse myelopathy secondary to C_1–C_2 subluxation lead to considerable disability. Joint replacement, particularly of the hips, has been beneficial in several forms. Cervical fusion should be considered whenever upper motor neuron signs appear, a particular concern in types IH, IV, and VI. Stiff joints are a more or less striking feature of all except type IV. Like other somatic features, such as coarse facies, reduced joint mobility is less striking in type III. In type IS, stiff hands, hip arthropathy, and clouding of the cornea produce the main disabilities. Carpal tunnel syndrome contributes to disability in all types. The major life-threatening problems in types II mild, IV, and VI are valvular heart disease and progressive narrowing of the middle and lower airways. The latter frequently presents as obstructive sleep apnea or complications with general anesthesia.

Genetic disturbances of mucopolysaccharide metabolism without mucopolysacchariduria include the mucolipidoses. Type II is also called I-cell disease because of conspicuous inclusions in cultured cells, and is a severe disorder similar to Hurler syndrome. Type III, also called pseudo-Hurler polydystrophy, has stiff joints, cloudy corneae, carpal tunnel syndrome, short stature, coarse facies, and sometimes mild mental retardation, and is compatible with survival to adulthood (37). Neither shows mucopolysacchariduria despite lysosomal storage of mucopolysaccharide and a demonstrable defect in degradation of mucopolysaccharides. Both are autosomal recessive and genetically heterogeneous. The basic biochemical defect (Table 42–3) is an enzyme responsible for post-translational modification of lysosomal enzymes. This defect results in multiple enzyme deficiencies and accumulation in tissues of both mucopolysaccharides and mucolipids.

Mucopolysacchariduria can be identified by several standard screening tests, at least one of which is part of the standard battery performed when a metabolic screen is ordered. Fractionation and characterization of the urinary mucopolysaccharides are useful in separating the types of disorders, but enzymatic assay may be needed for diagnostic confirmation. Prenatal diagnosis by biochemical or molecular genetic methods is possible.

Like other lysosomal disorders, the mucopolysaccharide and mucolipid disorders share distinctive characteristics: 1) intracellular storage occurs; 2) the storage material is heterogeneous because the degradative enzymes are not strictly specific; 3) deposition is vacuolar on electron microscopy; 4) many tissues are affected; and 5) the disorders are clinically progressive. Therapy by replacement of the deficient enzyme is possible, but technically difficult and of transient benefit. Bone marrow transplant is clearly effective in the disorders lacking central nervous system involvement, and is still being investigated in patients with mental retardation (38).

PSEUDOXANTHOMA ELASTICUM

The cardinal features of pseudoxanthoma elasticum occur in the eyes, blood vessels, and skin (Fig. 42–2). Although the most easily recognized finding in the ocular fundus is the angioid streak due to a break in Bruch's membrane, progressive visual loss occurs from retinal hemorrhages. The media of muscular arteries develops degeneration of the elastic fibers and a histologic pattern similar to Mönckeberg arteriolarsclerosis. Peripheral pulses are gradually lost and intermittent claudication is common. Myocardial infarction, stroke, and gastrointestinal hermorrhage are also complications of vascular involvement and the leading causes of death. The condition gets its name from the characteristic skin lesions that develop in flexural folds and resemble plucked chicken skin. The skeleton and joints are not usually involved. The basic defect is unclear. Elastic fibers throughout the body show calcification. Genetic heterogeneity is evident by both autosomal recessive (the most common form) and autosomal dominant inheritance.

FIBRODYSPLASIA OSSIFICANS PROGRESSIVA

Fibrodysplasia ossificans progressiva is characterized by progressive ossification of ligaments, tendons, and aponeuroses. An inexorable, progressive course begins in the first year or so of life, usually with a seemingly inflammatory process and nodule formation on the back of the thorax, neck, or scalp. Local heat, leukocytosis and elevated sedimentation rate are observed at this stage, and acute rheumatic fever is sometimes diagnosed. A valuable clue to the correct diagnosis is a short great toe with or without a short thumb. Fibrodysplasia ossificans progressiva is the leading cause of congenital hallux valgus. Most cases of this autosomal dominant disorder are the consequence of new muta-

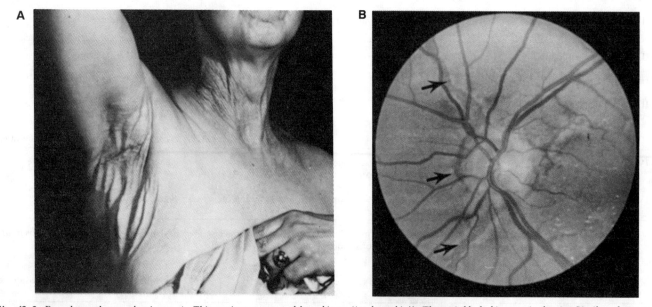

*Fig. 42–2. Pseudoxanthoma elasticum. A. This patient compared her skin to "turkey skin". The wrinkled skin was inelastic. Similar changes were noted in other flexural folds. B. Angioid streaks (**arrows**) in the left retina of a sister of the patient whose axilla is shown in A. This woman had no visual complaints.*

tion. Life expectancy is considerably reduced, with progressive restriction in lung capacity contributing to respiratory insufficiency and terminal pneumonia (39).

Reed E. Pyeritz, MD, PhD

1. Beighton P, de Paepe A, Hall JG, et al: Molecular nosology of heritable disorders of connective tissue. Am J Med Genet 1992, 42:431–488
2. Ala–Kokko L, Baldwin CT, Moskowitz RW, et al: Single base mutation in the type II procollagen gene (COL2A1) as a cause of primary osteoarthritis associated with a mild chondrodysplasia. Proc Natl Acad Sci USA 87:6565–6568, 1990
3. Kuivaniemi H, Tromp G, Prockop DJ: Mutations in collagen genes: causes of rare and some common diseases in humans. FASEB J 5:2052–2060, 1991
4. Kontusaari S, Tromp G, Kuivaniemi H, et al: A mutation in the gene for type III procollagen (COL3A1) in a family with aortic aneurysms. J Clin Invest 86:1465–1473, 1990
5. Beighton P, de Paepe A, Danks D, et al: International nosology of heritable disorders of connective tissue, Berlin, 1986. Am J Med Genet 29:581–594, 1988
6. Rimoin DL: International nomenclature of constitutional diseases of bone: Revision—May, 1977. Birth Defects 14(6B):39–45, 1978
7. Pyeritz RE: Heritable and developmental disorders of connective tissues and bone, Arthritis and Allied Conditions, 11th ed. Edited by McCarty DJ. Philadelphia, Lea & Febiger, 1989, pp 1332–1359
8. Pyeritz RE: Marfan syndrome: guidelines for recognizing an elusive disorder. J Musculoskel Med 7:21–35, 1990
9. Dietz HC, Cutting GR, Pyeritz RE, et al: Defects in the fibrillin gene cause the Marfan syndrome: linkage evidence and identification of a missense mutation. Nature 352:337–339, 1991
10. Kainulainen K, Steinmann B, Collins F, et al: Marfan syndrome: no evidence for heterogeneity in different populations and more precise mapping of the gene. Am J Hum Genet 49:662–667, 1991
11. Pyeritz RE, Murphy EA, Lin SJ, et al: Growth and anthropometrics in the Marfan syndrome, Endocrine Genetics and Genetics of Growth. Edited by CJ Papadatos, Bartsocas CS. New York, Alan Liss, 1985, pp 355–366
12. Arn PH, Scherer LR, Haller JA Jr, et al: Clinical outcome of pectus excavatum in the Marfan syndrome and in the general population. J Pediatr 115:954–958, 1989
13. Kuhlman JE, Scott WW Jr, Fishman EK, et al: Acetabular protrusion in the Marfan syndrome. Radiology 164:415–417, 1987
14. Hall J, Pyeritz RE, Dudgeon DL, Haller JA, Jr: Pneumothorax in the Marfan syndrome: prevalence and therapy. Ann Thorac Surg 37:500–504, 1984
15. Pyeritz RE, Fishman EK, Bernhardt BA, et al: Dural ectasia is a common feature of the Marfan syndrome. Am J Hum Genet 43:726–732, 1988
16. Gott VL, Pyeritz RE, Cameron DE, et al: Composite graft repair of Marfan aneurysm of the ascending aorta: results in 100 patients. Ann Thorac Surg 52:38–45, 1991
17. Mudd SH, Levy HL, Skovby F: Disorders of transsulfuration, Metabolic Basis of Inherited Disease, 7th ed. Edited by Scriver CR, Beaudet AL, Sly WS, Valle D. New York, McGraw-Hill, 1993
18. Mudd SH, Skovby F, Levy HL, et al: The natural history of homocystinuria due to cystathionine beta-synthase deficiency. Am J Hum Genet 36:1–31, 1985
19. Herrmann J, France TD, Spranger JW, et al: The Stickler syndrome (hereditary arthroophthalmopathy). Birth Defects 11(2):76–103, 1975
20. Francomano CA, Liberfarb RM, Hirose T, et al: The Stickler syndrome: evidence for close linkage to the structural gene for type II collagen. Genomics 1:293–296, 1987
21. Byers PH: Disorders of collagen biosynthesis and structure, Metabolic Basis of Inherited Disease. 6th ed. Edited by Scriver CR, Beaudet AL, Sly WS, Valle D. New York, McGraw-Hill, 1989, pp 2805–2842
22. Beighton P: The Ehlers–Danlos syndrome, McKusick's Heritable Disorders of Connective Tissue. Edited by P. Beighton. St. Louis, CV Mosby, 1992, in press
23. Pyeritz RE. Genetics and cardiovascular disease, Heart Disease, 4th ed. Edited by Braunwald E. Philadelphia, WB Saunders, 1992, pp 1622–1655
24. Elsas LJ II, Miller RL, Pinnell SR: Inherited human collagen lysyl hydroxylase deficiency: ascorbic acid response. J Pediatr 92:378–384, 1978
25. Horton WA, Collins DL, DeSmet AA, et al: Familial joint instability syndrome. Am J Med Genet 6:221–228, 1980
26. Latta RJ, Graham GB, Aase J, et al: Larsen's syndrome. A skeletal dysplasia with multiple joint dislocations and unusual facies. J Pediatr 78:291–298, 1971
27. Byers PH: Brittle bones-fragile molecules: disorders of collagen gene structure and expression. Trends Genet 6:293–300, 1990
28. Rimoin DL, Lachman RS: The chondrodysplasias, Principles and Practice of Medical Genetics, 2nd ed. Edited by Emery AE, Rimoin DL. New York, Churchill Livingston, 1990, pp 895–932
29. Nicoletti B, Kopits SE, Ascani E, McKusick VA (eds): Human Achondroplasia. New York, Plenum, 1988
30. Wynne–Davies R, Hall CM, Apley AG: Atlas of Skeletal Dysplasias. Churchill Livingstone, Edinburgh, 1985
31. Scott CR: Achondroplastic and hypochondroplastic dwarfism. Clin Orthopaedics 114:18–45, 1976
32. Pyeritz RE, Sack GH Jr, Udvarhelyi GB: Thoracolumbosacral laminectomy in achondroplasia: Long-term results in 22 patients. Am J Med Genet 28:433–444, 1987
33. Aryanpur J, Carson B, Hurko O, et al: Craniocervical decompression for cervicomedullary compression in pediatric patients with achondroplasia. J Neurosurg 72:375–382, 1990
34. Horton WA, Hall JG, Scott CI, et al: Growth curves for height for diastrophic dysplasia, spondyloepiphyseal dysplasia congenita, and pseudoachondroplasia. Am J Dis Child 136:316–319, 1982
35. Lee B, Vissing H, Ramirez F, et al: Identification of the molecular defect in a family with spondyloepiphyseal dysplasia. Science 244:978–980, 1989
36. Neufeld EF, Muenzer J: The mucopolysaccharidoses, Metabolic Basis of Inherited Disease. 6th ed. Edited by Scriver CR, Beaudet AL, Sly WS, Valle D. New York, McGraw-Hill, 1989, pp 1565–1587
37. Kelly TE, Thomas GH, Taylor HA Jr, et al: Mucolipidosis III (pseudo-Hurler polydystrophy): Clinical and laboratory studies of 12 patients. Johns Hopkins Med J 137:156–175, 1975
38. Lenarsky C, Kohn DB, Weinberg KI, et al: Bone marrow transplantation for genetic diseases. Hematol Oncol Clin N Am 4:589–602, 1990
39. Connor JM, Evans DAP: Fibrodysplasia ossificans progressiva: the clinical features and natural history of 34 patients. J Bone Joint Surg 64B:76–83, 1982

43. MISCELLANEOUS SYNDROMES INVOLVING SKIN AND JOINTS

This chapter covers several unrelated dermatoses, each of which can involve the joints.

LOBULAR PANNICULITIS

Several inflammatory diseases primarily affect cutaneous fat lobules. Two of these, Weber–Christian disease and pancreatic panniculitis, are associated with joint manifestations.

Weber–Christian disease is characterized by recurrent crops of erythematous nodules and plaques over the lower extremities, arms, trunk, face, breasts, and buttocks. It is seen especially in young to middle-aged women. Systemic involvement of the mesentery, heart, lungs, kidneys, liver, spleen, adrenal glands, bone marrow, and central nervous system can occur. Development of skin lesions may be associated with fever, malaise, nausea, vomiting, abdominal pain, weight loss, hepatomegaly, and arthralgias. Painful osteolytic lesions have been reported (1). The prognosis is usually good, with gradual spontaneous resolution of the attacks, but the systemic form is occasionally fatal (2). Major causes of death are sepsis, hepatic failure, hemorrhage, and thrombosis.

Diagnosis of Weber–Christian disease requires a skin biopsy that includes fat. An α-1-antitrypsin level should be obtained to rule out a deficiency, although lesions seen in α-1-antitrypsin deficiency are clinically somewhat different, with frequent ulceration and oozing (3).

The etiology is unknown. High levels of circulating immune complexes have been reported. Treatment includes nonsteroidal antiinflammatory drugs (NSAIDs), corticosteroids, antimalarials, and immunosuppressive drugs.

Pancreatic panniculitis occurs in patients with either pancreatitis or pancreatic cancer of the acinar cells (4,5). Tender, red nodules commonly appear in the pretibial region, but also on the thighs, buttocks, and other areas. The skin lesions are often associated with arthralgias, especially in the ankles. These arthralgias are due to periarticular fat necrosis. Arthritis occurs in approximately 60%, and fever, osteolytic bone lesions, pleuritis, pericarditis, or synovitis can occur (6).

Skin or synovial biopsies show very characteristic areas of fat necrosis, with ghost-like fat cells. Basophilic deposits of calcium may be seen. Synovial fluid may be creamy with lipid droplets. Pathogenesis may be related to the release of pancreatic enzymes such as trypsin, amylase, and lipase. Increased lipase and amylase levels have been found in fluid aspirated from skin lesions and in pleural, pericardial, and ascitic fluid (4). Eosinophilia can occur. Treatment is directed at the pancreatic disease.

ERYTHEMA NODOSUM

Erythema nodosum is a syndrome of inflammatory cutaneous nodules, often found on the extensor surface of the lower legs. It can be acute, chronic, or migratory, occurs three times more frequently in women, and has a peak incidence between the ages of 20 and 30 years. Often the disease is self-limited and resolves in three to six weeks. There are a number of conditions associated with erythema nodosum (Table 43-1). The triad of bilateral hilar lymphadenopathy, erythema nodosum, and polyarthralgias-arthritis is called Lofgren's syndrome. One-half of these patients have acute sarcoidosis, and the other half have an infection. The arthralgias can persist after resolution of skin lesions. Histology shows inflammation and thickening of the septae in the fat.

Work-up usually should include a full-thickness skin biopsy. Other tests that may be helpful on initial work-up, but that should be individualized to the patient, include complete blood count with differential, antistreptolysin titer, chest roentgenogram, pharyngeal culture, and intradermal skin tests for tuberculosis, coccidiodomycosis, blastomycosis, and histoplasmosis. Virologic and *Yersinia* titers may be helpful (7,8).

The pathogenesis is unknown, but may be related to circulating immune complexes. Isolated cases have been seen with IgA nephropathy and cryoglobulinemia, both of which are associated with circulating immune complexes.

Treatment of any underlying condition is helpful. Bed rest, NSAIDs, potassium iodide, and occasionally oral glucocorticoids can be helpful.

ACNE SYNDROMES

Acne vulgaris is a common abnormality that involves the sebaceous follicle. The type of acne lesion depends on the depth of inflammation into the dermis. More severe forms of acne have deeper subcutaneous invasion, leading to nodules and cysts. The more severe acne syndromes discussed below are associated with musculoskeletal abnormalities.

Acne conglobata includes polyporous comedones, cysts, deep abscesses, draining sinuses, and bridging scars occurring on the buttocks, thighs, and upper arms, as well as the face, posterior neck, back, and chest. Although most patients with acne conglobata are Caucasian, the associated musculoskeletal syndrome occurs mostly in black men over the age of 22. Musculoskeletal involvement is associated with skin flares and includes sacroiliitis with or without a peripheral arthropathy (9,10). Peripheral joint involvement is symmetric 60% of the time, and arthralgias can be present. The disease is recurrent and episodic. The radiologic abnormalities include soft tissue swelling, periarticular osteoporosis, cartilage loss with joint space narrowing, erosions, periostitis, new bone formation, and alignment abnormalities. Coarse paravertebral ossifications, hyperostoses, smooth anterior syndesmophyte formations with corner erosions and sclerosis, and calcified tendons also have been reported. There are no consti-

tutional symptoms. The follicular occlusion triad includes acne conglobata, hidradenitis suppurativa, and dissecting cellulitis of the scalp, and has similar patient characteristics and musculoskeletal symptoms to acne conglobata alone.

Acne fulminans is a rare form of acne seen mostly in Caucasian male adolescents who experience a sudden onset of nodulocystic and ulcerated cysts on the face, back, chest, and shoulders. Acne vulgaris precedes acne fulminans, and exacerbation occurs with viral illness, stress and fatigue, or onset of isotretinoin treatment. It is associated with fever, weight loss, myalgias, myositis, elevated erythrocyte sedimentation rate (ESR), leukocytosis, anemia, osteoarthritis, and sterile osteolytic bone lesions. Circulating immune complexes have been seen in several cases. The bone lesions can be painful and occur most often in the clavicles and metaphyses of long bones. They tend to flare with the skin lesions and can be detected by bone scan. Ninety percent of symptomatic bone lesions are seen on roentgenograms. Arthritis is present in one-third of patients with the acne fulminans-associated musculoskeletal syndrome. Arthralgias and myalgias of the hips and shoulders are common. Myositis, associated with muscle weakness, normal muscle enzymes, and abnormal EMGs occurs rarely. The arthritis is nondeforming, self-limited, and often involves the knees. Small joint involvement and sacroiliitis are relatively uncommon. Sterile osteolytic bone lesions of the clavicles and metaphysis of long bones have been seen (11). Radiographs of large joints can show diffuse areas of demineralization, periosteal new bone formation, and transverse bands of radiolucency. Biopsy of synovium has shown mild hyperplasia with moderate numbers of lymphocytes and plasmacytes. Treatment includes isotretinoin, dapsone, oral corticosteroids, and azathioprine. Even with treatment, the prognosis is variable. Some patients experience recurrent episodes of arthritis, arthralgias, and myalgias for years. Acne fulminans leaves cutaneous scars.

The pathogenesis of these acne-associated musculoskeletal syndromes is unclear. Some acne fulminans patients have an exaggerated response to intradermal *P acnes* antigen. Patients with acne conglobata have increased lymphocyte proliferation in response to *P acnes*, but not to phytohemagglutinin. Some acne conglobata patients develop antibodies against *P acnes*. The musculoskeletal abnormalities vary with the various syndromes (Table 43-2).

In 27% of patients, isotretinoin use is associated with mild transient myalgias and arthralgias that do not require stopping the treatment. About 10% of patients with these symptoms develop asymptomatic, small, hyperostotic lesions of the spine. Other isotretinoin-associated abnormalities include soft tissue calcification of tendons and ligaments and arthritis (12).

SWEET'S SYNDROME

Sweet's syndrome is otherwise known as acute febrile neutrophilic dermatosis. It is usually seen in middle-aged women and presents with tender, red-blue papules and plaques on the face, neck, and arms (Fig. 43-1). Pustules and bullae may be present. There are often systemic symptoms, including fever, malaise,

Table 43-1. *Associations with erythema nodosum*

Medications:		Sulfonamides, estrogen, oral contraceptives
Infections:	Bacterial	Streptoccus, tuberculosis, Yersinia, leprosy, leptospirosis, tularemia, Cat-scratch disease
	Fungal	Coccidioidomycosis, blastomycosis, histoplasmosis, dermatophytes
	Viruses	Paravaccinia, infectious mononucleosis
Sarcoidosis		
Inflammatory bowel disease		
Malignancy:		Lymphoma and leukemia, postradiation therapy
Behcet's syndrome		
Pregnancy		

Table 43-2. *Characteristics of musculoskeletal syndromes associated with acne**

Characteristic	AC**	AF†	Isotretinoin
Age (years)	>22	≤22	≥15
Gender (F:M)	1:4	1:37	1:1
Race	black	white	
Constitutional symptoms	−	+	−
Myalgias	−	+	+
Myositis	−	+	−
Arthralgias	+	+	+
Arthritis	+	+	−
Bone lesions	−	+	−
Skeletal hyperostoses	−	−	+

* Adapted from reference 9.
** AC = Acne conglobata
† AF = Acne fulminans

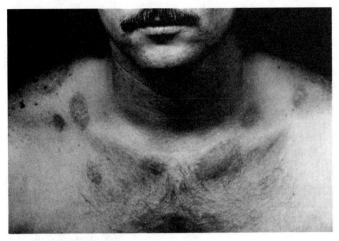

Fig. 43–1. Typical cutaneous plaques of Sweet's syndrome. (Illustration provided by Dr HR Schumacher, Jr.)

conjunctivitis, iridocyclitis, proteinuria, oral ulcerations, arthralgias, and arthritis (13). Approximately 20% to 25% of patients have an acute self-limited polyarthritis involving the hands, wrists, ankles, and knees that occur with the skin eruption (14). Elevated ESR and alkaline phosphatase are common. Sterile osteomyelitis may occur, though rarely (11). Idiopathic Sweet's syndrome resolves spontaneously in one to three months if untreated, and 30% have recurrences.

Skin pathology reveals a neutrophilic infiltrate with leukocytoclasis and edema of the papillary dermis. There is no evidence of vasculitis.

Sweet's syndrome is associated with underlying hematologic malignancies, particularly acute myeloid and myelomonocytic leukemia, which occur 10% of the time. It has also been seen after respiratory tract illnesses, inflammatory bowel disease, pregnancy, and connective tissue diseases. Approximately 50% of patients have a coexisting underlying condition (13).

The etiology of Sweet's syndrome is unknown, but some clinical aspects suggest that it is due to an immunologic reaction. Orally administered glucocorticoids are usually effective. Other treatments include aspirin, indomethacin, colchicine, and potassium iodide.

PUSTULOSIS PALMARIS ET PLANTARIS

Pustulosis palmaris et plantaris is a chronic, relapsing pustular eruption of the palms and soles. The pustules are seen mainly on the thenar eminence, mid palm, heel, and instep. It has been associated with chronic recurrent multifocal osteomyelitis and sternocostoclavicular hyperostosis. Chronic recurrent multifocal osteomyelitis begins with an insidious pain and swelling of the affected bones, most commonly the medial ends of the clavicles and the distal metaphyses of long bones. It usually occurs in children and young adults, affecting females more than males. Diagnosis is made by radiography, showing the acute changes of lytic lesions with sclerotic rims adjacent to the growth plate and dense sclerosis in the chronic stage. Bone scans are more sensitive than roentgenograms. Twenty percent of those with chronic recurrent multifocal osteomyelitis develop palmoplantar pustulosis. Laboratory tests show a mild leukocytosis and elevated ESR. Rare complications include premature closure of the epiphyses, bony growth abnormalities, and thoracic outlet syndrome. The natural history of chronic recurrent multifocal osteomyelitis is recurrent exacerbations over months to years. Treatment with oral glucocorticoids is effective, but relapse after stopping the drug is common (11).

Palmoplantar pustulosis affects 9.4% of patients with sternocostoclavicular hyperostosis. This is seen mostly in Japan in men and women between age 30 and 60, with resolution usually occurring by age 60. Sternocostoclavicular hyperostosis causes pain and swelling in the upper anterior chest wall. Some patients have arthritis, with 23% having ankylosing spondylitis and 25% sacroiliitis (15). Associated psoriatic skin lesions are common. It

appears to start in the soft tissue and secondarily involve bone. Complications rarely include subclavian compression and thrombophlebitis.

PYODERMA GANGRENOSUM

Pyoderma gangrenosum is an uncommon ulcerative skin condition that is associated with underlying systemic diseases in about 50% of patients. The clinical appearance includes painful ulcers, commonly found on the legs, with well-defined, undermined borders with a surrounding erythema (Fig. 43–2). Lesions often begin as pustules. Healing of ulcers results in atrophic and cribiform scars. A superficial ulcer with bullous borders has been seen in association with preleukemic or leukemic conditions. Some patients with pyoderma gangrenosum get arthralgias and a progressive, erosive arthritis that is independent of any associated rheumatoid arthritis (RA).

Pyoderma gangrenosum is associated with inflammatory bowel disease (both Crohn's disease and ulcerative colitis), RA, seronegative arthritis, and hematologic diseases (myelocytic leukemias, hairy cell leukemia, and myelofibrosis) (16). The inflammatory bowel disease can be asymptomatic and detected only by radiography. The course of the skin disease can be independent of the activity of the bowel disease or RA.

There is no diagnostic histology of pyoderma gangrenosum, but biopsies need to be done to rule out other causes of ulcers, such as vasculitis or infection. A monoclonal gammopathy is seen in 10% to 20% of cases, usually IgA, but occasionally IgG or IgM. Work-up of suspected pyoderma gangrenosum should include a careful history and physical exam, skin biopsy for routine pathology and culture, gastrointestinal tract studies, serum protein electrophoresis, immunoelectrophoresis, and complete blood count. Immunofixation electrophoresis has shown to be sensitive in detecting the associated monoclonal gammopathies (17).

Pathogenesis is unknown, but numerous immunologic abnormalities have been described. Granulocyte abnormalities involving chemotaxis, migration, defective bactericidal capacity, and oxidative burst have been described. Abnormalities in cell-mediated immunity have also been noted. Treatment includes proper management of any underlying systemic disease, local therapy, sulfa and sulfones (dapsone, sulfasalazine, sulfapyridine), topical or intralesional glucocorticoids, oral and/or pulse intravenous prednisone, hyperbaric oxygen, clofazimine, minocycline, rifampin, cytotoxic drugs (azathioprine, cyclophosphamide, chlorambucil), and cyclosporine.

LICHEN MYXEDEMATOSUS

Lichen myxedematosus (scleromyxedema or papular mucinosis) is a rare fibromucinous disorder first described in 1954 by Gottron. The skin findings include waxy papules, sclerosis, and induration of the skin involving the hands, arms, face, trunk, and legs. There are some features of scleroderma, such as acroscle-

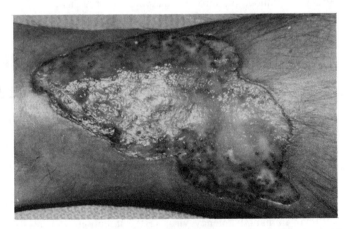

Fig. 43–2. Typical leg ulcer of pyoderma gangrenosum in a patient with ulcerative colitis.

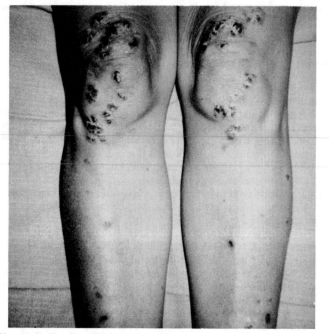

Fig. 43–3. *Tender skin nodules due to the cutaneous vasculitis of erythema elevatum diutinum (illustration courtesy of Dr HR Schumacher, Jr).*

ERYTHEMA ELEVATUM DIUTINUM

Erythema elevatum diutinum is a rare disease. Clinical features include multiple persistent erythematous plaques and nodules often located over extensor surfaces of joints on the hands, arms, and legs (Fig. 43–3). The lesions can be pruritic or painful, especially after exposure to cold, and early lesions can be bullous or vesicular. An association with RA has been reported (19). There are often arthralgias of the associated joint.

Biopsy of early lesions shows a leukocytoclastic vasculitis with a dense neutrophilic dermal infiltrate. Later biopsies show fibrosis. Paraproteinemias, especially IgA, have been reported.

The etiology is unknown, but it is thought that immune complexes are involved, similar to mechanisms seen in other forms of leukocytoclastic vasculitis. Intradermal injection of streptococcal antigen in patients with erythema elevatum diutinum has induced characteristic lesions (20).

Victoria Werth, MD

1. Pinals RS: Nodular panniculitis associated with an inflammatory bone lesion. Arch Dermatol 101:359–363, 1970
2. Ciclitira PJ, Wight DGD, Dick AP: Systemic Weber–Christian disease. Br J Dermatol 103:685–692, 1980
3. Smith KC, Su WPD, Pitelkow MR, et al: Clinical and pathologic correlations in 96 patients with panniculitis, including 15 patients with deficient levels of alpha₁-antitrypsin. J Am Acad Dermatol 21:1192–1196, 1989
4. Mullen GT, Caperton EM Jr, Crespin SR, et al: Arthritis and skin lesions resembling erythema nodosum in pancreatic disease. Ann Intern Med 68:75–87, 1968
5. Schrier RW, Melman KL, Fenster LF: Subcutaneous nodular fat necrosis in pancreatitis. Arch Intern Med 116:832, 1965
6. van Klaveran RJ, de Mulder PHM, Boerbooms AMT, et al: Pancreatic carcinoma with polyarthritis, fat necrosis, and high serum lipase and trypsin activity. Gut 31:953–955, 1990
7. Schorr–Lesnick B, Brandt LJ: Selected rheumatologic and dermatologic manifestations of inflammatory bowel disease. Am J Gastro 83:216–223, 1988
8. White JW: Erythema nodosum. Dermatol Clin 3:119–127, 1985
9. Knitzer RH, Needleman BW: Musculoskeletal syndromes associated with acne. Seminars in Arthr Rheum 20:247–255, 1991
10. Bookbinder SA, Fenske NA, Clement GB, et al: Clavicular hyperostosis and acne arthritis. Ann Intern Med 97:615–616, 1982
11. Sofman MS, Prose NS: Dermatoses associated with sterile lytic bone lesions. J Am Acad Dermatol 23:494–498, 1990
12. Pittsley RA, Yoder FW: Retinoid hyperostosis: skeletal toxicity associated with long-term administration of 13-cis-retinoic acid for refractory ichthyosis. N Engl J Med 308:1012–1014, 1983
13. Kemmett D, Hunter JAA: Sweet's syndrome: a clinicopathologic review of twenty-nine cases. J Am Acad Dermatol 23:503–507, 1990
14. Krauser RE, Schumacher HR: The arthritis of Sweet's syndrome. Arthritis Rheum 18:35–41, 1975
15. Sonozaki H, Kawashima M, Hongo O, et al: Incidence of arthroosteitis in patients with pustulosis palmaris et plantaris. Ann Rheum Dis 40:554–557, 1981
16. Callen JP: Pyoderma gangrenosum and related disorders. Med Clin N Am 73:1247–1261, 1989
17. Prystowsky JH, Kahn SN, Lazarus GS: Present status of pyoderma gangrenosum. Arch Dermatol 125:57–64, 1989
18. Gabriel SE, Perry HO, Oleson GB, et al: Scleromyxedema: a scleroderma-like disorder with systemic manifestations. Medicine 67:58–65, 1988
19. Yiannias JA, El-Azhary RA, Gibson LE: Erythema elevatum diutinum: a clinical and histopathologic study of 13 patients. J Am Acad Dermatol 26:38–44, 1992
20. Wolff HH, Scherer R, Maciejewski W, et al: Erythema elevatum diutinum. II. Immunoelectronmicroscopical study of leukocytoclastic vasculitis within the intracutaneous test reaction induced by streptococcal antigen. Arch Dermatol Res 261:17–26, 1987

rosis, flexion contractures, and decreased oral orifice. On skin biopsy there is mucin in the dermis, diffusely thickened skin, and an increased number of large, stellate, fibroblasts associated with irregular collagen bundles. There is usually an associated monoclonal IgG lambda gammopathy. Other associations include multiple myeloma, Waldenstrom's macroglobulinemia, non-Hodgkins lymphoma, esophageal aperistalsis, inflammatory myopathy, erosive arthritis, median neuropathy, and sicca complex (18). The myopathy is commonly associated with dysphagia, and elevations in muscle enzymes and abnormal EMGs are frequent. Raynaud's phenomenon, calcinosis cutis, telangiectasiae, pulmonary diffusion abnormalities and hypertension, and digital ulcers are rare. Systemic disease with muscle weakness, dysphagia, and weight loss can occur. The course of the disease is variable, with reports of some patients having spontaneous resolution and others a stable uncomplicated course.

Treatment with melphalan, prednisone, and cytoxan has been used. Melphalan carries a risk of sepsis and hematologic malignancies.

The etiology of scleromyxedema is unknown. Serum from patients with lichen myxedematosus can stimulate proliferation of normal human skin fibroblasts in culture. It is possible that certain IgG lambda paraproteins activate the fibroblast.

44. AIDS AND OTHER IMMUNODEFICIENCY DISEASES

Inflammatory musculoskeletal manifestations have long been recognized and are relatively common during the course of immunodeficiency states. Defects in both humoral and cell-mediated immunity can lead to the development of joint inflammation.

HUMAN IMMUNODEFICIENCY VIRUS INFECTION

Human immunodeficiency virus (HIV) infection is currently the most common and important acquired immune deficiency state. First recognized in 1981, it has reached epidemic proportions with devastating consequences in terms of public health and health care expenditures. During the early stages, HIV infection produces minimal or no symptomatology. As the disease progresses, a variety of constitutional symptoms occur, including fever, weight loss, anorexia, lymphadenopathy, and the development of infections (primarily *Pneumocystis pneumoniae* and *Candida*) and Kaposi's sarcoma. Later stages are characterized by profound disturbances of cell-mediated immune function with lymphopenia, diminished T cells, depressed lymphocyte proliferation, and inversion of the T-cell helper to suppressor/cytotoxic ratio—the so-called acquired immunodeficiency syndrome, or AIDS (1,2). The etiologic agent responsible for AIDS is the well-defined HIV retrovirus (3).

Since the initial description, the Centers for Disease Control (CDC) estimates that approximately one million individuals in the USA are currently infected with HIV, and the World Health Organization estimates from 5–10 million people worldwide are infected. As of December 31, 1991, a total of 206,392 cases of AIDS in the USA had been reported to the CDC, and 133,232 of these patients are now dead. Worldwide, 418,403 cases of AIDS had been reported. The musculoskeletal syndromes associated with HIV infection have become more clearly defined (4). Since the original report by Winchester et al (5) of Reiter's syndrome in patients with AIDS, a wide spectrum of other rheumatic disorders have been described. These include psoriatic arthritis, undifferentiated spondylarthropathy, oligo- and polyarthritis, dermatopolymyositis, Sjogren's-like syndrome, lupus-like syndrome, septic arthritis, vasculitis and others.

Pathogenesis

Human immunodeficiency virus is a RNA retrovirus that belongs to the family *Retroviridae* (or retrovirus) and the subfamily *Lentivirinae*. All retroviruses share a common set of three genes designated *gag*, *pol*, and *env*.

The retrovirus proviral genome is 9 kilobases in length and comprises the flanking long terminal repeat sequences that contain regulatory segments for viral replication as well as other structural and regulatory genes (6).

The CD4 receptor expressed predominantly by T-helper/inducer lymphocytes and, to a lesser extent, by monocytes and macrophages, has a high affinity for the gp120 glycoprotein antigen of the envelope membrane of HIV. These CD4-positive cells play a critical role in the complex regulation of the immune system; thus, their depletion and dysfunction, as seen in HIV infection, leads to the occurrence of opportunistic infection and malignancies.

Available evidence suggests multifactorial mechanisms contribute to the pathogenesis of AIDS, including direct and indirect effects of retrovirus infection, and additional reactive or immunologically mediated mechanisms (7,8).

A direct role for HIV in the mediation of rheumatic manifestations is not conclusively proven. Human immunodeficiency virus is seldom isolated from synovial fluid aspirates or the synovial membrane. Furthermore, in caprine arthritis encephalitis virus (CAEV) infection, the titers of coculturable CAEV in the synovial fluid and synovial fluid cells of infected goats disappear several months after infection, and before the onset of arthritis. There are, however, occasional reports describing the isolation and detection of HIV and human T-cell lymphotropic virus (HTLV-1) from synovial fluid aspirates, and muscle of affected patients. In addition, polymyositis is seen in 50% of monkeys infected with simian immunodeficiency virus, and the retrovirus can be isolated from affected muscle.

Increased production of pro-inflammatory cytokines including interleukin–1, tumor necrosis factor, and gamma-interferon (IFN-γ) in both experimental animal models and human retroviral infection provides support for an indirect effect of retrovirus infection in the pathogenesis of observed rheumatic manifestations. Some of these mediators, particularly IFN-γ, enhance the expression of class II major histocompatibility complex antigens on several cell types, including epidermal Langerhans, synovial, and muscle cells (9). Growth factors induced by HIV appear to play a role in the pathogenesis of Kaposi's sarcoma. The role of similar growth factors in the pathogenesis of the various rheumatic complications of AIDS deserves further consideration.

The role of reactive and autoimmune mechanisms merits consideration. In general, autoantibodies directed against nuclear or cytoplasmic antigens have not been identified in affected individuals. Occasionally low titer antinuclear antibodies are reported in HIV-infected patients. The presence, however, of antiphospholipid antibodies including VDRL, anticardiolipin, and lupus anticoagulant, are frequently described in HIV patients. Clinical complications attributed to the presence of these antibodies have

not been reported. This suggests that their presence, as well as the presence of circulating immune complexes, may be related to the underlying presence of HIV or opportunistic infection in this population.

Any of the opportunistic or superimposed infections seen during the course of HIV infection may trigger a reactive arthritis. This is an attractive hypothesis to explain the increased incidence of Reiter's syndrome in black Zimbabwean patients, despite the fact that they lack the presence of HLA–B27 (10). Moreover, the recent observation that co-infection with *Mycoplasma fermentans* (incognitus strain) enhances the cytopathic ability of HIV provides further support for a possible role of opportunistic or superimposed infection in the pathogenesis of AIDS and its rheumatic manifestations.

A variety of HIV antigens, including p24, gp41, and gp120, have been demonstrated in tissues of patients with HIV infection. All of these tissues harbor immune effector cells capable of reacting to foreign antigenic stimuli. Consequently, triggering of an immune reaction leading to tissue damage might result from stimulation of these cells by HIV antigens.

Epidemiology

The exact prevalence of rheumatic complaints in patients with HIV infection is uncertain. To date, only a few prospective studies have examined this issue. Berman et al (4) first studied in a prospective manner a large number of HIV patients to ascertain the frequency and clinical spectrum of rheumatic manifestations. Subsequent studies have conclusively shown a high prevalence and wide spectrum of rheumatic manifestations in HIV-infected patients. A summary of these studies indicate that as many as 70% of HIV patients develop some type of rheumatic complaint (11).

Clinical Syndromes

A broad array of rheumatic syndromes is associated with HIV infection, ranging from arthralgia to reactive arthritis, and more severe necrotizing vasculitis (Table 44–1). Arthralgia can be the first rheumatic manifestation and can occur at any stage of HIV infection. They are usually of moderate intensity, intermittent, and oligoarticular. Large joints, including knees, shoulders, and elbows, are most commonly involved. In approximately 10% of patients, arthralgia may be severe and are unresponsive to conventional analgesic medication—the so-called "painful articular syndrome" (4,12). Arthralgia in this syndrome is excruciating and debilitating, necessitating emergency care or hospitalization for the use of intravenous narcotic medication.

Reiter's syndrome was the first distinct rheumatologic disorder described in association with HIV infection (5). The onset of

Table 44–1. Rheumatic manifestations associated with HIV infection

Articular:	Arthralgias
	Reiter's syndrome
	Psoriatic arthritis
	Undifferentiated spondylarthritis
	HIV-associated arthritis
Muscular:	Myalgias
	Polymyositis—Dermatomyositis
	—HIV induced
	Myopathy:
	—AZT induced
	Pyomyositis
Sjogren's-like syndrome	
Lupus-like syndrome	
Vasculitis	
Miscellaneous:	Fibromyalgia
	Hypertrophic osteoarthropathy
	Osteonecrosis of bone
	Soft tissue involvement: i.e. bursitis, tendinitis, Dupuytren's contractures

Reiter's syndrome may precede by up to 2 years, occur concomitantly, or most commonly follow the appearance of clinical evidence of immunodeficiency. Therefore, a high index of suspicion is needed when examining individuals that belong to a high risk group for HIV infection and who present with Reiter's syndrome.

Most patients develop the incomplete form with typical articular and some extraarticular features, but absence of urethritis and conjunctivitis. The usual articular symptoms are asymmetric oligoarthritis of large joints (most frequently knees), enthesopathy, and other extraarticular manifestations, such as circinate balanitis, keratoderma blennorrhagica, stomatitis, or uveitis. Clinical and radiologic evidence of spinal or sacroiliac joint involvement may be seen, and HLA-B27 antigen positivity is found in up to two-thirds of patients. The clinical course of HIV-associated Reiter's syndrome is variable, from a mild or moderate course of a transient nature, to a rapidly deforming, disabling and incapacitating course refractory to conventional antiinflammatory medication.

Psoriasis and its related arthritis are present with increased prevalence in HIV-infected patients. A variety of psoriatic rashes can occur in HIV infection, including vulgaris, guttate, sebopsoriasis, pustular, and exfoliative erythroderma. Single or combination forms may be seen in a given individual. Nail changes are common, and range from pitting to severe onycholysis. Nail changes are frequently confused with fungal infection or pyogenic paronychia, but potassium hydroxide and culture examination are negative. Psoriasis and psoriatic arthritis may precede or follow the clinical onset of immunodeficiency. Sacroiliac and spinal involvement may also occur, as well as enthesopathy and dactylytis. The clinical course is variable, with a tendency to follow a progressive course refractory to conventional therapy in a majority of patients; erosions and crippling deformities may develop in a relatively short period (13).

The association of HIV infection with undifferentiated spondylarthropathy is well established. These patients do not develop sufficient clinical manifestations to be classified as having Reiter's syndrome, psoriatic arthritis, or ankylosing spondylitis. Enthesitis, oligoarthritis, dactylytis, onycholysis, conjunctivitis, and spondylitis are the presenting manifestations. Bilateral sacroiliitis can be seen.

Infected patients appear to develop an otherwise unexplained distinct inflammatory articular syndrome. The HIV-associated arthritis tends to be oligoarticular in approximately one-half of patients, with mono- and polyarticular forms being equally distributed in the remainder. Polyarthritis is asymmetric, involving large, weight bearing joints such as knees and ankles. An occasional patient may present with a clinical picture similar to rheumatoid arthritis (RA), but lacking joint erosions and rheumatoid factor. Patients with HIV-associated arthritis do not exhibit any extraarticular manifestation suggestive of Reiter's syndrome, psoriatic arthritis, or other spondylarthropathy. Tests for HLA-B27 are negative, and HLA-DR typing has not revealed any unusual increased prevalence of a particular antigenic specificity. Most patients are in late stages of HIV infection, and the average duration is four weeks.

Muscle involvement is common. Myalgias, usually generalized but occasionally localized, are the most common symptom. They are transient, recurrent, and usually respond to analgesic therapy. Muscle atrophy is also relatively common. Dermatomyositis and polymyositis may also be associated with HIV infection. The clinical picture is identical to the idiopathic forms, with proximal muscle weakness that may precede or follow the appearance of immunodeficiency. Elevation of muscle enzymes and electromyographic and histologic findings are also identical.

Other types of muscle involvement include zidovudine-induced myopathy, muscle infection (pyomyositis), and myositis ossificans (14,15). Proximal muscle weakness most commonly follows zidovudine (AZT) therapy (14). This condition is distinct from HIV-associated myopathy, and a rapid improvement follows AZT withdrawal. A direct zidovudine-induced toxic mitochondrial myopathy with the appearance of "ragged red fibers," indicative of abnormal mitochondrial with paracrystalline inclusions, is responsible for this disorder.

A Sjogren's-like syndrome, with xerophthalmia, xerostomia, and parotid gland enlargement, is associated with HIV infection (16). In contrast to the idiopathic form, this Sjogren's-like syndrome or "diffuse infiltration lymphocytosis syndrome" occurs predominantly in men, and is characterized by prominent parotid gland swelling or large neck masses, absence of arthritis, impressive extra-salivary lymphoid infiltration, lack of Ro(SS-A) and La(SS-B) antibodies and rheumatoid factor, and a predominance of CD8$^+$ lymphocytes. The frequency of HLA-B5 is elevated in black patients. Of interest, recent reports have demonstrated the presence of serum antibodies against HIV p24 antigen, and retroviral particles antigenically related to HIV in lymphoblastoid indicator cells incubated with homogenates of salivary tissue obtained from patients with idiopathic Sjogren's syndrome.

Several vasculitic syndromes also are associated with HIV infection (17). A polyarteritis nodosa-like syndrome with vasculitis of medium-sized blood vessels involving skin, nerve, and muscle, is most commonly seen. Mononeuritis is also a frequent finding.

The HIV infection may mimic other connective tissue disorders, particularly systemic lupus erythematosus (SLE), RA, and polymyositis. Of interest, patients with the idiopathic form of SLE or RA who become infected with HIV may enter into clinical remission. A recent report, however, described a patient with coexistent RA and HIV infection, whose disease activity did not remit (18,19).

Septic arthritis is a relatively unusual complication, and only isolated cases of septic arthritis and bursitis have been reported. Hemophiliac and intravenous drug abuser patients are at a high risk for septic arthritis. Osteomyelitis may be present alone or coexistent with septic arthritis.

Fibromyalgia has been reported in approximately 30% of HIV-infected patients (20). Hypertrophic osteoarthropathy, multiple sites of aseptic bone necrosis, and a variety of soft tissue involvements including Dupuytren's contracture, capsulitis of the shoulder, rotator cuff lesions, tennis elbow, carpal tunnel syndrome, and osteochondritis may also occur.

Rheumatic Complaints Associated with HTLV

The etiologic agent of adult T-cell leukemia, HTLV-1, is also associated with rheumatic syndromes including polymyositis, polyarthritis, and Sjogren's syndrome. Polymyositis associated with HTLV-1 is identical in its clinical presentation to the idiopathic and HIV-associated forms. The arthropathy is usually oligoarticular, affecting weight-bearing joints such as the knees, and runs a chronic course with an occasional flare. Polyarthritis may be seen occasionally. Large joints, including shoulders, wrists, and knees, are preferentially affected. The erythrocyte sedimentation rate is usually elevated, and rheumatoid factor positivity is observed in one-half of patients. No clinical signs of leukemia or AIDS are detected in patients with HTLV-1 joint involvement. Anti-HTLV-1 antibodies are detected in sera and synovial fluid. Synovial fluid analysis reveals lymphocytosis, with "flower" cells or atypical lymphocytes being a characteristic finding.

Recently, an HTLV-1 transgenic mouse model has been developed, which spontaneously develops a similar type of arthritis as that seen in humans (21).

Enthesitis was recently reported in a 26-year old woman, native of Cabo Verde, Africa, who was positive for HTLV-II. No co-infection with another retrovirus was detected.

Laboratory Findings in HIV Infection

Several abnormal laboratory findings are seen in patients with HIV infection. Polyclonal hypergammaglobulinemia is the most common abnormality, although a few cases of hypo- or agammaglobulinemia have been described. Circulating immune complexes, often containing IgA, and antiphospholipid antibodies, particularly IgG, are common in HIV infected patients. Synovial effusions are present in about one-third of affected patients. These effusions are small (5–10 ml), and inflammatory in character with white cell counts ranging from 2000–14,500/mm^3 and containing predominantly polymorphonuclear cells. Typically, the involved synovial membrane exhibits mild to moderate non-specific proliferative changes, and HIV p24 antigen can be demonstrated in cells of the synovial lining layer and mononuclear cells of the subsynovial space. Radiologic evidence of joint involvement includes soft tissue swelling, joint space narrowing, erosions, whittling, osteolytic lesions, periostitis, sacroiliac joint space widening, erosions, and syndesmophyte formation.

Therapy

Most patients respond to antirheumatic therapy with a combination of analgesics and nonsteroidal antiinflammatory medications. Phenylbutazone and sulfasalazine are highly effective in patients with Reiter's syndrome and psoriatic arthritis (22). Some patients, especially those with Reiter's syndrome and psoriatic arthritis, may be refractory to therapy. In these patients, immunosuppressive drugs such as cyclosporin and methotrexate have been beneficial (11). The use of immunosuppressive therapy should be carefully monitored because of the possibility of worsening the immunodeficiency state as well as the possible development of Kaposi's sarcoma and full-blown AIDS.

Topical steroids are effective in patients with uveitis. Local steroid injection is useful in treating severely inflamed joints and tendons. Prednisone, alone or in combination with methotrexate and/or AZT, is useful in the management of polymyositis. Doses ranging from 30–60 mg/day are effective.

Improvement of psoriasis and psoriatic arthritis may occur with AZT and antibiotic treatment (trimethaprin/sulfamethoxazole or co-trimoxazole). Appropriate physical therapy and occupational rehabilitation are also indicated in the overall management of HIV-infected patients.

OTHER IMMUNODEFICIENCY STATES

Inflammatory musculoskeletal involvement is not unusual in primary deficiency states, including immunoglobulin and complement component deficiencies.

Primary Immunodeficiency

Rheumatic symptoms develop in approximately 15% to 20% of patients with common variable immunodeficiency (CVID) or agammaglobulinemia. The most characteristic presentation is a chronic rheumatoid arthritis-like clinical picture, which is somewhat atypical because it is oligoarticular and affects large weight bearing joints, particularly knees, with a relative sparing of small joints. Rheumatoid factor is usually absent. The synovial membrane exhibits mild, nonspecific synovitis, with mononuclear cell infiltration, and often a significant number of plasma cells (23). An infectious etiology for the arthritis in some cases is suggested by the fact that infectious organisms have been isolated from the synovial fluid and membrane of several patients. The prevalence and severity of this complication have greatly diminished with the use of immunoglobulin therapy (24,25).

Several other forms of autoimmune diseases have been reported in association with CVID, including hemolytic anemia, thrombocytopenia, chronic active hepatitis, parotitis, progressive systemic sclerosis, dermatomyositis, SLE, and Sjogren's syndrome. Arthritis has also been described in patients with selective IgA deficiency that may be difficult to differentiate from juvenile rheumatoid arthritis (JRA). The problem is compounded by the increased prevalence (4%) of IgA deficiency in patients with JRA. Patients with selective IgA deficiency should not be given gammaglobulin therapy or plasma, because they may react to the foreign IgA and develop severe hypersensitivity reactions (25).

Complement Deficiencies

A variety of rheumatic disorders are associated with inherited and acquired deficiencies of the complement system. The most common complement component deficiency by far is C2 deficiency, associated with a variety of rheumatic disorders including SLE, discoid lupus and subcutaneous lupus erythematous, dermatomyositis and polymyositis, vasculitides, JRA, glomerulonephritis, and inflammatory bowel disease. C1q, C1r, C1s, C4 and CIINH deficiencies have each been associated with the development of SLE.

Luis R. Espinoza, MD
Marta Lucia Cuéllar, MD

1. Siegal FP, Lopez C, Hammer GS, et al: Severe acquired immunodeficiency in male homosexuals, manifested by chronic perianal ulcerative herpes simplex lesions. N Engl J Med 305:1439–1444, 1981
2. Brennan TA: The acquired immunodeficiency syndrome (AIDS) as an occupational disease. Ann Intern Med 107:581–583, 1987
3. Barre–Sinoussi F, Chermann JC, Rey F, et al: Isolation of a T-lymphocyte retrovirus from a patient at risk for acquired immunodeficiency syndrome (AIDS). Science 220:868–871, 1983
4. Berman A, Espinoza LR, Diaz JD, et al: Rheumatic manifestations of human immunodeficiency virus infection. Am J Med 85:59–64, 1988
5. Winchester R, Bernstein DH, Fischer HD, et al: The co-occurrence of Reiter's syndrome and acquired immunodeficiency. Ann Intern Med 106:19–26, 1987
6. Greene WC: The molecular biology of human immunodeficiency virus type 1 infection. N Engl J Med 324:308–317, 1991
7. Fauci AS: The human immunodeficiency virus: infectivity and mechanisms of pathogenesis. Science 239:617–622, 1988
8. Espinoza LR, Aguilar JL, Berman A, et al: Rheumatic manifestations associated with human immunodeficiency virus infection. Arthritis Rheum 32:1615–1622, 1989
9. Illa I, Nath A, Dalaka M: Immunocytochemical and virological characteristics of HIV-associated inflammatory myopathies: similarities with seronegative polymyositis. Ann Neurol 29:474–481, 1991
10. Davis P, Stein M, Latif AS, et al: Acute arthritis in Zimbabwean patients: possible relationship to human immunodeficiency virus infection. J Rheumatol 16:346–348, 1989
11. Espinoza LR, Jara LJ, Espinoza CG, et al: Association between HIV infection and spondyloarthropathies. Rheum Dis Clin NA 1992;18:257–266
12. Winchester R: AIDS and the rheumatic diseases. Bull Rheum Dis 39:1–10, 1990
13. Espinoza LR, Berman A, Vasey FB, et al: Psoriatic arthritis and acquired immunodeficiency syndrome. Arthritis Rheum 31:1034–1040, 1988
14. Espinoza LR, Aguilar JL, Espinoza CG, et al: Characteristics and pathogenesis of myositis in human immunodeficiency virus infection—distinction from azidothymidine-induced myopathy. Rheum Dis Clin 17:117–129, 1991
15. Victor G, Branley J, Opal SM, et al: Pyomyositis in a patient with the acquired immunodeficiency syndrome. Arch Intern Med 149:704–709, 1989
16. Itescu S, Brancato LJ, Buxbaum J, et al: CD8 lymphocytosis syndrome in human immunodeficiency virus (HIV) infection: a host immuno response associated with HLA–DR5. Ann Intern Med 112:3–10, 1990
17. Calabrese LH, Estes M, Yen–Liebermann B, et al: Systemic vasculitis in association with human immunodeficiency virus infection. Arthritis Rheum 32:569–576, 1989
18. Jaffe IA: Rheumatoid arthritis and AIDS (letter). J Rheumatol 1989;16:845
19. Kerr LD, Spiera H: The coexistence of classic RA and AIDS. (letter). J Rheumatol 1991;18:1739–1740
20. Buskila D, Gladman D, Langevitz P, et al: Fibromyalgia in human immunodeficiency virus infection. J Rheumatol 1990;17:1202–1206
21. Iwakura Y, Tosu M, Yoshida E, et al: Induction of inflammatory arthropathy resembling rheumatoid arthritis in mice transgenic for HTLV-1. Science 253:1026–1029, 1991
22. Youssef PP, Bertouch JV, Jones PD: Successful treatment of human immunodeficiency virus-associated Reiter's syndrome with sulfasalazine (concise communication). Arthritis Rheum 35:723–724, 1992
23. Lee AH, Levinson AI, Schumacher Jr HR: Hypogammaglobulinemia and rheumatic disease. Semin Arthritis Rheum 22:250–264, 1993
24. Good RA, Rotstein J, Mazzitello WF: The simultaneous occurrence of rheumatoid arthritis and agammaglobulinemia. J Lab Clin Med 249:343–357, 1957
25. Preston SJ, Buchanan WW: Rheumatic manifestations of immune deficiency. Clin Exp Rheumatology 7:547–555, 1989

45. HYPERTROPHIC OSTEOARTHROPATHY

Hypertrophic osteoarthropathy (HOA) or *achropachy* is a syndrome characterized by excessive proliferation of skin and bones at the distal parts of the extremities. Its most conspicuous clinical feature is a unique bulbous deformity of the tips of the digits, conventionally known as *clubbing* (Fig. 45–1). In advanced stages, periosteal proliferation of the tubular bones and synovial effusion become evident (1).

PATHOLOGY AND PATHOGENESIS

The bulbous deformity of the digits is due to edema and excessive collagen deposition. Vascular hyperplasia with endothelial damage is another prominent feature. Parallel events may occur at the joints (2) and at the tubular bones where excessive fibroblast proliferation elevates the periosteum and new osteoid matrix is deposited.

Recent studies of patients with cyanotic heart diseases have yielded data that may explain the pathogenesis of HOA. These patients are an excellent model for the study of hypertrophic osteoarthropathy since all of them have the lifelong presence of clubbing, and over one-third display the fully developed syndrome. No other internal illness is so highly associated with acropachy. Patients with cardiogenic HOA frequently develop thrombocytopenia due to an increased peripheral destruction of platelets. In addition, these patients have a bizarre platelet population characterized by the presence of macrothrombocytes with aberrant volume distribution curves. These features suggest that in cases with right-to-left shunts of blood, large platelets, which normally would break up in the highly dichotomized pulmonary vascular bed, would instead gain direct access to the systemic circulation, reach its most distal sites in axial streams, and interact with endothelial cells, with the subsequent release of fibroblast growth factor(s) thus inducing acropachy (3). It also has been demonstrated that not only patients with cardiogenic HOA but also those with the primary form of the syndrome have raised circulating levels of von Willebrand factor antigen (4). These data suggest that cardiogenic HOA develops as a result of platelet/endothelial cell activation localized at the distal parts of the extremities with the ensuing release of fibroblast growth factor(s).

Similar mechanisms may be operative in other conditions associated with HOA. Lesser degrees of right-to-left shunts are evident in lung cancer, intestinal polyposis, and in the hepatopulmonary syndrome of liver cirrhosis. Endothelial cell activation is a prominent feature of endarteritis or endocarditis of infective etiology. There is homology between platelet-derived growth factor (PDGF) and the simian sarcoma virus, an agent implicated in the etiology of lung cancer, suggesting a theoretical source of a PDGF-like material. It has been shown that in pulmonary fibrosis the infiltrating cells produce excessive amounts of PDGF. All this new information needs to be confirmed by further studies.

CLINICAL FEATURES

Some patients may be asymptomatic and unaware of the deformity of their digits. Other patients, particularly those with malignant lung tumors, may suffer incapacitating bone pain (2). Characteristically, this pain is deep-seated, more prominent in the lower extremities, and is aggravated by dependency of the limbs. Physical examination is the key to the diagnosis since the bulbous deformity of the digits is unique (Fig. 45–1). The increase in soft tissue typically molds the fingernail into a "watch crystal" convexity, and the nailbed rocks when palpated. Toes are also affected, but early changes are more difficult to discern.

The digital index provides a practical bedside method to measure clubbing. With the use of a non-elastic string, the perimeter of each finger is measured at the nailbed (NB) and at the distal interphalangeal joint (DIP) levels. If the sum of the 10 NB/DIP ratios is more than 10, clubbing is most likely present (5). Loss of the normal angle between the nail and the swollen bed is also a useful clinical sign.

When the complete features of HOA are evident, thickening of the bones may be appreciated in areas of the extremities not covered by muscles such as ankles and wrists. The ankle, the site of the periostosis, is sometimes surrounded by cylindric soft tissue swelling. Periostosis is usually accompanied by tenderness of the affected area. Effusions into the large joints is a frequent but by no means universal finding. At palpation there is no detectable hypertrophy of the synovial capsule. Other features include the following: 1) range of motion of the joints may be slightly decreased; 2) arthrocentesis yields a clear viscous fluid with little inflammatory cell exudation; and 3) leucocyte counts are usually less than 1,000 cells/mm^3. These features reflect the fact that at least in early stages HOA is not an inflammatory or proliferative synovial disease (2,6).

There are clinical findings associated with particular types of secondary HOA. In most instances HOA involves the four extremities, but forms localized to one or two limbs may be seen. The majority of the latter occur as a reaction to prominent endothelial injury of that particular limb, such as aneurysms and infective endarteritis (7), or may be associated to patent ductus arteriosus with reversal of flow.

Primary HOA is characterized by a clearcut hereditary predisposition. One-third of these cases recognize a close relative with the same illness. There is male prevalence (9:1). Primary cases are prone to display a generalized skin hypertrophy, thus the term *pachydermoperiostosis*. This overgrowth roughens the facial features and can reach the extreme of cutis verticis gyrata, which is the most advanced stage of cutaneous hypertrophy. Also, they frequently demonstrate cutaneous glandular dysfunction manifested as hyperhydrosis, seborrhea, or acne (6,8).

LABORATORY TESTS AND IMAGING

Aside from the abnormal platelet population observed in patients with cardiogenic HOA, there are no other distinctive abnormalities in the laboratory examination. An array of biochemical alterations may be found that reflect the underlying illness, such as elevated sedimentation rates related to malignancies.

Plain radiology of the extremities may reveal abnormalities in an asymptomatic patient. Longstanding clubbing can produce acroosteolysis, although distal finger tuft hypertrophy may be observed in some chronic cases. Periostosis evolves in an orderly manner. When mild, it involves few bones (usually tibias and fibulas), periosteal apposition is limited to the diaphysis, and it has a monolayer configuration. Severe periostosis affects all tubular bones, spreads to metaphyses and epyphyses, and generates an irregular configuration. Also typical of HOA is preserva-

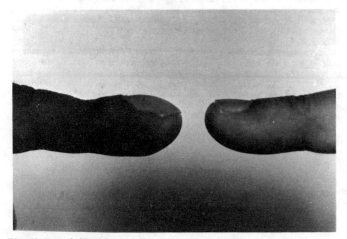

Fig. 45–1. A clubbed finger on the left compared with a normal one on the right.

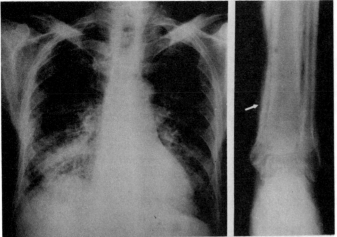

Fig. 45–2. *Radiographs of a 67-year old man with bronchogenic carcinoma. Periostosis of tibia and fibula is evident.*

tion of joint space and absence of erosions or paraarticular osteopenia (9) (Fig. 45–2). Radiographic changes are symmetric and affect first the distal parts of the lower extremities and then evolve in a centripetal fashion. Radionuclide bone scanning is a sensitive method for demonstrating periosteal involvement and may show abnormalities before radiographs.

DIAGNOSIS

In some cases of lung cancer, painful arthropathy may be the presenting manifestation of the syndrome, occuring even without detectable clubbing. Such patients could be misdiagnosed as having an inflammatory type of arthritis (1). Important clinical features in the differential diagnosis are the location of pain—in HOA not only is the joint involved but also the adjacent bone. Rheumatoid factor is usually absent, and there is only sparse inflammatory cell infiltration in the synovial fluid. There are instances of HOA in which the exuberant skin hypertrophy could be confused with acromegaly.

Patients should be classified as having the primary form of the syndrome only after a careful scrutiny fails to disclose any underlying illness. If in a previously healthy individual any of the manifestations of HOA become evident, a thorough search for an underlying illness should be undertaken. On the other hand, if clubbing appears in a patients previously diagnosed with any of the chronic illnesses listed in Fig. 45–3, it usually represents a bad prognostic sign. Clubbing in a patient with known rheumatic heart disease or intravenous drug addiction may indicate infective endocarditis. A similar consideration applies to the patients

Fig. 45–3. *Classification of hypertrophic osteoarthropathy.*

			DIGITAL CLUBBING			
		HYPERTROPHIC OSTEOARTHROPATHY				
PRIMARY			SECONDARY			
		GENERALIZED		LOCALIZED		
			Hemiplegia	Aneurysm	Infective arteritis	Patent ductus arteriosus
PULMONARY	CARDIAC	HEPATIC	INTESTINAL	MEDIASTINAL		MISCELLANEOUS
Cystic fibrosis	Congenital cyanotic diseases	Cirrhosis	Crohn's disease	Esophageal carcinoma		Graves's disease
Pulmonary fibrosis	Infective endocarditis	Carcinoma	Ulcerative colitis	Thymoma		Thalassemia
Chronic infections			Chronic infections	Achalasia		Diverse malignancies
Cancer: primary or metastatic			Laxative abuse			Others
A-V fistulae			Polyposis			
Mesothelioma			Malignant tumors			

with history of prosthetic vascular surgery who develop periostosis of a limb.

TREATMENT

Apart from the unsightliness, clubbing is usually asymptomatic and does not require therapy. Patients with painful osteoarthropathy generally respond best to nonsteroidal antiinflammatory drugs. Correction of a heart malformation, removal of a lung tumor, and successful treatment of endocarditis can produce a rapid regression of all symptoms.

Manuel Martínez–Lavín, MD

1. Marie P: De l'osteo-arthropathie hypertrophiante pneumique. Rev Med 10:1–36, 1891
2. Schumacher HR: Articular manifestations of hypertrophic pulmonary osteoarthropathy in bronchogenic carcinoma. Arthritis Rheum 19:629–635, 1976
3. Vazquez–Abad D, Martínez–Lavín M: Macrothrombocytes in the peripheral circulation of patients with cardiogenic hypertrophic osteoarthropathy. Clin Exp Rheumatol 9:59–62, 1991
4. Matucci–Cerinic M, Martínez–Lavín M, Rojo F, et al: Increased plasma levels of von Willebrand factor antigen in patients with hypertrophic osteoarthropathy. J Rheumatol 19:765–767, 1992
5. Vazquez–Abad D, Pineda C, Martínez–Lavín M: Digital clubbing; a numerical assessment of the deformity. J Rheumatol 16:518–520, 1989
6. Martínez–Lavín M, Pineda C, Valdez T, et al: Primary hypertrophic osteoarthropathy. Semin Arthritis Rheum 17:156–162, 1988
7. Stiles R, Resnick D, Sartoris D, et al: Unilateral lower extremity hypertrophic osteoarthropathy associated with aortic graft infection. South Med J 81:788–791, 1988
8. Matucci–Cerinic M, Lotti T, Jajic I, et al: The clinical spectrum of pachydermoperiostosis (primary hypertrophic osteoarthropathy) Medicine 91:208–214, 1991
9. Pineda C, Fonseca C, Martínez–Lavín M: The spectrum of soft tissue and skeletal abnormalities of hypertrophic osteoarthropathy. J Rheumatol 17:773–778, 1990

46. BONE AND JOINT DYSPLASIAS

The term *dysplasia* is a generic one, which over the years has been more or less appropriately applied to a number of entities within the realm of connective tissue disease. In many cases, the only feature the disorders have in common (other than their occurrence in bones and joints) is the appellation "dysplasia". This chapter includes discussions on the juvenile osteochondroses, hip dysplasia in infancy and childhood, and slipped capital femoral epiphysis and its complication, chondrolysis.

THE JUVENILE OSTEOCHONDROSES

The term *juvenile osteochondroses* (or osteochondritides) embraces a series of regionally located clinical entities, all described in the early years of radiography. These disorders (or as will be shown for some, non-disorders) were originally placed in one

group based chiefly on the prevailing albeit erroneous view that they share a common pathogenesis (1). The osteochondroses occur primarily in children, affect the epiphyseal and apophyseal centers, and have somewhat similar roentgenographic characteristics, which were thought to represent forms of localized osteonecrosis.

Because tuberculosis and osteomyelitis were prevalent enough to dominate orthopedic thought in the early years of the 20th century, the osteochondroses were singled out as being not of septic origin and hence were classified as *aseptic necrosis*, a term which is still encountered. A critical appraisal of these conditions has led to their separation into two major groups: 1) *true osteonecrosis* of an apophyseal or epiphyseal center; and 2) *non-necrotic abnormalities* of ossification, either genetic or traumatic in origin.

True Osteonecrosis

Legg–Calve–Perthes Disease. Coxa plana or idiopathic osteonecrosis of the proximal femoral capital epiphysis is usually designated by all three or just the last of the names of the three individuals who described it. The disorder occurs principally in boys ages 3 to 12 years, and is much more common in Caucasians than in blacks. The disease is bilateral in approximately 15% of the patients, and is associated with modest degrees of retardation of skeletal maturation (2). It is occasionally preceded by one or more episodes of transient synovitis (3).

The clinical findings include a slowly evolving painless limp, often in association with limitation of abduction and internal rotation, and a modest to moderate fixed flexion deformity (2). Although trauma, endocrine abnormality and infection have been proposed, no data exist to support these etiologic hypotheses. The cause of the abnormality remains obscure. Children with this disorder show a modest retardation in growth but no other clinical abnormalities, and specifically thyroid function is normal. Legg–Calve–Perthes disease must be distinguished from cretinoid dysgenesis, which may produce a similar radiographic image.

Biopsy specimens from affected femoral heads obtained early in the course of the disease show osteonecrosis, while those obtained at later intervals show progressive revascularization. Monitoring by roentgenographic studies or magnetic resonance imaging (MRI) reveals that the disease progresses through phases indicating death of the bone, fragmentation, gradual revascularization, and restoration of structure (2,4). The images initially show increased bone density and subsequent alteration in bony epiphyseal contour, irregularity, and lateral displacement of the femoral head (Fig. 46–1). Over a period of three to five years, a slow restoration to normal bone structure occurs, but often with development of a large, flat femoral head with a wide short neck (coxa magna et plana). By the time symptoms are sufficient to seek medical attention, the revascularization process is often well advanced, as evidenced by increased activity on bone scan or MRI (5).

Treatment of Legg–Calve–Perthes disease is based in part on the estimated prognosis and natural history. Children in whom the process only affects the anterior aspect of the epiphysis, sparing the weight-bearing area, and those who are very young have an excellent prognosis; for the most part, the treatment need only be minimal (2). For those who are older and have complete lesions, avoidance of full weight bearing and increasing the coverage afforded by the acetabulum are the treatment goals. These may be achieved by either bracing or by surgical realignment of the femoral or acetabular structures using osteotomies (6). Late osteoarthritis (OA) is a common result in untreated cases.

Freiberg's Disease. Osteonecrosis of the epiphysis of the second, or occasionally third, metatarsal head in the growing child is designated by the eponym Freiberg's disease or infraction. A rare disorder, which occurs most frequently in children ages 10 to 14 years, the syndrome is believed to result from acute or chronic trauma, an epiphyseal slip, or a stress fracture (7). The condition is associated with local pain and tenderness, and a roentgenogram shows flattening, increased density, and progressive fragmentation of the epiphyseal center. The condition is self-limited, but may over time progress to a minor deformity of the toe and later, to OA. Shoe inserts that transfer the weight to the adjacent metatarsal necks often relieve symptoms.

Kienbock's Disease. Idiopathic osteonecrosis of the carpal lunate occurs more frequently in adults than in children and is more common than most of the other lesions, except perhaps, Legg–Calve–Perthes disease. The disorder is more clearly related to trauma than the other forms of osteonecrosis, in that it can occur directly following dislocations or direct injury (8). Variation in ulnar length and alterations in osseous vascularity have been implicated as predisposing to Kienbock's disease (9). Patients with this disorder often complain of pain in the mid wrist, particularly with active usage of the hand. Roentgenograms show an early increase in density of the bone, followed fairly rapidly by irregularity of contour, cyst formation, and fragmentation (Fig. 46–2), but early diagnosis can now be achieved using MRI (10). Often resection, or reconstructive surgery, is required to relieve symptoms (8,9).

Preiser's, Panner's and Friedrich's Diseases. Preiser's disease is similar to Kienbock's disease but affects the carpal scaphoid. It is much less frequent, and its cause is even more obscure (11). Panner's disease, osteonecrosis of the capitellar epiphyseal center of the distal humerus, is a rarely seen lesion in children. It is probably caused by or at least associated with trauma occurring as a result of a fall on the outstretched hand. Friedrich's disease is a similar condition affecting the medial end of the clavicle. The cause is obscure (12).

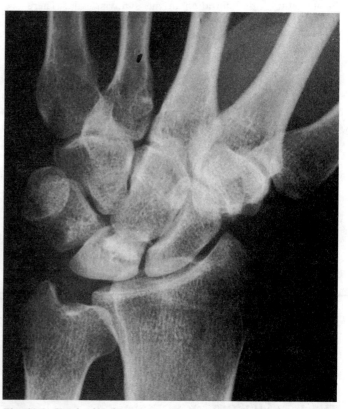

Fig. 46–2. Kienbock's disease in a 36-year-old male who did not recall any specific trauma to the wrist. Note on the anteroposterior radiograph of the carpus that the lunate is more dense than normal and irregular in contour and trabecular architecture. The center most portion of the bone shows a marked increase in density and a surrounding zone of radiolucency.

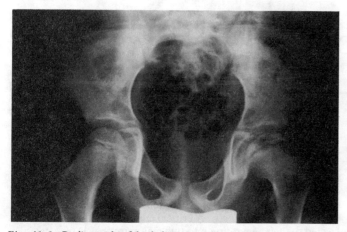

Fig. 46–1. Radiograph of both hips in a 10-year-old boy with Legg–Calve–Perthes disease. The unaffected hip (L) shows normal contours. The affected right side shows enlargment and flattening of the femoral head, irregularity of ossification, and partial fragmentation.

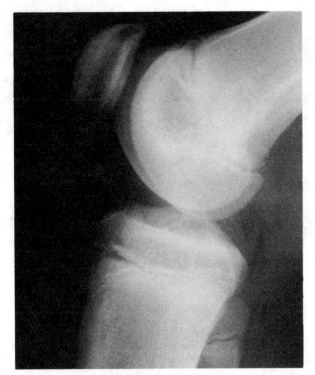

Fig. 46–3. Osgood–Schlatter's disease in a 12-year-old boy who complained of pain and mild swelling in the region of the tibial tubercle. Note the slight irregularity of ossification of the anterior portion of the epiphysis (arrow). This finding is often associated with deep soft tissue swelling, not evident on these films.

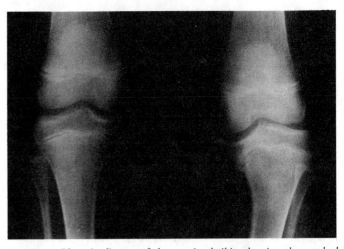

Fig. 46–4. Blount's disease of the proximal tibia showing the marked degree of medial bowing and distortion of the medial tibial condyle. Note especially the irregularity of the epiphyseal plate, which is presumed to be responsible for the deformity.

Non-necrotic Abnormalities

Osgood–Schlatter Disease. Idiopathic osteochondrosis of the tibial tubercle, known as Osgood–Schlatter disease, is not a true osteonecrosis but probably represents a partial avulsion of the tibial tubercle as a result of muscle pull of the quadriceps expansion through the short broad patellar tendon. The disorder is seen especially in boys between 10 to 16 years of age, and is characterized by pain, prominence, and tenderness over the region of the patellar tendon insertion into the distal extension of the proximal tibial epiphysis.

The clinically evident soft-tissue swelling can be easily seen on roentgenograms in the lateral view. The studies may also demonstrate irregularities of the physeal plate and adjacent epiphysis and metaphysis (Fig. 46–3). Ultrasonography appears to be a competent method of diagnosis (13). As the disorder progresses, small fragments of bone may be seen in the tendon, which may persist into adult life. The disorder is self-limited, with a cure usually occurring within one to two years, at the time of termination of length growth and closure of the physis. The adult patient is often left, however, with striking but asymptomatic knobby knees (14). In rare cases, the acute symptoms are severe enough to require limiting the child's activities to control pain. Although rarely performed, operative procedures have been described that prematurely close the plate in order to reduce disability.

Blount's Disease. Tibia vara, or Blount's disease, appears to result from a selective abnormality of chondroepiphyseal growth of the medial side of the proximal tibial physis (1). The lateral side of the same growth plate and the child's remaining skeletal parts appear to be normal. The disorder, almost always bilateral, may be present early in life (infantile form) or develop later (adolescent form). In either case, however, the growth of the medial physis is slowed and distorted, causing a progressively severe bow leg (tibia vara) (15). As the process evolves, the lateral collateral ligament and cruciate ligaments become less competent so that the deformity is much more severe on standing than when lying down.

Radiographic examination shows irregularity of the medial portion of the epiphyseal line, an abnormal slope to the medial tibial (and in late cases, femoral) epiphyses and an irregular "beak" on the metaphyseal side of the plate (15) (Fig. 46–4). Bow legs in infancy may occur on the basis of nutrition (mild rickets) or physiologically (more frequent in blacks and self-limited in extent), but neither of those are as progressive or develop the extreme degree of deformity or anatomic changes seen in Blount's disease. For that reason, it is essential to recognize the disorder and treat it early by either bracing, which is often helpful, particularly in the infantile form of the disease, or by surgical procedures. Stapling of the epiphysis, repeated osteotomies or in extreme cases, intra-epiphyseal corrective realignment may be necessary (15).

Sever's Disease. A lesion very similar to Osgood–Schlatter disease, Sever's disease occurs in the growing child at the insertion of the Achilles tendon into the posterior apophysis of the os calcis. Children usually aged 6 to 10 complain of pain in the heel(s), frequently worse with prolonged walking, and show a modest edema and some tenderness over the tendinous insertion.

Roentgenographic study shows a sometimes startling increase in the density and seeming fragmentation of the apophysis. This finding is not due to osteonecrosis and may be truly nonpathologic, representing a phase of ossification of the apophyseal center for certain individuals. The important issue in relation to this disease is not to overtreat. The disorder is certainly self-limited, and the symptoms often respond to slightly increasing the heel height. A similar traction apophysitis occurring at the base of the fifth metatarsal is known as Iselin's disease (16).

Osteochondritis Dissecans. Although the term *osteochondritis* implies an inflammatory cause, osteochondritis dissecans, particularly of the knee joint, is probably traumatic in origin. It may result simply from a shearing fracture of the subchondral bone, which initially does not disturb the overlying cartilage. The natural history of such an injury is for the segment to work loose, fracture the cartilage, and eventually be discharged into the joint where without a blood supply it becomes necrotic. The cartilage, on the other hand, needs no blood supply when bathed in synovial fluid, so that it continues to not only survive, but for some unexplained reason, may show a proliferation creating a free body or *joint mouse*.

Osteochondritis dissecans classically occurs in the knee joint of young men, ages 10 to 20. The symptoms are initially vague, consisting of mild aching pain and intermittent swelling. As the disorder progresses, the symptoms become accentuated, and with discharge of the free body, crepitus and mechanical locking may ensue. The most frequent site for the development of the lesion is the lateral face of the medial condyle often slightly posteriorly. Roentgenograms clearly demonstrate the lesion, but MRI is useful and diagnostic (17).

Treatment of osteochondritis dissecans is often unnecessary in children under 12 years of age in whom the radiographic appearance may result from an abnormality of epiphyseal ossification, rather than being a real lesion. In older individuals, however, a surgical approach, either by arthroscopy or arthrotomy, is most often required. The body can at times be fixed in situ and will heal, but on occasion it may have to be removed and the bony base drilled. In some cases the defect can be treated by allograft implantation (17).

Scheuermann's Disease. Adolescent round back or kyphosis, epiphysitis of the spine, and osteochondritis deformans juvenilis dorsi are all synonyms for this obscure entity, which is characterized by its occurrence in the dorsal spine and prevalence among adolescent males (1). No known cause has been identified, and indeed the pathologic definition of the disease and its relationship to the ring apophyses have not been fully explained. The child with this disorder is often asymptomatic but occasionally complains of mild pain in the dorsal spine. A kyphosis is noted along with a progressive limitation of extension in some patients. The round back deformity often remains stationary and ceases to be problem with skeletal maturity, but in some patients may continue to gradually increase to a point where bracing or surgery is required.

Roentgenographic studies are frequently diagnostic. Irregularities and scalloping of the anterior margin of most or all of the thoracic vertebrae on lateral view are the earliest findings. In cases in which the lesions progress, the vertebrae are seen to become wedge-shaped, such that the normal thoracic kyphosis is increased to a pathologic degree.

Less Common Osteochondroses. Numerous additional osteochondroses were described in the first three decades of the twentieth century. These include Calve's disease, osteochondrosis, and collapse of the vertebral body to produce *wafer vertebra* or *vertebra plana*. Evidence now exists to support the proposition that all such lesions are pathologic fractures, mostly on the basis of eosinophilic granuloma, or occasionally other such infiltrative marrow lesions such as leukemia or Gaucher's disease. Kohler's disease of the tarsal navicular may on rare occasions represent a true osteonecrosis of that bone. In most of the patients in whom one sees a markedly dense and seemingly fragmented bone on roentgenogram, however, the lesion represents a normal variant of ossification, which is verifiable in many cases by obtaining a roentgenogram of the opposite foot. The same may be said for other such lesions, which have met with varying degrees of acceptance among the pediatric orthopedists over the years. These include such conditions as Kohler's disease of the primary patellar center, Sinding–Larsen's and Larsen–Johannson's disease of the secondary patellar centers, Van Neck's disease of the ischial pubic synchondrosis, Milch's disease of the iliac apophysis, Buchman's disease of the iliac crest, Pierson's disease of the symphysis pubis, and Mandl's disease of the trochanter (1).

HIP DYSPLASIA IN INFANCY AND CHILDHOOD

Developmental dislocation or dysplasia of the hip (DDH) is one of the most prevalent causes of hip disability in children and of subsequent OA in later life (18). Although the cause of the condition is not known, a genetic factor is clearly operative, based on the frequency with which the disorder occurs in families as well as the sex and race distribution. Dysplasia of the hip is six times more frequent in girls than in boys and over 30 times more common in Caucasians than blacks. The rates for individuals from northern Italy and Scandinavia are among the highest in the world; those for children from the Orient are among the lowest. The left side is affected 1.5 times more frequently than the right. When the disease is bilateral, approximately 30% of the time, the left side is usually more severely involved (18).

The anatomic abnormalities in children with DDH, and in adults who have been inadequately or untreated, have been well described, although some controversies exist. The acetabulum is oblique, shallow, and directed anteriorly. The bony buttress on the lateral acetabular wall is insufficient in size and magnitude to provide coverage for the femoral head, particularly in adduction and external rotation. The femoral head and neck are almost

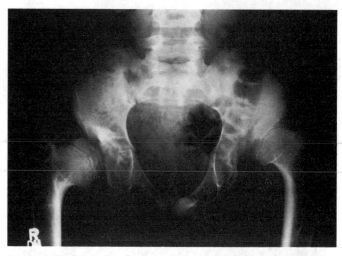

Fig. 46–5. *Radiographs of a 6-year-old child with the late results of an inadequately treated developmental dislocation of the hip. Note that the left hip is high riding and dislocated. The left shows a poorly developed acetabulum with a deformed femoral head and wide neck.*

always anteverted in relation to the femoral shaft, and the head is small and often deformed (Fig. 46–5). The limbus has been described by some as thickened, folded, and interposed, and the capsule as loose and redundant. The iliopsoas tendon has been implicated in some cases as a deforming force, and many of the patients have significant contractures of the adductor muscle groups.

Ideally the condition is recognized at birth on the basis of the finding of an abnormal "click", which may be palpated over the hip region as the infant's hip is abducted and adducted. Within a few weeks, the click can no longer be elicited. The diagnosis is then dependent on the findings of limitation of abduction, shortening of the femur, instability of the hip, abnormally placed thigh creases, and on widening of the perineum in bilateral cases. The diagnosis is readily confirmed by roentgenographic demonstration of an abnormal position of the ossified portions of the femur in relation to the bony pelvis. Computed tomography (CT) and presumably MRI have made this diagnosis more secure, since these newer imaging techniques provide information regarding the soft tissues in addition to the bone. In recent years ultrasonography has added a new dimension, particularly for diagnosis in children under six months of age (19).

If treatment can be started in the nursery or in the first few weeks of life, splinting in abduction carries a low morbidity and the prognosis for full restoration to normal anatomy is excellent. The longer DDH is left untreated, however, the longer the treatment period and the less sure the result. Furthermore, later discovery may require more complex treatment protocols including open reduction, femoral varus, and derotation or innominate osteotomy. The treatment must be carefully done since osteonecrosis may result and complicate the picture. If the patient is untreated or inadequately treated in childhood, the likelihood is high that they will develop OA relatively early in life. Pain, progressive limp, a Trendelenburg gait, shortening of the leg, and limitation of movement gradually increase over time until the patient becomes incapacitated and in many cases requires total hip replacement.

SLIPPED CAPITAL FEMORAL EPIPHYSIS

For most individuals, the proximal femoral (capital) epiphysis unites to the neck of the femur between the ages of 16 and 19 years. Just prior to this event, the physeal plate may become acutely or chronically susceptible to shear, and the head may slip, displacing medially and posteriorly in relation to the shaft of the femur and producing an adduction, lateral rotation, and extension deformity (1) (Fig. 46–6). Slipping of the capital femoral epiphysis (SCFE), known otherwise as adolescent coxa vara or proximal femoral epiphyseolysis, is a common problem in pedi-

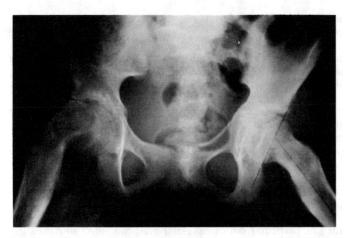

Fig. 46–6. *Slipped capital femoral epiphysis in an 11-year-old child. Note that the hip on the right shows a medial and posterior displacement of the femoral head in relation to the neck. The neck is already somewhat wide, and there is some disuse osteoporosis of the pelvis, suggesting that the slip has been present for some time. The opposite side shows a slight degree of distortion of the normal head-neck relationship suggesting that an early slip may be present.*

pins, which remain the safest system of treatment. More severe slips may require osteotomies or osteoplastic procedures on the femoral neck. If the patient is seen early in the course and treated effectively, the prognosis is generally good. If the patient is seen late and the slip is more severe, the correction obtained is usually less anatomic, and the likelihood of a late onset OA is markedly increased. If closely studied, large numbers of patients formerly thought to have idiopathic or primary OA show roentgenographic signs of an old, mild SCFE.

One of the major complications of SCFE is *chondrolysis*. For reasons as yet not understood, some patients with moderate or severe slips develop progressive limitation of movement of the hip, despite adequate treatment. They go on to demonstrate an autolysis of the acetabular and femoral cartilage, evidenced by extraordinary narrowing of the joint space on roentgenograms (20). Several recent studies have implicated pin protrusion into the acetabulum as a cause of this syndrome (21). The disorder is more frequent in women (the opposite of the SCFE syndrome, which is far more frequent in men) in blacks and Hispanics on the U.S. mainland, and in nonwhites on Hawaii. If untreated, the process goes on to a progressive failure of the hip. Surprisingly, if the patients are placed on limited weight bearing, about 40% recover at least partially.

Henry J. Mankin, MD

1. Siffert RS: Classification of the osteochondroses. Clin Orthop 158:10–18, 1981
2. Catterall A: Legg–Calve–Perthes' syndrome. Clin Orthop 158:41–52, 1981
3. Landin LA, Danielsson LG, Wattsgard C: Transient synovitis of the hip: its incidence, epidemiology and relation to Perthes' disease. J Bone Joint Surg 69B: 238–242, 1987
4. Bos CF, Bloem JL, Bloem RM: Sequential magnetic resonance imaging in Perthes' disease. J Bone Joint Surg 73B:219–224, 1991
5. Ranner G, Ebner F, Fotter R, et al: Magnetic resonance imaging in children with acute hip pain. Pediatr Radiol 20:67–71, 1989
6. Thompson GH, Salter RB: Legg–Calve–Perthes' disease: current concepts and controversies. Orthop Clin North Am 18:617–635, 1987
7. Binek R, Levinsohn EM, Bersani F, et al: Freiberg disease complicating unrelated trauma. Orthopedics 11:753–757, 1988
8. Beckenbaugh RD, Shives TC, Dobyns JH, et al: Kienbock's disease: the natural history of Kienbock's disease and consideration of lunate fractures. Clin Orthop 149:98–106, 1980
9. Almquist EE: Keinbock's disease. Clin Orthop 202:68–78, 1986
10. Trumble TE, Irving J: Histologic and magnetic resonance imaging correlations in Keinbock's disease. J Hand Surg 15:879–884, 1990
11. Ferlic DC, Morin P: Idiopathic avascular necrosis of the scaphoid: Preiser's disease? J Hand Surg 14:13–16, 1989
12. Macule F, Ferreres A, Palliso F, et al: Aseptic necrosis of the sternal end of the clavicle Friedrich's disease. Acta Orthop Belg 56:613–655, 1990
13. Lanning P, Heikkinen E: Ultrasonic features of the Osgood–Schlatter lesion. J Pediatr Orthop 11:538–540, 1991
14. Krause BL, Williams JP, Catterall A: Natural history of Osgod–Schlatter disease. J Pediatr Orthop 10:65–68, 1990
15. Langenskiold A: Tibia vara: osteochondrosis deformans tibiae. Blount's disease. Clin Orthop 158:77–82, 1981
16. Canale ST, Williams KD: Iselin's disease. J Pediatr Orthop 12:90–93, 1992
17. Garrett JC: Osteochondritis dissecans. Clin Sports Med 10:569–593, 1991
18. Coleman SS: Congenital Dysplasia and Dislocation of the Hip. St. Louis, CV Mosby Co., 1978
19. Millis MB, Share JC: Use of ultrasonography in dysplasia of the immature hip. Clin Orthop 274:160–171, 1992
20. Carney BT, Weinstein SL, Noble J: Long-term follow-up of slipped capital femoral epiphysis. J Bone Joint Surg 73:667–674, 1991
21. Riley PM, Weiner DS, Gillespie R, et al: Hazards of internal fixation in the treatment of slipped capital femoral epiphysis. J Bone Joint Surg 72:1500–1509, 1990

atric patients. The onset is often insidious and the presentation subtle; although in a small percentage of the patients the event is preceded by an acute trauma to the hip.

The disorder is considerably more frequent in boys than girls (2:1), and approximately 50% of the cases are bilateral, with one side slipping somewhat earlier than the other. The child sometimes complains of pain in the hip, often referred to the medial side of the knee. On physical examination, the patient may have some shortening, an abnormal gait (usually with a Trendelenburg component), limitation of abduction, medial rotation, and flexion. The diagnosis is best made by standard anteroposterior and especially lateral roentgenograms, which usually clearly demonstrate the slip, even when it is minimal. The degree of slip is important in establishing prognosis and determining treatment. It can usually be assessed by determining the percentage of medial, or posterior displacement, or both, either on roentgenograms or on CT (20). Patients with SCFE have recently been noted to have a greater than average retroversion at the neck–shaft angle, which may be a factor in pathogenesis.

The origin of the problem is obscure. Aside from the sex predilection, two somatotypes appear to be more frequently affected: the short obese boy with poorly developed secondary sex characteristics and the extremely tall and lean child. The oblique angle assumed by the femoral neck at this age coupled with the increased retroversion suggest increased susceptibility to physeal shear. An inherent factor in the epiphyseal plate may also weaken the structure at the age of susceptibility. The possibility of some genetic, hormonal, or autoimmune factors have been proposed, but only limited data have been developed in support of these contentions.

Minimal slips are best treated by fixation in situ with threaded

47. DISORDERS OF THE BACK AND NECK

Back or neck pains are the chief complaint of a considerable percentage of the patients presenting in a primary care setting. They are a major challenge for occupational medicine and rheumatology (1).

Defining the cause of a pain of the axial skeleton involves among other things the process of exclusion (2). Since these complaints are so prevalent and systemic diseases that present

with axial pain so rare, the exercise of exclusion is seldom productive.

There are several red flags in a patient's history however, that should alert the physician to the possibility of a systemic disease presenting with axial symptoms. Almost all axial regional musculoskeletal illnesses force the patient to seek a static posture that unloads the involved region. Recumbency, erect seating, and static standing postures are sought. Axial pain with movement, even writhing, characterizes vascular problems such as aortic dissection or visceral diseases involving the retroperitoneum and obstructive uropathies, among others.

Bone pain from metastatic infection or neoplasia characteristically is accentuated at night, and causes the patient to pace and fidget. Most, but not all, of these patients have systemic symptoms such as fever or weight loss. Also, most have an elevated erythrocyte sedimentation rate (ESR) if not anemia and other laboratory abnormalities associated with the particular process. Metastatic infections tend to localize to the disc or the epidural space. The illness is subacute and, in the latter case (which is a surgical emergency), often characterized by localizing radicular signs. Metastatic tumors can compromise spine stability or encroach on roots or structures within the canal. Both are indications for emergent radiation therapy or, because of increasing success, surgical extirpation and stabilization.

Primary tumors do occur within the canal as well. Extradural tumors present with pain, often at rest and often radicular, with a less prominent mechanical component. Intradural tumors are more insidious; pain is less localizing and neurologic signs more prominent. Cauda equina tumors present as poorly localizing low back pain, often causing the patient to sit in a chair (when not pacing the floor at night) rather than choose recumbency. Neurologic compromise from any destructive process of the cauda equina places sphincter control at risk and can cause saddle anaesthesia.

These are the settings where axial imaging should be pursued; scintiscanning, particularly if sensitivity is enhanced by the SPECT technique, has near perfect sensitivity for any of the processes that impinge on bony structures. Both computed tomography (CT) and magnetic resonance imaging (MRI) approach this sensitivity, and have great specificity for all infectious and neoplastic processes of the axial skeleton. Furthermore, CT-guided tissue biopsy is usually feasible, safe, and diagnostic.

LOW BACK PAIN

Diagnosis

Low back pain is the most frequent musculoskeletal complaint and the most frequent musculoskeletal illness at all ages and in all strata of the population. The treating physician can make the generic diagnosis of regional low back pain by exclusion of other illnesses that present with low back pain. Some physical findings such as spinal range of motion and distraction can be rendered reliable with effort. Most signs that involve prodding and probing the low back are unreliable, and all signs are nonspecific in the setting of regional low back pain.

Imaging techniques have proven even more disappointing. Contemporary imaging modalities can provide detailed anatomic definition which, in the adult, offers nothing for the differential diagnosis of regional low back pain. In other words, any degenerative image found by any modality in a population with regional low back illness can be found in a pain-free population matched for all other parameters with sufficient likelihood to render pathogenetic inferences effete (3,4). An equally cogent deduction is that any degenerative change discerned does not alter the likelihood of remission of the symptom of low back pain. Finally, any degenerative change discerned will persist even after the symptoms have subsided. Imaging for regional low back pain is counterproductive both in time and in physician's ability to promote in the patient a perception that regional low back pain is an intermittent and remittent illness and not a reflection of a bad back. Promulgating this perception of healing should color the entire interaction with the patient and is the logical conclusion of the process of history and physical examination. In the history little is dissuasive of this conclusion, aside from the features discussed above and those that might suggest an inflammatory spondylarthropathy. The physical examination is critical only in that the physician can be reassured regarding major neurologic compromise and relevant underlying diseases such as pelvic or prostatic pathology.

Regional backache is a diagnosis with inherent uncertainty as to the specific cause of the discomfort, but it is not an assertion of ignorance. The diagnosis offers assurance regarding systemic disease and allows the physician to draw prognostic inferences and to offer counseling regarding the extensive menu of therapeutic alternatives. The diagnosis of regional backache offers far more intellectual and therapeutic satisfaction than such traditional heuristic assertions as disc disease or facet arthritis.

Further, the diagnosis of a regional backache is more likely to lead to a therapeutic interaction if the physician and the patient can be made cognizant of the following reasoning: given the frequency and universal prevalence of regional musculoskeletal predicaments, it behooves the treating physician to consider why any particular individual would choose to seek medical recourse for this particular musculoskeletal predicament. Sometimes the explanation is consonant with the tradition of scientific medicine; this person has chosen to be a patient because the predicament was too unfamiliar, too painful, or too prolonged. However, from multiple studies (5), it is becoming clear that such constrained pathophysiologic inferences serve the chief complaint poorly. The decision to be a patient is often tempered by the psychosocial setting in which the musculoskeletal predicament is experienced. Sometimes, the musculoskeletal illness even serves as a surrogate complaint. It is an easier conceptualization than the realization that some other force in life, such as job or marital dissatisfaction, is compromising the ability to cope with the musculoskeletal predicament. Regional musculoskeletal illnesses are often confounded in this fashion and are never well managed unless the confounders are recognized early.

Anatomy of the Lumbosacral Spine

Clinicians are better able to advise patients with low back pain if they understand the functional anatomy of the low back region and appreciate how it changes with aging. The detailed pathoanatomy is interesting, relevant to the surgeon and investigator, and is the traditional prerequisite for a discussion of therapy. However, while interesting pathoanatomy is highly prevalent, its definition offers little likelihood of insight into the cause of the pain in a particular patient. Therefore, this chapter will substitute biomechanical considerations (6) for the traditional pathoanatomic discourse.

The spine is a multi-curved flexible column comprised of linked and interdependent motion segments. Each segment is comprised of adjacent vertebrae articulated at two posterior diarthrodial apophyseal (facet) joints and a single anterior complex synarthrosis, the disc (Fig. 47–1). The consequence of force applied to the spine is a function of the integrated biomechanical response of the motion segments and their associated musculature. In most postures, force is directed to the intervertebral disc. When erect, the force transduced through the L3 disc approaches the weight of the upper half of the body. Deviation from the erect posture will add to stress measurable at the disc. For example, sitting increases strain compared to the erect posture, as does forward flexion when seated or standing. In most postures, the anterior abdominal musculature and the facet joints are under considerably less strain than discal structures. The facet joints constrain torsion and extension. These simple principles are the basis for advising the patient regarding the role of biomechanics in management.

Treatment for Acute Low Back Pain

The mainstay of therapy of the acute backache is to de-medicalize the event. In all likelihood, the process is self-limited; some 80% of patients are well or nearly so in two weeks and at least 90% in two months. Further, although there is considerable likelihood of recurrence, nearly all are left no worse for wear. Finally, with certain exceptions, the natural history cannot be meaningfully altered by interventions. Patients should be made to use their own best judgement. Educating patients and dissuading them from this traditional algorithm is a challenging yet critical

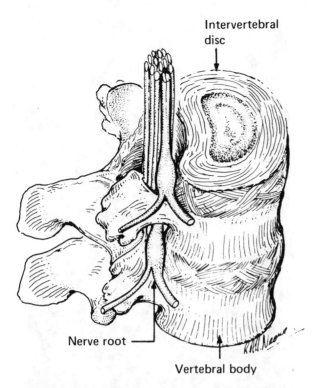

Fig. 47–1. The lumbar spine showing the arrangement of the intervertebral disc between the vertebral bodies, with a central nucleus pulposus surrounded by the annulus fibrosus. The nerve roots emerge through the intervertebral foramina in close relationship to the posterolateral margins of the disc (courtesy of Ciba-Geigy).

undertaking (7). Most patients with backache bring to the medical interaction presuppositions and expectations that initiate this algorithm; therefore, they must be disabused.

Nearly all available interventions have been subjected to clinical trials. Few of these trials escape critical review unscathed; many are uninterpretable. Nonetheless, there is more than enough information to place most of the therapeutic options for acute low back pain into perspective (8,9).

Rest. Rest was a mainstay of therapy for many illnesses in the early decades of this century. For most conditions, it has been discarded. It can be discarded as well for acute low back pain. Certainly recumbency unloads the lumbosacral spine, but only if the patient is fully recumbent. The patient is better off standing, or sitting erect, than propping up in bed. Besides it has not been possible to demonstrate enhanced healing rates with prescribed bed rest—only increased absenteeism from work (10). Suggesting postures to avoid, based on the biomechanical considerations introduced above, such as slouching forward over a desk, for example, is far more sensible than proscribing motion or function.

Pharmacologic Agents. There are over a dozen controlled trials incorporating various analgesics, nonsteroidal antiinflammatory drugs (NSAIDs), benzodiazepines, colchicine, and narcotics. The agents are more consistent and impressive in their toxicities than in differential benefit. The case is easily made for empathy, reassurance, psychological support and a mild analgesic such as acetaminophen along with warm showers.

Exercise. There are advocates for flexing, and there are advocates for extending. There are advocates for isotonic exercises and advocates for combinations. Each has a theory, each is offered with zeal and each has a following. Several regimens are supported by trials showing a degree of benefit; however, two trials demonstrate harm from exercise regimens for acute low back pain. For that reason, an easily defensible approach is to suggest exercises ad lib, postures to avoid, and returning to full function, even to work, as early as possible even before complete remission.

Physical Modalities. Most of the physical modalities have escaped critical testing. Some of the various forms of needling are carried along by dint of precedent; others such as facet joint injections are performed in spite of trials that demonstrate lack of benefit (11). Benefit from spinal manipulation is demonstrable but only for one subset of uncomplicated low back pain—younger individuals hurting for at least two weeks but no more than four—and even then the benefit is modest at best (12). Another newer modality, the use of a transcutaneous electrical nerve stimulation (TENS) unit, has performed poorly in one trial for chronic low back pain (13), but has not been adequately studied for acute low back pain. Various forms of traction have been subjected to trials, most of which are difficult to interpret. In overview, traction is unimpressive if not useless beyond enforcing bed rest and rendering the patient totally passive and nonfunctional.

Structured Programs of Education and Therapy. As previously discussed, acute low back pain challenges the resources of all health care providers. It would make sense to be proactive, offering to all patients at the initiation of the illness access to advice and conservative interventions. In the industrial setting, where clinical improvement can be measured in terms of time lost from work, such programs have been shown to be useful. In the setting of a health maintenance organization (HMO), symptomatic benefit has proven elusive.

Surgery. All forms of surgical intervention have nothing to offer the patient with acute low back pain. Most surgical interventions for low back pain have never been subjected to any systematic assessment. Those that have, such as laminectomy with or without fusion, have fared poorly.

NECK PAIN

Neck pain rivals low back pain in incidence and prevalence; however, neck pain is less likely to cause patients to seek medical attention. For regional musculoskeletal illness of the neck, medical consultation is sought if the pain is perceived as too intense, too prolonged, or associated with disability, such as difficulty seeing over the shoulder when driving a car in reverse. The quality of the discomfort is what would be expected for regional musculoskeletal illness elsewhere: use-associated pain, restriction in motion, relief with unloading, and abruptness of onset. Associated neurologic or systemic symptoms raise the spectre of other causes, as is the case for low back pain. Likewise, cervical pain can herald visceral catastrophe, particularly cardiovascular catastrophe. Neck pain can be an anginal equivalent, a manifestation of temporal arteritis, and a classic presentation for aortic dissection. In these instances, range of motion is not compromised, and the discomfort is likely to present more in the anterior neck and throat. Further, neck pain becomes as confounded an illness as low back pain if it is associated with work incapacity.

Cervical Anatomy

Although it bears little on the clinical algorithm for regional neck pain, cervical anatomy is important in the consideration of other cervical syndromes. The cervical roots exit nearly immediately and emerge essentially surrounded by the fibrous capsules contributed by uncovertebral, facet, and disc joints. The joints of Luschka or uncovertebral joints are small diarthrodial joints located on hooklike projections of the posterolateral margin of the bodies of cervical vertebrae contributing to all cervical foramina except those of the first two roots. The roots are covered by a sheath of dura as they course to the foramen. The dura then forms the dentate ligaments which anchor the cord near the posterior longitudinal ligament (Fig. 47–2). More than any other segment, the normal cervical cord nearly fills the canal and is tethered. In flexion, the normal cord is stretched as much as 2 cm. Most rotation of the neck occurs at the craniocervical junction; most flexion/extension at C5–C6. The intervertebral discs normally comprise one-third of the length of the cervical spine, which explains the extraordinary pliancy of this segment. Even so, these discs are small; the largest is C6–C7, which approaches a total volume of 1.5 ml and a nucleus pulposus volume of 0.25 ml. Neck motion reflects the extensibility of the discs and the impressive range of the facet joints, which easily override, par-

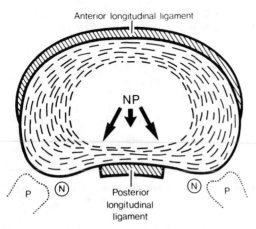

Anterior longitudinal ligament

NP

P   N   N   P

Posterior longitudinal ligament

Fig. 47–2. *Vertebral landmarks in sagittal section. N designates the nerve root, NP = nucleus pulposus, P = pedicle.*

ticularly during extension, and thereby diminish the area of the neural foramen.

Degenerative changes of the vertebral column are lumped under the term *spondylosis*. Cervical spondylosis involves the ligaments lining the canal and the structures that define the neural foramen: the pedicles, the discs, the end-plates, the joints of Luschka, and the apophyseal or facet joints. Spondylosis is common, involves all these structures, and becomes ubiquitous in the later decades. It is easily demonstrated by all imaging techniques and reflected in progressive restriction in range of motion. As a result, the specificity of all forms of cervical spondylosis for a particular episode of regional neck pain is so low as to render attempts at specific diagnosis futile; aggressive imaging is meaningless at best. Exuberant cervical osteophytosis is said to occasionally cause dysphagia. However, exuberant osteophytosis and calcification of spinal ligaments is ubiquitous in the elderly so that attributing any symptoms to such changes is a tenuous exercise.

One pattern of spondylosis is sufficiently distinctive and radiologically dramatic as to warrant special recognition. Diffuse idiopathic skeletal hyperostosis (DISH) is also called ankylosing hyperostosis or Forestier/Rotes–Querol disease and is apparent on spine roentgenograms in as many as 10% of the elderly. The physician sees flowing calcification and ossification along the anterolateral aspect of at least four contiguous vertebral bodies. Unlike the more usual pattern of spondylosis, disc height is relatively normal. Furthermore, as opposed to the inflammatory spondylarthropathies, there is no sacroiliitis or apophyseal joint ankylosis. The radiographic appearance can be striking (Fig. 47–3). In the dorsal spine the changes are characteristically contralateral to the heart.

The involvement of the spine is associated with osteophytes and ligamentous calcifications elsewhere: calcification of the sacrotuberous and iliolumbar ligaments in the pelvis; paraacetabular bony outgrowths; and olecranon, calcaneal, and patellar hypersotoses. As dramatic as these radiographic and pathologic changes may be, it is not clear they predispose the elderly to any special morbidity (14).

Neck pain rarely localizes just to the neck. Peculiar radiations to the shoulder, suboccipital, and inter-scapular regions are common and often overshadow the pain in the neck itself. This panoply of discomfort must reflect the complex and redundant neuroanatomy of the cervical spine. Even the vertebral arteries are susceptible to impingement and compromise from various osteophytes as they traverse their bony foramina, resulting in the rare but distinctive *vertebral artery syndrome* characterized by dizziness, tinnitus, occasional retroorbital headaches, and fleeting blurred vision associated with neck motion. Finally, there are the torticollis or wry neck syndromes. Usually, this is associated with pain and reflects guarded motion in the setting of regional musculoskeletal disease. Painless torticollis has been observed in all age groups, mimicking the movement disorder so typical of phenothiazine toxicity. The etiology is hotly debated with some

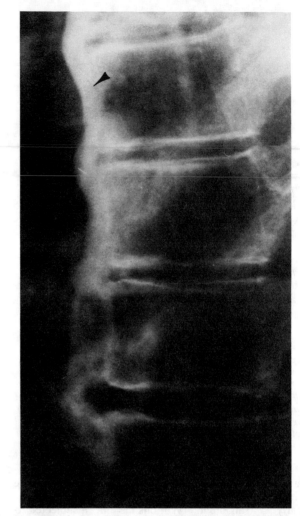

Fig. 47–3. *Spinal abnormalities in DISH. A lateral radiograph of the thoracic spine reveals ossification along the anterior aspect of the vertebral bodies (arrow). Observe the bumpy spinal contour, radiolucent extensions at the level of the intervertebral disc, and a linear radiolucency between the deposited bone and the anterior surface of the vertebra. The intervertebral discs are mildly narrowed (illustration provided by Dr D Resnick).*

advocating pharmacologic intervention for a neuromuscular disease and others for a psychiatric disorder.

Treatment

A discussion of management of neck pain is on far shakier ground than for low back pain because of a relative dearth of clinical investigation. Nonetheless, the natural history of acute neck pain is similar to that for acute backache; at least 80% are well within a month.

The mainstays of therapy are reassurance and support, including promulgating a decision-making role for the patient. Most patients with cervical pain will spontaneously posture in slight forward flexion and resist deviation in any plane, thereby placing least stress on cervical structures while maintaining erect posture. This is to be encouraged. A soft cervical collar provides no more than a reminder at the cost of considerable nuisance. In a multicenter British trial, about 75% of all subjects were well or nearly so in one month, regardless of exposure to physical modalities such as a collar or traction or to placebo events. It has not been possible to demonstrate benefit from spinal manipulation for neck pain, and there is a risk of doing considerable violence to the neural structures. The experience with surgery for neck pain is at least as disappointing as for low back pain; in most series (none of which are controlled) some 50% of patients are no better off for the experience.

Table 47–1. *Signs and symptoms of cervical radiculopathies*

Root	Pain Numbness	Sensory Loss	Motor Loss	Reflex Loss
C3	Occipital region	Occiput	None	None
C4	Back of neck	Back of neck	None	None
C5	Neck to outer shoulder and arm	Over shoulder	Deltoid	Biceps supinator
C6	Outer arm to thumb and index fingers	Thumb and index fingers	Biceps (triceps) and wrist extensors	Triceps supinator biceps
C7	Outer arm to middle finger	Index and middle fingers	Triceps	Triceps
C8	Inner arm to fourth and fifth fingers	Fourth and fifth fingers	Intrinsics, extrinsics	None

RADICULOPATHY

Given the architecture of neural foramina and the likelihood of spondylotic changes in the anatomic components, it is remarkable that all of us do not suffer radiculopathies. It is even more remarkable that most radiculopathies are intermittent and remittant illnesses implying that some components of the spondylotic process, quite likely in associated soft tissues, are reversible.

There are two major reasons for considering radiculopathy as a separate clinical issue: one benefits the physician and the other the patient. For the physician, there is the intellectual satisfaction of localization. We may not be able to define the pathophysiology but at least we know its location with some reliability. For the patient, radiculopathy portends peripheral damage, provokes a special anxiety since the experience of referred pain appears to defy reason, and offers some specific therapeutic options.

Localization

Table 47–1 presents the traditional symptoms and signs associated with compromise of each cervical root. Table 47–2 does likewise for the lumbar radiculopathies. The categorization is clinically useful but far from completely valid or reliable. Generalization of symptoms and signs, beyond a single root, is not unusual and probably reflects some multiplicity of innervation peripherally and dispersion of input at the level of the cord. Further, some presentations are confounded by coincidental neuropathies; for example, nearly 10% of elderly lack at least one Achilles' reflex, further comprising the specificity of this neurologic sign for radiculopathy. A coincident cervical radiculopathy can render subclinical entrapment neuropathies overt. The so-called *double crush syndrome* is an experimental reality, but has more clinical advocacy than is justified by supporting clinical data.

Nonetheless, localizing information is forthcoming from careful elicitation of symptoms and inspection to note focal atrophy, as well as mobility, muscle, and reflex testing and discernment of sensory deficits. For lumbar radiculopathies, there are *tension signs* as well. For cervical radiculopathies, there are advocates of compression and distraction tests, which have been shown to correlate with myelographically demonstrable root compression, but are low in sensitivity (15) and difficult to perform reliably. The history can be structured and rendered more reliable by the use of pain diagrams and questionnaires. All signs can be rendered more reliable if examinations are standardized and practiced; however, this additional effort is more appropriate for clinical investigation than it is useful in clinical practice.

Tension or stretch signs can be elicited in the lower extremity and are probably more sensitive to radiculopathy than the signs elaborated in Table 47–2. Straight-leg raising takes up the slack on the lower lumbar roots that contribute to the sciatic nerve; by 30°, the nerve is taut. The normal nerve can withstand further flexion at the hip with the knee extended. Resistance to such movement is the traditional Lesegue's sign for sciatica. Many variations on this theme have proponents. There are even those who are convinced that the crossed straight-leg raising test is more specific for sciatica caused by discal protrusion. Here, elevating the asymptomatic leg provokes discomfort in the symptomatic leg. The specificity of this test has not been established; its sensitivity is low. The other commonly employed stretch test is the femoral stretch accomplished by flexing the knee with the patient prone. This tests for compromise in the roots contributing to the femoral nerve.

Treatment

Localization allows the physician an opportunity for a palliative explanation of the illness. Unfortunately, this does not alter therapeutic considerations from those that pertain to neck and low back pain without radiculopathy. There is some evidence that surgery for a lumbar radiculopathy, such as for sciatica, may afford the patient a higher likelihood of relief than conservative management (8). However, this benefit has not been demonstrated for acute illness (less than six weeks) or for chronic illness (greater than six months). Other invasive modalities, including percutaneous discectomy and chymopapain, are of unprovable benefit for radiculopathy. In fact, there is no substantive support for the former and little for the latter for backache, let alone sciatica.

In the occasional patient, radiculopathy presents with more neurologic compromise than impairment of deep tendon reflexes. The innervated musculature is at risk, and weakness and atrophy are the unfortunate outcome. Such is exceptional; however, any evidence of overt weakness or atrophy is a mandate for surgical consultation. Surgical intervention is an empiric option and surgical judgement a prerequisite. The likelihood of success increases if imaging the relevant spinal segment documents correlative discal pathology.

LUMBAR SPINAL STENOSIS

The cardinal symptom of lumbar spinal stenosis is neurogenic claudication. This is the experience of aching pain with or without paresthesia in the buttock, posterior thigh, or calf precipitated by walking or even assuming an erect posture. Typically, the symptoms are bilateral, and sphincter function is not impaired. The patient assumes a characteristic bent gait, the so-called *simian stance*, to postpone the onset of symptoms with ambulation. Often they will choose to ambulate assisted by a walker or shopping cart over which they can stoop without falling forward. Likewise, sitting is more likely to offer rapid palliation than recumbency. It is because this syndrome is so distinctive that lumbar stenosis survives as a clinical entity. The differential

Table 47–2. *Signs and symptoms of lumbar radiculopathy*

Root	Pain Numbness	Sensory Loss	Motor Loss	Reflex Loss
L4	anterior thigh and medial leg	medial leg to medial malleolus	anterior tibialis	patellar
L5	lateral leg and dorsum of the foot	lateral leg and dorsum of the foot	extensor hallucis longus	posterior tibial
S1	lateral foot	lateral foot	peroneus longus and brevis	Achilles reflex

diagnosis is limited to atypical presentations of vascular claudication and, more remotely, mass lesions encroaching on the cauda equina. Stenosis seldom provokes the cramping pain that is the hallmark of vascular claudication.

Nearly one-half of patients with symptomatic stenosis have a reduced or absent Achilles reflex, one-third have objective lower extremity weakness, and one-fifth have diminished or absent knee jerk reactions. Suggestions of polyradiculopathy are discernible by careful electrodiagnostic testing in the vast majority. The population at greatest risk is the elderly, particularly elderly men. Therein lies the diagnostic dilemma: well over 10% of all elderly lack Achilles reflexes. The prevalence of low back pain of some type and degree approaches 50%. And finally, the presence of degenerative changes, including some degree of compromise in the dimensions of the lumbar canal, is nearly ubiquitous. The false-positive rate for images of the lumbar spine to diagnose stenosis varies from 9% to 35% depending on the criteria employed.

In view of these considerations, the diagnosis of lumbar stenosis as a cause of low back pain is based on the stereotypical nature of the symptoms (16). It is not an anatomic diagnosis, nor is its pathophysiology certain. Further, the experience following surgical decompression of the cord is anything but impressive. Perhaps one-third of patients subjected to these extensive procedures clearly benefit from them. Patients need a thoughtful and circumspect assessment; surgery is an option of desperation. Prior to surgery, myelographic documentation of complete or near-complete obstruction of the caudal subarachnoid space is prudent.

LUMBOSACRAL AND PELVIC INSUFFICIENCY FRACTURES

Insufficiency fractures are spontaneous linear disruptions of cortical and subadjacent trabecular bone without displacement. The classic example is the *march* or stress fracture of the metatarsal in the healthy foot thought to reflect forces in usage that exceed the resilience of the bone. In the elderly or the osteoporotic patient, pelvic structures are similarly susceptible (17). Spontaneous fractures of the pubic rami and the ribs are well described and are common in the setting of steroid-induced osteoporosis where they may be asymptomatic and heal with exuberant callus formation. They also occur without hypercorticism and without exuberant callus. Such fractures are being recognized more frequently. Aching pain that is prominent at rest and exacerbated by weight bearing more than movement is suggestive. Pubic rami, sacrum and iliac wings are all susceptible, as are tibial plateaus. At the outset, the fracture is typically subradiographic, suggesting other possible causes of bone pain, including neoplasia. They are often demonstrable by scintiscanning although the physician must remain cognizant of the limited specificity of this technique. These fractures are diagnosed by exclusion of other possibilities and by the confidence gained in demonstrating linearity by CT or MRI imaging and by documenting healing radiographically.

DISABLING BACKACHE

By definition, regional backache interferes with function. Attempts to lean forward, even while seated, exacerbate the pain. Lifting is problematic and more so when the object cannot be held close to the body. The challenge is not just to the worker faced with materials handling. All of us face the potential for the illness of work incapacity.

The United States provides two programs of recourse. The first is available to everyone and is administered by the Social Security Administration as Social Security Disability Insurance (SSDI) for those who have had considerable employment experience and Supplemental Security Insurance (SSI) for everyone else. The intent is to insure Americans against poverty as a consequence of the illness of work incapacity, whatever its cause. To qualify, the patient must no longer be employed and must be deemed incapable of any employment that can earn even minimum wage. The criteria for award are stringent and stated; nonetheless, imple-

mentation has proven difficult since the program was formulated in the 1950s.

There is another program administered on a state-by-state basis relevant to regional backache. If the backache is deemed to be an injury that arises out of and in the course of employment and occurs by accident, the patient is entitled to coverage under workers' compensation insurance. These policies not only provide all medical care, they supplement income until the employee is as well as possible. Then the policy provides fiscal compensation for compromised wage earning capacity or for the actual decrement in wages earned as a consequence of any persisting disability. The workers' compensation model is no fault in design, and has largesse that far outstrips SSDI/SSI. Workers' compensation programs are efficient in providing benefits (and, to a lesser extent, in monitoring safety) with regard to injuries that are a consequence of discrete traumatic events involving external forces; these comprise over 80% of the claims. The bulk of the remainder of claims relate to regional backache. These are responsible for over 80% of the cost of this system.

The role of the treating physician with respect to the administration of these insurance programs is quite circumscribed. For SSDI/SSI, the treating physician provides a database which, when adequate, is the basis for an award by the staff employed on behalf of the Secretary of Health and Human Services. For workers' compensation programs, the role of the treating physician is less passive. In treating any patient under such coverage, the physician or surgeon is tacitly certifying that the backache is a compensable injury. If the patient does not return to full health rapidly, the policy encourages and indemnifies attempts on the part of the treating physicians and surgeons to aggressively intervene. This accounts for intervention rates that, while they vary from place to place in the U.S., far outstrip the experience with the management of regional backache in circumstances other than those covered by workers' compensation. Further, surgical intervention rates in the U.S. far outstrip those for compensable backache in other industrialized nations. If the patient still is not well, the treating physician will participate in determining the likelihood of further improvement and the advisability of further intervention.

Both SSDI/SSI and workers' compensation administrative algorithms relentlessly converge on disability determination; the decision that the illness or injury renders the worker less competent to work. In the U.S. this determination pivots on the quantity of documented and demonstrable pathology—the concept of impairment-based disability determination. This precept holds that if there is sufficient pathology, the illness will include the illness of work incapacity. The precept has administrative appeal. However, for regional backache, measurement of impairment is of limited reliability and abysmal validity. As discussed above, the demonstration of pathology at the axial skeleton is almost totally nonspecific; therefore, many people who are disabled by backache will lack putatively determinative pathology. Nonetheless, the SSDI/SSI algorithm procures nearly 300,000 contracted examinations annually and the workers' compensation algorithm procures at least as many independent medical examinations in quest of pathologic documentation. The claimant is beleaguered if not demoralized by the demand that he or she prove illness beyond any preconception regarding the prerequisite magnitude of pathology. All too often the outcome is escalating illness behavior, a litigious contest, and an inexorable degradation of the claimant's humanity resulting in recourse to pain clinics for redress (18). The treating physician should become familiar with the sociopolitical context into which the patient's illness of work incapacity will be thrust, to understand the pitfalls in order to provide competent advice and guidance and to offer to their communities insights that may shape future policies less flawed.

Nortin M. Hadler, MD, FACP

1. Hadler NM: Occupational Musculoskeletal Diseases. New York, Raven Press, 1993
2. The Adult Spine. Volumes I and II. Edited by Frymoyer JW, Decker TB, Hadler NM, et al. New York, Raven Press, 1991
3. Wiesel SW, Tsourmas N, Feffer HL, et al: A study of computer-assisted

tomography. 1. The incidence of positive CAT scans in an asymptomatic group of patients. Spine 9:549–551, 1984

4. Boden SD, Davis DO, Dina TS, et al: Abnormal magnetic resonance scans of the lumbar spine in asymptomatic subjects. J Bone Joint Surg (Am). 72-A:403–408, 1990

5. Bigos SJ, Battié MC, Spengler DM, et al. A prospective study of work perceptions and psychosocial factors affecting the report of back injury. Spine 16:1–6, 1991

6. Pope MH, Wilder DG, Krag MH: Biomechanics of the lumbar spine. The Adult Spine. Edited by Frymoyer JW, Ducker TB, Hadler NM, et al. Raven Press, New York. 1991. pp 1487–1501

7. Hadler NM: The predicament of backache. J Occup Med 30:449–450, 1988

8. Frymoyer JW: Back pain and sciatica. N Engl J Med 318:291–300, 1988

9. Quebec Task Force on Spinal Disorders. Scientific approach to the assessment and management of activity-related spinal disorders. Spine 12 (Suppl 1):S1–S59, 1987

10. Deyo RA, Diehl AK, Rosenthal M: How many days of bed rest for acute low back pain? A randomized clinical trial. N Engl J Med 315:1064–1070, 1986

11. Carette S, Marcoux S, Truchon R, et al: A controlled trial of corticosteroid injections into facet joints for chronic low back pain. N Engl J Med 325:1002–1007, 1991

12. Hadler NM: The chiropractic and me. Whither? Whether? J Occup Med 33:1209–1211, 1991

13. Deyo RA, Walsh NE, Martin DC, et al. A controlled trial of transcutaneous electrical nerve stimulation (TENS) and exercise for chronic low back pain. N Engl J Med 322:1627–1634, 1990

14. Hutton C: DISH . . . a state not a disease? Brit J Rheum 28:277–278, 1989

15. Viikari–Juntura E, Porras M, Laasonen EM: Validity of clinical tests in the diagnosis of root compression in cervical disc disease. Spine 14:253–257, 1989

16. O'Duffy JD: Spinal stenosis. The Adult Spine. Edited by Frymoyer JW, Ducker TB, Hadler NM, et al. New York, Raven Press, 1991, pp 1801–1810

17. Stroebel RJ, Ginsburg WW, McLeod RA: Sacral insufficiency fractures: an often unsuspected cause of low back pain. J Rheumatol 18:117–119, 1991

18. Hadler NM: Back pain and the vortex of disability determination. Semin Spine Surg 4:35–41, 1992

48. OSTEONECROSIS

Osteonecrosis is a generic term used to describe the death of the cellular elements of bone. This term is preferred to those of ischemic bone necrosis, avascular necrosis, aseptic necrosis, and osteochondritis dissecans, although this last term has a somewhat different meaning, implying the presence of a loose body of dead bone in the articular cavity. Osteonecrosis has been described in a variety of clinical settings associated with a disease (Gaucher's disease), a medication (corticosteroids), a physiologic process (pregnancy), a pathologic process (embolism), or in the absence of any apparent predisposing factor or condition (truly idiopathic) (1,2). Osteonecrosis occurs in individuals of both sexes and all age groups. It occurs, for the most part, in the epiphysis of long bones such as the femoral and humeral heads, but other bones can also be affected. The femoral head is the most common site of osteonecrosis. It can occur in more than one bone, with the multiple bones affected sequentially or simultaneously. The availability of better imaging techniques, particularly magnetic resonance imaging (MRI), permits diagnosis of osteonecrosis at a very early stage, before radiographic changes occur, and even before clinical manifestations are present (3,4).

To best understand and compare the literature on osteonecrosis, one should examine how the diagnosis was made, the classification used for staging this disorder, details of the therapeutic intervention, and the criteria used to measure treatment success and failure (5).

PATHOGENESIS

Bone death occurring as the result of altered arterial blood supply is easily understood and can be systematically reproduced in experimental animals. If blood supply is completely interrupted and not promptly restored, bone death inevitably ensues. The final outcome depends on the size of the affected area and the magnitude of the reparative process, that is, viable bone cells replacing necrotic or nonviable bone. Failure to revitalize the involved area leads to bone collapse, followed by some degree of joint incongruity and the occurrence of secondary osteoarthritis (OA).

Prolonged ischemia may also lead to osteonecrosis. It may occur as a result of intra- or extravascular pathology occurring within the bone. Small vessel vasculitis, intravascular arteriolar thrombosis, venous occlusion, and microembolism are all well-recognized causes of ischemia. Proliferative processes such as Gaucher's disease indirectly alter the vascular supply by compressing the sinusoids. The direct toxic effect of some substances on different cell populations of the bone can also lead to osteonecrosis. Alcohol, for example, even if consumed in moderation (6), and corticosteroids, endogenous or exogenous, are toxic to lipocytes (7).

It has been postulated that the common pathway for the occurrence of osteonecrosis is that of increased intraosseous pressure (IOP), either as a primary (proliferative process) or a secondary (altered blood supply) event (8). Increased IOP in an organ essentially incapable of expanding results in compromise of blood supply to the bone and development of ischemia and cell damage. The presence of increased IOP in osteonecrosis has, in fact, been used as an aid for early diagnosis.

Although it is likely that increased IOP plays an important role in the pathogenesis of osteonecrosis, other factors such as cytotoxicity may be equally important. Moreover, increased IOP is not the *sine qua non* of osteonecrosis, since it may occur in other pathologic processes such as OA where osteonecrosis does not occur (9). Likewise, increased IOP has not been found in histologically proven, experimentally induced osteonecrosis in rabbits (10). The pathogenesis is likely to be better understood as it becomes possible to study pre-radiologic and even pre-clinical stages of the disease. Correlative histopathologic and imaging studies also may shed light on the pathogenesis. In summary, this condition develops in a variety of well-recognized clinical settings, which predispose to bone ischemia and cellular damage initially, and which may be followed by bone death, bone collapse, and joint incongruity (1,2).

CLINICAL FEATURES

The first clinical manifestation of osteonecrosis is the relatively abrupt onset of severe pain occurring initially only during weight bearing and later during non-weight bearing and even while at rest. In the early stages of osteonecrosis, decreased range of motion is primarily related to the presence of pain (1,2). The existence of a pre-clinical stage of osteonecrosis has been demonstrated in MRI studies (1–3,8,11). In some patients, pain becomes unbearable as osteonecrosis progresses, whereas in other patients with similar radiographs it does not. Some degree of bone remodeling can occur, allowing some patients to remain very functional despite decreased range of motion. A significant proportion of patients, however, have persistent and worsening pain, progressive loss of range of motion, and significant loss of function. In these patients, the time from onset of symptoms to the development of disability varies from months to years.

The most common clinical presentations encountered by rheumatologists are of young women with systemic lupus erythematosus who appear to be Cushingoid and have received high doses of corticosteroids; the average dose, cumulative dose, and duration of corticosteroid use appear to be less important. Other conditions associated with osteonecrosis are listed in Table 48–1.

DIAGNOSIS

For years, patients with osteonecrosis have been staged using plain roentgenograms. Although there are several classifications, the one most commonly used has four stages originally described by Arlet and Ficat (12) and a fifth stage, 0, added to include

Table 48–1. *Diseases or conditions with reported association with osteonecrosis*

1). Trauma
    Hip dislocation
    Hip fracture
    Post-arthroscopy
	8). Corticosteroids (exogenous and
	       endogenous)
	    Asthma
	    Aplastic anemia
	    Leukemias and lymphomas
	    Inflammatory bowel disease
	    Cushing's syndrome
	    Organ transplantation
	    Intraarticular and pulse intravenous
	       administration

2). Connective Tissue Disorders*
    Systemic lupus erythematosus
    Rheumatoid arthritis
    Vasculitis	

3). Hematologic Disorders
    Sickle cell disease
    Sickle - C disease
    Thalasemia minor
	9). Cytotoxics
	    Vinblastine
	    Vincristine
	    Cisplatin (intraarterial)
	    Cyclophosphamide
	    Bleomycin
	    5-fluorouracil

4). Proliferative Disorders
    Gaucher's disease
    Solid tumors	

5). Metabolic Disorders Gout	10). Alcohol

6). Disorders associated with fat necrosis
    Pancreatitis
    Pancreatic carcinoma
	11). Radiation
	
	12). Pregnancy

7). Embolism Decompression sickness	

* Almost all CTDs have been reported to be associated with ON; corticosteroids have been used in the majority, but not in all, patients.

asymptomatic patients with normal roentgenograms (11). These stages are defined in Table 48–2.

Procedures currently used to diagnose osteonecrosis include: 1) plain roentgenograms (1,2,11), neutral anteroposterior and frog views in the case of the hips, useful only in stages II, III, and IV (Fig. 48–1A); 2) bone scintigraphy (11), either qualitative, comparing the uptake of the radiopharmaceutical in the same joint on both sides of the body, or quantitative, measuring the actual uptake; 3) single photon emission computerized tomography (13), the usefulness of which is yet to be determined as this is a relatively new technique; and 4) MRI (2–4,11), proven to be of value in the diagnosis of pre-radiologic (stage I) or even pre-clinical (stage 0) disease.

Procedures less often used include: 1) physiologic invasive studies, measuring the IOP at baseline and after the injection of 5 ml of saline, the so-called stress test (an IOP > 30 mm Hg at baseline, and a 10 mm increase with the stress test diagnostic of osteonecrosis); 2) venography, usually done in conjunction with the measurement of IOP and also found to be abnormal in early stages of osteonecrosis; and 3) conventional tomograms, useful for staging, but not for diagnosis of early disease (1,2,8).

Although osteonecrosis can be regarded as a histopathologic diagnosis, bone biopsies are not recommended for diagnostic purposes. Histopathology can be used, however, to confirm the diagnosis of osteonecrosis in patients subjected to a surgical intervention. Characteristic histopathologic findings include marrow fibrosis, fat cell necrosis, necrotic bone, and some evidence of a reparative process.

The sensitivity, specificity, predictive negative, and predictive positive values of the above diagnostic procedures are not available in a single published study. It is unlikely that all could be compared because, as noted, some procedures are no longer in use. Moreover, since the gold standard—histologically proven dead bone—is not obtained in the majority of patients, these data are not available. Magnetic resonance imaging appears to be both very sensitive and specific for the diagnosis of osteonecrosis. By MRI, it is possible to distinguish normal bone and marrow, unrepaired dead bone and marrow, unrepaired dead bone with marrow replaced by debris, and zones of repair (3,4,11). Necrotic marrow and necrotic bone produce a high signal intensity in both T1 and T2 images; subchondral bone appears as dark striations. The combined appearance of these signals gives the characteristic, well-described serpiginous pattern (Fig. 48–1B).

TREATMENT

As noted, there is a need to establish outcome criteria if the success and failure of different treatment modalities are to be adequately compared. Such criteria have been developed by Stulberg et al (14) and are noted in Table 48–3.

There are two treatment alternatives for stages O-II: conservative treatment and core decompression. A conservative treatment program includes the following elements: 1) the judicious use of analgesics, 2) maintaining muscle strength and preventing contractures, and 3) the use of assistive devices to help pain for non-weight bearing ambulation. Patients who experience persistent and intractable pain and progressive functional loss should be considered for an arthroplasty, which ideally should be done before there is total collapse of the femoral head. The failure rate for hip arthroplasties in patients with osteonecrosis is much higher than in patients with other arthritides. This has been attributed to young age, poor bone quality, active lifestyle, and oftentimes bilateral hip involvement. Thus, patients age 40 or less

Table 48–2. *Staging in osteonecrosis**

Stage 0: Clinical manifestations absent; normal radiographs**.
Stage I: Clinical manifestations present; normal radiographs†.
Stage II: Areas of osteopenia and osteosclerosis in radiographs.
Stage III: Early bone collapse manifested as the "crescent sign" (translucent subcortical bone delineates the area of dead bone).
Stage IV: Late bone collapse manifested as flattening of the articular surface with or without joint incongruity.

* After Ficat and Arlet (12).
** Diagnosis made by magnetic resonance imaging.
† Diagnosis made by invasive physiological studies in published literature.

Table 48–3. *Recommended criteria in determining treatment outcome in osteonecrosis**

1. Clinical improvement as determined by a valid instrument (i.e. Harris hip scale).
2. Radiographic stabilization.
3. Bone survival (i.e. femoral head survival).

*After Stulberg et al (14).

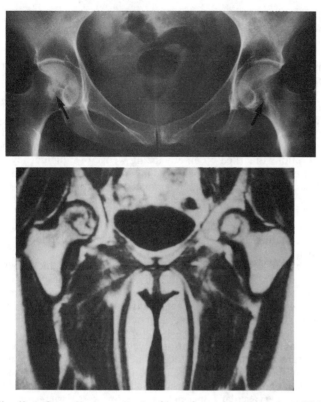

Fig. 48–1. *Stage II osteonecrosis of both femoral heads. A. (top) Plain film of the pelvis and both hips shows patchy foci of increased density (arrows) characteristic of stage II osteonecrosis; there is no collapse of the femoral heads. B. (bottom) T1-weighted coronal MRI shows curvilinear areas of low signal in both femoral heads typical of osteonecrosis (courtesy of WK Bernreuter, MD).*

with stage III osteonecrosis may receive osteotomies and bone-grafting (15). For osteotomies to be successful, prolonged non-weight bearing is essential. Long-term follow-up of these patients is needed before these procedures can be recommended for all young patients with stage III osteonecrosis. The value of bone grafting in halting disease progression in these patients needs to be determined. Patients with osteonecrosis of non-weight bearing joints may not require any intervention, as they may have little pain and limited but tolerable functional loss.

Core decompression was first used in France by Arlet and Ficat, and later in the United States by Zizic and Hungerford (16,17). The rationale for core decompression is reducing IOP, reestablishing the blood supply, and allowing living bone adjacent to dead bone to contribute to the reparative process (17). In the published experience of these authors, good to excellent results have been obtained in the majority of patients with stages I and II osteonecrosis and even in a significant proportion of patients with stage III disease. Stulberg (14) randomized 50 hips (31 patients) with stages I–III osteonecrosis (stages 0 and IV were not studied) to either conservative (non-weight bearing) or surgical (core decompression) treatment. Decompression more predictably reduced pain and changed the indications for further surgery than did conservative treatment in stage I and II patients; clinical stabilization was achieved in 90% of stages I and II. In a study by Chan et al (18), core decompression (and bone grafting) was shown to halt disease progression in patients with early disease. In contrast, patients with advanced disease and with a large area of involved bone showed clinical and radiographic evidence of disease progression. Finally, Warner et al (19) studied 39 hips in 25 patients. Seventy percent of stages I and II osteonecrosis experienced stabilization, whereas only 13% of stages III and IV did so. From the combined experience reviewed, core decompression could be considered for patients in the early stages of osteonecrosis.

In contrast to these positive results, Camp and Colwell (20) and Hopson and Siverhus (21) reported the failure of core decom-

pression in achieving clinical stabilization, even in patients in the early stages of osteonecrosis. Camp and Colwell were impressed by the morbidity of the procedure (subtrocanteric fractures). They strongly recommend abandoning this procedure, arguing that there is no evidence that core decompression achieves a decreased IOP for any length of time. They further recommend conservative treatment (non-weight bearing) for stages 0–II, and arthroplasty or osteotomies for stages III and IV. As noted before, the indications for a major surgical procedure include not only evidence of radiographic progression, but worsening pain and incapacitation. It seems likely that a variety of alternative approaches will continue to be proposed until more definitively effective regimens are established.

The roles of electric stimulation and pulse electromagnetic fields in the management of stages 0–II osteonecrosis are of questionable value. Bone grafting may be tried as an intermediate approach between purely conservative treatment and more extensive surgery, although its value in halting disease progression is not uniformly accepted. Arthroscopy can be considered for removal of loose bodies in the knee and shoulder.

PROGNOSIS

The diagnosis of very early cases of osteonecrosis using available technology should result in better outcomes. Purely conservative treatment may conceivably prove to be all that is required for some patients with stages 0 and I disease. A combination of factors, such as the size of the area involved, degree of bone collapse, and underlying disorder, likely explains the lower success rate of arthroplasty in osteonecrosis patients as compared to patients with other disorders, specifically OA. Adequate follow-up of patients increases the likelihood of making proper and prompt management decisions.

Graciela S. Alarcón, MD, MPH

1. Steinberg ME, Steinberg DR: Osteonecrosis. Textbook of Rheumatology. Edited by Kelley WN, Harris ED, Ruddy S, Sledge CB, 4th ed. Philadelphia, WB Saunders, 1993, pp 1628–1650
2. Mankin HJ: Nontraumatic necrosis of bone (osteonecrosis). N Engl J Med 326:1473–1479, 1992
3. Jergesen HE, Heller M, Genant HK: Magnetic resonance imaging in osteonecrosis of the femoral head. Orthop Clin North Am 16:705–716, 1985
4. Jergesen HE, Lang P, Moseley M, et al: Histologic correlation in magnetic resonance imaging of femoral head osteonecrosis. Clin Orthop Rel Res 253:150–163, 1990
5. Stulberg BN, Bauer TW, Belhobek GH, et al: A diagnostic algorithm for osteonecrosis of the femoral head. Clin Orthop 249:176–182, 1989
6. Hungerford DS, Zizic TM: Alcoholism associated ischemic necrosis of the femoral head. Early diagnosis and treatment. Clin Orthop 130:144–153, 1978
7. Zizic TM, Marcoux C, Hungerford DS, et al: Corticosteroid therapy associated with ischemic necrosis of bone in systemic lupus erythematosus. Am J Med 79:596–604, 1985
8. Zizic TM, Marcoux C, Hungerford DS, et al: The early diagnosis of ischemic necrosis of bone. Arthritis Rheum 29:1177–1186, 1986
9. Colwell CW Jr: The controversy of core decompression of the femoral head for osteonecrosis. Arthritis Rheum 32:797–800, 1989
10. Warner JJP, Philip JH, Brodsky GL, et al: Studies of nontraumatic osteonecrosis. Manometric and histologic studies of the femoral head after chronic steroid treatment: an experimental study in rabbits. Clin Orthop 225:128–140, 1987
11. Lee MJ, Corrigan J, Stack JP, et al: A comparison of modern imaging modalities in osteonecrosis of the femoral head. Clin Radiol 42:427–432, 1990
12. Arlet J, Ficat P: Diagnostic de l'osteonecrose femorocapitale primitive au stade I (stade preradiologic): [The diagnosis of stage I (pre-radiologic) primary osteonecrosis of the femoral head]. Rev Chir Orthop 54:637–648, 1968
13. Gupta SM, Foster CR, Kayani N: Usefulness of SPECT in the early detection of avascular necrosis of the knees. Clin Nucl Med 12:99–102, 1987
14. Stulberg BN, Bauer TW, Belhobek GH: Making core decompression work. Clin Orthop 261:186–195, 1990
15. Scher MA, Jakim I: Interthrocanteric osteotomy and autogenous bone-grafting for avascular necrosis of the femoral head. J Bone Joint Surg 75A:1119–1132, 1993
16. Zizic TM: Osteonecrosis. Curr Opin Rheumatol 3:481–489, 1991
17. Hungerford DS: Response: the role of core decompression in the treatment of ischemic necrosis of the femoral head. Arthritis Rheum 32:801–806, 1989
18. Chan TW, Dalinka MK, Steinberg ME, et al: MRI appearance of femoral head osteonecrosis following core decompression and bone grafting. Skeletal Radiol 20:103–107, 1991
19. Warner JJP, Philip JH, Brodsky GL, et al: Studies of nontraumatic osteonecrosis of the femoral head. Clin Orthop 225:104–127, 1987
20. Camp JF, Colwell CW: Core decompression of the femoral head for osteonecrosis. J Bone Joint Surg 68A:1313–1319, 1986
21. Hopson CN, Siverhus SW: Ischemic necrosis of the femoral head. J Bone Joint Surg 70A:1048–1051, 1988

49. PAGET'S DISEASE OF BONE

Paget's disease of bone (osteitis deformans) is a disorder of unknown etiology characterized initially by excessive bone resorption and subsequently by excessive bone formation, culminating in a mosaic pattern of lamellar bone associated with extensive local vascularity and increased fibrous tissue in adjacent marrow (1). Paget's disease of bone is a focal disorder since some bone is always spared, no matter how widespread the pagetic process.

In the United States, Paget's disease is estimated to occur in approximately 1% to 3% of persons over age 45 and is usually polyostotic. Men tend to predominate, and the disease is almost always first detected after the age of 40. Familial clustering may take place.

The primary event in Paget's disease is probably a focal, intense resorption of bone (osteolytic phase), leading to the formation of typical resorption lacunae filled with osteoclasts. The osteoclasts may assume bizarre shapes and contain as many as 100 nuclei, a feature not seen normally or in other pathologic states. Pagetic osteoclasts have been found to contain nuclear and cytoplasmic inclusions that resemble viral nucleocapsids and express paramyxoviral antigens and transcripts. It has thus been suggested, although not established, that the disorder is a late manifestation of infection with viruses such as measles, respiratory syncytial, or canine distemper virus (1,2). Osteoclasts are derived from hematopoietic precursor cells of the mononuclear phagocyte lineage. Increased numbers of osteoclast-like cells are generated in long-term marrow cultures from Paget's disease compared to normals. Increased levels of the cytokine interleukin-6 (IL-6) are produced by the pagetic cells suggesting that IL-6 could be an autocrine/paracrine factor for pagetic osteoclasts (3).

Early in the disease, osteolysis is accompanied by some element of repair, usually observed in focal regions near the excessive resorption. The newly deposited bone comprises woven as well as lamellar bone. The local fatty or hematopoietic marrow is replaced by a loose, fibrous connective tissue stroma that frequently appears hypervascular.

The pagetic process occurs in both cancellous and cortical bone. The characteristic and diagnostic mosaic pattern of Paget's disease results from the abnormal deposition of lamellar bone. The so-called cement lines are formed at sites where these lamellae are joined.

In some patients the rate of resorption diminishes, whereas bone formation continues, resulting in an increased mass of bone per unit volume (osteoblastic or sclerotic phase). In general, however, in this disease a close coupling between formation and resorption is observed, even though formation may appear excessive and involved bones may be larger than normal.

Overall, enormous increases may occur in rates of resorption and formation of bone that involve increased fluxes of mineral ions from resorbing bone into newly forming bone. Bone matrix is resorbed, as reflected in the increased urinary excretion of hydroxyproline-containing peptides, which may exceed 1,000 mg of hydroxyproline/24 hours. The increased bone accretion and the increased local vascularity account for the increased uptake by pagetic lesions of bone-seeking isotopes, as detected by scanning procedures.

Levels of alkaline phosphatase activity in the serum are characteristically elevated in patients with Paget's disease of bone. These increased levels reflect the osteoblastic activity, which is essential for bone formation, and generally correlate with the extent and activity of the pagetic process. In rare instances, roentgenographically typical Paget's disease of bone may be associated with a normal level of alkaline phosphatase activity but only when a small bone or portion of a bone is involved.

Levels of alkaline phosphatase activity tend to rise gradually, often reaching a plateau characteristic for each individual, although in some patients wide fluctuations are seen, with decreases associated with immobilization or intercurrent infections. In the rare individuals who develop sarcoma at the site of pagetic involvement, an explosive rise in alkaline phosphatase levels may be seen.

The roentgenographic appearance of pagetic bone reflects the predominant pathologic process and the stage of the disorder. The initial lesion is a focal area of radiolucency, particularly evident in the skull where the term *osteoporosis circumscripta* is used. In long bones, especially the tibia and the femur, the resorption is marked by an advancing wedge of radiolucency.

Attempts at repair are observed as islands of increased density or as coarsened trabecula. In some instances, the dimensions of the involved bone may increase, and thickening of the cortex results, progressing to a sclerotic appearance. Thickening of the pelvic brim or iliopectineal line (brim sign) is a helpful finding in differentiating Paget's disease from metastatic carcinoma of bone.

The most common sites of involvement are the spine, pelvis, skull, femur, and tibia, and in individuals with widespread disease, almost every bone may be involved, including the small ones. In most instances, Paget's disease of bone is asymptomatic. The disorder becomes apparent clinically when the involvement results in pain, gross deformity, compression of neural structures, fracture of an involved bone, alteration of joint structure and function, or locally increased vascularity. When bone of the appendicular skeleton is involved, the overlying skin may be abnormally warm. Occasionally the excessive circulation in the hypervascular bone and surrounding soft tissues contributes to the development of high output cardiac failure.

Specific features are associated with each site of involvement (1,2). Skull involvement may produce obvious enlargement of the head with increased frontal bossing and dilated, pulsating, superficial vessels. If the facial bones are affected, a leonine appearance may result. Deafness is the consequence of involvement of the ossicles, the temporal bone, or compression of neural elements.

Symptomatic spinal involvement can produce pain directly or as a result of neural compression. Spinal cord compression is a rare complication. Pain in the limbs may be localized over the lesion or result from nerve root compression or associated joint disease. Hip disease secondary to involvement of the subchondral bone of the femoral head or acetabulum is common in Paget's disease and may be associated with a striking degree of protrusio acetabuli (Fig. 49-1). A similar arthropathy may occur in knees due to involvement of the distal femurs or patellas. Hyperuricemia and gout may occur more often than expected by chance (1,4). Causes of this association have not been defined.

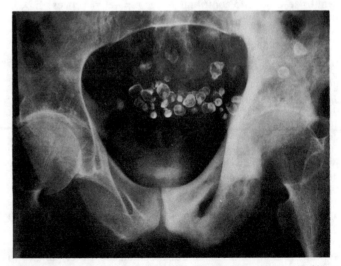

Fig. 49-1. *Pelvis of an 82-year-old man who had Paget's disease of bone for at least 10 years. The joint (cartilage) space of the left hip joint is severely narrowed and the iliopectineal line is thickened (brim sign), as evidenced by comparison with the opposite side.*

The dread complication of Paget's disease of bone is osteosarcoma, which fortunately occurs in fewer than 1% of patients. Other associated neoplasms include giant cell tumors and nonneoplastic granulomas. Malignant tumors occasionally metastasize to pagetic bone.

Metabolic complications usually result from some interruption of the mechanisms that control the close bone formation-resorption coupling. Immobilization or fracture may lead to hypercalciuria, or rarely, hypercalcemia.

Since Paget's disease of bone is frequently asymptomatic and does not result in significant clinical disability, in many instances no therapy is indicated (1,2,4–6,7). In symptomatic individuals, specific therapy is available, but careful clinical evaluation is essential to determine the nature of the pain or disability. Nonsteroidal antiinflammatory agents such as aspirin or indomethacin may suppress pain, although in doses commonly used these drugs do not affect the biochemical abnormalities. Other agents can suppress pagetic bone resorption (decrease urinary hydroxyproline excretion) and subsequently produce a decrease in bone formation (decrease serum alkaline phosphatase levels) accompanied by lessening of pain and improvement in function.

Synthetic salmon calcitonin administered subcutaneously usually results in clinical improvement within several weeks. When therapy is discontinued, symptoms usually return. Some patients may experience a plateau in the response, or symptoms may return and alkaline phosphatase levels increase despite continued therapy. Neutralizing antibodies to salmon calcitonin are responsible for the refractory state in some patients; the latter can still respond to human calcitonin.

The only bisphosphonate compound currently approved for use in the United States is disodium etidronate. It is administered orally in dosages of 5 to 10 mg/kg/day for courses of no longer than six months to decrease bone resorption. Clinical and biochemical improvement may first become evident after the drug has been discontinued; improvement may last longer than six months. Some individuals experience a temporary paradoxical increase in bone pain and a mineralization defect in involved bone. So-called second-generation bisphosphates, available in Europe for more than a decade, are now undergoing therapeutic trials in this country. Several of these bisphosphonates are more effective than disodium etidronate, induce long-term remissions and do not produce mineralization defects. There is no longer a role for mithramycin in the treatment of Paget's disease.

If irreversible damage in joints such as hips and knees has taken place joint replacement can be very effective. Results are excellent in approximately three-quarters of the patients reported. It is worthwhile to administer calcitonin before surgery to reduce the activity of the disease and decrease local vascularity.

Steven M. Krane, MD

1. Singer FR, Krane SM: Paget's disease of bone. Metabolic Bone Disease and Clinically Related Disorders. Edited by Avioli LV, Krane SM. Philadelphia, Penn. W.B. Saunders & Co. 1990, pp 546–615
2. Rebel A (ed): Symposium on paget's disease. Clin Ortho Rel Res 217:1–170, 1987
3. Roodman GD, Kurihara N, Ohsaki Y, et al. Interleukin-6. A potential autocrine/paracrine factor in Paget's disease of bone. J Clin Invest 89:46–52, 1992
4. Paget's Disease of Bone. Edited by Singer FR, Wallach S. New York, NY Elsevier, 1991, pp 1–313
5. Bijvoet OLM, Vellenga CJLR, Harinck HIJ: Paget's disease of bones: Assessment, therapy, and secondary prevention. Clinical Disorders of Bone and Mineral Metabolism. Edited by Kleerekoper M, Krane SM. New York, NY, Mary Ann Liebert, 1989, pp 525–542
6. Krane SM: Paget's disease of bone. Current Therapy in Endocrinology and Metabolism. Edited by Bardin CW. Philadelphia, Penn., B.C. Decker, Inc., 1991, pp 456–460

50. REGIONAL RHEUMATIC PAIN SYNDROMES

The regional rheumatic pain syndromes, because of their prevalence, complexity, and lack of diagnostic laboratory tests, present a challenge to the clinician. Yet success in diagnosis and treatment is most gratifying. The conditions discussed in this chapter include disorders involving muscles, tendons, entheses, joints, cartilage, ligaments, fascia, bone and nerve. A working knowledge of regional anatomy and an approach utilizing a regional differential diagnosis will help to obtain a specific diagnosis (1).

A precise history is needed to identify the conditions present; often more than one syndrome can occur concomitantly. A complete neuromusculoskeletal examination should be performed emphasizing careful palpation, passive range of motion (ROM), and active ROM alone and sometimes with resistance. Some guidelines for the management of these conditions is provided in Table 50–1.

CAUSATIVE FACTORS

Many syndromes of the neuromusculoskeletal system are the result of injury from a specific activity or event, ranging from only one episode to repetitive overuse, especially when abnormal body position or mechanics is present. With aging, tendons become less flexible and elastic, making them more susceptible to injury. Also with aging and with disuse atrophy, the muscles become weaker and exhibit less endurance and bulk, resulting in a decrease in muscle absorption of mechanical forces otherwise transmitted to joints, tendons, ligaments, and entheses. A shortened musculotendinous unit from lack of stretching is more prone to injury. A genetic predisposition to certain regional syndromes exists resulting from variations in anatomy and abnormal biomechanics. Systemic inflammatory diseases may have characteristic local manifestations. Unfortunately, causative factor(s) often are not identified.

Table 50–1. Guidelines for management of regional rheumatic pain syndromes

1. Exclude systemic disease and infection by appropriate methods. Diagnostic aspiration is mandatory in suspected septic bursitis. Gram stain, culture, and sugar determination on the bursal fluid provide prompt diagnosis of a septic bursitis
2. Teach the patient to recognize and avoid aggravating factors that cause recurrences
3. Instruct the patient in self-help therapy including the daily performance of mobilizing exercises
4. Provide an explanation of the cause for pain, thus alleviating concern for a crippling disease. When the regional rheumatic pain syndrome overlies another rheumatic problem, the clinician must explain the contribution each disorder plays in the symptom complex and then help the patient deal with each one
5. Provide relief from pain with safe analgesics, counterirritants (heat, ice, vapocoolant sprays) and if appropriate, intralesional injection of a local anesthetic or anesthetic with depository corticosteroid agent
6. Provide the patient with an idea of the duration of therapy necessary to restore order to the musculoskeletal system Symptomatic relief often corroborates the diagnosis

GENERAL CONCEPTS OF MANAGEMENT

Drug Therapy

Oral medications, including nonsteroidal antiinflammatory drugs (NSAIDs) and analgesics, play a role in management of regional musculoskeletal disorders. The NSAIDs help reduce inflammation and pain. For additional pain relief, analgesics such as acetaminophen can be added. Tricyclic antidepressants such as amitriptyline may also be useful in chronic pain and neurogenic or myofascial pain.

Comprehensive management of these regional syndromes should be undertaken rather than relying on oral medications alone. The causative aspects, as noted above, should be evaluated, and activity modification should be advised as needed. Local injections and physical therapy also can be useful components of treatment as described below.

Intralesional Injections

After specific diagnosis of a regional rheumatic pain syndrome, local injection with lidocaine, corticosteroids, or both is often of benefit (2). In fact, the immediate pain relief from a properly directed injection into a tendon sheath, bursa, enthesis or nerve area, for a specific problem, further validates the diagnosis. Injection of an area of nonspecific muscle tenderness with a corticosteroid preparation should be discouraged.

Basic principles of intralesional injections include aseptic technique and use of small needles (25-gauge 5/8" or 1 1/2" or a 22-gauge 1 1/2"). The use of separate syringes for lidocaine and corticosteroid avoids mixing of the two substances, and permits infiltration of lidocaine beginning intracutaneously with a small wheal and continuing to the site of the lesion. This method helps make the injection relatively painless. When the needle reaches the desired site, the syringe is changed with the needle left in place, and the corticosteroid is then injected. This technique helps avoid possible subcutaneous and skin atrophy secondary to corticosteroid use. When injecting a tendon sheath, the needle should be placed parallel to the tendon fibers and not into the tendon itself. In many instances, using a more water-soluble corticosteroid is preferable to lessen the possibility of corticosteroid-induced tendon weakness or post-injection flare.

Physical Therapy

The goals of therapeutic exercise are to increase flexibility by stretching, increase muscle strength by resistive exercises, and improve muscle endurance by some repetitive regimen. The physician should become knowledgeable about exercise prescriptions for the various conditions (3). For example, older women tend to have tight calf muscles, which predispose to calf cramps, Achilles tendon problems, or other ankle and foot disorders. Tight quadriceps, hamstring, and iliopsoas muscles are related to problems in the low back, hip, and knee regions. Exercise to stretch these muscles can be taught by the physician. Instruction for quadriceps strengthening, especially by straight leg raising from the sitting position, and for pelvic tilt exercise can be given in the office (4).

Heat or cold modalities provide pain relief and muscle relaxation and serve as a prelude to an exercise regimen. They are of doubtful benefit when used alone over an extended period.

DISORDERS OF THE SHOULDER REGION

Shoulder pain is one of the most common musculoskeletal complaints in people over age 40. In younger people athletic injuries are a frequent source of such pain. The shoulder itself is a remarkable ball and socket joint, which allows for considerable motion. This mobility, however, is accompanied by some instability, from which shoulder problems can result. Many shoulder conditions have similar precipitating factors and symptoms, and multiple lesions involving different structures around the joint may be present in the same shoulder. Understanding the anatomy is important to diagnosis and management (see Chapter 2).

The glenohumeral, acromioclavicular, sternoclavicular, and scapulothoracic joints all work synchronously to achieve the desired motion. Important shoulder ligaments include the acromioclavicular capsular, coracoacromial, coracoclavicular (trapezoid and conoid), coracohumeral, sternoclavicular, and glenohumeral ligaments. The subacromial bursa, which is inferior to the acromion, is contiguous with the subdeltoid bursa and covers the humeral head. Overlying the bursa is the deltoid muscle. The rotator cuff comprises the tendons of the supraspinatus, infraspinatus, teres minor, and subscapularis muscles and attaches at the humeral tuberosities. The rotator cuff provides internal and external rotation of the shoulder, and fixes the humeral head in the glenoid fossa during abduction to counteract the pull of the

deltoid, which tends to displace the humeral head from the glenoid. The mechanism whereby the deltoid muscle and the downward-acting short rotators combine to produce abduction is called *force-couple*. After 30° of abduction, a constant 1:2 ratio exists between movement of the scapular articulation and the glenohumeral joint, with a combined movement known as *scapulohumeral rhythm*.

Pain may be referred to the shoulder from the cervical region due to cervical spondylosis, from the thorax due to a Pancoast tumor, from the abdomen area secondary to gallbladder or hepatic lesions, or from the diaphragm.

Rotator Cuff Tendinitis

Rotator cuff tendinitis, or impingement syndrome, is the most common cause of shoulder pain. Tendinitis (and not bursitis) is the primary cause of pain but secondary involvement of the subacromial bursa occurs in some cases. The condition may be acute or chronic and may or may not be associated with calcific deposits within the tendon. The key finding is pain in the rotator cuff on active abduction, especially between 60° and 120°, and sometimes when lowering the arm. In more severe cases, however, pain may begin on initial abduction and continue throughout the ROM. In acute tendinitis pain comes on more abruptly and may be excruciating. Such cases tend to occur in younger patients and are more likely to have calcific deposits in the supraspinatus tendon insertion (Fig. 50–1). The deposits are best seen on roentgenogram in external rotation, appearing round or oval and several centimeters in length. These deposits may resolve spontaneously over a period of time. A true subacromial bursitis may also be present when calcific material ruptures into the bursa.

The more typical chronic rotator cuff tendinitis manifests as an ache in the shoulder, usually over the lateral deltoid, and occurs on various movements, especially on abduction and internal rotation. Other symptoms include difficulty in dressing oneself and night pain arising from difficulty in positioning the shoulders. Tenderness on palpation and some loss of motion may be evident on examination. The initial movement to detect rotator cuff tendinitis is to determine whether pain is present on active abduction of the arm in the horizontal position. Passive abduction is then carried out. Usually in rotator cuff tendinitis, less pain is present on passive abduction than active abduction. Conversely, pain may be increased on active abduction against resistance. The

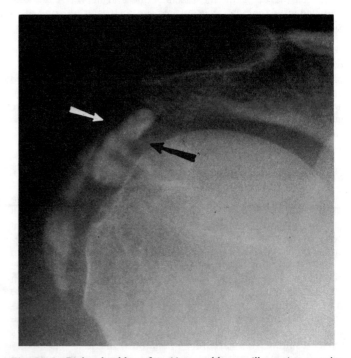

*Fig. 50–1. Right shoulder of a 44-year-old man illustrating massive calcareous deposits in the supraspinatus tendon (**white arrow**) and subdeltoid bursa (**black arrow**).*

impingement sign is nearly always positive. This maneuver is performed with one hand of the examiner raising the patient's arm in forced flexion while the other hand prevents scapular rotation (5). A positive sign occurs if pain develops at or before 180° of forward flexion. Another useful test to confirm rotator cuff disease is the impingement test, performed by injecting 2–5 ml of 2% lidocaine into the subacromial bursa. Pain relief on abduction following the injection denotes a positive impingement test. The same test can be used in another way to determine whether apparent shoulder weakness is due to pain. Once pain is eliminated with the injection, the arm is retested for weakness. If the weakness is still present, the result is again considered positive.

The causes of rotator cuff tendinitis are multifactorial, but relative overuse, especially from overhead activity causing impingement of the rotator cuff, is commonly implicated. Compression of the rotator cuff occurs above by the edge and under surface of the anterior third of the acromion and the coracohumeral ligament and below by the humeral head. There is also age-related decrease in vascularity and degeneration of the cuff tendons and reduction of strength of the cuff muscles due to aging or decline in use. Osteophytes on the inferior portion of the acromioclavicular joint or acute trauma to the shoulder region contribute to development of tendinitis. An inflammatory process such as rheumatoid arthritis (RA) can also cause rotator cuff tendinitis independent of impingement. Treatment consists of rest and modalities such as hot packs, ultrasound, or cold applications, with specific ROM exercises as soon as tolerated. Nonsteroidal antiinflammatory drugs are often beneficial; however, the most frequent treatment is injection of a depot corticosteroid into the subacromial bursa, the floor of which is contiguous with the rotator cuff.

Rotator Cuff Tear

Generally, an acute tear of a rotator cuff after trauma is easily recognized. The trauma may be superimposed on an already degenerative and possibly even partially torn cuff. In trauma, especially falls, resulting in a ruptured cuff, fractures of the humeral head and dislocation of the joint should also be considered. However, at least one-half of patients with a tear recall no trauma. In these cases, degeneration of the rotator cuff gradually occurs, finally resulting in a complete tear. Rotator cuff tears are classified as small (1 cm or less), medium (1–3 cm), large (3–5 cm), or massive (>5 cm) (6). Shoulder pain, weakness on abduction, and loss of motion occur in varying degrees, ranging from severe pain and mild weakness to no pain and marked weakness. A positive drop-arm sign with inability to actively maintain 90° of passive shoulder abduction may be present in large or massive tears. Surgical repair is indicated in the younger patient.

Less easily diagnosed is the smaller, chronic complete tear of the rotator cuff or a partial (incomplete) tear. Pain on abduction, night pain, weakness, loss of abduction, and tenderness on palpation can be present in both of these types of tears. A small complete tear, however, can exist despite fairly good abduction. Tears of the rotator cuff may also occur as a result of the chronic inflammation in RA, and is often present with cystic swelling around the shoulder.

The definitive diagnosis of a ruptured rotator cuff is established by an abnormal arthrogram showing a communication between the glenohumeral joint and the subacromial bursa. In a partial tear, in which an intact layer of rotator cuff tissue still separates the joint space from the subacromial bursa, a small ulcer-like crater is seen on the arthrogram. Diagnostic ultrasonography or magnetic resonance imaging (MRI) are also helpful in identifying rotator cuff tears (7). Small complete tears and incomplete tears of the rotator cuff are treated conservatively with rest, physical therapy, and NSAIDs. Although their role has not yet been established by careful studies, subacromial injections of a steroid may be of benefit in relieving pain.

Bicipital Tendinitis

This condition is manifested by pain, most often in the anterior region of the shoulder and occasionally more diffusely. The pain may be acute, but is usually chronic and is related to impingement of the biceps tendon by the acromion. Tenosynovitis of the long head of the biceps is present, and the tendon may be frayed and fibrotic. Palpation over the bicipital groove reveals localized tenderness. The patient's response should be compared with palpation of the opposite side, since this tendon has normal tenderness. Pain may be reproduced over the bicipital tendon in some cases by supination of the forearm against resistance (Yergason's sign), shoulder flexion against resistance (Speed's test), or by extension of the shoulder. Bicipital tendinitis and rotator cuff tendinitis may occur at the same time. Treatment of bicipital tendinitis consists of rest, hot packs, ultrasound, and as pain subsides, passive then active ROM exercises. Nonsteroidal antiinflammatory drugs may be helpful, and occasionally a small amount of corticosteroid carefully injected in the tendon sheath may be of benefit (8).

Subluxation of the bicipital tendon is manifested as a sensation of pain with the shoulder going out and then popping back in. Tenderness may be present over the bicipital tendon, and a snap over the tendon may be noted in the shoulder when the arm is passively abducted to 90° and moved from internal to external rotation and back. Rupture of the biceps tendon occurs at the superior edge of the bicipital groove. Full rupture of the long head of the tendon produces a characteristic bulbous enlargement of the lateral half of the muscle belly. Generally, these two latter conditions of the biceps tendon are treated conservatively.

Adhesive Capsulitis

Known also as *frozen shoulder* or *pericapsulitis*, adhesive capsulitis is associated with generalized pain and tenderness with severe loss of active and passive motion in all planes. It is rare before age 40 and may be secondary to any type of shoulder problem. Muscle atrophy may occur early in the course. Every stiff and painful shoulder, however, is not necessarily adhesive capsulitis. In addition to local shoulder problems leading to adhesive capsulitis, inflammatory arthritis and diabetes may also be causes. Additional factors such as immobility, low pain threshold, depression, and neglect or improper initial treatment also favor the development of a frozen shoulder. Many cases, however, are idiopathic. The joint capsule adheres to the anatomic neck, and the axillary fold binds to itself, causing restricted motion. The capsule becomes thickened and contracted.

Arthrography helps confirm this diagnosis by showing a decrease in volume of the shoulder joint capsule with loss of the normal axillary pouch and often absence of dye in the biceps tendon sheath. The joint may accept as little as 0.5–3.0 ml of dye or occasionally up to 10 ml, whereas a normal shoulder joint has a capacity of 28–35 ml. A frozen shoulder is best treated with a comprehensive program involving NSAIDs and corticosteroidal injections into the glenohumeral joint and the subacromial bursa (9). Physical therapy consists of ice packs, ultrasound, transcutaneous electrical nerve stimulation (TENS), and gentle ROM exercises—beginning with pendulum exercises and wall climbing with the fingers—and finally active ROM and strengthening exercises. Rarely manipulation under anesthesia may be needed in resistant cases.

Suprascapular Neuropathy

The suprascapular nerve, which innervates the supraspinatus and infraspinatus, may be damaged by trauma, overactivity of the shoulder, local ganglion, or a fracture of the scapula. The nerve may be compressed at the suprascapular notch. The condition is marked by weakness on abduction and external rotation. In chronic cases atrophy of the supraspinatus and infraspinatus muscles may be seen. Electrodiagnostic studies help confirm the diagnosis. Treatment generally consists of physical therapy and may include a local corticosteroid injection into the area of the suprascapular notch. In some chronic cases, surgical decompression is needed.

Long Thoracic Nerve Paralysis

Injury to the long thoracic nerve produces weakness of the serratus anterior muscle, resulting in a winged scapula. Pain along the base of the neck and downward over the scapula and deltoid region may be felt, along with fatigue on elevation of the arm. The winging of the scapula becomes apparent when the patient pushes against the wall with arms outstretched. Trauma and diabetes seem to be common causes of this disorder, but it is often idiopathic and usually self-limited.

Brachial Plexopathy

Brachial plexopathy presents with a deep, sharp shoulder pain of rapid onset made worse by abduction and rotation and followed by weakness of the shoulder girdle. An electromyogram helps confirm this diagnosis by demonstrating positive sharp waves and fibrillations in the involved muscles. Recovery may take from one month to several years. Brachial plexopathy can result from trauma, tumor, radiation, inoculation neuritis, diabetes, infection, or median sternotomy done for cardiac surgery, or it can be idiopathic.

Thoracic Outlet Syndrome

A constellation of symptoms resulting from compression of the neurovascular bundle, where the brachial plexus and subclavian artery and vein exit beneath the clavicle and subclavius muscle is known as the thoracic outlet syndrome. The neurovascular bundle is bordered below by the first rib, anteriorly by the scalenus anterior muscle, and posteriorly by the scalenus medius muscle. The clinical picture depends on which component is compressed—neural, vascular, or both. Neurologic symptoms predominate in most patients. Pain, paresthesia, and numbness are the principal symptoms, radiating from the neck and shoulder down to the arm and hand, especially distributing to the ring and little fingers. Symptoms are worsened by activity. Weakness and atrophy of intrinsic muscles may be seen as a late finding. Vascular symptoms consist of discoloration, temperature change, pain on use, and Raynaud's phenomenon.

The differential list is large, so the diagnosis is arrived at in part by exclusion. Women outnumber men in incidence. Inquiries about the relationship of symptoms to activities must be made, since shoulder abduction may initiate or worsen symptoms. A careful neurologic examination and evaluation for arterial and venous insufficiency and postural abnormalities should be done. The Adson test, in which the patient holds a deep breath, extends his neck, and then turns his chin toward the side being examined, is positive when the radial pulse becomes extremely weak or disappears. Many normal people may have this finding, but if the maneuver reproduces the patient's symptoms, it is more significant. With the hyperabduction maneuver, the radial pulse is monitored when the patient raises an arm above the head. A reduction in the radial pulse strength may indicate arterial compression. Again, this test may be positive in normal people. A chest roentgenogram should be obtained to look for a cervical rib, an elongated transverse process of C7, or healing fractures or exostoses. Because of the difficulty in measuring nerve conduction velocity of the involved nerves, results of these tests have been somewhat inconsistent, but in capable hands they furnish additional supporting information. Somatosensory evoked potentials have also been used successfully. An angiogram or venogram can be obtained in cases of suspected arterial or venous compression.

In general, management of thoracic outlet syndrome is conservative. Good posture is emphasized. Stretching of the scalene and pectoral muscles, together with scapula mobilization and strengthening of the shoulder girdle musculature, is beneficial. A local anesthetic injection into the scalene anticus muscle, if a trigger point is present, may be helpful as well. In resistant or severe cases of thoracic outlet syndrome, the first rib and the scalene muscle may be resected.

DISORDERS OF THE ELBOW REGION

Olecranon Bursitis

The subcutaneous olecranon bursa is frequently involved with bursitis, either secondary to trauma or as an idiopathic condition. The bursa is characteristically swollen and tender on pressure, but pain may be minimal and generally no motion is lost. Aspiration may yield clear or blood-tinged fluid, having a low viscosity, or grossly hemorrhagic fluid. Aspiration alone and protection from trauma are generally sufficient to resolve the condition. A small dose of corticosteroid may be injected, but the physician must be aware of the possibility of secondary infection, skin atrophy, or chronic local pain that apparently results from subclinical skin atrophy (10). Inflammatory olecranon bursitis may be due to gout, RA, or calcium pyrophosphate deposition disease. Olecranon bursitis has also been seen in uremic patients undergoing hemodialysis. With septic olecranon bursitis, localized erythema is the major clue. Heat, pain, and a positive culture are also frequently present. The condition is treated by aspiration and drainage and the administration of appropriate antibiotics. Surgical excision is occasionally needed.

Lateral Epicondylitis

Lateral epicondylitis, or tennis elbow, is a common condition in those who overuse their arms. Localized tenderness directly over or slightly anterior to the lateral epicondyle is the hallmark of this disorder. Pain may occur during handshakes, lifting a briefcase, or other similar activities. Probably less than 10% of patients actually acquire lateral epicondylitis through playing tennis; rather, job and recreational activities, including gardening and other athletics, are the usual causes. Pathologically, the condition consists of degeneration of the common extensor tendon, particularly of the extensor carpi radialis brevis tendon. Tendon tears may be the cause of chronic cases.

Treatment of lateral epicondylitis is aimed at altering activities and preventing overuse of the forearm musculature. Ice packs, heat, and NSAIDs are of some benefit. A forearm brace can also be used. A local steroid injection with a 25-gauge needle over the lateral epicondyle often produces satisfactory initial relief. Isometric strengthening is important as the initial part of a rehabilitation program.

Evaluation of chronic cases should include a roentgenogram to check for calcification, exostosis, or other bony abnormalities. Entrapment of the radial nerve at the elbow can also cause discomfort and a vague aching at that site. Forced forearm supination against resistance seems to aggravate the symptoms of a neural entrapment more than the symptoms of lateral epicondylitis, in which resisted wrist extension aggravates the pain.

Medial Epicondylitis

Medial epicondylitis, or golfer's elbow, which mainly involves the flexor carpi radialis, is less common and less disabling than lateral epicondylitis. Local pain and tenderness over the medial epicondyle are present, and resistance to flexion of the wrist exacerbates the pain. Alteration of activities and NSAIDs usually alleviate the problem, although occasionally a local corticosteroid injection is required.

Tendinitis of Musculotendinous Insertion of Biceps

Tendinitis of the distal insertion of the biceps (lacertus fibrosus) may cause dull pain throughout the antecubital fossa of the elbow (11). Palpation confirms the source of pain, and mild swelling may be present. Heat, NSAIDs, rest, and occasionally a local injection of corticosteroids generally are beneficial in this self-limiting condition.

Ulnar Nerve Entrapment

Entrapment of the ulnar nerve at the elbow produces numbness and paresthesia of the little finger and adjacent side of the ring finger and aching of the medial aspect of the elbow. Hand clumsiness can be present. Tenderness may be elicited when the ulnar nerve groove, located on the posteroinferior surface of the medial epicondyle, is compressed. The little finger may have decreased sensation and weakness on abduction and flexion. Elevating the hand by resting the forearm on the head for one minute may produce paresthesia. In long-standing cases, atrophy and weakness of the ulnar intrinsic muscles of the hand occur. A positive Tinel's sign by tapping the nerve at the elbow is often present. Similar symptoms may result from subluxation of the nerve.

Ulnar nerve entrapment has multiple causes, including external compression from occupation, compression during anesthesia, trauma, prolonged bed rest, earlier fractures, and arthritis. A nerve conduction test that shows slowing of ulnar motor and sensory conduction and prolonged proximal latency aids in confirming the diagnosis. Avoiding pressure on the elbow and repetitive elbow flexion may be all that is necessary, but in severe persistent cases, surgical correction is needed.

DISORDERS OF THE WRIST AND HAND

Ganglion

A ganglion is a cystic swelling arising from a joint or tendon sheath that occurs most commonly over the dorsum of the wrist. It is synovial lined and contains thick jelly-like fluid. Ganglia are generally of unknown cause but may develop secondary to trauma or prolonged wrist extension. Usually, the only symptom is swelling, but occasionally a large ganglion produces discomfort on wrist extension. Treatment, if indicated, consists of aspiration of the fluid, with or without injection of corticosteroid. Use of a splint may help prevent recurrence. In severe cases, the whole ganglion may be removed surgically.

De Quervain's Tenosynovitis

De Quervain's tenosynovitis may result from repetitive activity involving pinching with the thumb while moving the wrist. It has been reported to occur in new mothers and as a complication of pregnancy. The symptoms are pain, tenderness, and occasionally swelling over the radial styloid. Pathologic findings include inflammation and narrowing of the tendon sheath around the abductor pollicis longus and extensor pollicis brevis. A positive Finkelstein test result is usually seen: pain increases when the thumb is folded across the palm and the fingers are flexed over the thumb as the examiner passively deviates the wrist toward the ulnar side. Treatment involves splinting, local corticosteroid injection, and NSAIDs as indicated. Rarely, surgical removal of inflamed tenosynovium is needed.

Tenosynovitis of the Wrist

Tenosynovitis occurs in other flexor and extensor tendons of the wrist in addition to those involved in De Quervain's tenosynovitis (12). The individual tendons on the extensor side that may be vulnerable are the extensor pollicis longus, extensor indicis proprius, extensor digiti minimi, and extensor carpi ulnaris, and on the flexor side, the flexor carpi radialis, flexor carpi ulnaris, flexor digitorum superficialis, and flexor digitorum profundus.

The findings vary depending on which tendon is involved. Localized pain and tenderness are usually present, and there is sometimes swelling. Pain on resisted movement is often seen. The tenosynovitis may be misinterpreted as arthritis of the wrist.

This problem may be due to repetitive use, a traumatic episode, inflammatory arthritis, or may be idiopathic. The treatment consists of avoiding overuse, splinting, and NSAIDs. A local corticosteroid injection into the tendon sheath, avoiding direct injection into the tendon itself, is usually of benefit.

Pronator Teres Syndrome

An uncommon condition, pronator teres syndrome is not easy to diagnose, because it has some features similar to carpal tunnel syndrome. In this case, however, the median nerve is compressed at the level of the pronator teres muscle. The patient may complain of aching in the volar aspect of the forearm, numbness in the thumb and index finger, weakness on gripping with the thumb, and writer's cramp. The most specific finding is tenderness of the proximal part of the pronator teres, which may be aggravated by resistive pronation of the forearm. Pronator compression often produces paresthesia after 30 seconds or less. In some patients, a positive Tinel's sign is found at the proximal edge of the pronator teres. Unlike carpal tunnel syndrome, nocturnal awakening and numbness in the morning are absent. Pronator teres syndrome is thought to result from overuse by repetitive grasping or pronation, trauma, or a space-occupying lesion.

Although they often fail to localize the lesion, electrodiagnostic studies may reveal signs of denervation of the forearm muscles supplied by the median nerve but sparing the pronator teres. If the condition does not improve with alteration of activities and with time, exploratory surgery may be undertaken. Fibrous or tendinous bands or a hypertrophied pronator muscle may be found.

Anterior Interosseous Nerve Syndrome

Compression of the anterior interosseous nerve near its bifurcation from the median nerve produces weakness of the flexor pollicis longus, flexor digitorum profundus, and pronator quadratus muscles. Sensation is not affected, but a person with this syndrome cannot form an "O" with the thumb and index finger because motion is lost in the interphalangeal (IP) joint of the thumb and the distal interphalangeal (DIP) joint of the index finger. Electromyography may help confirm the diagnosis. Repetitive overuse, trauma, and fibrous bands are the principal causes of this syndrome. Protection from trauma usually results in improvement; if not, surgical exploration may be undertaken.

Radial Nerve Palsy

The most common type of radial nerve palsy is the spiral groove syndrome, or bridegroom palsy, in which the radial nerve is compressed against the humerus. The most prominent feature is a wrist-drop with flexion of the metacarpophalangeal (MCP) joints and adduction of the thumb. Anesthesia in the web space and hypesthesia from the dorsal aspect of the forearm to the thumb, index, and middle fingers may be present. If the radial nerve is compressed more proximally through improper use of crutches or prolonged leaning of the arm over the back of a chair ("Saturday night palsy"), weakness of the triceps and brachioradialis muscles may also occur. Compression injuries generally heal over a period of weeks. Splinting the wrist during this recovery time prevents overstretching of the paralyzed muscles and ligaments. Electrodiagnostic studies are helpful in determining the specific point of compression.

Posterior Interosseous Nerve Syndrome

Posterior interosseous nerve entrapment in the radial tunnel produces discomfort in the proximal lateral portion of the forearm. The fingers cannot be extended at the MCP joints. Because the posterior interosseous nerve, a branch of the radial nerve, is primarily a motor nerve, sensory disturbances are rare. Occupational or recreational repetitive activity with forceful supination, wrist extension, or radial deviation against resistance may be a factor. Direct trauma and such nontraumatic conditions as a ganglion also have been implicated. Interestingly, this syndrome has been seen in RA due to synovial compression of the nerve and, therefore, must be distinguished from a ruptured extensor tendon.

Superficial Radial Neuropathy (Cheiralgia Paresthetica)

A lesion of this sensory nerve is more common than previously thought and causes symptoms of a burning or shooting pain and sometimes numbness and tingling over the dorsoradial aspect of the wrist, thumb, and index fingers. Hyperpronation and ulnar wrist flexion may be provocative. Decreased pin prick sensation and a positive Tinel's sign may be seen. Electrodiagnostic studies are helpful in the diagnosis.

Tight wrist restraints from handcuffs or watch bands are well-known causes. Trauma to the area, repetitive wrist motion, diabetes, ganglion cyst, venipuncture, and local surgical procedures, are other possible etiologies. The neuropathy may resolve with time. Treatment consists of splinting, NSAIDs, local corticosteroid injection, or surgical neurolysis in some cases.

Carpal Tunnel Syndrome

Carpal tunnel syndrome is the most common cause of paresthesias in the hands. The median nerve and flexor tendons pass through a common tunnel at the wrist whose rigid walls are bounded dorsally and on the sides by the carpal bones, and on the volar aspect by the transverse carpal ligament (Fig. 50–2). Any process encroaching on this tunnel compresses the median nerve, which innervates the thenar muscles (for flexion, opposition, abduction); the radial lumbricales; and the skin of the radial side of the palm, thumb, second and third fingers, and the radial half of the fourth finger.

Symptoms are variable, but episodes of burning pain or tingling in the hand are common, often occurring during the night and relieved by vigorous shaking or movement of the hand. Numbness is a common complaint, affecting the index and middle fingers, radial side of the ring fingers, and occasionally the thumb. Some patients experience only numbness, without much pain. Numbness may also occur with activities such as driving or holding a newspaper or book. The patient may have a sensation of hand swelling when in fact no swelling is visible. Occasionally the pain spreads above the wrist into the forearm or, rarely, even above the elbow and up the arm. Bilateral disease is common.

A positive Tinel's sign or Phalen's sign may be present. Phalen's test is performed by holding the flexed wrists against each other. Loss of sensation may be demonstrated in the index, middle, or radial side of the fourth finger. Weakness and atrophy of the muscles of the thenar eminence may gradually appear in chronic cases. Confirmation of the diagnosis can be obtained by demonstrating prolonged distal latency times during electrodiagnostic studies.

A variety of disorders may cause carpal tunnel syndrome, including edema from pregnancy or trauma, osteophytes, ganglia related to tenosynovial sheaths, lipomata, and anomalous muscles, tendons, and blood vessels that compress the median nerve. Carpal tunnel syndrome has been observed in various infections such as tuberculosis, histoplasmosis, sporotrichosis, coccidioidomycosis, and rubella. Rheumatoid arthritis, gout, pseudogout, and other inflammatory diseases of the wrist can cause compression of the median nerve. Amyloid deposits of the primary type or in association with multiple myeloma can occur at this site, and carpal tunnel syndrome may be the initial manifestation of the disease. The syndrome has also been reported to occur in myxedema and acromegaly. In many cases, however, no obvious cause can be found or a nonspecific tenosynovitis is evident. Many of the idiopathic cases may be due to occupational stress.

In milder cases, splinting the wrist in a neutral position may relieve symptoms. Local injections of corticosteroids into the carpal tunnel area, using a 25-gauge needle, are helpful for nonspecific or for inflammatory tenosynovitis. The benefit, however, may be only temporary depending upon the degree of compression and the reversibility of the neural injury. When conservative treatment fails, surgical decompression of the tunnel by release of the transverse carpal ligament and removal of tissue compressing the median nerve is often beneficial. Even with surgery, however, symptoms may sometimes recur.

Ulnar Nerve Entrapment at the Wrist

The ulnar nerve can be entrapped at the wrist proximal to Guyon's canal, in the canal itself, or distal to it (13). Guyon's canal is roughly bounded medially by the pisiform bone, laterally by the hook of the hamate, superiorly by the volar carpal ligament (pisohamate ligament), and inferiorly by the transverse carpal ligament. Because the ulnar nerve, on entering the canal, bifurcates into the superficial and deep branches, the clinical picture may vary having only sensory, only motor, or both sensory and motor findings.

The complete clinical picture includes pain, numbness, and paresthesias of the hypothenar area, clumsiness, and a weak hand grip, including difficulty using the thumb in a pincher type movement. Pressure over the ulnar nerve at the hook of the hamate may cause tingling or pain. Atrophy of the hypothenar and intrinsic muscles can occur. Clawing of ring and little fingers may be seen, resulting from weakness of the third and fourth lumbricales. Loss of sensation occurs over the hypothenar area.

If the superficial branch alone is involved, then only numbness, pain and loss of sensation occurs. Entrapment of the deep branch produces only motor weakness of the ulnar innervated muscles. The sites of motor weakness depend on the exact location of nerve compression; for example, if the compression is more distal, then the hypothenar muscles and intrinsics may be spared, causing weakness and atrophy of only the adductor pollicis, deep head of the flexor pollicis brevis, and first dorsal interosseous muscles. The causes of ulnar neuropathy at the wrist include trauma, ganglia, bicycling, inflammatory arthritis, flexor carpi ulnaris hypertrophy, fractures, neuroma, lipomata, and diabetes.

The diagnosis is assisted by electrodiagnostic studies, indicating a prolonged distal latency of the ulnar nerve at the wrist and denervation of the ulnar innervated muscles. Treatment includes rest from an offending activity, splinting, or a local corticosteroid injection; however, surgical exploration and decompression may be necessary.

Volar Flexor Tenosynovitis

Inflammation of the tendon sheaths of the flexor digitorum superficialis and flexor digitorum profundus tendons in the palm is extremely common but often unrecognized. Pain in the palm is felt on finger flexion, but in some cases the pain may radiate to the proximal interphalangeal (PIP) and MCP joints on the dorsal side, thus misleading the examiner. The diagnosis is made by palpation and identification of localized tenderness and swelling of the volar tendon sheaths. The middle and index fingers are most commonly involved, but the ring and little fingers can also be affected. Often a nodule composed of fibrous tissue can be palpated in the palm just proximal to the MCP joint on the volar side. The nodule interferes with the normal tendon gliding and can cause a triggering or locking, which may be intermittent and produces an uncomfortable sensation. Similar involvement can occur at the flexor tendon of the thumb. Volar tenosynovitis may be part of inflammatory conditions, such as RA, psoriatic arthritis, or apatite crystal deposition disease. It is seen frequently in conjunction with osteoarthritis (OA) of the hands. The most

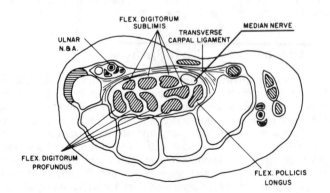

Fig. 50–2. Cross-section of wrist illustrating the position of the transverse carpal ligament (flexor retinaculum) and the structures occupying the osseous-fibrous carpal tunnel.

common cause is overuse trauma of the hands from gripping with increased pull on the flexor tendons. Injection of a long-acting steroid into the tendon sheath usually relieves the problem (14), although surgery on the tendon sheath may be needed in unremitting cases.

Infection of the tendon sheaths in the hand requires drainage and antibiotics. People with drug addictions and diabetes may be at increased risk for such infections. Atypical mycobacterium or fungal infections also cause a chronic tenosynovitis in the hands. *Mycobacterium marinum*, which is found in infected fish, barnacles, fish tanks, and swimming pools, is a common culprit (15).

Dupuytren's Contracture

In Dupuytren's contracture a thickening and shortening of the palmar fascia occurs. In established cases the diagnosis is obvious with typical thick, cord-like superficial fibrous tissue felt in the palm causing a contracture, usually of the ring finger. The fifth, third, and second fingers are involved in decreasing order of frequency. Initially, a mildly tender fibrous nodule in the volar fascia of the palm may be the only finding leading to a confusion with volar flexor tenosynovitis. Dimpling or puckering of the skin over the involved fascia helps identify the early Dupuytren's contracture. The initial nodules probably result from a contraction of proliferative myofibroblasts. The tendon and tendon sheaths are not implicated, but the dermis is frequently involved, resulting in fixation to the fascia. The progression of the disease varies, ranging from little or no change over many years to rapid progression and complete flexion contracture of one or more digits.

The cause of this condition is unknown, but a hereditary predisposition appears to be present. Some patients also have associated plantar fasciitis, knuckle pads, and fibrosis in the shaft of the penis. The disorder is about five times more frequent in men, occurs predominately in Caucasians, and is more common in Europe. A gradual increase in incidence of the disease occurs with age. An association exists between Dupuytren's contracture and chronic alcoholism, epilepsy, and diabetes.

Treatment depends entirely on the severity of the findings. Heat, stretching, ultrasound, and intralesional injection of corticosteroids may be helpful in early stages. When actual contractures occur, surgical intervention may be desirable. Limited fasciectomy is effective in most instances, but more radical procedures, including digital amputation, may rarely be necessary. Palmar fasciotomy is a useful and more benign procedure, but if the disease remains active, recurrence is likely.

DISORDERS OF THE HIP REGION

Trochanteric Bursitis

Although common, trochanteric bursitis frequently goes undiagnosed. It occurs predominantly in middle-aged to elderly people, and somewhat more often in women than men. The main symptom is aching over the trochanteric area and lateral thigh. Walking, various movements, and lying on the involved hip may intensify the pain. Onset may be acute, but more often is gradual with symptoms lasting for months. In chronic cases the patient may fail to adequately locate or describe the pain, or the physician may fail to note the symptoms or interpret them correctly. Occasionally the pain may have a pseudoradiculopathy quality, radiating down the lateral aspect of the thigh. In a few cases the pain is so severe that the patient cannot walk and complains of a diffuse pain of the entire thigh.

The best way to diagnose trochanteric bursitis is to palpate over the trochanteric area and elicit point tenderness. In addition to specific pain on deep pressure over the trochanter, other tender points may be noted throughout the lateral aspect of the thigh muscle. Pain may be worse with external rotation and abduction against resistance. Although bursitis is generally considered to be the principal problem, the condition may actually arise at the insertions of the gluteus maximus and gluteus medius tendons. Local trauma and degeneration play a role in the patho-

genesis. In some cases calcification of the trochanteric bursa is seen. Conditions that may contribute to trochanteric bursitis, apparently by adding stress to the area, include OA of the lumbar spine or of the hip, leg-length discrepancy, and scoliosis. Treatment consists of local injection of depot corticosteroid using a 22-gauge, 3 1/2″ needle to ensure that the bursal area is reached (16). Nonsteroidal antiinflammatory drugs, weight loss, and strengthening and stretching of the gluteus medius muscle and iliotibial band help in overall management.

Iliopsoas (Iliopectineal) Bursitis

The iliopsoas bursa lies behind the iliopsoas muscle, anterior to the hip joint and lateral to the femoral vessels. It communicates with the hip in 15% of the cases. When the bursa is involved, groin and anterior thigh pain are present. This pain becomes worse on passive hip hyperextension and sometimes on flexion, especially with resistance. Tenderness is palpable over the involved bursa. The patient may hold the hip in flexion and external rotation to eliminate pain and may limp to prevent hyperextension. The diagnosis is more apparent if a cystic mass, which is present in about 30% of the cases, is seen; however, other causes of cystic swelling in the femoral area must first be excluded. A bursal mass may cause femoral venous obstruction or femoral nerve compression. As with most bursitis, acute or recurrent trauma and inflammatory conditions like RA may be a cause. The diagnosis is confirmed by plain roentgenogram and injection of a contrast medium into the bursa, or by computed tomography (CT) or MRI. Iliopsoas bursitis generally responds to conservative treatment including corticosteroid injections. With recurrent involvement, excision of the bursa may be necessary.

Ischial (Ischiogluteal) Bursitis

Ischial bursitis is caused by trauma or prolonged sitting on hard surfaces as evidenced by the name, *weaver's bottom*. Pain is often exquisite when sitting or lying down. Because the ischiogluteal bursa is located superficial to the ischial tuberosity and separates the gluteus maximus from the tuberosity, the pain may radiate down the back of the thigh. Point tenderness over the ischial tuberosity is present. Use of cushions and local injection of a corticosteroid are helpful.

Piriformis Syndrome

Piriformis syndrome is not well recognized and incompletely understood, even though it was first described in 1928 (17). The main symptom is pain over the buttocks, often radiating down the back of the leg as in sciatica. A limp may be noted on the involved side. Women are more often affected, and trauma plays a major role. Tenderness of the piriformis muscle on rectal or vaginal examination is of help in diagnosis. Pain is evident on internal rotation of hips against resistance. Pain and weakness have also been noted on resisted abduction and external rotation. A carefully done local injection of lidocaine and corticosteroid into the piriformis muscle may help.

Meralgia Paresthetica

The lateral femoral cutaneous nerve (L2–L3) innervates the anterolateral aspect of the thigh and is a sensory nerve. Compression of the nerve causes a characteristic intermittent burning pain associated with hypesthesia and sometimes numbness of the anterolateral thigh. Extension and abduction of the thigh or prolonged standing and walking may make symptoms worse, whereas sitting may relieve the pain. Touch and pin-prick sensation over the anterolateral thigh may be decreased. Pain may be elicited by pressing on the inguinal ligament just medial to the anterior superior iliac spine. This syndrome is seen more commonly in people who have diabetes, are pregnant, or are obese. Direct trauma, compression from a corset, or a leg-length discrepancy may also be factors. Nerve conduction velocity studies help confirm the diagnosis. Weight loss, heel correction, and time generally alleviate the problem. Because entrapment of the nerve often occurs just medial to the anterior superior iliac spine, a local injection of a corticosteroid at that site may help.

DISORDERS OF THE KNEE REGION

Popliteal Cysts

Popliteal cysts, also known as *Baker's cysts*, are not uncommon, and the clinician should be well aware of the possibility of dissection or rupture. A cystic swelling with mild or no discomfort may be the only initial finding. With further distention of the cyst, however, a greater awareness and discomfort is experienced, particularly on full flexion or extension. The cyst is best seen when the patient is standing and is examined from behind. Any knee disease having a synovial effusion can be complicated by a popliteal cyst. A naturally occurring communication may exist between the knee joint and the semimembranosus–gastrocnemius bursa, which is located beneath the medial head of the gastrocnemius muscle. A one-way valvelike mechanism between the joint and the bursa is activated by pressure from the knee effusion. An autopsy series has shown that about 40% of the population have a knee joint–bursa communication.

Popliteal cysts are most common secondary to RA, OA, or internal derangements of knees. There are a few reported cases secondary to gout and Reiter's syndrome. A syndrome mimicking thrombophlebitis may occur resulting from cyst dissection into the calf or actual rupture of the cyst. Findings include diffuse swelling of the calf, pain, and sometimes erythema and edema of the ankle. An arthrogram of the knee will confirm both the cyst and the possible dissection or rupture. Ultrasound is also useful in making a diagnosis and monitoring the course. History of a knee effusion is often a hint that a dissected Baker's cyst is the cause of the patient's swollen leg. If necessary, a venogram can also be done to exclude the possibility of concomitant thrombophlebitis. A cyst related to an inflammatory arthritis is treated by injecting a depot corticosteroid into the knee joint, and possibly into the cyst itself, which usually resolves the problem. If the cyst results from osteoarthritis or an internal derangement of the knee, surgical repair of the underlying joint lesion is usually necessary to prevent recurrence of the cyst.

Anserine Bursitis

Seen predominantly in overweight, middle-aged to elderly women with big legs and OA of the knees, anserine bursitis produces pain and tenderness over the medial aspect of the knee about 2″ below the joint margin. The pain is worse on stair climbing. The pes anserinus (Latin for "goose foot") is composed of the conjoined tendons of the sartorius, gracilis, and semitendinosus muscles. The bursa extends between the tendons and the tibial collateral ligament. The diagnosis is made by eliciting exquisite tenderness over the bursa and by relief with a local lidocaine injection. The treatment is rest, stretching of the adductor and quadriceps muscles, and a corticosteroid injection into the bursa.

Anserine bursitis is often overlooked since it frequently occurs concomitantly with OA of the knee, which when present is the assumed cause of pain; however, in some cases of dual involvement, anserine bursitis is the principal source of pain.

No Name, No Fame Bursitis

An unnamed bursa is located between the superficial and deep portions of the medial collateral ligament. When inflamed, pain and point tenderness over the area occur (18). Pain is noted particularly when the knee is flexed at 90°. A local corticosteroid injection into the bursa usually alleviates the symptoms.

Prepatellar Bursitis

Manifested as a swelling superficial to the kneecap, prepatellar bursitis results from trauma such as frequent kneeling, leading to the name *housemaid's knee*. The prepatellar bursa lies anterior to the lower half of the patella and upper half of the patellar ligament. The pain is generally slight unless pressure is applied directly over the bursa. The infrapatellar bursa, which lies between the patellar ligament and the tibia, is also subject to trauma and swelling. Chronic prepatellar bursitis can be treated by protecting the knee from the irritating trauma.

Septic prepatellar bursitis should also be considered when swelling is noted in this area. Generally, erythema, heat, and increased tenderness and pain are present. Often a history of trauma to the knee with puncture or abrasion of the skin overlying the bursa is obtained. The bursal fluid should be aspirated and cultured, and treatment with appropriate antibiotics should be instituted if infection is demonstrated.

Medial Plica Syndrome

A plica is a synovial fold in the knee joint, and infrapatellar, suprapatellar, and medial plicae have been identified. The medial plica can sometimes cause knee symptoms (19). Patella pain can be the predominant complaint, and snapping or clicking of the knee, a sense of instability, and possible pseudolocking of the knee may be seen. The plica can become symptomatic through any traumatic or inflammatory event in the knee. Diagnosis and treatment are made through arthroscopy, in which a thickened, inflamed, and occasionally fibrotic medial patella plica, leading to a bowstring process, is seen.

Popliteal Tendinitis

Pain in the posterolateral aspect of the knee may occur secondary to tendinitis of the popliteal tendons (hamstring and popliteus). With the knee flexed at 90°, tenderness on palpation may be found. Straight leg raising with or without palpation may cause pain. Running downhill increases the strain on the popliteus and can lead to tendinitis. Rest and conservative treatment are indicated, although occasionally a corticosteroid injection may be beneficial.

Pellegrini–Stieda Syndrome

Pellegrini–Stieda syndrome, which generally occurs in men, is thought to result from trauma and is followed by an asymptomatic period. Later, the symptomatic stage of medial knee pain and progressive restriction of knee movement coincides with the beginning of calcification of the medial collateral ligament, typically appearing as an elongated, amorphous shadow on roentgenogram (20). The pain is self-limited, and improvement usually occurs within several months.

Patellar Tendinitis

Patellar tendinitis, or *jumper's knee*, is seen predominantly in athletes engaging in activities such as repetitive running, jumping, or kicking. Pain and tenderness are present over the patellar tendon. Treatment consists of rest, NSAIDs, ice, knee bracing, and stretching and strengthening of the quadriceps and hamstring muscles. Corticosteroid injections have been reported to be contraindicated because of risk of rupture. In some chronic cases surgery is needed.

Rupture of Quadriceps Tendon and Infrapatellar Tendon

When the tendons around the patella rupture, the quadriceps tendon is involved about 50% of the time; otherwise, the infrapatellar tendon is involved. Quadriceps tendon rupture is generally caused by sudden violent contractions of the quadriceps muscle when the knee is flexed. A hemarthrosis of the knee joint may follow. Rupture of the infrapatellar tendon has been associated with a specific episode of trauma, repetitive trauma from sporting activities, and systemic diseases. Patients with chronic renal failure, RA, hyperparathyroidism, and gout, and systemic lupus erythematosus patients on steroids have been reported to have spontaneous ruptures of the quadriceps tendon. The patient experiences a sudden sharp pain and cannot extend the leg.

Roentgenograms may show a high riding patella. The tendon is generally found to be degenerated, and surgical repair is necessary.

Peroneal Nerve Palsy

In peroneal nerve palsy, a painless foot drop with a steppage gait is usually evident. Pain sensation may be slightly decreased along the lower lateral aspect of the leg and the dorsum of the foot. Direct trauma, fracture of the lower portion of the femur, compression of the nerve over the head of the fibula, and stretch injuries are all causes of this palsy. Generally, the common peroneal nerve is compressed, affecting the muscles innervated by the superficial peroneal nerve (which supplies the everters), and the deep peroneal nerve (which supplies the dorsiflexors of the foot and toes). An electromyogram is helpful in demonstrating slowing of nerve conduction velocities. Treatment consists of removing the source of compression and use of an ankle–foot orthosis if necessary. Occasionally, surgical exploration is needed.

Patellofemoral Pain Syndrome

This syndrome consists of pain and crepitus in the patellar region (21). Stiffness that occurs after prolonged sitting is alleviated by activity; overactivity involving knee flexion, particularly under loaded conditions such as stair climbing, aggravates the pain. On examination, pain occurs when the patella is compressed against the femoral condyle or when the patella is displaced laterally. Joint effusions are uncommon and usually small. The symptoms of patellofemoral pain syndrome are often bilateral and occur in a young age group. This syndrome may be caused by a variety of patellar problems such as patella alta, abnormal quadriceps angle, and trauma. The term *chondromalacia patellae* has been used for this syndrome, but patellofemoral pain syndrome is preferred by many. Treatment consists of analgesics, NSAIDs, ice, rest, and avoidance of knee overuse. Isometric strengthening exercises for the quadriceps muscles are of benefit. In some patients, however, surgical realignment may be tried.

DISORDERS OF THE ANKLE AND FOOT REGION

Achilles Tendinitis

Usually resulting from trauma, athletic overactivity, or improperly fitting shoes with a stiff heel counter, Achilles tendinitis can also be caused by inflammatory conditions such as ankylosing spondylitis, Reiter's syndrome, gout, RA, and calcium pyrophosphate deposition disease. Pain, swelling, and tenderness occur over the Achilles tendon at its attachment and in the area proximal to the attachment. Crepitus on motion and pain on dorsiflexion may be present. Management includes NSAIDs, rest, shoe corrections, heel lift, gentle stretching, and sometimes a splint with slight plantar flexion. The Achilles tendon is vulnerable to rupture, and the tendon itself must not be injected with a corticosteroid.

Retrocalcaneal Bursitis

The retrocalcaneus bursa is located between the posterior surface of the Achilles tendon and the calcaneus. The bursa's anterior wall is fibrocartilage where it attaches to the calcaneus, whereas its posterior wall blends with the epitenon of the Achilles tendon. Manifestations of bursitis include pain at the back of the heel, tenderness of the area anterior to the Achilles tendon, and pain on dorsiflexion. Local swelling is present, with bulging on the medial and lateral aspects of the tendon. Retrocalcaneal bursitis, also called sub-Achilles bursitis, may coexist with Achilles tendinitis, and distinguishing the two is sometimes difficult. This condition may be secondary to RA, spondylitis, Reiter's syndrome, gout, and trauma. Treatment consists of administra-

tion of NSAIDs, rest, and a local injection of a corticosteroid carefully directed into the bursa.

Subcutaneous Achilles Bursitis

A subcutaneous bursa superficial to the Achilles tendon may become swollen in the absence of systemic disease. This bursitis, known as *pump-bumps*, is seen predominantly in women and results from pressure of shoes, although it can also result from bony exostoses. Other than relief from shoe pressure, no treatment is indicated.

Calcaneal Bursitis and Plantar Fasciitis

The terms *calcaneal bursitis* and *plantar fasciitis* to some extent have been used interchangeably to describe the symptoms of pain on the plantar surface of the heel with weight bearing and tenderness on palpation. This overlapping of terms has led to some confusion, making it difficult to differentiate these conditions. Calcaneal bursitis seems to occur in older people who already have a calcaneal spur and then have some trauma resulting in bursitis. The trauma is usually from athletic activity, prolonged walking, improper shoes, or striking the heel with some force. Plantar fasciitis may be idiopathic; on the other hand, it also is more likely to be present in younger patients with spondylarthritis. Sometimes periosteal proliferation occurs at the calcaneus, resulting in a heel spur. In both conditions NSAIDs, use of heel cup orthoses, arch support, or local injection with a corticosteroid may help.

Achilles Tendon Rupture

Spontaneous rupture of the Achilles tendon is well known and occurs with a sudden onset of pain during forced dorsiflexion. An audible snap may be heard, followed by difficulty in walking and standing on toes. Swelling and edema over the area usually develop. Diagnosis can be made with the Thompson test, in which the patient kneels on the chair with the feet extending over the edge, and the examiner squeezes the calf and pushes toward the knee. Normally this produces plantar flexion, but in a ruptured tendon no plantar flexion occurs. Achilles tendon rupture is generally due to athletic events or trauma from jumps or falls. The tendon is more prone to tear in these having preexisting Achilles tendon disease or in those on corticosteroids. Orthopedic consultation should be obtained, and immobilization or surgery may be selected, depending on the situation.

Tarsal Tunnel Syndrome

In the tarsal tunnel syndrome the posterior tibial nerve is compressed at or near the flexor retinaculum. Just distally, the nerve divides into the medial plantar, lateral plantar, and posterior calcaneal branches. The flexor retinaculum is located posterior and inferior to the medial malleolus. Numbness, burning pain, and paresthesias of the toes and sole extend proximally to the area over the medial malleolus. Nocturnal exacerbation may be reported. The patient gets some relief by leg, foot, and ankle movements. A positive Tinel's sign may be elicited on percussion posterior to the medial malleolus, and loss of pin prick and two-point discrimination may be present. Women are more often affected than men. Trauma to the foot, especially fracture, valgus foot deformity, hypermobility, and occupational factors may relate to acquisition of tarsal tunnel syndrome. An electrodiagnostic test may show prolonged motor and sensory latencies and slowing of the nerve conduction velocities. In addition, a positive tourniquet test and pressure over the flexor retinaculum can induce symptoms. Shoe corrections and steroid injection into the tarsal tunnel may be of benefit, but often surgical decompression is needed.

Posterior Tibial Tendinitis

Pain and tenderness just posterior to the medial malleolus occur in posterior tibial tendinitis. This can be due to trauma,

RA, or spondylarthropathy. Extension and flexion may be normal, but pain is present on resisted inversion or passive eversion. The discomfort is usually worse after athletic events, and swelling and localized tenderness may be present. Treatment usually includes rest, NSAIDs, and possibly a local injection of a corticosteroid. Immobilization with a splint is sometimes needed.

Peroneal Tendon Dislocation and Peroneal Tendinitis

Dislocation of the peroneal tendon may occur from a direct blow, repetitive trauma, or sudden dorsiflexion with eversion. Sometimes a painless snapping noise is heard at the time of dislocation. Other patients report more severe pain and tenderness of the tendon area that lies over the lateral malleolus. The condition may be confused with an acute ankle sprain. Conservative treatment with immobilization is often satisfactory since the peroneal tendon usually reduces spontaneously. If the retinaculum supporting the tendon is ruptured, however, surgical correction may be needed. Peroneal tendinitis can also occur and be manifested as localized tenderness over the lateral malleolus. Conservative treatment is usually indicated.

Hallux Valgus

In hallux valgus, deviation of the large toe lateral to the midline and deviation of the first metatarsal medially occurs. A bunion (adventitious bursa) of the head of the first metatarsophalangeal (MTP) joint may be present, often causing pain, tenderness, and swelling. Hallux valgus is more common in women. It may be caused by a genetic tendency and wearing pointed shoes, or it can be secondary to RA or generalized OA. Stretching of shoes, use of bunion pads, or surgery may be indicated. Metatarsus primus varus, a condition in which the first metatarsal is angulated medially, is seen in association with or secondary to the hallux valgus deformity.

Bunionette

A bunionette, or *tailor's bunion*, is a prominence of the fifth metatarsal head resulting from the overlying bursa and a localized callus. The fifth metatarsal has a lateral (valgus) deviation.

Hammer Toe

In hammer toe, the PIP joint is flexed and the tip of the toe points downward. The second toe is most commonly involved. Calluses may form at the tip of the toe and over the dorsum of the IP joint, resulting from pressure against the shoe. Hammer toe may be congenital or acquired secondary to hallux valgus and may result from improper footwear. When the MTP joint is hyperextended, the deformity is known as *cocked-up toes*. This may be seen in RA.

Morton's Neuroma

Middle-aged women are most frequently affected by Morton's neuroma, an entrapment neuropathy of the interdigital nerve occurring most often between the third and fourth toes. Paresthesia and a burning, aching type of pain is experienced in the fourth toe. The symptoms are made worse by walking on hard surfaces or wearing tight shoes or high heels. Tenderness may be elicited by palpation between the third and fourth metatarsal heads. Occasionally, a neuroma is seen between the second and third toes. Compression of the interdigital nerve by the transverse metatarsal ligament and possibly by an intermetatarsophalangeal bursa or synovial cyst may be responsible for the entrapment. Treatment usually includes a metatarsal bar or a local steroid injection into the web space. Ultimately, surgical excision of the neuroma and a portion of the nerve may be needed.

Metatarsalgia

Pain arising from the metatarsal heads, known as metatarsalgia, is a symptom resulting from a variety of conditions. Pain on

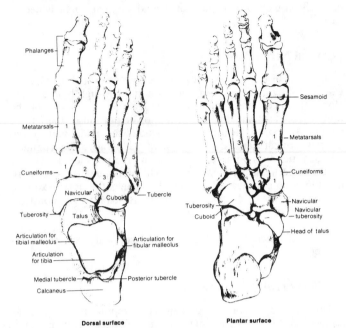

Fig. 50–3. Bones of the feet (illustration provided by Dr JJ Calabro).

standing and tenderness on palpation of the metatarsal heads are present. Calluses over the metatarsal heads are usually seen. The causes of metatarsalgia are many, including foot strain, use of high heels, everted foot, trauma, sesamoiditis, hallux valgus, arthritis, foot surgery, or a foot with a high longitudinal arch. Flattening of the transverse arch and weakness of the intrinsic muscles occur, resulting in a maldistribution of weight on the forefoot. Treatment is directed at elevating the middle portion of the transverse arch with an orthotic device, strengthening of the intrinsic muscles, weight reduction, and use of metatarsal pads or metatarsal bar.

Pes Planus

Pes planus, or "flat foot," is often asymptomatic, but may cause fatigue of the foot muscles and aching with intolerance to prolonged walking or standing. There is loss of the longitudinal arch on the medial side and prominence of the navicular and head of the talus (Fig. 50–3). The calcaneus is everted (valgus), and out-toeing can be seen on ambulation. The tendency for this condition is largely inherited and is seen with generalized hypermobility. A Thomas heel, firm shoes, and grasping exercises to strengthen the intrinsic muscles are helpful. A shoe orthosis may be needed for more severe cases. The asymptomatic flat foot is left untreated.

Pes Cavus

In contradistinction to pes planus, pes cavus, or *claw foot*, is characterized by an unusually high medial arch, and in severe cases, a high longitudinal arch, resulting in shortening of the foot. These abnormally high arches further result in shortening of the extensor ligaments, causing dorsiflexion of the PIP joints and plantar flexion of the DIP joints, thus giving a claw-like appearance to the toes. The plantar fascia may also be contracted. Generally, a tendency to pes cavus is inherited, and in a high percentage of cases an underlying neurologic disorder is present. Although pes cavus can cause foot fatigue, pain, and tenderness over the metatarsal heads with callus formation, it may also be asymptomatic. Calluses generally develop over the dorsum of the toes. Use of metatarsal pads or a bar is helpful, and stretching of the toe extensors is usually prescribed. In severe cases surgical correction may be needed.

Posterior Tibialis Tendon Rupture

The rupture of the posterior tibialis tendon, which is not commonly recognized, is a cause of progressive flat foot (22). It may be caused by trauma, chronic tendon degeneration, or RA. An insidious onset of pain and tenderness may be noted along the course of the tendon just distal to the medial malleolus, along with swelling medial to the hindfoot. The unilateral deformity of hindfoot valgus and forefoot abduction is an important finding. The forefoot abduction can best be seen from behind; more toes are seen from this position than would be seen normally. The result of the single heel rise test is positive when the patient is unable to rise onto the ball of the affected foot while the contralateral foot is off the floor. Orthopedic consultation should be obtained to determine whether the rupture should be treated conservatively with NSAIDs and casting or with a surgical repair.

DISORDERS OF THE ANTERIOR CHEST WALL

Chest wall pain of a musculoskeletal origin is fairly common. It must be differentiated from chest pain of a cardiac nature, which is the usual main concern, or from pulmonary or gastrointestinal disease. Pain can also radiate to the chest as a result of cervical or thoracic spine disease. The musculoskeletal syndromes usually associated with chest wall pain are Tietze's syndrome and costochondritis. Both conditions are characterized by tenderness of one or more costal cartilages, and the terms have sometimes been used interchangeably. The two disorders, however, are generally separated by the presence of local swelling in Tietze's syndrome but not in costochondritis (23).

Tietze's syndrome is much less common than costochondritis and is of unknown etiology. Its onset may be gradual or abrupt with swelling usually occurring in the second or third costal cartilage. Pain, which ranges from mild to severe, may radiate to the shoulder and be aggravated by coughing, sneezing, inspiration, or by various movements affecting the chest wall. Tenderness is elicited on palpation, and approximately 80% of patients have a single site.

Costochondritis is much more common and is associated with pain and tenderness of the chest wall, without swelling. Tenderness is often present over more than one costochondral junction, and palpation should duplicate the described pain. In one study of 100 patients with non-cardiac chest pain, 69% were found to have local tenderness on palpation and in 16% the palpation elicited the typical pain (24). Other names attached to costochondritis include anterior wall syndrome, costosternal syndrome, parasternal chondrodynia, and chest wall syndrome. Some individuals with chest wall pain are found to have fibromyalgia or localized myofascial pain. Chest wall pain can also complicate heart or lung disease, so its presence does not exclude more serious problems.

Xiphoid cartilage syndrome or xiphoidalgia, also known as *hypersensitive xiphoid* or *xiphodynia*, is characterized by pain over the xiphoid area and tenderness on palpation. Pain may be intermittent and brought on by overeating and by various twisting movements.

These three conditions are often self-limiting. Treatment consists of reassurance, heat, stretching of chest wall muscles, or local injections of lidocaine, corticosteroid, or both.

In addition, a number of other disorders may produce chest wall pain. Sternocostoclavicular hyperostosis is manifested by a painful swelling of the clavicles, sternum, or ribs and may be relapsing. It is associated with an elevated sedimentation rate, pustules on the palms and soles, and progression to ossification of the chest wall lesions. Condensing osteitis of clavicles is a rare, benign condition of unknown etiology, occurring primarily in women of child-bearing age. It is characterized by sclerosis of the medial ends of the clavicles without involvement of the sternoclavicular joints. Pain and local tenderness are present.

Any condition involving the sternoclavicular joint, including spondylarthropathy, OA, and infection, can cause chest wall pain. Stress fracture of the ribs, cough fracture, herpes zoster of the thorax, and intercostobrachial nerve entrapment are other causes of chest pain.

Thorough palpation of the chest wall must be done including the sternoclavicular joint, costochondral junctions, sternum, and chest wall muscles. Maneuvers such as crossed-chest adduction of the arm and backward extension of the arm from 90° of abduction help in elucidating whether chest pain is of a musculoskeletal origin. Imaging studies may include plain roentgenogram of the ribs, special roentgenogram of the sternoclavicular joint, tomogram, and bone scan. A CT scan or MRI provide the most detail of the sternoclavicular joint.

Joseph J. Biundo, Jr., MD

1. Shoen RP, Moskowitz RW, Goldberg VM: Soft Tissue Rheumatic Pain: Recognition, Management, Prevention. Philadelphia, Penn. Lea & Febiger, 1988
2. Petri M, Dobrow R, Neiman R, et al: Randomized double-blind placebo controlled study of the treatment of the painful shoulder. Arthritis Rheum 30:1040–1045, 1987
3. Kisner C, Colby LA: Therapeutic Exercise: Foundations and Techniques, 2nd ed., Philadelphia FA Davis, 1990
4. Biundo JJ, Hughes GM: Rheumatoid arthritis rehabilitation: practical guidelines, Part I. J Musculoskeletal Med 8(8):85–96, 1991
5. Neer CR: Impingement lesions. Clin Orthoped 173:70–77, 1983
6. Post M, Silver R, Singh M: Rotator cuff tear: diagnosis and treatment. Clin Orthop Rel Res 173:78–91, 1983
7. Crass JR, Craig EV, Thompson RC, et al: Ultrasonography of the rotator cuff: surgical correlation. J Clin Ultrasound 12:487–492, 1984
8. Neviaser RJ: Lesions of the biceps and tendinitis of the shoulder. Orthop Clin N Am 11:343–348, 1980
9. Steinbrocker O, Arojyros TG: Frozen shoulder: treatment by local injections of depot corticosteroids. Arch Phys Med Rehab 55:209–213, 1974
10. Weinstein PS, Canoso JJ, Wohlgethan JR: Long-term follow up of corticosteroid injection for traumatic olecranon bursitis. Ann Rheum Dis 43:44–46, 1984
11. Cyriax J: Diagnosis of soft tissue lesions, Textbook of Orthopaedic Medicine, Vol. 1. London, Bailliere Tindall, 1982, pp 173
12. Stern PJ: Tendinitis, overuse syndromes, and tendon injuries. Hand Clinics 6(3):467–475, 1990
13. Wu JS, Morris JD, Hogan GR: Ulnar neuropathy at the wrist: Case report and review of the literature. Arch Phys Med Rehabil 66:785–788, 1985
14. Anderson B, Kaye, S: Treatment of flexor tenosynovitis of the hand ("Trigger finger") with corticosteroids. Arch Intern Med 151:153–156, 1991
15. Williams CS, Riordan DC: Mycobacterium mariunum infections of the hand. J Bone Joint Surg 55A:1042–1050, 1973
16. Ege Rasmussen KJ, Farro N: Trochanteric bursitis, treatment by corticosteroid injection. Scand J Rheumatol 14:417–420, 1985
17. Wyant GM: Chronic pain syndromes and their treatment. III. The piriformis syndrome. Can Anaesth Soc J 26:305–308, 1979
18. Stuttle FL: The no-name and no-fame bursa. Clin Orthoped 15:197–199, 1959
19. Galloway MT, Jokl P: Patella plica syndrome. Ann Sports Med 5:38–41, 1990
20. O'Donoghue DH: Treatment of Injuries to Athletes, 4th ed. Philadelphia, WB Saunders, 1984, pp 509–510
21. Cox JS: Chondromalacia of the patella: a review of update - Part 1. Comtemp Orthop 6:17–31, 1983
22. Rosenberg ZS, Cheung Y, Jahss MH, et al: Rupture of posterior tibial tendon: CT and MR imaging with surgical correlation. Radiology, 169:229–235, 1988
23. Calabro JJ: Costochondritis. N Engl J Med 296:946–947, 1977
24. Wise CM, Semble L, Dalton CB: Musculoskeletal chest wall syndromes in patients with noncardiac chest pain: a study of 100 patients. Arch Phys Med Rehabil 72:147–149, 1992

51. REFLEX SYMPATHETIC DYSTROPHY SYNDROME AND TRANSIENT REGIONAL OSTEOPOROSIS

REFLEX SYMPATHETIC DYSTROPHY SYNDROME

The reflex sympathetic dystrophy syndrome (RSDS) is characterized by severe, unrelenting pain affecting a distal extremity. Typically, the whole hand or foot is affected. Occasionally more proximal areas, such as the knee, patella, or one or more digits may be involved. Pain is often characterized as burning, and patients find that wrapping the affected part with moist applications provides relief.

Clinical Features

A distinctive complex of signs and symptoms may accompany the pain syndrome and is characterized by some or all of the following features: tenderness, swelling, vasomotor and sudomotor changes, and dystrophic skin changes. Patients may report exquisite sensitivity to touch such as with clothing or bedclothes (*allodynia*) or severe pain with repetitive touch or gentle pressure (*hyperpathia*). These patients often will appear to overreact, since they may refuse the physician an opportunity to examine the affected part. The features of RSDS are described in Table 51–1 (1).

Men and women are equally affected. There is no predilection for the dominant side. Reflex sympathetic dystrophy syndrome is thought to occur more frequently in older adults, but a number of recent reports have emphasized occurrence of the disease in children. Trauma is the most common precipitating event. This may be as minor as hitting the hand against the edge of a table or as major as a crush injury or fracture. The likelihood of developing RSDS is not related to the severity of the injury or the intensity of associated pain. Hemiplegia, myocardial ischemia, peripheral nerve injury, or exposure to certain drugs such as barbiturates or anti-tuberculosis drugs also have been associated with RSDS.

Steinbrocker and Argyros divided the syndrome into three stages (2). The first, or acute, stage is characterized by burning pain, tenderness, swelling, and vasomotor and sudomotor changes that may persist for three to six months. The second, or dystrophic, stage, which may persist an additional three to six months, is characterized by persistent aching or burning pain, swelling with induration, and dystrophic skin and nail changes. The final, or atrophic stage, evolves gradually and is characterized by skin and subcutaneous atrophy and the development of

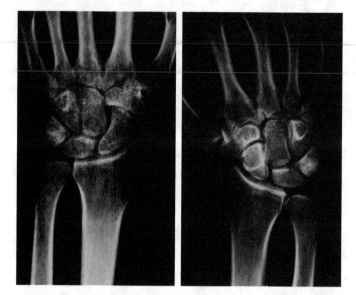

Fig. 51–1. *Radiographs of the hands of a 42-year-old woman with RSDS of the left hand. The affected hand (A) demonstrates patchy osteopenia. The normal opposite hand (B) is shown for comparison. These changes developed within two months of onset of symptoms.*

contractures resembling Dupuytren's contractures in the hand or foot. Pain persists and tends to ascend the extremity to the shoulder and shoulder girdle or to the buttock and back. The hand may become a claw-like, useless structure.

Radiologic changes are present in up to 85% of patients. The plain radiograph may reveal a diffuse, patchy osteopenia (Fig. 51–1) initially; later the osteopenia has a ground-glass appearance. Patchy osteopenia is not pathognomonic of RSDS as it may occur with disuse or immobilization, but its presence should always raise the question of RSDS. The three phase bone scan is more helpful and specific for RSDS (Fig. 51–2). The first (radionuclide blood flow) and second (blood pool) phases typically show asymmetric blood flow and pooling. Increased flow and pooling are present in approximately 50% of patients, and diminished flow and uptake are seen in 15% to 20% of patients with RSDS. Approximately 85% of patients have an abnormal third (bone scan) phase in which increased uptake in periarticular structures is present (3,4).

Pathogenesis

The pathogenesis of RSDS is poorly understood. Several hypotheses have been proposed, although none completely explains the syndrome. They may be arbitrarily divided into those favoring dysfunction in the peripheral nervous system or in the central nervous system (5). Disruption of peripheral nerve pathways as a result of trauma may promote formation of synapses between efferent and afferent nerves. These are termed *ephapses* and can be demonstrated in experimental models of peripheral nerve injury. They may cause an RSDS-like syndrome by short-circuiting normal control mechanisms. Alternatively, sensitization of peripheral mechano- (and possibly pain-) receptors has been implicated as a cause of RSDS and has special appeal since it may explain the presence of allodynia and hyperpathia. A role for the central nervous system in the development of RSDS has been favored by other investigators. Early theories focused primarily on regulatory centers in subcortical gray matter. More recently, Roberts has argued persuasively that sensitization of

Table 51–1. *Major clinical features of RSDS*

Symptom	Description
Severe pain	Usually burning in character, but may be described as aching, boring, or throbbing among others
Tenderness	Affected extremity usually demonstrates diffuse tenderness, which is more prominent in periarticular structures but also present in interarticular tissues
Allodynia	Touch sensitivity. Light touch, such as clothes or bedclothes at night, may evoke pain response, and patients may pull away from examiner
Hyperpathia	Severe pain with repetitive mild or moderate stimuli
Dystrophic skin	Shiny skin with loss of normal wrinkling. Often fine scaling is present, and the skin has a doughy consistency
Swelling	May be pitting or non-pitting
Vasomotor changes	Changes in temperature (usually cool or cold, but may be warm) and color (usually dusky purple)
Sudomotor changes	Changes in sweat and hair apparatus, usually consisting of hyperhidrosis and hypertrichosis

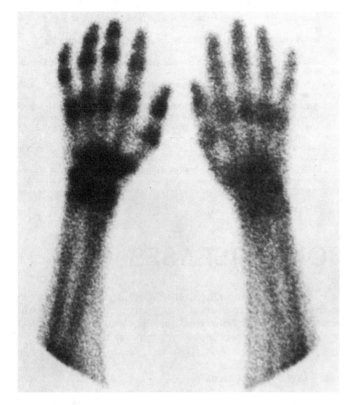

Fig. 51–2. Bone scan (phase 3) in a patient with RSDS demonstrating enhanced radionuclide uptake in periarticular tissues in the affected left hand.

wide dynamic neurons in the spinal cord best explains the findings in RSDS (6). These issues are more fully discussed elsewhere (7).

Reflex sympathetic dystrophy syndrome was first recognized as a distinct clinical entity by Silas Weir Mitchell and his colleagues during the American Civil War when they established the first field hospital to care for injured soldiers. In 1872 Mitchell used the term *causalgia* to describe the characteristic burning pain often present. Since then, a family of interrelated conditions has been described, including major and minor causalgia, Sudeck's atrophy, shoulder–hand syndrome, and algodystrophy among many others (1).

Diagnosis

The clinician should suspect RSDS when persistent or disproportionately severe pain occurs following trauma surgery or certain painful medical problems (Table 51–2). Laboratory studies are normal or negative unless related to an underlying or associated condition. Radiographic or scintigraphic findings often will help confirm the diagnosis. Thermographic abnormalities also may be a useful diagnostic adjunct when performed by experienced thermographers and interpreted cautiously. The presence

Table 51–2. *Conditions associated with RSDS*

Trauma, major or minor
Peripheral nerve injury, including entrapment
Cervical or lumbar radiculopathy
Cervical spondylosis
Cerebrovascular accident
Hemiplegia
Neoplasm
Drugs (barbiturates, anti-tuberculous)
Arthroscopy of the knee
Venous thrombophlebitis
Arterial thrombosis

of allodynia or hyperpathia is considered to be diagnostic of the condition.

Treatment

Treatment of RSDS must be initiated as early as possible. The likelihood of a good or excellent outcome worsens rapidly following any delay. Analgesic or nonsteroidal antiinflammatory drugs and physiotherapy should be started immediately. More aggressive therapy is warranted unless substantial improvement occurs within two weeks. Systemic corticosteroids or sympathetic blocks may be given at this time. Unfortunately, there are no specific guidelines available to assist in choosing between these alternatives.

Systemic steroids are useful in a number of patients with RSDS (8). Generally, these are given over a four week period; for example, starting with 15 mg/4 times daily for four to five days, then gradually tapering the dose. Treatment should not be extended beyond this time as there is no evidence of improved outcome, and the risk of adverse reaction increases. Symptomatic benefit is often delayed until the third or fourth week of treatment, and there may be a mild, transient increase in symptoms on completion of the regimen. Local intravenous administration of corticosteroids using a Bier Block technique may also be of benefit (9).

Sympathetic blockade is an important diagnostic and therapeutic technique in RSDS. Most, but not all, patients with RSDS will experience pain relief transiently following a sympathetic block. Response to such blocks is not diagnostic of RSDS, nor should the physician exclude this diagnosis in patients who do not respond. A series of three to five sympathetic blocks may be required to see a response, and the duration of pain relief may increase with each successive block. A small percentage of patients will have permanent pain relief from sympathetic blocks; others may require surgical sympathectomy for permanent relief. While response to blocks is essential before patients are subjected to surgery, the success of the surgery is variable and unpredictable.

Sympathetic blocks are usually performed by administering 10 to 30 ml of local anesthetic (lidocaine or bupivocaine) in the area of the stellate ganglion for upper extremity RSDS and in the lumbar sympathetic ganglia for lower extremity disease. It is critical to ascertain that the block is technically successful by demonstrating a temperature increase, erythema, vasodilation, and in the upper extremity, a Horner's syndrome. Sympathetic blocks also may be done by epidural administration of anesthetic or by regional intravenous infusion of guanethidine, bretylium, or reserpine. The latter requires use of a Bier block technique in which the affected arm or leg is exsanguinated by elevation or use of compressive bandages and a tourniquet placed on the part proximal to the affected area to prevent venous outflow. Guanethidine or a similar agent is infused into the affected extremity and allowed to bind to sympathetic receptors for 10–20 mins before the tourniquet is released.

Many other treatments have been advocated for RSDS. The effectiveness of measures such as transcutaneous nerve stimulation, acupuncture, calcium channel blockers, alpha- or beta-adrenergic blocking agents, griseofulvin, and hypnosis have not been documented to be effective, however. In Europe calcitonin has been widely used, and several reports have demonstrated excellent outcome (5). Other therapies have not been widely studied.

TRANSIENT REGIONAL OSTEOPOROSIS

The syndrome(s) of transient regional osteoporosis or partial transient osteoporosis bears a striking similarity to RSDS and may be one of the RSDS variants or an incomplete form of RSDS. The lower extremity is most commonly affected (95%), and the hip joint is at greatest risk (10). Pain is the presenting problem, but there are usually no or few abnormal physical findings. Laboratory studies, including the erythrocyte sedimentation rate, are usually normal or negative. Osteopenia is present in virtually all cases, and there is increased radionuclide uptake on bone scan. There is no clear response to systemic steroids or sympathetic blockade. Usually the disorder resolves spontaneously within 12 months, but it may persist for several years.

Franklin Kozin, MD

1. Kozin F, McCarty DJ, Sims J, et al: The reflex sympathetic dystrophy syndrome. I. Clinical and histological studies. Amer J Med 60:321–330, 1976
2. Steinbrocker O, Argyros TG: The shoulder-hand syndrome: present status as a diagnostic and therapeutic entity. Medical Clin North Amer 42:1533–1553, 1958
3. Kozin F, Genant HK, Bekerman C, et al: The reflex sympathetic dystrophy syndrome. II. Roentgenographic and scintigraphic evidence of bilaterality and of periarticular involvement. Amer J Med 60:332–338, 1976
4. Macinnon SE, Holder LE: The use of three-phase radionuclide bone scanning in the diagnosis of reflex sympathetic dystrophy syndrome. J Hand Surg 9A:556–563, 1984
5. Kozin F: Reflex sympathetic dystrophy syndrome. Bulletin Rheum Dis 36:1–7, 1986
6. Roberts J: A hypothesis on the physiological basis for causalgia and related pains. Pain 24:297–311, 1986
7. Payne R: Neuropathic pain syndromes, with special reference to causalgia and reflex sympathetic dystrophy. Clin J Pain 2:59–73, 1986
8. Kozin F, Ryan LM, Carrera GF, et al: The reflex sympathetic dystrophy syndrome. III. Scintigraphic studies and further evidence for the therapeutic efficacy of systemic corticosteroids and proposed diagnostic criteria. Amer J Med 70:23–30, 1981
9. Poplawski ZJ, Wiley AM, Murray JF: Posttraumatic dystrophy of the extremities. J Bone Joint Surg 65A:642–655, 1983
10. Lakhanpal S, Ginsberg WW, Luthra HS, Hunder GG: Transient regional osteoporosis: a study of 56 cases and review of the literature. Ann Intern Med 106:444–450, 1987

52. METABOLIC BONE DISEASES

Metabolic bone diseases are manifested by bone pain or fractures that are the result of generalized abnormalities of the bone tissue, which in turn are caused by disturbances of serum minerals, calcium-regulating hormones, bone growth factors, cytokines, or agents that interfere with mineralization or resorption. When bone resorption and formation are both markedly increased, as in hyperparathyroidism or Paget's disease, the rapidly formed new bone is structurally abnormal. In osteomalacia, mineralization is abnormal and unmineralized osteoid accumulates, leading to bone pain and fractures. In some bone diseases, there is an imbalance between resorption and formation, which can lead to rapid loss; for example, with corticosteroids bone resorption is increased but formation is decreased. The most common metabolic bone disease is osteoporosis, which usually results from a small, life-long imbalance between resorption and formation. On the other hand, several rare diseases cause increased bone density, either because osteoclasts do not function (osteopetrosis) or because formation exceeds resorption (osteosclerosis).

DIAGNOSTIC TESTS

Standard serum levels of calcium, phosphate, magnesium, acid-base status, renal function, and liver function are necessary to help characterize bone disease. A 24-hour urine collection for calcium excretion is often helpful in evaluating calcium balance, and very low levels suggest intestinal malabsorption. Alkaline phosphatase is produced by osteoclasts and increases when bone formation is increased. Since this enzyme is produced in several tissues, the bone-specific assays are most useful in evaluating bone disease. Osteocalcin (bone gla protein) is secreted only by osteoblasts; serum assays for this recently-discovered protein correlate with increased osteoid formation (1). Urine hydroxyproline has been widely used to assess bone resorption, but it is not sensitive, not specific, and can be increased by protein in the diet. Newer assays for collagen cross-links (urine pyridinoline and urine N-telopeptide) are both sensitive and specific for bone resorption (2).

A serum 25-hydroxy-vitamin D level should be used to detect vitamin D deficiency, which may occur with levels in the low-normal range. Measurement of 1,25-dihydroxyvitamin D is expensive and should be used in patients with renal dysfunction or suspected vitamin D abnormalities (Table 52-2). In the past, there were several methods of measuring parathyroid hormone (PTH), but the double-site immunometric assay that measures the intact hormone is more sensitive and specific, even in renal failure, than all the previous methods. In cases of hypercalcemia of malignancy, the intact PTH is usually decreased (3).

Standard radiographs can evaluate severity of vertebral compression fractures. They also can be diagnostic of Paget's disease, and occasionally can show pseudofractures of osteomalacia or the subperiosteal bone resorption of hyperparathyroidism. The trabecular patterns of the hip can help assess bone loss, but the bone density is more accurate. "Demineralization" may be the result of over-exposure of roentgenograms in patients with normal bone. On the other hand, patients who have lost 30% of bone mineral may have normal roentgenograms.

Bone Mass Measurements

The only reliable way to ascertain the bone mineral density is to measure it directly. Large errors are found if bone density is estimated from the clinical history (4). Bone densitometry is indicated in patients who have fractures with minimal trauma or in persons who have risk factors for developing osteoporosis. The short-term precision represents the average error when a person is measured twice; this is important when following the course of an individual patient. The bone density must change by 2.8 times the precision to be significant. For example, with dual energy x-ray absorptiometry of the hip (precision 2%) the measured densities will change by up to 5.6% just by walking around the room and repeating the measurement. Long-term precision errors can also be seen when the hardware is altered. Because bone loss is slow compared with the precision of the densitometers, it usually takes several years to determine the rate of change of an individual patient.

Single photon absorptiometry has been used for two decades, but it is limited to the radius or heel and has precision of about 2%. Quantitated computed tomography measures the volumetric density of trabecular bone in the vertebral bodies, but the precision is about 5%. Dual energy x-ray absorptiometry can be used at the spine, hip, radius, or total body (precision 1%, 2%, 2%, and 1%, respectively). This noninvasive technique has a very low radiation exposure and takes only about 10 minutes per measurement. Currently, the spine measurement is the most precise method of assessing trabecular bone. In patients with osteoarthritis or scoliosis, however, the spine measurement may be falsely elevated.

The different bone mass measurements all yield similar results when comparing normal women with those who have osteoporosis (5). The relative risk for future fractures is about two for each standard deviation decrease in bone mass compared with age-matched persons (6,7) (Fig. 52–1). No technique has been shown to be superior at predicting fractures in general, although the hip measurement is slightly better at predicting hip fractures in elderly individuals (8).

OSTEOPOROSIS

Osteoporosis is by far the most common metabolic bone disease. It is characterized by decreased bone mineral density (osteopenia) and ultimately fractures. Fractures that are commonly associated with osteopenia include vertebral compression, Colles', and hip (9).

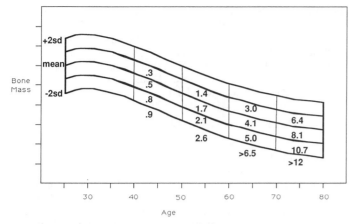

Fig. 52–1. Risk of non-spine fracture, %/yr

Epidemiology

The prevalence of vertebral compression fractures is about 20% in postmenopausal Caucasian women. The incidence of hip fractures increases exponentially after age 50 in women and after age 60 in men. One-third of all Caucasian women over the age of 80 will have a hip fracture; a woman's lifetime risk of hip fracture is 15%. With the trend toward aging in our society, as well as a slight secular trend toward increased fracture rate, the number of patients with hip fractures is steadily increasing. Caucasians and Asians have a higher prevalence than blacks.

Whether a bone will fracture depends on the nature of the trauma sustained as well as the strength of the bone, which in turn depends on the quantity and quality of bone (Fig. 52–2). In elderly persons, hip fractures usually occur after a fall. Sedative or diuretic drugs, alcohol use, slippery rugs, high-heeled shoes, and unprotected bathrooms can all lead to falls. The propensity to fall is an important factor that deserves more emphasis; some of these factors are more reversible than bone mass. The gait speed may play a role, because the forward momentum in the normal gait will aid in recovering from a fall, whereas with a slow gait a woman might drop right on her hip. Padding of the bone may also reduce the impact, so that extra fat may add some protection (10).

Risk Factors and Differential Diagnosis

Table 52–1 lists the common risk factors for osteoporosis. In normal persons, age is the most important factor in predicting bone density, and it is associated independently with fracture risk (6). In women from age 40 to 80, every decade doubles the risk of getting an osteoporotic fracture. Bone density increases until about age 30, then it starts its universal and inexorable decline. Women also experience a rapid loss of bone for approximately six years after menopause. From age 30 to 80 the total body calcium decreases from 840 g to 680 g (a 20% decrease), and the trabecular bone of the spine shows a 60% decrease. Hereditary factors account for 80% of an individual's peak bone mass, and they probably influence the rate of loss as well. It is not known why black people have higher bone density, but they have both a higher bone mass and a decreased bone turnover when they are older; these changes may relate to increased body fat. Black girls gain more bone during puberty. Women have lower bone density than men, and they also lose bone rapidly at menopause.

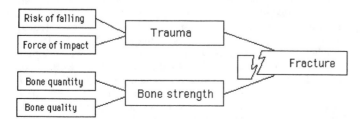

Fig. 52–2. Risk factors for osteoporotic fractures

Table 52–1. Risk factors for osteoporosis

Age
Heredity
Sex
Hormonal factors
    (decreased estrogen, testosterone)
Associated diseases
    (renal, hepatic, myeloma, hypercalciuria)
Drugs (steroids, thyroid, heparin)
Nutritional factors
Weight (fat protective)
Activity
Cigarette smoking
Alcohol

Hormonal factors are very important. Estrogen or testosterone deficiency is the most common contributing cause to post-menopausal osteoporosis. Even irregular menstrual cycles are associated with decreased bone density (11). Other causes include renal or hepatic failure, multiple myeloma, hypercalciuria, inflammatory arthritis, hyperthyroidism, intestinal malabsorption, mastocytosis, and Cushing's disease. Some of these may also cause osteomalacia, which can clinically mimic osteoporosis. Inherited diseases of collagen production usually present as osteogenesis imperfecta, but mild cases are clinically indistinguishable from osteoporosis. Hyperparathyroidism causes osteitis fibrosis, which may also present with low bone density and fractures.

Drugs associated with bone loss include corticosteroids, thyroid hormone (in doses that suppress thyroid-stimulating hormone), heparin, gonadotropin-releasing hormone agonists, and possibly furosemide. Thiazide diuretics appear to protect bone mass (12). The importance of nutritional factors is still controversial. Calcium deficiency contributes to low bone density, especially if there is a lifetime habit of poor calcium intake. Although heavy caffeine use or protein intake can cause statistically significant increases in urine calcium, they probably do not cause major bone loss. Weight is a positive risk factor, which may be related to higher estrogen levels in women with more body fat. Although bone loss with complete immobilization is rapid and severe, ordinary inactivity is only a modest risk factor. Smoking and heavy alcohol use cause bone loss.

Bone Quality

The quality of the bone helps determine whether it will fracture. The micro-architecture of normal bone consists of connected plates. In osteoporotic bones, these turn to disconnected plates and rods, and the bone loses its structural integrity. Women with equal bone density but a more intact trabecular architecture are less prone to fracture. Other aspects of bone quality are not well understood but include ability to repair microfractures, strength of the crystalline structure, and integrity of the underlying collagen matrix.

Prevention and Treatment

Many cases of osteoporosis could be prevented by giving women estrogen replacement at the time of menopause. This may reduce the incidence of hip fractures by 50% (13). The dose required to prevent bone loss is 0.625 mg/day of conjugated estrogens; the route of administration does not seem to matter (14). There is no convincing evidence that progesterone has any additive effect to estrogen. Upon discontinuing estrogen therapy, bone is lost rapidly, so that long-term replacement is necessary. The decision to take estrogen must depend on the individual patient, because the skeletal system is only one aspect of health in a postmenopausal woman. Estrogens are associated with risks, such as increased uterine cancer and gallstones, but these do not cause major increases in mortality. There may be a slight increase in the risk of breast cancer after long-term estrogen therapy. Estrogens probably decrease the incidence of cardiovascular disease, which is the most common cause of mortality. Currently, large scale studies are in progress to define these risks and benefits.

Treatment of osteoporosis is difficult and there are many areas of uncertainty (15). Although no treatment programs have been definitely shown to be effective at reducing fractures, a modest inhibition of bone resorption will likely be beneficial to most patients. Many studies are in progress to establish the optimal treatment programs. The agents that block bone resorption (estrogen, calcitonin, bisphosphonates) also eventually decrease bone formation. The bone density improves most rapidly in the first 6 to 12 months and then reaches a plateau. The overall increase in bone density is limited by the initial bone formation rate, and gains above 5% to 10% are rarely seen. None of the studies have been large enough to determine the effect of this modest increase on the fracture incidence. Agents that increase bone formation (fluoride, PTH) are not yet successful. Fluoride causes dramatic increases in the bone density, but the bone is of abnormal quality, and there are substantially more fractures, especially in the hip and long bones. Parathyroid hormone has been studied in only a few patients, in whom the spine bone improves, but the cortical bone deteriorates.

The intestinal absorption of calcium is less efficient in postmenopausal women than in younger women. Calcium supplements are beneficial to women with osteoporosis, especially if they were initially consuming less than 600 mg/day (16). An intake of 1,000 to 1,500 mg/day should be the first step in any treatment regimen. The only risk is in the small group of patients with absorptive hypercalciuria. Calcium from dairy products or supplements are equally well absorbed provided the calcium supplement is chewable or dissolvable and is taken with food. Calcium helps prevent further bone loss (17).

In addition to preventing osteoporosis, estrogen is currently the best drug for treating postmenopausal osteoporosis. In perimenopausal women, it abolishes the rapid bone loss, and in older women, it causes a small increase in bone mass. Estrogen blocks bone resorption (14), and the magnitude of increase in bone density is similar to that seen with other anti-resorbing agents. Doses are the same as for preventing osteoporosis. In elderly women, gradual increase in the dose of estrogen starting at 0.3 mg/day, may help alleviate breast tenderness. Regimens that do not result in menses, such as continuous daily medroxy progesterone 2.5 mg/day with conjugated estrogen, 0.625 mg/day, can improve compliance.

In women who cannot or will not take estrogens, other antiresorptive therapies can be used. Calcitonin, which acts by directly inhibiting osteoclastic resorption, currently must be given by subcutaneous injection, and is quite expensive. A reasonable dose range is 50–100 units three times a week. Often, patients will experience flushing or gastrointestinal (GI) side effects, which may respond to dose reductions. Calcitonin is most effective in patients with high bone resorption rates (18). When it is discontinued, the bone density decreases.

The bisphosphonates are analogs of pyrophosphate, and they bind avidly to calcium apatite. Their mechanism of action is obscure, but they result in decreased bone turnover, with lower resorption and formation. Etidronate, the first bisphosphonate available in the United States, increases the bone density by about 5% (19). It is important to realize that continuous etidronate can result in osteomalacia and mineralization defects. The dose used in the clinical trials of postmenopausal osteoporosis is 400 mg/day for two weeks, repeated every three months. Occasional GI upset was noted, without any other serious side effects. The bisphosphonates are poorly absorbed from the GI tract, and in the presence of calcium, absorption is even worse. Etidronate has not been approved by the US Food and Drug Administration for the treatment of osteoporosis, because the long-term effect of fractures is unknown.

Vitamin D is necessary for healthy bones. In elderly patients, formation of vitamin D in the skin is impaired, so that dietary intake of at least 400 units/day becomes necessary (20). Large doses of vitamin D (25,000 units/week) can be toxic and actually worsen bone loss. The effectiveness of calcitriol (1,25-dihydroxyvitamin D) is controversial. Calcitriol does not increase bone density (21). One study suggested that calcitriol might reduce the number of spine fractures (22). This form of vitamin D is powerful and can easily increase the serum or urine calcium to danger-ous levels. Children treated with calcitriol for several years (for hypophosphatemic rickets) develop nephrocalcinosis (23); therefore, calcitriol should be used only in patients with low calcitriol levels or in women who have renal failure or malabsorption.

Patients should be encouraged to walk and keep active. Back extension exercises may be helpful. Measures to prevent falls are important, especially in the elderly.

CORTICOSTEROID-INDUCED OSTEOPOROSIS

Corticosteroids have several unfortunate effects on bone metabolism (24). They increase bone resorption (in part by increasing osteoclast affinity for mineral) and decrease bone formation (by directly inhibiting osteoblasts). Intestinal calcium absorption is directly inhibited, and often mild secondary hyperparathyroidism may result. Hypercalciuria is frequently found and may be caused by renal tubular effects. Despite this, about 50% of patients on long-term corticosteroids for asthma have normal bone density measurements. Bone density measurements can thus be helpful in monitoring patients who must receive chronic steroids. Treatment of these patients is difficult and is based on scarce data. The available agents are the same as those for osteoporosis. Since bone formation is usually decreased, drugs that block resorption would theoretically not work as well in steroid-induced osteoporosis as in postmenopausal osteoporosis. Hypercalciuria can be treated with thiazide diuretics. Calcium supplementation should be given to help overcome the decreased calcium absorption. Vitamin D treatment has been suggested, but should be used with caution in patients who already have hypercalciuria.

PRIMARY HYPERPARATHYROIDISM

Primary hyperparathyroidism is a common disorder, especially in postmenopausal women. About 28 new cases per 100,000 persons are diagnosed each year. A solitary parathyroid adenoma is usually the cause of the excess secretion of PTH. The classic symptoms of primary hyperparathyroidism can be described by the old rhyme: "Bones, stones, abdominal moans, and psychiatric groans." In its advanced state, the disease presents with pathologic bone fractures, and the bone histology shows osteitis fibrosis with excessive resorption as well as formation. The bone loss is more marked in the cortical bone than in the trabecular bone. Kidney stones result from the hypercalciuria. Stomach ulcers and depression are also associated with the disease. Laboratory abnormalities include elevated serum PTH levels (the intact hormone should be measured), hypercalcemia, increased urine calcium and cyclic adenosine monophosphate, and low serum phosphate. Often 1,25 dihydroxyvitamin D levels are increased. It has become common practice for many physicians to check chemistry panels containing calcium as part of routine screening of their patients. Many cases have been discovered that would previously have gone undetected. Whether these asymptomatic patients should undergo parathyroidectomy is the subject of debate (25).

OSTEOMALACIA

Osteomalacia is characterized by excessive unmineralized osteoid. Whereas normal bone has less than 5% osteoid, in some cases this can increase to 40% to 50%. This reduces bone strength and also causes pain. Fractures are common. The growth plates of bones are particularly affected in growing children, who may have rickets with bowed legs, and deformed skulls and ribs. The causes of rickets or osteomalacia and some of the associated laboratory findings are shown in Table 52–2. The old terminology of some of these diseases is bracketed by quotation marks, because it is confusing and reflects the lack of knowledge about vitamin D when these diseases were named. Most cases are caused by decreased serum mineral levels or by toxins. In the presence of ultraviolet light, vitamin D is manufactured in skin from cholesterol precursors. The liver hydroxylates at the 25 position and then the kidney at the 1 position to form 1,25-dihydroxyvitamin D (calcitriol), which is the active metabolite. It is a steroid hormone with cellular receptors, and

Table 52–2. *Osteomalacia*

	Ca	PO4	25-D	1,25-D	Other
Vitamin D abnormalities					
D-deficiency	↓	↓	↓	↓	↑ PTH & Alk Phos
Liver disease	↓	↓	↓	↓	↑ PTH & Alk Phos
Renal disease	↓	↑	N	↓	↑ PTH & Alk Phos
1 α hydroxylase deficiency ("vitamin D dependent rickets type I")	↓		N	↓	↑ PTH & Alk Phos
Vitamin D resistance due to abnormal receptor ("vitamin D dependent rickets type II")	↓	↓	N	↑	↑ PTH & Alk Phos
x-linked hypophosphatemic rickets ("vitamin D resistant rickets")	± ↓	↓	N	N	1,25-D inappropriately normal
Hypophosphatemia					
Renal phosphate loss	N	↓	N	N	
Excessive antacid intake	N	↓	N	± ↑	
Hereditary hypophosphatemia with hypercalciuria	N	↓	N	↑	↑ urine calcium
Toxicities					
Fluoride	N	N	N	N	
Etidronate	N	± ↑	N	N	
Parenteral aluminum	N	N	N	± ↓	↓ PTH
Other					
Hypophosphatasia	N	N	N	N	↓ Alk Phos
Acidosis	N	N	N	N	
Oncogenic osteomalacia	± ↓	↓	N	↓	↑ PTH & Alk Phos

families have been described with various abnormalities in the receptor number or function.

RENAL OSTEODYSTROPHY

Patients with end-stage renal disease who need dialysis rarely have normal bones. Their bone disease is extremely variable, and ranges in severity from asymptomatic to life-threatening. There are several patterns of bone disease in these patients. The most common is secondary hyperparathyroidism. Since the damaged kidneys do not make enough 1,25(OH)2-vitamin D, the serum calcium is low. The serum phosphate, however, is elevated, because the kidneys do not excrete it. The high serum phosphate inhibits what little renal hydroxylation of vitamin D remains. This increases the PTH and bone resorption ensues in an attempt to normalize the serum calcium. In addition, the parathyroid gland is not as sensitive to serum calcium in renal patients as in normal patients, which further encourages excessive PTH. The increased PTH stimulates both bone formation and resorption, and the final result may vary from patient to patient (26).

If the serum phosphate becomes too high, metastatic calcifications will result. To prevent this, many patients have been treated with oral aluminum-containing antacids. This will control the phosphate by preventing intestinal absorption, but some of the aluminum may be absorbed. Aluminum is toxic to both osteoblasts and parathyroid cells. Patients with markedly elevated aluminum levels will have osteomalacia and low PTH. Patients on chronic dialysis may also have acidosis, corticosteroid therapy, hypogonadism, iron accumulation, or deficiencies of growth factors. Thus, the spectrum of bone disease in these patients is complex. Often a bone biopsy is the only way to establish the correct diagnosis. β_2-microglobulins accumulate after years of dialysis; this leads to amyloidosis which is found especially in the bones and joints (27).

Susan M. Ott, MD

1. Delmas PD, Christiansen C, Mann KG, et al: Bone Gla protein (osteocalcin) assay standardization report. J Bone Miner Res 5:5–11, 1990
2. Hanson DA, Weis MA, Bollen AM, et al: A specific immunoassay for monitoring human bone resorption: quantitation of type I collagen cross-linked N-telopeptides in urine. J Bone Miner Res 7:1251–1258, 1992
3. Nussbaum SR, Potts JT Jr: Immunoassays for parathyroid hormone 1–84 in the diagnosis of hyperparathyroidism. J Bone Miner Res 6 Suppl 2:S43–50, 1991
4. Slemenda CW, Hui SL, Longcope C, et al: Predictors of bone mass in perimenopausal women: a prospective study of clinical data using photon absorptiometry. Ann Intern Med 112:96–101, 1990
5. Ott SM, Kilcoyne RF, Chesnut CH: Ability of four different techniques of measuring bone mass to diagnose vertebral fractures in postmenopausal women. J Bone Mineral Res 2:201–210, 1987
6. Hui SL, Siemenda CW, Johnston CC: Age and bone mass as predictors of fracture in a prospective study. J Clin Invest 81:1804–1809, 1988
7. Cummings SR, Black DM, Nevitt MC, et al: Appendicular bone density and age predict hip fracture in women. JAMA 263:665–668, 1990
8. Cummings SR, Black DM, Nevitt MC, et al: Bone density at various sites for prediction of hip fractures. The Study of Osteoporotic Fractures Research Group. Lancet 341(8837):72–75, 1983
9. Raisz LG: Local and systemic factors in the pathogenesis of osteoporosis. New Engl J Med 318:818, 1988
10. Melton LJ, Cummings SR: Heterogeneity of age-related fractures: implications for epidemiology. Bone and Mineral 2:321–331, 1987
11. Drinkwater BL, Bruemner B, Chesnut CH: Menstrual history as a determinant of current bone density in young athletes. JAMA 263:545–548, 1990
12. LaCroix AZ, Wienpahl J, White LR, et al: Thiazide diuretic agents and the incidence of hip fracture. N Engl J Med 322:286–290, 1990
13. Barzel US: Estrogens in the prevention and treatment of postmenopausal osteoporosis: a review. Am J Med 85:847–850, 1988
14. Lufkin EG, Wahner HW, O'Fallon WM, et al: Treatment of postmenopausal osteoporosis with transdermal estrogen. Ann Intern Med 117:1–9, 1992
15. Riggs BL, Melton LJ: The prevention and treatment of osteoporosis. N Engl J Med 327:620–627, 1992
16. Dawson–Hughes B: Calcium supplementation and bone loss: a review of controlled clinical trials. Am J Clin Nutr 54:274, 1991
17. Reid IR, Ames RW, Evans MC, et al: Effect of calcium supplementation on bone loss in postmenopausal women. N Engl J Med 328:460–464, 1993
18. Civitelli R, Gonnelli S, Zacchei F, et al: Bone turnover in postmenopausal osteoporosis: effect of calcitonin treatment. J Clin Invest 82:1268–1274, 1988
19. Watts NB, Harris ST, Genant HK, et al: Intermittent cyclical etidronate treatment of postmenopausal osteoporosis. N Engl J Med 323:7, 1990
20. Chapuy MC, Arlot ME, Duboeuf F, et al: Vitamin D3 and calcium to prevent hip fractures in elderly women. N Engl J Med 327:1637–1642, 1992
21. Ott SM, Chesnut CH: Calcitriol treatment is not effective in postmenopausal osteoporosis. Ann Intern Med 110:267–274, 1989
22. Tilyard MW, Spears GFS, Thomson J, et al: Treatment of postmenopausal osteoporosis with calcitriol or calcium. N Engl J Med 326:357–362, 1992
23. Verge CH, Lam A, Simpson JM, et al: Effects of therapy in x-linked hypophosphatemic rickets. N Engl J Med 325:1843–1848, 1991
24. Lukert BP, Raisz LG: Glucocorticoid-induced osteoporosis: pathogenesis and management. Ann Intern Med 112:352, 1990
25. Potts JT (ed): Proceedings of the NIH consensus development conference on diagnosis and management of asymptomatic primary hyperparathyroidism. J Bone Mineral Res 6 (suppl 2):S1–S165, 1991
26. Slatopolsky E: The interaction of parathyroid hormone and aluminum in renal osteodystrophy. Kidney International 31:842, 1987
27. Drueke TB, Zingraff J, Noel LH, et al: Amyloidosis and dialysis: pathophysiological aspects. Contrib–Nephrol 62:60–66, 1988

53. FOREIGN BODY SYNOVITIS

The penetration of a foreign body into a joint, tendon sheath, or periarticular soft tissue can induce monarticular synovitis, tenosynovitis, or cellulitis around joints (1). Foreign bodies most commonly described in association with synovitis include different plant thorns, wood splinters, and sea urchin spines, all of which can easily break inside the articular cavity. Less often fish bones, chitin fragments, silica, silicone, metals, plastics, rubber, and gravel have been found to cause foreign body synovitis (1–5).

Also, patients with silicone or metallic prostheses may develop detritic synovitis with synovial proliferation and formation of foreign body granulomas (6). Metallic, silicone, and cement particles may be found in synovial fluid and inflamed synovium (4). Lead projectiles that penetrate into major joints may cause not only synovitis, but also systemic manifestations of lead toxicity, as synovial fluid serves as a solvent of lead (7). An acute necrotizing dactylitis that might be confused with synovitis also occurs as a result of high pressure gun injuries or when grease or paint are accidentally injected into a finger tip (4). This type of injury requires immediate surgical drainage and debridement.

CLINICAL FEATURES

Most patients may recall localized acute pain at the time of the injury, which is often followed by an asymptomatic period, usually lasting a few days, or more rarely lasting weeks or months. Not infrequently the initial injury is forgotten by the patient or missed when history is elicited. After the latent period, signs of acute or chronic synovitis become apparent (4).

Most often, the synovitis follows a subacute or cyclic course with periods of remission of pain and partial resolution of the inflammatory changes (4,10). In a few patients, the synovitis subsides spontaneously or after administration of antibiotics or nonsteroidal antiinflammatory agents (4). The intensity of the articular inflammation associated with foreign body penetration probably depends on the nature of the foreign body, type of coating with different toxic proteins, degree of bacterial contamination, and surface charge of the particles (4).

The joints most commonly affected are those unprotected by clothing such as the knee and finger joints. Affected joints present variable degrees of periarticular swelling, synovial thickening, and joint effusion. Fever is characteristically absent or low grade, except in those patients with synovitis due to sea urchin spines or other foreign bodies of animal origin, who may present with fever, myalgias, lymph node enlargement, and synovitis of surrounding joints (10). Professional fishing and diving, other marine recreational activities, farming, and gardening are well-recognized risk factors (1,4,8,9). Differential diagnosis must include other causes of acute and chronic inflammatory monarthritis, such as septic arthritis, tuberculosis, osteomyelitis, monarticular juvenile rheumatoid arthritis, and different types of dactylitis (erysipeloid, atypical mycobacteria, psoriasis, and seal finger) (10,11). When the initial injury is missed and subchondral bone changes are present, foreign body synovitis may be confused with a bone tumor (4).

LABORATORY, RADIOLOGIC, AND PATHOLOGIC FINDINGS

White cell count and differential are usually normal, and erythrocyte sedimentation rate can be mildly increased. The synovial fluid is cloudy or bloody. Analysis reveals leukocyte counts ranging from 10,000–60,000 cells/mm³ (4,13). Polymorphonuclear cells may predominate even in the absence of infection. Cultures for bacteria and fungi are sterile, except when an infectious agent has been introduced along with the foreign body. Fresh preparations of synovial fluid only occasionally reveal birefringent fragments of plant thorn, non-birefringent plastic, or dark metallic particles or needle-shaped fiberglass (12). Particles are much more often embedded in synovium. Radiologic studies detect only radiodense foreign bodies such as metal, fish bone,

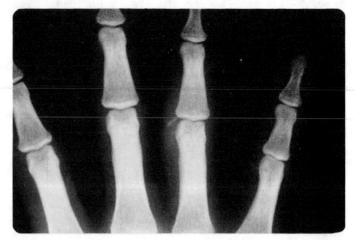

Fig. 53–1. *Soft tissue swelling surrounding a radio-opaque sea urchin spine in a patient with foreign body synovitis.*

and sea urchin spines (calcium carbonate), and usually miss plant thorns, wood, and plastic (Fig. 53–1). Most roentgenograms reveal only soft tissue swelling of the affected joint without associated bone changes. Less often, periarticular demineralization is present, and occasionally there are focal areas of osteolysis, osteonecrosis, periosteal new bone formation, or periarticular calcification. These changes may mimic those seen in osteomyelitis or bone tumor (4,11,12).

Ultrasound has been shown to be sensitive enough to detect small pieces of non-metallic foreign bodies, such as wood, plastic, and glass in the skin. Computed tomography has been useful in identification of plant thorns in isolated cases (14). The role of

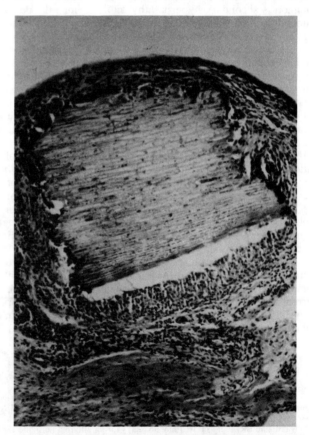

Fig. 53–2. *Photomicrograph of synovium of a proximal interphalangeal joint of a patient with foreign body synovitis. Note the characteristic plant thorn fragment surrounded by giant cells and a mononuclear cell infiltrate.*

nuclear magnetic resonance imaging has not been fully explored in the clinical detection of foreign bodies in joints. In a study performed on experimentally induced foreign body injuries in cadaver hands, nuclear magnetic resonance and computed tomography were the preferred methods to detect plastic wood fragments when plain films were unrevealing (15). Arthroscopy has been helpful in identifying foreign bodies only in isolated cases, because foreign bodies are easily fragmented and often lie deep in the inflamed synovium (4).

Excisional biopsy of articular and periarticular tissues with pathologic and bacteriologic studies is usually required for adequate diagnosis and treatment of most patients (4). Synovium usually reveals synovial lining cell proliferation and diffuse infiltrates of lymphocytes and plasma cells with focal polymorphonuclear cell infiltrates. These local infiltrates are similar to those seen in Reiter's syndrome and in chronic septic arthritis and contrast with the marked diffuse polymorphonuclear infiltrates seen in acute septic arthritis. Inflammation is often accentuated around the foreign body (Fig. 53–2). Giant cell formation in synovium is prominent in patients with foreign bodies inside joints (4), but can be minimal or absent in those patients with foreign bodies in the periarticular tissues (11). Polarized light microscopy also can help identify the birefringence of plant thorns or of crystals of calcium carbonate in patients with sea urchin spine-induced synovitis (4,8). Granulomas similar to those seen in sarcoidosis are seen in patients with sea urchin synovitis (4,8).

TREATMENT

In about 30% of patients, foreign body synovitis will resolve spontaneously in a matter of weeks to months. The remaining patients with chronic synovitis require excisional biopsy, exten-sive synovectomy, and articular lavage to remove the foreign bodies (4,16). After surgery, resolution of joint swelling may be slow in some patients in association with periosteal new bone formation.

José Luis Ferreiro-Seoane, MD

1. Kelly JJ: Blackthorn inflammation. J Bone Joint Surg 48B:474–478, 1966
2. Goodnough CP, Frymoyer JW: Synovitis secondary to non-metallic foreign bodies. J Trauma 15:960–965, 1975
3. Sugarman M, Stobie DG, Quismorio FP, et al: Plant thorn synovitis. Arthritis Rheum 20:1125–1128, 1977
4. Reginato AJ, Ferreiro JL, O'Connor CR, et al: Clinical and pathologic studies of twenty-six patients with penetrating foreign body injury to the joint, bursae, and tendon sheaths. Arthritis Rheum 33:1753–1762, 1990
5. Schumacher HR, Majno G: Thorns in the skin and joints of the monkey. Arch Path 84:536–538, 1967
6. Christie A, Pierret G, Levitan J: Silicone synovitis. Semin Arthritis Rheum 19:166–171, 1989
7. Windler EC, Smith RB, Bryan WJ, et al: Lead intoxication and traumatic arthritis of hip secondary to retained bullet fragments: a case report. J Bone Joint Surg 60:254–255, 1978
8. Daupleix D, Dreyfus P, Bovier F, et al: Les arthritis a piquants d'oursin: a propos de deux nouveaux cas. Rev Rhum Mal Osteoartic 51:333–335, 1984
9. Cracchiolo A, Goldberg L: Local and systemic reactions to puncture injuries by the sea urchin spine and date palm thorn. Arthritis Rheum 20:1125–1128, 1977
10. Lazaro MA, Garcia Morteo D, Benycar MA, et al: Lymphadenopathy secondary to silicone hand joint prosthesis. Clin Exp Rheumatol 8:17–22, 1990
11. O'Connor CR, Reginato AJ, DeLong W: Foreign body reaction simulating acute septic arthritis. J Rheumatol 15:1568–1571, 1988
12. Goupille P, Fouquet B, Favard L, et al: Two cases of plant thorn synovitis: difficulties in diagnosis and treatment. J Rheumatol 17:252–254, 1990
13. Schumacher HR, Reginato AJ: Atlas of Synovial Fluid and Crystal Analysis. Chapter 22. Lea & Febiger, Philadelphia, 1991
14. Little CL, Parker MG, Callowich MC, et al: The ultrasonic detection of soft tissue foreign bodies. Invest Radiol 21:275–277, 1986
15. Russell RC, Williamson DA, Sullivan JW, et al: Detection of foreign body in the hand. J Hand Surg Am 16A:2–11, 1991
16. Dominguez JJ, Dalisme C: Artritis de tobillo por cuerpo extrano de origen vegetal. Rev Ortop Traum 24:287–290, 1990

54. SPORTS AND OCCUPATIONAL INJURIES

Injuries occur in all sports and vigorous occupations. The frequency and type of injury are activity-related (1,2) and are of two types, acute and chronic.

Acute injuries result from direct trauma to a muscle, bone, or ligament and include pulled muscles, fractures, and ligamentous sprains or tears. Acute injuries occur at an identifiable point in time. *Chronic* injuries are overuse injuries as a result of repetitive microtrauma to the musculoskeletal system, which exceeds the body's adaptive or healing capabilities.

SPORTS INJURIES

Muscle and Tendon Injuries

A soft tissue injury from direct trauma may result in a muscle hematoma, manifested by localized tenderness, swelling, and pain when the damaged muscle is stretched. Treatment should consist of cold applications, rest, and compression followed by a rehabilitation program of stretching and strengthening. Aspiration of a liquified hematoma may relieve some symptoms. If an early return to the sport is desired, the patient should wear protective padding and minimize the chance of reinjury and muscle tears, thus decreasing the risk of myositis ossificans. Heat should not be used during rehabilitation, because it has been associated with an increased incidence of myositis ossificans.

Muscle tears are common, especially in middle-aged athletes, often occurring after inadequate warm-up or stretching prior to participating in rigorous sports. Muscle injuries occur in activities of long duration characterized by relative high intensity and involving ballistic activity and eccentric contractions. A prodrome of aching and soreness at the muscle–tendon junction after activity often precedes the acute injury. The onset is usually sudden, characterized by a stabbing pain and the inability to use the affected extremity against resistance. The involved muscle may have a palpable defect. Treatment consists of ice, rest, and splinting in a position of muscle relaxation for mild to moderate tears. In severe cases with complete loss of muscle continuity, operative repair should strongly be considered. After the pain subsides, rehabilitation should begin for mild to moderate tears with stretching, strengthening, and gradual return to sports. Delayed treatment or undertreatment may hamper return to activity or produce prolonged impairment of performance. The most common locations for these injuries are the medial head of the gastrocnemius in tennis players, quadriceps in sprinters, and hamstrings and biceps in weight lifters.

Failure may also occur within the tendinous portion of the muscle. Rupture is usually the result of a sudden contraction of the muscle. Local corticosteroid injections have been associated with subsequent predisposition to rupture (3,4). The most common example of this injury is Achilles tendon rupture, which occurs with the sudden contraction of the gastrocnemius and soleus complex (see Chapter 50). The tendon usually ruptures in midsubstance, but the rupture may also be found at the bony insertion or at the musculotendinous junction. A prodrome of aching may precede failure. The onset of pain is sudden, followed by swelling, a marked weakness, and often absence of active joint motion with inability to plantar flex the foot. Treatment consists of ice and immobilization in plantar flexion. For the competitive athlete, surgical repair may offer the best treatment (5). Rehabilitation involves slowly restoring dorsiflexion of the foot with the use of consecutively smaller heel lifts, followed by a stretching program. Isokinetic training is useful in restoring the athlete to full function.

Other tendons commonly affected by rupture are the long head of the biceps, the distal biceps insertion, insertion of the flexor tendons into the fingers, and the quadriceps tendon at both the tibia and the superior pole of the patella.

Table 54–1. *Classification and treatment of ligament tears*

	1st Degree	2nd Degree	3rd Degree
Injury	Minimal tear	Partial tear	Complete tear
Laxity	None	Mild-moderate	Unstable
Treatment	Ice with rehabilitative and supportive care	Ice, muscle rehabilitation, functional bracing, possible cast	Ice, splint Possible surgery
Prognosis	Excellent	Good	Variable

Ligament Injuries

Ligament injuries can occur at bony insertions or in midsubstance. The pattern of injury is dependent on the rate at which the ligament is loaded. At high speeds, failure occurs in midligament, whereas at low speeds, failure occurs as a bony avulsion (6). The ligament at risk depends on the direction of force and the position of the joint at the time of injury. Ligamentous injuries can be classified according to severity of injury. Treatment of these injuries is described in Table 54–1.

Fractures

Fractures usually result from a direct blow over the involved site or in conjunction with ligamentous injuries causing a bony avulsion. Care should be taken not to ignore pain away from the site of direct trauma, because a force strong enough to break bones can be transmitted. For example, a clavicular fracture can result from falling on an outstretched hand. Symptoms of a fracture are acute pain, point tenderness, and swelling. Deformity or instability may or may not be present. Careful examination of the overlying skin should be made because treatment of open fractures requires debridement, irrigation, and parenteral antibiotics to avoid the complication of osteomyelitis. Treatment usually consists of immobilization for six to eight weeks in a cast or splint or open reduction and internal fixation. Joint motion is best preserved with early mobilization and fracture bracing whenever possible. Rehabilitation consists of establishing full motion and muscle strength prior to returning to rigorous sporting activity.

Stress Fractures

Stress fractures differ from acute traumatic fractures, because they result from repetitive muscular action that exceeds the bone's strength and capacity for normal remolding. In people with normal bones, these fractures occur with either new or accelerated vigorous activity. A detailed history is essential to discover a recent change in shoes or intensity or frequency of activity (7). Insufficiency or fatigue fractures commonly follow relatively normal stress on abnormal bone, as seen in Paget's disease, hyperparathyroidism, osteoporosis, rheumatoid arthritis (RA), and irradiation therapy. Fatigue fractures are not uncommon following surgical procedures that produce increased stress or altered muscular biomechanics on normal or abnormal bone (8).

A clinical examination for stress fractures is done in the patient giving a history of pain related to activity that is relieved by rest. Often there is point tenderness and occasionally a palpable mass over the fracture. The site of pain is often characteristic for the activity history (Table 54–2). Initial roentgenograms are usually negative. Stress fractures show on roentgenograms 2 to 17 weeks after the onset of pain (9). Bone scans are usually positive early, showing an oval, well-marginated area of uptake in the cortex (10).

Differential diagnosis includes shin splints, osteomyelitis, eosinophilic granuloma, osteoid osteomas for chronic stress fractures, and malignant bone tumors. These lesions can be differentiated from the more common stress fracture by tomograms, computed tomography (CT) scans and a repeat roentgenogram to observe for callus as part of the fracture healing of the cortical defect.

Table 54–2. *Location of stress fracture by activity**

Location	Activity
Sesamoids of metatarsals	Prolonged standing or jumping activity
Metatarsal shaft	Marching; stamping on ground; prolonged standing; ballet; postoperative bunionectomy
Navicular	Stamping on ground; marching; long distance running
Calcaneus	Jumping; parachuting; prolonged standing; recent immobilization
Tibia	
Mid and distal shaft	Long distance running
Proximal shaft (children)	Running
Fibula	
Distal shaft	Long distance running
Proximal shaft	Jumping; parachuting
Patella	Hurdling
Femur	
Shaft	Ballet; long distance running
Neck	Ballet; marching; long distance running; gymnastics
Pelvis, obturator ring	Stooping; bowling; gymnastics
Lumbar vertebra (pars interarticularis)	Ballet; weight lifting; scrubbing floors; gymnastics
Lower cervical, upper thoracic spinous process	Clay shoveling
Ribs	Carrying heavy pack; golf; coughing; tennis
Clavicle	Postoperative radical neck surgery
Coracoid of scapula	Trap shooting
Humerus, distal shaft	Throwing a ball
Ulna	
Coronoid	Pitching a ball
Shaft	Using a pitchfork; propelling wheelchair
Hook of hamate	Swinging golf club; tennis racquet; baseball bat

* Modified from reference 8.

Treatment involves resting the involved area and modifying activity. Analysis of provoking activity and gradual resumption of training after pain subsides are essential to prevent a recurrence. A recurrence of pain with resumption of activity should alert the patient and physician to the probability of a recurrence of the fracture. Stress fractures of the hip may require operative stabilization to prevent displacement and possible avascular necrosis.

Shin Splints

Shin splints describe a syndrome of chronic anterior tibial compartment pain that is most common along the medial border of the tibia. The pain is exacerbated by exercise, particularly running, may not be relieved by rest, and may last hours to days. Roentgenograms typically show no abnormality, and the bone scan may be consistent with periostitis. Debate persists as to whether this is a chronic enthesitis or whether an element of chronic exercise-induced compartment syndrome is present. Recent work by Garth and Miller (11) has proposed that this is an overuse syndrome of the flexor digitorum longus, which is overused to maintain the toes flat on the ground until toe-off is achieved. They suggest treating this syndrome with metatarsal pads. The treatment otherwise is rest, ice, and supportive taping.

Table 54–3. *Chronic overuse syndromes*

Grade	Symptoms	Treatment
I	Pain after activity only	Ice
II	Pain during and after activity but no significant interference with performance	Ice and 10% to 25% decrease in activity
III	Pain during and after activity with interference with performance	Ice, 25% to 75% decrease in activity, antiinflammatory agents
IV	Constant pain that interferes with activities of daily living	Ice, complete rest of involved area, antiinflammatory agents

Chronic Overuse Syndromes

Chronic overuse injuries are the result of stresses that exceed the body's adaptive or healing capabilities. All are characterized by the same constellation of symptoms, pathophysiology, and treatment principals (Table 54–3). They can occur in bone as stress fractures, tendons as tendinitis, and muscle–tendon–bone junctions as lateral epicondylitis or tennis elbow (see Chapter 50). Overuse injuries have a changing spectrum with advancing age. Athletes over the age of 50 have more complaints of metatarsalgia, plantar fasciitis, and meniscal injuries than those under 30. The younger group has a high incidence of stress fractures, periostitis, and patellar pain.

The pattern of chronic injury is one of inflammation and repair. The constant repetitive stresses of the body during strenuous exercise lead to adaptive changes that enhance performance—"the training effect". In some cases, however, this training leads to microscopic tears in the muscle–tendon bone units. These microscopic lesions trigger an inflammatory response.

The initial response to injury consists of pain, edema, erythema, and warmth. This phase is followed by a reparative phase of fibroblast proliferation, collagen deposition (scar), regeneration, and remodeling. As the healing process proceeds, there is tissue contraction as the collagen matures and contracts, leading to a loss of motion.

Treatment is based on the stage at which the patient is seen. In general, it involves the early use of cold applications, antiinflammatory medications, modification of activity, and then strengthening, and a gradual return to activity. Surgery is rarely indicated.

Knee Injuries

The knee is a frequently injured joint because of its position and vulnerability during sporting activities and deserves special attention. All of the preceding descriptions apply to injuries of the bone and soft tissue around the knee. Internal derangements of the knee are a common problem. An effusion soon after an injury should be aspirated and the fluid analyzed. Further diagnostic studies may be indicated, depending on the clinical picture and the fluid characteristic. The most common cause of an acute hemarthrosis is an anterior cruciate ligament tear (12), which often is seen in conjunction with other injuries such as meniscal tears and collateral ligament disruptions. Other injuries associated with acute hemarthrosis are subchondral fractures, dislocation of the tibia, and loose bodies (13). Other diseases, such as pigmented villonodular synovitis or coagulation disorders may also cause a hemarthrosis.

The knee menisci are at high risk for a tearing injury during rotation of the knee, especially when the knee is in flexion. The symptoms include pain over the joint line, swelling with bloody or clear fluid, and a history of locking and giving way. The McMurray test may produce painful clicking in the knee during flexion and extension while the medial or lateral joint space is compressed. Magnetic resonance imaging (MRI) is helpful, but there is a wide range of diagnostic accuracy depending on the reader and MRI quality. In the most experienced hand, an MRI

Table 54–4. *Some professions at risk for occupational overuse syndromes (usually a cervicobrachial syndrome)**

Professions	Risk (%)
Keypunch operators	16–28
Typists	13
Calculator operators	10
Cash register operators	11–16
Packing machine operators	12
Assembly line operators	16

* Modified from reference 21.

reporting a medial meniscal tear will be 89% accurate when compared with arthroscopic findings. Reported variability in MRI accuracy ranges from 65% to 95% for medial meniscal pathology. Also, MRIs tend to over-read pathology, and clinical correlation is important (14). If the injury is within the vascularized zone of the meniscus, operative repair should be considered (15). In patients with suspected internal derangements of the knee, roentgenograms are recommended to exclude fractures or unsuspected findings such as bone tumors (16).

OCCUPATIONAL INJURIES

Occupational Overuse Injuries

There are three main causes of occupational overuse injuries: 1) rapid, repetitive movements such as typing; 2) less frequent but more forceful movements such as in an assembly line; and 3) static loading, especially of the upper extremity as in typists and welders (Table 54–4). Frequently encountered problems include bicipital tendinitis, carpal tunnel syndrome, and de Quervain's tendinitis (16). Musicians and other performing artists are increasingly recognized as victims of similar overuse syndromes (17).

Often patients do not present with a clear-cut tendinitis or bursitis but have general complaints of aching muscle groups. It is necessary to obtain a detailed account of the activities that provoke the pain and posture used at that time. Often simple interventions, such as changing the height of a keyboard or the viewing angle of the video display terminal, will markedly improve symptoms (18). Other recommendations include reducing the work rate, with more frequent hourly breaks and scheduled stretching (19). A graded part-time resumption of the job should be followed to allow time for conditioning. Relaxation exercises are sometimes beneficial.

Occupational Osteoarthritis

Certain occupations are associated with increased stress and trauma to joints (20,21). The pathophysiology is not clear but may be related to bone fatigue with repeated insults, leading to microfractures, collapse, cyst formation, and degeneration. Ligamentous injury also leads to abnormal joint alignment and biomechanics. Vascular injuries or spasm-promoting activities may

Table 54–5. *Occupation-related arthritis*

Occupation	Site of osteoarthritis
Ballet dancers	Ankles and feet
Lacrosse players	Ankles, knees, and feet
Soccer players	Ankles, knees, and feet
Cyclists	Patellofemoral joint
Farmers	Hips
Miners	Elbows
Riveters	Elbows
Metal workers	Elbows
Pneumatic tool operators	Hands and wrists; also osteoporosis, cystic carpal bones, osteonecrosis, and osteolysis (Raynaud's phenomenon also reported)
Cotton mill workers	Interphalangeal joints
Coal miners	Knees, lumbar spine

* From reference 21.

promote osteonecrosis. Table 54–5 lists various occupations with their commonly associated patterns of arthritis. The syndrome of low back pain is commonly encountered and attributed to occupational factors. It is discussed in Chapter 47.

Sally Pullman, MD
Pekka Mooar, MD

1. Garrick J, Regua R: Injury in high school sports, Pediatric 61:465–469, 1978
2. Graham GP, Bruce PJ: Survey of intercollegiate athletic injuries to women. Res Q Am Assoc Health Phys Educ 48:217–220, 1977
3. Lee HB: Avulsion and rupture of the tendocalcaneous after injection of hydrocortisone. Br Med J 2:395, 1957
4. Noyes FR, Grood ES, Nussbaum NS, et al: Affect of intraarticular corticosteroid injections on ligamentous properties: a biomechanical and histological study in Rhesus knee. Clin Orthop 123:197–209, 1977
5. DeStefano V, Nixon JE: Ruptures of the achilles tendon. J Sports Med Phys Fitness 1:34–37, 1975
6. Noyes FR, DeLucas JL, Torbick PJ: Biomechanics of anterior cruciate ligament failure: an analysis of strain-rate sensitivity and mechanisms of failure in primates. J Bone Joint Surg Am 56:236–253, 1974
7. Jackson DW, Strizak AM: Stress fractures in runners, excluding the foot, AAOS Symposium on the Foot and Leg in Running Sports. Edited by Mack R. St. Louis, Mo., CV Mosby, 1982, pp 109–122
8. Resnick D, Niwayama G: Physical injuries, Diagnosis of Bone and Joint Disorders, Edited by Resnick D, Niwayama G. Philadelphia, Penn., WB Saunders, 1981, pp 2241–2326
9. Roub LW, Gumerman LW, Hanley EN Jr, et al: Bone stress: a radionuclide imaging perspective. Radiology 132:431–438, 1979
10. Daffner RH, Martinez S, Gehweiler JA: Stress fractures in runners. JAMA 247:1039–1041, 1982
11. Garth WP Jr, Miller ST: Evaluation of claw toe deformity, weakness of the foot intrinsics, and posteromedial shin pain. Am J Sports Med 17:821–827, 1989
12. Noyes F, Basset R: Arthroscopy in acute traumatic hemarthrosis of the knee. J Bone Joint Surg 52A:687–695, 1980
13. Jain AS, Swanson AJG, Murdoch G: Hemarthrosis of the knee. Injury 15:178–181, 1983
14. Fischer SP, Fox JM, DelPisso W, et al: Accuracy of diagnosis from MRI of the knee: A multicenter analysis of 1014 patients. J Bone Joint Surg 73A:2–10, 1991
15. Cassidy RE, Shaffer AJ: Repair of peripheral meniscus tears. Am J Sports Med 9:209–214, 1987
16. Joyce JM, Mankin HM: Caveat arthroscopes: extra-articular lesions of bone simulating intra-articular pathology of the knee. J Bone Joint Surg 65A:289–292, 1983
17. Hoppmann RA, Patrone NA: Musculoskeletal problems in instrumental musicians. Textbook of Performing Arts Medicine. Edited by RT Satloff, et al. New York: Raven Press, 1991, pp 71–109
18. Hadler M: Industrial rheumatology. Arthritis Rheum 20:1019–1025, 1977
19. Stone E: Repetitive strain injuries. Med J Aust 2:616–618, 1983
20. Maeda K, Hunting W, Grandjean E: Localized fatigue in accounting-machine operators. J Occup Med 22:810–816, 1980
21. McDermott F: Repetition strain injury: a review of current understanding. Med J Aust 14:196–200, 1986

55. NONSTEROIDAL ANTIINFLAMMATORY AGENTS AND CORTICOSTEROIDS

The rheumatic diseases are characterized by varying degrees of tissue damage, inflammation, and loss of normal function, and may be associated with annoying rashes, disabling arthritis, or lethal nephritis or cerebritis. Although scores of distinct rheumatic diseases and syndromes are outlined in this *Primer*, only a few classes of drugs are available to treat them. This chapter will discuss two relatively fast-acting classes of drugs used extensively in the treatment of inflammatory rheumatic diseases: the nonsteroidal antiinflammatory drugs (NSAIDs), including aspirin and other salicylates, and corticosteroids.

Inflammation is the normal protective response to tissue injury and consists of a sequence of events that results in elimination of the injurious agent, healing of the damaged tissue, and restoration of normal function. With a chronic disease such as rheumatoid arthritis (RA), normal inflammation is unable to eliminate the cause of the disease, which is unknown. The inflammatory process is amplified by the products of injured tissue, and possibly by the loss of inhibitory mechanisms, resulting in continued inflammation, progressive tissue injury, disease manifestations, and increasing loss of function (1).

Corticosteroids and NSAIDs differ in the scope and degree to which they inhibit the chronic inflammatory process. By impairing the activity of various natural mediators of inflammation, such as bradykinins, prostaglandins, leukotrienes, and oxygen radicals, NSAIDs and low doses of corticosteroids partially prevent the final expression of inflammation. Because they are acting on terminal events in the inflammatory cascade (see Chapter 7), the benefits of these drugs are quickly evident. If too effective (as with high doses of corticosteroids), their use may be complicated by infections, impaired wound healing, and a general inability of the patient to cope with the environmental insults that are normally controlled by inflammatory mechanisms.

Since these drugs do not prevent tissue injury, it is not surprising that joint damage and other evidence of organ damage may progress during therapy. Although disease modifying properties are sometimes ascribed to corticosteroids, it is generally accepted that their large side effect profile limits long-term use. In this chapter, only the antiinflammatory properties of corticosteroids will be addressed. Sustained drug-induced remission is generally not expected with the short-acting antirheumatic agents, which act distally in the inflammatory cascade.

NONSTEROIDAL ANTIINFLAMMATORY DRUGS

Aspirin is the prototype of the NSAIDs. These agents reduce, but do not completely eliminate, the signs and symptoms of established inflammation. The presence of drug in the blood is associated with a rapid onset of benefit, but exacerbation of signs and symptoms occurs quickly after metabolism or excretion of the drug. Nonsteroidal antiinflammatory drugs have no major effect on the underlying disease process. In addition to their antiinflammatory effects, NSAIDs decrease pain, suppress fever, and decrease platelet adhesiveness, leading to a multitude of short-term and long-term, prescribed and nonprescribed uses. In the United States, available NSAIDs include aspirin, salicyl salicylate, magnesium choline salicylate, other salicylates, ibuprofen, phenylbutazone, indomethacin, sulindac, naproxen, tolmetin, fenoprofen, meclofenamate sodium, diflunisal, piroxicam, ketoprofen, diclofenac, flurbiprofen, etodolac, ketorolac, nabumetone, and oxoprozin (Table 55–1). Many others are under development or available elsewhere (2). Although ketorolac may be given parenterally and indomethacin is also marketed in a rectal suppository form, all other available NSAIDs are administered orally.

With the exception of nabumetone, a pro-drug that is administered as a base, NSAIDs are organic acids and are highly bound to plasma proteins. These properties may enhance drug concentrations in inflamed tissues, which are more permeable to plasma proteins and tend to have a lower pH. These drugs may be classified by their chemical structure, but it is more useful to remember their plasma half-life, which is related to the frequency of administration and in some instances to the occurrence of adverse reactions, especially in the elderly (Table 55–1). They have a broad range of pharmacologic activities. Nonsteroidal antiinflammatory drugs inhibit cyclooxygenase, the enzyme that transforms arachidonic acid via endoperoxides to prostaglandins, prostacyclin, and thromboxanes. Currently available drugs have little effect on lipoxygenase, which transforms arachidonic acid to leukotrienes, although the next generation of NSAIDs may possess this property. Diclofenac has an indirect inhibitory effect on lipoxygenase by stimulating uptake of arachidonic acid into triglycerides, but is predominantly a cyclooxygenase inhibitor. Nonsteroidal antiinflammatory drugs also have been demonstrated to suppress bradykinin release, alter lymphocyte responses, and decrease granulocyte and monocyte migration and

Table 55–1. *Some nonsteroidal antiinflammatory drugs*

Drug	Dose range (mg/day)	Half-life (h)	Doses per day	Gastrointestinal adverse effects*
Hetero carboxylic acids				
Aspirin (acetylsalicylic acid)	1000–6000	4–15	2–4	+++
Magnesium choline salicylate	1500–4000	4–15	2–4	+
Salsalate	1500–5000	4–15	2–4	+
Diflunisal	500–1500	7–15	2	+++
Meclofenamate sodium	200–400	2–3	4	++
Phenylacetic acids				
Ibuprofen	1200–3200	2	3–6	++
Fenoprofen	1200–3200	2	3–4	++
Ketoprofen	100–400	2	3–4	++
Diclofenac	75–150	1–2	2–3	++
Flurbiprofen	100–300	3–4	2–3	++
Naphthaleneacetic acids				
Naproxen	250–1500	13	2	++
Indoleacetic acids				
Indomethacin	50–200	3–11	2–4	+++
Sulindac	300–400	16	2	+++
Etodolac	600–1200	7	3–4	+**
Pyrrolealkanoic acids				
Tolmetin	800–1600	1	4–6	++
Pyrazolidinediones				
Phenylbutazone	200–800	40–80	1–4	++
Oxicams				
Piroxicam	20	30–86	1	+++
Pyrrolo-pyrrole				
Ketorolac (oral and parenteral)	15–150	4–6	4	?†
Naphthylalkanone				
Nabumetone	1000–2000	~24	1–2	+**
Oxazolepropionic acid				
Oxaprozin	600–1200	21–25	1	?**

* + = Mild, no change in drug regimen required; ++ = frequent, may need to add gastro-protective agent; +++ = more frequent and/or severe, often requires withdrawal of the drug.
** Risk not fully established.
† Risk not fully established for parenteral or oral preparations.

phagocytosis, under certain laboratory conditions. Advances in knowledge about specific elements of the inflammatory process now permit the selection of compounds for their ability to suppress specific elements such as cyclooxygenase or lipoxygenase.

Adverse Effects

Although NSAIDs are generally well tolerated, they are associated with a wide spectrum of potential clinical toxicities. None of the NSAIDs is completely safe. The major toxicities occur in the gastrointestinal (GI) tract, central nervous system, hematopoietic system, kidney, skin and liver. Generally, side effects tend to be dose related (3).

Gastrointestinal Effects. Perhaps because of their effects on prostaglandin synthesis, NSAIDs as a group tend to cause gastric irritation and to exacerbate peptic ulcers (4). Suppression of prostaglandin synthesis induced by NSAIDs increases gastric acid production, decreases the production of gastric mucus and bicarbonate, and decreases the rate of cellular proliferation of the gastric mucosa, impairing the normal protective mechanisms of the stomach. They worsen GI bleeding, both by increasing acid production in the stomach and by decreasing platelet adhesiveness. Indomethacin, sulindac, and meclofenamate sodium have an extensive enterohepatic recirculation, which increases GI exposure to these drugs and enhances their toxicity. Firmly compressed regular aspirin tablets may dissolve slowly in the stomach, causing irritation and superficial ulceration of gastric mucosa directly under the undissolved tablet. Ion-trapping of weak organic acids, such as NSAIDs in mucosal cells, leads to back diffusion of hydrogen ions and may result in mucosal damage.

Anticoagulant Effects. Nonsteroidal antiinflammatory drugs may produce two types of anticoagulant effects. Platelet adhesiveness is decreased by inhibiting a prostaglandin-initiated sequence that is necessary for platelet activation. Because platelets lack mitochondria and are unable to synthesize additional cyclooxygenase, acetylation of this enzyme by aspirin irreversibly

decreases platelet aggregation in response to various stimuli. This effect persists for about 10–12 days until the acetylated platelets are replaced by newly produced platelets that have not been exposed to aspirin. This property has led to the use of aspirin in dosages as low as 80 mg/day to prevent platelet aggregation and emboli in patients prone to transient ischemic attacks, but it is also responsible for aspirin-induced enhancement of bleeding due to peptic ulcers or other causes. Cyclooxygenase inhibition by other NSAIDs is reversible. Their platelet effects also are reversible and persist only as long as the drug is present. The second type of anticoagulant effect occurs when protein-bound NSAIDs displace warfarin from plasma protein-binding sites, thus increasing warfarin's anticoagulant effect. This is clinically significant only for phenylbutazone and for salicylates in toxic concentrations.

To avoid excessive bleeding at surgery, aspirin should be stopped two weeks preoperatively, but other NSAIDs need be stopped only long enough to allow for their complete excretion. For example, tolmetin and ibuprofen can be stopped 24 hours preoperatively, because they will be completely excreted and have no effect on platelet adhesiveness at the time of the surgery. Because the nonacetylated salicylates are poor inhibitors of cyclooxygenase, they have little or no effect on platelets and sometimes may be used when other NSAIDs are contraindicated by an excessive risk of bleeding.

Hepatic Effects. Reversible hepatocellular toxicity, characterized by elevations of one or more liver enzymes, has been observed in up to 15% of patients treated with NSAIDs and has been emphasized with diclofenac (5). Transaminase elevations usually revert to normal after discontinuation of the drug and sometimes become normal even when the drug is continued. Rarely, NSAID-induced hepatic dysfunction may be more severe, causing elevation of bilirubin or prolonged prothrombin times, in which case discontinuation of the drug is mandatory. Phenylbutazone-induced hepatocellular cholestasis, and granulomatous hepatitis may be fatal in some patients. In the case of benoxaprofen, failure to recognize early evidence of hepatic toxicity led to fatal hepatorenal syndrome in some patients, resulting in withdrawal of the drug from marketing. Fatal fulminant hepatitis has occurred rarely with other NSAIDs, emphasizing that serum transaminase levels should be checked on a regular basis during treatment with NSAIDs.

Renal Effects. Nonsteroidal antiinflammatory drugs may decrease creatinine clearance and increase creatinine concentrations in some patients predisposed by hypovolemia, impaired renal function, or decreased renal blood flow, probably by suppressing the vasodilatory function of renal prostaglandins. These creatinine elevations sometimes revert to normal even with continued use of the drug, but NSAIDs should be used cautiously in patients with conditions that may impair renal perfusion or function, in patients with decreased circulating blood volume, and in the elderly who are predisposed to these conditions. Use of NSAIDs in rheumatic diseases associated with a high incidence of renal involvement, such as scleroderma and systemic lupus erythematosus (SLE), also deserves caution. Acute interstitial nephritis and the nephrotic syndrome rarely occur with NSAIDs, but the greatest number of cases have been reported with fenoprofen. Most patients recover when the drug is discontinued, but occasionally dialysis or high-dose corticosteroid therapy has been needed to support the patients prior to recovery of renal function (6).

Other Adverse Effects. Other fairly common side effects include various types of skin reactions and rashes (3). Hypersensitivity responses include an aspirin-associated syndrome of rhinitis, nasal polyposis, and asthma. Anaphylaxis has been associated with tolmetin and zomepirac, but it occasionally has occurred with other NSAIDs. Agranulocytosis and aplastic anemia have been reported rarely with a number of NSAIDs, but appear to be more frequent with phenylbutazone and have resulted in a number of deaths, particularly in women over 60 years of age. Salicylates cause blood level-related tinnitus and hearing loss, and overdoses can cause numerous central nervous system manifestations including coma. Headaches occur with indomethacin, and confusion may appear in elderly patients treated with indomethacin, naproxen, or ibuprofen. Aseptic meningitis has occurred rarely in patients with SLE or mixed connective tissue disease who were treated with ibuprofen or other NSAIDs (3).

Pharmacokinetics

In general, currently available NSAIDs are readily and completely absorbed after oral administration, unless enteric coating (to decrease gastric irritation) or encapsulation (to produce sustained release) is used. Aspirin and sulindac have active metabolites with longer half-lives than the parent drugs. Indomethacin, meclofenamate sodium, and sulindac display enterohepatic recirculation. Salicylate and diflunisal exhibit Michalis–Menton kinetics; consequently, the plasma half-life of the drug increases as the plasma concentration increases. Thus, doses need be given less frequently when plasma concentrations are high, and toxic concentrations take much longer to clear than would be anticipated. Nabumetone is a poor inhibitor of prostaglandin synthesis but is rapidly transformed by the liver to an acidic metabolite with potent inhibitory effects. Essentially all available NSAIDs ultimately are converted to inactive metabolites by the liver and are excreted predominantly in urine, although sulindac may also be converted to an inactive metabolite by the kidney. Biliary excretion occurs with some NSAIDs and NSAID metabolites, thus moderate decreases in creatinine clearance prolong plasma clearance of active drug less markedly than would be the case if unmetabolized active drug or active metabolite were cleared only by renal excretion. Nevertheless, dosage reduction and extra care are advisable if NSAIDs are used in elderly patients or those with impaired renal function (2,3).

Aspirin and NSAID Use

It is important to individualize treatment with aspirin and other NSAIDs. Substantial individual variability is present with respect to the pharmacology and pharmacokinetics of these drugs, which also vary in effectiveness in different disorders. In addi-

tion, the optimum dosage varies from one disorder to the next. Simple acute headaches or muscle aches, for example, can be treated with intermittent low or moderate doses of acetaminophen, aspirin, or ibuprofen, which are available without prescription. Similar dosing with ibuprofen is particularly useful for menstrual cramps. Osteoarthritis may require more prolonged therapy, but generally moderate doses are sufficient. Patients with RA or other types of chronic inflammatory arthritis usually need prolonged treatment with maximum tolerated doses and receive little or no benefit from acetaminophen.

The NSAIDs are usually thought to be more effective than the salicylates for acute gout, acute bursitis, and spondylarthropathies such as ankylosing spondylitis and Reiter's syndrome. Indomethacin is often tried first in these conditions and is usually remarkably effective, although relatively high doses are needed and intolerance is fairly common. Other NSAIDs are also effective, but phenylbutazone is used only if the others fail, because of its greater risk of potentially fatal bone marrow suppression. As potential second-line agents for the treatment of spondylarthropathies become available, such as sulfasalazine, the role of phenylbutazone will become minimal.

Aspirin or NSAIDs are commonly used in the treatment of RA. The selection of a particular agent depends on a patient's medical history, such as a history of bleeding or of GI intolerance, and on the personal preference of the prescribing physician. Enteric-coated aspirin and nonacetylated salicylates tend to be better tolerated than plain aspirin. When salicylates are used, dose is adjusted to achieve a serum salicylate level of 20–30 mg/dl (200–300 mcg/ml); however, drug levels of other NSAIDs are rarely used. If the patient has insufficient benefit or intolerable toxicity to a specific NSAID, another NSAID is often substituted, usually at a moderate dose to establish tolerance. The dose is then cautiously increased to the maximum recommended or tolerated level and continued for at least two weeks at that dose. Insufficient efficacy or intolerance may prompt additional therapeutic trials of other NSAIDs until the patient has achieved satisfactory control of the inflammation with tolerable side effects (2).

There is little evidence to suggest that combinations of salicylate and NSAIDs, or one NSAID with another, are more beneficial than single drug therapy. Furthermore, toxicity is probably additive (7).

Caution is advised in prescribing NSAIDs to the elderly; to patients with peptic ulcer disease, impairment of renal or hepatic function, congestive heart failure, or hypertension; and to those being treated with anticoagulants, oral hypoglycemics, or other drugs that may interact with the NSAID. Patients should be followed especially closely during introduction of an NSAID, when doses are increased, or when the patient's condition changes (3).

Even optimal use of NSAIDs does not completely suppress all evidence of inflammation, particularly in chronic RA. If the patient with RA does not develop a spontaneous remission within a number of months, a slow-acting antirheumatic drug should be added to the continuing NSAID therapy (see Chapter 10C).

CORTICOSTEROIDS

Immune-driven inflammation underlies most of the clinical manifestations of rheumatic disease. Therapeutic administration of corticosteroid produces rapid, potent, and reliable (albeit evanescent) suppression of inflammation, the extent and duration of which depends on the dose, dosing schedule, and length of treatment. The marked attenuating effect of corticosteroids on inflammation had led at one time to the mistaken conclusion that corticosteroids were a cure for RA. This unsurpassed short-term efficacy and versatility have made corticosteroids a key element in the treatment of many rheumatic diseases.

Pharmacology and Mechanisms of Action

Orally administered corticosteroids are well absorbed, although prednisone and cortisone require activation by the liver. In plasma, corticosteroids bind primarily to the alpha-globulin transcortin, while a small portion binds to albumin. Corticosteroids enter target cells and couple with a specific cytoplasmic receptor before transfer to the nucleus where the corticosteroid-receptor complex binds to chromatin and modulates protein synthesis (8). Corticosteroids decrease collagen synthesis and impair wound healing; augment hepatic gluconeogenesis and glycogen deposition, while inhibiting the action of insulin; impair lipogenesis and stimulate lipolysis in adipose tissue; and increase liver synthesis of protein while enhancing peripheral catabolism. Corticosteroids have a profound effect on bone metabolism through interference with intestinal absorption of calcium, inhibition of osteoblast collagen synthesis, elevation of parathyroid hormone levels resulting in amplification of osteoclast bone resorption, and enhanced renal calcium excretion.

The mechanism by which corticosteroids achieve a profound short-term effect on inflammation is not completely understood, but they may interrupt the inflammatory and immune cascade at several levels including: 1) impairment of antigen opsonization; 2) interference with inflammatory cell adhesion and migration through vascular endothelium; 3) interruption of cell–cell communication by alteration of release or antagonism of cytokines; 4) impairment of leukotriene and prostaglandin synthesis; and 5) inhibition of neutrophil superoxide production (9). Corticosteroids decrease immunoglobulin generation, inhibit immune clearance of sensitized erythrocytes, and impair the transit of immune complexes across basement membranes (10).

Physiologic corticosteroid production and release by the adrenal glands is one mechanism by which the body contains the inflammatory cascade. In a way, the clinical application of corticosteroids to inflammatory disease is an effort to imitate the mediating effects of endogenous corticosteroid production. Based on animal models of arthritis, some investigators have hypothesized that abnormal function of the pituitary–adrenal axis may be a factor in susceptibility to some forms of inflammatory arthritis (11).

Imprecision exists in our current techniques of corticosteroid use. Pharmacologic corticosteroids are mono-agents with a fixed ratio of various effects on mineral and glucose metabolism and on inflammation, whereas adrenal output has multiple control facets and a level of responsiveness that is not achievable by exogenous means. Since we lack the ability to fine-tune corticosteroid delivery, the dose required to abate an inflammatory process in the body might be substantially lower if corticosteroids could be delivered in a short burst to appropriate sites at critical points in the propagation of inflammation. Even in an individual with rheumatic disease, however, inflammation is important in the repair and defense mechanisms of the body. The lack of precision in prescribing corticosteroids and the consequent administration of higher than necessary doses for long periods of time leads to generalized suppression and the development of unwanted side-effects.

Pharmacodynamics

Cortisol, a 17-hydroxy corticoid compound secreted by the adrenal cortex, is the prototype for the available synthetic corticosteroids. Minor structural modifications of this parent hormone have led to the creation of a panel of drugs with a wide spectrum of plasma half-lives, antiinflammatory potency, and mineralocorticoid effect (Table 55–2). Unlike NSAIDs in which plasma half-life correlates well with dosing and side effects, corticosteroids have biologic half-lives that are 2–36 times longer than their plasma half-lives. In addition, the onset of biologic effect lags behind peak plasma levels. Corticosteroids are rapidly and widely distributed in tissues. They cross the placenta poorly with fetal concentrations varying between approximately 10%, for prednisone and prednisolone, to 30%, for betamethasone and hydrocortisone, of that in the maternal circulation (12).

Corticosteroids may increase the clearance of aspirin (13) and occasionally increase the dose of warfarin needed for therapeutic anticoagulation; consequently, during corticosteroid tapering, dose reductions for both medications may be necessary. Diuretics and amphotericin may augment the potassium-wasting effect of corticosteroids. Since a portion of circulating corticosteroid is bound with low affinity to albumin, the development of hypoal-

Table 55–2. Characteristics of some available corticosteroid preparations

Drug	Relative Antiinflammatory Potency	Equivalent Dose (mg)	Sodium Retaining Potency	Biologic Half-life (hours)
Short-acting				
Hydrocortisone	1	20	2+	8–12
Cortisone	0.8	25	2+	8–12
Prednisone	4	5	1+	12–36
Prednisolone	4	5	1+	12–36
Methylprednisolone	5	4	0	12–36
Triamcinolone	5	4	0	12–36
Long-acting				
Betamethasone	20–30	0.6	0	36–54
Dexamethasone	20–30	0.75	0	36–54

buminemia can be associated with elevations in free plasma corticosteroid and potentially increased efficacy and toxicity. Drugs that stimulate hepatic enzymes may decrease the half-life of corticosteroids. Corticosteroids may interfere with vaccination therapy resulting in a truncated antibody response to inactivated vaccines, or in the case of live attenuated vaccines, to growth of the organism in the patient. Because delayed hypersensitivity type reactions are impaired, skin testing to antigens such as tuberculosis may be falsely negative.

Dosing Regimens

Because of the multitude of corticosteroid preparations and dosing regimens and the great variety of clinical applications, significant medical art is required to sagely prescribe corticosteroids in rheumatic disease. Several different strategies exist, and many preparations with various half-lives are available. In general, increasing doses and dosing frequencies of corticosteroids correspond to enhanced inflammatory suppression, more rapid onset of therapeutic benefit, and increased side effects. Thus doses given several times a day are more potent than once-a-day dosing, which is in turn more efficacious than every other day use. Intramuscular and intravenous corticosteroid preparations are used initially to circumvent delayed absorption following oral administration. Choices of therapeutic regimen are often made in an attempt to minimize toxicity while providing sufficient antiinflammatory effect to modify disease activity. When disease control is required in a timely but non-urgent manner, daily oral dosing, given in the morning to minimize adrenal suppression, is adequate. In the face of active rheumatic disease requiring more rapid but non-emergent control, administration of daily corticosteroid in a split dose given 2 to 4 doses per day yields a more rapid onset and greater degree of antiinflammatory effect. If the dosing interval is substantially longer than the biologic half-life, as when prednisone is given every 48 hours, nearly normal hypophyseal–pituitary–adrenal function is maintained, avoiding some of the risks of daily therapy. Alternate-day prednisone often can be used to maintain disease suppression in chronic therapy, but more intensive dosage schedules are usually required initially to achieve control of the disease process.

In rheumatic diseases that require rapid amelioration of damaging inflammation, treatment can be initiated with a short course or even single treatment of high-dose corticosteroid. Pulse therapy with intravenous methylprednisolone, 1000 mg infused over 30–45 minutes, given daily for one to three days has proven efficacy in the treatment of SLE, vasculitis, and RA (14,15). At such suprapharmacologic doses, profound effects on lymphocyte function may occur leading to a prolonged effect on disease activity. By virtue of this purported durable effect, lower oral daily or alternate-day corticosteroid may be acceptable in maintaining disease suppression than would otherwise be necessary. Furthermore, repeated pulses given once a month, may allow oral maintenance corticosteroid to be more efficiently reduced. A three-day course of daily intravenous methylprednisolone given once a month during the initial phases of life- or organ-threatening diseases, such as vasculitis and SLE, is often useful in bringing about rapid control and in lowering maintenance corticoste-

Table 55–3. *Corticosteroid dosing regimens*

Regimen	Indication	Rationale	Relative Efficacy*	Relative Side-Effects*
Oral				
Once daily low dose (≤10 mg prednisone)	Maintenance therapy	"Physiologic" dose Suppress symptoms	+	+
Alternate day moderate dose (>10 mg prednisone)	Non-symptomatic manifestations of mild to moderate disease; maintenance therapy	Some adverse reactions lessened Less adrenal suppression	+ +	+
Once daily moderate† to high dose	Control of active disease	Effective in many rheumatic diseases Less adverse reactions than split dose	+ +	+ +
Split daily dose	Rapid control of active disease	Increased efficacy over equivalent single dose	+ + +	+ + +
'Mini-pulse'‡	Rapid control of severe disease	More rapid control Possibly allows lower maintenance	+ + +	+ +
Parenteral				
Intramuscular Depo-steroids	Limited use as rescue (targeted injections preferred)	Temporary disease control	+ +	+ +
Intravenous pulse	Severe/emergent life or organ-threatening disease	Rapid control of severe disease; possibly decreases maintenance	+ + + +	+ + + +

* Efficacy and side effects vary with the dose given
† Given in morning to minimize adrenal suppression
‡ e.g. 100–200 mg/day prednisone for 2 to 5 days

roid. High-dose corticosteroid pulses have additional or more frequent toxicities that need to be considered in the evaluation of an individual. Alternatively, the use of mini-pulses of oral prednisone (100 mg–200 mg/day) for several days at the beginning of treatment or with subsequent flares may also expedite disease control (16). Table 55–3 provides a summary and an interpretation of the different corticosteroid regimens.

Adverse Reactions

As might be expected when a hormone with many potential target organs is used at pharmacologic doses, wide-spread unwanted effects are encountered (17). The severity of these side effects depends on the maximum dose, duration of treatment or cumulative dose, and on the type of corticosteroid used.

Available corticosteroid preparations all affect bone metabolism by decreasing calcium absorption from the GI tract and by inhibiting osteoblast collagen production leading to loss of bone mass. Especially in the context of rheumatic diseases, which hasten calcium loss from bone by virtue of disuse and immobilization, juxtaarticular hyperemia, and the release of various cytokines, accelerated osteoporosis with pathologic fractures can occur. Supplemental calcium and vitamin D may slow this process, but cannot prevent it. New preparations of corticosteroids currently under development such as deflazacort may prove to offer long-term antiinflammatory benefit with less risk of steroid-induced osteoporosis (18). Alternate-day corticosteroids probably do not decrease the risk of osteoporosis, cumulative dose being equal.

Exogenous administration of corticosteroids can shut down native adrenal corticosteroid production through effects on the pituitary–adrenal axis. Without the ability to increase corticosteroid production in the face of stressors, such as injury, infection, or surgery, Addisonian crisis and shock may develop. The chances of developing adrenal suppression increase as 1) doses exceed the average daily equivalent output of the adrenal glands of 5.0–7.5 mg prednisone, 2) therapy continues for more than a few weeks or months, 3) doses are given late in the day or in split doses, or 4) with the use of long-acting corticosteroid preparations. Alternate-day dosing with prednisone or prednisolone does lessen the risk of adrenal suppression, but cases exist of adrenal insufficiency developing in patients on alternate-day treatment.

Similarly, adrenal suppression can sometimes develop with short courses and low doses of corticosteroid. If doubt exists, an adrenocorticotropic hormone stimulation test, metapyrone test, or other endocrinologic assays may be useful in determining if pituitary and adrenal functions are preserved, before discontinuation of corticosteroid treatment.

The inhibitory effect of corticosteroids on inflammatory and immune responses, which makes them so efficacious in the treatment of autoimmune driven inflammatory disease, also results in increased risk of bacterial and opportunistic infections such as tuberculosis, *pneumocystis carinii*, and fungi. Effects on glucose and protein metabolism may cause hyperglycemia, centripetal fat deposition leading to rounded facies and a cervical fat pad, and hyperlipidemia. Corticosteroids, especially those preparations with significant mineralocorticoid effect (Table 55–2) or any used in high dosages can create electrolyte abnormalities such as hypokalemia; fluid retention causing edema; and hypertension. Cutaneous problems include capillary fragility resulting in petechiae and easy bruisability, acne, hirsutism, impaired wound healing, hyperhidrosis, and striae. Glaucoma and cataract formation complicate corticosteroid use.

Long-term treatment may lead to weakness from steroid myopathy that can be confused with reactivation of disease in myositis patients. Gastric ulcer and gastritis are significant risks with high-dose or long-term corticosteroid use, and may be synergistic with NSAIDs. Pancreatitis can also occur. In pediatric cases, long-term daily corticosteroid use adversely affects growth through inhibition of growth hormone production and antagonism of its actions. Accelerated atherosclerosis is a significant long-term problem as corticosteroid therapy stretches into years or even decades, and may especially develop at sites of vascular endothelial damage induced by vasculitis or SLE.

Often adverse reactions of corticosteroids, which may be more prominent with high-dose and intravenous pulse therapy, include dissemination of previously localized infections, osteonecrosis, psychiatric disturbances, and bowel or diverticular perforations. Sudden death ensuing after high-dose intravenous corticosteroids may be related to unrecognized electrolyte imbalances and rapid shifts of ions. High-dose corticosteroids can mask the symptoms of other inflammatory processes, such as abscesses or bowel perforation, making diagnosis difficult.

Corticosteroid Use

Once the decision to use corticosteroids is made, the treatment regimen derives from a consideration of the individual patient, the specific disease process being treated, and concomitant illnesses, for example, diabetes or hypertension, as well as the relative advantages and disadvantages of the various corticosteroid preparations and dosing regimens. For self-limited processes such as allergic reactions, the choice and tapering schedule are not as vital as with chronic rheumatic diseases. In attempting to balance the untoward effects of long-term corticosteroid use with effective and prolonged suppression of rheumatic disease, some key points need to be kept in mind. The desired dose is the minimum necessary to suppress disease activity; however, this value may not be readily apparent, especially as disease activity fluctuates and the duration of therapy lengthens. Occasionally changes in laboratory parameters such as erythrocyte sedimentation rate as in polymyalgia rheumatica, creatine kinase as in polymyositis, or anti-double-stranded-DNA and complement levels as in SLE may be harbingers of rising disease activity, but usually it is the physician's clinical impression that must be utilized.

Tapering should be gradual to avoid major flares of disease that would necessitate an increase in corticosteroid dose or frequency, thus negating previous gains in lowering the corticosteroid dose. In this way, overzealous dose reductions may result in a paradoxical prolongation of corticosteroid treatment, increasing its toxicity. Abrupt decreases or withdrawal of corticosteroids from RA patients who are on even minimal doses is frequently marked by a flare of arthritis. At the upper levels of corticosteroid doses (>40 mg/day prednisone or equivalent), dose reductions can be made in decrements of 10 mg every few days to weeks, whereas such rapid decrements when the dosage is below 40 mg/day, and especially below 20 mg/day, could invite exacerbation. Consequently, serial reductions of 2.5–5.0 mg/day every few weeks to months (even 1.0–0.5 mg decrements in RA patients) should be chosen in certain chronic inflammatory diseases when daily doses drop below 20 mg/day. In general, dose reduction should not be more frequent than the time required to detect a steroid dose-related exacerbation of disease activity; this can be as short as a few days with RA, or as long as one to two months with polymyositis or lupus nephritis. With doses below 10 mg/day, the reduction interval must be long enough to allow recovery of adrenal function, and the interval increases with the duration of corticosteroid therapy.

Occasionally, alternate-day dosing can be initiated from the outset (19) or rapidly achieved by only reducing the alternate-day dose, such as tapering from 60 mg/day to 60 mg every other day, if disease is easily controlled. This is a preferable dose schedule since the risks of adrenal suppression, growth retardation, and Cushingoid changes are lessened (19); however, alternate-day dosing is generally utilized later in the treatment course, after initial control of acute inflammation. A clue that alternate-day dosing may be inadequate for a given patient is the subjective report by the patient that symptoms worsen at the end of the day when no corticosteroid is taken.

Concomitant illnesses or previous adverse reactions may further direct corticosteroid choice and dosing schedule. A patient with diabetes may experience less hyperglycemia on an alternate-day schedule. A patient with known hypertension may better tolerate a corticosteroid that has lower mineralocorticoid effect. High doses of corticosteroid or pulses may be relatively contraindicated in a patient with osteonecrosis or in someone with recent surgical wounds in the process of healing.

Given the diversity of the recognized rheumatic diseases, treatment approaches have arisen that are tailored to each disease entity. Specific corticosteroid treatment approaches for each rheumatic disease are discussed in individual chapters dealing with each disorder.

Harold E. Paulus, MD
Ken J. Bulpitt, MD

1. Paulus HE: Antirheumatic drugs, Internal Medicine, 3rd ed. Edited by Stein JH. Boston, Little Brown, 1990, pp 1789–1795
2. Paulus HE, Furst DE: Aspirin and other nonsteroidal antiinflammatory drugs, Arthritis and Allied Conditions, 11th ed. Edited by McCarty Jr DJ. Philadelphia, Lea and Febiger, 1989, pp 507–543
3. Schlegel SI, Paulus HE: Nonsteroidal antiinflammatory drugs—use in rheumatic disease, side effects and interactions. Bull Rheum Dis 36:1–8, 1986
4. Schoen RT, Vender RJ: Mechanisms of nonsteroidal antiinflammatory drug-induced gastric damage. Am J Med 86:449–458, 1989
5. Katz LM, Love PY: NSAIDs and the liver, Clinical Applications of NSAIDs, Subpopulation Therapy and New Formulations. Edited by Famaey JP, Paulus HE. New York, Marcel Dekker, 1992, pp 247–263
6. Blackshear JL, Napier JS, Davidman M, et al: Renal complications of nonsteroidal antiinflammatory drugs. Arch Intern Med 143:1130–1134, 1985
7. Furst DE, Blocka K, Cassell S, et al: A controlled study of concurrent therapy with a nonacetylated salicylate and naproxen in rheumatoid arthritis. Arthritis Rheum 30:146–154, 1987
8. Chan L, O'Malley BW: Steroid hormone action: recent advances. Ann Intern Med 89:694–701, 1978
9. Weiss MM: Corticosteroids in rheumatoid arthritis. Semin Arthritis Rheum 19:9–21, 1989
10. Parrillo JE, Fauci AS: Mechanisms of glucocorticoid action on immune processes. Ann Rev Pharmacol Toxicol 19:179–201, 1979
11. Wilder RL, Sternberg EM: Neuroendocrine hormonal factors in rheumatoid arthritis and related conditions. Curr Opin Rheumatol 2:436–40, 1990
12. Turner ES, Greenberger PA, Patterson R: Management of the pregnant asthmatic patient. Ann Intern Med 6:905–918, 1980
13. Furst DE: Clinically Important interactions of nonsteroidal antiinflammatory drugs with other medications. J Rheumatol 15(suppl 17):58–62, 1988
14. Ballou SP, Khan MA, Kushner I: Intravenous pulse methylprednisolone followed by alternate day corticosteroid therapy in lupus erythematosus: a prospective evaluation. J Rheumatol 12:944–948, 1985
15. Neumann V, Hopkins R, Dixon J, et al: Combination therapy with pulsed methylprednisolone in rheumatoid arthritis. Ann Rheum Dis 44:747–751, 1985
16. Iglehart IW, Sutton JD, Bender JC, et al: Intravenous pulsed steroids in rheumatoid arthritis: a comparative dose study. J Rheumatol 17:159–162, 1990
17. Gallant C, Kenny P: Oral glucocorticoids and their complications. J Am Acad Dermatol 14:61–177, 1986
18. Gray ES, Doherty SM, Galloway J, et al: A double-blind study of deflazacort and prednisone in patients with chronic inflammatory disorders. Arthritis Rheum 34:287–295, 1991
19. Axelrod L: Glucocorticoids, Textbook of Rheumatology, 4th ed. Edited by WN Kelley, ED Harris Jr, S Ruddy, CB Sledge. Philadelphia, WB Saunders, 1993, pp 779–796

56. SLOW-ACTING ANTIRHEUMATIC DRUGS AND CYTOTOXIC AGENTS

The treatment of rheumatoid arthritis (RA) and other systemic rheumatic diseases has changed significantly over the last 20 years. The variety of drugs available has increased dramatically, and in RA there is a greater appreciation of the need to treat early before cartilage damage occurs (see Chapter 10). The appreciation that these erosions occur early in the disease (1) has led to a much more aggressive approach to treatment with the early use of slow-acting antirheumatic drugs (SAARDs) (2).

Especially if SAARDs are to be used at an early stage in disease, however, it is important that their potential adverse effects are recognized. Treatment should be chosen to provide maximum benefit to the patient without harm. In using SAARDs and cytotoxic therapies, it is important to try to answer three questions: 1) What drugs are available? 2) Is there a rationale for choosing one drug over another? 3) How do we tell whether the drug is working or producing adverse reactions?

The question of which drug to use in an individual will be influenced by a number of factors. For example, rheumatoid patients with low-grade early synovitis will often be started on antimalarials or sulfasalazine, while those with more aggressive disease (such as synovitis plus extraarticular manifestations) might be started on low-dose methotrexate or gold. Patients with

Table 56–1. *Some mechanisms of action of SAARDs*

Antimalarials	Inhibition of lysosomal enzymes
Chloroquine	Inhibits PMN and lymphocyte responses (in vitro)
Hydroxychloroquine	Inhibits IL–1 release (in vivo)
Sulfasalazine	Inhibits PMN migration
	Reduces lymphocyte responses
	Inhibits angiogenesis
D-Penicillamine	Inhibits neovascularisation (in vitro)
	Inhibits PMN myeloperoxidase
	Scavenges free radicals
	Inhibits T cell function
	Impairs antigen presentation
Gold	Inhibits PMN function
	Inhibition of T and B cell activity
	Inhibits macrophage activation (in vitro)
Methotrexate	Decreases thymiolate synthetase
	Activity and subsequent DNA synthesis
	Diminishes PMN chemotaxis
Azathioprine	Interferes with DNA synthesis
	Inhibits lymphocyte proliferation
Cyclophosphamide	Crosslinks DNA leading to cell death
	Decreases circulating T and B cells
Chlorambucil	Similar to cyclophosphamide
Cyclosporin A	Blocks synthesis/release of IL–1 and IL–2

systemic lupus erythematosus (SLE) who have predominantly skin and joint problems generally will start on antimalarials with an effort to avoid corticosteroids and cytotoxics. Sulfasalazine may be an initial choice more often in reactive arthritis. Felson et al (3) has recently reported a meta-analysis of randomized controlled trials of SAARDs in RA demonstrating little difference in efficacy between methotrexate, injectable gold, D-penicillamine and sulfasalazine. Auranofin and hydroxychloroquine, on the other hand, were significantly less effective.

Some rheumatologists are using SAARDs with corticosteroids early in RA, hoping to reduce or cease the corticosteroid once synovitis is controlled. Although these approaches seem theoretically sensible, efficacy and safety of these regimens remain unproven due to the lack of controlled studies. The following is a discussion of the clinical pharmacology of commonly used individual agents. Their mechanisms of action are complex, and none has a single effect (Table 56–1).

ANTIMALARIALS

Hydroxychloroquine and chloroquine have been used in the treatment of connective tissue diseases since the early 1950s. The pharmacokinetics of both are characterized by extensive accumulation in tissues and large volumes of distribution leading to very long half-lives. It might take three to four months before steady state plasma concentrations are reached, which may explain some of the delayed action (3). The optimal therapeutic concentration for hydroxychloroquine has not yet been established, although plasma concentrations in RA of 700–2,100 ng/ml have been proposed. Antimalarials have been shown to be effective in RA and to suppress both musculoskeletal and systemic manifestations of systemic lupus erythematosus (4). Chloroquine seems to be no different from hydroxychloroquine in reducing symptoms, but is associated with a higher incidence of side effects. Major adverse reactions include indigestion, skin rash, visual disturbance, and retinopathy, although retinal toxicity is extremely rare at currently recommended doses (5 mg/kg/day chloroquine diphosphate and 7.5 mg/kg/day hydroxychloroquine sulfate). Fundoscopic examination and visual field testing are recommended every six months (Table 56–2). Quinacrine is another antimalarial most often used for cutaneous SLE.

D-PENICILLAMINE

D-penicillamine forms disulfides and acts as a metal chelator. Its multiple mechanisms of action include reduction in immunoglobulin synthesis by monocytes and lymphocytes, inhibition of

polymorphonuclear leucocyte and T lymphocyte function, and possible protection of tissues through oxygen radical damage (5). D-penicillamine is rapidly absorbed and converted into disulfides or inorganic sulphates. The oral bioavailability is decreased by food, antacids, and iron supplements. The drug has a relatively short half-life of between two and seven hours. D-penicillamine is effective in RA in doses between 600–1500 mg/day, although the higher dose is associated with a significant increase in side effects. There is conflicting data as to whether D-penicillamine prevents joint erosions in RA. More than 25% of patients taking D-penicillamine will have to discontinue the drug because of side effects within the first 12 months. The major adverse reactions include skin rashes, proteinuria, hematuria, neutropenia, thrombocytopenia, and a variety of autoimmune phenomena including the induction of antinuclear antibodies and drug-induced lupus, Goodpasture's syndrome, and myasthenia gravis. Some of these adverse reactions are seen more frequently in patients who demonstrate slow sulfoxidation. Also, there may be some association with HLA–DR3 and –B8. D-penicillamine should be started in doses of between 125–250 mg/day and increased to a maximum of 750 mg/day over a period of a few months. When disease is controlled the dose can be reduced, but most patients will suffer an exacerbation of their symptoms if the drug is stopped (6). While taking D-penicillamine, patients need to have regular blood and urine tests as outlined in Table 56–2.

SULFASALAZINE

Although sulfasalazine was initially developed as an antirheumatic drug, it was not until the last 10 years that efficacy in RA and the seronegative spondylarthropathies was recognized (7). Sulfasalazine interferes with a variety of cellular and mediator aspects of inflammation. The drug is split by colonic bacteria into its two component parts—sulfapyridine and 5–amino salicyclic acid (5–ASA). 5–ASA is poorly absorbed, while sulfapyridine (the active component) is metabolized in the liver by acetylation. In the treatment of RA, sulfasalazine is significantly better than placebo, and there is some suggestion that it may slow the development of bony erosions. Sulfasalazine would seem to have similar efficacy to gold and D-penicillamine, although comparative clinical trials have not been of sufficient power to demonstrate differences. Up to 50% of patients on sulfasalazine develop side effects and, in the majority of cases, these occur within the first four months of treatment (8). In only one-half of these cases, however, will the adverse effect be sufficient to discontinue the drug. Side effects include skin rashes, nausea, abdominal pain, hepatic enzyme abnormalities, central nervous system disturbances, and blood dyscrasias, particularly in patients who have

Table 56–2. *Suggested regimen for monitoring SAARD therapy*

Antimalarials	Regular visual assessment—fundoscopic examination, visual field evaluation or use of AMSLER grid
Sulfasalazine	CBC, LFTs, biweekly to monthly for three months, then every 1 to 3 months
D-Penicillamine	CBC and urinalysis biweekly on initiating or changing dose, then 1–3 monthly
Gold compounds—	
Injectable	CBC, urinalysis prior to each injection initially, then prior to every second or third injection. Urinalysis monitored by patient.
Oral	CBC, urinalysis biweekly to monthly.
Methotrexate	CBC, LFTs biweekly, then 1–3 monthly.
Cyclophosphamide	CBC and urinalysis monthly after initial weekly tests.
Azathioprine	CBC 1–2 weekly initially, then 1–3 monthly LFTs 1–3 monthly
Chlorambucil	CBC biweekly to monthly initially, then 3 monthly
Cyclosporin A	CBC, serum creatinine, blood pressure weekly, then 2–4 weekly on maintenance dose.

Table 56–3. *Predominant toxicities associated with SAARDs*

	Mucocutaneous	Hematologic	Gastrointestinal	Hepatic	Renal	Lung	Malignancy
Hydroxychloroquine	+	+	++	–	–	–	–
Sulfasalazine	++	++	++	++	–	–	–
D-penicillamine	+++	++	++	+	++	+	–
Oral Gold	+	+	+++	+	+	–	–
Parenteral Gold	+++	++	+	+	++	+	–
Azathioprine	+	++	++	++	–	–	+
Methotrexate	–	+	+++	++	–	+	–
Cyclophosphamide	–	+++	++	–	–	–	++
Chlorambucil	–	+++	+	–	–	–	++
Cyclosporin	–	+	+++	+	++	–	?

N.B. – → +++ = No association → Strong association

glucose-6 phosphate dehydrogenase deficiency. Oligospermia also occurs as does discoloration of urine and sweat. Monitoring of liver function and blood counts need to be much more vigilant during the first three to four months of therapy (Table 56–2).

GOLD

Sulfydryl-containing organic gold compounds have been used since the early 1920s for the treatment of RA. They are also effective in juvenile chronic arthritis and psoriatic arthritis. The gold complexes fall into two major groups: water soluble thiolates or the fat soluble phosphine derivative (9). The chemistry of gold compounds is complex; it is still not quite clear in what form gold circulates in the body. Gold compounds interfere with lymphocyte, monocyte, and neutrophil function, as well as with immunoglobulin and antibody production. The metabolites of gold compounds circulate in the blood primarily bound to plasma proteins, but significant concentrations of gold also are found within the red cells. Gold is eliminated very slowly from the body, with significant tissue concentrations being found 20 years after the last dose.

Plasma concentrations vary significantly between patients, but are of the order of 300 μg/100 ml when patients are stabilized on a 50 mg/week regimen. Aurothioglucose (an oily complex) is absorbed slightly more slowly than aurothiomalate following intramuscular injection. Gold is taken up more quickly by inflamed tissues, particularly the macrophage. The half-life of both oral and intramuscular gold compounds is long (Table 56–3), but accumulation of gold in patients on auranofin is slightly less than those on intramuscular gold. Injectable gold complexes have been shown to be significantly better than placebo in patients with RA, although the change in disease activity measures such as functional capacity, grip strength, and active joint count are relatively modest (10). Injectable gold compounds are of similar efficacy to other SAARDs, including D-penicillamine, sulfasalazine, azathioprine, and methotrexate (11). Few patients remain on gold therapy for longer than five years, due to lack of or loss of efficacy and adverse reactions. Auranofin has been shown to be better than placebo but slightly less effective than injectable gold complexes, D-penicillamine, methotrexate, and sulfasalazine. However, it has a lower incidence of toxicity. Injectable gold complexes are used in doses of between 10–50 mg/week. Frequency of injections is reduced once a total dose of 1 g has been given. Doses of auranofin are between 3–6 mg/day with side effects being dose-related.

Adverse reactions to gold complexes are major reasons for discontinuation of therapy. Auranofin has few serious adverse reactions, although diarrhea is dose-related. Mucocutaneous reactions, proteinuria, and thrombocytopenia are also seen. Skin rashes and mouth ulcers are also commonly seen with intramuscular gold, while blood dyscrasias, proteinuria, and pulmonary complications are rare but potentially lethal. Patients on intramuscular gold treatment should be monitored very carefully for hematologic and renal adverse events with a complete blood count and urinalysis for protein and blood being done at regular intervals, if not before each injection. Eosinophilia may predict adverse reactions. A significant number of people developing severe blood dyscrasias on gold therapy show a progressive fall in their white cell or platelet count prior to developing a signifi-

cant problem. There is still wide variation in the practice of rheumatologists regarding monitoring strategies. Liang and Fries (12) have suggested the following strategy: 1) patient to fill in questionnaire on side effects prior to each injection; 2) weekly white cell and platelet count with monthly complete blood count; 3) dip stick urinalysis for blood and protein (performed by patient before each injection); and 4) monthly review by physician.

In a recent survey of the efficacy of gold compounds (9), Champion, et al concluded that doses in the range 10–50 mg/week for one to two years are more effective than placebo, and that dose response relationships in the range of 10–150 mg/week have not been established. The most commonly used regimen after test doses is 50 mg/week up to a total of 1,000 mg or dramatic improvement. Doses are spread out when apparent maximum improvement is achieved. Excellent clinical response occurs in 20% to 35% of patients and peaks at 6–12 months, but only one-half of these patients maintain this response after 12 months.

METHOTREXATE

Methotrexate is an analogue of folic acid and aminopterin and inhibits dihydrofolate reductase thereby impairing DNA synthesis (13). Low doses are rapidly absorbed after oral administration. The parent compound and metabolites circulate bound to serum albumin. Methotrexate is oxidized to an active metabolite 7-hydroxy methotrexate, and metabolites and parent drug accumulate in the liver as polyglutamates. Methotrexate is eliminated from the body by the kidneys and through biliary excretion in the feces. In doses of 7.5–20 mg/week methotrexate has been shown to be better than placebo and equal to or slightly better than azathioprine, penicillamine, antimalarials, and gold. Tugwell et al (14) have performed a meta-analysis of clinical trials with methotrexate showing that the drug works relatively rapidly (within one to two months) with peak efficacy at six months. Recent studies suggest that patients with RA will remain on methotrexate for a longer period of time than with other SAARDs (15).

Adverse effects provide the major concern with long-term methotrexate use (Table 56–4). Anorexia and nausea, particularly in the 24 hours after dosing, are quite common, but can be reduced or eliminated without affecting antiinflammatory activities by co-prescribing folic acid. Liver enzymes show transient elevation in up to 60% of cases, but this does not correlate with the development of hepatic fibrosis. Although the incidence of moderate fibrosis is very low, there is still some concern with long-term use since fibrosis does seem to correlate with the concentration of methotrexate and its metabolites in hepatic tissues. The question of when, or if, to biopsy the liver in patients on long-term methotrexate has still not been answered. The decision has to be made on an individual basis and determined by previous hepatic disease, length of time on and dose of methotrexate, and other risk factors. Pulmonary hypersensitivity associated with severe hypoxia has been reported and is usually reversible on drug withdrawal. Patients taking methotrexate should have regular liver function tests and complete blood counts.

Table 56-4. *Side effects of methotrexate*

	Frequency	Management
Gastrointestinal		
Abdominal Pain	+++	Temporary withdrawal
Nausea	+++	Usually allows tolerance at a
Diarrhea	+	lower dose in addition to
Stomatitis	+++	folate therapy
Hepatotoxicity		
Abnormal Enzymes	+++	Temporary withdrawal
Hepatic Fibrosis	+	
Hematologic		
Macrocytosis	+++	
Neutropenia	+	Cease
Pancytopenia	+	Cease
Skin		
Alopecia/Rash	++	Dose modification
Renal		
Proteinuria	+	
Respiratory		
Pneumonitis	+	Withdraw
Risk of Infection		
Herpes Zoster	+	

N.B. + = Rare <5%
++ = 5-15%
+++ = >15%

AZATHIOPRINE

Azathioprine is an oral purine analogue that interferes with the synthesis of adenosine and guanine. It has to be metabolized to an active component that interferes with DNA synthesis, particularly in rapidly dividing cells. Approximately one-half of the oral dose is absorbed. Azathioprine has a plasma half-life of approximately 60 to 90 minutes resulting from renal excretion, cellular uptake, and metabolism. Controlled clinical trials have demonstrated azathioprine to be better than placebo and to have a significant steroid-sparing effect. It has been shown to be beneficial in the treatment of RA, SLE, and a variety of other connective tissue diseases. Comparative studies against hydroxychloroquine, D-penicillamine, intramuscular gold, and cyclophosphamide in RA have shown it to be no different from these SAARDs but slightly more likely to produce side effects (16). In RA, the efficacy of azathioprine is greater with doses of 2.5 mg/kg/day than with a lower dose of 1.25 mg/kg/day. Nausea, vomiting, and diarrhea occur relatively frequently, but do not usually cause cessation of treatment. Bone marrow suppression and hepatitis can also occur, but the real risk with azathioprine is an increase in the incidence of lymphoproliferative malignancies after long-term treatment (17).

ALKYLATING AGENTS

Nitrogen mustard, chlorambucil, and cyclophosphamide will substitute alkyl radicals into other molecules such as DNA and RNA. Chlorambucil is rapidly absorbed and has a half-life of approximately two hours (18). It has been used in doses of between 0.5 and 0.2 mg/kg/day for the treatment of RA, juvenile chronic arthritis, vasculitis, and systemic sclerosis. Chlorambucil is particularly beneficial in reducing the severity and incidence of amyloidosis complicating RA, juvenile chronic arthritis, and ankylosing spondylitis (16). Chromosomal damage can be induced, and the major adverse reaction is an increased risk of leukemia and other malignancies.

Cyclophosphamide is a derivative of nitrogen mustard and can be taken orally or intravenously. The drug has a plasma half-life of between 2 and 10 hours and is metabolized primarily by the liver with a small contribution by the kidney and the lung (16). Cyclophosphamide itself is inactive but is converted into the active metabolite that produces the immunosuppressive effect and also causes bladder toxicity. Cyclophophamide has been shown to be effective in the treatment of severe RA, systemic vasculitis, and SLE. The usual oral dose of cyclophosphamide is 50-150 mg/day (0.7-3 mg/kg/day). In many clinical situations, however, it is now possible to substitute lower total dose (and, therefore, less toxic) regimens of intermittent intravenous bolus (0.5-1 g/meter^2/body surface area) every four to six weeks. Adverse events are frequent with cyclophosphamide and include hemorrhagic cystitis with the potential for bladder carcinoma; immunosuppression leading to increased risk of infection, particularly herpes zoster; suppression of gonadal function in both women and men; and long-term effects of immunosuppression with an increased incidence of lymphoma and other hematologic malignancies.

CYCLOSPORIN

Cyclosporin A is a new immunomodulating agent believed to selectively block the synthesis and release of interleukin-1 from monocytes and interleukin-2 from T-helper cells. Absorption of cyclosporin A is slow, often incomplete, and is reduced by food. The drug is highly bound to plasma protein, particularly the lipoproteins. Cyclosporin undergoes extensive metabolism, primarily in the liver, and has a terminal elimination half-life of six hours (in healthy volunteers) to 20 hours (in patients with severe liver disease) (18). Cyclosporin has been shown to be effective in comparison to placebo in patients with RA and to have similar efficacy to azathioprine and D-penicillamine. The major problem with use of cyclosporin is that the majority of patients have a significant decrease in renal function and increase in blood pressure while on the drug. This occurs with higher doses but occasionally even at relatively low doses (<5 mg/kg/day) even though renal function returns to normal once the drug is stopped (19).

Peter Brooks, MD

1. Brook A, Corbett M: Radiographic change in early rheumatoid disease. Ann Rheum Dis 36:71–73, 1971
2. Wilske KR, Healey LA: Remodeling the pyramid—a concept whose time has come. J Rheumatol 16:565–567, 1989
3. Tett S, Cutler D, Day RO: Antimalarials in rheumatic diseases. Clinical Rheumatol 4:467–489, 1990
4. The Canadian Hydroxychloroquine Study Group: A randomized study of the effect of withdrawing hydroxychloroquine sulphate in systemic lupus erythematosus. New Engl J Med 324:150–154, 1991
5. Joyce DA: D-penicillamine. Clinical Rheumatol 4:553–574, 1990
6. Ahern MJ, Hall ND, Case K, et al: D-penicillamine withdrawal in rheumatoid arthritis. Ann Rheum Dis 84:213–217, 1984
7. Porter DR, Capell HA: The use of sulphasalazine as a disease modifying antirheumatic drug. Clinical Rheumatol 4:535–551, 1990
8. Donovan S, Hawley S, MacCarthy J, et al: Tolerability of enteric coated sulfasalazine in rheumatoid arthritis: results of a co-operative clinical study. Brit J Rheumatol 29:201–204, 1990
9. Champion GD, Graham GG, Ziegler JB: The gold complexes. Clinical Rheumatol 4:491–534, 1990
10. Clark P, Tugwell P, Bennett K, et al: Meta-analysis of injectable gold in rheumatoid arthritis. J Rheumatol 16:442–447, 1989
11. Furst DE: Rational use of disease modifying anti-rheumatic drugs. Drugs 39:19–37, 1990
12. Liang MH, Fries JF: Containing costs in chronic disease: monitoring strategies in the gold therapy of rheumatoid arthritis. J Rheumatol 5:241–244, 1978
13. Songsiride JN, Furst DE: Methotrexate—a rapidly acting drug. Clinical Rheumatol 4:575–593, 1990
14. Tugwell P, Bennett K, Ghent M: Methotrexate in rheumatoid arthritis. Ann Intern Med 107:358–366, 1987
15. Wolfe F, Hawley DJ, Lathem MA: Termination of slow acting antirheumatic therapy in rheumatoid arthritis: a 14-year prospective evaluation of 1,017 consecutive starts. J Rheumatol 17:994–1002, 1990
16. Luqmani RA, Palmer RG, Bacon PA: Azathioprine, cyclophosphamide, and chlorambucil. Clinical Rheumatol 4:595–619, 1990
17. Silman AJ, Petrie J, Hazleman B, et al: Lymphoproliferative cancer and other malignancies in patients with rheumatoid arthritis treated with azathioprine: a 20-year follow-up study. Ann Rheum Dis 47:988–992, 1988
18. Kahan BD: Drug therapy: cyclosporin. New Engl J Med 321:1725–1738, 1989
19. Tugwell P, Bombardier C, Gent M, et al: Low-dose cyclosporine versus placebo in patients with rheumatoid arthritis. Lancet 335:1051–1056, 1990

57. BIOLOGIC AGENTS AS POTENTIAL NEW THERAPIES FOR AUTOIMMUNE DISEASES

There is no convincing evidence that any of the currently employed therapeutic agents substantially alter the long-term destructive course of rheumatoid arthritis (RA). Although the etiology of RA remains unknown, several immune and inflammatory pathways that contribute to cartilage and bone destruction have been identified. There is now early experience with the use of biologic agents directed against some of these pathways in humans, as well as data obtained from the use of these agents in animal models of autoimmune disease. Therapies with monoclonal antibodies (MAbs) directed against several cell surface constituents and cytokine inhibitors have been shown to be safe and possibly efficacious in early open trials. These are now being more rigorously tested in double-blind placebo controlled trials (1). In addition, experimental studies with "blocking peptides" and immunization with autoreactive T cell receptor peptides have implications for therapy in RA. Biologic agents that have been used, or are currently in early trials in patients with RA, are summarized in Table 57–1 (1).

There is considerable evidence supporting the importance of immune processes in the pathogenesis of RA (2). Antigen-activated T cells infiltrate the synovial membrane (3). This leads to a series of inflammatory processes resulting in vascular and synovial cell proliferation with resorption of cartilage and bone. Nonimmunologic pathways also may contribute to tissue injury and destruction in established RA (4). Degradation of articular extracellular matrix components is a hallmark of RA, and is likely mediated by neutral proteinases such as collagenase, stromelysin, elastase, and cathepsin G. A schematic diagram of cellular and humoral pathways implicated in the pathogenesis of chronic inflammation is presented in Fig. 57–1. The model suggests sites for therapeutic interruption that could be exploited in treating autoimmune disorders such as RA.

T CELLS AS A FOCUS OF THERAPY

Attempts to deplete lymphocytes as a therapeutic maneuver is not a new approach in the treatment of RA. Methods to remove T cells (or ablate their function) have ranged from thoracic duct drainage in the 1970s to the use of MAbs to specific T cell surface markers in the 1990s. Lymphapheresis, thoracic duct drainage, and total lymphoid irradiation have all been employed in an effort to eliminate lymphocytes in patients with refractory RA. Each of these methods has been reported to have some beneficial effect. However, these approaches also have proven to be impractical or associated with significant morbidity, such as infectious complications.

CD5 is a 67 kDa surface glycoprotein found on most T cells (helper and cytotoxic) and a B cell subset. The exact function of CD5 is not known. In an attempt to increase the potency of MAb therapy directed against CD5, a murine MAb to CD5 was conju-

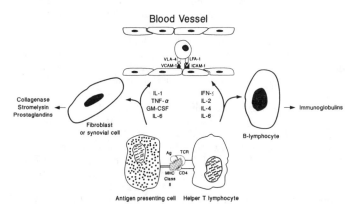

Fig. 57–1. Schematic illustrating the cellular and humoral pathways implicated in the pathogenesis of rheumatoid arthritis. Il–1 = interleukin–1; TNF–α = tumor necrosis factor - α; GM–CSF = granulocyte-macrophage-colony stimulating factor; IL–6 = interleukin-6; IFN–γ = interferon-γ; IL–2 = interleukin-2, IL–4 = interleukin–4; IL–6 = interleukin–6; Ag = antigen; TCR = T cell receptor; MHC = major histocompatability complex; VLA–4 = very late antigen–4; VCAM–1 = vascular adhesion molecule–1; LFA–1 = lymphocyte-function associated antigen–1; ICAM–1 = intercellular adhesion molecule-1 (reproduced from reference 1 with permission).

gated to a potent plant toxin, the A chain of ricin, that inhibits protein synthesis and causes death of the targeted cell. In early Phase I and Phase II trials in which RA patients have received the anti-CD5 immunoconjugate (10–25 mg/day for 5 days), the agent reversibly depleted circulating T cells and reversibly decreased T cell proliferative responses to antigens and mitogens (5). The most common side effects were fatigue, fever, malaise, nausea, vomiting, rash, peripheral edema, hypoalbuminemia, and elevations of hepatic transaminase levels. In addition, immune responses directed against the murine anti-CD5 MAb were often observed; however, this has not been associated with significant clinical problems following retreatment with the anti-CD5 toxin. Improvements in tender and swollen joint counts were noted more frequently in patients with earlier disease compared to those with longstanding disease.

Monoclonal antibody therapy directed against CD3+ (used primarily in transplant rejection) and CD5+ T cells has shown promise in suppressing T cell function; however, it may be more appropriate to selectively target T-cell subsets, such as CD4+ T cells, that are implicated in pathogenetic immune responses in RA (Fig. 57–1). Efficacy of anti-CD4 MAb therapy in several animal models of human autoimmune disease, including collagen arthritis, murine systemic lupus erythematosus, murine myasthenia gravis, murine experimental allergic encephalomyelitis, murine diabetes mellitus, murine thyroiditis, and murine uveitis supports the role of CD4+ T cells as playing a central role in the pathogenesis of these disorders.

There are several mechanisms by which anti-CD4 MAb might exert an effect in autoimmune disorders. Treatment with the MAb may cause immunosuppression by depleting CD4+ T cells, either by directly killing the cells (either complement mediated or by inducing apoptosis) or by clearing antibody-coated CD4+ T cells (by complement and Fc mechanisms). Antibody-dependent cellular cytotoxicity may also contribute to CD4+ T cell depletion. Alternatively, binding of the anti-CD4 MAb to helper T cells might inhibit major histocompatibility complex (MHC) class II-dependent T cell responses by blocking the interaction of CD4+ T cells with the antigen presenting cell (APC). Finally, anti-CD4 MAb therapy may transmit an inhibitory signal to the CD4+ T cells.

Pilot studies in patients with RA have been conducted with murine anti-CD4 MAbs (6). Fever and chills have been noted in

Table 57–1. Biologic agents studied in persons with rheumatoid arthritis

Biologic Agent	Target Antigen/Cytokine
Murine anti-CD5 ricin toxin MAb	CD5
Humanized campath 1-H MAb	CDw52
Murine anti-CD4 MAb	CD4
Chimeric or humanized anti-CD4 MAb	CD4
Diphtheria-IL-2 fusion toxin	IL-2 receptor
IL-1 receptor antagonist	IL-1
Soluble IL-1 receptor	IL-1
Recombinant IFN-γ	IFN-γ
Chimeric anti-TNF-α MAb	TNF-α
Murine anti-ICAM-1 MAb	ICAM-1 (CD54)
Soluble TNF receptor	TNF-α
Murine anti-IL-6 MAb	IL-6
Chimeric anti-CD7 MAb	CD7

some patients and may be related to transient cytokine release. Human anti-murine responses were common in these patients; however, retreatment with murine anti-CD4 was generally well tolerated with the exception of a mild anaphylactic reaction in one patient.

There are potential problems with murine MAbs in the treatment of autoimmune diseases. First, the recipient's humoral response to the murine MAb potentially may result in toxicity or neutralize the efficacy of the MAb. In an effort to overcome this problem, chimeric and humanized MAbs have been developed that exhibit lower immunogenicity compared to the parent murine MAb. Chimeric antibodies consist of human immunoglobulin constant region fused to the variable region of the murine MAb, whereas humanized antibodies contain only a portion of the murine variable region (generally the hypervariable segments. A second potential problem with available MAbs to T cells is undesirable suppression of normal immune function. In mice, treatment with an anti-CD4 MAb (L3T4) results in depletion of CD4+ T cells, blocks primary and secondary humoral immune responses, and inhibits the generation of cellular immune responses. These effects are reversible; however, the return of CD4+ T cells is gradual and immune suppression may persist for prolonged periods following treatment.

A Phase I trial using a chimeric MAb to CD4 (cM-T412) in patients with refractory RA has recently been completed (7). Infusion with cM-T412 induced an immediate rapid decline in CD4+ T cells; circulating CD4+ T cells remained depressed in many patients even six months after treatment. Proliferative responses of peripheral blood lymphocytes to phytohemagglutinin, concanavalin A, pokeweed mitogen, purified protein derivative, and tetanus toxoid were low immediately following infusion compared to pre-treatment responses, but returned to near pre-treatment responses by day 60. Adverse experiences were minimal; symptoms suggestive of a mild cytokine release syndrome (fever, myalgias, malaise) were noted in 19 of the 25 patients and were frequently accompanied by transient elevations of serum IL-6 levels. No significant human antibody response to the cM-T412 variable region was detected, suggesting there may be less human immune response to this chimeric MAb than to murine anti-CD4 MAbs. Significant clinical improvement, was noted in 43% of patients at five weeks and 33% at six months following the chimeric MAb infusion; however, the study was open-label and medication changes were permitted during the trial. Phase II double-blind placebo controlled trials are now in progress in RA patients in the United States and Europe.

CDw52 (CAMPATH antigen) is present on all lymphocytes (B and T cells) and some monocytes. CAMPATH 1H, a humanized IgG directed against CDw52 rat MAb is being tested in Phase I trials in RA patients. Early results indicate that this MAb also depletes circulating lymphocytes, primarily CD4+ T cells.

To more specifically target T cells involved in the perpetuation of potentially pathogenic immune responses, MAbs directed against cell surface antigens expressed on activated T cells have been developed. When T cells become activated they express high affinity IL-2 receptors (IL-2R), not expressed on resting T cells (8). The expression of IL-2R during the course of a normal immune response has been extensively studied. Activation antigens such as IL-2R represent attractive targets for selectively abrogating active immune responses without interfering with resting T cells. Monoclonal antibodies to the IL-2R have been shown to suppress rodent allograft rejection, murine lupus nephritis, and collagen induced arthritis.

DAB_{486} IL-2, an IL-2R specific cytotoxin, is a fusion protein encoded by a hybrid gene that consists of the coding sequence for the enzymatically active fragment A of diphtheria toxin (DT) and the membrane-translocating portion of DT fragment B fused together with the gene for human IL-2 (9). DAB_{486} IL-2 binds avidly to IL-2R and is rapidly internalized via receptor-mediated endocytosis. Once the fusion protein is internalized, the enzymatically active fragment A portion is released into the cytosol and inhibits protein synthesis via fragment A-catalyzed ADP-ribosylation of elongation factor 2, ultimately resulting in cell death. DAB_{486} IL-2 has been shown to be effective in treating rat adjuvant arthritis. Clinical improvement has been reported in 9 of

19 refractory RA patients in a Phase I trial using DAB_{486} IL-2 (10). Phase II double-blind placebo controlled trials in RA using the IL-2 diphtheria fusion toxin are in progress.

More specific approaches to immunotherapy of autoimmune diseases necessitate identification of T cell receptor (TCR) gene products expressed by pathogenetic autoantigen reactive T cell clones in these diseases in humans. This approach is based on the hypothesis that receptors on T cells specific for an inciting autoantigen share variable region determinants not expressed by most T cells. Most T cells express the α/β form of the T cell receptor on their surface. The individuality of T cell clones is based on distinct amino acid sequences in the variable regions of the constituent TCR α and β chains. Analysis of T cell repertoires in autoimmune diseases is an area of intense scientific interest since MAbs to specific autoreactive T cells could potentially be effective in treating autoimmune diseases.

Recently, disease-associated TCRs have been identified for some animal models of autoimmunity, such as experimental allergic encephalomyelitis (EAE). The development of murine EAE has been linked to two TCR β variable (Vβ) region families, Vβ8.2 and Vβ13, which are present in a minority (10%) of the total T cell repertoire. Therapy with MAbs directed against these TCR Vβ families protects against the development of EAE, even if treatment is begun after the onset of neurologic disease.

There has been considerable interest in identifying disease-related TCR variable regions in patients with RA. In adjuvant arthritis, an animal model of RA, the disease can be transferred with T cell clones specific for the inciting antigen. Small numbers of T cells are required, illustrating that very few antigen-specific T cells are required to initiate and maintain chronic arthritis. In type II collagen-induced arthritis, a model of RA, TCR Vβ families have been identified that appear to contribute to the pathogenesis of this disease. Administration of MAbs to Vβ2, Vβ5, or Vβ8 suppressed type II collagen induced arthritis, whereas the administration of MAbs to other Vβ regions was ineffective.

Although findings have varied, one recent report suggests that in activated synovial T cells there is evidence of oligoclonality of the TCR; isolated IL-2R+ T cells from the synovium of 5 RA patients had Vβ3, Vβ14, and Vβ17 expressed in the majority of samples (11). Dominant rearrangements were observed within these three Vβ families consistent with limited oligoclonal expansion of activated T cells. The TCR α/β repertoire in RA synovial tissue is unlikely to be static as the disease evolves; indeed, recent evidence indicating greater TCR diversity with increasing disease duration supports this hypothesis (12).

Vaccination using autoreactive T cells has been shown to be effective in preventing arthritis in the rat adjuvant arthritis model and murine collagen-induced arthritis. T cell vaccination in rat adjuvant arthritis not only protected animals from developing the disease, but also induced remission of established disease. Vaccination with disease-associated TCR variable region peptides in an EAE model has also been shown to be effective in preventing the neurologic disease in these animal models. Synthetic TCR V region peptides have been safely administered (intradermally) to patients with multiple sclerosis; an immune response to these TCR peptides was induced in some patients. A major problem with vaccination with TCR-derived peptides in human RA at this time is the lack of information concerning the nature of putative pathogenic T cells in RA.

B CELLS AS A FOCUS OF THERAPY

The antigen receptor on B cells is the immunoglobulin molecule itself. Immunoglobulins consist of constant regions that are shared by several antibodies of a particular isotype and variable regions that include unique determinants called idiotypes. Immunoglobulins that react with the same antigen may express shared idiotypes. Therefore, B cells bearing the relevant cell surface idiotype may be targeted with an anti-idiotype MAb and their function modulated. The potential therapeutic usefulness of antiidiotypic MAbs is suggested by studies in which an anti-idiotype MAb to anti-DNA was used to successfully suppress nephritis in B/W mice.

ANTIBODIES TO ANTIGEN-PRESENTING CELLS

Activation of specific T cells by APCs can also be prevented by agents that block recognition structures on the APC. A reasonable target for this approach in RA would be MHC class II antigens (Fig. 57–1). Certain MHC class II alleles are associated with autoimmunity, for example, HLA–DR1 and HLA–DR4 with RA. The response of CD4+ T cells to antigen with the development of cellular and humoral immunity requires that antigen be presented as peptides to T cells in a complex with MHC class II gene products on APCs. MAbs directed against appropriate disease-related MHC class II allelic products have been tested in several animal models of human autoimmune diseases. The mechanism underlying the apparent therapeutic effectiveness of MAbs directed against disease-related MHC class II molecules is unclear, but it seems unlikely this can be entirely ascribed to physical blockade of the MHC class II molecule targeted, because effects are observed long after the antibody has been administered. MAbs directed against MHC class II molecules might also deplete B cells (and perhaps other MHC class II bearing cells) that could result in generalized, rather than selective, immunosuppression. An alternative approach is the construction of "designer peptides" that will block specific antigen presentation without depleting B cells. Such an approach has successfully prevented EAE.

CYTOKINES AND CYTOKINE INHIBITORS

Several cytokines have immunoregulatory properties; the precise roles of many cytokines in autoimmune diseases is still being investigated. Interleukin-1 likely contributes to the pathogenesis of RA (Fig. 57–1) by virtue of its capacity to induce the release of metalloproteinases from chondrocytes and prostaglandin E2 and collagenase production by synovial cells (13). In addition, IL–1 stimulates bone resorption, T cell activation, and the expression of adhesion molecules such as lymphocyte function-associated antigen-1 (LFA-1) and intercellular adhesion molecule-1 (ICAM-1). Therefore, inhibition of IL–1 activity is a logical strategy in an attempt to down-regulate the inflammatory process of RA.

A naturally occurring inhibitor of IL–1, interleukin–1 receptor antagonist (IL–1ra), has been identified, the protein sequenced, and its gene cloned (14). Recombinant IL–1ra (rIL–1ra) blocks IL–1-induced synovial cell prostaglandin E_2 and collagenase secretion by chondrocytes; blocks IL–1 induced degradation of proteoglycans and inhibition of glycosaminoglycan synthesis in bovine nasal cartilage explants; and has been shown to reduce the severity of joint lesions in rat adjuvant arthritis, streptococcal cell-wall induced arthritis, and collagen-induced arthritis. Recombinant IL–1ra given as daily subcutaneous injections has been used in a Phase I trial in RA patients. Double-blind placebo controlled Phase II trials in RA patients are in progress.

Soluble IL–1 receptors represent an alternative approach to IL–1 inhibition (15). The soluble IL–1 receptor binds IL-1 and inhibits binding of IL–1 to cell surface receptors. In the rat model of EAE, soluble IL–1 receptor antagonist resulted in a significant delay in the onset of EAE, reduced the severity of paralysis and shortened the duration of disease.

Interferon–γ (IFN–γ) is a cytokine with immunomodulatory and antiproliferative effects secreted by activated T cells. The ability of IFN–γ to induce and enhance the expression of class II MHC antigens on cells may be a factor in the pathogenesis of autoimmune disorders such as RA. However, little or no IFN–γ is present in the rheumatoid synovium or synovial fluid. Based on the assumptom that the negligible levels of IFN–γ in the synovial fluid of patients with RA reflects a clinically relevant defect, several clinical trials have been undertaken to determine the efficacy of recombinant IFN–γ (rIFN–γ) in the treatment of RA (16). Potential mechanisms by which rIFN–γ may work in treating RA include suppression of B cells, decrease in the number of circulating neutrophils, inhibition of release of certain cytokines, as well as other antiproliferative mechanisms. Overall, minimal clinical improvement was noted except in one study. It should be noted that administration of rIFN–γ in multiple sclerosis resulted in disease exacerbation in several patients. A similar exacerba-

tion of disease with rIFN–γ treatment has been reported in one patient with SLE. In addition, in the (NZB/NZW) F1 model of lupus nephritis, treatment with rIFN–γ accelerated the development of glomerulonephritis, whereas administration of an anti-IFN–γ MAb resulted in substantial clinical improvement characterized by marked decreases in proteinuria, delay in DNA antibody production, and increased survival.

Other cytokines, such as TNF–α and IL-6, may also be appropriate targets for therapeutic manipulation. Monoclonal antibodies directed against IL-6 and TNF–α are being evaluated in patients with RA, as is a recombinant solubilized TNF-α receptor.

ADHESION MOLECULES AS TARGETS OF THERAPY

Expression of cell adhesion molecules on endothelial cells and complementary ligands on the surfaces of circulating leukocytes (Fig. 57–1) appears to play a critical role in determining the site of leukocyte emigration from the intravascular space and the nature of the leukocyte populations attracted into the ensuing inflammatory lesion. A three-step model has recently been proposed to account for leukocyte–endothelial cell recognition: primary adhesion that is intrinsically unstable, leukocyte activation, and activation-dependent binding (more stable) with subsequent transmigration of the leukocyte (17). This model implies that the specificity of endothelial leukocyte interactions is determined by unique combinations of adhesion molecule–ligand interactions at each step. Isolated RA synovial endothelial cells constitutively express the selectin designated endothelial leukocyte adhesion molecule type–1 (ELAM–1) and up-regulate expression of this selectin following exposure to IL–1.

With regard to lymphocytes, the precise sequence of events involved in endothelial cell binding and transmigration has not been established. There is evidence that interaction of the β_2 integrin LFA–1 with its ligand, ICAM–1, is capable of mediating transendothelial migration of T cells. ICAM–1 is also expressed on RA synovial endothelial cells and is regulated by IL–1.

Murine MAbs to LFA–1 β chain (anti-CD18) and to ICAM–1 (anti-CD54), administered to rabbits with phorbol myristic acetate induced lung inflammation and inhibited neutrophil migration into the lungs. Anti-CD18 has been shown to inhibit the inflammatory response in a rabbit model of antigen-induced arthritis (18). Treatment with anti-CD54 MAb also resulted in a significant amelioration of chronic inflammation in this animal model. This same MAb has shown promising therapeutic effects in an open-label Phase I trial in RA.

Larry W. Moreland, MD
William J. Koopman, MD

1. Moreland LW, Heck LW, Sullivan W, et al: New approaches to the therapy of autoimmune diseases: rheumatoid arthritis as a paradigm. Am J Med Sci 305:40–51, 1993
2. Harris ED: Rheumatoid arthritis: pathophysiology and implications for therapy. N Engl J Med 322:1277–1289, 1990
3. Panayi GS, Lanchbury JS, Kingsley GH: The importance of the T-cell in initiating and maintaining the chronic synovitis of rheumatoid arthritis. Arthritis Rheum 35:729–735, 1992
4. Koopman WJ, Gay S: Do nonimmunologically mediated pathways play a role in the pathogenesis of rheumatoid arthritis? Rheum Dis Clin N Am 19:107–122, 1993
5. Strand V, Lipsky PE, Cannon GW, et al: Effects of administration of an anti-CD5 plus immunoconjugate in rheumatoid arthritis. Results of two phase II studies. Arthritis Rheum 36:620–630, 1993
6. Horneff G, Burmester GR, Emmrich F, Kalden JR: Treatment of rheumatoid arthritis with an anti-CD4 monoclonal antibody. Arthritis Rheum 34:1209–1240, 1991
7. Moreland LW, Bucy RP, Tilden A, et al: Use of a chimeric monoclonal anti-CD4 antibody in patients with refractory rheumatoid arthritis. Arthritis Rheum 36:307–318, 1993
8. Rubin LA, Nelson DL: The soluble interleukin-2 receptor: biology, function, and clinical application. Ann Int Med 113:619–627, 1990
9. Bacha P, Williams DP, Waters C, et al: Interleukin-2 receptor-targeted cytotoxicity: interleukin–2 receptor-mediated action of a diphtheria toxin-related interleukin-2 fusion protein. J Exp Med 167:612–622, 1988
10. Sewell KL, Trentham DE: Rapid improvement in refractory rheumatoid arthritis by an interleukin–2 receptor targeted immunotherapy. (Abstract) Clin Res 39:314A, 1991
11. Howell MD, Diively JP, Lundeen KA, et al: Limited T-cell receptor B-chain heterogeneity among interleukin–2 receptor-positive synovial T-cells suggests a role for superantigen in rheumatoid arthritis. Proc Nat Acad Sci USA 88:10921–10925, 1991
12. Bucht A, Oksenberg JR, Lindblad S, et al: Characterization of T-cell receptor

αβ repertoire in synovial tissue from different temporal phases of rheumatoid arthritis. Scand J Immunol 35:159–165, 1992

13. Dinarello CA: Interleukin–1 and interleukin–1 antagonism. Blood 77:1627–1652, 1991

14. Arend WP: Interleukin–1 receptor antagonist: a new member of the interleukin family. J Clin Invest 88:1445–1451, 1991

15. Jacobs CA, Baker PE, Roux ER, et al: Experimental autoimmune encephalomyelitis is exacerbated by IL–1α and suppressed by soluble IL–1 receptor. J Immunol 146:2983–2989, 1990

16. Cannon GW, Pincus SH, Emkey RD, et al: Double-blind trial of recombinant gamma-interferon versus placebo in the treatment of rheumatoid arthritis. Arthritis Rheum 32:964–973, 1989

17. Butcher EC: Leukocyte-endothelial cell recognition: three (or more) steps to specificity and diversity. Cell 67:1033–1036, 1991

18. Jasin HE, Lightfoot E, Davis LS, et al: Amelioration of antigen-induced arthritis in rabbits treated with monoclonal antibodies to leukocyte adhesion molecules. Arthritis Rheum 35:541–549, 1992

58. THERAPEUTIC INJECTION OF JOINTS AND SOFT TISSUES

After more than 40 years of use and many concerns regarding efficacy and toxicity, there is ample controlled and anecdotal evidence for the therapeutic value of intraarticular and soft tissue injection in various rheumatic diseases. Although a few other substances have been utilized, such as ^{90}yttrium, radioactive gold and cytotoxic agents, it is the corticosteroids that continue to be used. When used properly, there is little support for the statement that these agents destroy cartilage or bone, but there is similarly no evidence that they prevent ongoing joint destruction. Corticosteroid injection can improve quality of life by suppressing joint inflammation and pain, increasing function and facilitating exercise programs (Table 58–1). Judicious use can result in a systemic *steroid-sparing effect* when injecting a recalcitrant joint in rheumatoid arthritis (RA) and can eliminate the need for a larger oral dose of prednisone. Many opportunities for justified cost savings exist, such as results from a favorable response to wrist injection for carpal tunnel syndrome and avoiding a surgical release of the transverse carpal ligament. Injecting one or multiple metacarpophalangeal joints in RA to temporarily relieve pain and restore lost function can decrease the need for aggressive physical medicine treatments and facilitate a more rapid return to a more normal functional state.

The use of this therapeutic modality should be within the purview of the primary care physician. Although absent from many training programs, the technique for intraarticular and soft tissue injection can be easily mastered. When the diagnosis is in doubt, or the value of injection is being considered, the rheumatology consultant will be a valuable asset. Routes for arthrocentesis of some joints are shown in Chapter 8. Discussions of the techniques for injection and of the medications used are available in standard rheumatology texts (1).

GENERAL THERAPEUTIC CONCERNS

Corticosteroid injection is an outpatient office procedure, requiring familiarity with the anatomy of the region to be injected. A sterile surgical pack is not required, but use of gloves by the operator is recommended and is now mandated by OSHA regulations. No one corticosteroid has been proven more effective than others, but the least soluble preparation, triamcinolone, may give the most prolonged relief. Some experienced clinicians routinely dilute the corticosteroid with local anesthetic while others maintain that in doing so the therapeutic benefit is also being diluted. Although complications of corticosteroid injections are rarely seen, concerns such as osteopenia, a Charcot joint secondary to masking of pain by the injection and subsequent joint overuse, a post-injection flare (possibly due to the injected crystalline steroid material), tendon rupture, and localized dermal, subcutaneous, or fat necrosis necessitate cautious use of injection therapy. The rarely (if ever) seen corticosteroid-induced arthropathy should not discourage proper use of this very effective therapeutic modality (2). No area should be injected more often than 3 or 4 times per year. Although some have recommended non-weight bearing for several days after injection (3), other controlled studies do not support the need for such a conservative approach, and normal, non-strenuous activity is often permitted (4). Vigorous exercise may speed resorption of steroid from the joint. Generalized corticosteroid toxicity is not a concern with infrequent use of local injections, although evidence for systemic absorption is the not-infrequent comment by the patient of feeling better globally shortly after the injection. Iatrogenic joint sepsis following an injection is a potential concern, but this is rarely seen in the hands of experienced clinicians (2,5).

INDICATIONS FOR INJECTION

Rheumatoid Arthritis

The antiinflammatory and immunosuppressive actions of corticosteroids are effective whether injected into a joint or soft tissues of a patient with RA or used systemically. Inhibition of collagenase, gene expression (6), decrease in leukotriene and prostaglandin synthesis, inhibition of neutrophil and monocyte-generated superoxide anion radicals, suppression of interleukin-1 synthesis and antagonism of its action, and antagonism of macrophage inhibition factor (7) are among the demonstrated effects that translate into clinical effectiveness. Decrease in joint pain, swelling, and heat can be seen in one or two days after intraarticular injection; these benefits often persist for weeks or months thereafter. Classic reports by Hollander (5) and McCarty (8) support these observations. The often dramatic effect of intraarticular corticosteroids, however, can lead to an overdependence on this approach that results in excessive use and unfortunate neglect of other forms of therapy. Extraarticular sites of involvement may also respond to local use of corticosteroids as seen with nerve entrapment at the wrist (carpal tunnel), ankle (tarsal tunnel) and elbow (ulnar nerve). Painful rheumatoid nodules may shrink in size after local infiltration with corticosteroids.

Osteoarthritis

Although traditionally considered to be degenerative, osteoarthritic joints will also respond temporarily to intraarticular corticosteroid. Recent evidence in laboratory animals indicates that the progression (9) of osteoarthritic lesions can be slowed and the severity of cartilage lesions and osteophyte formation may also be affected (10,11). Corticosteroid injected into the frequently symptomatic first carpometacarpal joint or into the knee, especially if combined with joint aspiration, can result in rapid pain relief.

Table 58–1. Some major benefits of intraarticular and soft tissue injection

1) Alleviate pain and suppress inflammation in a joint or tendon or bursa which is:
   a) Inflamed out of proportion to other areas
   b) Not responsive to non-invasive anti-inflammatory therapy.
2) Avoid institution of, or increase in dose of systemic corticosteroid therapy ("steroid sparing").
3) Decrease swelling of inflamed soft tissue to relieve nerve entrapment, e.g. carpal tunnel syndrome, tarsal tunnel syndrome.

Acute Crystalline and Other Arthropathy

Gout and pseudogout will respond to intraarticular corticosteroid injection, although usually oral nonsteroidal antiinflammatory drug (NSAID) therapy will be adequate and certainly less traumatic for the patient with an exquisitely painful joint who does not have some contraindication to NSAID use (12). In this situation, as in any acute arthritis, joint sepsis must be excluded by appropriate studies on the aspirated synovial fluid (see Chapter 8C). The immediately available results of these studies, plus clinical judgment, only rarely warrants delaying corticosteroid injection until complete bacteriologic studies are reported (7).

Acute bouts of arthritis seen in systemic lupus erythematosus, Reiter's syndrome, psoriasis, ankylosing spondylitis, and inflammatory bowel disease will also benefit from intraarticular corticosteroids.

SOFT TISSUE INJECTION

Corticosteroid injection at sites of soft tissue inflammation can be equally as effective as in the intraarticular areas already discussed and is, in many instances, technically less demanding. Among the common problems that respond well are the carpal tunnel syndrome (13), tendinitis and bursitis at the shoulder and elbow, and trochanteric bursitis (14) (see Chapter 50).

Stenosing tenosynovitis of the hand including de Quervain's disease (15) can benefit from local injection (16). Olecranon bursitis, prepatellar bursitis, anserine bursitis of the medial knee, ischial bursitis, Achilles tendinitis and calcaneal bursitis all will respond favorably to injection. Although debate will certainly continue, a recent controlled trial of corticosteroid injection into facet joints for chronic low back pain concluded that there was little value in this procedure (17). The "tender points" of fibromyalgia and myofascial syndromes are discussed in Chapter 41; these can generally be managed without injections.

Herbert Kaplan, MD

1. Owen DS Jr: Aspiration and injection of joints and soft tissues. Textbook of Rheumatology. 4th Ed. Edited by WN Kelley, ED Harris Jr, S Ruddy, CB Sledge. WB Saunders, 1993, pp 545–561

2. Gray RG, Tenenbaum J, Gottlieb NL: Local corticosteroid injection treatment in rheumatic disorders. Semin Arthritis Rheum 10:231–254, 1981

3. Neustadt DH: Intra-articular therapy in rheumatoid synovitis of the knee: effects of post injection rest regimen. Clin Rheumatol Practice 3:65–68, 1985

4. Chatham WW, Williams GV, Moreland LW, et al: Intra-articular injections: should you rest joints? Arthritis Rheum 32(Suppl 1):R45, 1989

5. Hollander JL: Intrasynovial corticosteroid therapy in arthritis. Maryland State Med J 19:62–66, 1969

6. Grant EN, Bellamy N, Fryday-Field K, et al: Double-blind randomized controlled trial and six-year open follow-up of yttrium-90 radiosynovectomy versus triamcinolone hexacetonide in persistent rheumatoid knee synovitis. Inflammopharmacol 1:231–238, 1992

7. Weiss MM: Corticosteroids in rheumatoid arthritis. Semin Arthritis Rheum 19:9–21, 1989

8. McCarty DJ: Treatment of rheumatoid joint inflammation with triamcinolone hexacetonide. Arthritis Rheum 15:157–173, 1972

9. Pelletier JP, Martel-Pelletier J: The therapeutic effects of NSAIDs and corticosteroids in osteoarthritis: to be or not to be. J Rheumatol 16:266–269, 1989

10. Williams JM, Brandt KD: Triamcinolone hexacetonide protects against fibrillation and osteophyte formation following chemically induced articular cartilage damage. Arthritis Rheum 28:1267–1274, 1985

11. Pelletier JP, Martel-Pelletier J: Protective effects of corticosteroids on cartilage lesions and osteophyte formation in the Pond–Nuki dog model of osteoarthritis. Arthritis Rheum 32:181–193, 1989

12. Groff GD, Franck WA, Raddatz DA: Systemic steroid therapy for acute gout: a clinical trial and review of the literature. Arthritis Rheum 19:329–336, 1990

13. Phalen GS: The carpal tunnel syndrome: 17 years' experience in diagnosis and treatment of 654 hands. J Bone Joint Surg 48:211–228, 1966

14. Shapira D, Nahir M, Scharf Y: Trochanteric bursitis: a common clinical problem. Arch Phys Med Rehabil 67:815–817, 1986

15. Anderson BC, Manthy YR, Brouns MC: Treatment of de Quervain's tenosynovitis with corticosteroids. Arthritis Rheum 34:793–798, 1992

16. Gunther SF, Marks MR, Gunther BB: Efficacy of cortisone injection for trigger finger and thumbs. Arthritis Rheum 32:(Suppl 4):S71, 1989

17. Carette S, Marcoux S, Truchon R, et al: A controlled trial of corticosteroid injections into facet joints for chronic low back pain. N Engl J Med 325:1002–1007, 1991

59. THE SURGICAL TREATMENT OF ARTHRITIS

Patients with arthritis, especially those with rheumatoid arthritis (RA), often have special needs at surgery because of multiple joint involvement. They should be treated by a multidisciplinary team composed of an arthritis surgeon, rheumatologist, nurses, therapists, and social workers. Surgical candidates with RA are frequently weak and discouraged. They face the prospect of a series of operations before achieving reasonable functional independence. In spite of this, patients may have unrealistic expectations regarding the outcome of the surgery. By participating in the planning and timing of surgical events, patients can better comprehend the duration of treatment, understand the necessity of prolonged physical therapy, and develop realistic goals for the procedures. Because pain relief is the most attainable result of reconstructive surgery, pain is the primary indication for most operations. Restoration of motion and function is less predictable and careful preoperative assessment of each patient's disability must be performed before improvement can be anticipated. Certainly, the major single advance in recent years in the care of patients with arthritis has been the development of total joint replacement.

In patients with osteoarthritis (OA), there are numerous alternatives to joint replacement, many of which are preferable, especially in younger patients. For patients with RA, procedures such as arthrodesis, synovectomy, repair of ruptured tendons, and other nonprosthetic procedures still play an important role for relief of pain and restoration of function. Joint replacement surgery, however, has revolutionized the outlook for patients with multiple joint involvement.

PREOPERATIVE EVALUATION

Medical Considerations

The first consideration is whether a painful joint requires surgery. Treatment of synovitis with medication and physical modalities is usually appropriate. If structural damage to the joint is the problem, then it is unrealistic to expect that medication will be sufficient. However, it is better to perform surgery as indications arise rather than wait until the patient has many severely involved joints requiring longer periods of hospitalization and rehabilitation.

General operative risk should be assessed, including the systemic manifestations of rheumatic disease. Patients should be taking the lowest possible dose of corticosteroids. In addition, patients should be examined for carious teeth and signs and symptoms of urinary tract infection or prostatic hypertrophy as these could increase the risk of postoperative infection. Women should have a preoperative urine culture because they frequently will have asymptomatic bactiuria.

Patient Cooperation

It is important to evaluate the patient's motivation and ability to participate in postoperative rehabilitation. Often, preoperative assessment and instruction by physical therapists and occupational therapists are helpful. Instruction in crutch ambulation may facilitate postoperative training.

If multiple procedures are necessary, it may be helpful to

perform surgery such as foot surgery or hip reconstruction first, because the demands of postoperative rehabilitation are less with these procedures. This will aid in predicting the response to a procedure such as total knee replacement, which requires more active rehabilitation on the part of the patient.

DISEASE-RELATED FACTORS

Rheumatoid Arthritis

Patients with inflammatory rheumatic disease pose certain problems that can influence the results and risks of surgery. In addition to the systemic problems presented by patients with RA, multiple joint involvement often creates special difficulties. Crutches are necessary after lower extremity surgery, therefore, it is essential to evaluate the patient's ability to use crutches before the operation. If there is extensive involvement at the shoulder, elbow, or wrist, axillary crutches may not be appropriate. Forearm crutches are an alternative, particularly if involvement of the wrist or elbow makes the use of axillary crutches painful. It may be necessary to perform arthrodesis of the wrist before operating on the lower extremities, so that the patient will be able to use forearm crutches in the postoperative period. In addition, patients who do not have 100° of knee flexion find it difficult to arise from a seated position without applying major forces to the upper extremity. If the upper extremities can not cope with these forces, maximal hip and knee flexion must be obtained after surgery to minimize the need for upper extremity assistance. The cervical spine is involved significantly in 30% to 40% of patients with RA (1). Although this usually is not apparent to the patient, it should be considered in the preoperative evaluation to avoid the potentially disastrous consequences of excessive manipulation of the neck during intubation or positioning for spinal anesthetic.

Much has been written about the increased susceptibility to infection in RA. These patients have been shown to be at higher risk for infection following total joint replacement (2). Postoperatively, antibiotic prophylaxis is recommended for dental procedures, cystoscopy, and other procedures likely to result in transient bacteremia because these could lead to a secondary prosthetic joint infection (3).

Approximately 10% of patients with RA are on corticosteroids when undergoing surgery, and they are probably at increased risk of infection. Because steroids can produce friable skin, patients must be handled carefully while sedated or anesthetized. Increased doses of steroids will be required in the perioperative period.

Aspirin and other nonsteroidal antiinflammatory drugs (NSAIDs) may produce bleeding tendencies due to platelet inhibition. Therefore, these agents should be discontinued up to 1 week prior to surgery and replaced with nonacetyl salicylates or pure analgesics. The effect of immunosuppressive drugs on infection must be considered. Although controversy exists concerning the effect of penicillamine on wound healing, many arthritis surgeons believe that healing is delayed in those patients taking penicillamine. There are conflicting reports concerning the effects of methotrexate on wound healing and infection during the perioperative period. Currently, many rheumatologists recommend temporarily discontinuing methotrexate during the immediate preoperative and postoperative period (4).

Juvenile Rheumatoid Arthritis

Patients with juvenile arthritis present certain challenges that may directly influence the results of surgical intervention. The temporomandibular joint is frequently involved in juvenile arthritis as well as in adult RA. In the child, temporomandibular joint dysfunction combined with micrognathia may cause difficulties with intubation and respiration following extubation. Careful preoperative analysis by the anesthesiologist will prevent some of these difficulties, and fiber-optic intubation will minimize trauma and postoperative laryngeal edema.

The range of motion achieved after arthroplasty in juvenile rheumatoid arthritis is generally less than would be predicted from that achieved at the time of surgery. Special measures such as serial casting may be necessary following total knee replacement to correct flexion contracture. The young age at which some patients with juvenile arthritis undergo arthroplasty exposes their prosthetic joints to both greater functional demands and a longer period of exposure to late complications, such as infection and loosening.

Ankylosing Spondylitis

Patients with ankylosing spondylitis have diminished chest excursion and are, therefore, at greater risk for postoperative pulmonary problems. Because of cervical spine rigidity, intubation may be extremely difficult. Sometimes preoperative tracheostomy is required before an anesthetic agent can be delivered. Ossification in the anulus fibrosus and spinal ligaments can create great difficulty in carrying out spinal anesthesia. Careful assessment by the anesthesiologist is useful in choosing the appropriate type and route of anesthetic and in anticipating difficulties.

Following total hip replacement, patients with ankylosing spondylitis frequently fail to regain the same range of motion achieved by patients with RA or OA (5). Although the range of motion achieved may be only 65° to 75° of hip flexion, this often leads to a significant improvement in function and independence. This limited motion is due not only to the increased involvement of the periarticular soft tissues seen in this disease, but may also be due to an increased frequency of heterotopic ossification in the muscles and capsules surrounding the hip joint, although this increased risk of heterotopic ossification has been challenged (6). Indomethacin or postoperative irradiation have been used to decrease heterotopic bone formation. If advised of this preoperatively, the patient can make a more informed decision regarding the desirability of surgery and is less likely to experience disappointment in the postoperative period.

Psoriatic Arthritis

Patients with psoriatic arthritis sometimes have skin involvement in the area of the proposed surgical incision. Contamination of psoriatic skin by microorganisms may lead to an increased risk of infection following incision through such skin. Clearing up the skin at the operative site by appropriate local therapy before surgery is desirable.

Enteropathic Arthropathy

The arthropathies related to chronic inflammatory intestinal disease also pose a special threat of postoperative infection because of both late hematogenous seeding from a focus of infection in the bowel and the occasional source of contamination from the colostomy in proximity to the incision for hip replacement.

Systemic Lupus Erythematosus

Patients with systemic lupus erythematosus (SLE) who develop osteonecrosis of the femoral head or other sites (see Chapter 48) present a very difficult problem for the physician. The patients are often young and treated with large doses of corticosteroids when they develop osteonecrosis. Implanting a prosthetic joint in a young patient invites long-term failure related to wear and loosening; to do so in a patient on long-term treatment with corticosteroids may also add the risk of infection. In young patients with SLE, prosthetic replacement may well be justified to relieve pain and improve the quality of life; it is likely that revision arthroplasty may be required at some future time (7,8). Osteonecrosis of a femoral condyle at the knee may be treated by osteotomy as well as by arthroplasty.

Although total joint arthroplasty has dramatically improved the function of patients with arthritis, its applicability is not universal. An abiding principle of reconstructive surgery is that preservation of bone stock by timely early performance of nonprosthetic procedures is preferable to joint replacement, particularly in younger, active patients.

SURGICAL INTERVENTION SITES

Cervical Spine

Posterior cervical fusion remains the most commonly performed surgical procedure for pain and neurologic compromise secondary to cervical instability from RA. Because many patients may have significant atlantoaxial instability (subluxation or impaction) without symptoms, it is often unclear whether these patients should have prophylactic surgical stabilization. Due to the reported high postoperative complication rate (early postoperative mortality of 27% in one study), most surgeons use progressive neurologic deterioration and pain not controlled with non-operative management as indications for surgery. Using these criteria, excellent results without significant morbidity or mortality have been reported (9).

The most commonly performed procedures include atlantoaxial fusion and occipitocervical fusion for atlantoaxial subluxation and atlantoaxial impaction (upward migration of the dens). Nonunion rates range from 0% to 50% for occipitocervical fusions. Postoperative mortality rates from 0% to 33% have been noted. Subaxial subluxations are stabilized by posterior fusions, and debate continues as to whether laminectomy should also be performed in the subaxial region.

Shoulder

More than two-thirds of adult patients with RA have shoulder pain from the glenohumeral joint, the acromioclavicular joint, or the subacromial space (10). The acromioclavicular joint can be treated by excision of the end of the clavicle with the addition of an anterior acromioplasty and subacromial decompression if indicated. Rotator cuff tears may be repaired with standard techniques; however, the tears are often irreparable because of their size and the poor quality of tendons.

Most rheumatoid shoulder surgery is directed toward treatment of the glenohumeral joint. Synovectomy may be performed for synovitis unresponsive to medical management if the articular surfaces are congruent and smooth. Pain can be relieved and range of motion temporarily improved with a well-performed synovectomy. Although successful results from glenohumeral arthrodesis have been reported in RA patients, most surgeons would not recommend this procedure because of multiple joint involvement.

Glenohumeral arthroplasty is now widely accepted in the surgical treatment of RA (11,12). Although some report good results from replacement of only the humeral head, most surgeons recommend replacement of both the glenoid and the humeral head if the rotator cuff is intact. Early surgical referral may lead to better results if arthroplasty is performed prior to significant rotator cuff disease. Some would suggest a hemiarthroplasty if the cuff is torn and irreparable, while others recommend a constrained arthroplasty. Pain relief is predictable following total shoulder replacement, but significant increase in range of motion is less predictable.

Elbow

A number of surgical procedures have been described for the treatment of RA of the elbow (13) but synovectomy and total elbow arthroplasty are the most common. Synovectomy may be done arthroscopically or by more traditional open methods. Open synovectomy may also include excision of the radial head.

There are two main types of elbow replacement commonly used. The unconstrained prosthesis is for use in patients without gross instability or severe destruction. Patients with RA respond very well to this procedure. Eighty-seven percent good and excellent results were reported in 64 patients at an average follow-up of 3.5 years. The semi-constrained designs provide some inherent stability to the prosthetic elbow but allow for some laxity. Morrey has reported good results with this design; 40% to 50% of the replacements in his large series were for RA. In RA patients, often both the shoulder and elbow are involved and the question arises as to which joint should be replaced first. A review of 35 patients suggests that the more painful and limiting joint should be repaired first. If equally involved, the elbow should be replaced first (14).

Wrist and Hand

A number of soft tissue and bone procedures have been described for the rheumatoid wrist and hand (15). Severe arthritis of the wrist may be treated with arthroplasty or arthrodesis. Commonly performed arthroplasties include the silicone flexible implant by Swanson, and various other metal/polyethylene designs. While an excellent result from arthroplasty is better than an excellent result from arthrodesis, arthrodesis is performed more commonly due to complications and the early failure rate of replacement arthroplasty. In patients with RA, it is relatively easy to obtain an arthrodesis and relief of pain is long-lasting. Patients may even function well with bilateral wrist arthrodesis if both are fused in neutral alignment or with one in slight flexion and one in mild extension.

Metacarpophalangeal arthroplasty is the most commonly performed replacement arthroplasty for the rheumatoid hand. Swanson and others have reported excellent pain relief but only modest improvements in grip and pinch strength. Thumb fusion or arthroplasty can be critical to maintain pinch.

Hip

The early experience with hip replacements was plagued by a number of problems that no longer exist as major impediments to long-term success. The first was infection. Although early hip replacements had a high incidence of infection, improvements in the operating room environment and the use of prophylactic antibiotics have substantially reduced the incidence of infection to less than 1%. Currently, particulate debris from cement or polyethylene causing loosening is seen as the major problem in total hip replacement (16,17).

The rate of aseptic loosening requiring revision is estimated at approximately 1% per year; long-term follow-ups at 10 to 15 years have reported a revision rate of approximately 10% to 15%. Roentgenographic analyses, however, suggest an increasing loosening rate with time, with significant signs of loosening in 30% to 40% of femoral components. However, 10-year follow-ups of femoral components cemented with modern technique show 97% are stable (18). Hybrid total hip replacement (cemented femoral stem and uncemented acetabulum) may lead to improved long-term results.

The results of cemented implants in revision of total hip replacement demonstrate diminished longevity. An increased interest has, therefore, arisen in alternative methods of treating failed aseptic total hip replacement, which has brought forth new efforts in the use of cementless components and the increasing use of bone graft to restore lost bone stock. Based on long-term follow-up studies from the first generation of total hip replacements, it appears that conventional hip replacement, while one of the most successful operations devised, has limitations and should be considered in younger, heavier, more active patients only in the absence of suitable alternatives.

Knee

The principles of reconstructive surgery in the knee are similar to those in the hip. The technical goals are maximum conservation of bone stock, restoration of function, and diminution of pain. In unicompartmental disease of the knee in the young active patient, osteotomy may be the procedure of choice. The principle is to unload the affected compartment and have the load shared with the opposite compartment. In the older patient with unicompartmental disease and a satisfactory patellofemoral articulation, unicompartmental arthroplasty may be an alternative to total knee replacement (TKR) (19).

Fixed deformities become worse with time. While all nonsurgical measures should be tried, it is important not to allow deterioration to proceed to the extent that an appropriate alternative has been missed. In both osteotomy and unicompartmental arthroplasty, the more normal the remainder of the joint and the better the range of motion preoperatively, the better the functional result. The earlier the rheumatologist and orthopedic surgeon confer on a problem, the more likely the appropriate procedure will be performed at the proper time.

Modern TKR resurfaces the distal femur and proximal tibia with minimal bone resection. Modern prosthetic designs seek to reproduce the normal anatomy and allow normal kinematics of the knee. The technical goal of knee arthroplasty is to place these components in anatomic alignment and to restore proper ligament and muscle tension by appropriate soft tissue releases. By so doing, shear forces on prosthetic fixation are minimized, and ligaments participate in load sharing. Excellent results are now attainable in OA and RA patients (20). There is a need to be selective in choosing patients for TKR, however, because these replacements are mechanical devices with a finite "life". Clearly, the results of revision TKR do not approach those of primary replacement (21).

Arthroscopic debridement of the knee is indicated in early degenerative arthritis if symptoms are thought to be worsened by internal derangement. Debate continues as to the benefit of arthroscopic debridement or lavage for osteoarthritic knees in the absence of meniscal pathology (22). Arthroscopy can also be helpful in diagnosing and, at times, treating inflammatory arthritis. Synovial biopsy for diagnosis and arthroscopic synovectomy for early disease can be helpful in the short-term management of RA. Knee joint lavage through large bore needles without arthroscopy may also decrease the synovitis of RA when accompanied by steroid injection. Radiation synovectomy has also produced early good results in the management of inflammatory arthritis (23), but is not widely available in the USA.

Foot and Ankle

The forefoot and hindfoot are commonly involved in RA. Patients commonly develop metatarsalgia and are noted to have prominent metatarsal heads and an associated hallux valgus deformity. Surgical procedures include arthrodesis of the first metatarsophalangeal (MTP) joint and resection of the second to fifth metatarsal heads, resection of all five metatarsal heads, replacement arthroplasty of the first MTP joint, isolated osteotomies, or a combination of the above procedures. The hindfoot often shows involvement of the posterior tibial tendon and early arthritic changes at the talo-navicular joint. If the talo-navicular symptoms do not respond to conservative management with medication and orthotic support, early talo-navicular fusion while the foot remains flexible has produced pain relief in greater than 80% of patients. If the hindfoot is passively uncorrectable or unstable, a double or triple arthrodesis may be necessary.

Ankle arthrodesis is the most consistent method of alleviating ankle pain, and numerous techniques have been described. Unfortunately, arthrodesis may be difficult to obtain, and complications are common (24). Although attempts have been made at total ankle arthroplasty, the complication and early failure rates are high. There may, however, be an indication for total ankle replacement in the severely involved RA patient who has significant arthrosis or arthrodesis of the remaining hindfoot. Some have reported good results in selected patients, and newer designs may be more promising.

C. Lowry Barnes, MD
Clement B. Sledge, MD

1. Collins DN, Barnes CL, FitzRandolph RL: Cervical spine instability in rheumatoid patients having total hip or knee arthroplasty. Clin Orthop 272:127–135, 1991
2. Wilson MG, Kelley K, Thornhill TS: Infection as a complication of total knee-replacement arthroplasty. Risk factors and treatment in sixty-seven cases. J Bone Joint Surg 72A:878–883, 1990
3. Sullivan PM, Johnston RC, Kelley SS: Late infection after total hip replacement caused by an oral organism after dental manipulation: a case report. J Bone Joint Surg 72A:121–123, 1990
4. Weinblatt ME: Methotrexate. Textbook of Rheumatology, 4th ed. Edited by Kelley WN, Harris ED, Ruddy S, Sledge CB, Philadelphia, WB Saunders, 1993, pp 767–778
5. Walker LG, Sledge CB: Total hip arthroplasty in ankylosing spondylitis. Clin Orthop 262:198–204, 1991
6. Kilgus DJ, Namba RS, Gorek JE, et al: Total hip replacement for patients who have ankylosing spondylitis: the importance of the formation of heterotopic bone and of the durability of fixation of cemented components. J Bone Joint Surg 72A:834–839, 1990
7. Bergman NR, Rand JA: Total knee arthroplasty in osteonecrosis. Clin Orthop 273:77–82, 1991
8. Johnston RA, Kelly IG: Surgery of the rheumatoid cervical spine. Ann Rheum Dis 49 Suppl 2:837–844, 1990
9. Lipson SJ: Rheumatoid arthritis of the cervical spine. Clin Orthop 239:121–127, 1989
10. Kelly IG: Surgery of the rheumatoid shoulder. Ann Rheum Dis 49 Suppl 2:824–827, 1990
11. Barrett WP, Thornhill TS, Thomas WH: Nonconstrained total shoulder arthroplasty in patients with polyarticular rheumatoid arthritis. J Arthroplasty 4:91, 1989
12. Thomas BJ, Amstutz HC, Cracchiolo A: Shoulder arthroplasty for rheumatoid arthritis. Clin Orthop 265:125–128, 1991
13. Souter WA: Surgery of the rheumatoid elbow. Ann Rheum Dis 49 Suppl 2:871–882, 1990
14. Friedman RJ, Ewald FC: Arthroplasty of the ipsilateral shoulder and elbow in patients who have rheumatoid arthritis. J Bone Joint Surg 69A:661–666, 1987
15. Norris SH: Surgery for the rheumatoid wrist and hand. Ann Rheum Dis Suppl 2:1990
16. Maloney WJ, Jasty M, Harris WH, et al: Endosteal erosion in association with stable uncemented femoral components. J Bone Joint Surg 72A:1025–1034, 1990
17. Schmalzried TP, Kwong LM, Jasty M, et al: The mechanism of loosening of cemented acetabular components in total hip arthroplasty. Clin Orthop 274:60–78, 1992
18. Mulroy RD Jr, Harris WH: The effect of improved cementing techniques on component loosening in total hip replacement: an 11-year radiographic review. J Bone Joint Surg 72B:757–760, 1990
19. Scott RD, Cobb AG, McQueary FG, et al: Unicompartmental knee arthroplasty: eight to twelve year follow-up with survivorship analysis. Clin Orthop 271:96–100, 1991
20. Harris WH, Sledge CB: Total hip and total knee replacement (Second of two parts). New Engl J Med 323:801–807, 1990
21. Friedman RJ, Hirst P, Poss R, et al: Results of revision total knee arthroplasty performed for aseptic loosening. Clin Orthop 255:235–241, 1990
22. Livesley PJ, Doherty M, Needoff M, et al: Arthroscopic lavage of osteoarthritic knees. J Bone Joint Surg 73B:922–926, 1991
23. Sledge CB, Zuckerman JD, Shortkroff S, et al: Synovectomy of the rheumatoid knee using intra-articular injection of Dysprosium-165-ferric hydroxide macroaggregates. J Bone Joint Surg 69A:970–975, 1987
24. Scranton PE: Anoverview of ankle arthrodesis. Clin Orthop 268:96–101, 1991

60. REHABILITATION OF PATIENTS WITH RHEUMATIC DISEASES

Rehabilitation and prevention of deformity are cooperative processes by which patients, health care providers, and families support patients in reaching their maximal potential for function. A team of rehabilitation specialists can provide evaluation of function, with treatment aimed at preserving, restoring, or preventing its decline. The specialists most often consulted include physiatrists, physical and occupational therapists, social workers, vocational counselors, and speech pathologists.

People with rheumatic diseases often need the use of rehabilitation techniques because their disease course is typically chronic—waxing and remitting—and often interferes with function, resulting in disability (1). Evaluation of the functional status of patients with arthritis is important in planning a comprehensive treatment program and in identifying and implementing those interventions that may minimize disability. Functional status must be evaluated in the context of the patient's usual activity.

Function is the result of processes responding to interactions between organ systems and body parts, the entire body and the environment, and the individual and society. Function is often not predictable from simply identifying anatomic or physiologic deficits. It is influenced by motivation and is often determined by beliefs and expectations about diseases and their consequences.

Difficulties in performing the usual activities of daily life, such as dressing, grooming, feeding, and preparing food, are common problems for patients with arthritis. In addition, social and sexual relationships, vocational and avocational activities, and psychological difficulties should be evaluated. Often patients will comment that they are too tired to get out or that they are worried about fertility. These comments may indicate more significant problems and should be further explored. Alternatively, patients may be referred to an occupational therapist or social worker for in-depth assessments. An example of a screening tool designed to evaluate these problems is presented in Fig. 60–1.

Patients with pain, fatigue, weakness, and difficulty in performing their usual daily activities are most likely to benefit from rehabilitation. Sources of pain in patients with rheumatic diseases include joint pain and stiffness; soft tissue inflammation including tendinitis, bursitis, fasciitis and fibromyalgia; and neuropathic pain, most commonly secondary to nerve root compression or peripheral nerve entrapment. However, muscle itself may be a source of pain as is seen in polymyalgia rheumatica and polymyositis. Pain management often includes the use of heat, cold, splinting, walking aids, and transcutaneous nerve stimulation.

Many instruments have been developed to measure function. These are multidimensional questionnaires assessing performance (such as activities of daily living and mobility), pain, global ratings of clinical status, and fatigue (2–6). Physicians caring for people with rheumatic diseases should use these tools and be familiar with criteria and processes that are used in evaluating work disability.

In obtaining a pain history, the patients' selection of words is often a clue to the origin of pain. For example, ''boring'' or ''burning'' frequently reflects pain of neurologic origin; ''stiffness'' or ''tightness'' often describes pain of inflammatory origin.

Fatigue is a hallmark of chronic inflammatory diseases. Its causes are varied and may result from physiologic or psychologic causes. Care should be taken to fully evaluate the probable cause of fatigue. Assessments should include determination of aerobic capacity, sleep history, mood, muscle strength, and muscle endurance. Patterns of motion should be considered in an effort to determine if substitution patterns are energy draining.

The appropriate use of heat, cold, exercise, rest, traction, splints, orthoses, adaptive equipment, and education may help restore and maintain function, and are considered standard rehabilitation treatments. These interventions are most likely to be successful in modulating symptoms rather than controlling the disease process. Rehabilitation treatments should be individualized for patients' needs, must be practical, and should produce an outcome that is valuable and noticeable to patients.

PHYSICAL MODALITIES

Patients with rheumatic disease often need pain control as well as assistance in increasing motion. Nonmedicinal interventions commonly used in rehabilitative practice to relieve pain include both heat and cold. In general, heat is effective in relieving joint pain and stiffness. Specifically, it is useful in the chronic or subacute situations in which joint inflammation and swelling are minimal, and contracture, muscle spasm, or adhesive capsulitis are seen. Heat is a useful adjunct to a stretching program. Superficial heat can be delivered using hot packs, infrared, and hydrotherapy; none of these penetrate the joint to raise intraarticular temperature. Heat can raise the pain threshold and produce sedation and anesthesia. Deep heat is delivered by ultrasound or microwave. Ultrasound can raise intraarticular temperatures and may be useful as an adjunct to stretching techniques, because it increases the plastic stretch of ligamentous structures placed under tension.

Cold, whether delivered by ice packs or topical sprays, can decrease muscle spasm, decrease spasticity, raise pain threshold, provide good local analgesia, and slow down the metabolic rate. Historically, ice has been believed to cause more symptoms of stiffness in patients with rheumatoid arthritis (RA); but some clinical trials suggest that ice may have a beneficial effect in RA. There is evidence to suggest that cold is equally as effective as heat when used adjunctively in range of motion (ROM) programs designed to treat soft tissue problems or degenerative joint disease.

Several studies have explored the combined use of heat or cold and exercise, comparing the results to exercise alone. These modalities seem to enhance the efficacy of exercise programs, perhaps by their analgesic effects. Questions remain about the mechanism of heating versus cooling in treating musculoskeletal problems. Deep heat raises the intraarticular temperature, while superficial heating can actually lower the intraarticular temperature. This seeming paradox is explained by noting that dissipation of joint heat may require vasodilatation, and the vasoconstriction

---

BRIEF INTERVIEW REFERRAL QUESTIONNAIRE

1. Do you have any physical problems that prevent you from doing what you wish or need to do on a daily basis?

2. Do you have the stamina to perform your daily routines or an unexpected activity?

3. In which role do you spend most of your time? Has this recently changed?

4. What do you do for pleasure or recreation? How often do you do these activities?

5. Do you feel in control of your life with respect to decision making, daily activity and routines, and responding to needs and requests of others?

A ''yes'' response to question #1 should prompt the interviewer to question further and suggest a referral to either the physical therapist or the occupational therapist.

A ''no'' response to questions #2 or #5 should generate a referral.

If questions #3 and #4 are answered in a fashion that indicates the patient is inactive or isolated, a referral to a rehabilitation professional is appropriate.

Fig. 60–1. An example of a brief interview referral questionnaire used to help evaluate whether referral is advised.

produced by superficial cold may inhibit or decrease the heat loss. In general, superficial heat rather than deep heat is thought to be the treatment of choice in reducing pain around an inflamed joint, but neither heat nor cold has been shown to influence the progression of these diseases. No beneficial influence of superficial heat on the inflammatory processes has been demonstrated in RA. In fact, increasing the temperature might increase the metabolic rate and potentiate the inflammatory process (7).

Low frequency current has been used to provide analgesia to soft tissues and joints as well as to stimulate muscle contraction. Transcutaneous electrical nerve stimulation (TENS) is the most commonly used electrotechnique. This is a low voltage AC or DC system delivered in pulsed form. It is thought to control perceived pain by stimulating sensory afferents. Neuromuscular stimulation may be delivered in low voltage DC or AC, or high DC, and stimulates the motor neuron. Controlled studies are done relatively rarely in evaluating the efficacy of electric current in the treatment of arthritic pain. The several studies that have been reported suggest that TENS is of unproven benefit (7).

Rest has been shown to be beneficial in the treatment of several arthritic conditions. Most of the clinical studies have looked at its efficacy in patients with RA. Rest, either local or systemic, reduces inflammation and relieves pain. Rheumatoid nodules and roentgenographic joint destruction do not develop when limbs are immobile. Bed rest reduces inflammation and corrects hematologic abnormalities (8). These others have confirmed finding and have noted that patients had decreased pain without loss of strength over the short term.

Casts and splints can be used to reduce local swelling and are most frequently applied to the wrists, hands, and knees. Ample data support the belief that reduction of pain and inflammation occurs; neither strength nor motion at the wrist are lost when the splint is used for less than eight weeks (9).

Rest and splinting have demonstrated efficacy. Their drawbacks primarily are atrophy and joint stiffness. The stiffness usually can be reversed with a vigorous passive ROM exercise program. Bed rest is associated with a decrease in lean body mass and bone mass even after only 2 weeks of rest. In addition, deconditioning occurs with bed rest after one to two weeks. Loss of strength occurs, but at a slower rate than the cardiovascular deconditioning. Local and systemic rest therapies should be monitored to assure maximal benefits and lowest risks (10).

EXERCISE

Fatigue and decreased endurance are frequent symptoms in patients with rheumatic diseases. Treatment of fatigue, weakness, and decreased stamina usually includes exercise. Goals of exercise include increased muscle strength, improved stamina, and increased ROM. Exercise is also prescribed to assist in weight reduction and promote a feeling of well being. Exercise prescriptions are varied and should be specific enough to identify the goal as well as the form and the frequency the exercise should take.

Exercise may be either passive, active, or active-assisted. Passive exercise refers to movement performed by someone other than the patient, such as the physical therapist, or with the use of a device. In active exercise, the patient does the movement. Active-assisted exercise means that the patient moves the limb with support or assistance from the therapist or device.

Active exercise is further classified by how the muscle functions. Isotonic exercise, which is performed in most everyday activities, involves muscle contraction at variable rates and strength with motion of the limb. Isometric exercise employs active muscle contraction during which the muscle length does not shorten and the limb does not move. Isokinetic exercise involves an active contraction as the limb moves at a specified rate against a fixed resistance. Resistive exercise refers to active exercise performed against resistance. Contractions may be concentric (shortening) or eccentric (lengthening); for example, the quadriceps muscle contracts concentrically and the hamstring eccentrically at knee extension.

Exercise should be prescribed for specific purposes, as well as to assist patients in reaching personal goals. Some forms of exercise are preferable for a given problem and disease (see below). Even passive ROM exercise, for example, increases joint temperature and white cell counts in crystalline arthropathy. Isometric exercise maintains strength without causing disease flares in patients with RA (11).

Endurance. Endurance is a measure of the ability to sustain a given static or dynamic task. Static endurance is the duration of a force sustained by a muscle that isometrically contracts. Dynamic endurance requires repetitive movement of muscle. Training in one form of exercise may not be transferable to another. An improvement in isotonic performance, for example, may not result in a commensurate improvement in isometric performance; the reverse may also be true. For patients with minimal joint pain and good functional strength, low-resistance, high-repetition exercise is appropriate. A number of investigators have demonstrated improved cardiovascular function and mobility following bicycling, jogging, skiing, and riding a stationary bicycle in patients with RA. Other benefits from this type of exercise include improved function in activities of daily living, less sick leave, and less bone demineralization in postmenopausal women (12).

Muscle Strengthening Exercise. Muscle atrophy often accompanies the inflammatory arthritides. Reasons for this include disuse, bed rest, use of splints, local inflammation or vascular events, and drug effects. A muscle can lose 30% of its bulk in 1 week. Loss of muscle bulk is associated with functional decline.

Muscle-strengthening exercises are useful for muscles that are weak but not inflamed and should be instituted in a graduated program to allow for weakness, pain tolerance, and functional needs. Isometric exercises restore and maintain strength in patients with inflammatory disease without producing an increase in synovitis. Because resistive exercises are often associated with increased intraarticular pressures and temperatures, they should be discouraged in patients with highly active inflammatory arthritis.

The anatomic areas most likely to need isometric strengthening exercises include neck flexors and extensors, especially when weaning from a soft collar; the shoulder rotator cuff muscles, deltoid, triceps, and biceps; abdominal muscles and back extensors; and the quadriceps, posterior tibialis, toe extensors, and flexors. Techniques for strengthening include positioning the limb in a supported pain-free position and providing instruction for isometric contraction. A device to offer resistance, such as a belt, rubber tubing, floor, or door, may be used when pain and inflammation resolve. The efficacy of strengthening exercises for the hand and wrist remains unproven.

Isotonic exercise with low-weight resistance may be initiated when the isometric program has been well established, the patient is pain-free during exercise, and additional strengthening is needed. Isokinetic exercise is rarely used for people with arthritis.

Rest. Activity and specific muscle-group exercises must be balanced with rest. Patients with inflammatory arthropathy have sleep–wake cycle disruption, as do patients with soft tissue syndromes such as fibromyalgia. Medications used in treating these syndromes and diseases, including nonsteroidal antiinflammatory agents and corticosteroid preparations, also may disrupt natural sleep patterns. These alterations can result in chronic fatigue. Relaxation techniques and exercise may help restore a more normal sleep pattern.

Periodic recumbency during the day has been advocated as a strategy for improving performance. If one can balance strenuous activity with rest, exhaustion is prevented. Recumbency permits a fully supported posture that relieves the force of gravity, permitting muscles to rest. One study suggests that interrupting physical activity with rest results in more total hours of physical activity over a 24-hour period (13). This theory of energy conservation further suggests that adaptive aids, proper posture, and properly designed and fitted splints and orthoses can help sustain maximal functional performance by minimizing energy-inefficient postures, patterns of movement, and environments.

Recreational Activity. People with both RA and osteoarthritis (OA) often seek advice about suitable recreational activities. Since most patients are in fact deconditioned, aerobic exercise is often recommended. The use of low impact aerobic activity is also beneficial in the treatment of soft tissue rheumatism and fibromyalgia. Clinical wisdom teaches that low-resistance exercise is generally well tolerated. In addition, activities in which the limb is fixed at the distal end of the lever (closed kinetic chain exercises) produce significantly higher peak torque at joints, while the shear forces are reduced when compared to open kinetic chain activities. Closed kinetic chain activity includes running, walking, and jumping. Open kinetic chain activity includes cycling and swimming. Characteristically, patients with arthritis do best with reduced load closed kinetic chain activity (walking rather than running) and low resistance open kinetic chain activity (stationary bicycle with low pedal resistance). When possible, it is good to identify those activities that are enjoyable to patients rather than exclusively "good for them". The former are likely to be continued over time.

Maintaining Function. The maintenance of functional ROM is necessary for daily activity and efficiency of movement. Critical ranges necessary for normal ambulation have been carefully determined. This is not true for functional activity of the upper extremity, because a greater variation in patterns of motion and substitutions can be made without significant loss of function. In general, the ability to flex the fingers, supinate the hand, flex the elbow more than 90°, and abduct the shoulder to 90° are essential for self-care and household activities.

To preserve critical function, a ROM program employing a stretch at the end of the pain-free range of motion is desirable. Active and active-assisted ROM are the preferred forms of stretch. When weakness precludes active motion, joint mobility should be preserved using passive ROM or devices and gravity to maintain motion. For example, a pulley or pendulum can be used for circular exercises of the shoulder.

Stretching exercises are particularly helpful in the shoulder following episodes of adhesive capsulitis, calcific tendinitis, and referred pain from cervical radiculopathy. Other examples of such interventions include active-assisted ROM of wrist into extension, maintaining intrinsic muscle length in the fingers and toes, reducing flexion contractures of the knees, and increasing hip extension. Much controversy surrounds the proper stretching techniques for low back pain. The traditional management includes flexion exercises and abdominal strengthening. More recently, extension exercise in an attempt to correct postural abnormalities has been acknowledged to be clinically useful. Both techniques have their place in a clinical management program. The use of extension exercises is specifically recommended for patients with spondylitis. Adjunctive use of heat prior to stretch followed by cold application is often useful in gaining ROM. Evidence suggests that passive stretch may provide significant improvement in range and function in some patients with ankylosing spondylitis (7).

Manipulation is the movement of joints through a range that is greater than their normal range by a few degrees. Occasionally this is done under local anesthesia, as in frozen shoulder, apparently with good results. However, the efficacy of manipulation has not been firmly documented.

Massage, which may use a stroking, kneading, or tapping technique, is primarily used for muscle and general relaxation. No evidence supports the use of massage as a method to stretch or strengthen muscles.

Traction has been used to decrease contractures in the peripheral joints, especially the knee, hip, wrist, and elbow, and to relieve pain caused by compression on the nerve roots by protruded intervertebral discs. More than 25 pounds is needed to increase the interspace distance between cervical vertebrae, and several hundred pounds are needed to do the same for the lumbar spine. Data support the clinical efficacy of traction in cervical radiculopathy.

SPLINTS AND ORTHOSES

A static splint or orthosis is a device used to support a weak or unstable joint, immobilize and rest a joint for pain relief, or maintain a body segment in a functional alignment. Dynamic splints can help create motion of a body part. This type of splint has traditionally been used in managing postoperative hands. The most commonly used splints for the hand are the finger ring splints to inhibit hyperextension of the proximal interphalangeal (PIP) joint in people with swan neck deformities, thereby placing the finger in a more functional position closer to 30° of flexion. Such splints stabilize the lax proximal volar capsule and help with intrinsic muscle relaxation. By rotating the splint 180°, a boutonniere orthosis is created, which supports the dorsal capsule so that the extensor hood is not fully stretched. This permits interosseus and lumbrical muscles to extend the PIP joint. Typically, ring splints are fabricated out of thermoplastic materials. Recently, the use of silver for these splints has made them more cosmetically appealing and acceptable to patients. Patients with carpometacarpal joint disease can benefit from a thumb post splint to immobilize the thumb in flexion and abduction, hence reducing painful motion and permitting functional use of the thumb (Fig. 60–2).

Wrist splinting is helpful for painful arthritis or tendinitis. Resting wrist splints extend from the midforearm to the ends of fingers, and hence interfere with function. They may be clinically useful when worn at night to prevent cramping in flexion and stiffening of the hand and to relieve carpal tunnel symptoms. Functional wrist splints extend from forearm to midpalmar crease and permit full finger use while supporting the wrist.

Upper extremity orthotics are often custom made, although ready-made versions are available. The use of lightweight, heat moldable, washable plastic materials has made splinting readily available and acceptable.

Spinal orthoses are primarily used for relief of pain with the exception of a stabilizing halo or a SOMI (Suboccipital Metal Immobilizer), which may be needed in cases of severe cervical instability. Other spinal braces do not immobilize as effectively in all planes. For the patient with C1–C2 instability, only a halo will provide firm stability, but for those with C5–C6 foraminal encroachment or weakness of the extensors of the neck, a soft collar will support the head and reduce pain. The osteoporotic patient with pain from acute compression fractures and dorsal kyphosis will experience pain relief with temporary use of a brace or corset. The corset is more comfortable, but the thoracic brace

Anatomic Site	Problem	Splint
Wrist	Swelling Pain Carpal tunnel	Functional wrist splint " " " " " "
Hand	Swelling Pain	Resting hand splint " " "
	Swan neck Boutonnière	Finger ring splint
Thumb	Carpometacarpal pain Metacarpophalangeal pain Metacarpophalangeal instability	Thumb post splint " " " " " "

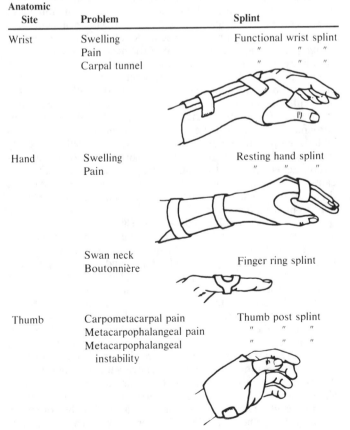

Fig. 60–2. A variety of hand and wrist splints used for patients with rheumatic disease.

may be needed for immobilization. The brace utilizes a three-point pressure system consisting of axillary, chest, and pelvic straps, an abdominal corset, and anterior forces from the uprights in the back. A variety of braces have been used to manage thoracic spine problems. The Jewett, Knight–Taylor, and Knight spinal are those most frequently used for thoracic stabilization. They do immobilize the patient somewhat, while they reinforce abdominal muscles. Often a corset is better tolerated than the thoracic extension braces and is as effective in management of thoracic spine pain associated with vertebral collapse. Thoraco-lumbar braces do not prevent vertebral compression fractures.

Lumbosacral bracing is used to relieve pain. The corset is the orthosis of choice, because it limits lordosis and supports the abdominal musculature with minimal limitations of motion. It is possible that osteoporosis or weakening of the abdominal musculature can occur with prolonged usage. Upright activity and abdominal strengthening exercises should be performed during the bracing period, and the corset should be discontinued at the earliest possible time.

No spinal orthosis has been shown to be effective in preventing deformity or relieving pain for patients with spondylarthropathy. These are, in fact, not recommended since they may increase osteoporosis.

Unlike the spinal and upper extremity orthoses, which are designed to decrease motion and provide local rest to painful anatomic areas, the lower extremity orthoses are often needed to correct a biomechanical problem or malalignment. They are designed to provide stability and proper alignment or to decrease weight on the limb. The only way to realign the hip (short of surgery) is to place it in a long leg brace with a pelvic band, in traction, or in a spica cast, all of which severely limit function. These methods are rarely used.

The knee can be orthotically aligned by any one of three different approaches. One is a long leg brace from midthigh to foot. This knee–ankle–foot orthosis can control flexion–extension or valgus–varus motion. A second type of knee brace controls rotation and valgus–varus motion. Examples of this brace include the Lennox Hill, Lerman, and Swedish Knee Cage (Fig. 60–3). The third approach is to position the foot in such a way as to create motion at the knee. If the foot is kept in 5° of plantar flexion throughout gait and dorsiflexion is blocked, a moment of force is created that favors knee extension. This helps compensate for a weak quadriceps muscle. A solid-ankle-cushion-heel design permits rapid compression of the heel, because it is made of polyurethane and favors knee extension.

An orthosis for the foot should be comfortable, transferrable to different shoes, and lightweight (Fig. 60–4). It should balance the foot with respect to the floor—that is, the foot should be parallel to the floor for stable, efficient walking, while the tibia remains perpendicular. Often, patients with inflammatory arthropathies will develop deformities that cannot be corrected, especially those where the joint fuses, as in psoriatic arthritis. Alternatively, severe ligamentous laxity may occur, so that the foot cannot be held in the corrected position, as in RA. In these cases, the orthosis should accommodate rather than correct the problem, to provide a comfortable gait.

Significant foot involvement occurs in 80% of patients with RA and in 50% of those with OA. The patient with RA may have forefoot problems of painful callosities, cock-toe deformity, subluxed metatarsophalangeal (MTP) joints, and hallux valgus. The patient with OA may develop mallet toes, hallux valgus, or hallux rigidus. These problems are easily accommodated by providing a deep, wide, soft leather shoe with a crepe sole that permits adequate toe clearance and a metatarsal pad or bar to remove weight from the MTP joints. A rocker sole can be used to facilitate roll off. Common hindfoot problems include heel pain, Achilles tendinitis, collapse of the medial arch, and pronation. These abnormalities are often associated with pain and instability, especially on uneven ground. Treatment requires a sturdy shoe that can accommodate an insert and has a firm medial counter, such as an extra-depth shoe, or a walking shoe or sturdy running shoe. The insert should incorporate a scaphoid pad to support the arch and may also need a more rigid orthosis that immobilizes the hindfoot. Occasionally, such an orthosis must be

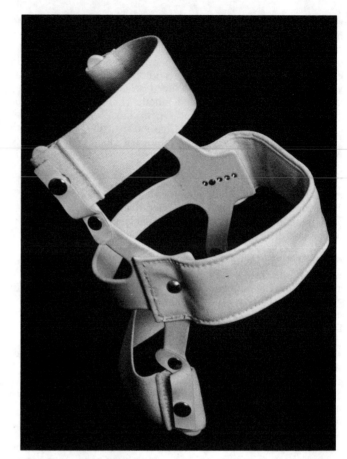

Fig. 60–3. *A Swedish knee cage.*

able to extend over the maleoli. Heel pain may respond to a soft or rigid heel cup and supination of the foot.

Evidence suggests that shoe modifications may be of some benefit for valgus or varus knee deformities, because the patient can shift the weight-bearing column medially or laterally as needed.

Plaster casting to immobilize painful joints has been successful in treating tendinitis of the elbow (tennis elbow), wrist and finger tendons (de Quervain's tendinitis), and Achilles tendon. Plaster casting has also been successfully used to stretch contractures, especially those of the elbow, knee, and heel cord. This is accomplished by recasting every few days while obtaining 1°–2°

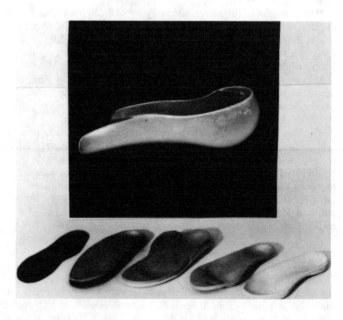

Fig. 60–4. *A variety of shoe inserts.*

more in the desired direction. A turnbuckle orthosis can also be used.

ADAPTIVE AIDS

To conserve energy, relieve pain, and promote maximal function, patients with arthritis may need an assistive device that can substitute for the absent or deficient function. Patients, however, must be willing to use the device.

Mobility aids include canes, crutches, and wheelchairs; motorized versions of wheelchairs have become more streamlined and affordable. The case is prescribed for balance and for partially relieving weightbearing (14). Crutches can almost completely unweight a limb. If there is a significant balance problem or if endurance is compromised, the wheelchair is the preferred device. Bathroom safety equipment such as grab bars, tub seats, and raised toilet seats can improve independence in self-care. Kitchen and self-care devices can significantly improve function, conserve energy, and reduce joint stress. Manuals listing these devices are readily available (15).

COMPREHENSIVE CARE

The interactions between chronic pain and medications, between functional loss and deformity, and between self-concept and appearance are complex. Interventions to treat all aspects of the disease and their psychologic impact are needed for the arthritis patient. The rehabilitation team, consisting of occupational and physical therapists and physicians, can help significantly by teaching patients how to evaluate and solve problems pertaining to mobility, self-care, and psychosocial function.

One area of need for support and counseling is that of sexual dysfunction. Sexual problems are common in the population in general but patients with arthritis, particularly those with hip dysfunction and juvenile onset arthritis, experience more frequent dysfunction. Mechanical problems associated with pain, stiffness, decreased ROM, fatigue, and family problems related to role disruption and drug-related mood changes have all been recognized as contributors to sexual problems. A pamphlet published by the Arthritis Foundation is available with suggestions for relieving pain and dysfunction associated with sexual activity (16).

Inability to work in the home, school, or work site is a major problem for people with arthritis. Musculoskeletal disorders are the second most frequent cause of work disability; people with RA and OA have the highest disability rates (17). Rehabilitation treatments are associated with improved functional level and economic independence (18), and patients with such problems should be referred for therapy.

Vocational or job counseling should begin with a determination of the patient's level of function, the ergonomics or energy requirements to perform the job, and an evaluation of the work site with respect to architectural barriers. If adjustments can be made in the work setting or home, this is the desired course. The patient who has the ability to control working conditions—hours, pace, team activity—is more likely to continue working (19).

Lynn Gerber, MD

1. Colvez A, Blanchet M: Disability trends in the US population 1966–1976: analysis of reported causes. Am J Public Health 71:464–471, 1981
2. Fries JF, Spitz P, Kraines RG, et al: Measurement of patient outcome in arthritis. Arthritis Rheum 23:137–145, 1980
3. Jette AM: Functional capacity evaluation: an empirical approach. Arch Phys Med Rehabil 61:85–89, 1980
4. Meenan RF, Gertman PM, Mason JH: Measuring health status in arthritis: the arthritis impact measurement scales. Arthritis Rheum 23:146–152, 1980
5. Liang MH: The historical and conceptual framework for functional assessment in rheumatic diseases. J Rheum 155:2, 1987
6. Pincus T, Summey JA, Soraci SA, et al: Assessment of patient satisfaction in activities of daily living using a modified standard health assessment questionnaire. Arthritis Rheum 26:1346, 1983
7. Michlovitz SL: Thermal Agents in Rehabilitation, 2nd ed. Philadelphia, Penn., Davis, 1990
8. Backman CL, Deitz JC: Static wrist splint: its effect on hand function in 3 women with RA. Arthritis Care Res 1:151, 1988
9. Gault SJ, Spyker JM: Beneficial effect of immobilization of joints in rheumatoid and related arthritides: a splint study using sequential analysis. Arthritis Rheum 12:34–44, 1969
10. Drinkwater BL, Horvath SM: Detraining effects on young women. Med Sci Sports 4:9105, 1972
11. Machover S, Sapecky AJ: Effect of isometric exercise on the quadriceps muscle in patients with rheumatoid arthritis. Arch Phys Med Rehabil 47:737–741, 1966
12. Nordemar R: Physical training in rheumatoid arthritis: a controlled long term study II. Functional capacity and general attitudes. Scand J Rheumatol 10:25–30, 1981
13. Gerber L, Furst G, Shulman B, et al: Patient education program to teach energy conservation behaviors to patients with rheumatoid arthritis: a pilot study. Arch Phys Med Rehabil 68:442–445, 1987
14. Blount WP: Don't throw away the cane. J Bone Joint Surg 38A:695–698, 1956
15. Guide to Independent Living for People with Arthritis. Atlanta, Ga., Arthritis Foundation, 1988
16. Living and loving with arthritis: information on sex and arthritis. Atlanta, Ga., Arthritis Foundation, 1991 (pamphlet)
17. Kramer J, Yelin E, Epstein W: Work disability in rheumatoid arthritis: effects of disease, social and work factors. Ann Intern Med 93:551–556, 1980
18. Spiegel JS, Spiegel TM, Ward NB, et al: Rehabilitation for rheumatoid arthritis: a controlled trial. Arthritis Rheum 29:628–637, 1986
19. Walliston KA, Kaplan GD, Mardes SA: Development validation of the health focus of control (HLC) scale. J Consult Clin Psychol 4:530–535, 1976

61. PSYCHOSOCIAL FACTORS AND ARTHRITIS

A wide variety of psychological and environmental variables may be affected by and may influence health status. Most of the literature regarding the psychosocial dimensions of arthritis has been based on the responses of adult patients with rheumatoid arthritis (RA), although psychosocial factors are an important variable in most, if not all, rheumatic conditions.

ENVIRONMENTAL STRESS

Most studies indicate that arthritis is associated with a variety of stressors that may adversely affect patients. Patients with RA commonly report that stress often precedes flare-ups in disease activity (1). There also is some evidence that neural structures (such as the hypothalamus) associated with stress responses may be involved in the inflammatory process in RA (2). Recently, investigators have begun to examine relationships between stress, the immune system, and other biologic variables. It has been reported, for example, that frequent daily stresses are associated with high proportions of B cells relative to T cells (3) and high erythrocyte sedimentation rates (4). More complex relationships also have been found in which daily stresses are associated with mood disturbances that, in turn, are related to decreases in soluble interleukin-2 receptor levels and increases in joint pain (5).

DEPRESSION AND ANXIETY

Studies of the emotional reactions associated with arthritis primarily have used standardized measures such as the Minnesota Multiphasic Personality Inventory (MMPI), Beck Depression Inventory (BDI), Center for Epidemiologic Studies–Depression scale (CES–D), the Anxiety and Depression subscales of the Arthritis Impact Measurement Scales (AIMS) (see Chapter 8F), and structured psychiatric interviews. Most investigations have found that patients with RA and fibromyalgia (FM) show elevated levels of depression and anxiety relative to healthy controls or other patient groups. For example, the frequency with which depression and anxiety disorders are diagnosed among RA patients has been found to range from 14% to 42% (6). The frequency of these disorders among FM patients has been found to range from 20% to 86% (7). No studies have examined the frequency of mood and anxiety disorders among large samples of patients with osteoarthritis (OA).

Psychological distress has been shown to be associated with high levels of medical service utilization among patients with RA (8). Thus, early identification and effective treatment of psychological distress might reduce patients' health care costs and improve their well-being. It should be noted, however, that some of the measures that are used to evaluate psychological distress, such as the MMPI and BDI, contain items that are biased because they refer to physical symptoms associated with arthritis or other chronic diseases. As a result, a patient with arthritis might produce elevated scores on the MMPI Depression scale by responding "false" to an item such as, "I am about as able to walk as I ever was." Nevertheless, elevated levels of depression and anxiety have been found among patients with RA and FM even when relatively uncontaminated measures, such as the CES-D and structured psychiatric interviews, have been used (6).

Several recent longitudinal investigations have examined changes in anxiety and depression among RA patients. It has been reported that anxiety and depression levels show only modest change over periods ranging from 6 months to 5 years (9). Two of these studies have revealed that increases in the number of tender or painful joints tend to be accompanied by increases in anxiety and depression (10). However, it also has been shown that pain severity, age, lack of satisfaction with current life style, and degree of functional impairment are better predictors of depression and anxiety than are joint counts and other measures of disease activity (11). It is possible that disease activity would be a more powerful predictor of psychological distress if patients were studied intensively over short time periods in order to eliminate inaccurate recall of subjective events. Indeed, in a recent study of 54 patients with RA followed daily for 75 consecutive days, it was found that age, neuroticism, and chronic pain were independent predictors of daily mood states, such as depression, anxiety, and hostility (12). Disease activity failed to predict daily mood. The lack of association between disease activity and affective distress may seem surprising. However, the potential effects of disease activity on patients' psychological reactions may be modified by cognitive and behavioral factors, such as patients' perceptions of helplessness, control, and self-efficacy as well as their coping strategies.

COGNITIVE AND BEHAVIORAL FACTORS THAT INFLUENCE PSYCHOLOGICAL REACTIONS

Learned Helplessness and Perceptions of Control

Learned helplessness refers to a phenomenon characterized by emotional, motivational, and cognitive deficits in adaptive coping with stressful situations. The deficits are produced by an individual's perception that no viable solutions are available to eliminate or reduce the source of stress. It has been suggested that learned helplessness might underlie a portion of the psychological distress and behavioral disabilities shown by patients with arthritis. That is, many patients may develop the belief that their diseases are beyond their effective control because the diseases are of unknown causes, have no cures, and have chronic and unpredictable courses. This perception of uncontrollability may cause the patients to experience anxiety and depression (emotional deficits) that, in turn, may lead to increased pain and reduced attempts to engage in activities of daily living (motivational deficits) or to develop new means of adapting to their disabilities and distress (cognitive deficits).

The importance of perceptions of helplessness in adaptation to arthritis has been confirmed in many studies. All of these investigations have used various forms of a self-report measure, the Arthritis Helplessness Index (AHI), to assess the extent to which individuals believe they can control their arthritis symptoms. It has been shown, for example, that high levels of helplessness among patients with RA are associated with low self-esteem, use of maladaptive coping strategies, high levels of pain and depression, and high levels of functional impairment (13,14). Moreover,

a three-year longitudinal study has shown that disease severity and helplessness are the best predictors of future disability in physical functioning (15). These investigations suggest that improved perceptions of control over symptoms are desirable for patients with RA. Nevertheless, a recent study has demonstrated that patients who believe they can control their symptoms suffer psychological distress in response to increased pain unless they cognitively restructure their pain experiences, such as adopting the belief that pain has made life more precious (16).

Self-Efficacy

Another cognitive factor closely related to perceptions of helplessness or control is self-efficacy. In contrast to perceptions of control of numerous symptoms, self-efficacy represents a belief that one can perform specific behaviors or tasks to achieve specific health-related goals. There may be great variation for any individual in self-efficacy for different behaviors. For example, an individual with RA may have high self-efficacy for pacing daily activities to reduce pain and fatigue but may have low self-efficacy for performing exercises to improve physical function.

Self-efficacy tends to predict health status if individuals believe that the relevant behaviors will lead to improved health and if they value improved health status. Lorig and coworkers reported that high baseline levels of self-efficacy for pain and functional ability were strongly associated with low levels of pain, disability, and depression at the initial assessment and at a four-month follow-up assessment (17). An independent investigation found that high self-efficacy for pain was significantly correlated with low frequencies of observable displays of pain behavior among persons with RA even after controlling for demographic factors and disease severity (18).

Coping Strategies

The coping process is comprised of several stages. These are: 1) appraisal of the threat associated with a particular stressor; 2) performing behaviors (coping strategies) that may control the impact of the stressor; and 3) evaluating the outcomes produced by the behaviors and, if necessary, performing alternative coping responses.

Studies of coping among patients with various forms of arthritis primarily have used three instruments: the Ways of Coping Scale, the Coping Strategies Questionnaire, and the Vanderbilt Pain Management Inventory. Despite the use of different instruments, it has been found consistently that passive coping strategies, such as escapist fantasies (hoping that pain will get better someday) and catastrophizing (believing that no coping strategy will effectively control symptoms) are associated with high levels of psychological distress and high levels of pain among patients with RA (19). Conversely, psychological adjustment and relatively low levels of pain and functional impairment have been found to be associated with strategies such as attempts to derive personal meaning from the illness experience, seeking information about arthritis, focusing on positive thoughts during pain episodes, and infrequent catastrophizing.

Nearly all studies have consisted of cross-sectional examinations of the relationships between coping strategies and health status. A recent longitudinal investigation, however, used causal modeling to examine predictors of psychosocial adaptation to RA (20). It was found that high baseline levels of perceived competence (a construct similar to self-efficacy) and low helplessness contributed directly to low future levels of depression. In addition, initial levels of helplessness interacted with passive pain coping strategies so that the presence of one of these factors led to an increase in the other. Passive coping strategies, in turn, contributed directly to high future levels of impairment in psychosocial functions, such as family and social relationships and work. These data represent the first evidence of causal links between perceptions of control, self-efficacy, coping strategy use, and psychosocial adaptation to RA.

PSYCHOSOCIAL INTERVENTIONS

Given the strong relationships between health status and cognitive and behavioral factors, attention recently has been devoted to testing psychosocial interventions that may improve patients' pain, emotional states, or function. The major psychosocial interventions can be classified according to the factors that the interventions were intended to modify in order to improve patient health status. Nevertheless, many of the interventions share common treatment components. It should be noted that these interventions do not include protocols that are intended only to increase patient knowledge, exercise, or adherence with treatment regimens.

Control and Self-Efficacy Interventions

Several investigators have examined the effects of group therapy interventions on patients' perceptions of symptom control and health status. For example, Bradley and colleagues evaluated a biofeedback-assisted group therapy intervention that trained patients with RA and their family members in relaxation and behavioral problem-solving skills. The intervention, relative to attention-placebo and no adjunct treatment conditions, produced significant reductions in pain behavior and disease activity at posttreatment. A one-year follow-up showed that patients who received the intervention reported lower levels of pain and depression than those who received no adjunct treatment (21). Contrary to expectations, however, neither perceptions of control nor functional ability were influenced by the intervention.

In contrast to interventions designed to increase perceptions of symptom control, treatments that emphasize self-efficacy have tended to produce better maintenance of treatment gains. Lorig et al. (22) recently reported that the Arthritis Self-Management Program (ASMP) produced significant increases in self-efficacy for pain and other symptoms as well as significant reductions in pain ratings and arthritis-related physician visits among patients with RA and OA. Moreover, these improvements were maintained for four years after treatment initiation. Estimated net four-year savings in health care costs were $648 for each patient with RA and $189 for each patient with OA. However, the ASMP did not alter functional ability among the patients.

Coping Skills Training

All of the studies of coping skills training have been conducted with OA patients. Keefe et al (23,24) compared the effects of a coping skills training program, relative to arthritis education and standard care, in patients with OA of the knee. Coping skills training produced significant reductions in patients' ratings of pain and psychological disability. These effects generally were maintained at six-month follow-up. In addition, patients who received coping skills training reported significant reductions in physical disability from posttreatment to follow-up.

Education and skills training delivered to patients by telephone may represent a cost-effective method for improving patient adherence with treatment and health status. Weinberger and colleagues recently examined the outcomes produced by a telephone intervention, delivered by lay personnel, for patients with OA. This intervention provided education, reviewed medications and clinical problems with the patients, and taught strategies for increasing patient involvement during physician encounters. The telephone intervention produced significant improvements in patients' reports of pain and functional ability and did not substantially increase patients' health care costs (25). Several reanalyses of the data revealed that the beneficial effects of the intervention could not be attributed to enhanced social support, satisfaction with care, morale, medication adherence, or intensified medical treatment (26,27). It remains to be determined if the beneficial effects of telephone counseling may be replicated by other investigators and if the factors that mediate these effects may be identified.

FUTURE DIRECTIONS

There are complex relationships between patients' cognitive and behavioral responses to their illnesses and their well-being. Psychosocial interventions produce reliable improvements in patients' pain and emotional states. The effects of these interventions on functional abilities, however, is variable.

It is anticipated that several issues will receive greater attention from future investigators. First, there will be increased emphasis on longitudinal studies of the relationships among patients' responses to their illnesses and their well-being and health status. The intensive daily study methodology is an especially useful method for understanding these complex relationships. Second, there will be greater use of large data bases and multivariate methods of analysis to better identify causal associations among medical status variables, demographic and psychosocial factors, well-being, and health status. Third, more effort will be devoted to understanding the relationships among patients' environments, thoughts, behaviors, and immune system responses. There also will be attempts to determine the influence of these associations on clinical status and long-term outcomes. Finally, two important concerns will be addressed in studies of psychosocial interventions. There will be modifications of current psychosocial interventions so that they may have greater impact on patients' functional abilities. In addition, attention will be devoted to helping patients maintain their improvements following treatment. This will include training family members and patients to better recognize events that lead to relapses in coping skill usage, and development of skills to respond constructively to these events.

Laurence A. Bradley, PhD

1. Affleck GA, Pfeiffer C, Tennen H, et al: Attributional processes in rheumatoid arthritis patients. Arthritis Rheum 30:927–931, 1987
2. Chikanza IC, Petrou P, Kingsley G, et al: Defective hypothalamic response to immune and inflammatory stimuli in patients with rheumatoid arthritis. Arthritis Rheum 35:1281–1288, 1992
3. Zautra AJ, Okun M, Robinson SE, et al: Life stress and lymphocyte alterations among patients with rheumatoid arthritis. Health Psychol 8:1–14, 1989
4. Thomason BT, Brantley PJ, Jones GN, et al: The relation between stress and disease activity in rheumatoid arthritis. J Behav Med 15:215–220, 1992
5. Harrington L, Affleck G, Urrows S, et al: Temporal covariation of soluble interleukin-2 receptor levels, daily stress, and disease activity in rheumatoid arthritis. Arthritis Rheum 36:199–203, 1993
6. Ahles TA, Khan S, Yunus MB, et al: Psychiatric status of patients with primary fibromyalgia, patients with rheumatoid arthritis, and subjects without pain: a blind comparison of DSM-III diagnoses. Am J Psychiat 148:1721–1726, 1991
7. Hudson JI, Goldenberg DL, Popo HG, et al: Comorbidity of fibromyalgia with medical and psychiatric disorders. Am J Med 92:363–367, 1992
8. Katz PP, Yelin EH: Prevalence and correlates of depressive symptoms among persons with rheumatoid arthritis. J Rheumatol 20:790–796, 1993
9. Wolfe F, Hawley DJ, Cathey MA: Clinical and health status measures over time: prognosis and outcome assessment in rheumatoid arthritis. J Rheumatol 18:1290–1297, 1991
10. Parker J, Smarr K, Anderson S, et al: Relationship of changes in helplessness and depression to disease activity in rheumatoid arthritis. J Rheumatol 19:1901–1905, 1992
11. Hawley DJ, Wolfe F: Anxiety and depression in patients with rheumatoid arthritis: a prospective study of 400 patients. J Rheumatol 15:932–941, 1988
12. Affleck G, Tennen H, Urrows S, et al: Neuroticism and the pain-mood relation in rheumatoid arthritis: insights from a prospective daily study. J Consult Clin Psychol 60:119–126, 1992
13. Nicassio PM, Wallston KA, Callahan LF, et al: The measurement of helplessness in rheumatoid arthritis: the Arthritis Helplessness Index. J Rheumatol 12:462–467, 1985
14. DeVellis RF, Callahan LF: A brief measure of helplessness in rheumatic disease: the helplessness subscale of the Rheumatology Attitudes Index. J Rheumatol 20:866–869, 1993
15. Lorish CD, Abraham N, Austin J, et al: Disease and psychosocial factors related to physical functioning in rheumatoid arthritis. J Rheumatol 18:1150–1157, 1991
16. Tennen H, Affleck G, Urrows S, et al: Perceiving control, construing benefits, and daily processes in rheumatoid arthritis. Can J Behav Sci 24:186–203, 1992
17. Lorig K, Chastain RL, Ung E, et al: Development and evaluation of a scale to measure perceived self-efficacy in people with arthritis. Arthritis Rheum 32:37–44, 1989
18. Buescher KL, Johnston JA, Parker JC, et al: Relationships of self-efficacy to pain behavior. J Rheumatol 18:968–972, 1991
19. Keefe FJ, Brown GK, Wallston KA, et al: Coping with rheumatoid arthritis pain: catastrophizing as a maladaptive strategy. Pain 37:51–56, 1989
20. Smith CA, Wallston KA: Adaptation in patients with chronic rheumatoid arthritis: application of a general model. Health Psychol 11:151–162, 1992
21. Bradley LA, Young LD, Anderson KO, et al: Effects of cognitive-behavioral therapy on rheumatoid arthritis pain behavior: one-year follow-up. Pain Research

and Clinical Management, vol 3 (edited by R Dubner, G Gebhart, M Bond). Amsterdam: Elsevier, 1988, pp. 310–314

22. Lorig KR, Mazonson PD, Holman HR: Evidence suggesting that health education for self-management in patients with chronic arthritis has sustained health benefits while reducing health care costs. Arthritis Rheum 36:439–446, 1993

23. Keefe FJ, Caldwell DS, Williams DA, et al: Pain coping skills training in the management of osteoarthritic knee pain: a comparative study. Behav Ther 21:49–62, 1990

24. Keefe FJ, Caldwell DS, Williams DA, et al: Pain coping skills training in the management of osteoarthritic knee pain-II: follow-up results. Behav Ther 21:435–447, 1990

25. Weinberger M, Tierney WM, Cowper PA, et al: Cost-effectiveness of increased telephone contact for patients with osteoarthritis: a randomized, controlled trial. Arthritis Rheum 36:243–246, 1993

26. Weinberger M, Tierney WM, Booker P, et al: The impact of increased contact on psychosocial outcomes in patients with osteoarthritis: a randomized, controlled trial. J Rheumatol 18:849–854, 1991

27. Rene J, Weinberger M, Mazzuca S, et al: Reduction of joint pain in patients with knee osteoarthritis who have received monthly telephone calls from lay personnel and whose medical treatment regimens have remained stable. Arthritis Rheum 35:511–515, 1992

62. THE ECONOMIC IMPACT OF ARTHRITIS

ESTIMATING THE COST OF ILLNESS

Health economists traditionally divide the economic costs of illness into two components: *direct costs*, defined as the cost of treating the illness, and *indirect costs*, or those costs due to lost productivity as a result of morbidity or mortality. The direct costs of an illness are estimated from the perspective of the society as a whole, even though insurance or free care may buffer the individual with illness from those costs. Indirect costs include the lost wages of those people forced to leave the labor force or to reduce their work time, the equivalent in wages of homemakers' activities when they can no longer function fully in that role, and the value individuals place on non-work (or non-homemaking) activities they must forego as a result of the illness. In practice, estimates of the wage-loss costs are more precise than those of homemaker's losses, because it is difficult to price the latter in the marketplace. Furthermore, estimates of homemaker's losses are more precise than those placed on non-work activities.

Estimates of direct and indirect costs of illness are sensitive to the prices placed on health care services and to the real value of wages. In a period of rapid inflation in medical care costs, illnesses with high health care costs will appear to be more burdensome even though what is done on behalf of people with those illnesses has not changed. Likewise, when real wages grow, illnesses associated with a high prevalence of work disability appear to be more burdensome even though the prevalence of work disability has not increased. The estimates of the economic impact of arthritis is affected by both of these dynamics. Because arthritis is a frequent cause of work disability and wages have been relatively stagnant, and because arthritis is generally not a high-cost condition while medical care inflation has been rampant, estimates of the impact of arthritis show a slight decrease over time. This decrease in estimates of cost have occurred despite the increasing prevalence of the condition due to population aging and to apparently increased work disability rates.

THE ECONOMIC IMPACT OF ARTHRITIS

Three comprehensive studies of the national cost of illness have been performed by Rice and colleagues for the years 1962, 1972, and 1980 (1–4); Table 62–1 summarizes the results of these studies. In 1962 when the total cost of arthritis was approximately $4 billion, one-half was accounted for by direct medical expenditures and one-half was due to indirect costs. The 1960s may have been the best decade for the United States in terms of economic growth, with real wages rising by 3% per year during

that time. By 1972, the proportion of the total cost of arthritis due to lost wages grew to 60%, even though the absolute direct cost of treating this group of conditions increased by 100%, to $4 billion. After wages stagnated in 1973 in the face of medical care inflation, the proportion of all costs due to direct medical care expenditures increased to 62%, even though the wage loss portion increased in absolute terms from $5 to $8 billion. The real value of the medical care expenditures grew from 0.3% to 0.5% of gross national product (GNP), while the real value of the indirect costs receded, from 0.4% to 0.3% of GNP.

During the years studied, the total cost of arthritis ranged from 0.7% to 0.8% of GNP. When GNP declines by this much, the economy can be said to be in a mild to moderate recession. Thus, the economic cost of arthritis every year approximates the impact of the recent economic downturn. Because the costs accrue in every year, however, they are not noticed.

WORK DISABILITY DUE TO ARTHRITIS

As stated earlier, accounting methods, particularly high rates of medical care inflation in a time of stagnant wages, reduce estimates of the total costs of arthritis. Table 62–2 displays cross-sectional data of the prevalence of work disability among people with arthritis. Only rheumatoid arthritis (RA) has been studied in clinical samples. In the RA studies (5–8), from 51% to 59% of people who had worked prior to onset of the disease were no longer employed; among all people with RA, 49% were not working. In a community-based sample, the diagnosis is not verified by physicians. In this study, the proportion not working varied from 36% among those reporting arthritis symptoms without having received a definitive diagnosis from their physician, to 53% among those with osteoarthritis, to 72% (among those with RA) (8,9).

TRENDS IN WORK DISABILITY DUE TO ARTHRITIS

As evidenced by the data in Table 62–2, a high proportion of working age people with arthritis report that they are out of the labor force due to their condition. Yelin and Katz (10) recently evaluated the trend in work disability among such people. Table 62–3 summarizes the data from their study. They found that the proportion of working age people with arthritis in the work force declined overall by 16% between 1970–1975 and 1982–1987. The decline was especially steep among those 55–64 years of age with arthritis (35%). Thus, the access of people with arthritis to jobs seems to have diminished with the passage of time.

Table 62–1. *The economic cost of arthritis in the United States: 1962, 1972, and 1980*

Year	Direct Costs			Indirect Costs			Total		
	Billions	% Total	% GNP	Billions	% Total	% GNP	Billions	% Total	% GNP
1962	2	50	0.3	2	50	0.3	4	100	0.7
1972	4	44	0.3	5	56	0.4	9	100	0.7
1980	13	62	0.5	8	38	0.3	21	100	0.8

Source: references 1–4. GNP gross national product.

Table 62–2. *Work disability rate among persons with arthritis, by study type*

Study	Type of Sample	Condition	Group Studied	Work Disability Rate
Yelin, et al, 1980	Clinical	RA	Worked before onset	59%
Reisine, et al	Clinical	RA	Worked before onset	57%
Yelin, et al, 1987	Clinical	RA	Worked before onset	51%
Yelin, et al, 1987	Clinical	RA	All working age persons	49%
Pincus, et al	Community	RA	All working age persons	72%
Pincus, et al	Community	OA	All working age persons	53%
Pincus, et al	Community	Arthritis, not specified	All working age persons	36%

Source: Reference 8

SUMMARY

Studies of the economic impact of arthritis indicate a small increase between the years 1962 and 1980, due to sharply rising medical care costs for this set of conditions and little change in the indirect costs with the wage stagnation after the early 1970s. At any one point, the absolute impact of arthritis is roughly equivalent to the impact of a mild to moderate recession, just under 1% of GNP; however, these estimates are sensitive to changes in the relative prices of medical care and wages. While studies of the economic impact indicate stagnancy in the indirect cost of arthritis, studies of the time trend in the work disability rate due to this condition show a rising prevalence of work loss. Thus, if wages had continued their historic climb, the great prevalence of work disability due to arthritis would have yielded much larger and growing estimates of their impact. Other dynamics yield a downward bias in estimates of the economic impact of arthritis. This is so, because arthritis disproportionately affects

the elderly who are less often expected to work, and non-work losses are not well estimated by current methods. In addition, arthritis disproportionately affects women whose work is either not remunerated (in the case of homemakers) or poorly remunerated (in the case of most female workers). Thus, although the economic impact of arthritis approaches 1% of GNP—a large sum in and of itself—according to current methods of accounting, the true economic cost is no doubt much larger.

Edward Yelin, PhD

1. Rice D: Estimating the Cost of Illness. National Center for Health Statistics, Health Economics Series, No. 6, 1966
2. Cooper B, Rice D: The Economic Costs of Illness Revisited. Soc Security Bull 39:21–35, 1976
3. Rice D, Hodgson T, Kopstein A: The Economic Costs of Illness: A Replication and Update. Health Care Financing Rev 7:61–80, 1985
4. Yelin E, Felts W: A summary of the impact of the musculoskeletal conditions in the United States. Arthritis Rheum 33:750–755, 1990
5. Yelin E, Meenan R, Nevitt M, et al: Work disability in rheumatoid arthritis: effects of disease, social, and work factors. Ann Intern Med 93(4):551–556, 1980
6. Reisine S, Grady K, Goodenow C, et al: Work disability among women with rheumatoid arthritis: the relative importance of disease, social, work and family factors. Arthritis Rheum 32:539–543, 1989
7. Yelin E, Henke C, Epstein W: The work dynamics of the person with rheumatoid arthritis. Arthritis Rheum 30:507–512, 1987
8. Felts W, Yelin E: The economic impact of the rheumatic diseases in the United States. J Rheumatol 16:867–884, 1989
9. Pincus T, Mitchell J, Burkhauser R: Substantial work disability and earnings losses in individuals less than 65 with osteoarthritis: comparisons with rheumatoid arthritis. J Clin Epidemiol 42:449–457, 1989
10. Yelin E, Katz P: Labor force participation among persons with musculoskeletal conditions, 1970–1987: national estimates derived from a series of cross-sections. Arthritis Rheum 34:1361–1370, 1991

Table 62–3. *Proportion of persons with arthritis in laborforce in the United States: 1970–1975 versus 1982–1987*

Year	Age 18–44	45–54	55–64	All
1970–1975	72%	70%	55%	67%
1982–1987	73%	61%	37%	56%
Change	+1%	−13%	−33%	−16%

Source: Reference 10

63. NONTRADITIONAL REMEDIES

"All who drink of this remedy are cured, except those who die. Thus, it is effective for all but the incurable."

Galen

The use of unproven remedies is widespread in the United States. Indeed a recent *Time* magazine cover feature discussed "the new age of alternative medicine" (1). Most rheumatic disease patients, regardless of socioeconomic or educational background, try a number of unproven remedies at an economic cost of many billions of dollars annually (2).

Why? Perhaps because "the quack sells hope" (3). Rheumatic diseases are still largely chronic and incurable. Many of our conventional therapies are not really very acceptable. Also, we probably have overestimated our ability to alleviate our patients' suffering (4). The notion that there may be cheap, safe, simple, and potentially effective alternatives is one that is seductive to patients who may feel helpless in the face of unpredictable but often relentlessly progressive and disabling disease. And our explanations of why patients are sick are often inadequate. Thus therapies that promise to empower with control of their illness—such as wearing a copper bracelet or minding their diets—offer a powerful attraction indeed.

What then is the harm? It has been argued that expenditures on unproven remedies divert scarce health care resources from more appropriate areas. It seems doubtful, however, that pa-

tients would be likely to invest these dollars in the traditional health care budget even if they were dissuaded from unproven remedies. Alternative medicine offends and angers many of us. We have been rigorously trained in science. We often have little sympathy for patients who question our wisdom and appear so foolish as to seek alternatives to our recommendations. We may have underestimated patient dissatisfaction with long waits, short visits, brusque answers, inadequate explanations, frequent drug side effects, persistent symptoms, and high charges. A serious worry is that patients seeking alternative remedies will inappropriately neglect their illness. Despite the recognized limitations of our therapeutic interventions, we clearly have much to offer our patients (4,5). We certainly want to offer these patients the best we have. The greatest danger is that some alternative therapies are not innocuous but, in fact, may be harmful. There are well-documented instances of patients receiving drugs other than those promised with very adverse results, such as marrow aplasia or serious infections from contaminants, including death (6).

Yet, despite our impressive scientific advances, we must concede the limits of our understandings of rheumatic diseases and the empiricism of our therapies. For example, we use gold because it was employed for tuberculosis and because we thought the pathogenesis of rheumatoid arthritis (RA) was similar to tuberculosis. We use hydroxychloroquine, which worked for malaria, and methotrexate, which derived from management of psoriasis. Is it less rational to consider other new possible therapies that seem unusual today?

We, as physicians, pride ourselves on our intellectual curiosity and honesty, and we recognize that novel ideas and insights may emanate from unsuspected sources. Indeed, the study of certain unconventional therapies, such as antimicrobials, diet and nutrition, and exercise, has been enlightening.

PLACEBO THERAPY

It is appropriate to begin discussion of specific nontraditional therapies with placebo. Placebo derives from the Hebrew *et-ha-lech* (I shall walk) (Psalm 116:9), which was translated into the Septuagint Greek as *euarestiso* and then into the Latin as *placebo* (I shall please). It was not until the 18th century that the term was associated with make-believe medicine (7). Placebo therapy can be remarkably effective, with salutary effects in up to 45% of arthritis patients (8). Reasons for this are unclear, but may include psychological conditioning, neurohumoral, neuroimmunologic, and other factors. We need to be reminded of this powerful potential effect as we evaluate therapies.

ANTIMICROBIAL THERAPIES

Nitroimidazole antimicrobial drugs have been used to treat patients with RA. Their use was predicated on the efficacy of another imidazole derivative, levamisole, and on the unproven notion that RA is caused by *Amoeba limax* and could thus be treated with these agents. Controlled studies concluded that the benefit afforded was not dramatic and was attended by a large number of side effects (2). Agents in this class of drugs include metronidazole and clotrimazole. Unsubstantiated claims of efficacy are still made for these drugs.

Rifamycin is an antibiotic that blocks DNA-dependent RNA polymerase and inhibits cellular protein synthesis. It has been administered intraarticularly to treat rheumatoid synovitis of the knee. Controlled studies have indicated clinical benefit with few adverse effects and with diminished pathologic abnormalities for IV rifamycin; benefit was inconsistent when the drug was given orally (2,9). It was speculated that rifamycin might act as an antimitotic agent.

Tetracycline was proposed for treating patients with RA many years ago based on the unproven hypothesis that the disease was caused by mycoplasma infection. Examination of the possible efficacy of this antibiotic (1 g 4 times/day for 52 weeks) for patients with established RA found no differences compared with placebo controls, and no patients experienced remissions. These observations were interpreted as indicating that organisms sensitive to tetracycline did not play an active role in advanced RA (2). More recent work has found that tetracyclines, particularly minocycline, reduced collagenase activity, impaired bone resorption, affected T-cell and neutrophil function, and were antiproliferative, antiinflammatory, and antiarthritic in animal models of chronic arthritis. Recent uncontrolled observations suggest modest antirheumatic effect for minocycline in patients with RA (10). A large, controlled multicenter trial sponsored by the National Institutes of Health is underway to evaluate potential utility of minocycline in RA.

Several other antimicrobials have been considered for arthritis therapy. To assess whether patients with chronic inflammatory arthritis and antibody titers to *Borrelia burgdorferi* of 1:64 or greater might respond to antibiotic therapy, subjects were randomized to placebo or ceftriaxone (2 gm/day intravenously for 2 weeks) in a double-blind trial (11). Results were encouraging in about 40% of patients. A study of ampicillin, 3 gm/day for 3 months during the first year of disease, followed by traditional drugs (mainly gold or antimalarials) for seropositive RA patients, was associated with retardation of disease progression in 58% of patients and complete remission in 16% up to 4½ years later (12). In a small, brief, double-blind, placebo-controlled trial, the antiviral agent amantadine was reportedly beneficial to a group of patients with teenage-onset juvenile rheumatoid arthritis who had elevated antibody titers to influenza A and who were born in a year of influenza epidemic (13). These are interesting observations which, if confirmed, could be interpreted as consistent with the hypotheses that chronic arthritis in some patients results from bacterial, spirochete, or viral infection(s), that antimicrobials are antirheumatic, or both.

PHARMACOLOGIC THERAPIES

Dapsone has been used in the treatment of patients with RA, and others with certain inflammatory skin diseases based on its immunomodulatory effects in vitro (inhibition of the alternate complement pathway and neutrophil cytotoxicity). Several and its effecuncontrolled and controlled studies have shown significant improvement of clinical and laboratory parameters of RA. Despite potentially serious adverse effects, including anemia, headache, and possible agranulocytosis, dapsone was well tolerated. This drug has been favorably compared with the slower-acting, second-line antirheumatic drugs (2). More data are needed before its status as a major antirheumatic drug can be accepted.

Since the successful introduction of penicillamine as an antirheumatic drug, other effective but less toxic sulfhydryl-containing compounds have been sought. In response to this search, pyrithioxine, tiopronin, and 5-thiopyridoxine have been studied. Tiopronin, like penicillamine, dissociated rheumatoid factor in vitro and has now been studied in four trials in patients with RA. Tiopronin seemed more effective than penicillamine (although differences did not reach statistical significance) and it had comparable adverse reactions. Unless tiopronin is shown to be effective at lower doses with less toxicity, its use will be limited. 5-Thiopyridoxine is a structural analog of vitamin B_6 with a sulfhydryl group, like penicillamine, at the 5 position. It was effective in treating cold agglutinin disease and in reducing cold agglutinin titers, and was therefore studied in patients with RA. Treated patients demonstrated significant improvement, but side effects were frequent. 5-Thiopyridoxine, like tiopronin, is very similar to penicillamine. Unfortunately, its potential value seems limited. Certainly, an effective, tolerable penicillamine-like (sulfhydryl) compound would be desirable as an alternative to penicillamine.

Beta-adrenergic blockers have been found to suppress cellular release of rheumatoid factor in vitro, formation of human EA-rosettes, and lymphocyte proliferation. Based on these data and on anecdotal observations of benefit, clinical studies of the effect of propranolol on RA were carried out. Findings did not document a significant antirheumatic effect (2). Beta blockers have not found a role in therapy for rheumatic disease.

Haloperidol, a major tranquilizer, was shown to increase serum protein sulfhydryl levels in patients with RA, as did the slow-acting antirheumatic drugs. Twelve patients with RA who received haloperidol showed a significant increase in serum sulfhydryl levels and clinical improvement; extra-pyramidal side effects were mild (2). More observations are necessary.

Ethylenediaminetetraacetate (EDTA) was used in an uncontrolled fashion to treat patients with RA, and the responses were alleged to be good to excellent. Toxic reactions included nausea and potassium loss (2). Available information was insufficient to regard this substance as antirheumatic.

Other pharmacologic agents have been used to treat RA. Most represent preliminary, unconfirmed, and often uncontrolled studies. These include captopril and cisretinoic acid for which data are incomplete (2). Thalidomide has been useful in the treatment of erythema nodosum leprosum, which may have some clinical and immunologic similarities to RA. Open studies of thalidomide for RA and cutaneous lupus suggested promise (14). Isoprinoside is an antiviral, immunostimulatory drug that increases interleukin–2 production, stimulates T cell differentiation, increases natural killer cell function, improves monocyte chemotaxis, and induces lymphocyte surface markers. It has been used to promote pharmacologic immunoenhancement in the elderly and to treat patients with RA; results have been inconsistent (15). Amiprilose hydrochloride is a novel, synthetic carbohydrate with antiinflammatory and immunomodulatory properties. It appeared promising in trials for RA (16).

BIOLOGIC AGENTS

Thymopoietin, a polypeptide isolated from thymus gland extracts, is immunologically active. It induced early T cell differentiation, inhibited B cell differentiation, and affected functions of mature lymphocytes. The pentapeptide, corresponding to certain thymopoietin residues, retained biologic activity and was examined in several clinical trials. Patients with RA who were treated with certain dosages showed significant clinical benefit, with several adverse effects (2). Further trials are underway to better define any potential role of this material in the therapy of RA.

Several groups tried transfer factor therapy for small numbers of patients with RA. The rationale for use was its ability to confer antigen-specific (and perhaps antigen-nonspecific) immunity to immunodeficient hosts. Unfortunately, it is unclear what, if any, is the critical immunodeficiency in RA, what antigen-specific response would be desirable to confer, and from which donors transfer factor should be prepared. Perhaps these considerations contributed to the inability to document convincingly the clinical efficacy of transfer factor for patients with the disease (12).

Placental factor therapy has been used to treat patients with RA, based on the rationale that since pregnancy is known to ameliorate the symptoms of RA, the placental membrane may be immunomodulatory. Preliminary reports of placental-eluted gammaglobulins suggested clinical and immunologic improvement, usually accompanied by mild side effects (2). This experience has evolved into therapeutic use of gammaglobulins.

Bee, ant, and other venoms have been considered for treating patients with RA. Bee venoms are rich in phospholipase and other antiinflammatory substances. They have been shown to suppress the development of experimental arthritis, but have not been proven to affect disease in humans. Moreover, the estimated therapeutic dose of bee venom would now be prohibitively expensive. Purified extracts from *Pseudomyrmex*, an ant species, were clinically effective in treating patients with RA, and the extracts showed in vitro anticomplementary and lymphocyte-inhibitory effects (2). Snake venoms have been promoted for treating arthritis, presumably also based on the presence of potentially potent antiinflammatory substances. Little or no clinically relevant scientific data are available on their use. The ant and perhaps other venom studies are of interest. Some may eventually provide a novel and useful mode of antirheumatic therapy.

A Chinese herbal remedy, *Tripterygium Wilfordii* hook F, has been studied in a prospective, controlled, double-blind fashion in patients with RA. Results indicated significant improvement in clinical parameters (joint tenderness and swelling, morning stiffness, grip strength, and walking time) and immunologic measures (erythrocyte sedimentation rate, C-reactive protein, and Ig levels) after one month of therapy. Adverse experiences included diarrhea, vaginal hemorrhage, and anorexia. An extract of this substance was found to be potently immunosuppressive, with effects including inhibition of T cell and B cell proliferation, interleukin–2 elaboration, and immunoglobulin production. This might explain the antirheumatic effect (17).

The lay press has featured claims that sex hormone therapy (progesterone and estrogen for women, and testosterone and progesterone for men) resulted in dramatic cures for patients with osteoarthritis and RA. Little objective data exists to substantiate these claims.

Considerable enthusiasm has been generated for fever-producing bacterial vaccine therapy for RA. Controlled studies have not been performed and no definitive study of bacterial vaccine therapy has yet been conducted.

TOPICAL THERAPIES

Dimethyl sulfoxide (DMSO) has a structure similar to sulindac and possesses unique solvent properties. Usually applied topically, the properties of DMSO include membrane penetration, antiinflammatory effects, scavenging of oxygen free radicals, nerve blockade, bacteriostasis, diuresis, and vasodilation. Dimethyl sulfoxide has not been found to be effective for digital ulcers in patients with systemic sclerosis or for RA. Indeed, one report associated DMSO therapy with worsening of experimental arthritis in animals (2). It has received considerable publicity, which may contribute to its popularity, and is sought by many frustrated patients. More than a few patients travel abroad for DMSO therapy, particularly to certain clinics in Mexico. It has been repeatedly documented that these clinics have misrepresented medications, dispensed potentially hazardous drugs, and have not provided DMSO to patients. In fact, patients have been given corticosteroids, diazepam, phenylbutazone, or dipyrone (18). Dimethyl sulfoxide is also widely available in this country in an impure form for veterinary use.

Several topical creams are now available that have little scientific support for their efficacy. A recent study compared 10% triethanolamine salicylate (contained in various over-the-counter creams) with placebo for osteoarthritic knees. No clinical benefit was apparent from treatment (2). Creams containing capsaicin, to deplete neural substance P and promote analgesia appear promising; lotions containing gold are marketed, but are not known to be of proven efficacy.

MECHANICAL AND INSTRUMENTAL THERAPIES

The lay press has reported that hyperbaric oxygen may benefit those with arthritis. A rationale for using this therapy in RA was based on findings of low pH, low synovial fluid pO_2, increased oxygen uptake, elevated lactate production, and relatively inadequate blood flow in inflamed joints. Experimentally, hyperbaric oxygen had immunosuppressive and antiarthritic effects. However, patients who were given hyperbaric oxygen for RA or for other reasons have not experienced improvement of their arthritis.

Laser irradiation to soft tissues and joints has immunologic effects, and uncontrolled studies of patients with RA have reported benefits. Confirmation and extension of these observations is needed. Intraarticular use of laser for synovectomy is also of interest.

Few published studies on the effectiveness of acupuncture exist. The mechanisms by which insertion of fine needles into predetermined anatomic locales can induce anesthesia and relieve pain remain obscure. Placebo, hypnotic, and endorphin-like effects have been suggested. Adjunctive benefit has been suggested for RA, but no benefit was demonstrated for osteoarthritis, chronic shoulder pain, or low back pain (2).

Photopheresis has been used in pilot studies for RA and appears promising (19). Therapy involves extra corporeal photoactivation of biologically inert methoxysalen (8–methoxypsoralen) by ultraviolet A energy to a form that covalently cross links lymphocyte DNA and subsequent reinfusion of injured cells into patients. This form of therapy has been successful for cutaneous T-cell lymphoma.

NUTRITIONAL THERAPY

A relationship between nutrition and rheumatic disease may occur through two possible mechanisms that are not mutually exclusive. Nutritional modification might alter immune responsiveness, thereby affecting manifestations of rheumatic disease. Rheumatic disease may also be a manifestation of food hypersensitivity in the same manner as more traditionally recognized forms of food allergies, such as eczema, urticaria, asthma, and gastrointestinal problems.

Modification of the Immune Response

Nutritional status exerts a profound influence on immune responsiveness. Protein or protein-calorie malnutrition, fasting, caloric restriction, and qualitative changes in dietary intake were associated with altered immune responses in animals and humans and, in some instances, affected the expression and evolution of autoimmune disease. For example, NZB/NZW F_1 hybrid mice with systemic lupus erythematosus (SLE) who were fed coconut oil (a diet deficient in essential fatty acids) or given prostaglandin E_1 survived longer than control animals or those fed a safflower oil-rich diet (rich in essential fatty acids). Experimental mice with SLE fed a Menhaden oil diet rich in eicosapentaenoic acid (a naturally occurring, substituted, polyunsaturated fatty acid analog), lived longer than control mice. Benefit was achieved if the diet was begun after onset of clinical SLE. Similar diets have ameliorated collagen-induced arthritis in animals in some but not all experimental circumstances. Clinical trials for patients with RA (20) but not SLE (21) thus far suggested modest decreases in certain symptoms. These observations suggest that dietary factors, which modified the generation of arachidonic acid-derived prostaglandins or leukotrienes, affect inflammatory and immunologic responses and may potentially ameliorate symptoms of rheumatic diseases (3).

Vitamins and Minerals

Ascorbic acid has interesting immunoenhancing effects and was found at reduced levels in joints and blood of patients with RA, who have impaired immune responses. There is, however, no clinical evidence that vitamin C has therapeutic effects for RA (2).

Copper bracelets were used by the ancient Greeks for their mysterious power to relieve aches and pains. Copper salts have been used more recently concurrent with the development of gold salt therapy for RA. Patients with rheumatic diseases were treated in open trials with copper compounds, achieving generally favorable results but also many adverse effects. Copper in bracelets is absorbed through the dermis. Patients wearing copper bracelets experienced more subjective improvement than did those wearing identical-appearing placebo aluminum bracelets. Although of interest, copper salts have not achieved an important role in rheumatic disease therapy.

Oral zinc therapy has been tried in patients with RA. The rationale was based on the following observations: 1) serum zinc levels are low in RA, 2) zinc promotes wound and ulcer healing, 3) D-penicillamine enhances intestinal absorption of zinc, 4) zinc is antiinflammatory in vitro, and 5) zinc is necessary for the maintenance of certain cellular immune responses. Zinc-deficient mice or cattle had impaired T cell mediated immune responses, and zinc deficiency was found in some children with common variable immunodeficiency. Immune responses could be restored with zinc. Elderly subjects also displayed significant improvement in RA when given zinc sulfate. One study of zinc in RA indicated that, at certain intervals, the zinc-treated group fared better than did the placebo-treated patients. Improvement was not quantitatively great, was not consistent at all evaluation times, and was not confirmed in several other studies (2).

L-Histidine, available in health food stores, has been used to treat patients with RA. Possible benefit was seen in only a small subgroup of patients. Serum histidine, but not other amino acids, was decreased in patients with RA compared with normal subjects, patients' family members, and other individuals. Serum levels correlated with clinical features of disease, and histidine–cystine–copper inhibited in vitro heat-induced aggregation of human IgG. A prospective randomized, placebo-controlled trial suggested benefit in patients over 45 years of age with more active and prolonged RA.

Food Allergy

Food antigens may cross the gastrointestinal mucosal barrier, enter the circulation in antigenic form, circulate as immune complexes, and sensitize cells, and may therefore be pathogenic. The gastrointestinal tracts of patients with RA might be more penetrable to food antigens than those of normal individuals, although this hypothesis has not been confirmed. While adverse food reactions have traditionally been associated with gastrointestinal, respiratory, or cutaneous manifestations, they have also been linked with many other symptoms (3). Both IgE- and non-IgE-mediated immunologic mechanisms are important.

Physicians and patients have been intrigued for many years with the idea that arthritis might in some instances be the result of hypersensitivity to foods or food-related products. Certain observations suggest relationships between foods and rheumatic

diseases. These include largely uncontrolled reports of palindromic rheumatism associated with sodium nitrate hypersensitivity; Behcet's syndrome with black walnuts; lupus with canavanine in alfalfa (which may crossreact with native DNA or activate B lymphocytes), and hydrazine; and RA with alternaria, house dust, tobacco smoke, petrochemicals, tartrazine, dairy products, wheat, corn, beef, and other foods. Since some of these patients had circulating immune complexes containing IgE–IgG–anti-IgE, it was proposed that these related to pathogenesis of symptoms (3). Rheumatoid-like synovitis in rabbits has been induced by substituting cows' milk for water in the diet. Recent careful double-blinded, prospective, placebo-controlled studies confirmed that, for a very few selected patients, inflammatory arthritis may be associated with certain foods and that some of these patients had evidence of immunologic reactivity to these food antigens. These observations supported the suggestion that individualized dietary manipulations may prove to be beneficial for certain patients with rheumatic disease (3).

Our traditional view that patients with rheumatic diseases should follow a sound, balanced diet and that no further relationship exists between food and symptoms is changing. Provocative experimental and clinical observations suggest that nutritional modulation might affect autoimmunity and clinical disease. Certain patients may have food sensitivity as a basis for their symptoms.

OTHER THERAPIES

Biofeedback improved the symptoms of patients with RA and compared favorably with physiotherapy. Larger studies over long periods of time are needed before an adjunctive therapeutic role for biofeedback is clear.

The number of potential unproven remedies for arthritis is probably limited only by the imagination. Claims of efficacy have been made for many remedies, usually in the lay or popular literature or by word of mouth, but not in peer-reviewed, scientific literature. Such remedies include burial in horse manure; yucca tablets; cocaine; buckeyes; horse chestnuts; potatoes; mussel extracts; immune milk; Chinese herbal remedies, which have been found to be adulterated with corticosteroids; topical oils, such as snake, cod liver, olive, peanut, and motor; and topical applications of brake fluid, gasoline, kerosene, lighter fluid, corncob particles, and aloe vera.

Gadgets and devices have also been popular. These include an "inductoscope" (allegedly of magnetic induction), a "solarama board" (to align mixed-up electrons), an earthboard or "vitalator" (to produce rejuvenating electrons), a "vrilium tube" (containing barium chloride in a brass tube), an "oxydonor" (to "reverse the death process into life process" and cure arthritis), a "polorator" (purported electric heat-shocking machine), and vibrators. "Radon pads," said to emit radioactive materials, and sitting in an inactive uranium mine have also been promoted for arthritis therapy, without evident substantiation of efficacy (2).

CONCLUSIONS

The prevalence of nontraditional remedies should be considered a reminder of the limitation of our understanding of rheumatic disease and of our ability to satisfactorily alleviate the suffering of our patients. That we consider them seriously is an indication of our open-mindedness and intellectual curiosity.

Some nontraditional arthritis remedies have been used safely and effectively, some are undergoing serious evaluation, and a few are of theoretical interest and may find future utility in treating patients with rheumatic disease. Others are best left to folklore.

Use of unproven remedies is widespread and costly. Educating colleagues, patients, and the public as to proper or inappropriate use of such remedies poses a difficult challenge, but is one that must be met, with appropriate understanding and sympathy for our patients, if we are to protect our patients from unnecessary hazards, maximize available health care resources, and ultimately better care for our patients.

" 'I didn't say it was good for you' the King replied. 'I said there was nothing like it.' "

Lewis Carroll
Through the Looking Glass

Richard M. Panush, MD

1. Wallis C: Why new age medicine is catching on. Time, Nov 4, 1991, pp 68–76
2. Panush RS: Controversial arthritis remedies. Bull Rheum Dis 34:1–10, 1984
3. Panush RS, editor: Nutrition and Rheumatic Diseases. Rheum Dis Clinics 17:xiii–447, 1991
4. Panush RS: What we don't know about rheumatoid arthritis and its therapy, Mediguide for Inflammatory Diseases, Edited by Goodwin JS, New York, NY Lawrence Dellacorte Publications, 9(1):1–3, 1990
5. Hochberg MC, Paul E, Aristidou M: Increase correlation of "avoidable mortality" from musculoskeletal disease and rheumatology manpower: a measure of effectiveness of subspecialty care. Arthritis Rheum 31:S36, 1988
6. Kraus A, Guerra–Bautista G, Alarcon–Segovia D: *Salmonella arizona* arthritis and septicemia associated with rattlesnake ingestion by patients with connective tissue diseases: a dangerous complication of folk medicine. J Rheumatol 18:1328–1331, 1991
7. Lasagna L: The placebo effect. J Allergy Clin Immunol 78:161–165, 1986
8. Weinblatt ME, Maier AL, Emery P: Substantial placebo response in active rheumatoid arthritis (RA). Arthritis Rheum 33:S152, 1990
9. Gabriel SE, Conn DL, Luthra H: Rifampin therapy in rheumatoid arthritis. J Rheumatol 17:163–166, 1990
10. Breedveld FC, Bijmans BAC, Mattie H: Minocycline treatment for rheumatoid arthritis; an open dose finding study. J Rheumatol 17:43–46, 1990
11. Caperton EM, Heim–Duthoy K, Matzke GR, et al: Ceftriaxione therapy of chronic inflammatory arthritis. Arch Intern Med 150:1677–1682, 1990
12. Wawrzynska–Pagowska J, Brzezinska B: A trial of ampicillin in the treatment of rheumatoid arthritis. Results of long-term observations indicating the possibility of inhibiting the progression of bone deformity. Rheumatologia 22:1–10, 1984
13. Pritchard MH, Munro J: Preliminary report: successful treatment of juvenile chronic arthritis with a specific antiviral agent. Br J Rheumatol 28:521–524, 1989
14. Gutierrez-Rodriquez O, Starusta–Bacal P, Guiterrez–Montes O: Treatment of refractory rheumatoid arthritis—the thalidomide experience. J Rheumatol 16:158–163, 1989
15. Brezeski M, Madhok R, Hunter JA, et al: Randomized, double-blind, placebo controlled trial of inosine pranobex in rheumatoid arthritis. Ann Rheum Dis 49:293–295, 1989
16. Riskin WG, Gillings DB, Scarlett JA: Amiprilose hydrochloride for rheumatoid arthritis. Ann Intern Med 111:455–465, 1989
17. Tao X, Davis LS, Lipsky PE: Effect of the chinese herbal remedy *Triptergium Wilfordii* Hook F on human immune responsiveness. Arthritis Rheum 34:1274–1281, 1991
18. Dlesk A, Ettinger MP, Longley S, et al: Unconventional arthritis therapies. Arthritis Rheum 25:1145–1147, 1982
19. Malawista SE, Trock DH, Edelson RC: Treatment of rheumatoid arthritis by extra corporeal photochemotherapy: a pilot study. Arthritis Rheum 34:646–654, 1991
20. Kremer JM, Lawrence D, Jubiz W, et al: Dietary fish oil and olive oil supplementation in patients with rheumatoid arthritis: clinical and immunological effects. Arthritis Rheum 33:810–820, 1990
21. Moore GE, Yarboro C, Sedving NG, et al: Eicosapentaenoic acid (EPA) in the treatment of systemic lupus erythematosus (SLE). Arthritis Rheum 30:533, 1987

APPENDICES

1. The American Rheumatism Association 1987 revised criteria for the classification of rheumatoid arthritis

Critierion	Definition
1. Morning stiffness	Morning stiffness in and around the joints, lasting at least 1 hour before maximal improvement
2. Arthritis of 3 or more joint areas	At least 3 joint areas simultaneously have had soft tissue swelling or fluid (not bony overgrowth alone) observed by a physician. The 14 possible areas are right or left PIP, MCP, wrist, elbow, knee, ankle, and MTP joints
3. Arthritis of hand joints	At least 1 area swollen (as defined above) in a wrist, MCP, or PIP joint
4. Symmetric arthritis	Simultaneous involvement of the same joint areas (as defined in 2) on both sides of the body (bilateral involvement of PIPs, MCPs, or MTPs is acceptable without absolute symmetry)
5. Rheumatoid nodules	Subcutaneous nodules, over bony prominences, or extensor surfaces, or in juxtaarticular regions, observed by a physician
6. Serum rheumatoid factor	Demonstration of abnormal amounts of serum rheumatoid factor by any method for which the result has been positive in <5% of normal control subjects
7. Radiographic changes	Radiographic changes typical of rheumatoid arthritis on posteroanterior hand and wrist radiographs, which must include erosions or unequivocal bony decalcification localized in or most marked adjacent to the involved joints (osteoarthritis changes alone do not quality)

*For classification purposes, a patient shall be said to have rheumatoid arthritis if he/she has satisfied at least 4 of these 7 criteria. Criteria 1 through 4 must have been present for at least 6 weeks. Patients with 2 clinical diagnoses are not excluded. Designation as classic, definite, or probable rheumatoid arthritis is *not* to be made.

2. Criteria for determination of progression and remission of rheumatoid arthritis and of functional capacity of patients with the disease

Classification of Progression of Rheumatoid Arthritis (1)

Stage I, Early
*1. No destructive changes on roentgenographic examination
2. Roentgenologic evidence of osteoporosis may be present

Stage II, Moderate
*1. Roentgenologic evidence of osteoporosis, with or without slight subchondral bone destruction; slight cartilage destruction may be present
*2. No joint deformities, although limitation of joint mobility may be present
3. Adjacent muscle atrophy
4. Extraarticular soft tissue lesions, such as nodules and tenosynovitis may be present

Stage III, Severe
*1. Roentgenologic evidence of cartilage and bone destruction, in addition to osteoporosis
*2. Joint deformity, such as subluxation, ulnar deviation, or hyperextension, without fibrous or bony ankylosis
3. Extensive muscle atrophy
4. Extraarticular soft tissue lesions, such as nodules and tenosynovitis may be present

Stage IV, Terminal
*1. Fibrous or bony ankylosis
2. Criteria of stage III

*The criteria prefaced by an asterisk are those that must be present to permit classification of a patient in any particular stage or grade.

1. Steinbrocker O, Traeger CH, Batterman RC: Therapeutic criteria in rheumatoid arthritis. JAMA 140:659–662, 1949

Proposed Criteria for Clinical Remission in Rheumatoid Arthritis* (1)

Five or more of the following requirements must be fulfilled for at least two consecutive months:
1. Duration of morning stiffness not exceeding 15 minutes
2. No fatigue
3. No joint pain (by history)
4. No joint tenderness or pain on motion
5. No soft tissue swelling in joints or tendon sheaths
6. Erythrocyte sedimentation rate (Westergren method) less than 30 mm/hour for a female or 20 mm/hour for a male

* These criteria are intended to describe either spontaneous remission or a state of drug-induced disease suppression, which simulates spontaneous remission. To be considered for this designation a patient must have met the ARA criteria for definite or classic rheumatoid arthritis at some time in the past.
No alternative explanation may be invoked to account for the failure to meet a particular requirement. For instance, in the presence of knee pain, which might be related to degenerative arthritis, a point for "no joint pain" may not be awarded.
Exclusions: Clinical manifestations of active vasculitis, pericarditis, pleuritis or myositis, and unexplained recent weight loss or fever attributable to rheumatoid arthritis will prohibit a designation of complete clinical remission.

1. Pinals RS, et al: Preliminary criteria for clinical remission in rheumatoid arthritis. Arthritis Rheum 24:1308–1315, 1981

American College of Rheumatology revised criteria for classification of functional status in rheumatoid arthritis (1)*

Class I: Completely able to perform usual activities of daily living (self-care, vocational, and avocational)
Class II: Able to perform usual self-care and vocational activities, but limited in avocational activities
Class III: Able to perform usual self-care activities, but limited in vocational and avocational activities
Class IV: Limited in ability to perform usual self-care, vocational, and avocational activities

* Usual self-care activities include dressing, feeding, bathing, grooming, and toileting. Avocational (recreational and/or leisure) and vocational (work, school, homemaking) activities are patient-desired and age- and sex-specific.

1. Hochberg MC, Chang RW, Dwosh I, et al: The American College of Rheumatology 1991 revised criteria for the classification of global functional status inrheumatoid arthritis. Arthritis Rheum 35:498–502, 1992

3. Revised criteria for the classification of systemic lupus erythematosus

1982 Revised criteria for classification of systemic lupus erythematosus*

Criterion	Definition
1. Malar rash	Fixed erythema, flat or raised, over the malar eminences, tending to spare the nasolabial folds
2. Discoid rash	Erythematous raised patches with adherent keratotic scaling and follicular plugging; atrophic scarring may occur in older lesions
3. Photosensitivity	Skin rash as a result of unusual reaction to sunlight, by patient history or physician observation
4. Oral ulcers	Oral or nasopharyngeal ulceration, usually painless, observed by a physician
5. Arthritis	Nonerosive arthritis involving two or more peripheral joints, characterized by tenderness, swelling, or effusion
6. Serositis	a) Pleuritis—convincing history of pleuritic pain or rub heard by a physician or evidence of pleural effusion *OR* b) Pericarditis—documented by ECG or rub or evidence of pericardial effusion
7. Renal disorder	a) Persistent proteinuria greater than 0.5 grams per day or greater than 3+ if quantitation not performed *OR* b) Cellular casts—may be red cell, hemoglobin, granular, tubular, or mixed
8. Neurologic disorder	a) Seizures—in the absence of offending drugs or known metabolic derangements; e.g., uremia, ketoacidosis, or electrolyte imbalance *OR* b) Psychosis—in the absence of offending drugs or known metabolic derangements, e.g., uremia, ketoacidosis, or electrolyte imbalance
9. Hematologic disorder	a) Hemolytic anemia—with reticulocytosis *OR* b) Leukopenia—less than 4,000/mm^3 total on two or more occasions *OR* c) Lymphopenia—less than 1,500/mm^3 on two or more occasions *OR* d) Thrombocytopenia—less than 100,000/mm^3 in the absence of offending drugs
10. Immunologic disorder	a) Positive LE cell preparation *OR* b) Anti-DNA: antibody to native DNA in abnormal titer *OR* c) Anti-Sm: presence of antibody to Sm nuclear antigen *OR* d) False positive serologic test for syphilis known to be positive for at least 6 months and confirmed by *Treponema pallidum* immobilization or fluorescent treponemal antibody absorption test
11. Antinuclear antibody	An abnormal titer of antinuclear antibody by immunofluorescence or an equivalent assay at any point in time and in the absence of drugs known to be associated with "drug-induced lupus" syndrome

*The proposed classification is based on 11 criteria. For the purpose of identifying patients in clinical studies, a person shall be said to have systemic lupus erythematosus if any four or more of the 11 criteria are present, serially or simultaneously, during any interval of observation.

1. Tan EM, Cohen AS, Fries JF, et al: The 1982 revised criteria for the classification of systemic lupus erythematosus (SLE). Arthritis Rheum 25:1271–1277, 1982

4. Preliminary criteria for classification of systemic sclerosis (scleroderma)

For the purposes of classifying patients in clinical trials, population surveys, and other studies, a person shall be said to have systemic sclerosis (scleroderma) if the one major or two or more minor criteria listed below are present. Localized forms of scleroderma, eosinophilic fasciitis, and the various forms of pseudoscleroderma are excluded from these criteria.

A. Major criterion

Proximal scleroderma: Symmetric thickening, tightening, and induration of the skin of the fingers and the skin proximal to the metacarpophalangeal or metatarsophalangeal joints. The changes may affect the entire extremity, face, neck, and trunk (thorax and abdomen).

B. Minor criteria

1. *Sclerodactyly*: Above-indicated skin changes limited to the fingers

2. *Digital pitting scars or loss of substance from the finger pad*: Depressed areas at tips of fingers or loss of digital pad tissue as a result of ischemia

3. *Bibasilar pulmonary fibrosis*: Bilateral reticular pattern of linear or lineonodular densities most pronounced in basilar portions of the lungs on standard chest roentgenogram; may assume appearance of diffuse mottling or "honeycomb lung." These changes should not be attributable to primary lung disease.

1. Masi AT, Rodnan GP, Medsger TA Jr, et al: Preliminary criteria for the classification of systemic sclerosis (scleroderma). Arthritis Rheum 23:581—590, 1980

5. Jones criteria for guidance in the diagnosis of rheumatic fever

Jones criteria (revised) for guidance in the diagnosis of rheumatic fever* (1)

Major manifestations	Minor manifestations
Carditis	Clinical
Polyarthritis	Fever
Chorea	Arthralgia
Erythema marginatum	Previous rheumatic fever
Subcutaneous nodules	or rheumatic heart disease

Plus

Supporting evidence of preceding streptococcal infection:
Increased ASO or other streptococcal antibodies
Positive throat culture for group A streptococcus
Recent scarlet fever

*The presence of two major criteria, or of one major and two minor criteria, indicates a high probability of the presence of rheumatic fever if supported by evidence of a preceding streptococcal infection. The absence of the latter should make the diagnosis suspect, except in situations in which rheumatic fever is first discovered after a long latent period after the antecedent infection (e.g., Sydenham's chorea or low-grade carditis).

1. Stollerman GH, Markowitz M, Taranta A, et al: Jones criteria (revised) for guidance in the diagnosis of rheumatic fever. Circulation 32:664–668, 1965

6. Criteria for the diagnosis of juvenile rheumatoid arthritis

I. General

The JRA Criteria Subcommittee in 1982 again reviewed the 1977 Criteria (1) and recommended that *juvenile rheumatoid arthritis* be the name for the principal form of chronic arthritic disease in children and that this general class should be classified into three onset subtypes: systemic, polyarticular, and pauciarticular. The onset subtypes may be further subclassified into subsets as indicated below. The following classification enumerates the requirements for the diagnosis of JRA and the three clinical onset subtypes and lists subsets of each subtype that may be useful in further classification.

II. General criteria for the diagnosis of juvenile rheumatoid arthritis:

  A. Persistent arthritis of at least six weeks duration in one or more joints

  B. Exclusion of other causes of arthritis (see list of exclusions)

III. JRA onset subtypes

The onset subtype is determined by manifestations during the first six months of disease and remains the principal classification, although manifestations more closely resembling another subtype may appear later.

  A. Systemic onset JRA: This subtype is defined as JRA with persistent intermittent fever (daily intermittent temperatures to 103°F or more) with or without rheumatoid rash or other organ involvement. Typical fever and rash will be considered probable systemic onset JRA if not associated with arthritis. Before a definite diagnosis can be made, arthritis, as defined, must be present.

  B. Pauciarticular onset JRA: This subtype is defined as JRA with arthritis in four or fewer joints during the first six months of disease. Patients with systemic onset JRA are excluded from this onset subtype.

  C. Polyarticular JRA: This subtype is defined as JRA with arthritis in five or more joints during the first six months of disease. Patients with systemic JRA onset are excluded from this subtype.

  D. The onset subtypes may include the following subsets:

    1. Systemic onset (SO)
      a. Polyarthritis
      b. Oligoarthritis
    2. Oligoarthritis (OO) (Pauciarticular onset)
      a. Antinuclear antibody (ANA) positive-chronic uveitis
      b. Rheumatoid factor (RF) positive
      c. Seronegative, B27 positive
      d. Not otherwise classified
    3. Polyarthritis (PO)
      a. RF positivity
      b. Not otherwise classified

IV. Exclusions

  A. Other rheumatic diseases
    1. Rheumatic fever
    2. Systemic lupus erythematosus
    3. Ankylosing spondylitis
    4. Polymyositis and dermatomyositis
    5. Vasculitic syndromes
    6. Scleroderma
    7. Psoriatic arthritis
    8. Reiter's syndrome
    9. Sjögren's syndrome
    10. Mixed connective tissue disease
    11. Behçet's syndrome
  B. Infectious arthritis
  C. Inflammatory bowel disease
  D. Neoplastic diseases including leukemia
  E. Nonrheumatic conditions of bones and joints
  F. Hematologic diseases
  G. Psychogenic arthralgia
  H. Miscellaneous
    1. Sarcoidosis
    2. Hypertrophic osteoarthropathy
    3. Villonodular synovitis
    4. Chronic active hepatitis
    5. Familial Mediterranean fever

V. Other proposed terminology

Juvenile chronic arthritis (JCA) and juvenile arthritis (JA) are new diagnostic terms currently in use in some places for the arthritides of childhood. The diagnoses of JCA and JA are not equivalent to each other, nor to the older diagnosis of juvenile rheumatoid arthritis or Still's disease. Hence reports of studies of JCA or JA cannot be directly compared with one another nor to reports of JRA or Still's disease. Juvenile chronic arthritis is described in more detail in a report of the European Conference on the Rheumatic Diseases of Children (2) and juvenile arthritis in the report of the Ross Conference (3).

1. JRA Criteria Subcommittee of the Diagnostic and Therapeutic Criteria Committee of the American Rheumatism Association: Current proposed revisions of the JRA criteria. Arthritis Rheum 20(Suppl)195–199, 1977
2. Ansell BW: Chronic arthritis in childhood. Ann Rheum Dis 37:107–120, 1978
3. Fink CW: Keynote address: Arthritis in childhood, Report of the 80th Ross Conference in Pediatric Research. Columbus, Ross Laboratories, 1979, pp 1–2

7. The American College of Rheumatology 1990 criteria for the classification of fibromyalgia (1)

1. History of widespread pain

   Definition. Pain is considered widespread when all of the following are present: pain in the left side of the body, pain in the right side of the body, pain above the waist, and pain below the waist. In addition, axial skeletal pain (cervical spine or anterior chest or thoracic spine or low back) must be present. In this definition, shoulder and buttock pain is considered as pain for each involved side. "Low back" pain is considered lower segment pain.

2. Pain in 11 of 18 tender point sites on digital palpation.

   Definition. Pain, on digital palpation, must be present in at least 11 of the following 18 tender point sites:
   Occiput: bilateral, at the suboccipital muscle insertions.
   Low cervical: bilateral, at the anterior aspects of the intertransverse spaces at C5–C7.
   Trapezius: bilateral, at the midpoint of the upper border.
   Supraspinatus: bilateral, at origins, above the scapula spine near the medial border.
   Second rib: bilateral, at the second costochondral junctions, just lateral to the junctions on upper surfaces.
   Lateral epicondyle: bilateral, 2 cm distal to the epicondyles.
   Gluteal: bilateral, in upper outer quadrants of buttocks in anterior fold of muscle.
   Greater trochanter: bilateral, posterior to the trochanteric prominence.
   Knee: bilateral, at the medial fat pad proximal to the joint line.

   Digital palpation should be performed with an approximate force of 4 kg.
   For a tender point to be considered "positive" the subject must state that the palpation was painful. "Tender" is not to be considered "painful."

For classification purposes, patients will be said to have fibromyalgia if both criteria are satisfied. Widespread pain must have been present at least 3 months. The presence of a second clinical disorder does not exclude the diagnosis of fibromyalgia.

1. Wolfe F, Smythe HA, Yunus MB, et al: The American College of Rheumatology 1990 Criteria for the classification of fibromyalgia. Report of the multicenter criteria committee. Arthritis Rheum 33:160–172, 1990

8. The American College of Rheumatology criteria for the classification and reporting of osteoarthritis of the hand (1), hip (2), and knee (3)

Classification criteria for osteoarthritis of the hand, traditional format*

Hand pain, aching, or stiffness
   and
3 or 4 of the following features:
   Hard tissue enlargement of 2 or more of 10 selected joints
   Hard tissue enlargement of 2 or more DIP joints
   Fewer than 3 swollen MCP joints
   Deformity of at least 1 of 10 selected joints

* The 10 selected joints are the second and third distal interphalangeal (DIP), the second and third proximal interphalangeal, and the first carpometacarpal joints of both hands. This classification method yields a sensitivity of 94% and a specificity of 87%. MCP = metacarpophalangeal.

Combined clinical (history, physical examination, laboratory) and radiographic classification criteria for osteoarthritis of the hip, traditional format*

Hip pain
   and
At least 2 of the following 3 features
   ESR <20 mm/hour
   Radiographic femoral or acetabular osteophytes
   Radiographic joint space narrowing (superior, axial, and/or medial)

* This classification method yields a sensitivity of 89% and a specificity of 91%. ESR = erythrocyte sedimentation rate (Westergren).

Criteria for classification of idiopathic osteoarthritis (OA) of the knee*

Clinical and laboratory	Clinical and radiographic	Clinical†
Knee pain +	Knee pain +	Knee pain +
at least 5 of 9:	at least 1 of 3:	at least 3 of 6:
Age >50 years	Age >50 years	Age >50 years
Stiffness <30 minutes	Stiffness <30 minutes	Stiffness <30 minutes
Crepitus	Crepitus	Crepitus
Bony tenderness	+	Bony tenderness
Bony enlargement	Osteophytes	Bony enlargement
No palpable warmth		No palpable warmth
ESR <40 mm/hour		
RF <1:40		
SF OA		
92% sensitive	91% sensitive	95% sensitive
75% specific	86% specific	69% specific

* ESR = erythrocyte sedimentation rate (Westergren); RF = rheumatoid factor; SF OA = synovial fluid signs of OA (clear, viscous, or white blood cell count <2,000/mm^3).

† Alternative for the clinical category would be 4 of 6, which is 84% sensitive and 89% specific.

1. Altman R, Alarcón G, Appelrouth D, et al: The American College of Rheumatology criteria for the classification and reporting of osteoarthritis of the hand. Arthritis Rheum 33:1601–1610, 1990

2. Altman R, Alarcón G, Appelrouth D, et al: The American College of Rheumatology criteria for the classification and reporting of osteoarthritis of the hip. Arthritis Rheum 34:505–514, 1991

3. Altman R, Asch E, Bloch G, et al: Development of criteria for the classification and reporting of osteoarthritis: classification of osteoarthritis of the knee. Arthritis Rheum 29:1039–1049, 1986

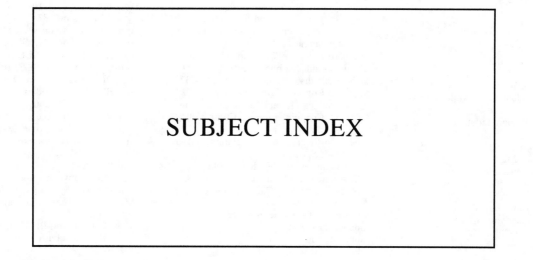

SUBJECT INDEX

Antinuclear antibodies (ANA) (cont'd)
  in systemic sclerosis, 121
Antiphospholipid syndrome, 111, 117–119
  clinical features of, 117–118
  etiology of, 117
  differential diagnosis of, 118
  laboratory tests in, 118
  pathogenesis of, 117
  pregnancy loss in, 117
  prognosis of, 118
  thrombosis in, 117
Antistreptolysin, 2
Antistreptolysin O and rheumatic fever, 170
Apatite crystals, 222–224
  and CREST syndrome, 223
  and dialysis, 246
  and disease associations with, 223
  identification of, 222–223
  miscellaneous, 224–225
  pathogenesis of, 222–223
  principles of, 222–223
Apatite crystal deposition disease,
  and volar flexor tenosynovitis, 283
Aplastic bone disease, 246
ARA; See American Rheumatism Associa-
    tion
Arachidonic acid metabolites, 56–57
Arterial form of Ehlers–Danlos syndrome,
    250
Arteritis
  cranial, giant cell, 4, 141–142
  of temporal vessels, 141–142
Arthralgias
  in HIV infection, 259–260
Arthritis;
  See also Rheumatic diseases associated
    with intestinal bypass,
  atrophic, 2
  bacterial, 192–197
  Barmah Forest virus and, 199
  Brucella, 200
  Candida, 200
  crystal-induced; See Crystal-induced ar-
    thritis
  deformans, 2
  economic impact of, 322–324
  See also Enteropathic arthritis
  See also Exercise for patient with, fungal,
  gonococcal; See Gonococcal arthritis
  and hyperlipoproteinemia, 244–245
  hypertrophic, 2
  infectious; See Infectious arthritis
  occupation-related, 298
  proliferative, 2
  psoriatic; See Psoriatic arthritis
  and psychosocial factors; See Psychosocial
    factors
  reactive; See Reactive arthritis
  septic; See Septic arthritis
  surgical treatment of, 312–315
  therapeutic injections for, 311
  tuberculous, See Tuberculous arthritis
Arthritis Foundation,
  guidelines for JRA treatment plans, 174
Arthrocentesis, 67–70
  complications of, 69–70
  indications for, 67–68
  technique of, 68–69
  therapeutic value of, 67
Arthropathies
  angioimmunoblastic lymphadenopathy, 234
  associated with endocrine diseases, 242–
    243
  associated with hematologic diseases
    and malignant disorders, 231–234
  carcinoma polyarthritis, 233
  hemophilic, 231–232

Arthropathies (cont'd)
  leukemia, 233–234
  lymphoma, 234
  metastatic carcinomatous, 241
  myelomatosis, 233
  of sickle cell disease, 232
  of thalassemia, 233
  of Waldenstrom's macroglobulinemia, 233
  of Wilson's disease, 228
Arthroplasty
  elbow, 313
  fingers, 314
  for osteonecrosis, 275
  for Paget's disease, 277
  shoulder, 313
  thumb, 314
  wrist, 314
Arthroscopy, 73–74
  for osteoarthritis, 189–190
  for osteonecrosis, 274–275
Articular cartilage, 8–11
  anchorin CII, as a protein in, 10
  basement membrane in, 19
  biglycan in, 10
  chondrocytes in, 9
  chrondron, 10
  chrondronectin, as a protein in, 10
  collagen, type of; See Collagen
  composition of, 9
  decorin in, 10
  definition of, 8
  degradation of, 10–11
  dermatan sulphate in, 10
  insulin-like growth factor, 10
  Interleukin-1 in, 10
  markers of, 10–11
  matrix turnover in, 10
  metalloproteinases in, 10
  and osteoarthritis, 10–11
  proteoglycans, 8–9
  and RA, 11
  structure of, 8–9
  tumor necrosis growth factor-α in, 10
  tumor necrosis growth factor-β in, 10
Articular infections, See Infectious arthritis
Articular surface, abnormalities in, 76
Aschoff nodule, 1
Aschoff, Ludwig, 1
Ascorbic acid; See also Vitamin C and
    ochronosis,
  and RA, 326
Aseptic necrosis, 264
Aspirin, 300–304
  adverse effects of, 301
  dosage of, 301
  enteric coated, 301
  for JRA, 173–174
  for Kawasaki disease, 176
  for use with NSAIDs, 300–301
  for Paget's disease, 277
  for RA, 97
  and Reye's syndrome, 173–174
  surgery and, 312
  for Sweet's syndrome, 257
Assistive devices, See Adaptive aids
Asymptomatic CPPD crystal deposits, 220
Asymptomatic gout, 213
Atlantoaxial subluxation, treatment of, 100
Auranofin; See also Gold for psoriatic arthri-
    tis,
  for RA, 98
Aurothioglucose; See Gold
Aurothiomalate; See Gold
Auspitz, Heinrich, 3
Autoantibodies; See also Antibodies
  anticentromere, 42
  autoantigen, targets of, 42

Autoantibodies; See also Antibodies (cont'd)
  genetic orgins of associated diseases, 41
  laboratory tests for, 65–66
  MHC molecules and expression of, 42
  molecular biology of, 40–43
  regulated V region, genes and natural, 41
  T cells and response, 42
  Tolerance and response, 42
Autoimmune disorders, 34
  organ specific versus generalized, 34
Autoimmunity, avoidance of, 32
Avascular necrosis
  and gout, 215
  and osteoarthritis, 189
Azathioprine, 306; See also SAARDs
  for Bechet's syndrome, 207
  mechanisms of action, 304
  monitoring of, 305
  for RA, 98
  for SLE, 115
  toxicity of, 305
AZT, for HIV infection, 261

B

B. abortus, 200
B. canus, 200
B. melitensis, 200
B. suis, 200
B$_2$ macroglobulin
  amyloid, 236–237
  in dialysis, arthropathy and, 246
B cells
  and antigen processing, 28
  function of, 30
  genetics of, 30
  in immune response, 28, 30
  and immune tolerance, 32
  and immunoglobulins, 30
  and Lyme disease, 202
  as new therapy, 309
  and proteoglycans, 27
  receptors, variable regions of, 31
  and Sjogren's syndrome, 135
  in SLE, 105–106
B lymphocytes; See B cells in immune re-
    sponse,
Back
  disorders of, 268–273
  low, pain in; See Low back pain
Back pain; See also Low back pain
  causes of, 268
  disabling, 272–273
  in lumbar spinal stenosis, 272
Bacterial arthritis, 192–197;
  See also Infectious arthritis
Bacteroides fragilis and bacterial arthritis,
    195
Baehr, George, 3
Baillie, Matthew, 1
Baillou, Guillaume (Ballonius), 1
Bagratuni, L., 4
Baker's cysts, 284
Bannatyne, Gilbert A., 2
Barber, Stuart, 4
Barmah Forest virus and arthritis, 199
Basement membrane, in articular cartilage,
    19
Bechterew, Vladimir von, 2, 3
Bed rest and pain management, 316
Behavioral factors
  influencing psychosocial reactions
    to rheumatic diseases, 320–322;
  See also Cognitive factors
Behcet's syndrome, 206–207
  and association with HLA allele, 206, 207

Behcet's syndrome (cont'd)
  in children, 177
  clinical features of, 206–207
  diagnostic criteria for, 206
  immunopathogenesis of, 207
  pathology of, 207
  treatment of, 207
Benign hypermobility form of Ehlers–Danlos syndrome, 250
Benign neoplasms, 238–240
Benign rheumatoid nodules, 180
Betahemolytic streptococcus, in rheumatic fever, 2
Bernstein, L., 3
Bicipital tendinitis, 279, 297
Billings, Frank, 2
Biologic agents, as potential new therapies, 307–310
  Adhesion molecules, 310
  Antibodies to antigen-presenting cells, 309
  B cells, 309
  Cytokines, 309
  Cytokine inhibitors, 309
  T cells, 307–309
Biologic therapies, nontraditional, 325
Biopsy, synovial, 72
Blastomycosis, 200
Block, O.J., 3
Blood transfusion and hemochromatosis, 226
Blount's disease, 265
Boldero, Harold E., 2
Bone disease and dialysis patients
  Aluminum-induced, 245
  Aplastic, 246
Bone remodeling
  cellular events in, 12
  collagen, type I and, 12
  cytokines and, 12
  osteoclasts in, 12; See also osteoclasts
  osteoclasts, precursors and, 12; See also osteoclasts
  1,25 dihydroxyvitamin D and, 12
  Haversian canals in cortical bone, 12
  hematopoietic precursors and, 12
  Interleukin-1 and, 12
  Interleukin-6 and, 12
  parathyroid hormones and, 12
  pluripotent precursors and, 12
  systemic hormones and, 12
Bones
  cancellous, 11, 12
  cells in, 12–13; See also Cells
  cortical, 11, 12
  density and mass of, and osteoarthritis, 184
  dysplasias of, 263–267
  formation of, 11–14
  infection of, in hemodialysis, 246
  marrow, abnormalities in, 78
  measurement of mass, 290–291
  metabolic disease of, 290–294
  Paget's disease of, 276–277
  remodeling of, 11–12; See also Bone remodeling
  resorption and cytokines, 13–14
  resorption, control of, 13
  tumors of and joint involvement, 233–234
  sex hormones and, 14
Boorde, Andrew, 1
Borrelia burgdorferi and Lyme disease, 201–203
Borrelia garini and Lyme disease, 201
Bouchard, Charles, 3
Bouchard's nodes, 3
  definition of, 63
  in osteoarthritis, 108
Bouillaud, Jean-Baptiste, 1

Boutonniere deformities, 63
Braces, for thoracic spine problems; See Orthotics
Brewerton, Derek, 3
Brodie, Benjamin, 2, 4
Brucella arthritis, 200
Brucellosis, 200
Brucella
  osteomyelitis, 200
  spondylitis, 200
Buchman's disease, 266
Bunionette, 286
Bursitis
  anserine, 284
  calcaneal, 285
  iliopectineal, 283
  iliopsoas, 283
  ischial, 283–284
  ischiogluteal, 283–284
  no name, no fame, 284
  olecranon, 280
  prepatellar, 284
  retrocalcaneal, 285
  trochanteric, 283
Butterfly rash of SLE, 107
Bywaters, Eric L., 2

C

C-reactive protein
  and P component in amyloid, 205
  in Kawasaki disease, 176
  in rheumatic fever, 170
  in RA, 91
  in SLE, 110–111
Calcaneal bursitis, 285
Calcification; See Apatite crystals
Calcitonin
  in bone remodeling, 12
  for osteoporosis, 292
  synthetic salmon, for Paget's disease, 277
Calcium
  in corticosteroid-induced osteoporosis, 292
  deficiency of, in secondary hyperparathyroidism, 293
  and effects of corticosteroids, 292
  for osteomalacia, 293
  in prevention of osteoporosis, 292
Calcium crystal deposition diseases, 224
Calcium oxalate crystal deposition and dialysis, 246
Calcium pyrophosphate crystals
  and hemochromatosis, 226
  in ochronosis, 237
  in Wilson's disease, 228
Calcium pyrophosphate dihydrate and osteoarthritis, 191
Calcium pyrophosphate dihydrate
  deposition disease (CPPD), 219–222
  and apatite crystals, 224
  chondrocalcinosis in, 219
  clinical features of, 219–220
  crystal clearance from joints in, 221–222
  etiologic classification of, 219
  and hemochromatosis, 226
  and hypothyroidosis, 226
  pathogenesis of crystal deposition, 222
  pathogenesis of inflammation, 220–221
  radiologic features of, 220
  synovial fluid PPi in, 221
  treatment of, 222
Calve's disease, 226
Cancer, and arthritis; See Malignancy
Candida and HIV infection, 258
Candida arthritis, 200
Capsulitis, adhesive, 279–280
Carcinoma, polyarthritis of, 233

Cardiac manifestations
  of RA, 95
  of SLE, 110
Carpal tunnel syndrome, 282
  and myelomatosis, 233
  and occupational injuries, 297
  and pronator teres syndrome, 281
Cartilage, articular; See Articular cartilage
Cartilage erosion, mechanisms of, 90
Casts and pain management, 316
Cathepsin G, substrates of, 53
Causalgia, in reflex sympathetic dystrophy syndrome, 289
Cazenave, Pierre, 3
CD2 cells, 28, 29
CD3 cells, 29
CD4 cells, 28, 29, 34, 259
CD8 cells, 28, 29, 34
CD11 cells, 28
CD19 cells, 29
Cecil, Russell, 2
Ceftriaxone and Lyme disease, 203
Cefuroxime and Lyme disease, 203
Cells
  A, 6
  antibody-mediated effects on, 34
  antigen-presenting, 28
  B; See B cells
  natural killer; See Natural killer cells
  osteoblast, 12
  osteoblast precursors, 12
  osteoclasts, 12
  osteocytes, 13
  synovial lining, 5
  T; See T cells
Cellular reactivity, as immunopathologic mechanism, 34
Central nervous system, in SLE, 108–109
Cervical anatomy, 270
Cervical orthoses, 318
Cervical spine, as surgical site, 313
Charcot, Jean-Martin, 2
Charcot joint, 190, 243
  See also Neuropathic osteoarthropathy and osteoarthritis,
Cheiralgia paresthetica, 282
Chest wall, anterior, rheumatic pain syndromes in, 287
Chauffard, Anatole, 4
Chikungunya virus, and arthritis, 198
Childhood dermatomyositis, 178–179
Chlamydia in Reiter's syndrome, 160, 161
Chlorambucil,
  for Behcet's syndrome, 207
  mechanism of action, 304
  monitoring of, 305
  for RA, 99
  toxicities of, 305
Chloroquine
  mechanism of action, 304
  monitoring of, 305
  for RA, 99, 304
  for sarcoidosis, 205
  for SLE, 114
  toxicities of, 305
Chondrocalcinosis, 219
  See also Calcium pyrophosphate dihydrate deposition disease
  in alkaptonuria, 227
  in hemochromatosis, 226
Chondrocytes, in articular tissues, 9
Chondroitin sulfates in connective tissue, 23–24
Chondrolysis of hip, acute, in children, 267
Chondroma, intracapsula solitary, 240
Chondromalacia patellae
  in children, 188

Paget's disease of bone (cont'd)
  clinical features of, 277
  radiologic findings in, 276–277
  and osteoporosis circumscripta, 276
Pain; *See* Regional rheumatic pain syndromes
Paine, Alexander, 2
Palindromic rheumatism, 208
  and RA, 208
Pancreatitis, and panniculitis, 256
Panner's disease, 264
Panniculitis syndrome
  lobular, 255–256
  pancreatic, 256
  in Weber–Christian disease, 255–256
Paracelsus, 1
Parathyroid hormone; *See also* Hormones
  in bone remodeling, 12
Partial transient osteoporosis, 290
Parvovirus, 197
  B19, 197
  B19 and fibromyalgia, 197
Pasteurella multicida and joint infection, 194
Patellar tendinitis, 285
Patellofemoral pain syndrome, 285
Patient
  education in SLE, 113
  education in fibromyalgia, 249
  evaluation of, 60–66
Paulley, J.W., 4
Pediatric rheumatic diseases, 171–182;
  See also individual disease entries
  Behcet's syndrome, 177
  benign rheumatoid nodule, 180
  chronic, infantile, neurologic, cutaneous,
    and articular syndrome, 181
  chronic recurrent multifocal osteomyelitis,
    181
  dermatomyositis, 178–179
  discitis, 181
  granuloma annulare, 180
  Henoch–Schonlein purpura, 177
  infantile chronic hyperostosis, 181
  juvenile rheumatoid arthritis, 172–174
  juvenile spondylarthropathies, 174–175
  Kashin–Beck disease, 181
  Kawasaki disease, 175–176
  Moya Moya, 177–178
  Mseleni disease, 181
  Mucha–Habermann disease, 177–178
  neonatal SLE, 178
  neuroblastoma, 181
  nonarticular rheumatism, 172
  overlap syndromes, 179–180
  polyarteritis nodosa, 177
  reflex sympathetic dystrophy syndrome,
    180
  SLE, 178
  systemic sclerosis, 180
  Takayasu arteritis, 177
  transient or toxic synovitis of hip, 180
  vasculopathies, 177
  vasculitis, 177
  Wegener's granulomatosis, 177
Pellegrini–Stieda syndrome, 285
Pelvic insufficiency fracture, 272
Penicillamine, *See also* SAARDs
  adverse effects of, 304–305;
  D-penicillamine, 304–305
  and gold, 304
  for JRA, 174
  for palindromic rheumatism, 208
  pharmacology of, 304–305
  for RA, 99
  for Wilson's disease, 228
Penicillin
  for Lyme disease, 203

Penicillin (cont'd)
  and pediatric Henoch–Schonlein purpura,
    177
  resistance to, in gonococcal infection, 196
  for rheumatic fever, 171
Penicillin-resistant gonococcal strains and
    disseminated gonococcal infection, 196
Periarticular, abnormalities in, 79
Pericapsulitis, 279–280
Pericarditis, in SLE, 109
Periodic syndromes, 207–209
  intermittent hydrarthrosis, 208
  Familial Mediterranean fever, 208
  palindromic rheumatism, 208
Peripheral nervous system, inflammatory response to, 90
Peroneal nerve palsy, 285
Peroneal tendinitis, 286
Peroneal tendon dislocation, 286
Pes cavus, 286
Pes planus, 286
Petrone, Luigi, 4
Phagocytosis, 44, 299
Phalen's sign, 282
Pharmacologic therapies, nontraditional, 325
Phenylacetic acids, 299
Phenylbutazone; *See also* NSAIDs
  adverse effects of, 299–300
  for ankylosing spondylitis, 158
  dosage of, 299
Phlebotomy therapy for hemochromatosis,
    226
Physical examination, of patient with rheumatic disease, 61–64
Physical therapy, for osteoarthritis, 189
Pierson's disease, 266
Pigmented villonodular synovitis, 238–239
  diffuse, 238–239
  localized nodular tenosynovitis, 239
  localized nodular synovitis, 239
  and osteoarthritis, 189
Piriformis syndrome, 285
Piroxicam; *See also* NSAIDs
  adverse effects of, 299–300
  dosage of, 299
Pitcairn, David, 1
Pituitary disorders, arthropathy of, 243
Placebo therapy, nontraditional, 324
Plantar fasciitis, 285
Plasma exchange, 116; *See also* Lymphapheresis;
Plasmin, substrates of, 45
Plasmin activators, 53
Plaster casting for painful joints, 319
Platelet activating factor (PAF),
  as mediator of inflammation, 45, 58–59
Platelet-derived growth factor
  and inflammation, 45, 47
  and hypertrophic osteoarthropathy, 262
Plicamycin, and bone remodeling, 12
Plotz, Charles, 2
Pneumocystic pneumoniae and HIV infection, 259
POEMS syndrome, 233
Polyarteritis nodosa
  in children, 177
  clinical features of, 142
  diagnosis of, 143
  laboratory tests for, 142
  treatment, 147
Polyarthritis
  in carcinoma, 233
  in gonococcal infection,
  juvenile, chronic, 2, 181
  in rheumatic fever, 169
Polychondritis
  corticosteroids for, 303

Polychondritis (cont'd)
  relapsing, 149–151
Polyclonal activation,
  as mechanism of autoimmunity, 33
Polymorphism
  in articular infection, 192
  in Behcet's syndrome, 206
  in vasculitis, 139
Polymorphonuclear leukocytes in connective
    tissue, 43
Polymorphonuclear leukocytes elastase, 53
Polymyalgia rheumatica
  association with giant cell arteritis, 149
  clinical picture of, 149
  corticosteroids for, 149
  history of, 4
  treatment of, 149
Polymyositis, 127–131
  See also Dermatomyositis anti-Jo-1 antibodies in, 128
  classification of, 128
  clinical features of, 129–130
  corticosteroids for, 303
  differential diagnosis of, 128
  etiology and pathogenesis of, 128–129
  history of, 129
  laboratory findings in, 130
  pathology of, 130
  prognosis of, 131
  treatment of, 130–131
  and undifferentiated connective tissue diseases, 136
Polymyositis/dermatomyositis; *See also* Dermatomyositis;
Popliteal cyst, 284
Popliteal tendinitis, 284–285
Posterior interosseous nerve syndrome, 282
Posterior tibial tendinitis, 286
Posterior tibialis tendon rupture, 287
Pott's disease, 199
Poynton, Frederick, 2
Praetorius and Poulsen, 1
Prednisolone; *See* Corticosteroids
Pregnancy
  in osteonecrosis, 273
  in SLE, 112, 113, 116
Preiser disease, 264
Prepatellar bursitis, 264
Primary bone tumors, involvement of joints,
    241
Primary generalized osteoarthritis, 188
Primary malignant tumors, 240
Primary osteoarthritis, 188
Probenecid
  and uric acid levels, 218
  for gout, 218
Procainamide-induced lupus, antibodies in,
    111
Progressive systemic sclerosis, 3; *See* Systemic sclerosis
Pronator teres syndrome, 281
Prosthetic joint infections, 194–195
Proteins
  AA in amyloidosis, 237
  AL in amyloidosis, 236
  anchorin CII, in articular cartilage, 10
  chondronectin, in articular cartilage, 10
  core, of cartilage proteoglycan, 9
  G1a (osteocalcin), 12, 113
  links of cartilage proteoglycan, 9
  measurement of, in synovial fluid, 72
Proteinases,
  activation, control of, 55
  aspartic, 52
  cysteine, 52
  extraarticular matrix-degrading, 52–55
  gene expression, control of, 55

Proteinases (cont'd)
and tissue injury, 52–56
Proteoglycans
biglycan in, 10
cartilage, 9–10
cell-associated, 24–25
collagen, interaction with, 26
composition of, 9–10
core protein in, 9, 25
decorin in, 10
definition of, 23
glycosaminoglycans in, 23–24, 26–27
hyaluronic acid, interact with, 25–26
as immunogens, 27
structural domains of, 9; *See also* Globular domains
Pseudogout, 219
Pseudomonas aeruginosa, and bacterial arthritis, 194
Pseudoneurotrophic joints, 220
Pseudo-osteoarthritis, 220
Pseudorheumatoid arthritis, 219–220
Pseudoxanthoma elasticum, 254–255
Psoriasis; *See* Psoriatic arthritis
Psoriatic arthritis, 161–163
association with HLA allele, 162
in children, 175
Class II, 162
clinical features of, 162
corticosteroids for, 163
dermatologic features of, 162
etiology of, 161–162
and HIV infection, 162, 220
laboratory findings in, 162–163
NSAIDs for, 163
and osteoarthritis, 189
pathogenesis of, 161–162
radiologic findings in, 162–163
rheumatoid factor in, 162
surgery for, 313
and synovial biopsy, 162–163
treatment of, 163
and volar flexor tenosynovitis, 283
Psoriatic skin lesions, and pustulosis palmaris et plantaris, 257
Psychogenic rheumatism, and fibromyalgia, 247–248
Psychosocial factors and arthritis, 320–322
anxiety, 320
depression, 320
future directions, 322
Psychosocial interventions, factors in, 320–322
Control and self-efficacy, 321
Coping skills training, 321
Psychosocial reactions, factors in, 320–322
behavioral, 320
cognitive, 320
Pulmonary manifestations, in SLE, 110
Pump bumps, 285
Pustulosis palmaris et plantaris, 257
Pyoderma gangrenosum, 164, 257
Pyrazolidinediones, 299
Pyrrolealkanoic acids, 299
Pyrrolo-Pyrole, 299

Q

Q fever, 2
Quadriceps tendon, rupture of, 296
Quinidine, and pediatric Henoch–Schonlein purpura, 177
Quinine, and pediatric Henoch–Schonlein purpura, 177

R

RA; *See* Rheumatoid arthritis
RA cells; *See* Rheumatoid arthritis cells

Radial nerve palsy, 282
Radiculopathy, 270–272
localization of, 271
treatment of, 272–272
Radiologic findings; *See* individual disease entries
Ragan, Charles, 2
Rash, butterfly, of SLE, 107
Raynaud, Maurice, 3
Raynaud's phenomenon
and apatite crystals, 223
in systemic sclerosis, 121–122
and thoracic outlet syndrome, 280
in undifferentiated connective tissue syndromes, 233
Reactants, acute phase, 64–65
Reactive arthritis, 153–154; *See also* Infectious arthritis
and *Chlamydia trachomatis*, 153
after infectious disease, 153–154
and HLA-B27, 153–154
and *Salmonella* species, and association with HLA allele, 153–154
and *Shigella flexneri*
and association with HLA alleles, 153–154
and *Yersinia* species
and association with HLA alleles, 153–154
and yersinial arthritis, 153–154
Reactive arthritis after infectious enteritis, 167–168
and antibodies, 167
clinical features of, 167
and HLA-B27 allele, 167
pathogenesis of, 167
treatment of, 167
Reflex sympathetic dystrophy syndrome, 288–290
in children, 180
clinical features of, 288
diagnosis of, 288–289
pathogenesis of, 288–289
treatment of, 289–290
Regional rheumatic pain syndromes, 277–288
ankle, 285–287
anterior chest wall, 287–288
causative factors, 278
elbow region, disorders of, 278–280
feet, 285–287
general concepts for management of, 277
hand, 281–283
hip, 283–284
shoulder region, disorders of, 280–281
Rehabilitation, definition of, 315
Rehabilitation, of patients
with rheumatic diseases, 315–320
adaptive aids, 319
comprehensive care, 319
exercise, 316–317
physical modalities, 316
orthoses, 317–319
splints, 317–319
Rehabilitation specialists, 315–316
Reiter, Hans, 4
Reiter's syndrome, 159–161
antinuclear antibody in, 160
BASE syndrome and, 159
in children, 159, 175
Chlamydia and, 160, 161
clinical features of, 159–160
corticosteroids, topical for, 161
course and prognosis of, 161
epidemiology of, 159
European Spondylarthropathy Study Group and, 159
eye and, 160

Reiter's syndrome (cont'd)
gastrointestinal tract and, 160
heart and, 160
history of, 4, 159
and HIV virus, 160, 259–260
and HLA alleles, 159
HLA-B27 in, 159–161
immunopathology of, 33
laboratory findings in, 160
mucous membrane and, 160
musculoskeletal features in, 159
NSAIDs for, 161
and osteoarthritis, 189
and psoriatic arthritis, 162
radiologic features of, 160
rheumatoid factor in, 160
and *Salmonella*, 159–160
and sexually acquired reactive arthritis, 159
Shigella and, 159–160
and skin, 160
treatment of, 161
urogenital tract features in, 159–160
Relapsing polychondritis, 149–151
diagnosis of, 151
management of, 151
musculoskeletal symptoms of, 151
ocular symptoms of, 150
otorhinolaryngeal disease and, 150
respiratory disease and, 150
Remodeling of bone, 11–12; *See also* Bone remodeling
Renal crisis in systemic sclerosis, 124–125
Renal disease, in gout, 212–214
Renal effects of NSAIDs, 300
Renal failure end-stage, in SLE, 108
Renal osteodystrophy, 245, 293
Repetitive stress, and osteoarthritis, 184–185
Reticuloendothelial system and SLE, 110
Reye's syndrome, and aspirin, 173–174
Rheumatic diseases; *See also* individual disease entries
classification of, 82–86
evaluation of patient with symptoms of, 60–82
history of, 1–4
and HLA alleles, 39–40
laboratory evaluation strategy for, 64
nontraditional remedies for, 324–327
nutrition, as therapy for, 326
patient history, 60–64
pediatric, 179–182
physical examination for, 60–64
psychosocial aspects of, 320–322
synovial fluid in, 70–72
Rheumatic fever,
clinical aspects of, 169–170
clinical consequences of, 170
diagnosis of, 170
epidemiology of, 168
history of, 1–2
Jones criteria for diagnosis of, 170
laboratory findings in, 170
pathogenesis of, 168–169
synovial biopsy in, 170
treatment of, 171
Rheumatic heart disease, 170
Rheumatic pain syndromes, regional, 277–288;
See also Regional rheumatic pain syndromes
Rheumatism; *See also* Arthritis
nonarticular, pediatric, 172
Rheumatoid arthritis,
and acetaminophen, 97–98; *See also* NSAIDs
ankles in, 94

Transforming growth factor-beta, and bone remodeling, 12
Transient regional/partial osteoporosis, 290
Trauma, and osteoarthritis, 184–185
Triple helix of collagen, 16
True osteonecrosis, 264
Tuberculosis arthritis, 199
Tumor growth factor
    in amyloid, 237
    in articular cartilage, 10
    in inflammation, 47
Tumor necrosis factor
    in articular infections, 192
    in bone remodeling, 12
    and gouty inflammation, 212
    and HIV infection, 259
    and inflammation, 45
Type II hyperlipoproteinemia, 244–245
    xanthomas in, 244–245
Type IV hyperlipoproteinemia, 244–245
    arthropathy of, 244–245
    radiologic findings in, 244–245
    xanthomas in, 244–245
Type V hyperlipoproteinemia, skeletal lesions in, 244

U

UCTS; *See* undifferentiated connective tissue syndromes
Ulcerative colitis
    axial involvement, 164
    extra articular symptoms, 164–165
    and HLA allele, 164
    extra intestinal symptoms, 164–165
    intestinal symptoms, 164
    peripheral arthritis in, 164
    and pyoderma gangrenosum, 257
    spondylitis in, 164
Ulnar nerve entrapment
    elbow, 281
    wrist, 282–283
Ultrasonography, 74
Ultrasound, for pain management, 316
Undifferentiated connective tissue syndromes (UCTS), 135–137
Undulent fever, 200
Unverricht, Heinrich, 4
Urate crystal deposition, pathogenesis of, 212
Uric acid
    overproduction and underexcretion of, 211–212
    and renal disease, 214
    serum levels of, 209
    urinary, assays of, 1
Uricosuric drugs, for treatment of gout, 218

V

van Neck's disease, 266
van Leeuwenhoek, Antonj, 1
Vascular addresses, 89
Vasculitis
    association with rheumatic diseases, 144
    central nervous system and, 144
    in children, 137
    chronic therapy, 148
    corticosteroids for, 303
    endotheial cells, 140
    epidemiology of, 141–146
    and HIV infection, 259–260
    hypersensitivity, 145
    immune complexes in, 139
    immunotherapy and biologic agents for, 148
    initial therapeutic interventions for, 147–148
    laboratory tests in, 143
    pathology of, 137–139
    pathogenesis of, 139–141
    lympocytes in, 140
    in RA, 144
    in SLE, 144
    treatment of, 146–148
Vasoactive amines, in inflammation, 59
Vertebra plana, 266
Vertebral artery syndrome, 270
Vidal, Emil, 4
Viral arthritis, 197–198
    Adenovirus, 199
    Alphavirus, 198–199
    coxsackieviruses, 199
    Hepatitis A, B, C, 198
    HIV, 198
    Parvovirus B19, 197–198
Viral hepatitis, 298
Virchow, Rudolf, 2
Viscosity of synovial fluid, 71
Vitamins, as treatment, 326
Vitamin D
    for corticosteroid-induced osteoporosis, 292
    for osteomalacia, 293
    in prevention of osteoporosis, 292
    for secondary hyperparathyroidism, 293
von Willebrand's disease, and hemophilic arthropathy, 231
von Willebrand factor and inflammation, 45

W

Wafer vertebra, 266
Wagner, Ernst, 4
Waldenstrom's macroglobulinemia, 233

Water, in articular cartilage, 10
Weaver's bottom, 283
Weber–Christian disease, 283
Wegener, Friedrich, 4
Wegener's granulomatosis
    in children, 177
    clinical findings in, 143
    diagnosis of, 144
    laboratory tests in, 144
    treatment of, 147
Weiss, Soma, 3
Wells, William, 1
Westphal, Carl, 3
Whatley, Thomas, 4
Whipple's disease
    clinical features of, 165
    and HLA allele, 165
    laboratory findings in, 165
    treatment of, 165
    Tropheryma whippelli in, 165
Wilson's disease, 277–228
Winterbauer, Robert, 5
Wollaston, William, 1
World Health Organization, 82
    classification of lupus nephritis, 101
Wright-Schober test, 156
Wrists
    anatomy of, 62–63
    and De Quervains tenosynovitis, 281
    exercises for, 317
    ganglion in, 281
    physical examination of, 62–63
    splinting of, 318
    surgery for, 314
    tenosynovitis in, 281
    ulnar nerve entrapment in, 282–283

X

Xanthomas
    in hyperlipoproteinemia, 244
    inhibitors, for gout, 218
Xerostomia in Sjogren's syndrome, 132–133
Xiphoid, hypersensitive, 287
Xiphoidalgia, 287
Xiphodynia, 287

Y

Yersinia
    enterocolitica, 170, 182
    and erythema nodosum, 256
    and hemochromotosis, 226

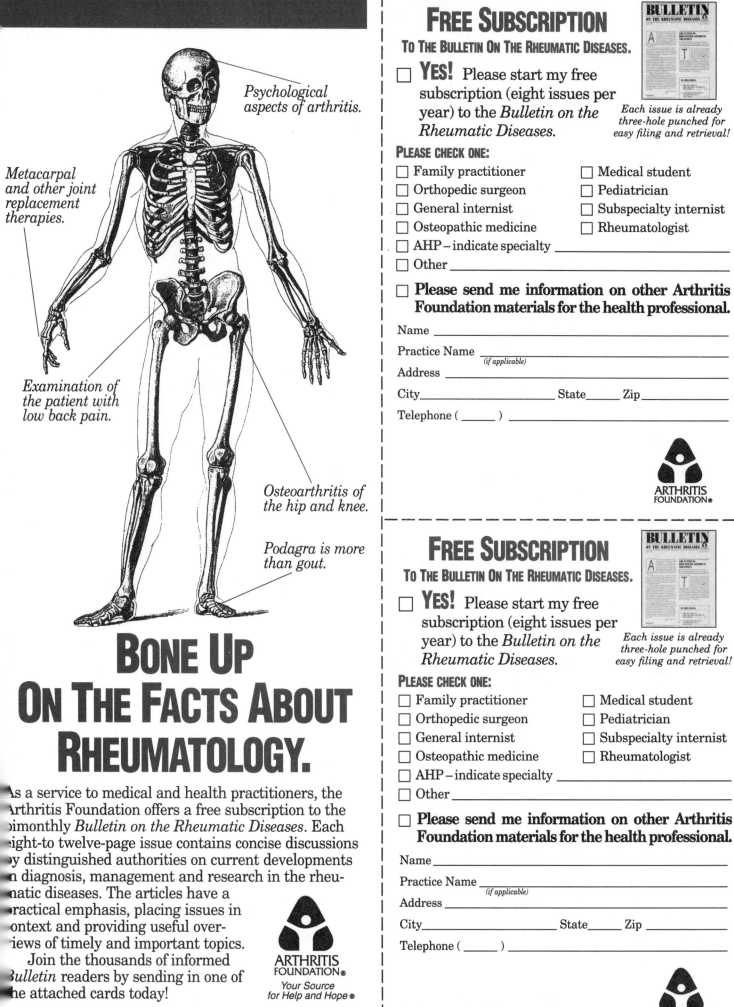

Psychological aspects of arthritis.

Metacarpal and other joint replacement therapies.

Examination of the patient with low back pain.

Osteoarthritis of the hip and knee.

Podagra is more than gout.

BONE UP ON THE FACTS ABOUT RHEUMATOLOGY.

As a service to medical and health practitioners, the Arthritis Foundation offers a free subscription to the bimonthly *Bulletin on the Rheumatic Diseases*. Each eight-to twelve-page issue contains concise discussions by distinguished authorities on current developments in diagnosis, management and research in the rheumatic diseases. The articles have a practical emphasis, placing issues in context and providing useful overviews of timely and important topics.

Join the thousands of informed *Bulletin* readers by sending in one of the attached cards today!

ARTHRITIS FOUNDATION®
Your Source for Help and Hope®

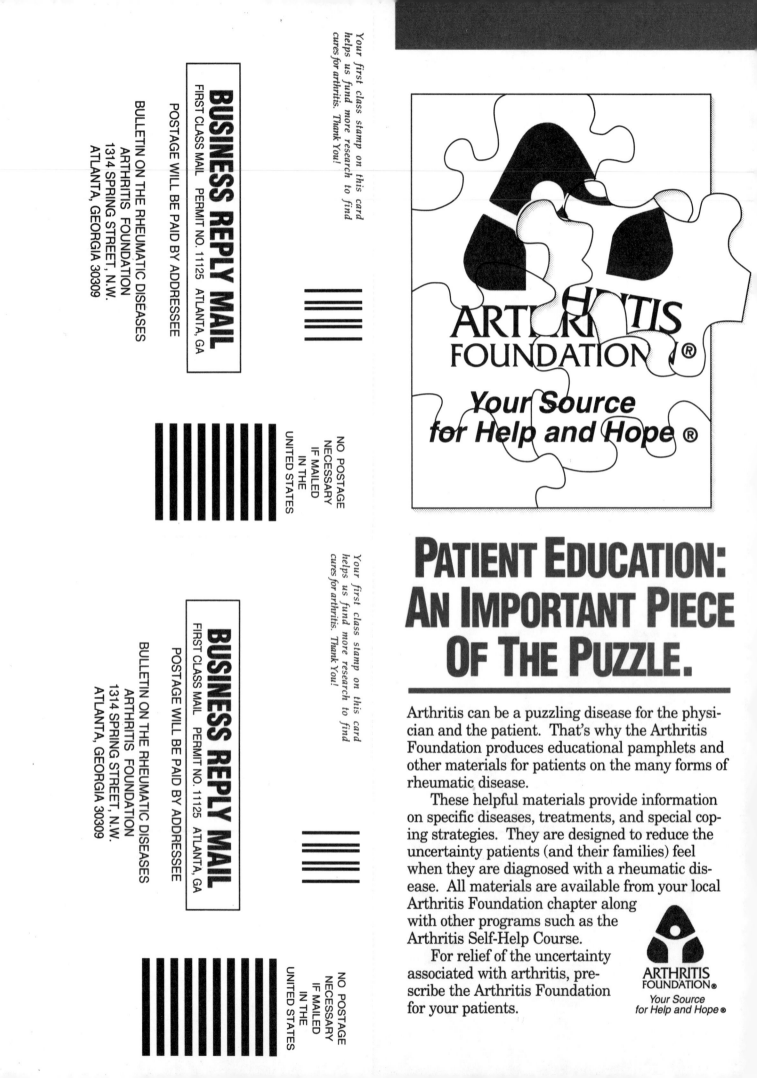

ARTHRITIS FOUNDATION ®

Your Source for Help and Hope ®

PATIENT EDUCATION: AN IMPORTANT PIECE OF THE PUZZLE.

Arthritis can be a puzzling disease for the physician and the patient. That's why the Arthritis Foundation produces educational pamphlets and other materials for patients on the many forms of rheumatic disease.

These helpful materials provide information on specific diseases, treatments, and special coping strategies. They are designed to reduce the uncertainty patients (and their families) feel when they are diagnosed with a rheumatic disease. All materials are available from your local Arthritis Foundation chapter along with other programs such as the Arthritis Self-Help Course.

For relief of the uncertainty associated with arthritis, prescribe the Arthritis Foundation for your patients.

ARTHRITIS FOUNDATION ®
Your Source for Help and Hope ®

Your first class stamp on this card helps us fund more research to find cures for arthritis. Thank You!

NO POSTAGE
NECESSARY
IF MAILED
IN THE
UNITED STATES

BUSINESS REPLY MAIL
FIRST CLASS MAIL   PERMIT NO. 11125   ATLANTA, GA

POSTAGE WILL BE PAID BY ADDRESSEE

BULLETIN ON THE RHEUMATIC DISEASES
ARTHRITIS FOUNDATION
1314 SPRING STREET, N.W.
ATLANTA, GEORGIA 30309

Your first class stamp on this card helps us fund more research to find cures for arthritis. Thank You!

NO POSTAGE
NECESSARY
IF MAILED
IN THE
UNITED STATES

BUSINESS REPLY MAIL
FIRST CLASS MAIL   PERMIT NO. 11125   ATLANTA, GA

POSTAGE WILL BE PAID BY ADDRESSEE

BULLETIN ON THE RHEUMATIC DISEASES
ARTHRITIS FOUNDATION
1314 SPRING STREET, N.W.
ATLANTA, GEORGIA 30309